HANDBOOK OF PSYCHOPATHY

Edited by

CHRISTOPHER J. PATRICK

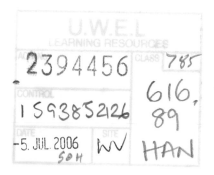
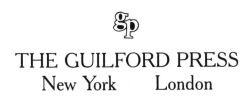

THE GUILFORD PRESS
New York London

Library of Congress Cataloging-in-Publication Data

Handbook of psychopathy / edited by Christopher J. Patrick.
    p. cm.
  Includes bibliographical references and index.
  ISBN 1-59385-212-6 (alk. paper)
  1. Antisocial personality disorders—Handbooks, manuals, etc.   I. Patrick,
Christopher J.
  RC555.H357 2006
  616.89—dc22

2005005954

To my brother, David,
my father, Donald,
and my mother, Susan

About the Editor

Christopher J. Patrick, PhD, is Starke R. Hathaway Distinguished Professor and Director of Clinical Training in the Department of Psychology at the University of Minnesota. He has published extensively in the areas of psychopathy, antisocial behavior, and substance use and abuse. Dr. Patrick's other research interests include emotion, personality, psychophysiology, and cognitive neuroscience. He is the recipient of Distinguished Early Career Contribution awards from the American Psychological Association (1995) and the Society for Psychophysiological Research (1993). He is currently a consulting editor for *Psychological Assessment* and for the *Journal of Abnormal Psychology*, as well as a former associate editor of *Psychophysiology*.

Contributors

Stephen D. Benning, MA, Department of Psychology, University of Minnesota, Minneapolis, Minnesota

Ronald Blackburn, PhD, Department of Clinical Psychology, University of Liverpool, Liverpool, United Kingdom

R. J. R. Blair, PhD, Mood and Anxiety Disorders Program, National Institute of Mental Health, Bethesda, Maryland

David J. Cooke, PhD, Douglas Inch Centre and Department of Forensic Clinical Psychology, Glasgow Caledonian University, Glasgow, United Kingdom

Karen J. Derefinko, MS, Department of Psychology, University of Kentucky, Lexington, Kentucky

Lilian Dindo, MA, Department of Psychology, University of Iowa, Iowa City, Iowa

Kevin S. Douglas, PhD, Department of Psychology, Simon Fraser University, Burnaby, British Columbia, Canada

John F. Edens, PhD, Department of Psychology, Southern Methodist University, Dallas, Texas

David P. Farrington, PhD, Department of Criminology, Cambridge University, Cambridge, United Kingdom

Katherine A. Fowler, MA, Department of Psychology, Emory University, Atlanta, Georgia

Don C. Fowles, PhD, Department of Psychology, University of Iowa, Iowa City, Iowa

Paul J. Frick, PhD, Department of Psychology, University of New Orleans, New Orleans, Louisiana

Jean-Pierre Guay, PhD, Department of Psychology, Brandeis University, Waltham, Massachusetts

Jason R. Hall, BA, Department of Psychology, University of Minnesota, Minneapolis, Minnesota

Robert D. Hare, PhD, Department of Psychology, University of British Columbia, Vancouver, British Columbia, Canada

Grant T. Harris, PhD, Research Department, Mental Health Centre, Penetanguishene, Ontario, Canada

Stephen D. Hart, PhD, Department of Psychology, Simon Fraser University, Burnaby, British Columbia, Canada

Kristina D. Hiatt, MS, Department of Psychology, University of Wisconsin, Madison, Wisconsin

William G. Iacono, PhD, Department of Psychology, University of Minnesota, Minneapolis, Minnesota

Raymond A. Knight, PhD, Department of Psychology, Brandeis University, Waltham, Massachusetts

David S. Kosson, PhD, Department of Psychology, Rosalind Franklin University of Medicine and Science, Chicago, Illinois

Robert F. Krueger, PhD, Department of Psychology, University of Minnesota, Minneapolis, Minnesota

Alan R. Lang, PhD, Department of Psychology, Florida State University, Tallahassee, Florida

Scott O. Lilienfeld, PhD, Department of Psychology, Emory University, Atlanta, Georgia

David T. Lykken, PhD, Department of Psychology, University of Minnesota, Minneapolis, Minnesota

Donald R. Lynam, PhD, Department of Psychology, University of Kentucky, Lexington, Kentucky

Angus W. MacDonald, III, PhD, Department of Psychology, University of Minnesota, Minneapolis, Minnesota

Monica A. Marsee, MS, Department of Psychology, University of New Orleans, New Orleans, Louisiana

Christine Michie, BSc, Department of Psychology, School of Life Sciences, Glasgow Caledonian University, Glasgow, United Kingdom

Michael J. Minzenberg, MD, UC Davis Imaging Research Center, UC Davis Health System, Sacramento, California

Craig S. Neumann, PhD, Department of Psychology, University of North Texas, Denton, Texas

Joseph P. Newman, PhD, Department of Psychology, University of Wisconsin, Madison, Wisconsin

Christopher J. Patrick, PhD, Department of Psychology, University of Minnesota, Minneapolis, Minnesota

John Petrila, PhD, Department of Mental Health Law and Policy, University of South Florida, Tampa, Florida

Stephen Porter, PhD, Department of Psychology, Dalhousie University, Halifax, Nova Scotia, Canada

Norman G. Poythress, PhD, Department of Mental Health Law and Policy, University of South Florida, Tampa, Florida

Vernon L. Quinsey, PhD, Department of Psychology, Queen's University, Kingston, Ontario, Canada

Adrian Raine, PhD, Department of Psychology, University of Southern California, Los Angeles, California

Soo Hyun Rhee, PhD, Department of Psychology, University of Colorado at Boulder, Boulder, Colorado

Marnie E. Rice, PhD, Research Department, Mental Health Centre, Penetanguishene, Ontario, Canada

Robert D. Rogers, PhD, Department of Psychiatry, Warneford Hospital, Oxford University, Oxford, United Kingdom

Randall T. Salekin, PhD, Department of Psychology, University of Alabama, Tuscaloosa, Alabama

Michael C. Seto, PhD, Law and Mental Health Program, Centre for Addiction and Mental Health, Toronto, Ontario, Canada

Larry J. Siever, MD, Department of Psychiatry, Mount Sinai School of Medicine, New York, New York

Jennifer L. Skeem, PhD, Department of Psychology and Social Behavior, School of Social Ecology, University of California, Irvine, California

Elizabeth A. Sullivan, MS, Department of Psychology, Rosalind Franklin University of Medicine and Science, Chicago, Illinois

Jeanette Taylor, PhD, Department of Psychology, Florida State University, Tallahassee, Florida

Edelyn Verona, PhD, Department of Psychology, University of Illinois at Urbana–Champaign, Champaign, Illinois

Gina M. Vincent, PhD, Department of Psychiatry, University of Massachusetts Medical School, Worcester, Massachusetts

Jennifer Vitale, PhD, Department of Psychology, Hampden–Sydney College, Hampden–Sydney, Virginia

Irwin D. Waldman, PhD, Department of Psychology, Emory University, Atlanta, Georgia

Thomas A. Widiger, PhD, Department of Psychology, University of Kentucky, Lexington, Kentucky

Michael Woodworth, PhD, Department of Psychology, University of British Columbia–Okanagan, Kelowna, British Columbia, Canada

Yaling Yang, BS, Department of Psychology, University of Southern California, Los Angeles, California

Preface

We are all fascinated by illusions, by things that differ from how they seem. The syndrome of psychopathy is inherently fascinating for this reason: It represents a severe form of psychopathology that is concealed by an outer facade of normalcy—what Hervey Cleckley described as a "convincing mask of sanity." Like *Amyciaea lineatipes*, a species of arachnid that mimics the physical appearance of ants on which it preys, psychopathic individuals readily gain the trust of others because they come across on initial contact as likeable, adjusted, and well meaning. It is only through continued interaction and observation that the psychopath's true, "darker" nature is revealed.

I began my research on this intriguing subject 20 years ago as a graduate student in clinical psychology at the University of British Columbia (UBC). At the time, I was interested in how well lie detector (polygraph) tests work—in particular, factors that might lead innocent persons to fail such tests and factors that might allow guilty suspects to "beat" them. One major question I set out to test was whether individuals diagnosed as psychopathic, because of their skills at lying and deception and their reputed absence of nervousness or guilt, might be able to defeat a lie detector test. I began by reading Cleckley's (1941) seminal monograph on psychopathy and found myself captivated by his case illustrations and his account of psychopaths as "color blind" with respect to normal emotional experience. I read Lykken's landmark study from 1957 in which he used experimental tasks and physiological measurement to test the hypothesis that psychopaths are deficient in anxiety response. I enrolled in a seminar course offered by one of my professors at UBC, Robert Hare, in which I gained exposure to other key empirical studies in this area, including those conducted by Hare and his colleagues. Through contact with Hare's lab group, I also learned how to diagnose psychopathy in criminal offenders using a criterion-based rating system they had developed, adapted from the work of Cleckley—a system that would evolve into Hare's Psychopathy Checklist—Revised (PCL-R; 1991).

These experiences provided me with the clinical and conceptual background I needed to undertake the study I had conceived of—a study in which I arranged for psychopathic and nonpsychopathic prisoners to be tested by professional polygraph examiners to determine whether they had committed a simulated ("mock") crime within the walls of the prison. In the course of this study, I completed diagnostic assessments on over 100 prisoners and I monitored the autonomic reactions of about 50 of these on a laboratory polygraph set up to record physiological responses concurrently with the field polygraph machine used by the examiner. I learned a variety of things from this experience. I learned that not all individuals classified as psychopathic according to Hare's diagnostic criteria presented the same way clinically: Some impressed as charming, gregarious, and witty; others as brash, arrogant, and abrasive; and others as cold and menacing. I learned that not all individuals diagnosed as psychopathic reported a lack of anxiousness in the polygraph test situation. I also learned that individuals classified as psychopaths varied in their physiological reactions on the polygraph test: Some showed very low resting levels of electrodermal and cardiovascular activity and small phasic responses to test questions, whereas others showed high levels of resting activity and pronounced reactions to test questions. Moreover, contrary to the primary hypothesis of the study, I found that very few of the guilty psychopaths succeeded in beating the lie detector test! In summary, I learned from my experiences in this research project that there was still much to be learned about the nature and underlying mechanisms of psychopathy.

In the years since I completed this initial study, a vast amount of new knowledge has in fact been gained regarding the construct of psychopathy. In particular, the publication of Hare's PCL-R in 1991 and its recent second edition (2003) has led to a surge of interest and activity in this area that has greatly advanced our understanding of the disorder, while at the same time highlighting important challenges that remain to be addressed. A new generation of researchers has risen to the fore, representing interests in distinctive facets and subtypes of psychopathy; affiliated personality traits; patterns of diagnostic comorbidity; underlying cognitive and affective mechanisms; developmental processes; phenotypic variation related to age, gender, ethnicity, culture, and other factors; and connections between psychopathy and salient clinical phenomena such as violence, substance abuse, suicide, sexual offending, recidivism, and amenability to treatment. The past several years have also witnessed the emergence of exciting new research paradigms and methods such as cognitive and affective neuroscience, molecular genetics, and advanced quantitative analysis techniques that hold great potential to elucidate unresolved questions in this area.

As a function of these developments, there exists a need for a detailed overview of where the field of psychopathy stands at present and where it appears to be headed in the future. The current handbook was designed to fill this need. It includes contributions from the world's foremost scientific experts on the topic. It highlights key conceptual and practical issues in the field and provides comprehensive coverage of published empirical work relevant to these issues. In addition, it provides coverage of new research methods and theoretical perspectives that hold promise for advancing understanding in this area. Because the PCL-R has emerged as the dominant assessment instrument in this area, special emphasis is placed on the conceptualization of psychopathy embodied in the PCL-R. However, limitations of this approach and alternative models and assessment techniques are considered in detail.

A challenge in an edited volume of this kind is to provide a comprehensive, integrative overview of existing knowledge in the area, as well as to identify priorities for future research in a coordinated way. It is often the case in edited books that chapters cover specific topics related to the research priorities of individual contributors, reviewed within a specific theoretical perspective. This can lead to fractionation as well as redundancy in coverage. To deal with this, contributors were sought for the current volume who were willing to provide a broad review of material within a designated content area without committing to a narrow theoretical perspective (i.e., the emphasis in the book is on descriptive summaries of empirical findings, theories are discussed to the extent that particular lines of work derive from them, and alternative interpretative frameworks are considered). For each of the chapters, a description of the desired content coverage was provided to the contributor, and based on a review of initial drafts of chapters, suggestions were offered as to additional published work that might be incorporated.

Chapters are organized into five broad thematic sections: (1) an initial section that reviews basic terms and influential theories, and which introduces the model of psychopathy embodied in the PCL-R; (2) a section on conceptualization and assessment that highlights recent findings on components (facets) of the psychopathy construct, self-report assessment of psychopathy, relationships with normal personality and disorders listed in the *Diagnostic and Statistical Manual of Mental Disorders*, and phenotypic variants ("subtypes"); (3) a section on etiology, emphasizing cognitive, affective, and behavioral processes and their neurobiological underpinnings, as well as developmental processes, that are relevant to an understanding of psychopathy; (4) a section on special populations, including coverage of psychopathy in children and adolescents, women, diverse ethnic and cultural groups, and noncriminals; and (5) a section focusing specifically on clinical and applied issues, including psychopathy in distinct clinical samples (violent offenders, individuals with substance abuse problems, and sexual offenders), prediction, treatment, and legal/ethical issues. In addition, Parts II–V each include a final integrative chapter that comments on key themes emerging from chapters within that section, and that highlights key priorities for future research. In the closing chapter of the book, I discuss fundamental unanswered questions in the field from the perspective of Cleckley's classic conceptualization of psychopathy—which served as the foundation for modern research on the topic—and suggest strategies by which these questions might be resolved empirically.

In comparison with other existing books on this topic, the current volume is unique in the scope, comprehensiveness, and currency of its coverage. Because of its focus on empirical research findings, the book will be of particular interest to academics and their students as well as researchers in other settings who are interested in crime, antisocial behavior, violence, and substance abuse. In addition, because of its in-depth coverage of issues related to clinical assessment, specialized populations, and intervention, the volume will serve as a valuable resource for psychologists, psychiatrists, and counselors working with criminal offenders and clients with substance abuse problems, and for correctional psychologists and staff. As a function of its emphasis on assessment and coverage of important legal and ethical issues, the book will also be of value to forensic psychologists and psychiatrists and criminal law professionals.

A volume of this kind entails an enormous investment of effort, energy, and patience over an extended period of time, and I owe a debt of thanks to many people for their assistance along the way. My work on this project was supported by the National Institute of Mental Health (Grant Nos. MH52384 and MH65137), by the National Institute on Alcohol Abuse and Alcoholism (Grant No. R01 AA12164), and by funds from the Hathaway Endowment at the University of Minnesota.

I am grateful to my editor at The Guilford Press, Jim Nageotte, for his wise counsel throughout. My thanks go out as well to my colleagues here at the University of Minnesota—William G. Iacono, Robert F. Krueger, David T. Lykken, and Angus W. MacDonald, III—for their contributions as authors, and for providing scholarly input at various stages. I am grateful also to the many other esteemed individuals who contributed to this volume. On the home front, I owe a special debt of gratitude to my wife, Deb, and my daughter, Sarah, who both sacrificed greatly for the sake of this project. Finally, I wish to thank my parents, Don and Susan, and my brother, Dave, for serving as inspiration to me in this and other ongoing efforts.

Many years have now passed since I undertook my first study in this area, but the phenomenon of psychopathy is one that continues to fascinate me. While much remains to be learned, significant advances have been made toward answering many of the questions that arose in my mind at the time I completed my initial study. I hope this book will serve to inspire and point the way for a new generation of researchers in this area—as I myself was inspired early on by the work of Cleckley, Lykken, and Hare.

REFERENCES

Cleckley, H. (1941). *The mask of sanity*. St. Louis, MO: Mosby.

Hare, R. D. (1991). *The Hare Psychopathy Checklist—Revised*. Toronto, ON, Canada: Multi-Health Systems.

Hare, R. D. (2003). *The Hare Psychopathy Checklist—Revised* (2nd ed.). Toronto, ON, Canada: Multi-Health Systems.

Lykken, D. T. (1957). A study of anxiety in the sociopathic personality. *Journal of Abnormal and Clinical Psychology, 55,* 6–10.

Contents

III. ETIOLOGICAL MECHANISMS

IV. PSYCHOPATHY IN SPECIFIC SUBPOPULATIONS

‘

I

THEORETICAL AND EMPIRICAL FOUNDATIONS

1

Psychopathic Personality

The Scope of the Problem

DAVID T. LYKKEN

The term "psychopathic personality," so awkward etymologically in its current usage, was an appropriate choice when first introduced in the late 1800s, for then it embraced a broad group of behavior pathologies suggestive of psychopathology but unclassifiable in any of the categories of mental disorder than current. In 1930, Partridge reviewed that literature and identified a subgroup for whom difficulty (or refusal) to adapt to the demands of society is the pathognomic symptom, and he named this disorder "sociopathic personality." For the next 50 years or so, dangerous or persistent lawbreakers were labeled variously as psychopaths or sociopaths with negligible diagnostic consistency or clarity. Psychiatric diagnosis was an impressionistic art form and even experienced practitioners often could not agree in classifying the same patients except in a very general way (e.g., "psychotic"). Diagnoses sometimes were based on highly subjective inferences about the patient's unconscious impulses and motivations or on the clinician's unsystematic and even quirky observations accumulated over years of practice.

The American Psychiatric Association (APA) published its first *Diagnostic and Statistical Manual of Mental Disorders (DSM)* in 1952 but it was not until the third edition, DSM-III, appeared in 1980 that some mea-

sure of diagnostic consistency was finally achieved. This was accomplished in DSM-III and in DSM-IV, published in 1994, by formulating diagnostic criteria that were relatively objective and noninferential. For the most part, the criteria were arrived at by consensus of committees of clinicians rather than by statistical analysis of empirical data. To be diagnosed with antisocial personality disorder (APD), an individual must show:

A. . . . A pervasive pattern of disregard for and violation of the rights of others occurring since age 15 years, as indicated by three (or more) of the following:

(1) failure to conform to social norms with respect to lawful behaviors as indicated by repeatedly performing acts that are grounds for arrest

(2) deceitfulness, as indicated by repeated lying, use of aliases, or conning others for personal profit or pleasure

(3) impulsivity or failure to plan ahead

(4) irritability and aggressiveness, as indicated by repeated physical fights or assaults

(5) reckless disregardful for safety of self or others

(6) consistent irresponsibility, as indicated by repeated failure to sustain consistent work behavior or honor financial obligations

(7) lack of remorse, as indicated by being in-

different to or rationalizing having hurt, mistreated, or stolen from another

B. The individual is at least age 18 years.
C. There is evidence of Conduct Disorder . . . with onset before age 15 years.
D. The occurrence of antisocial behavior is not exclusively during the course of Schizophrenia or a Manic Episode. (American Psychiatric Association, 1994, pp. 649–650)

No special psychiatric knowledge or insight was required to make a diagnosis on the basis of these guidelines, a fact that no doubt accounts for the good reliability or interrater agreement achieved by DSM-IV. The cookbook-like, relatively objective character of this list of criteria is obvious; what is not so apparent is the fact that there is no theoretical or empirical basis for supposing that this scheme carves Nature at her joints. Because there may be a variety of psychological causes for a given action, classifying people by their actions rather than their psychological dispositions or traits, although natural for the purposes of the criminal law, is less useful for the purposes of psychiatry or science.

Note that the cutoff age of 18 years for the APD diagnosis makes more sense in legal rather than psychiatric terms. In most of the United States, 18 is the age of legal responsibility, although, of course, it is absurd to suppose that delinquent youth undergo some psychological transformation on their 18th birthdays. In view of the alarming recent increase in the number of homicides and other major crimes by youngsters under age 18, many of them now being tried as adults and incarcerated for long periods, it is noteworthy that none of them could be classified as APD.

As one might expect from reviewing these diagnostic criteria, however, a large proportion of those heterogeneous individuals whom we call common criminals could be classified as APD as well as many feckless citizens who do not commit serious crimes. Consider, for example, persons meeting Criteria A1, A2, A4, and A7; these might be the garden-variety criminals who populate most jails and prisons. Persons who meet Criteria A3, A5, and A6 but not the others might also be diagnosed APD, although they are not criminals but, rather, drifters or addicts or drunks. APD is plainly a heterogeneous category in respect to etiology and also in respect to the psychological characteristics that give rise to the varied patterns of socially deviant behavior that serve to meet the criteria. Identifying someone as "having" APD is about as nonspecific and scientifically unhelpful as diagnosing a sick patient as having a fever or an infectious or a neurological disorder.

In spite of the heterogeneity of the group classified by the DSM-IV criteria, APD does at least demarcate a category of individuals that is socially important because many of these people are the reasons why we lock our doors, stay off the streets at night, move out of the cities, and send our children to private schools. A majority of inmates in our prisons meet these criteria for the diagnosis of APD[1] so it is not unreasonable to conclude that they identify more than half of the men whom we normally refer to as common criminals. But these antisocial personalities are clearly diverse, not only in symptoms but also in etiology. I have proposed (Lykken, 1995) a diagnostic scheme in which APD is treated as a family of disorders, comprising two main genera, the psychopaths and the sociopaths, each of which contains several species that differ from each other in their underlying causes.

Species that I classify as *psychopaths* fail to become socialized primarily because of a genetic peculiarity, usually a peculiarity of temperament. A child who is relatively fearless, or unusually impulsive, or given to intense fits of rage, for example, may be too difficult for average parents to control and steer clear of trouble. The larger and most important genus of the APD family consists of those people whom I call *sociopaths*. Many of these people might have become law-abiding and productive citizens had they been reared by healthy, competent, and socialized parents. Because their actual parents were incompetent and/or unsocialized themselves, however, sociopaths are likely not only to have been untrained, neglected, or abused but also to have inherited some of the same temperamental problems that kept their parents locked in the grim confines of the underclass.

The genus of sociopaths is the group that is growing—metastasizing—so rapidly that it already threatens to overwhelm our criminal justice system. Wolfgang and associates studied two cohorts of boys born in Philadelphia, the first in 1945 and the second in 1958 (Tracy, Wolfgang, & Figlio, 1990). Of the 1945 cohort, 6% became chronic criminals responsible for 61% of the Uniform Crime Report (UCR) Index Crimes (and from 69% to 82% of the violent crimes). Of the 1958 cohort, 8% were chronic recidivists, accounting for 68% of the UCR Index Crimes. Based on the 50% increase in the incidence of APD since 1984, we can estimate that perhaps 12% of the males born in Philadelphia in 1970 may be recidivist criminals by now. According to the broader Epidemiologic Catchment Area (ECA) study (Robins & Regier, 1991), the incidence of childhood conduct disorder (CD) among males born from 1961 to 1972 was nearly three times higher than the incidence among men born from 1926 to 1945 and the incidence of adult APD, which by definition must be preceded by CD, has increased in parallel.

IS THERE AN ANTISOCIAL PERSONALITY?

The Multidimensional Personality Questionnaire (MPQ; Tellegen & Waller, 1994) is a widely used self-report inventory with 11 factor-analytically derived scales plus three second-order factors defined by 10 of the 11 trait scales. The first factor, Positive Emotionality, is defined by the traits of Well-Being, Social Potency, Achievement, and Social Closeness. Negative Emotionality is defined by Stress Reaction, Alienation, and Aggression, while the third factor, Constraint, is made up of Control (vs. impulsiveness), Harm Avoidance, and Traditionalism.

We recently obtained scores on the MPQ from 67 inmates at Oak Park Heights,[2] Minnesota's maximum-security prison that receives offenders transferred primarily from other adult male institutions, men who are classified as extreme risks to the public. These inmates, most of whom would meet the criteria for APD, had been convicted of serious crimes; 31 are serving long terms for murder. The men in our sample were assured that neither the fact of their participation nor their resulting scores would become part of their prison records. The only incentive offered for participation was that they would be later given a computer-derived analysis of

the results and told how their scores compared with those of men in general.

Because the MPQ is a self-administered inventory and requires high school reading skills, a proportion of the inmate population could not be sampled, but there is no reason to think that the participants differed temperamentally from the nonreaders. We also collected MPQs from more than 850 male twins age 30 (Lykken, 2000) and used their scale means and standard deviations (SDs) to convert each inmate's scores into T scores, which have means equal to 50 and SDs equal to 10.

Figure 1.1 shows the MPQ T-score means for the 67 inmates. The profile has below-average scores on the scales that determine the Positive Emotionality superfactor of the MPQ; high scores on those comprising the Negative Emotionality superfactor; and reasonably average scores on the scales that comprise the third superfactor, Constraint.

However, the vertical dash-lines reveal that these serious criminals showed a great deal of variation on nearly all 10 traits. Some had really low scores on Well Being and Achievement, combined with frighteningly high scores on Alienation and Aggression. Many other inmates, serving equally long sentences, produced high scores on Positive

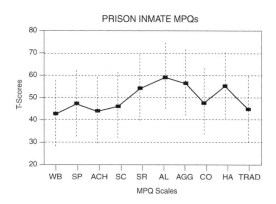

FIGURE 1.1. Mean scores of the 67 Oak Park inmates on 10 trait scales of the Multidimensional Personality Questionnaire. The vertical lines represent one standard deviation above and below each scale mean and reveal that this group of serious offenders was substantially more variable on nearly every scale than was the group of 850 noncriminal young men, for which the mean scores on this graph would be 50 and the standard deviation would be 10.

Emotionality, low scores on Negative Emotionality, and high scores on Control, Harm Avoidance, and Traditionalism. The behavior leading to a diagnoses of APD thus can result from a variety of genetic and/or experiential sources.

Figure 1.2 shows the MPQ *T* scores means for the 22 inmates scoring highest, and the 22 scoring lowest, on Harm Avoidance. The high scorers appear quite benign, deviating from average only in that elevated Harm Avoidance score indicating above-average fearfulness. I have previously argued (Lykken, 1957, 1995) that a boy who is innately relatively fearless will not react well to punishment or intimidation, the techniques most commonly relied on for the socialization of the young, and he may therefore be inclined to seek those peers in the street who admire his fearlessness and, in this way, to become a psychopath. Corroborating this idea, Figure 1.2 shows that the relatively fearless third of the inmate sample display the antisocial profile of high Negative Emotionality combined with low Positive Emotionality and low Constraint. Krueger, Caspo, Moffitt, Silva, and McGee (1996), in a longitudinal study of a normal birth cohort, found that this same pattern of temperament to be associated with antisocial deviance in adolescents.

Thus, while at least a third of these inmates show variants of an antisocial profile of MPQ scores, at least another third of these men, serving long terms in a maximum-security prison, show variants of normal, even harmless-looking, profiles. In fact, for 8 of the 10 MPQ scales in Figure 1.1, these 67 inmates show a within-group variance ranging from 40% to 340% higher than the norm group's variance on the same scales. Unless we are willing to suppose that a third of these prisoners were innocent and mistakenly convicted, this small data set demonstrates that even the persons who commit the most serious crimes are not all cut from the same cloth and, in fact, show wide within-group variations in their personality profiles.

SOCIALIZATION OF CHILDREN

How do most children avoid becoming social misfits? Probably in much the same way as the young of other social mammals learn the rules of their communities, through the monitoring and example of their elders. In southern Africa during the 1990s, the population of white rhinos was being depleted by violence. They were being murdered, not by poachers but by young male elephants who had been orphaned by culling operations in the Kruger National Park (Lemonick, 1997). The adults of the matriarchal herds had been shot and the baby elephants transported to other parks where they grew up without the normal years of parental supervision—and they grew up to be dangerous outlaws. The salvation of the white rhinos, it turned out, was to bring in a number of mature bull elephants, truly "big daddies," who could dominate and socialize these delinquent young males and teach them how a bull elephant is supposed to behave (Fager, 2000).

Our species ranks between the elephants and the great apes, toward the low end, and the ants and hymenoptera, at the high end, of the continuum of socialization. We are born with the capacity to develop a monitoring conscience that works to inhibit rule-breaking. We can learn to feel empathy for our fellow creatures and to take satisfaction in acts of altruism. Most of us develop a sense of responsibility to our families and our community, a desire to pull our own weight in the group effort for survival. We may be the only species with a strong, clearly differentiated self-concept so that we are motivated to emulate people whom we admire in order to feel good about ourselves.

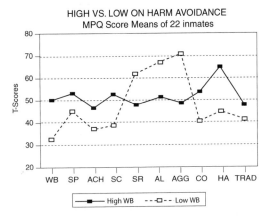

FIGURE 1.2. Mean MPQ scores for the 22 inmates scoring highest, and the 22 scoring lowest, on Harm Avoidance.

Unlike the hard-wired proclivities of the social insects, however, these prosocial inclinations do not emerge in us as well-formed instincts, but, like our inborn capacity for language, they must be elicited, shaped, and reinforced by our interactions with other, older humans during our early development. Our poor success in rehabilitating persons who have reached young adulthood still inadequately socialized suggests that, again like our language capacity, there may be a critical period for socialization. Unless it is evoked, sculpted, and made habitual in childhood, our human talent for socialization may wither and never develop.

WHEN SOCIALIZATION FAILS

Our ancient ancestors lived in relatively small, extended family groups in which grandparents, uncles, aunts, and older cousins all could and undoubtedly did participate in socializing the young. We know that this method of childrearing, the system to which we are evolutionarily adapted, worked because, in most of the traditional societies that still exist in the semiprivacy of our shrinking jungles, all or most adults are expected to cooperate in the rearing of all or most of the tribe's children, and although some of these societies are quite violent, they experience little intramural crime.

For example, in her important study of mental illness in primitive societies, Murphy (1976) found that the Yupic-speaking Eskimos in northwest Alaska have a name, *kunlangeta*, for the

> man who, for example, repeatedly lies and cheats and steals things and does not go hunting and, when the other men are out of the village, takes sexual advantage of many women—someone who does not pay attention to reprimands and who is always being brought to the elders for punishment. One Eskimo among the 499 on their island was called *kunlangeta*. When asked what would have happened to such a person traditionally, an Eskimo said that probably somebody would have pushed him off the ice when nobody else was looking. (p. 1026)

Because traditional methods of socialization are so effective in tribal societies, where the extended family rather than just a particular parent-pair participate in the process, the *kunlangeta* probably possesses inherent peculiarities of temperament that make him unusually intractable to socialization. Such a person I classify as a *psychopath*, an individual in whom the normal processes of socialization have failed to produce the mechanisms of conscience and habits of law-abidingness that normally constrain antisocial impulses.

Some 50 years ago, I conducted an experimental study of this type of antisocial character (Lykken, 1957). Since then, a substantial research literature on the psychopath has accumulated and, in this book, the authors summarize what we know now about these pathologic individuals whose character defects seem to have a biological basis. Yet, as one now surveys the current state of crime and violence in the United States, it is clear that the role played by the primary psychopath is only one small (but important) part of this broader picture.

In the West, and especially in Western urban society, the socialization of children is entrusted largely just to the parents, often to a single parent, and if the parents are overburdened or incompetent or unsocialized themselves then even a child of average temperament may grow up with the antisocial tendencies of a psychopath. I use the term "sociopath" to refer to persons whose unsocialized character is due primarily to parental failures rather than to inherent peculiarities of temperament. On the other hand, the psychopath is almost certain to be a bad parent and the child who receives from a parent both an unsocialized environment and a hard-to-socialize temperament is doubly handicapped.

IMPORTANCE OF FATHERS

There is a striking correlation, at least in the United States, between fatherless rearing and subsequent social pathology. Of the juveniles incarcerated in the United States for serious crimes during the 1980s, about 70% had been reared without fathers (Beck, Kline, & Greenfield, 1988; Sullivan, 1992). Of the antisocial boys studied at the Oregon Social Learning Center, fewer than 30% came from intact families (Forgatch, Patterson, & Ray, 1994). Of the more than 130,000 teenagers who ran away from home in the United States during 1994, 72% were leaving single-parent homes (Snyder & Sickmund, 1995). A 1994 study of "baby truants" in St. Paul, Minnesota—elementary school pupils who had more than 22 unexcused absences in the year—found that 70% were being reared by single mothers (Foster, 1994). Nationally, about 70% of teenage girls who have out-of-wedlock babies were raised without fathers (Kristol, 1994).

A survey by the county attorney in Minneapolis of 135 children who had been referred for crimes ranging from theft, vandalism, and burglary to arson, assault, and criminal sexual conduct—youngsters *ages 9 or younger*—found that 70% of these children were living in single-parent (almost always single-mother) homes (Wiig, 1995). If the baserate for fatherless rearing of today's teenagers is 30% (which is the best current estimate, although this rate is growing alarmingly), then one can calculate that the risk for social pathologies ranging from delinquency to death is about *seven times* higher for youngsters raised without fathers than for those reared by both biological parents. Calculation separately, on reasonable assumptions, for white and black youngsters, yields the same results for both (Lykken, 1995, p. 215).

Correlation does not, of course, prove a direct causal connection. Fatherless children may be at higher risk because single or divorced mothers tend to have to live in impoverished circumstances, often in bad neighborhoods. The biological parents of fatherless children may pass on to their offspring genetic disadvantages, lower IQs, or difficult temperaments. Women (and girls) who end up as single mothers may on average be less competent as parents, either because of their personal limitations or because parenting is simply too difficult and relentlessly demanding for most individuals to accomplish it successfully alone.

In an important recent paper, Harper and McLanahan (1998) analyzed the data from the National Longitudinal Survey of Youth (NLSY) to determine whether the increased crime rate among boys reared without fathers can be attributed to the fact that such children tend more often to be poor, to be black, to live in central cities, or to have been born to teenage mothers. Even after controlling for all of these factors, family structure remained the strongest predictor of the boy's incarceration by age 30. It is interesting that the presence of a stepfather did not decrease the risk associated with mother-only rearing, whereas boys reared by single fathers were no more at risk for serious delinquency—and subsequent sociopathy—than those brought up by both biological parents. This suggests that while the mother's role in childrearing is of central importance, the biological fathers function as an important socializing role model.

CAUSES OF CRIME

Gottesman and Goldsmith (1994) represented the probability of crime or antisocial behavior as a multiplicative function of genetic and environmental factors. Although one cannot argue with the descriptive truth of this formulation, I prefer not to conflate, as this scheme does, the early developmental environment, which is, or should be, dominated by parental interactions, with the current environment of neighborhood and peers. An alternative formulation, which I favor, is to think of antisocial behavior as a multiplicative function of antisocial proclivities or *criminality* interacting with the temptations or protections of the immediate environment. Then, criminality in turn can itself be thought of as a product of genetic factors interacting with early experience, especially experience with parental figures.

By claiming that criminality is a function of temperamental or other innate peculiarities combined with inadequate parenting, I seem to be asserting a leaden platitude. But it is a very important first principle that will point us in the right direction. Many social scientists, sociologists, and anthropologists assume something quite different. Anthropologists since Franz Boas have been "taught to hallow" the idea that "all human behavior is the result of social conditioning" (Freeman, 1992, p. 26). Some psychologists, like Mischel[3] and Haney and Zimbardo (1998), have assumed that behavior is primarily situational and that person-factors—individual differences in traits such as aggressiveness or fearlessness—are unimportant. The classical studies of Hartshorne and May (1928) left generations of psychologists with the belief that "honesty," which sounds very much like "socialization," is also situational, that honesty is not in fact a coherent trait. Sociological theories, like that of Sutherland and Cressey (1978) which dominated criminological thinking during much of the last century, held with Rousseau that crime is a violation of man's natural impulses and must be learned, and many people, including some psychologists, still subscribe to Rousseau's idea that the child is a kind of noble savage, naturally good until corrupted by social influences. Rousseau was able to maintain this inverted image of reality because he abandoned his own children to the care of their mother, but it is difficult to understand how anyone who has actually reared a little boy could sustain such a notion.

All these assumptions are violated in some degree by the contention that most important criminal behavior can be understood in terms of an acquired trait called conscientiousness interacting with the criminal impulse, which varies with both the individual and the situation. Yielding to criminal temptation means that, at least momentarily, the impulse is stronger than the forces of restraint. Children differ innately in characteristics that influence both sides of this equation. Fear of the consequences is an important restraining force and some children are innately more fearful than others. Relatively fearless children tend to develop an effective conscience less readily than most children do and therefore may be less constrained, not only by fear but also by guilt. Unusually impulsive children may act before they think about the consequences and thus fail to experience their internal restraints until it is too late.

Other innate differences among people influence the impulse side of the equation. A hot-tempered child is more sorely tempted to strike out than is one of a more placid disposition, and the newspapers daily report assaults and murders motivated solely by choleric temperament. Some sex criminals appear to possess a ravening, insatiable sex drive, whereas others seem to display a short-circuiting between the brain mechanisms for sex and aggression. For some people, risk itself is a powerful attraction because it can produce in them an excited "high" that is intensely gratifying—and many forms of criminal behavior provide this risk-produced high just as reliably as any

bungee jump. Unsocialized people tend to do a poor job of socializing their own children. For this reason, people with hard-to-socialize temperaments tend to produce children with a double liability, children with difficult temperaments whose parents are unable or unwilling to socialize them.

Figure 1.3 illustrates the differences between psychopathy and sociopathy and how these two troublesome syndromes are related to genetic factors and to parenting. The bell-shaped curve at the left of the figure indicates that most people are in the broad middle range of socialization with a few saintly people very high on this dimension whereas a few more, the criminals, are very low. The horizontal axis represents parental competence and the curve at the bottom assumes

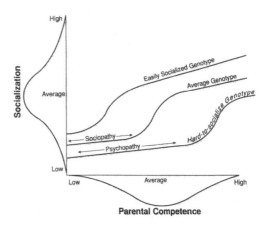

FIGURE 1.3. The socialization of three boys with different genotypes plotted as a function of parental competence. The top curve represents Pat, a boy with an easy-to-socialize temperament who is likely to make it even with relatively incompetent parents. Hard-to-socialize children like Mike, represented by the bottom curve, are likely to become psychopaths unless their parents are unusually skillful or unless strong socializing influences are provided from other sources in their rearing environments. The great majority of youngsters have average genotypes like Bill's, represented by the middle curve. If Bill's parents are average or better in their parenting skills, or if Bill's peer group is uniformly well socialized, then Bill will turn out all right. But if Bill's parents are incompetent and neither the extended family nor the peer group compensates for their ineptitude, then Bill is likely to become a sociopath. From Lykken (1995, p. 11). Copyright 1995 by Lawrence Erlbaum Associates, Inc. Reprinted by permission.

that most parents are average, some are incompetent, and a few are superparents.

The top curve in the body of the figure represents what might happen to a child, call him Pat, whose innate temperament makes him truly easy to socialize; he is bright, nonaggressive, moderately timid, with a naturally loving disposition. Like all little boys, he starts out life essentially unsocialized and, if his parents are totally incompetent, his neighborhood a war zone, and his peers all little thugs, Pat might remain marginally socialized. But boys like Pat tend to avoid conflict and chaos, they are attracted by order and civility, and they tend to seek out socialized mentors and role models. With even poor parenting, the Pats of this world tend to stay out of trouble.

The middle curve in Figure 1.3 represents Bill, a boy with an average genetic makeup, moderately aggressive, moderately adventurous. Because he is average, we can safely anticipate that average parents, living in an average neighborhood, will be able to raise Bill to be an average, law-abiding citizen. Incompetent parents, however, living in a disruptive neighborhood, will not succeed with Bill who will remain a sociopath.

Mike, the bottom curve in the figure, is really difficult to socialize; he may be fearless, impulsive, or hostile and aggressive. The great majority of parents would find Mike too much to cope with, a perennial source of worry and disappointment. Mike's curve goes up on the far right of the figure because really talented parents or, more likely, a truly fortuitous combination of parents, neighborhood, peer group, and subsequent mentors, can sometimes socialize even these hard cases. Mike, in all his interesting varieties, will be the principle subject of this volume.

SOME GENETIC RISK FACTORS ARE EMERGENIC

In the study of noncriminal 30-year-old male twins referred to earlier, MPQ data were obtained from both members of 189 monozygotic (MZ, or identical) twin pairs and from 141 dizygotic (DZ, or fraternal) pairs. The intraclass twin correlations for the DZ twins were less than half as large as those for the MZ twins for all the MPQ scales and superfactors and, as shown in Table 1.1, these MZ–DZ differences were especially marked for the Harm–Avoidance scale scores and for the Negative Emotionality and the Constraint superfactors. In another study of young male twins (Iacono & MacGue, 2002), 235 pairs of 17-year-old males who completed the MPQ produced similar MZ–DZ differences, also shown in Table 1.1.

As we saw in Figure 1.2, among male prison inmates whose average age was similar to that of these twins, those with the lowest scores on Harm Avoidance showed below-normal scores on Constraint generally and also strongly elevated scores on the Negative Emotionality factor, especially on Alienation and Aggression. Even among the noncriminal male twins, the 118 (25%) least-socialized twins (those who admitted the most illegal or antisocial acts) differed significantly ($p < 0.001$) from the remaining 352 twins on these same variables.

When the MZ twin correlation is substantial while the DZ correlation is near zero, it suggests that the genetic factors contributing to the variable in question combine interactively or configurally, rather than additively. Such traits, although half or more of their variance is genetically determined, tend not to

TABLE 1.1. Intraclass Correlations of 17-Year-Old and 30-Year-Old Male MZ and DZ Twins on Three crime-Relevant Traits Measured by the Multidimensional Personality Questionnaire

	17-year-old males		30-year-old males	
	MZs	DZs	MZs	DZs
Variable	158 pair	77 pair	189 pair	171 pair
Harm Avoidance Scale	0.48	0.02	0.63	0.06
Negative Emotion Factor	0.43	0.10	0.62	0.09
Constraint Factor	0.53	0.14	0.50	0.03

Note. Because the DZs are much less than half as similar, within pairs, as the MZs, these traits, each of which is a risk factor for antisocial behavior, while at least half their variance is genetically determined, do not tend to run in families.

run in families because even slight changes in the gene configuration may yield great differences in the traits, and even a traited parent is unlikely to pass on to an offspring all required components of the configuration in the random half of that parent's own genome.

Thus, if low Harm Avoidance or fearlessness is one source of primary psychopathy, and if this trait is emergenic (at least in younger males), then one can understand why primary psychopathy seems to occur almost as frequently in the offspring of well-socialized parents as it does among the underclass. Moreover, if Negative Emotionality and Constraint are also emergenic, at least among younger males, that fact may help explain why some children of even the most poorly socialized parents manage to find socialized mentors and rise out of the underclass (see Dash, 1996; Lykken, 2000).

NONCRIMINAL PSYCHOPATHY

How can a psychopath *not* be a criminal? Suppose Mike does have unusual parents who do not rely on threats and punishment but, instead, show Mike the joys of being treated with respect, with being loved; parents who find positive ways of eliciting socialized behavior and then rewarding that behavior with affectionate pride. If Mike's psychopathy is a result of one of the subtle brain malfunctions that are conjectured in later chapters, then even the most talented parents may be disappointed. But if Mike's "problem" is merely that he is relatively fearless, then those parents might produce a hero instead of a hoodlum. Some historical figures who, I believe, had the "talent" for psychopathy but who did not develop the full syndrome and achieved great worldly success include Winston Churchill (Carter, 1965; Manchester, 1986, 1988); the African explorer, Sir Richard Burton (Farwell, 1963; Rice, 1990); and Chuck Yeager, the first man to fly faster than sound (Wolfe, 1979; Yeager, 1985).

Even without such parents, if Mike is clever, he may avoid petty crimes and misdemeanors (or at least avoid getting caught) while boldly cultivating his innate charm and other talents to win success and status in legitimate society. If we can believe his biographer, Robert Caro (1982, 1988, 2002),

Lyndon Johnson exemplified this syndrome. He was relatively fearless, shameless, abusive of his wife and underlings, and willing to do or say almost anything required to attain his ends. Both Hitler and Stalin were relatively fearless, clever men, unconstrained by guilt or pity, whose ruthless rise to power would not have been possible had they felt normal degrees of caution or conscience. But politics is not the only legitimate profession in which the psychopath can shine. Psychopathic shortages of fear, conscientiousness, and altruism have been, alas, observed in businessmen, investment counselors, media personnel, actors, and entertainers, even in at least one former chief judge of the state of New York (Lykken, 1995, pp. 36–37).

As used by the media, *psychopath* conveys an impression of danger and implacable evil. Hervey Cleckley (1941, 1955, 1982), one of the first and best students of this syndrome, gave a more accurate picture of the psychopath's antisocialism: "Not deeply vicious, he carries disaster lightly in each hand" (1955, p. 33). Like the sociopath, the psychopath is characterized by a lack of the restraining influence of conscience and of empathic concern for other people. Unlike the ordinary sociopath, the primary psychopath has failed to develop conscience and empathic feelings, not because of a lack of socializing experience but, rather, because of some inherent psychological peculiarity which makes him especially difficult to socialize. An additional consequence of this innate peculiarity is that the psychopath behaves in a way that suggests that he is relatively indifferent to the probability of punishment for his actions. This essential peculiarity of the psychopath is not in itself evil or vicious, but, combined with perverse appetites, or with an unusually hostile and aggressive temperament, the lack of these normal constraints can result in an explosive and dangerous package. Perhaps the best collection of examples of criminal psychopaths and vignettes of psychopathic behavior can be found in Hare's (1993) excellent *Without Conscience*, where he asserts that psychopaths can be found "in business, the home, the professions, the military, the arts, the entertainment industry, the news media, academe, and the blue-collar world" (p. 57).

In marked contrast to these dangerous characters, and illustrative of why psychologists find such fascination in the psychopath, is the case of Oskar Schindler, the savior of hundreds of Krakow Jews whose names were on Schindler's list. Opportunist, bon vivant, lady's man, manipulator, unsuccessful in legitimate business by his own admission but wildly successful in the moral chaos of wartime, Schindler's rescue of those Jews can be best understood as a 35-year-old con man's response to a kind of ultimate challenge, Schindler against the Third Reich. Any swine could kill people under the conditions of that time and place; the real challenge—in the words that his biographer may have put in his mouth, the "real power"—lay in rescuing people, especially in rescuing Jews. Some parts of Stephen Spielberg's film *Schindler's List* (1993) do not fit with my diagnosis of Schindler as a primary psychopath, especially the scene near the end in which Schindler (portrayed by Oscar nominee Liam Neeson) breaks down and cries while addressing his Jewish workers. British film maker Jon Blair, whose earlier documentary film, *Schindler*, was truer to history than Spielberg's feature film, noted this same discrepancy: " 'It was slightly out of character, and, of course, it never actually happened,' Blair said" (in Richmond, 1994, p. 17).

NOTES

1. See Harpur, Hare, and Hakstian (1989, p. 9). The overlap of APD with criminality is much lower for women, perhaps because APD criteria are male-oriented: in the large Epidemiologic Catchment Area (ECA) study reported by Robins and Regier (1991), 55% of males but only 17% of females with APD were criminal.
2. I am indebted to Dr. Kenneth Carlson at Oak Park Heights Correctional Facility for collecting these data and sharing them with me.
3. "Imagine the enormous differences that would be found in the personalities of twins with identical genetic endowment if they were raised apart in two different families. . . . Through social learning vast differences develop among people in their reactions to most stimuli they face in daily life" (Mischel, 1981, p. 311).

REFERENCES

American Psychiatric Association. (1994). *Diagnostic and statistical manual of mental disorders* (4th ed.). Washington, DC: Author.

Beck, A., Kline, S., & Greenfeld, L. (1988). *Survey of youth in custody, 1987*. Washington, DC: Bureau of Justice Statistics.

Caro, R. A. (1982). *The path to power*. New York: Knopf.

Caro, R. A. (1988). *The years of Lyndon Johnson*. New York: Knopf.

Caro, R. A. (2002). *Master of the Senate*. New York: Knopf.

Carter, V. B. (1965). *Winston Churchill: An intimate portrait*. New York: Konecky & Konecky.

Cleckley, H. (1941). *The mask of sanity*. St. Louis, MO: Mosby.

Cleckley, H. (1955). *The mask of sanity* (3rd ed.). St. Louis, MO: Mosby.

Cleckley, H. (1982). *The mask of sanity* (rev. ed.). St. Louis, MO: Mosby.

Dash, L. (1996). *Rosa Lee: A generational tale of poverty and survival in urban America*. New York: Basic Books.

Fager, J. (2000, August 22). The delinquents. In *60 Minutes II*. New York: Columbia Broadcasting System.

Farwell, B. (1963). *Burton: A biography of Sir Richard Francis Burton*. New York: Holt, Rinehart & Winston.

Forgatch, M. S., Patterson, G. R., & Ray, J. A. (1994). Divorce and boys' adjustment problems: Two paths with a single model. In E. M. Hetherington, D. Reiss, & R. Plomin (Eds.), *Stress, coping, and resiliency in children and the family* (pp. 96–110). Hillsdale, NJ: Erlbaum.

Foster, E. (1994, April 7). Baby truants at record high in St. Paul. *Minneapolis Star-Tribune*, pp. 1, 8.

Freeman, D. (1992). Paradigms in collision. *Academic Questions, 5*, 23–33.

Gottesman, I. I., & Goldsmith, H. H. (1994). Developmental psychopathology of antisocial behavior: Inserting genes into its ontogenesis and epigenesis. In C. Nelson (Ed.), *Threats to optimum development: Biological, psychological and social risk factors* (pp. 69–104). Hillsdale, NJ: Erlbaum.

Haney, C., & Zimbardo, P. (1998). The past and future of U.S. Prison policy: Twenty-five years after the Stanford Prison Experiment. *American Psychologist, 53*, 709–727.

Hare, R. D. (1993). *Without conscience: The disturbing world of the psychopaths among us*. New York: Pocket Books.

Harper, C. C., & McLanahan, S. S. (1998). *Father absence and youth incarceration*. Paper presented at the 1998 annual meetings of the American Sociological Association, San Francisco.

Harpur, T. J., Hare, R. D., & Hakstian, A. R. (1989). Two-factor conceptualization of psychopathy: Construct validity and assessment implications. *Psychological Assessment, 1*, 6–17.

Hartshorne, H., & May, M. (1928). *Studies in the nature of character*. New York: Macmillan.

Iacono, W. G., & McGue, M. (2002). Minnesota Twin Family Study. *Twin Research, 5*, 482–487.

Kristol, I. (1994, November 3). Children need their fathers. *New York Times*, p. A15.

Krueger, R. F., Caspi, A., Moffitt, T. E., Silva, P. A., & McGee, R. (1996). Personality traits are differentially linked to mental disorders: A multi-trait, multi-diagnosis study of an adolescent birth cohort. *Journal of Abnormal Psychology, 105,* 299–312.

Lemonick, M. D. (1997). Young, single, and out of control. *Time, 150,* 68.

Lykken, D. T. (1957). A study of anxiety in the sociopathic personality. *Journal of Abnormal and Social Psychology, 55,* 6–10.

Lykken, D. T. (1995). *The antisocial personalities.* Mahwah, NJ: Erlbaum.

Lykken, D. T. (2000). The causes and costs of crime and a controversial cure. *Journal of Personality, 68,* 559–605.

Manchester, W. (1986). *The last lion: Winston Spencer Churchill; Visions of glory, 1874–1932.* New York: Little, Brown.

Manchester, W. (1988). *The last lion: Winston Spencer Churchill; Alone, 1932–1940.* New York: Little, Brown.

Mischel, W. (1981). *Introduction to personality* (3rd ed.). New York: Holt, Rinehart & Winston

Murphy, J. M. (1976). Psychiatric labeling in cross-cultural perspective. *Science, 191,* 1019–1028.

Murray, C. (1999). *The underclass revisited.* Washington, DC: AEI Press.

Partridge, G. E. (1930). Current conceptions of psychopathic personality. *American Journal of Psychiatry, 10,* 53–99.

Rice, E. (1990). *Captain Sir Richard Francis Burton.* New York: Scribner's.

Richmond, R. (1994, March 28). A look at the real Schindler tells the searing story. *Los Angeles Daily News,* p. 17.

Robins, L. N., & Regier, D. A. (1991). *Psychiatric disorders in America.* New York: Free Press.

Snyder, H. N., & Sickmund, M. (1995). *Juvenile offenses and victims: A national report.* Washington, DC: Office of Juvenile Justice and Delinquency Prevention.

Spielberg, S. (Director). (1993). *Schindler's list* [Film]. Los Angeles: Universal.

Sullivan, L. (1992, January 6). *Families in crisis* [Address by the then Secretary of Health and Human Services, delivered before the Council on Families in America of the Institute for American Values, p. 6].

Sutherland, E., & Cressey, D. (1978). *Principles of criminology* (10th ed.). Philadelphia: Lippincott.

Tellegen, A., & Waller, N. (1994). Exploring personality through test construction: Development of the Multidimensional Personality Questionnaire. In S. R. Briggs & J. M. Cheek (Eds.), *Personality measures: Development and evaluation* (Vol. 1, pp. 133–161). Greenwich, CT: JAI Press.

Tracy, P. E., Wolfgang, M. H., & Figlio, R. M. (1990). *Delinquency in two birth cohorts.* New York: Plenum Press.

Wiig, J. K. (1995). *Delinquents under 10 in Hennepin County.* Minneapolis, MN: Hennepin County Attorney's Office.

Wolf, T. (1979). *The right stuff.* New York: Farrar, Straus, Giroux.

Yeager, C. (1985). *Yeager: An autobiography.* New York: Bantam Books.

2

A Dual-Deficit Model of Psychopathy

DON C. FOWLES
LILIAN DINDO

Cleckley's classic description and interpretation of psychopathy, combined with the reference to insanity in the title of his book (*The Mask of Sanity*, 1941/1982), strongly encouraged the view that this form of antisocial behavior can be attributed to a deficit. Lykken's (1957) seminal paper articulating what has come to be called the "low fear hypothesis" of psychopathy initiated a now extensive literature on the nature of the deficit (see also Lykken, 1995, pp. 144–149, for a description of this study). Major developments in the past decade in both the adult psychopathy literature and the developmental psychopathology literature focused on antisocial behavior provide new insights into the contribution of low fear to the etiology of psychopathy. Interestingly, they also point to an important alternative pathway to psychopathy—one that has been especially prominent in the developmental psychopathology literature. This pathway involves an incompletely understood deficit that has been variously described as impulsivity, executive function deficits, poor emotion regulation, and so on.

The current standard for diagnosing psychopathy, Hare's (1991, 2003) Psychopathy Checklist—Revised (PCL-R), encompasses two, somewhat distinct dimensions. That is, factor analyses of the PCL-R item set yielded

evidence of two factors with a correlation of about .5 (Hare, 1991, 1998; Hare et al., 1990; Harpur, Hare, & Hakstian, 1989), characterized as affective–interpersonal or "core features" of psychopathy (Factor 1) and impulsive antisocial behavior (Factor 2) (Benning, Patrick, Hicks, Blonigen, & Krueger, 2003; Hare, 1991, 2003; Harpur et al., 1989). To anticipate comments to be made later, Factor 1 relates to the predatory inclinations and deficient emotional reactivity associated with psychopathy, whereas Factor 2 relates to impulsivity/disinhibition, early and chronic antisocial behavior, and a flavor of ineptness in the antisocial behavior (as opposed to competent, proactive predation). These factors also have been found in the Psychopathic Personality Inventory (PPI; Lilienfeld, 1990; Lilienfeld & Andrews, 1996). This self-report instrument, as discussed later, appears to validly assess these dimensions in normal populations. Alternative three- and four-factor models of the PCL-R have recently been proposed (see Hare & Neumann, Chapter 4; Cooke, Michie, & Hart, Chapter 5, this volume), but the validity of Factors 1 and 2 in relation to external criteria is much better documented. Consequently, the present discussion focuses on the broader factors embodied in the original two-factor model.

THE LOW-FEAR HYPOTHESIS

Lykken's Study

Lykken (1957) tested the low-fear hypothesis in three ways. First, he reasoned that the Taylor Manifest Anxiety Scale and the Welsh Anxiety Index from the Minnesota Multiphasic Personality Inventory (MMPI) more strongly reflect "neurotic self-description" (p. 7) or "neurotic maladjustment" (p. 8) or "negative emotionality" (Lykken, 1995, pp. 101–102). In contrast, he developed the Activity Preference Questionnaire (APQ; Lykken, 1995, p. 102) to assess "the extent to which anxiety *determines behavior choices*" (Lykken, 1957, p. 7, emphasis added) and found that it was negligibly correlated with the two neuroticism scales.

Lykken's view of the role of neuroticism in psychopathology is not entirely clear. In his 1995 extensive review and restatement of his position, he clearly referred to the APQ as measuring *fearfulness* (p. 150), and he commented that trait anxiety scales measure neuroticism (reflecting the high correlation between trait anxiety and neuroticism scales). At the same time, Lykken attributed the fearlessness in psychopaths to a deficit in an anxiety system that inhibits behavior (see "Gray's Theory Applied to Psychopathy," later). The fundamental distinction appears to be between the effects of anxiety/fear on *behavior* versus a cluster of characteristics including negative emotional *experience* and negative *self-descriptions*. Lykken does not appear to have been concerned with a major distinction between anxiety and fear that characterizes some of the recent literature on anxiety disorders.

Second, Lykken employed a classical conditioning paradigm in which electrodermal activity (EDA [the skin conductance response, or SCR, primarily a reflection of sweat gland activity; see Fowles, 1986]) constituted the conditioned response (CR) and unconditioned response (UCR), a buzzer served as the conditioned stimulus (CS), and electric shock served as the unconditioned stimulus (UCS). Finally, he created a "mental maze" with four response options at each choice point and 20 choice points. One response option was correct and advanced the subject to the next choice point. Of the three incorrect options, one resulted in shock. The instructed "manifest task" was to advance through the 20 choice points without errors, while the "latent task" was a presumably anxiety-mediated passive avoidance of the shocked response option at each choice point.

Two groups of psychopathic individuals were recruited from a local correctional facility to participate in the study. Primary psychopaths consisted of incarcerated individuals who most resembled Cleckley's prototype according to institutional psychologists. Inmates viewed as having psychopathic tendencies but not resembling the Cleckley prototype were designated neurotic psychopaths. Normal controls were recruited from a local high school.

The results were as predicted. The primary psychopaths had significantly lower APQ scores than the normal controls with the neurotic psychopaths intermediate but nearer to the controls. In contrast, the Taylor and Welsh anxiety scales showed a pattern in which the neurotic psychopaths were significantly *higher* than the normal controls with the primary psychopaths being intermediate and closer to the controls. The primary psychopaths showed poor electrodermal conditioning compared to the normal controls (but not compared to the neurotic psychopaths) and more rapid extinction of the electrodermal response to the CS compared to the neurotic psychopaths. In Lykken's mental maze task the primary psychopaths showed poor avoidance of the shocked error choices compared to normal controls, with the neurotic psychopaths at an intermediate position. Thus, Lykken's study portrayed the primary psychopath as suffering from a deficit in fear conditioning that could be assessed by a questionnaire designed to assess the effects of fear on behavior, electrodermal hyporeactivity during classical aversive conditioning, and poor passive avoidance of shock contingent on erroneous responses.

Replications of Lykken's Results

Of these three findings, electrodermal hyporeactivity in primary psychopaths has been the best replicated by far, as seen in an early review by Hare (1978). Numerous subsequent reviewers (Fowles, 1993; Fowles & Missel, 1994; Lykken, 1995, pp. 153–154, Raine, 1993, pp. 218–221; Siddle & Trasler,

1981; Zahn, Schooler, & Murphy, 1986) agreed.

Although not as robustly replicated, psychopaths' poor avoidance of punishment has received reasonable support. Schachter and Latané (1964) and Schmauk (1970) replicated Lykken's findings with shock as the punishment, as did an unpublished doctoral dissertation by Schoenherr (1964). An apparent challenge to the theory contained in Schmauk's results was dismissed for methodological reasons by Waid and Orne (1982). More results consistent with the hypothesis came from Newman, Widom, and Nathan (1985), who reported a deficit in passive avoidance of punishment for psychopaths with loss of money as the punishment in what they called a go/no-go task. Newman and Kosson (1986) replicated these results in a study that featured additional control conditions. In another study by Scerbo and colleagues (1990), psychopaths failed to show the expected excess of responding to response-contingent punishment but made more responses to the reward stimuli.

Psychopaths also have shown a deficit in avoiding response-contingent loss of money in a card-playing task developed by Siegel (1978) and modified by Newman, Patterson, and Kosson (1987). The probability of punishment, low at the beginning, increased with each block of 10 cards. Psychopaths continued to play the cards after the probability of punishment exceeded the probability of rewards, demonstrating insensitivity to response-contingent punishment. The card-playing task, adapted for children, has revealed response perseveration in children exhibiting conduct disorder (Daugherty & Quay, 1991; Fonseca & Yule, 1995; Shapiro, Quay, Hogan, & Schwartz, 1988), conduct problems with low anxiety (O'Brien & Frick, 1996; O'Brien, Frick, & Lyman, 1994), and conduct disorder combined with attention-deficit/hyperactivity disorder (Daugherty & Quay, 1991; Matthys, van Goozen, de Vries, Cohen-Kettenis, & van Engeland, 1998). Although the adult diagnosis of psychopathy is not applicable to child populations, these studies do suggest that insensitivity to response-contingent punishment may apply to some subset of antisocial children. Frick (e.g., Frick & Loney, 2000; Frick & Morris, 2004; O'Brien & Frick, 1996) suggested that this deficit especially characterizes those children high on the core features of psychopathy (Factor 1), labeled "Callous–Unemotional traits" in Frick's work with children (see "Factor 1 of Psychopathy in Childhood," later).

Replication of the APQ results has been less robust. Of five studies, three failed to discriminate psychopathic from nonpsychopathic prison inmates (Lykken, 1995, p. 149). On the other hand, when applied to college students, low APQ scores are associated with mild antisocial behaviors (speeding tickets, minor legal offenses, heavier drinking) and self-rated adjective descriptors that Lykken (1995, p. 150) sees as consistent with low fear (confident, daring, absence of nervousness, etc.).

Of considerable importance, the dimension assessed by the APQ is explicitly represented in Tellegen's (in press) Multidimensional Personality Questionnaire (MPQ), one of the influential exemplars of the three-factor approach to temperament. The MPQ consists of 11 first-order factors or primary trait dimensions that, in turn, define three major (orthogonal) second-order factors or superfactors: Negative Emotionality (cf. neuroticism) or NEM, Positive Emotionality (cf. extraversion) or PEM, and Constraint (cf. low disinhibition). The first two factors have a strong affective component, whereas Constraint refers more to the regulation of behavior. Some of the APQ items were used to construct the MPQ Harm Avoidance scale (Lykken, 1995, pp. 102, 150) that, along with Control and Traditionalism, defines the Constraint superfactor.

Clark and Watson (1999) describe this Disinhibition versus Constraint superfactor as "the tendency to *behave* in an undercontrolled versus overcontrolled manner . . . constrained individuals plan carefully, avoid risk or danger, and are controlled more strongly by the longer-term implications of their behavior" (p. 403, emphasis added). In contrast, worry and anxiousness (Tellegen, 1985) and general subjective distress (Clark & Watson, 1999) are associated with a separate NEM superfactor whose affective core on the MPQ is the Stress Reaction subscale. These results are consistent with Lykken's position that the *behavioral effects* of fear indexed by the APQ (and represented by Harm Avoidance and Constraint on the MPQ) are distinct from trait anxiety and neuroticism (represented by Stress Reaction and NEM on the MPQ). In addition, low scores on all three trait dimensions of the MPQ Constraint superfactor—Control, Harm Avoidance, and Traditionalism—were associated with life-course persistent delinquency (likely to include psychopaths) in a large, representative sample of male and female 18-year-olds (Krueger et al., 1994).

Gray's Theory Applied to Psychopathy

In 1970, Jeffrey Gray proposed an anxiety deficit in psychopathy conceptualized in terms of what he called the Behavioral Inhibition System (BIS), a construct derived from theories of animal learning and motivation supplemented by consideration of relevant neurobiological findings. The BIS can best be understood in relation to its counterpart, the Behavioral Approach System or Behavioral Activation System (BAS; e.g., Gray, 1978, 1979).

The BAS activates behavior in response to cues or CSs that signal response-contingent reward (simple approach paradigms) or safety and relieving nonpunishment (active avoidance paradigms). On the other hand, the BIS inhibits BAS-activated behavior in response to CSs for response-contingent punishment (passive avoidance) in an approach–avoidance conflict situation, or for frustrative nonreward in an extinction paradigm. From this theoretical perspective, a person with a weak BIS would be approach-dominant in conflict situations and slower to give up responding in extinction situations.

Gray's initial goal was to develop a model of the anxiolytic effects of anxiolytic drugs (alcohol, barbiturates, and minor tranquilizers). In an extensive review, Gray (1977) concluded that these drugs weaken the BIS—that is, reduce the ability to inhibit dominant but incorrect responses (Gray & McNaughton, 2000, p. 340). Considering that aversive stimuli (anticipation of punishment or frustration) activate the BIS and anxiolytic drugs weaken it, Gray concluded that the BIS mediates anxiety responses. Furthermore, he identified the septohippocampal system as the core neurobiological substrate for the BIS in the central nervous system, based on findings that the behavioral effects of lesions in this system paralleled the effects of anxiolytic drugs and that anxiolytic drugs raised the threshold for activating this system by electrical stimulation of the medial septal area.

Although Gray (1970) did not extensively discuss psychopathy, he did suggest that psychopaths seek rewards "with no fear of punishment" and that their persistent antisocial behavior reflects "a relative insensitivity to punishment" (p. 255)—implying a weak BIS combined with a normal (or possibly strong) BAS. Fowles (1980) underscored the match between predictions from the weak BIS hypothesis and the clinical features of psychopathy. The fundamental role of inhibition in Gray's work was relatively new in animal learning theory—for example, Hullian learning theory (1943, 1952) did not have a comparable construct—and was ideal to account for impulsivity in situations of response-contingent punishment and frustrative nonreward. Psychopaths should show weak behavioral inhibition (disinhibition) in passive avoidance and extinction situations.

In addition, whereas earlier formulations assumed that active avoidance is mediated by anxiety, the tradition embraced by Gray placed more emphasis on the anticipation of rewards: safety cues associated with avoidance of the punishment are viewed as the functional equivalent to reward cues and thus activate the BAS. As a result, Gray's theory predicted that psychopaths would have normal (or greater) active avoidance responses that would be more undersocialized. That is, some active avoidance responses are associated with a risk of punishment—for example, feigning remorse or lying to avoid blame for a misdeed and killing witnesses to reduce the chances of prosecution (represented in the animal literature in the two-way active avoidance paradigm; see Fowles, 1980). Such avoidance situations parallel approach–avoidance conflicts. The weak BIS hypothesis predicts that psychopaths would be less restrained by the potential punishments for making these active avoidance responses.

Finally, weak BIS activation in conflict situations predicts that psychopaths would be less anxious than other individuals in such contexts. Thus, the weak BIS hypothesis accounts for both the low anxiety and the behavioral disinhibition observed clinically in psychopaths (Cleckley, 1941/1982) and confirmed in laboratory investigations (Lykken, 1957). Lykken (1995) embraced this perspective (i.e., attributing the fear deficit in psychopathy to a weak BIS).

Gray's Theory Applied to Electrodermal Hyporeactivity

Fowles (1980) used the weak BIS hypothesis to account for discrepancies between heart rate and EDA in anticipation of shock. Hare's (1978) review concluded that, contrary to electrodermal hyporeactivity, psychopaths show normal or even larger cardiac increases in anticipation of punishment. Fowles (1980) proposed that EDA, at least under conditions of anticipation of punishment, reflects activity of the BIS. In contrast, heart rate is strongly tied to somatic activity in order to support metabolic demands, but in addition it reflects motivational processes associated with behavioral activation by the BAS. Given the normality of the BAS in psychopaths, this hypothesis of motivational specificity for heart rate and EDA accounted for the discrepant findings in anticipation of punishment. Gray's theory, thus, made predictions that fit both the clinical features of psychopathy and the psychophysiological findings during the anticipation of punishment.

Summary and Comment

To summarize, the original low-fear hypothesis was conceptualized as a deficit in fear/anxiety conditioning with an emphasis on the effects of fear/anxiety on behavior. Psychopaths were found to show poor aversive conditioning for EDA, to fail to inhibit punished behavior, and to score low on the APQ—a questionnaire designed to assess the effects of fear/anxiety on behavior. Many investigators have reported replications of the first finding and a reasonable number of the second finding. The third has not been well replicated with psychopaths, but a few results have suggested some validity for the APQ as an index of psychopathic features. Importantly, the APQ evolved into the Harm Avoidance scale of Tellegen's MPQ, which has been used extensively in the recent literature.

Patrick (personal communication, November 2004) noted that APQ items require a forced choice between dangerous versus *tedious/boring*, activities and, as a result, are more likely to reflect the "boredom susceptibility" component of the Sensation-Seeking Scale (SSS; see below and Zuckerman, 1991). Benning, Patrick, Blonigen, Hicks, and Iacono (2005, Tables 2 and 4) found that SSS–boredom correlates selectively with Factor 2 of the PPI (PPI-II), whereas the thrill-and-adventure-seeking (TAS) component of SSS correlates selectively with Factor 1 of the PPI (PPI-I). In support of this interpretation, Patrick's group has found that APQ-based items from the Harm Avoidance scale requiring a choice between risk and tedium correlate more with PPI-II, whereas non-APQ items that deal exclusively with attraction to danger seeking (e.g., "I think it would be fun and exciting to experience an earthquake") correlate more with PPI-I. Thus, Patrick suggested that although intended as an index of fearlessness, the APQ may be more an index of boredom aversion associated with psychopathy Factor 2.

Gray's proposal of a BIS deficit in psychopaths offered relatively good theoretical explanations for the clinical features of psychopaths and a way to account for the differences between EDA and heart rate in anticipation of punishment by attributing reactivity to BIS and BAS activity, respectively. In addition, Lykken (1995) reviewed an extensive literature in support of the low-fear hypothesis and found it to be consistent with the concept of a weak BIS. To anticipate issues to be discussed later, note that this formulation assumes that Harm Avoidance, BIS functioning, impulsivity, and the core features of psychopathy are functionally related and should show high correlations.

Over time, a number of issues have emerged that need to be addressed in the context of the low-fear hypothesis. For example, the current fundamental distinction between fear and anxiety at both a clinical and neurobiological level (e.g., Barlow, 2002; Butcher, Mineka, & Hooley, 2004, chap. 6; Gray & McNaughton, 2000, chap. 1; Lang, Davis, & Ohman, 2000) raises questions as to whether the deficit relates more to fear than anxiety, whether the BIS hypothesis is incompatible with a deficit in fear (as opposed to anxiety) conditioning, and whether Harm Avoidance relates to fear or anxiety. Other issues have emerged concerning the nature of the deficit and its relation to impulsivity (e.g., whether the impulsivity deficit relates to core features of psychopathy).

ANXIETY VERSUS FEAR

Considerable evidence at the clinical level points to a fundamental distinction between anxiety and fear (e.g., Barlow, 2000, 2002; Bouton, Mineka, & Barlow, 2001; Brown, Chorpita, & Barlow, 1998; Butcher et al., 2004, chap. 6; Mineka, Watson, & Clark, 1998). Within this framework, anxiety is more cognitive in nature, the defining feature being worry or anxious apprehension about inability to control potential *future* threats, combined with attentional hypervigilance regarding potential threat. Fear, in contrast, is said to constitute an activation of the fight–flight system with substantial autonomic arousal in order to deal with an *imminent* threat. Generalized anxiety disorder (GAD) is the prototype for anxiety, although in varying degrees anxiety is common to all anxiety disorders. Fear is the basis of phobic responses and of panic attacks, the latter being ostensibly uncued fear but often actually a fear response cued by internal (proprioceptive) stimuli.

Hierarchical and Tripartite Models

In the past two decades research has revealed considerable comorbidity between anxiety and depression and their related disorders and has identified neuroticism or negative affectivity as elevated in both. Two descriptive approaches, the tripartite model of Clark and Watson (1991) as recently modified (Mineka et al., 1998) and the hierarchical (latent structure) model of Barlow and his colleagues (e.g., Barlow, 2000, 2002; Brown et al., 1998) have yielded elegant and convergent conceptualizations of this comorbidity and related phenomena. A higher-order factor of negative affect is common to depression and the anxiety disorders, a higher-order factor of positive affect is specifically low in depression, and a lower-order factor of autonomic arousal is strongly related to panic disorder. Negative affectivity correlates strongly with neuroticism and trait anxiety measures.

Consistent with this model, an important twin study by Kendler, Neale, Kessler, Heath, and Eaves (1992) demonstrated a common genetic diathesis for GAD and major depression, with individual specific environment determining whether GAD or major depression develops. The authors suggested that this shared vulnerability to anxiety and depression consists of general distress reactivity, later found to be well indexed by neuroticism (Kendler, 1996). Similarly, other reviews have identified neuroticism as a major risk factor for anxiety and depression (Butcher et al., 2004, chap. 7; Clark, Watson, & Mineka, 1994; Klein, Durbin, Shankman, & Santiogo, 2002; Mineka et al., 1998).

From the perspective of psychopathy, this literature raises several overlapping questions. First, how can Gray's BIS as an *anxiety* system be understood in terms of the deficit in psychopathy, primarily conceptualized as low *fear*, and how does the BIS relate to measures of negative affect (NEM) versus Harm Avoidance? Second, how does the relatively strong distinction between anxiety and fear relate to the nature of the deficit in psychopathy? Third, how does Harm Avoidance relate to the anxiety-versus-fear distinction?

The BIS, Trait Anxiety, and Harm Avoidance

To a large extent, Gray's own views parallel the aforementioned picture (i.e., he drew a distinction between anxiety and fear and viewed neuroticism measures as an index of anxiety). He distinguished between anxiety and panic (e.g., Gray & McNaughton, 2000), with the BIS related to anxiety and the fight–flight system related to panic attacks. Furthermore, Gray and McNaughton (2000, pp. 34–35) characterized GAD as having strong cognitive-attentional components (an excessively strong focus on potential threats) that are manifestations of excessive activity in the BIS. At least in the past (see Gray & McNaughton, 2000), Gray viewed trait anxiety as strongly related to BIS reactivity. Thus, a hypothetical BIS deficit in psychopaths should relate to low scores on trait anxiety—contrary to the Harm Avoidance hypothesis that relates psychopathy to a component of disinhibition or low Constraint on Tellegen's MPQ.

In a major reevaluation of the theory, Gray and McNaughton (2000, p. 338) emphasized that the BIS is activated only when there is goal conflict. In their theoretical approach, *by definition*, only BIS activation constitutes "anxiety." In consequence, they suggest that neuroticism or trait anxiety may reflect "general sensitivity to threat" and that only a subset of threat-related stimuli (i.e., conflict-producing) increases anxiety as they define it. Consistent with this perspective, they use the terms "neuroticism" and "trait anxiety" to refer to "susceptibility to anxiety-related disorders" (p. 341). In spite of this conceptual distinction between trait anxiety and BIS reactivity, it appears that Gray and McNaughton view individual differences in BIS reactivity as a major contributor to trait anxiety. Nevertheless, important processes such as classical aversive conditioning or exposure to uncontrollable aversive stimuli, which do not involve motivational conflict, may affect susceptibility to anxiety disorders apart from BIS functioning.

Although not suggested by Gray and McNaughton, it is worth considering that the BIS may contribute significantly to Harm Avoidance (Fowles, 2000), consistent with Lykken's linkage of both the BIS and Harm Avoidance to psychopathy. The critical role of the BIS in inhibiting behavior in situations that involve danger or risk appears to fit Lykken's description of the APQ as reflecting the effects of fear/anxiety on behavior. Similarly, Clark and Watson's description (see previously) of the superfactor of Constraint as reflecting the inhibitory control over behavior to avoid immediate risk or danger and longer-term negative consequences seems parallel to the central role of the BIS in approach–avoidance conflict situations.

In contrast, Tellegen's (1985) description of NEM does not refer strongly to inhibition of behavior: "an appraisal of oneself as unpleasurably engaged, as stressed by one's own and others' actions and attitudes . . . a tendency to worry, to be anxious, to feel victimized and resentful, and to appraise generally in ways that foster negative emotional experiences" (p. 696). More generally, PEM and NEM strongly relate to *affect and cognitions*, whereas Harm Avoidance and the other Constraint factors have more to do

with inhibition of *behavior* that might lead to trouble. As a construct derived from animal paradigms having to do with inhibition of behavior rather than experienced affect, the BIS seems relevant to Harm Avoidance and Constraint. If so, the association of psychopathy and Harm Avoidance would fit with the BIS hypothesis. Although unfortunately this issue remains unresolved, this possibility at least is consistent with the view that psychopaths have a BIS deficit and are low on Harm Avoidance.

It should be kept in mind, however, that phenotypic, factor-analytically defined psychological traits are unlikely to map directly onto underlying brain systems (Lykken, 1971). Rather, it is more likely that underlying fear and anxiety systems interact with each other under many conditions and that both may contribute to components of the psychological traits of neuroticism/trait anxiety and Harm Avoidance or disinhibition. Thus, both a weak BIS and reduced cue-specific fear reactivity might contribute both to low Harm Avoidance and to lower scores on neuroticism/trait anxiety, perhaps in partially overlapping and partially specific ways. For example, Patrick (personal communication, November 2004) suggests that lesser cue-specific fear reactivity (associated with individual differences in fear-potentiated startle) is related to some aspects of both MPQ Stress reaction (e.g., vulnerability vs. insensitivity) and MPQ Harm Avoidance (i.e., pure enjoyment of dangerous activities, such as "I think I would enjoy the experience of an earthquake"), as opposed to preference for risk over tedium).

Fear Conditioning, the Amygdala, and the BIS

Gray and McNaughton (2000, p. 1) commented that current orthodoxy (other than their own work) views the amygdala rather than the septohippocampal system as the "key brain structure underlying anxiety." This comment refers to a large and elegant literature on the neural pathways involved in classical aversive fear conditioning, especially the work of Davis (e.g., Davis, Walker, & Lee, 1999; Lang et al., 2000) and LeDoux (e.g., 1995, 2000, 2002, pp. 212–229).

The (unconditioned) acoustic startle reflex in the rat is the point of departure for much of this literature. In particular, Davis's work on the potentiation of the startle reflex that occurs in the presence of a brief light (CS) previously paired with shock is of great interest, and the amygdala looms large in this effect. LeDoux's parallel work, which employs freezing rather than startle and a tone rather than a light CS, equally implicates the amygdala. Basic sensory information about the aversive CS is transmitted directly from the thalamus (basic sensory information) or indirectly via the cortex (more complex conditioned fear stimuli) to the lateral nucleus of the amygdala. As a result of the conditioning that has occurred to the CS, the lateral nucleus activates the central nucleus of the amygdala which, in turn, initiates the behavioral and physiological expression of fear.

Although at first glance this literature on *fear* conditioning appears unlikely to challenge a theory of *anxiety*, several issues arise from this work that are pertinent to Gray's theory and psychopathy. First, studies have suggested that the bed nucleus of the stria terminalis (seen as part of an "extended amygdala") plays a critical role in anxiety (Davis, 1998; Lang et al., 2000). Exposure to bright light for 5–20 minutes induces startle potentiation in rats similar to, but more prolonged than, that produced by fear CSs, as does injection of corticotropin-releasing hormone (CRH) into the ventricles. Ventricular CRH produces fear- and anxiety-like neuroendocrine and behavioral effects, and the anxiolytic drug chlordiazepoxide (as well as buspirone in the case of light) decreases both of these effects, suggesting that light and CRH exposure produce anxiety, which enhances the startle response. Various manipulations indicate that the bed nucleus of the stria terminalis, but not the central nucleus of the amygdala, is involved in this anxiety-like, longer-term potentiation of startle, but not in fear-potentiated startle. Conversely, the central nucleus of the amygdala is involved in fear-potentiated startle but not in the light- or CRH-potentiated startle effects.

A second finding in this amygdala/fear-reactivity literature distinguishes between explicit (e.g., tone–shock) fear conditioning and contextual fear conditioning (e.g., LeDoux, 1995, 2000, 2002). When animals are returned to the chamber in which explicit cue conditioning previously occurred, they freeze and act afraid in response to the environment. This *contextual conditioning* phenomenon depends on the hippocampus as well as the amygdala, the former presumably because of its "role in relational/configural/spatial processing" (LeDoux, 2002, p. 216); in contrast, the hippocampus is not involved in explicit cue conditioning. This view of the role of the hippocampus in the response to dangerous contexts overlaps to some extent with Gray's emphasis on the role of the septohippocampal system in passive avoidance conflict or in "facilitating entry into a dangerous situation" (Gray & McNaughton, 2000, p. 217; see also LeDoux, 1995; Patrick & Lang, 1999).

To accommodate this more recent research on fear conditioning and the amygdala, Gray and McNaughton (2000, pp. 281–284) modified the BIS to include the amygdala: Output from the septohippocampal system combined with activity in the amygdala constitutes anxiety, and the amygdala produces the increased nonspecific arousal and autonomic activity associated with BIS activity. With respect to the bed nucleus of the stria terminalis, Gray and McNaughton acknowledged the above findings but suggested that it is too early to conclude that the bed nucleus plays a critical role in anxiety.

With this modification of the theory of the BIS, there is somewhat less conflict with the amygdala literature, but Gray and McNaughton acknowledge that the BIS no longer is identified with a "neurally unified set of structures" (p. 284) as it was in the original theory. In any case, whatever the ultimate outcome of the septohippocampal system versus the extended amygdala as central to anxiety, the use of a classically conditioned fear CS to potentiate startle seems to reflect fear rather than anxiety.

PSYCHOPATHY AND THE STARTLE RESPONSE

The amygdala/fear research is important to psychopathy because it has inspired research on fear-potentiated eyeblink startle in humans (e.g., Bradley, Cuthbert, & Lang, 1999; Lang, Bradley, & Cuthbert, 1990) that has been applied to psychopathy. In general, induction of positive affect by exposure to positively valenced perceptual stimuli (e.g., pictures or sounds) attenuates the acoustic startle reflex, whereas induction of negative affect by exposure to negatively valenced stimuli potentiates startle.

Applying this paradigm, Patrick, Bradley, and Lang (1993) reported that psychopaths failed to show the normal potentiation of startle with negative pictures but did show normal attenuation of startle with positive pictures. The finding has been well replicated (Herpertz et al., 2001; Levenston, Patrick, Bradley, & Lang, 2000; Pastor, Molto, Vila, & Lang, 2003; Sutton, Vitale, & Newman, 2002; Vanman, Mejia, Dawson, Schell, & Raine, 2003). These results strongly support the *selective* fear deficit hypothesis, because positive pictures produced a normal attenuation of startle. They also point to the amygdala as a source of this deficit, because of the presumed role of the amygdala in the fear-potentiated startle phenomenon.

Consistent with this interpretation, attempts to identify subjects with stronger than normal potentiation of startle have been much more successful when subjects are selected for phobias rather than anxiety or high negative affect (Cook, 1999; Cuthbert et al., 2003). The strength of this perspective that amygdala dysfunction is central to psychopathy can be seen in Blair's (Chapter 15, this volume) proposal that punishment-based learning dependent on the amygdala is impaired.

The results of this psychopathy–startle work are theoretically important for another reason: The observed deficit in startle potentiation relates specifically to the affective–interpersonal factor (Factor 1) of the PCL-R (Patrick, Cuthbert, & Lang, 1994; Patrick et al., 1993), consistent with the idea that these core features of psychopathy reflect low fear (Lykken, 1995). In contrast, fear-potentiated startle appears to be unrelated to the impulsive antisocial behavior (Factor 2) component of psychopathy. This specificity challenges the assumption that low fear and impulsivity are two manifestations of the same underlying process, and it points to impulsivity as a second possible deficit. Indeed, Patrick and Lang (1999) and Patrick (in press) propose a similar dual-deficit model, suggesting that a deficit comparable to the effect of alcohol intoxication on higher cortical systems may be responsible for the impulsivity seen in connection with Factor 2.

PERSONALITY AND PSYCHOPATHY

Personality Inventories

The relevance of personality measures to psychopathy is obvious from the foregoing discussion regarding trait anxiety/neuroticism and Harm Avoidance/Constraint. Furthermore, Widiger (1998), Lynam and Derefinko (Chapter 7, this volume), and Krueger (Chapter 10, this volume) have proposed that psychopathy can be understood in terms of personality dimensions. The major approaches to personality include Tellegen's three-factor approach already mentioned, Eysenck's (1990) three factors of Neuroticism, Extraversion, and Psychoticism (the latter generally viewed as misnamed and reflecting disinhibition more than psychosis; Clark & Watson, 1999), and the five-factor model (FFM) of Costa and McCrae (1989). In addition, the EASI Temperament Inventory (EASI; Buss & Plomin, 1975, 1984), which indexes constructs of Activity, Sociability, and Emotionality (the latter encompassing correlated dimensions of Fearfulness, Anger, and Distress), has been employed in some studies.

As noted earlier, the MPQ Constraint dimension encompasses Harm Avoidance, Control, and Traditionalism components. MPQ PEM includes facets of Well-being, Social Potency, and Achievement, and MPQ NEM includes facets of Stress Reaction, Alienation, and Aggression. In addition, MPQ PEM has been subdivided into subdimensions reflecting distinctive interpersonal dispositions of "agency" and "communion" (Hicks, Markon, Patrick, Krueger, & Newman, 2004) or "affiliation" (Depue & Collins, 1999; Depue & Lenzenweger, 2001; Depue & Morrone-Strupinsky, in press).

Affiliation involves "enjoying and valuing close interpersonal bonds, and being warm and affectionate," whereas agency "reflects social dominance and the enjoyment of leadership roles, assertiveness, and a subjective sense of potency in accomplishing goals" (Depue & Morrone-Strupinsky, in press). These trait dimensions are essentially uncorrelated once the common element of well-being or positive affect has been eliminated from each. With regard to their association with psychopathy, the obvious prediction for primary psychopaths is low affiliation (lovelessness) combined with high agency.

The FFM factors are Neuroticism, Extraversion, Agreeableness (vs. Antagonism), Conscientiousness, and Openness to Experience. At the level of superfactors, FFM Neuroticism and Extraversion are highly similar to MPQ NEM and PEM. Conscientiousness and Agreeableness both correlate about .5 with MPQ Constraint, suggesting that they can be seen as components of Constraint, although each also has specific variance not found in Constraint (Clark & Watson, 1999). Considering the primary facets and citing Church (1994), Benning and colleagues (2003) identified the following as the strongest associations between the MPQ and FFM that are relevant to psychopathy: FFM (low) Agreeableness with the MPQ Aggression and Alienation facets of NEM, FFM Neuroticism with the MPQ Stress Reaction Facet of NEM, and FFM Conscientiousness with both the MPQ Control component of Constraint and the achievement facet of PEM. Thus, the Antagonism end of Agreeableness includes elements of MPQ NEM having less to do with stress reactivity, and Conscientiousness includes achievement or agentic elements of MPQ PEM.

Personality Correlates of the Psychopathy Factors

Recent research has considered the complex relationships of the two major components of psychopathy defined by the PCL-R with these personality dimensions. The correlation of about .5 between the PCL-R factors can result in two, quite different strategies (e.g., Krueger, Chapter 10, this volume)—either focusing on the variance in common or on the variance specific to each factor. In a critical decision, Patrick and his colleagues have examined the correlations for one factor after controlling for the variance common to both factors, thereby identifying the personality correlates of the variance *specific* to that factor. This strategy has been highly productive, and the results constitute much of the empirical core for the dual-deficit model of psychopathy embraced here.

Because of the complexity of the relationships among these different sets of broad superfactors and associated primary traits, the attempt to summarize the results discussed later is inherently difficult to follow. It may be useful to state the conclusions at the outset. The most important inferences to be drawn from the review below are that low fear and/or anxiety is specifically associated with affective–interpersonal dimension (Factor 1) of psychopathy and that impulsivity/disinhibition is specifically associated with the impulsive–antisocial behavior dimension (Factor 2). Several additional specific associations are important: (1) Factor 2 with externalizing disorder diagnoses, (2) Factor 1 with approach motivation (PEM) expressed as dominance rather than affiliation, and (3) Factor 2 with aggression, alienation, and antagonism (showing that lovelessness/poor attachments are not limited to Factor 1).

A summary of this literature by Patrick and his colleagues (Benning et al., 2003) concluded that neuroticism measures from several inventories correlated consistently and negatively with the unique variance in PCL-R Factor 1 but *positively* with the unique variance in PCL-R Factor 2. The negative correlations for Factor 1 reflect especially the distress, fear, and/or stress reaction components, whereas Factor 2 correlates positively with all facets of neuroticism (negative emotionality) (i.e., with anger, aggression, and alienation, as well as distress, fear, and stress reaction). Second, Factor 2, but not Factor 1, shows negative associations with the MPQ Constraint superfactor and the somewhat overlapping dimension of Conscientiousness from the FFM of Costa and McCrae (1989). Finally, MPQ Agentic PEM is correlated positively with PCL-R Factor 1 but negatively with Factor 2.

In a somewhat similar review of the psychopathy and personality literature that emphasized the FFM but employed only simple correlations between the PCL-R factors (i.e., not controlling for the overlap between the factors), Lynam and Derefinko (Chapter 7, this volume) found that a substantial negative correlation with Agreeableness for both PCL-R factors accounted for much of the correlation between those factors. Factor 1 correlated weakly and negatively with Conscientiousness but not at all with Neuroticism and Extraversion. Factor 2 showed a strong positive correlation with Neuroticism, a strong negative correlation with Conscientiousness, and a weak negative correlation with Extraversion. These findings are consistent with the summary by Benning and colleagues (2003) in showing that, at the level of the three-factor model superfactors, Factor 2 correlates strongly with Neuroticism. In addition, the Factor 2 negative correlation with FFM Conscientiousness is consistent with its negative associations with MPQ Constraint and MPQ agentic PEM. The positive correlation reported for Factor 2 with FFM Antagonism is consistent with Benning and colleagues' previously noted positive associations between PCL-R Factor 2 and the Aggression and Alienation scales of the MPQ, which are most related to FFM Agreeableness/Antagonism. The fact that both PCL-R factors showed negative associations with Agreeableness points to a strong common element of aggression and alienation that is not obvious for Factor 1 when only the specific variance is considered.

Because the PCL-R was developed on the basis of data from prisoner samples and is most appropriate for use in incarcerated populations, it is useful to consider other measures of the psychopathy construct appropriate for nonincarcerated samples. Probably the best such measure is the PPI (Lilienfeld & Andrews, 1996) mentioned earlier, which has shown robust associations with both factors of the PCL-R in incarcerated samples (Poythress, Edens, & Lilienfeld, 1998). Using a large, community-based male sample, Benning and colleagues (2003) found two dominant orthogonal (rather than correlated) factors in the PPI (labeled PPI-I and PPI-II) corresponding roughly to the PCL-R factors.

Using the MPQ, Benning and colleagues (2003) reported correlates of PPI-I and -II consistent with the aforementioned findings indicating that one component (PPI-I) of psychopathy is associated with low NEM and low stress reactivity and, more clearly than for the PCL-R factors, reduced effects of fear on behavior (i.e., low Constraint and low Harm Avoidance). Their results also supported the association of Factor 2 with high NEM, a strong negative orientation toward other people (high alienation and aggression, low social closeness), and impulsivity (low Control and Traditionalism but, importantly, not with Harm Avoidance). PPI-I was positively associated with agentic PEM and Social Potency. PPI-II was associated with a wide range of externalizing behaviors.

Dindo, McDade-Montez, and Watson (2005) have recently replicated Benning and colleagues' (2003) finding of two dominant factors for the PPI in a large group of undergraduate students. Furthermore, in this study, PPI-I was strongly and negatively correlated with several widely used trait measures of NEM and positively related to several measures of PEM. PPI-II showed opposing relations with NEM and PEM to those shown by PPI-I, and in addition showed positive associations with various indices of disinhibition and with various drinking and smoking behaviors.

Benning and colleagues (2005) evaluated the PPI factors in three diverse samples including young adults from the community, college students, and male prisoners. Consistent with findings for the PCL-R factors, their results emphasize that Factor 1 of the PPI is negatively related to anxiety and fear (anxiety, depression, trait anxiety, self-reported fear, social phobia, number of phobias), positively related to engagement in physically dangerous behavior and an egocentric interpersonal style, and generally unrelated to impulsivity and externalizing disorders. Similarly, as in previous studies, Factor 2 of the PPI was positively correlated with both internalizing (depression and anxiety) and externalizing disorders, impulsivity/disinhibition, trait anxiety, and anger, while being negatively correlated with prosocial attitudes toward others (sociability, empathy).

Summary

Overall, these results suggest the following: The unique variance in psychopathy Factor 1 shows a strong negative relation to the anxiety/fear components of neuroticism/NEM (fearfulness, distress, stress reaction, depression, phobias, trait anxiety) and little relation to alienation and aggression. PCL-R Factor 1 shows little unique relation to the Constraint superfactor, but PPI-I shows a positive correlation with engaging in dangerous behaviors (i.e., a negative correlation with Harm Avoidance, and a positive correlation with thrill and adventure seeking), as well as a dominant/exploitative orientation to others (agentic PEM, narcissism). Factor 1 appears to be unrelated to impulsivity/disinhibition (other than engaging in dangerous behavior) and to externalizing disorders.

In contrast, the unique variance in Factor 2 from both the PCL-R and the PPI tends to be positively correlated with neuroticism/NEM (anxiety, depression, fear, anger, alienation), impulsivity/disinhibition (i.e., negatively correlated with all aspects of Constraint), and the externalizing disorders, and it is negatively related to agentic PEM (in particular, its Achievement facet). Low FFM Agreeableness (high Antagonism) characterizes both factors for the PCL-R in prison males and is likewise associated with both factors of the PPI (Ross, Benning, Patrick, Thompson, & Thurston, 2005)—possibly because high Antagonism reflects both dominance (Factor 1) and Aggression (Factor 2).

Cluster Analysis of Psychopathy

Hicks and colleagues (2004) employed cluster analysis to identify subtypes among incarcerated PCL-R diagnosed psychopaths on the basis of the MPQ primary trait scales. As expected, the best-fitting cluster solution identified two subtypes with a strong resemblance to the specific correlates of PCL-R Factors 1 and 2 summarized earlier. Based on their most extreme trait scale scores, the subtypes were labeled "emotionally stable" (low Stress Reaction) and "aggressive" (high Aggression). In comparisons of the two subtypes on MPQ primary factors, the aggressive psychopaths were higher on Stress Reaction, Alienation, and Aggression and lower on Well-being, Achievement, and Control. In comparisons involving the MPQ superfactors, the emotionally stable psychopaths were higher on Agentic-PEM and Constraint, but lower on NEM.

Scores of the two subgroups on MPQ Social Closeness are of particular theoretical interest. Only the aggressive psychopaths were significantly lower than prisoner controls, with emotionally stable psychopaths being intermediate. Thus, although "lovelessness" has often been said to characterize primary psychopaths, only the aggressive (secondary) psychopaths showed significantly lower attachments (Social Closeness) than the controls.

Although the psychopathy subtypes clearly differed on personality traits in the directions suggested by the correlates of psychopathy Factors 1 and 2, it is of interest that the subtype groups differed significantly but only

"slightly" on Factor 2 and did not differ on Factor 1 scores. Also, as noted previously, all these subjects met the PCL-R criteria for psychopathy (i.e., overall PCL-R score > 30). Thus, from the perspective of the PCL-R as the operational definition of psychopathy, both subgroups must be considered "true" psychopaths.

A compelling explanation for the minimal factor differences (C. J. Patrick, personal communication, June 2004) is that there are two distinct etiological pathways to the high PCL-R phenotype with PCL-R Factors 1 and 2 representing imperfect indicators of the underlying trait dispositions associated with each. From this standpoint, Factor 1 reflects more a "fearless–dominant" trait disposition, and Factor 2 more an impulsive–antisocial behavior ("externalizing") disposition. However, because the items of the two PCL-R factors are rated substantially on the basis of overlapping, offense-related information, higher scores on one factor tend to be associated with higher scores on the other (i.e., there is a general element of criminal deviance that enters into the scoring of both factors).

Summary and Conclusions

Important theoretical inferences can be drawn from this literature with respect to the low-fear hypothesis. First, the low-fear/low-anxiety hypothesis clearly applies to PCL-R and PPI Factor 1 and the related emotionally stable subtype (from cluster analysis) with particularly strong evidence of a relation for Stress Reaction, but it does not apply to Factor 2, which is characterized by high levels of all aspects of NEM. Second, there is little indication that Factor 1 is more specifically related to low fear in the form of Harm Avoidance (engaging in dangerous behavior) than to low anxiety (anxiety, depression, trait anxiety, neuroticism, stress reactivity, etc.)—both appear to be strong correlates. Third, the impulsivity or disinhibition identified in the personality domain clearly applies to Factor 2 and the related aggressive subtype but not to Factor 1, for which the only component of impulsivity is low Harm Avoidance. Indeed, the emotionally stable psychopaths in Hicks and colleagues (2004) described themselves (in terms of their MPQ trait scores) as planful and unlikely to act without forethought. It appears, therefore, that the form of impulsivity associated with primary or Factor 1 psychopathy is one of willingness to take risks even after considering the consequences.

Fourth, Factor 2 and the aggressive subtype are more strongly associated with aggression and, to some extent, poor attachments or lovelessness in the form of high scores on anger, alienation, and antagonism. At the least, aggression and poor attachments are not specifically associated with emotionally stable psychopaths. In some respects, then, this group would be viewed by many as dangerous and severe "real" psychopaths, not as a group that is in some sense peripheral to the construct of psychopathy. Although the term "primary psychopath" traditionally has been applied to the emotionally detached group epitomized by Factor 1 features, it is unfortunate that such usage has tended to relegate the high negative affect, aggressive psychopaths (i.e., those epitomizing the Factor 2 features) to a category of lesser interest.

Fifth, emotionally stable psychopaths appear to be high in approach motivation (PEM), which is channeled into dominance and instrumental, controlling behavior rather than affiliation with others. Sixth, the identification of Factor 2 and aggressive psychopathy with the broad externalizing factor of psychopathology (see also Krueger, Chapter 10, this volume; Patrick, in press; Patrick, Hicks, Krueger, & Lang, 2005) identified in children and adults makes a connection to a very large developmental psychopathology literature on the etiology of externalizing disorders. Although a review of that literature is beyond the scope of this chapter, some major trends can be noted.

PSYCHOPATHY FACTORS IN CHILDHOOD

Factor 2 of Psychopathy and the Externalizing Disorders

Childhood disorders have long been characterized in terms of broad dimensions of internalizing—especially anxiety and depression—and externalizing psychopathology—especially attention-deficit/hyperactivity disorder (ADHD), oppositional defiant disorder (ODD), and conduct disorder (CD)—with antisocial behavior being strongly associated with externalizing disorders (e.g., Quay, 1986). Moffitt and Lynam (e.g., Lynam, 1998; Moffitt, 1993; Moffitt & Caspi, 2001; Moffitt & Lynam, 1994) have argued that early-onset ODD/CD, combined with hyperactivity (ADHD, but not the predominantly inattentive subtype) and neuropsychological deficits, frequently develops into adult psychopathy. A comprehensive review of this literature by Hinshaw and Lee (2003) found strong support for this perspective. In addition, Lynam (1998) found that adult psychopathy is predicted by this combination of ADHD symptomatology and aggressive behaviors. In other recent work, Krueger and colleagues (2002; see also Krueger, Chapter 10, this volume) demonstrated that the externalizing disorders share a latent vulnerability, largely reflecting genetic influence, that accounts for their comorbidity.

The general finding that psychopathy Factor 2 correlates strongly with impulsivity/disinhibition, combined with this factor's association with externalizing disorder symptoms and diagnoses (child/adult antisocial deviance, alcohol abuse/dependence, and drug abuse/dependence—see above and Krueger, Chapter 10, this volume), greatly strengthens the hypothesis that a subset of the comorbid ADHD–CD children develop into adult psychopaths. Thus, there is good evidence in support of an etiological pathway involving the specific features of Factor 2 or aggressive psychopathy by way of comorbid ADHD and antisocial behavior with an early onset. Not surprisingly, major theories concerning the deficit associated with ADHD focus on the concepts of impulsivity (Barkley, 1999) or dysfunction of regulatory or control processes (Douglas, 1999)—an admittedly complex and potentially vague concept akin to executive function deficits. Rather clearly, this etiological factor differs from the low fear/anxiety factor and thus constitutes a second important risk factor for psychopathy.

Factor 1 of Psychopathy in Childhood

For the researcher interested in the "classic," low fear, predatory psychopath, the ADHD antecedent to psychopathy that dominates the childhood literature does not appear to fit. The impulsivity and lack of emotional control of ADHD children have a negative impact on their social skills, making them socially inept and resulting in peer rejection (Hinshaw & Lee, 2003; Patterson, DeGarmo, & Knutson, 2000; Wicks-Nelson & Israel, 1997)—a picture inconsistent with the image of a cool predator. Frick's (Frick & Marsee, Chapter 18, this volume; Salekin, Chapter 20, this volume) relatively recent identification of a "callous–unemotional" (CU) dimension of antisocial behavior in children, designed to tap the PCL-R Factor 1 and found to be independent of ADHD, provides a possible solution to this theoretical difficulty. In general, Frick (e.g., 1998a, 1998b; Frick et al., 2003; Frick & Morris, 2004) has found strong support for the low fear hypothesis in this group.

DEFICITS, CORE FEATURES OF PSYCHOPATHY, AND DEVELOPMENT

Assuming that both low fear and impulsivity/executive function deficit pathways have been identified as contributing to the etiology of psychopathy, it is obvious that neither of these deficits per se fully embodies all the core features of clinically defined psychopathy. For example, lovelessness and guiltlessness are viewed as core features of psychopathy (e.g., McCord, 1982, pp. 24–27; McCord & McCord, 1964, p. 17), but neither are direct manifestations of either low fear or impulsivity. Instead, deficits of this kind are more appropriately viewed as risk factors creating developmental challenges or difficulties that may, in combination with environmental factors, contribute to the development of a negative interpersonal orientation and the failure to internalize conscience (e.g., Frick & Morris, 2004; Hinshaw & Lee, 2003). Three prominent research traditions have supported this model.

Developmental Theories of Antisocial Behavior

Patterson and his colleagues (e.g., Dishion, French & Patterson, 1995; Patterson et al., 2000; Patterson, Reid, & Dishion, 1992) have documented the importance of "coercive" parent–child interactions for the etiology of antisocial, aggressive behavior. The

child's coercive repertoire, in turn, ultimately generalizes to peers, teachers, and others. The poor reception by teachers and peers results in lessened engagement in school with subsequent academic failure, rejection by normal, nondeviant peers, and association with deviant peers, who contribute to the maintenance and further development of antisocial behavior.

Patterson's group (e.g., Patterson et al., 1992; especially Patterson et al., 2000) has emphasized the probable contribution of infant and child temperament: An extremely active and difficult infant in interaction with an insufficiently responsive parent results in distressed infant behavior that, by 24 months has escalated into the coercive behavior and lack of social skills that characterize both the hyperactive and the antisocial child and later often results in diagnoses of ADHD, ODD, and CD. Further, this process is seen as applicable to early starters for adult criminal careers, consistent with the ADHD/CD early-onset trajectory to psychopathy discussed earlier. This social learning model assumes that coercive parent–child relationships are incompatible with a mutually responsive, positive mother–child relationship (Dishion et al., 1995). In addition, the coercive process involves an antagonistic relationship in which coercion is employed to obtain things from others, and the negative reactions of others to the coercive child are likely to strengthen an antagonistic, loveless, exploitive interpersonal orientation.

An overlapping approach to temperament-based theories of the etiology of antisocial behavior, based more in developmental psychology, begins with the complex concept of the "difficult temperament" (especially, high negative affect strongly expressed; e.g., Campbell, 1998; Frick & Morris, 2004; Hinshaw & Lee, 2003). Infants with a difficult temperament represent a challenge to parenting that can promote poor parenting styles and maladaptive parent–child interactions. A number of investigators in this literature view the failure to develop "secure attachment" to the mother by age 1 year as a risk factor for later antisocial behavior. Although the correlations between infant difficult temperament and/or insecure attachment at age 1 year and later antisocial behavior are relatively modest (presumably because many other factors are important; Campbell, 1998, Hinshaw & Lee, 2003), this theoretical approach is noteworthy in the context of psychopathy for its emphasis on the attachment process, which conceptually is relevant to the development of a negative interpersonal orientation or lovelessness in adult psychopaths.

In the third relevant research tradition, Kochanska assessed the contributions of both impulsivity in the form of low inhibitory/effortful control and fearful temperament (constructs from Rothbart's three-factor model for children that parallel Tellegen's MPQ adult factors; Rothbart & Ahadi, 1994) on the later development of internalized conscience in young children. Kochanska and her colleagues (Kochanska, Murray, & Coy, 1997; Kochanska, Murray, Jacques, Koenig, & Vandegeest, 1996), using longitudinal designs, found that inhibitory/effortful control at toddler age has a direct effect on internalization of conscience at preschool and early school ages. Furthermore, effortful control was trait-like with robust longitudinal stability between toddlerhood and early school age ($r = .65$).

In contrast to the direct effect of inhibitory/effortful control, fearful temperament interacted with parenting style to predict the development of internalized conscience at ages 4 and 5 years (Kochanska, 1997, 2002). When children are divided into fearful and fearless temperament using a median split, internalized conscience is predicted by maternal gentle discipline (as opposed to harsher, power assertion discipline) for fearful but not fearless children. In contrast, internalization of conscience among fearless but not fearful children is predicted by a positive, mutually responsive mother–child relationship (i.e., a reward-based pathway). Thus, for a fearless child the punishment-based pathway is ineffective, leaving the parent with only a reward-based pathway.

Fowles and Kochanska (2000) assessed overall electrodermal reactivity in children from this longitudinal sample at age 4 and found the same pattern of results when this reactivity measure was substituted for the original measure of fearful temperament (with which it was uncorrelated). That is, using a median split on electrodermal reactivity, maternal gentle discipline predicted inter-nalized conscience for the reactive children, while attachment security (a substitute for a positive mother–child relationship) predicted internalized conscience for the nonreactive children. These findings suggested that electrodermal reactivity at an early age may reflect some aspects of temperament not captured by Kochanska's assessment of fearfulness based on behavioral observations and maternal ratings. It also suggests some continuity between her work and the adult psychopathy literature, because of the salience of electrodermal hyporeactivity in that literature. Also, Frick (e.g., Frick & Morris, 2004) cites Kochanska's research on fearful temperament as relating specifically to the CU subtype.

Deficits as Risk Factors for Core Features of Psychopathy

From the perspective of the etiology of psychopathy, a fearless temperament combined with a positive mother–child relationship results in a normal individual. On the other hand, the combination of fearlessness and the lack of a positive relationship results in a failure to internalize conscience and, presumably, an antisocial trajectory. Thus, the link between lovelessness and antisocial behavior could be conceptualized simply as the result of the combination of fearlessness and an inadequately positive mother–child relationship. More likely, given the other theories cited previously, fearlessness may make a positive relationship more difficult. In that case, the combination of fearlessness and lovelessness could be attributed to the absence of unusually skilled parenting in the face of a fearless child temperament (as suggested by Lykken, 1995)—similar to the outcomes in attachment theory and Patterson's social learning approach.

The major point to be made from these examples is that the deficits associated with psychopathy can be conceptualized primarily as risk factors for negative developmental trajectories. When they are combined with parenting that is insufficiently skilled to overcome or compensate for these challenges and other environmental adversities, an interpersonally negative, antisocial trajectory is initiated that can in some cases result in the development of psychopathy. The importance of interpersonal factors in this outcome is central in the attachment literature and in Kochanska's work, and their importance is implied in Patterson's work. From this standpoint, a loveless, guiltless orientation represents a developmental failure of the process of socialization. It also is noteworthy that the Patterson social learning and the attachment traditions are more identified with the ADHD–impulsivity pathway to psychopathy than with the low-fear pathway (Frick & Morris, 2004), suggesting that the core feature of lovelessness may be as integral to the impulsivity pathway as to the low-fear pathway.

SUMMARY AND DISCUSSION

Lykken's low-fear hypothesis has been supported in many respects in the recent literature, especially research by Patrick and his colleagues, as a process related primarily to the affective–interpersonal features of psychopathy embodied in PCL-R and PPI Factor 1 and to a subgroup of psychopaths whose description exemplifies the features of Factor 1. Research relating Factor 1 to poor potentiation of the startle response provides especially strong support, because of the critical role of conditioned fear in startle potentiation and the finding that enhanced startle potentiation is associated with selection of subjects for phobias more than for anxiety. The personality correlates of psychopathy also provide strong support, although they point to low anxiety as a factor as well.

Thus, it is not completely clear that the deficit in psychopathy is specifically one of low fear rather than a combination of low fear and low anxiety. An attractive possibility is that the most important contribution is poor fear conditioning and that low fear, in turn, makes anxiety less likely. That is, in the absence of conditioned fears, there is little for the future-oriented anxiety process to anticipate. Alternatively, perhaps the development of psychopathy in low-fear individuals is facilitated by low anxiety as well. Consistent with this possibility, Frick (1998) found that the presence of an anxiety disorder or trait anxiety reduced the severity and chronicity of conduct disorder. The same might be true of low-fear antisocial children: That is, normal or high levels of trait anxiety

may mitigate the effects of low fear in promoting antisocial behavior. In that case, low fear would still, in some sense, be a primary deficit but one made more severe by low anxiety.

If this analysis is correct, low fear and its antisocial outcome constitute a somewhat distinct process and aspect of psychopathology that has not been widely recognized. The internalizing disorders (anxiety and depression) have been found to reflect a shared genetic vulnerability to general distress reactivity, and the externalizing disorders are believed to reflect a vulnerability to impulsivity and/or executive function deficits. Low fear may not be merely the absence of anxiety, but rather it may represent a vulnerability somewhat distinct from anxiety. An attractive hypothesis is that it represents the low end of the autonomic arousal dimension identified in the tripartite model of Clark and Watson and the hierarchical (latent structure) model of Barlow and his colleagues discussed previously.

The impulsivity associated with psychopathy Factor 2 and its related subtype, combined with the identification of this factor as strongly related to the externalizing disorders, points to a separate deficit and an alternative etiological pathway to psychopathy. Indeed, this pathway, involving the combination of impulsive antisocial behavior and poor emotional control, has been highlighted much more in the childhood psychopathology literature.

The impulsivity associated with externalizing disorders involves a difficulty in inhibiting activated responses and acting without considering consequences. In contrast, the engagement in dangerous behaviors associated with low fear reflects a different process. Although it could be viewed as impulsive because of the associated risk taking, the individuals in question report that they take risks even after considering the consequences. At the least, two different types of impulsivity are involved.

In the context of the low-fear hypothesis, psychopaths who exemplify the features of PCL-R Factor 2 have not always been viewed as true psychopaths. Given that they meet PCL-R criteria for psychopathy and show strongly antagonistic, aggressive, alienated behavior, it seems legitimate to consider them true psychopaths but to keep in mind the different deficits and behavioral tendencies associated with the two types of psychopaths—or, perhaps more correctly, the two underlying etiological processes that confer risk to these variants of psychopathy.

We propose that the core features of psychopathy are not direct manifestations of either deficit identified here. Rather, they represent a developmental failure that is probabilistically associated with the deficits. This developmental process most likely begins with parent–child interactions, but it also involves interactions with peers, teachers, and others in the social environment. How "penetrant" the deficits are is difficult to ascertain. No neonatal characteristics have strong predictive value for adult antisocial behavior. Later assessments (e.g., of toddlers or preschoolers) already reflect the outcome of temperament by social environment interactions, making it difficult to claim that the temperament component is uncontaminated by early social environmental factors. It is noteworthy that only about 25% of children with ODD "mature" into conduct disorder over a 3-year period (Hinshaw & Lee, 2003). The most likely hypothesis is that temperamental deficits are significant contributors to the etiology of psychopathy but that many other factors also make a significant contribution.

Our conceptualization does not include a temperament directly related to lovelessness or lack of regard for others. However, attention should be directed to the possibility that such a temperament dimension exists. As noted previously, Depue and Morrone-Strupinsky (in press) propose a human trait of affiliation with temperament-like features that is a critical element in the formation and maintenance of affiliative bonds and social attachment. They argue that the experience of affection reflects the capacity to experience reward that is elicited by various affiliative stimuli and promotes affiliative bonding. Such a dimension of temperament could constitute a third etiological factor that would interact with the low-fear and impulsivity factors, especially with respect to the development of lovelessness or a callous orientation toward others. However, there is, at present, no clear information on the role of such a temperament in psychopathy.

REFERENCES

Barkley, R. A. (1999). Theories of attention deficit/hyperactivity disorder. In H. C. Quay & A. E. Hogan (Eds.), *Handbook of disruptive behavior disorders* (pp. 295–313). New York: Kluwer/Plenum Press.

Barlow, D. H. (2000). Unraveling the mysteries of anxiety and its disorders from the perspective of emotion theory. *American Psychologist, 55,* 1247–1263.

Barlow, D. H. (2002). *Anxiety and its disorders: The nature and treatment of anxiety and panic* (2nd ed.). New York: Guilford Press.

Benning, S. D., Patrick, C. J., Blonigen, D. M., Hicks, B. M., & Iacono, W. G. (2005). Estimating facets of psychopathy from normal personality Traits: A step toward community-epidemiological investigations. *Assessment, 12,* 3–18.

Benning, S. D., Patrick, C. J., Hicks, B. M., Blonigen, D. M., & Krueger, R. F. (2003). Factor structure of the Psychopathic Personality Inventory: Validity and implications for clinical assessment. *Psychological Assessment, 15,* 340–350.

Bouton, M. E., Mineka, S., & Barlow, D. H. (2001). A modern learning theory perspective on the etiology of panic disorder. *Psychological Review, 108,* 4–32.

Bradley, M., Cuthbert, B. N., & Lang, P. J. (1999). Affect and the startle reflex. In M. E. Dawson, A.M. Schell, & A.H. Bohmelt (Eds.), *Startle modification: Implications for neuroscience, cognitive science, and clinical science* (pp. 157–183). Cambridge, UK: Cambridge University Press.

Brown, T. A., Chorpita, B. F., & Barlow, D. H. (1998). Structural relationships among dimensions of the DSM-IV anxiety and mood disorders and dimensions of negative affect, positive affect, and autonomic arousal. *Journal of Abnormal Psychology, 107,* 179–192.

Buss, A. H., & Plomin, R. (1975). *A temperament theory of personality development.* New York: Wiley.

Buss, A. H., & Plomin, R. (1984). *Temperament: Early developing personality traits.* Hillsdale, NJ: Erlbaum.

Butcher, J. N., Mineka, S., & Hooley, J. M. (2004). *Abnormal psychology* (12th ed.). New York: Pearson Education.

Campbell, S. B. (1998). Developmental perspectives. In T. H. Ollendick & M. Hersen (Eds.), *Handbook of child psychopathology* (3rd ed., pp. 3–35). New York: Plenum Press.

Church, T. A. (1994). Relating the Tellegen and five factor models of personality structure. *Journal of Personality and Social Psychology, 67,* 898–909.

Clark, L. A., & Watson, D. (1991). Tripartite model of anxiety and depression; Psychometric evidence and taxonomic implications. *Journal of Abnormal Psychology, 100,* 316–336.

Clark, L. A., & Watson, D. (1999). Temperament: A new paradigm for trait psychology. In L. Pervin & O. P. John (Eds.), *Handbook of personality: Theory and research* (2nd ed., pp. 399–423). New York: Guilford Press.

Clark, L. A., Watson, D., & Mineka, S. (1994). Temperament, personality, and the mood and anxiety disorders. *Journal of Abnormal Psychology, 103,* 103–116.

Cleckley, H. (1982). *The mask of sanity* (6th ed.). St. Louis, MO: Mosby. (Original work published 1941)

Cook, E. W., III. (1999). Affective individual differences, psychopathology, and startle reflex modification. In M. E. Dawson, A. M. Schell, & A. H. Bohmelt (Eds.), *Startle modification: Implications for neuroscience, cognitive science, and clinical science* (pp. 187–208). Cambridge, UK: Cambridge University Press.

Costa, P. T., & McCrae, R. R. (1989). *NEO Personality Inventory—Revised.* Port Huron, MI: Sigma Assessment Systems.

Cuthbert, B. N., Lang, P. J., Strauss, C., Drobes, D., Patrick, C. J., & Bradley, M. M. (2003). The psychophysiology of anxiety disorder: Fear memory imagery. *Psychophysiology, 40,* 407–422.

Daugherty, T. K., & Quay, H. C. (1991). Response perseveration and delayed responding in childhood behavior disorders. *Journal of Child Psychology and Psychiatry, 32,* 453–461.

Davis, M. (1998). Are different parts of the extended amygdala involved in fear versus anxiety? *Biological Psychiatry, 44,* 1239–1247.

Davis, M., Walker, D. L., & Lee, Y. (1999). Neurophysiology and neuropharmacology of startle and its affective modification. In M. E. Dawson, A. M. Schell, & A. H. Boehmelt (Eds.), *Startle modification: Implications for clinical science, cognitive science, and neuroscience* (pp. 95–113). Cambridge, UK: Cambridge University Press.

Depue, R. A., & Collins, P. F. (1999). Neurobiology of the structure of personality: Dopamine, facilitation of incentive motivation, and extraversion. *Behavioral and Brain Sciences, 22,* 491–517.

Depue, R. A., & Lenzenweger, M. F. (2001). A neurobehavioral dimensional model. In W. J. Livesley (Ed.), *Handbook of personality disorders: Theory, research, and treatment* (pp. 136–176). New York: Guilford Press.

Depue, R. A., & Morrone-Strupinsky, J. V. (in press). A neurobehavioral model of affiliative bonding: Implications for conceptualizing a human trait of affiliation. *Behavioral and Brain Sciences.*

Dindo, L., McDade-Montez, L., & Watson, D. (2005). *Evidence for a two-factor model of psychopathy: Differential associations with personality, drug and alcohol use, and health-related behaviors.* Unpublished manuscript.

Dishion, T. J., French, D. C., & Patterson, G. R. (1995). The development and ecology of antisocial behavior. In D. Cicchetti & D. J. Cohen (Eds.), *Developmental psychopathology. Vol. 2: Risk, disorder, and adaptation* (pp. 421–471). New York: Wiley.

Douglas, V. (1999). Cognitive control processes in attention deficit/hyperactivity disorder. In H. C. Quay & A. E. Hogan (Eds.), *Handbook of disruptive behavior disorders* (pp. 105–138). New York: Kluwer/Plenum Press.

Eysenck, H. J. (1990). Biological dimensions of personality. In L. A. Pervin (Ed.), *Handbook of personality: Theory and research* (pp. 244–276). New York: Guilford Press.

Fonseca, A. C., & Yule, W. (1995). Personality and antisocial behavior in children and adolescents: An enquiry into Eysenck's and Gray's theories. *Journal of Abnormal Child Psychology, 23*(6), 767–781.

Fowles, D. C. (1980). The three arousal model: Implications of Gray's two-factor learning theory for heart rate, electrodermal activity, and psychopathy. *Psychophysiology, 17,* 87–104.

Fowles, D. (1986). The eccrine system and electrodermal activity. In M. G. H. Coles, S. W. Porges, & E. Donchin (Eds.), *Psychophysiology: Systems, processes, and applications* (Vol. 1, pp. 51–96). New York: Guilford Press.

Fowles, D. (1993). Electrodermal activity and antisocial behavior: Empirical findings and theoretical issues. In J.-C. Roy, W. Boucsein, D. Fowles, & J. Gruzelier (Eds.), *Progress in electrodermal research* (pp. 223–238). New York: Plenum Press.

Fowles, D. C. (2000). Electrodermal hyporeactivity and antisocial behavior: Does anxiety mediate the relationship? *Journal of Affective Disorders, 61,* 177–189.

Fowles, D. C., & Kochanska, G. (2000). Temperament as a Moderator of pathways to conscience in children: The contribution of electrodermal activity. *Psychophysiology, 37,* 788–795.

Fowles, D., & Missel, K. (1994). Electrodermal hyporeactivity, motivation, and psychopathy: Theoretical issues. In D. Fowles, P. Sutker, & S. Goodman (Eds.), *Progress in experimental personality and psychopathology research 1994: Special focus on psychopathy and antisocial behavior: A developmental perspective* (pp. 263–283). New York: Springer.

Frick, P. J. (1998a). Callous–unemotional traits and conduct problems: A two-factor model of psychopathy in children. In D. J. Cooke, A. Forth, & R. D. Hare (Eds.), *Psychopathy: Theory, research, and implications for society* (pp. 161–187). Dordrecht, The Netherlands: Kluwer.

Frick, P. J. (1998b). *Conduct disorders and severe antisocial behavior.* New York: Plenum Press.

Frick, P. J., Cornell, A. H., Bodin, S. D., Dane, H. A., Barry, C. T., & Loney, B. R. (2003). Callous–unemotional traits and developmental pathways to severe aggressive and antisocial behavior. *Developmental Psychology, 39,* 246–260.

Frick, P. J., & Loney, B. R. (2000). The use of laboratory and performance-based measures in the assessment of children and adolescents with conduct disorders. *Journal of Clinical Child Psychology, 29,* 540–554.

Frick, P. J., & Morris, A. S. (2004). Temperament and developmental pathways to conduct problems. *Journal of Clinical Child and Adolescent Psychology, 33,* 54–68.

Gray, J. A. (1970). The psychophysiological basis of intraversion–extraversion. *Behavior Research and Therapy, 8*, 249–266.

Gray, J. A. (1975). *Elements of a two-process theory of learning.* New York: Academic Press.

Gray, J. A. (1977). Drug effects on fear and frustration: Possible limbic site of action of minor tranquilizers. In L. L. Iversen, S. D. Iversen, & S. H. Snyder (Eds.), *Handbook of psychopharmacology: Vol. 8. Drugs, neurotransmitters, and behavior* (pp. 433–529). New York: Plenum Press.

Gray, J. A. (1978). The neuropsychology of anxiety. *British Journal of Psychology, 69*, 417–434.

Gray, J. A. (1979). A neuropsychological theory of anxiety. In C. E. Izard (Ed.), *Emotions in personality and psychopathology* (pp. 303–335). New York: Plenum Press.

Gray, J. A., & McNaughton, N. (2000). *The neuropsychology of anxiety: An enquiry into the functions of the septohippocampal system* (2nd ed.). Oxford, UK: Oxford University Press.

Hare, R. D. (1978). Electrodermal and cardiovascular correlates of psychopathy. In R. D. Hare & D. Schalling (Eds.), *Psychopathic behavior: Approaches to research* (pp. 107–144). New York: Wiley.

Hare, R. D. (1991). *Manual for the Revised Psychopathy Checklist.* Toronto, ON, Canada: Multi-Health Systems.

Hare, R. D. (2003). *The Hare Psychopathy Checklist—Revised, 2nd Edition.* Toronto, ON, Canada: Multi-Health Systems.

Hare, R. D. (1998). Psychopathy, affect, and behavior. In D. J. Cooke, A. E. Forth, & R. D. Hare (Eds.), *Psychopathy: Theory, research, and implications for society* (pp. 105–137). Dordrecht, Netherlands: Kluwer.

Hare, R. D., Harpur, T. J., Hakstian, A. R., Forth, A. E., Hart, S. D., & Newman, J. P. (1990). The Revised Psychopathy Checklist: Reliability and factor structure. *Psychological Assessment: A Journal of Consulting and Clinical Psychology, 2*, 338–341.

Harpur, T. J., Hare, R. D., & Hakstian, A. R. (1989). Two-factor conceptualization of psychopathy: Construct validity and assessment implications. *Psychological Assessment: A Journal of Consulting and Clinical Psychology, 1*, 6–17.

Herpertz, S. C., Werth, U., Lukas, G., Qunaibi, M., Schuerkens, A., Kunert, H., et al. (2001). Emotion in criminal offenders with psychopathy and borderline personality disorder. *Archives of General Psychiatry, 58*, 737–745.

Hicks, B. M., Markon, K. E., Patrick, C. J., Krueger, R. F., & Newman, J. P. (2004). Identifying psychopathy subtypes based on personality structure. *Psychological Assessment, 16*, 276–288.

Hinshaw, S. P., & Lee, S. S. (2003). Conduct and oppositional defiant disorders. In E. J. Mash & R. A. Barkley (Eds.), *Child psychopathology* (2nd ed., pp. 144–198). New York: Guilford Press.

Hull, C. L. (1943). *Principles of behavior.* New York: Appleton-Century-Crofts.

Hull, C. L. (1952). *A behavior system.* New Haven, CT: Yale University Press.

Kendler, K. S. (1996). Major depression and generalised anxiety disorder. Same genes, (partly) different environments—revisited. *British Journal of Psychiatry, 168*(Suppl. 30), 68–75.

Kendler, K. S., Neale, M. C., Kessler, R. C., Heath, A. C., & Eaves, L. J. (1992). Major depression and generalized anxiety disorder: Same genes, (partly) different environments. *Archives of General Psychiatry, 49*, 716–722.

Klein, D. N., Durbin, C. E., Shankman, S. A., & Santiogo, N. J. (2002). Depression and personality. In H. Gotlib & C. I. Hammen Eds.), *Handbook of depression* (pp. 115–140). New York: Guilford Press.

Kochanska, G. K. (1997). Multiple pathways to conscience for children with different temperaments: From toddlerhood to age 5. *Developmental Psychology, 33*, 228–240.

Kochanska, G. (2002). Mutually responsive orientation between mothers and their young children: A context for the early development of conscience. *Current Directions in Psychological Science, 11*, 191–195.

Kochanska, G., Murray, K., & Coy, K. C. (1997). Inhibitory control as a contributor to conscience in childhood: From toddler to early school age. *Child Development, 68*, 263–277.

Kochanska, G., Murray, K., Jacques, T. Y., Koenig, A. L., & Vandegeest, K. A. (1996). Inhibitory control in young children and its role in emerging internalization. *Child Development, 67*, 490–507.

Krueger, R. F., Hicks, B. M., Patrick, C. J., Carlson, S. R., Iacono, W. G., & McGue, M. (2002). Etiologic connections among substance dependence, antisocial behavior and personality: Modeling the externalizing spectrum. *Journal of Abnormal Psychology, 111*, 411–424.

Krueger, R. F., Schmutte, P. S., Caspi, A., Moffitt, T. E., Campbell, K., & Silva, P. A. (1994). Personality traits are linked to crime among men and women: Evidence from a birth cohort. *Journal of Abnormal Psychology, 103*, 328–338.

Lang, P. J., Bradley, M. M., & Cuthbert, B. N. (1990). Emotion, attention and the startle reflex. *Psychological Review, 97*, 377–395.

Lang, P. J., Davis, M., & Öhman, A. (2000). Fear and anxiety: Animal modes and human cognitive psychophysiology. *Journal of Affective Disorders, 61*, 137–159.

LeDoux, J. E. (1995). Emotion: Clues from the brain. *Annual Review of Psychology, 46*, 209–235.

LeDoux, J. E. (1996). *The emotional brain.* New York: Simon & Schuster.

LeDoux, J. E. (2000). Emotion circuits in the brain. *Annual Review of Neuroscience, 23*, 155–184.

LeDoux, J. E. (2002). *The synaptic self.* New York: Viking Penguin.

Levenston, G. K., Patrick, C. J., Bradley, M. M., & Lang, P. J. (2000). The psychopath as observer: Emotion and attention in picture processing. *Journal of Abnormal Psychology, 109*, 373–385.

Lilienfeld, S. O. (1990). *Development and preliminary validation of a self-report measure of psychopathic personality*. Doctoral dissertation, University of Minnesota.

Lilienfeld, S. O., & Andrews, B. P. (1996). Development and preliminary validation of a self report measure of psychopathic personality traits in noncriminal populations. *Journal of Personality Assessment, 66*, 488–524.

Lykken, D. T. (1957). A study of anxiety in the sociopathic personality. *Journal of Abnormal and Social Psychology, 55*, 6–10.

Lykken, D. T. (1971). Factor analysis. *Journal of Experimental Personality Research, 5*, 161–170.

Lykken, D. T. (1995). *The antisocial personalities.* Mahwah, NJ: Erlbaum.

Lynam, D. R. (1998). Early identification of the fledgling psychopath: Locating the psychopathic child in the current nomenclature. *Journal of Abnormal Psychology, 107*, 566–575.

Matthys, W., van Goozen, S.H. M., de Vries, H., Cohen-Kettenis, P. T., & van Engeland, H. (1998). The dominance of behavioural activation over behavioural inhibition in conduct disordered boys with or without attention deficit hyperactivity disorder. *Journal of Child Psychology and Psychiatry and Allied Disciplines, 39*, 643–651.

McCord, W., & McCord, J. (1964). *The psychopath: An essay on the criminal mind.* Princeton, NJ: Van Nostrand.

McCord, W. M. (1982). *The psychopath and milieu therapy.* New York: Academic Press.

Mineka, S., Watson, D., & Clark, L. A. (1998). Comorbidity of anxiety and unipolar mood disorders. *Annual Review of Psychology, 49*, 377–412.

Moffitt, T. E. (1993). Adolescence-limited and life-course-persistent antisocial behavior: A developmental taxonomy. *Psychological Review, 100*, 674–701.

Moffitt, T. E., & Caspi, A. (2001). Childhood predictors differentiate life-course persistent and adolescence-limited antisocial pathways among males and females. *Development and Psychopathology, 13*, 355–375.

Moffitt, T. E., & Lynam, D., Jr. (1994). The neuropsychology of conduct disorder and delinquency: Implications for understanding antisocial behavior. In D. Fowles, P. Sutker, & S. Goodman (Eds.), *Progress in experimental personality and psychopathology research 1994: Special focus on psychopathy and antisocial behavior: A developmental perspective* (pp. 233–262). New York: Springer.

Newman, J. P., & Kosson, D. S. (1986). Passive avoidance learning in psychopathic and nonpsychopathic offenders. *Journal of Abnormal Psychology, 95*, 252–256.

Newman, J. P., Patterson, C. M., & Kosson, D. S. (1987). Response perseveration in psychopaths. *Journal of Abnormal Psychology, 96*, 145–148.

Newman, J. P., Widom, C. S., & Nathan, S. (1985). Passive-avoidance in syndromes of disinhibition: Psychopathy and extraversion. *Journal of Personality and Social Psychology, 48*, 1316–1327.

O'Brien, B. S., & Frick, P. J. (1996). Reward dominance: Associations with anxiety, conduct problems, and psychopathy in children. *Journal of Abnormal Child Psychology, 24*, 223–240.

O'Brien, B. S., Frick, P. J., & Lynam, R. D. (1994). Reward dominance among children with disruptive behavior disorders. *Journal of Psychopathology and Behavioral Assessment, 16*, 131–145.

Pastor, M. C., Molto, J., Vila, J., & Lang, P. J. (2003). Startle reflex modulation. Affective ratings and autonomic reactivity in Spanish incarcerated psychopaths. *Psychophysiology, 40*, 934–938.

Patrick, C. J. (in press). Getting to the heart of psychopathy. In H. Herve & J. C. Yuille (Eds.), *Psychopathy: Theory, research, and social implications*. Hillsdale, NJ: Erlbaum

Patrick, C. J., Bradley, M. M., & Lang, P. J. (1993). Emotion in the criminal psychopath: Startle reflex modulation. *Journal of Abnormal Psychology, 102*, 82–92.

Patrick, C. J., Cuthbert, B. N., & Lang, P. J. (1994). Emotion in the criminal psychopath: Fear image processing. *Journal of Abnormal Psychology, 103*, 523–534.

Patrick, C. J., Hicks, B. M., Krueger, R. F., & Lang, A. R. (2005). Relations between psychopathy facets and externalizing in a criminal offender sample. *Journal of Personality Disorders, 19*, 339–356.

Patrick, C. J., & Lang, A. R. (1999). Psychopathic traits and intoxicated states: Affective concomitants and conceptual links. In M. E. Dawson, A. M. Schell, & A. H. Boehmelt (Eds.), *Startle modification: Implications for clinical science, cognitive science, and neuroscience* (pp. 209–230). Cambridge, UK: Cambridge University Press.

Patterson, G. R., DeGarmo, D. S., & Knutson, N. (2000). Hyperactive and antisocial behaviors: Comorbid or two points in the same process. *Development and Psychopathology, 12*, 91–106.

Patterson, G. R., Reid, J. B., & Dishion, T. J. (1992). *Antisocial boys*. Eugene, OR: Castalia.

Poythress, N. G., Edens, J. F., & Lilienfeld, S. O. (1998). Criterion-related validity of the Psychopathic Personality Inventory in a prison sample. *Psychological Assessment, 10*, 426–430.

Quay, H. C. (1986). Classification. In H. C. Quay & J. S. Werry (Eds.), *Psychopathological disorders of childhood* (3rd ed., pp. 1–34). New York: Wiley.

Raine, A. (1993). *The psychopathology of crime*. New York: Academic Press.

Ross, S. R., Benning, S. D., Patrick, C. J., Thompson, A., & Thurston, A. (2005). *Factors of the Psycho-*

pathic Personality Inventory: Criterion-related validity and relationships with the five-factor model of personality. Manuscript submitted for publication.

Rothbart, M. K., & Ahadi, S. A. (1994). Temperament and the development of personality. *Journal of Abnormal Psychology, 103,* 55–66.

Scerbo, A., Raine, A., O'Brien, M., Chan, C. J., Rhee, C., & Smiley, N. (1990). Reward dominance and passive avoidance learning in adolescent psychopaths. *Journal of Abnormal Child Psychology, 18*(4), 451–463.

Schachter, S., & Latané, B. (1964). Crime, cognition, and the autonomic nervous system. *Nebraska Symposium on Motivation, 12,* 221–273.

Schmauk, F. J. (1970). Punishment, arousal, and avoidance learning in sociopaths. *Journal of Abnormal Psychology, 76,* 325–335.

Schoenherr, J. (1964). *Avoidance of noxious stimulation in psychopathic personality.* Unpublished doctoral dissertation, University of California at Los Angeles. (University Microfilms No. 8334)

Shapiro, S. K., Quay, H. C., Hogan, A. E., & Schwartz, K. P. (1988). Response perseveration and delayed responding in undersocialized aggressive conduct disorder. *Journal of Abnormal Psychology, 97,* 371–373.

Siddle, D. A. T., & Trasler, G. (1981). The psychophysiology of psychopathic behaviour. In M. J. Christie & P. G. Mellett (Eds.), *Foundations of psychosomatics* (pp. 283–303). London: Wiley.

Siegel, R. A. (1978). Probability of punishment and suppression of behavior in psychopathic and nonpsychopathic offenders. *Journal of Abnormal Psychology, 87,* 514–522.

Sutton, S. K., Vitale, J. E., & Newman, J. P. (2002). Emotion among females with psychopathy during picture perception. *Journal of Abnormal Psychology, 111,* 610–619.

Tellegen, A. (1985). Structures of mood and personality and their relevance to assessing anxiety, with an emphasis on self-report. In A. H. Tuma & J. D. Maser (Eds.), *Anxiety and anxiety disorders* (pp. 681–706). Hillsdale, NJ: Erlbaum.

Tellegen, A. (in press). *Manual for the Multidimensional Personality Questionnaire.* Minneapolis: University of Minnesota Press.

Vanman, E. J., Mejia, V. Y., Dawson, M. E., Schell, A. M., & Raine, A. (2003). Modification of the startle reflex in a community sample: Do one or two dimensions of psychopathy underlie emotional processing? *Personality and Individual Differences, 35,* 2007–2021.

Waid, W. M., & Orne, M. T. (1982). Reduced electrodermal response to conflict, failure to inhibit dominant behaviors, and delinquency proneness. *Journal of Personality and Social Psychology, 43,* 769–774.

Wicks-Nelson, R., & Israel, A. C. (1997). *Behavior disorders of childhood.* Upper Saddle River, NJ: Prentice-Hall.

Widiger, T. A. (1998). Psychopathy and normal personality. In D. J. Cooke, A. E. Forth, & R. D. Hare (Eds.), *Psychopathy: Theory, research, and implications for society* (pp. 47–68). Dordrecht, Netherlands: Kluwer.

Zahn, T. P., Schooler, C., & Murphy, D. L. (1986). Autonomic correlates of sensation seeking and monoamine oxidase activity: Using confirmatory factor analysis on psychophysiological data. *Psychophysiology, 23,* 521–531.

Zuckerman, M. (1991). *Psychobiology of personality.* Cambridge, UK: Cambridge University Press.

3

Other Theoretical Models of Psychopathy

RONALD BLACKBURN

Psychological theories of psychopathy have always followed developments in the wider discipline. Early attempts at explanation appeared in the 1920s under the influence of psychoanalysis, but with the development of behaviorist learning theories, these gave way to alternative models. A summary of theories of psychopathy by Hare (1970) revealed the lingering influence of psychodynamic developmental models but also the emerging dominance of theories of socialization based on classical and instrumental conditioning and biologically based theories of emotion and motivation. With the subsequent "cognitive revolution," theorists attempted to identify possible mediators of psychopathy in information processing. Related developments in neuropsychology and more recently in cognitive neuroscience and evolutionary psychology have also had their influence.

Theories persist as long as they appear *plausible* to some investigators, and this is as much a matter of personal preference as of the supposed rationality of science. All the dominant traditions in psychology therefore continue to be represented in theories of psychopathy. The previous chapter discussed one of the more influential of these. This chapter describes alternative, though sometimes overlapping, models that have influenced recent research.

The chapter aims to summarize the main concepts of these theories and their current status. Because all research on psychopathy rests on theoretical assumptions, much of the research described in this handbook is linked to one or more of these theories. No attempt is therefore made to review the literature surrounding them, but relevant supporting evidence is described. Some theories were proposed prior to the development of the Psychopathy Checklist (PCL) and its revision (PCL-R; Hare, 1991; Hare & Neumann, Chapter 4, this volume), and tests of these have often used alternative questionnaire or rating scale measures. Some studies also equate psychopathy with the DSM-IV category of antisocial personality disorder (APD; American Psychiatric Association, 1994), but this does not adequately represent the construct as measured by the PCL-R. Where relevant, more recent studies are cited that have used the PCL or PCL-R, particularly the two subfactors, Factor 1 (callous, remorseless or detached) and Factor 2 (socially deviant or antisocial), in view of the common assumption that Factor 1 reflects the core attributes of psychopathy as currently conceptualized.

PSYCHOPATHY AND PSYCHOANALYTIC THEORY

The portrayal of the psychopath as an egocentric, impulsive, guiltless, and unempathic individual originates in psychodynamic thinking, and as Andrews and Wormith

(1989) note, most theories of psychopathy owe an intellectual debt to Freudian theory. Although Freud said little about crime, his theory of socialization aimed to explain the internalization of group standards in early childhood through the formation of the superego. This inner moral agency comprises moral rules in the form of the *conscience* and the positive values of the *ego-ideal*, and provides the standards by which the reality-oriented ego regulates behavior (Nass, 1966). Superego formation is held to depend on psychosexual and ego development through the child's fantasied and actual relations with its parents and is consolidated through the resolution of the Oedipal conflict. Impaired socialization results when parents fail to meet the child's emotional needs through rejection, neglect, or inconsistency.

Although Freud's theory has been criticized as untestable by many psychologists, the idea of a superego formed through relations with parents has been influential in thinking about antisocial behavior and psychopathy. Karpman (1948) argued for an etiological definition of psychopathy in terms of psychodynamics and distinguished *primary* or idiopathic psychopaths from *secondary* or symptomatic psychopaths. Only the former, who lack conscience, justify the diagnosis of psychopath (or "anethopath"). The latter exhibit antisocial behavior as a consequence of neurotic conflicts or prepsychotic disturbance. Observations of young offenders (e.g., McCord & McCord, 1964) also led to distinctions between those who are antisocial because of a harsh superego (neurotic delinquents), those with a deviant superego ("subcultural" or gang delinquents), and those deficient in superego (psychopathic delinquents).

Recent psychodynamic theorizing emphasizes early infant experiences and the evolution of *object relations*, the enduring patterns of interpersonal relationships derived from internal cognitive and affective representations. *Attachment theory* (Bowlby, 1969), for example, highlights the quality of infant–caregiver relationships during the first year of life as a determinant of later cognitive and social development. Kernberg (1996) proposed that disturbed early object relations are central to all personality disorders. Within this formulation, APD is equated with psychopathy as described by

Cleckley (1941/1982) and the PCL-R, and not the "diluted" version of DSM-IV, and falls within a "borderline personality organization" level. Borderline disorders display distortions in interpersonal relations and the control of affects as a result of disturbed object relations, but psychopaths are distinguished by the most severe level of superego disorganization within a spectrum of narcissistic disorders. Kernberg sees the psychopath as biologically predisposed to excessive aggressive drive, but this becomes dominant in response to traumatic experiences or distortions in early attachment arising from abuse and abandonment. Rage and envy thus become core affects, and the individual defends against a dangerous world through grandiosity and devaluation. The superego system is limited to primitive punitive prohibitions, being totally dependent on immediate external cues and crude self-interest for the regulation of interpersonal behavior.

Meloy and Giacono (1998) tested psychodynamic hypotheses using the Rorschach with antisocial children, adolescents, and inmates. The majority of subjects in each group displayed signs of attachment deficits. Also, psychopaths produced more borderline level object relations than nonpsychopaths and more signs of pathological narcissism, consistent with Kernberg's concept. However, samples were not random, and the validity of the Rorschach remains controversial.

Psychodynamic theories predict adverse developmental experiences in psychopaths, but evidence on the significance of early abuse is equivocal. A modest contribution is suggested in a prospective study by Luntz and Widom (1994), who found that abused males were more likely to meet criteria for DSM APD as adults than nonabused males, although this was not found for females. Another prospective study found that physical abuse and neglect, but not sexual abuse, in childhood increased the likelihood of APD in young adulthood (Johnson, Cohen, Brown, Smailes, & Bernstein, 1999). However, using the PCL-R in a retrospective study of young male offenders, Forth and Tobin (1995) found that a majority of both psychopaths and nonpsychopaths had experienced abuse, suggesting that traumatic childhood experience is not specific to psychopathy.

GOUGH'S ROLE-TAKING THEORY

Although not dismissing psychoanalytic developmental theory, Gough (1948) drew on the symbolic interactionist perspective of sociology in which self-concept and the capacity to look on oneself as an object emerge as the product of social interaction and communication. In taking the role of the other, a conception of the "generalized other" evolves from the integration of different conceptions of "me." The capacity to understand another's point of view, or *role-taking ability*, depends on the development of this conception. Role-taking ability enables sensitivity to the reactions of others and is basic to self-criticism and self-control.

Gough distilled a pattern of traits from the literature to distinguish psychopaths that closely coincides with Cleckley's (1941/1982) criteria, such as ignoring the rights of others, impulsivity, emotional poverty, and inability to form lasting interpersonal attachments. These behavioral manifestations could be accounted for by a pathological deficiency in role-taking ability. The psychopath is unable to foresee the consequences of his own acts because he does not know how to judge his own behavior from another's point of view.

This view of the psychopath as socially insensitive has some resemblance to Cleckley's view of psychopathy, but for Gough, the primary deficit is cognitive rather than affective. Inability to experience the social emotions of embarrassment, contrition and group loyalty, and lack of self-control are all a consequence of this deficit. While acknowledging possible genetic influences on psychopathy, he considers a developmental etiology more plausible (but see Schalling, 1978, for a biosocial interactional interpretation).

The ability to see oneself as a social object is basic to Gough's theory of socialization (i.e., the internalization of values, systems of control, and adaptive mechanisms required for compliance with societal norms). Socialization is construed as a personality dimension ranging from exemplary probity and rectitude at one extreme to an errant and rule-violating disposition at the other and is operationalized by the Socialization (*So*) scale (Gough, 1994). Although much of the research with *So* has been with offenders,

psychopathy is seen as an extreme of a continuum rather than a categorical entity and is not confined to adjudicated offenders. The construct and predictive validity of *So* is well supported. For example, the scale consistently discriminates delinquents from nondelinquents across gender and culture, and an early version of *So* involving 25 samples and over 10,000 individuals yielded a biserial correlation of .73 with the dichotomy of more versus less socialized.

Direct tests of Gough's theory of role-taking ability have, however, been few. Support was found in an analogue study by Reed and Cuadra (1957), who examined correlations of *So* with measures of perspective taking in 204 female student nurses. Students completed an adjective checklist describing themselves, other nurses in their working groups, and how they would be described by their peers. Accuracy of seeing the self as object, as measured by correspondence between peer descriptions and individual's own predictions of how they would be described correlated significantly (*r* = .41) with *So*. *So* also discriminated those nominated as most and least insightful in terms of understanding their own motives and awareness of the effects of their behavior on others.

Widom (1976) used Kelly's repertory grid to determine whether psychopaths construe situations differently from normals and whether their conceptualizations of how others construe these situations differ from their own. Clinical criteria were used to select primary and secondary psychopaths and both groups scored lower than normal controls on *So*. Although there were few differences between primary and secondary groups, when compared with controls, psychopaths made few distinctions between their own conceptualizations of situations and those of people in general, suggesting significant misperceptions of the perspective of others. In particular, they more frequently characterized situations as dull rather than exciting and construed people in general as similar to themselves in this respect. Widom did not examine psychopaths' perceptions of how others viewed their own behavior, but she considered this apparent deficiency in understanding the thinking of others to be consistent with Gough's concept of a role-taking deficiency.

Also consistent with a deficit in perspective taking are findings of an attentional deficit in undersocialized individuals (Kosson & Newman, 1989). While less and more socialized students were equally able to divide their attention between a visual and auditory task, incentives to focus on the visual task produced a greater decrement in responding to the secondary task in the undersocialized group, suggesting that they overfocus on events of immediate significance at the expense of peripheral information.

Doren (1987) suggests that Gough's theory cannot provide a comprehensive account of psychopathy, but Schalling (1978) presents evidence for its compatibility with several other theories and believes that *So* is the most salient self-report scale related to psychopathy. However, although *So* correlates moderately but significantly with Cleckley ratings of psychopathy and the PCL, correlations are mainly with Factor 2 (Hare, 1991). Low scores on *So* may not therefore tap the callous, unempathic traits identified by Factor 1. Nevertheless, Gough's account addresses significant aspects of social cognition in psychopaths.

LINGUISTIC AND EMOTIONAL PROCESSING IN PSYCHOPATHS

Cleckley's influential conceptualization portrayed the psychopath as emotionally and interpersonally shallow and behaviorally irresponsible and unreliable. Despite an outer mask of robust mental health, this was a "distinct clinical entity" in which the central feature was an impairment in appreciating what the most important emotional experiences of life mean to others. By analogy with semantic aphasia, he hypothesized that the psychopath's defect was a "deep," probably biologically based disorder disturbing the integration of experience and resulting in a pathological loss of meaning. An affective deficit has been widely accepted as central to psychopathy and is supported by studies of responses to aversive stimuli (e.g., Lykken, 1957, 1995; Patrick, 1994). The possible manifestation of this deficit in disordered language processing has been investigated over several years by Hare (1998).

In an early study of cerebral lateralization, Hare (1979) used tachistoscopic recognition of words presented to the left visual field (LVF) or right visual field (RVF) to test the

hypothesis of dominant (left) hemispheric dysfunction psychopaths. Because verbal information presented to the RVF (and hence the contralateral left hemisphere) is generally more readily identified than that presented to the LVF in right-handed males, less superior recognition of words presented in the RVF would suggest a dominant hemisphere dysfunction. Psychopaths showed the same degree of RVF superiority as nonpsychopaths, indicating no left-hemisphere dysfunction. However, Hare and Jutai (1988) subsequently extended the visual task from simple word recognition to abstract semantic categorization of words. Nonpsychopaths made fewer errors to RVF presentations of words than to LVF presentations, but the reverse was found for psychopaths, suggesting that the left hemisphere of psychopaths may be less specialized for linguistic processing.

Hare and McPherson (1984) examined cerebral lateralization further using recall of words presented simultaneously in pairs in a dichotic listening task. Psychopaths showed less right-ear (left-hemisphere) advantage than nonpsychopaths, suggesting less hemispheric specialization for language in psychopaths across auditory as well as visual modalities. However, Hiatt, Lorenz, and Newman (2002) failed to replicate this and noted that the impaired recognition of psychopaths is inconsistent with the findings of intact recognition of simple visual stimuli found in Hare's other studies. This study is considered further later. Nevertheless, taken together, Hare's results imply that some language processes may not be as strongly lateralized in psychopaths as in nonpsychopaths.

However, Hare, Williamson, and Harpur (1988) proposed that psychopaths may additionally be characterized by poor integration of the affective components of language due to impaired interhemispheric communication or inefficient distribution of processing resources. From evidence that the denotative (literal) and connotative meanings of words are mediated by the left and right hemispheres, respectively, they hypothesized that the affective deficits characterizing psychopaths reflect failure to extract connotative meaning from emotional words. In a study requiring grouping of words presented in a booklet according to similarity of meaning, psychopaths grouped words primarily on the basis of denotative meaning, whereas non-psychopaths grouped them primarily according to connotative meaning.

There is also evidence that in lexical decision tasks (deciding whether a string of letters makes up a word), affective words produce greater accuracy and faster recognition than neutral words in normals, and some data suggesting that affective words produce shorter latency electrocortical evoked potentials (ERPs). Arguing that psychopaths make less efficient use of affective information, Williamson, Harpur, and Hare (1991) predicted that psychopaths would differentiate less between affective and neutral words in a lexical decision task involving divided visual fields, and recorded reaction time (RT) and ERPs in small groups of psychopaths and nonpsychopaths. As predicted, nonpsychopaths made faster lexical decisions and showed larger ERPs to affective than to neutral words. Psychopaths failed to show this differentiation in either behavioral or electrocortical responses. No differential laterality effects between groups emerged, suggesting that anomalous processing of affective information is not simply a function of weak language lateralization in psychopaths.

More recently, Hare (1998) accounted for the processing anomalies of psychopaths in terms of the ineffective inter- and intra-hemisphere distribution of cognitive and affective resources controlling behavior and suggested that cerebral anomalies in psychopaths may be most pronounced in the frontal cortex. A study by Intrator and colleagues (1997) supports this. They examined the relative cerebral blood flow during a lexical decision task in psychopaths and nonpsychopaths using brain-imaging techniques. Contrary to expectation, psychopaths showed *greater* activation to emotional stimuli than nonpsychopaths or controls in bilateral frontotemporal and subcortical regions. The post hoc interpretation was that psychopaths require greater additional resources for emotional processing, which is more efficiently automated through learning experiences in nonpsychopaths. Alternative interpretations seem possible.

However, Day and Wong (1996) proposed a link between the weaker lateralization of language in psychopaths and differential processing of denotative and connotative meaning by left and right hemispheres. Supporting this, nonpsychopaths showed LVF (right-hemisphere) advantage in processing negative emotional words, whereas psychopaths did not. Although Hare (1998) criticizes these findings, pointing to inconsistent unpublished data, Hiatt and colleagues (2002) obtained some support for Day and Wong. They attempted to replicate Hare's findings of unusual language lateralization and also the findings on lateralization of emotion processing in psychopaths with a dichotic listening task requiring discrimination of words from emotion stimuli (words presented in emotional or neutral tones).

As noted earlier, contrary to the results of Hare and McPherson (1984), psychopaths showed the same degree of left-hemispheric lateralization for words as nonpsychopaths. Psychopaths did, however, show less lateralization than nonpsychopaths in processing emotion stimuli. Like Hare and Jutai (1988), Hiatt and colleagues suggest that abnormal asymmetries in psychopaths depend on task complexity, and that this increases demands on interhemispheric processing. The less lateralized emotion processing of psychopaths may equally reflect poor hemispheric integration and a greater distribution of functions that are normally lateralized in the right hemisphere. These suggestions are in agreement with Hare's recent views.

Hare's research has firmly established that there are idiosyncrasies in the linguistic and emotional processing of psychopaths that may well be central to their observed affective deficits. He sees this as the result of a functional deficit in brain functioning rather than structural damage, and as probably constitutional or "hard wired." This is speculative, and the extent to which this deficit involves subcortical as well as cortical systems is currently uncertain. However, as Hare acknowledges, his research program represents explorations in search of a theory rather than a fully formed theory of psychopathy.

PSYCHOPATHY, PERSONALITY, AND THE BIOLOGY OF SOCIALIZATION

Theories that link psychopathy to biological substrates of personality that may influence the socialization process owe their origins to attempts by early learning theorists to translate Freudian concepts of development and socialization into terms that can be examined through experimental studies. More recently, they draw on developments in theories of personality and emotion. This section focuses on the theories of Eysenck, Gray, and Quay.

Eysenck's Theory

Eysenck's theory of personality evolved over almost half a century. This discussion examines the theory of criminality and psychopathy originating in 1964 and subsequently developed by Eysenck (1977, 1996) and Eysenck and Gudjonsson (1989). Criminality is construed as a continuously varying disposition to commit crimes, ranging from "altruistic behaviour through normal conduct to victimless but possibly antisocial behaviour to victimful behavior in criminality" (Eysenck & Gudjonsson, 1989, p. 3). Although Eysenck acknowledges that criminals are heterogeneous and that criminality and psychopathy are not identical, his theory centers on "the actively antisocial, psychopathic criminal" (1977, p. 59) exemplifying the undersocialized extreme and seeks to explain why some people fail to comply with rules.

Attributes of criminals are deduced from three propositions. First, the structural model of personality relates temperament variations to three independent dimensions of Neuroticism–Stability (N), Psychoticism–Superego (P), and Extraversion–Introversion (E), commonly defined by the Eysenck Personality Questionnaire (EPQ), which also contains a Lie (L) scale. Second, N, E, and P have a biological basis. N reflects greater reactivity in the limbic and autonomic systems, resulting in stronger responses to stress, and higher levels of "drive." Underlying E is the level of cortical arousal or arousability, governed by corticoreticular circuits. Extraverts have low arousal relative to introverts, form conditioned responses less readily, and require more intense stimulation to maintain "hedonic tone" (i.e., pleasurable states of consciousness). More tentatively, P is also related to arousal (Eysenck, 1996).

Third, socialization entails the acquisition of restraints over natural hedonism in the form of "conscience" through classical conditioning. Cues associated with punishment of antisocial behavior by parents and others arouse an anticipatory conditioned aversive state of fear or anxiety, which is reduced and reinforced by an inhibitory response that avoids punishment, and "conscience is indeed a conditioned reflex" (Eysenck, 1977, p. 118). This is similar to Lykken's (1995) theory of socialization. Because extraverts form conditioned responses slowly, they will be less well socialized than introverts. This is the central explanatory component of the theory. Criminals as a group are predicted to be more extraverted, and to exhibit lower arousal and weaker conditionability, but because of high drive (N) they should also score highly on N. From the similarity of traits of P to those attributed to psychopaths (hostile, unempathic, impulsive, egocentric), criminals are further predicted to score highly on P. High P scores will characterize primary psychopaths, although secondary psychopaths will be high on N and E. As a group, however, psychopaths and criminals will have higher mean scores on N, E, and P.

Personality and Crime

In research on offenders with the EPQ, the most consistent findings are that P is related to both official and self-reported delinquency, but high P scores, rather than high E or N, characterize more serious and persistent offenders (see Blackburn, 1993). Strongest support for an association between E and antisocial behavior comes from self-report studies and the failure of E to discriminate official offenders with any consistency weakens the theory. Less evidence is available on psychopathy. Hare (1982) found significant though small correlations of the PCL with P (positive) and L (negative) in prison inmates, and this was replicated by Kosson, Smith, and Newman (1990) among white prison inmates but not among black inmates. Thornquist and Zuckerman (1995) also found a correlation of the PCL-R with P only among white inmates. Harpur, Hare, and Hakstian (1989) again found correlations of the PCL with EPQ P and L, but these were attributable to Factor 2. There were also small correlations of N with Factor 1 (negative) and Factor 2 (positive).

The five-factor model (FFM) identifies a Big Five rather than a "big three" personality structure, the main dimensions being neuroticism, extraversion, agreeableness, conscientiousness, and openness to experience. This preserves Eysenck's N and E, but P (and L reversed) is a composite of low agreeableness (i.e., antagonism) and low conscientiousness (Watson, Clark, & Harkness, 1994; Zuckerman, Kuhlman, Joireman, Teat, & Kraft, 1993). Widiger and Lynam (1998; see also Lynam & Derefinko, Chapter 7, this volume) hypothesized that Factor 1 of the PCL-R is primarily a measure of antagonism and Factor 2 a mixture of antagonism and low conscientiousness. This may accommodate findings on the relation of P to the PCL-R. Harpur, Hart, and Hare (2002) found some support for this hypothesis in prison and student samples, but no significant relationships were observed between the PCL-R and either N or E. Overall, the evidence does not support a clear relationship of E with psychopathy.

Arousal and Learning in Psychopaths

The theory that the substrate of N lies in thresholds of limbic system activation lacks firm support, and the proposed link of P to arousal remains to be investigated. Attempts to link E to cortical arousal using electroencephalogram (EEG) indices have also produced inconsistent results (Zuckerman, 1991). Clinical studies of psychopaths have often reported EEG abnormalities in the form of low frequency activity, consistent with low arousal, but in one study using Minnesota Multiphasic Personality Inventory (MMPI) measures, low EEG arousal was a characteristic of secondary but not primary psychopaths (Blackburn, 1979). The unitary concept of arousal has also been questioned, and any relationships of EEG indices to personality are more likely for specific traits than for broad personality dimensions (Zuckerman, 1991). Although differences in learning between introverts and extraverts have been shown under several conditions, these appear to reflect the influence of specific emotional systems rather than the differences in general arousal held by Eysenck to underlie E (see, e.g., Patterson & Newman, 1993).

There is, however, support for the prediction that psychopaths are underresponsive to punishment stimuli and acquire conditioned

responses to these stimuli more slowly. In his seminal study, Lykken (1957) found that primary psychopaths were deficient in learning passive avoidance of punished responses compared with controls and were slower to develop conditioned electrodermal responses (EDRs). Secondary psychopaths fell between primary psychopaths and controls on these measures. Although Eysenck does not clearly distinguish active from passive avoidance, these findings are consistent with the theory and a deficit in passive avoidance learning in psychopaths is an established finding (e.g., Newman & Kosson, 1986; Newman & Schmitt, 1998; Thornquist & Zuckerman, 1995). However, Newman and his colleagues find that passive avoidance deficits of psychopaths are confined to situations involving competing cues of both reward and punishment. This is not predictable from Eysenck's theory. (Newman's theory is discussed later.) Moreover, Thornquist and Zuckerman (1995) found that passive avoidance errors were uncorrelated with any scales of the EPQ, correlating significantly only with impulsivity and sensation seeking.

Weaker anticipatory anxiety or fear responses of psychopaths were further demonstrated by Hare (1965), who found poorer EDR conditioning to shock as an unconditioned stimulus. Subsequent findings, however, suggested that poorer autonomic conditionability is limited to EDRs and contradict the hypothesis of a generalized deficit in conditionability. Hare and Quinn (1971) recorded EDRs, digital vasomotor, and heart rate responses to an aversive stimulus (shock) and a pleasant stimulus (slide of a nude female). Psychopaths again exhibited smaller conditioned anticipatory responses to shock, though not to slides, but this applied only to EDRs. Other research also suggests that psychopaths are not autonomically underaroused or unresponsive to nonaversive stimulation or generally insensitive to punishment cues (Blackburn, 1993). The most reliable finding is that psychopaths display electrodermal hyporesponsiveness when anticipating or experiencing aversive stimulation. Although significant for the low-fear model of psychopathy (see Fowles & Dindo, Chapter 2, this volume), this provides equivocal support for Eysenck's theory.

A further prediction from the arousal postulate is that extraverts require more stimulation to support positive "hedonic tone" and thus have a higher optimal level of stimulation. Eysenck observes that delinquent activities often appear to stem from boredom and risk taking, and others also see stimulation seeking as a characteristic of psychopaths (see below). The links between extraversion, stimulation seeking, and arousal, however, are by no means clearly established. Optimal level of stimulation has commonly been operationalized by Zuckerman's Sensation-Seeking Scale (SSS; see Zuckerman, 1991), but research with these clearly indicates that stimulation seeking correlates primarily with impulsivity and Eysenck's P dimension. Together with undersocialization as measured by Gough's So scale, these variables define a factor of impulsive–sensation seeking (Imp–SSS) that is largely independent of extraversion as measured by EPQ E (Zuckerman, Kuhlman, & Camac, 1988). Eysenck (1996) has continued to assert that sensation seeking is one of the traits making up extraversion, but Zuckerman's findings question the postulated link between criminality, extraversion, and optimal level of stimulation.

Critiques of the Theory

There are several inconsistencies in Eysenck's theory (Blackburn, 1993), and his view that differences in arousal and conditionability underlie introversion–extraversion was criticized by Gray (1970, 1981). He argued that introverts form conditioned anxiety responses more readily because they are more susceptible to *fear* or punishment cues. N and E are derivatives of more basic and biologically causal forebrain systems subserving emotion. N reflects greater sensitivity to both reward and punishment, E the balance between sensitivity to reward and punishment. Gray suggests that rotation of Eysenck's N and E dimensions through 45° will yield dimensions of NI and NE, which he calls "anxiety" and "impulsivity." In his "conceptual nervous system," these are the dispositional expressions of activity in the behavioral inhibition system (BIS) and behavioral activation system (BAS), respectively. Applications of this theory to psychopathy focus on low anxiety and the BIS (see Fowles & Dindo, Chapter 2, this volume). Psychopaths are held to have a weak

BIS (low N, high E) being relatively insensitive to punishment cues. Gray subsequently incorporated Eysenck's P dimension into this system, suggesting that anxiety was a function of high N, low E, and low P (Gray, 1987). Psychopathy represents the opposite extreme (low N, high E, and high P). Impulsivity is a function of high levels of all three dimensions. This later model is discussed further below.

Blackburn (1987, 1993) also questioned Eysenck's differentiation of primary and secondary psychopaths on N and E. He describes a 45° rotation of MMPI indices of N and E giving rise to dimensions of *social* anxiety or withdrawal and impulsivity, but identifiable with Gray's dimensions. Blackburn equates psychopathy with this impulsivity dimension, and observer ratings support this (Blackburn, 1987, 1998). However correlations of impulsivity were stronger with PCL-R Factor 2 than with Factor 1.

An empirically derived personality typology based on these dimensions yielded two groups of mentally disordered offenders scoring highly on impulsivity but differentiated by the anxiety–withdrawal dimension. Highly impulsive–low anxious offenders appear to correspond to primary psychopaths, impulsive–highly anxious offenders to secondary psychopaths. This implies that primary psychopaths have an overreactive BAS and an underreactive BIS, while in secondary psychopaths, both systems will be overreactive. (Although the differentiation of primary and secondary [or "neurotic"] psychopaths was borrowed from Lykken [1957], Lykken [1995] now sees secondary psychopaths as having an overreactive BAS and a normal BIS). Primary psychopaths scored higher than secondary psychopaths on E, but lower on P, although the two groups were not distinguished by N (Blackburn, 1987). These patterns are inconsistent with Eysenck's proposals.

The theory of socialization has also been criticized. The claim that socialization is mediated through the conditioning of anxiety or fear is difficult to demonstrate, and it would require more precise parameters of timing and stimulus intensity than are likely under normal conditions. While the importance of punishment in child training is widely accepted, many argue that positive reinforcement of behavior incompatible with socially disapproved behavior is equally involved. Social learning theorists also emphasize the role of modeling in both prosocial and antisocial behavior, and the development of cognitive self-regulation in socialization (Bandura, 1986). Eysenck's theory has therefore been criticized for relying on a narrow concept of human development derived from animal laboratory studies (Passingham, 1972; Trasler, 1978).

Eysenck's theory of criminality and psychopathy is not, then, well supported. Although his dimensional system of personality is established at the descriptive level and provides a framework for further theoretical developments, support for the central theoretical links between extraversion, its physiological substrate, and the process of socialization is at best equivocal. Despite the empirically supported significance of P for psychopathy, in the absence of a theory linking P to socialization, this association currently lacks explanatory power.

Psychopathy as Pathological Stimulation Seeking

Quay (1965) proposed that the primary and distinctive features of psychopathy are impulsivity and lack of tolerance for sameness. Drawing on research demonstrating the motivating properties of sensory deprivation, he saw "much of the impulsivity of the psychopath, his need to create excitement and adventure, his thrill-seeking behavior, and his inability to tolerate routine and boredom as a manifestation of an inordinate need for increases or changes in the pattern of stimulation" (p. 181). Excessive stimulation seeking could also involve legal or moral transgressions. Possible mediators were low basal reactivity to sensory input or more rapid adaptation to stimulation resulting in a need for more intense and varied input. Quay saw this model as consistent with evidence for poor conditionability and avoidance learning in psychopaths and with Eysenck's theory of extraversion. A similar model of sensation seeking was developed independently by Zuckerman (1991).

Evidence favoring an association between heightened stimulation seeking and psychopathy has been consistent (Blackburn, 1978; Quay, 1977). For example, Skrzypek (1969) used a behavior rating scale developed by Quay to select psychopathic and neurotic delinquents. He found that brief exposure to unpatterned stimulation produced a greater increase in the preference for complex patterns in psychopaths. Studies using Zuckerman's SSS have also shown higher levels of sensation seeking in psychopaths (Harpur et al., 1989), although the associations are mainly with Factor 2 of the PCL. However, Levenson, Kiehl, and Fitzpatrick (1995) found that questionnaire scales of primary and secondary psychopathy did not correlate with all SSS subscales and suggest that thrill-seeking behavior, such as rock climbing, is not a necessary correlate of psychopathy or undersocialized behavior. Nevertheless, the finding of a single factor of impulsivity, poor socialization, and general sensation seeking (Zuckerman et al., 1988) lends further credence to Quay's model at the descriptive level. Zuckerman (1991) argues that this Imp–SSS factor is equivalent to Eysenck's P and is the dimension underlying psychopathy.

Evidence on the substrate of stimulation seeking suggested by Quay is more equivocal. As noted earlier, studies of autonomic reactivity to nonaversive stimulation have not confirmed a general hyporesponsiveness to sensory input in psychopaths. Limited data on habituation in peripheral autonomic responding to monotonous stimulation in psychopaths also contradicts Quay's hypothesis (Blackburn, 1978). Zuckerman (1991) has concluded that there is no evidence for a relationship between sensation seeking and low arousal and now sees sensation seeking in terms of an optimal level of catecholamine system activity.

There are other difficulties in attempting to link stimulation seeking to arousal or arousability. Like Eysenck, Quay assumes an optimal or preferred level of stimulation. Motivation for stimulus seeking or avoidance comes from the discrepancy between this preferred level and the current level of input, not the level of arousal per se. It is not obvious why a high preferred optimal level should be related to low rather than a high arousal level. Research on sensory deprivation demonstrated that what is reinforcing for stimulus-deprived subjects is the information content of sensory input, not stimulus intensity as such (Jones, 1969). Some theorists therefore propose that people seek an optimal level of uncertainty or incongruity (see Blackburn, 1978). Preference for a more incongruous or complex level of information might hence underlie the sensation seeking of psychopaths.

Gray's Biological Model of Emotion and Personality

The generality of Eysenck's N, E, and P dimensions is now established in personality research. As noted earlier, they are accommodated by (or accommodate, as Eysenck prefers) four of the Big Five dimensions, and are similar to what Tellegen (1985) identifies as Negative Emotionality, Positive Emotionality, and Constraint, respectively (see Lynam & Derefinko, Chapter 7, this volume). Gray's proposals regarding the personality dimensions associated with the BIS and BAS should therefore also apply to corresponding dimensions in other systems. Cloninger's dimensional system (Cloninger, 1987), which is based on Gray's model, also contains scales of Harm Avoidance and Novelty Seeking that purport to measure individual differences in the BIS and BAS, respectively.

Gray (1987) predicted that a weak BIS, which he viewed as central to psychopathy, is manifest in a combination of N–E+P+, and that the impulsivity of a high BAS is reflected in a combination of N+E+P+. Tests of these predictions in normal samples using self-report measures of the BIS and BAS and Cloninger's measures (e.g., Carver & White, 1994; Diaz & Pickering, 1993; Zuckerman & Cloninger, 1996) suggest that BIS scales correlate with N+E– and Cloninger's Harm Avoidance, but not with EPQ P. BAS measures correlate with P, E, Cloninger's Novelty Seeking, and lack of constraint, and also Zuckerman's Imp–SSS factor, but not with N as Gray proposed.

Although Zuckerman equates psychopathy with both Imp–SSS and P, he does not believe that Gray's emotional systems translate readily into personality dimensions. Nevertheless, on the basis of theoretical arguments and findings such as those above, Pickering and Gray (1999) proposed that a highly reactive BAS is indexed by high scores on inventories related to impulsive sensation seeking and by a combination of E and P. Diaz and Pickering (1993) also concluded that in

view of the lack of a relationship of P to BIS underreactivity, a weak BIS may be necessary but not sufficient for psychopathy, and that the risk taking element of psychopathy is represented independently by P. This suggests that psychopathy is related to both a weak BIS and a strong BAS, contrary to the proposals of Fowles (1980), who attributed psychopathy solely to a weak BIS.

However, the relation of anxiety to the BIS and psychopathy is unclear, partly as a result of Gray's broad conception of "anxiety" as a personality disposition. Although psychopaths are often said to exhibit little "anxiety or fear," these terms are not synonymous. Watson and Clark (1984) distinguish harm avoidance from anxiety or negative affect, and Depue and Lenzenweger (2001) cite animal and human research indicating that anxiety and fear (harm avoidance) are independent. Lykken (1995) identifies low fear as the substrate of primary psychopathy, and he equates it with harm avoidance. Harm avoidance in this context is a primary trait contributing to Tellegen's higher-order Constraint factor, unlike Cloninger's Harm Avoidance, which is clearly a measure of N+E–. Lykken also considers low fear and low Constraint to be closely related to sensation seeking. This is consistent with the association of Imp–SSS with P, the opposite of Constraint. However, given the proposed relationship of sensation seeking and low Constraint to the BAS (Pickering & Gray, 1999), it is also consistent with a view of primary psychopathy as a function of a strong BAS as much as a weak BIS.

Correlations of the PCL-R with personality questionnaire measures are generally weak but suggest, if anything, that psychopathy is related more to a strong BAS than a weak BIS. As noted earlier, a modest relationship of psychopathy to Eysenck's P is reasonably well established, but contrary to Gray's earlier views, P is not now considered to index a weak BIS (Diaz & Pickering, 1993). Similarly, the absence of a consistent relationship of the PCL-R with N and E also contradicts Gray's concept of psychopathy as entailing low anxiety.

Evidence for a relationship of psychopathy with other measures of negative affectivity is mixed. Harpur and colleagues (1989) found that of eight anxiety measures used, one correlated negatively with PCL total, six correlated significantly, and negatively, with Factor I, while one correlated positively with Factor 2. Comparable results were obtained by Patrick (1994). Total PCL-R was uncorrelated with measures of negative affectivity, but these correlated negatively with Factor 1 and positively and more strongly with Factor 2. Verona, Patrick, and Joiner (2001) found a *positive* correlation of total PCL-R with negative affectivity, but this was due largely to Factor 2. Schmitt and Newman (1999), however, found that neither total PCL-R nor Factors 1 and 2 were correlated with scales of neuroticism, anxiety, or neurotic introversion (BIS) or with Tellegen's Harm Avoidance or Constraint scales. Verona and colleagues also reported insignificant correlations of Tellegen's Constraint scales with Factor 1.

These correlational data provide equivocal support for the view that either lack of anxiety or fear and a weak BIS are intrinsic characteristics of psychopaths. Fowles (1987) suggested that psychopaths may report anxiety because their risky lifestyle generates stress. However, it is equally plausible that stress and anxiety in some psychopaths (possibly secondary psychopaths) are a consequence of traumatic emotional experiences earlier in life that contribute to their impulsivity. Moreover, measures of risk taking and impulsivity are uncorrelated with trait anxiety (Zuckerman et al., 1988), and high risk takers are not necessarily antisocial (Levenson et al., 1995). The strongest support for a weak BIS in psychopaths comes from laboratory measures of passive avoidance learning, but passive avoidance errors in psychopaths do not correlate with personality measures that Gray considers BIS indicators (Thornquist & Zuckerman, 1995). Their correlation with Imp–SSS implies rather a BAS involvement.

Despite the elegance and parsimony of Gray's model of psychopathy, his theoretical constructs simplify complex underlying physiological processes (Newman, 1997), and his personality theory has not gone unchallenged. Depue and Lenzenweger (2001) disagree with Gray, Zuckerman, and Cloninger on the causal biological lines of influence on personality. They suggest that behavioral inhibition is related to fear responsiveness and Constraint, not N or anxiety. Imp–SSS also represents an emergent

trait reflecting the interaction of two more fundamental neurobiological systems underlying E and Constraint. They nonetheless note that "argument far exceeds data" (p. 146). It would appear that the same applies to current attempts to link psychopathy to higher dimensions of personality on the one hand, and biological systems on the other. As Zuckerman (1991) has argued, it may be too optimistic to expect any simple isomorphism between personality structure at the phenotypic level and brain organization at the neural and biochemical level.

PSYCHOPATHY AS DEVELOPMENTAL DELAY

Theories relating psychopathy to failures of parental socialization view morality as the acquisition of conforming behavior through conditioning or other learning processes. Moral discriminations of right and wrong are primarily affective responses to the avoidance of punishment and moral action is irrational conformity to culturally relative standards (Gibbs & Schnell, 1985). Cognitive-developmental theorists, such as Piaget and Kohlberg, dispute this view of socialization and see morality as motivated by cognitive needs for the understanding of reality. Moral reasoning develops sequentially through universal stages of cognitive development, and it entails cognitive growth in which children actively construct moral judgments through social experiences and role-taking opportunities rather than passively internalizing the rules of socializing agents (Kohlberg, 1984).

Kegan (1986) proposed that psychopathy reflects a failure of cognitive development. Combining the stage theories of Piaget and Kohlberg with his own, he suggested that differentiation of self from the external world proceeds through parallel cognitive, sociocognitive, and affective changes. Prior to adolescence, the developing child has a concept of an independent self and is able to recognize that others have needs and take their role but is unable to coordinate personal needs and feelings with those of another. Right action is what meets one's own needs, and the child does not experience guilt as internal self-punishment.

This preadolescent stage corresponds to Piaget's stage of concrete operational thought and Kohlberg's preconventional stage, when moral and self-serving values are not differentiated, and Kegan suggests that psychopaths have a developmental delay at this stage. This is a disturbance in the ordinary process of growth resulting from a lack of familial and peer group support for development beyond the preadolescent state. Most of the criteria of psychopathy, such as lying, selfishness, callousness, and irresponsibility, reflect this failure to relate independent points of view.

Kegan's theory clearly overlaps with that of Gough, but evidence for it is limited. Kegan cites a number of studies indicating that delinquents, particularly recidivists, display lower moral reasoning, but it remains unclear whether a delayed stage of moral development characterizes psychopaths. Two early studies of psychopathic delinquents supported this (see Kegan, 1986). O'Kane, Fawcett, and Blackburn (1996) also found that scores of mentally disordered offenders on PCL-R total and on Factor 2 were negatively correlated with scores on the Defining Issues Test, a questionnaire of moral reasoning, but when IQ was partialed out, the relation of moral reasoning to psychopathy was no longer significant. Research has also indicated that the relation between moral thought and moral action is neither simple nor direct, and it is uncertain whether lower moral development could entirely account for the salient characteristics of psychopaths as Kegan suggests.

COGNITIVE THEORIES OF PSYCHOPATHY

Both Eysenck and Gray see psychopathy as the outcome of physiological differences in emotion systems that affect learning through classical conditioning. Many theorists, however, assign primacy in emotion, learning, and motivation to cognitive mediation. For example, research by Rescorla (1988) showed that classical conditioning in humans is influenced by awareness and motivation and entails the extraction of information about relations between environmental events rather than being a simple reflexive process.

Cognitive theories commonly employ the computer metaphor of information processing in which cognitive activities are construed in terms of the interplay between cognitive processes of decoding, encoding, retrieval, and attention, and cognitive structures that are the organized representations of stored information, including beliefs, schemas, and tacit assumptions (see e.g., Meichenbaum, 1993). Dysfunctions in cognition may represent deficiencies in cognitive processing or distortions or biases in the content of thinking arising from cognitive structures. Newman's theory of psychopathy emphasizes a cognitive deficit, while Beck's theory focuses on cognitive distortions.

Psychopathy as a Cognitive Deficit: Newman's Theory of Response Modulation

Impulsivity or lack of restraint is central to several conceptions of psychopathy. Newman and his colleagues (Gorenstein, 1991; Gorenstein & Newman, 1980; Newman, 1998; Patterson & Newman, 1993) attribute this lack of restraint to a deficit in cognitive processing that impairs the ability of psychopaths to accommodate the meaning of contextual environmental cues when engaged in goal-directed activity. The central concept is *response modulation*, a brief and relatively automatic shift of attention from goal-directed action in which a dominant response set is suspended to accommodate environmental feedback. In approach–avoidance situations, psychopaths fail to make this shift and are hence less likely to appreciate the consequences of their actions or to learn to modify their behavior.

The hypothesis originates in observations by Gorenstein and Newman (1980) that analogies to the disinhibited behavior of psychopaths and other groups are seen in the effects of lesions in the septohippocampal system in animals. Characteristic of the septal syndrome is a marked perseveration of goal-directed behavior and poor passive avoidance learning in the face of a punishment incentive to inhibit a rewarded response. Failure to modulate a dominant response might account for parallel characteristics of the human "disinhibitory syndrome," such as the poor passive avoidance learning of psychopaths.

Several experiments established the utility of the analogy. For example, Newman, Patterson, and Kosson (1987) found that psychopaths, as defined by Hare's PCL, exhibited perseveration for reward while engaged in a computerized card-turning task in which face cards produced monetary reward but number cards led to loss of money. The ratio of reward to punishment was high during initial trials to elicit a dominant response set, but rate of punishment increased with subsequent trials, until all cards elicited monetary loss. Psychopaths displayed a pronounced perseverative tendency, continuing to play cards long after the controls, despite losing money. However, perseveration was eliminated by increasing the intertrial interval and providing feedback about winnings, suggesting the importance of reflecting on the situation.

Newman and Kosson (1986) also demonstrated that the failure of psychopaths to inhibit punished responses may be limited to situations in which they are focused on rewarded behavior. Hypothesizing that psychopaths would show passive avoidance errors primarily when forming a dominant response set for reward at the outset, they observed performance in a go/no-go (inhibit) discrimination task in which response to the correct cue produced monetary reward, and failure to inhibit response to the incorrect cue resulted in punishment (loss of money). In a control task not producing a dominant response set, both failure to respond to the correct cue and response to the incorrect cue were punished. Psychopaths made more passive avoidance errors (commission errors) than nonpsychopaths in the reward and punishment condition. However, groups did not differ in response inhibition in the punishment-only condition or in failure to respond to the correct stimulus (omission errors). These results suggest that the passive avoidance learning deficit in psychopaths is context specific. Their ability to avoid punishment when there is no approach contingency or when the avoidance contingency is salient from the outset of the task was further shown by Newman, Patterson, Howland, and Nichols (1990). When the reward and punishment task was modified to minimize the formation of a dominant response set, psychopaths no longer showed deficient passive avoidance. Their poor passive avoidance

learning was also associated with less reflectivity (pausing) following the punishment stimulus, consistent with inadequate cognitive processing.

Patterson and Newman (1993) proposed a psychobiological model to account for these and related findings in which they identify four interdependent stages involving intra-individual and situational factors. In *Stage 1*, the opportunity for reward establishes an appetitive motivational state and a response set entailing allocation of attention to goal-relevant stimuli. Overfocus on the goal is affected by individual differences in ease of forming and maintaining approach response sets, as addressed by Gray's BAS concept. Following an aversive event that disrupts the approach response set, *Stage 2* entails automatic processing of the disruptive event and an increase in arousal as a result of a mismatch between expectation and reality. This is influenced by the reactivity to aversive events associated with the BIS.

Stage 3 calls for coping with the aversive event through effortful adaptive switching from an active response set to a passive, information-gathering set. Failure to shift from automatic processing to information processing results in facilitation of the dominant response rather than its inhibition. The critical individual difference variable is response modulation of the goal-directed response set. This may reflect the facilitating effects of BAS arousal on goal-directed motor behavior and BIS facilitation of cognitive processing. *Stage 4* involves associative learning necessary for developing predictability of the environment through retrospective reflection on the stimuli warning of aversive outcomes. Failure to reflect results in associative deficits that are a subsequent source of poor judgment and an impulsive cognitive style. The deficit in psychopaths is assumed to be a functional anomaly rather than a structural "organic" dysfunction and represents the extreme of a continuum of cognitive mediating processes in humans (Gorenstein, 1991).

While the model shares its major components with Gray's analysis of the BIS functions of the septohippocampal system, it is more specific in identifying interactions between BIS and BAS in accounting for disinhibited behavior. The model does not attribute deficient passive avoidance learning in psychopaths primarily to a weak BIS, as suggested by Fowles and Gray. Although failure to inhibit responses to punishment cues could arise from a weak BIS or a strong BAS, the response modulation hypothesis implies that neither of these is a necessary condition. However, findings on this issue have been inconclusive. Arnett, Smith, and Newman (1997) examined psychophysiogical responding during passive avoidance learning, recording heart rate and EDR to index BAS and BIS activity, respectively. They found greater heart rate and speed of response to reward in psychopaths relative to controls but no differences in EDR, consistent with hypersensitivity of the BAS. A comparison of psychophysiological and behavioral responses during active avoidance followed by a passive avoidance task proved inconclusive in supporting weak BIS, strong BAS, or response modulation models. However, Arnett and colleagues suggest that impulsivity, sensation seeking, delay of gratification, and poor moral reasoning may be better accounted for by hypersensitivity to reward than by insensitivity to punishment.

The model also differs from the low-fear hypothesis of passive avoidance learning in postulating an attentional rather than a motivational deficit. In Newman's studies using the PCL-R, comparisons have often been made between high- and low-anxious psychopaths and nonpsychopaths (e.g., Arnett, Howland, Smith, & Newman, 1993). He argues that the interaction of anxiety and psychopathy is important because low anxiety is considered a characteristic of primary psychopathy by Cleckley and others. This is not tapped by the PCL-R, which is independent of anxiety (Schmitt & Newman, 1999). Lykken (1995) suggests that low fear rather than low anxiety distinguishes primary psychopaths, and he questions the reliability of findings on the poor passive avoidance learning of low anxious psychopaths. However, Newman and Schmitt (1998) found that low-fear psychopaths were not distinguished in passive avoidance learning from low-fear controls.

The response modulation hypothesis also predicts that deficient processing of peripheral information in psychopaths is not limited to fear-related stimuli but should also be apparent with motivationally neutral cues. This was tested by Newman, Schmitt, and Voss (1997), who used a discrimination task

in which contextual cues normally interfere with performance, hence indicating the processing of contextual cues. The task provided incentives in order to facilitate a dominant response set, and as predicted, the motivationally neutral cues produced significantly less interference in performance in low-anxious psychopaths than in low-anxious controls. The finding that psychopaths are less sensitive than controls to affectively neutral stimuli is not easily accommodated by the low-fear hypothesis, nor by the view that the primary deficit of psychopaths is specific to affective responding.

Newman (1998) proposed that the failure of psychopaths to allocate processing resources to secondary tasks while engaged in goal-directed behavior accounts not only for their failure to profit from experience but may also disrupt major components of self-regulation, such as self-monitoring, self-evaluation, and self-control. Gorenstein (1991) similarly attributed the proposed cognitive processing deficit of psychopaths to a general inability to develop mental representations of contingencies between many kinds of events, including goals and intentions. These suggestions go beyond the data, and the research has so far not entailed direct examination of cognitive processing in psychopaths.

Failure to replicate the relationship of psychopathy to passive avoidance learning among African American offenders (Kosson et al., 1990; Newman & Schmitt, 1998; Thornquist & Zuckerman, 1995) also questions the generality of the relationship. Similarly, the focus on low-anxious psychopaths leaves the impulsive unsocialized behavior of high-anxious, "secondary" psychopaths unaccounted for. However, Newman (1998) notes that the response modulation deficit hypothesis generates testable predictions and provides a viable alternative to other hypotheses.

Psychopathy as Cognitive Distortion: Beck's Theory

Beck's theory of emotional disorders (Beck, 1976) drew on Lazarus's theory that both the arousal and experience of emotion are determined by cognitive appraisal of the situation (see Lazarus, 1991). Appraisal refers to a rapid preconscious cognitive process in which the situation is evaluated in terms of its meaning, meaning being governed by the relation of the situation to personal beliefs or expectations and goals. The kind of appraisal determines the nature of the emotion. Beck's theory relies on the concept of schema, central to which is the notion of the personal domain, which includes self-concept and values, as well as personal relationships and possessions. Following appraisal theory, he sees specific emotions as the consequence of specific cognitive appraisals about the effect of events on one's domain. For example, anger is the appraisal of unwarranted violation of one's domain. Because a schema represents knowledge derived from personal learning history, it is subject to biases or distortions in attention and judgment, such as arbitrary inferences, selective abstraction, or overgeneralization. These biases are a source of emotional dysfunction.

This theory was subsequently extended to a general theory of personality and personality disorder. The theory takes an evolutionary view and construes prototypical personality patterns as genetically determined strategies favored by natural selection to facilitate survival and reproduction. For example, the strategy of cheating and exploiting characteristic of psychopaths would have had survival value in earlier times. Affects related to pain and pleasure play a key role in the mobilization and maintenance of crucial strategies, but information processing is antecedent to the operation of these strategies, which are triggered by evaluation of situational demands. Evaluations depend on beliefs embedded in schematic structures that determine cognitive, affective, and motivational processes. Personality traits are the overt expression of these underlying cognitive structures and represent strategies resulting from the interaction of genetic predispositions and exposure to environmental influences.

Dysfunctional strategies are exaggerations of normal traits and reflect dysfunctional schemas of self and others. These give rise to distorted automatic self-evaluations, biased attributions of causality, and "if . . . then" conditionals (e.g., "If I don't exploit others, I will never get what I deserve."). Each personality disorder is characterized by a characteristic "cognitive profile," a composite of beliefs about the self and others, core beliefs, affects, and strategies.

In the case of the psychopath (which Beck accepts is broader than the DSM construct of APD), the view of self is that of a strong, autonomous loner, while others are seen as exploitative and deserving exploitation in return, or as weak and vulnerable and to be preyed upon. Core beliefs are to look out for oneself, to avoid victimization by being aggressor and exploiter, and an entitlement to break social rules, while conditional beliefs center on rules that getting one's deserts requires manipulating others. The typical strategy is to attack, rob, or cheat others, although a more subtle variant is to manipulate and defraud. Finally, the typical affect is likely to be anger over the injustice that others possess more than they do.

This characterization of the psychopath as a self-serving "cheater" with an egocentric level of moral development is consistent with most other conceptions, but the unique theoretical perspective is that these attributes are mediated by dysfunctional schemas about the self, the world, and the future that are maintained through selective, confirmatory experiences. An adequate test of the theory would require prospective demonstration that deviant schemas predict deviant behavior in psychopaths, but very few studies have examined the beliefs and evaluations of psychopaths.

Some findings are, however, consistent with cognitive distortions in psychopaths. For example, Widom's demonstration that psychopaths do not distinguish between their own construals and those of other people (Widom, 1976) suggests cognitive biases. Klass (1980) also used a repertory grid to assess self-evaluations of transgression in sociopathic (defined by antisocial history) and nonsociopathic methadone patients and students. Compared to the normal group, sociopaths showed less discrepancy between negative evaluations of harming a disliked as opposed to harming a liked victim and also construed harm-doing behavior as self-congruent, suggesting a deviant self-schema. However, differences between sociopaths and nonsociopaths were marginal. Evidence for deviant causal attributions was found by Serin (1991), who examined prison inmates divided into psychopaths and nonpsychopaths on the PCL. Although groups did not differ on the Novaco Anger Scale, psychopaths reported greater anger and more attributions of hostile intent than nonpsychopaths in response to vignettes of provocative situations.

PSYCHOPATHY AS INTERPERSONAL STYLE

Most theories attempt to account for psychopathy in terms of *intrapersonal* mediators, yet Cleckley and most writers emphasize *interpersonal* dysfunctions as the hallmark of psychopathy. Vaillant (1975), for example, suggested that psychopathy could not exist outside social structures such as in an isolated castaway on a desert island. As Fowles (1980) notes, the weak BIS model accounts for *some* observed attributes of psychopaths, but not for the interpersonal features of "lovelessness" or interpersonal conflict, which he suggests have more to do with learning history than with deficient learning mechanisms. However, Levenson (1992) argues that the "trivialisation of the other" (p. 62) is the central feature to be explained in psychopathy. Deficient socialization models also assume that psychopaths have simply failed to control natural impulses. They do not therefore address the motives or goals of psychopaths or the functions their behavior serves. This is directly addressed in the interpersonal theory originating with Leary (1957) and subsequently developed by others (e.g., Kiesler, 1996; Wiggins & Trapnell, 1996), which Blackburn (1998) developed into a cognitive-interpersonal model of psychopathy. This model proposes that central to psychopathy is a coercive style of relating to others that is supported by expectations of hostility.

Leary (1957) developed a structural model of interpersonal behavior that now has firm empirical support (Kiesler, 1996). This portrays interpersonal variables as blends of two orthogonal dimensions of power or control (dominance vs. submission) and affiliation (hostility vs. love or nurturance) that form the coordinates of a circular structure or circumplex known as the *interpersonal circle*. These dimensions represent the fundamental motivational concerns communicated in varying combinations in interpersonal transactions. Blame, for example, represents a blend of hostility and control, deference a blend of submission and affiliation. The circle also provides a map for identifying personality variation. Interpersonal style refers to regularities in managing interactions across social encounters and relationships, different styles reflecting an emphasis on different areas of the circle.

Rigid or inflexible styles characterize personality disorders. Leary (1957) saw psychopathy as represented by a hostile or aggressive–sadistic style, in which fear is inspired in others through subtle forms of critical, humiliating, and punitive interactions. Adjacent to this style in the circle is the hostile–dominant style represented by narcissistic personality, and reflected in self-love, arrogance, and exploitation. The former is motivated by desire to humiliate, the latter by a need for status. From findings with a rating scale, the Chart of Interpersonal Reactions in Closed Living Environments (CIRCLE), Blackburn (1998) suggested that the core features of psychopathy are exemplified by extreme interpersonal styles falling in the hostile–dominant quadrant of the circle. In CIRCLE, the *coercive* axis between hostility and dominance represents both the aggressive–sadistic and competitive styles described by Leary. However, primary psychopaths are expected to be more dominant, secondary psychopaths more hostile and submissive. Wiggins (Wiggins & Trapnell, 1996) argued that interpersonal dimensions represent the metaconcepts of agency (dominance) and communion (affiliation). In these terms, the hostile–dominant styles of psychopaths can be construed as interpersonal dispositions that communicate concerns about power and status in social hierarchies (agency), but also the rejection or avoidance of intimacy (communion).

Research supports the association of psychopathy with hostile dominance. Harpur and colleagues (2002) found that PCL total and Factor 1 and Factor 2 scores projected significantly onto the hostile–dominant quadrant of the circle as measured by both self- and observer ratings on an adjective checklist. In a small sample of prisoners, they also found that the Psychopathy Checklist: Screening Version (PCL:SV) was aligned closely with the hostile–dominant axis. Kosson, Steuerwald, Forth, and Kirkhart (1997) similarly found that among students, self- and observer ratings of dominance and hostility were significantly related to their scores on both Factor 1 and Factor 2 of the PCL-SV. Ratings of hostile–dominant verbal and nonverbal interactions during the assessment interview also correlated with PCL-R scores, particularly Factor 1, in prison inmates. Verona and colleagues (2001) also found that Factor 1 of the PCL-R correlated with the Social Potency scale of Tellegen's Multidimensional Personality Questionnaire (MPQ), while Factor 2 correlated with MPQ Aggression. Both MPQ scales correlated with total PCL-R score.

Recent studies with CIRCLE in forensic psychiatric patients also indicate a moderately strong relationship of a coercive style with PCL-R total scores ($r = .47$) and scores on both Factor 1 ($r = .46$) and Factor 2 ($r = .40$; Blackburn, 2005). A coercive style was highly predictive of future institutional misconduct and matched the predictive power of the PCL-R in this respect. Among non-mentally ill offenders, a coercive style was also strongly associated with a history of chronic offending (Blackburn, 1998).

Interpersonal theory conceptualizes interpersonal styles as modes of self-presentation that are maintained by the reactions they elicit from others. Different styles are hence underpinned by beliefs about the self and others. From a social cognitive perspective, Carson (1979) suggested that interpersonal styles function as self-fulfilling prophecies. For example, a hostile individual has learned to expect hostile reactions from others and behaves in ways that get them. Blackburn and Lee-Evans (1985) also suggested that the behavior of psychopaths may be accounted for by a cognitive bias to perceive malevolent intent in others. From the interpersonal model, it would therefore be predicted that psychopaths have hostile expectations of others and that their style induces hostile reactions.

There is some support for these predictions. Blackburn (1998) found that expectations of hostile dominance in others were significantly associated with a coercive style, but comparable associations with the PCL-R were not assessed. However, Serin's findings of an association of psychopathy with hostile attributions (Serin, 1991) support the model. Also consistent are findings of Kosson and colleagues (1997) that the emotional reactions of interviewers, such as avoidance of confrontation, trepidation, or lack of warmth, were significantly related to interviewees' scores on the PCL-R and to ratings of their hostile–dominant style.

The model therefore has empirical support, but it clearly does not account for all findings on psychopathy. It does not, for example, predict cognitive or neuropsychological deficits or a weak BIS, although it is not incompatible with intraindividual factors that may constrain early learning. However, because agreeableness–antagonism of the FFM coincides with the coercive axis of the interpersonal circle, the model converges with the proposal that psychopathy is linked to this dimension of the Big Five (Widiger & Lynam, 1998; Lynam & Derefinko, Chapter 7, this volume). It is similarly consistent with evolutionary perspectives (see below), and with Millon's view that the primary motivation of antisocial and narcissistic personalities is self-enhancement (Millon & Davis, 1996). Nevertheless, interpersonal theory attempts to explain surface dispositions or styles in terms of mediating cognitions that depend on interpersonal experiences (Carson, 1979). Like Beck's theory, the model therefore implies that the behavior of adult psychopaths is as much a product of their social learning histories as of predisposing genetic factors.

EVOLUTIONARY PERSPECTIVES ON PSYCHOPATHY

Evolutionary theory posits that the core of human nature consists of adaptations taking the form of evolved psychological mechanisms for solving specific problems of survival or reproduction (Buss, 1999). Specific motives, goals, and strivings emerged from these, the most universal being strivings for status in the competition for resources. Competition for resources, including mates, involves impeding others' chances of acquiring resources, and this may include stealing, cheating, attacking, humiliating, or ensuring compliance of the other. This increases the control of access to desired outcomes and reduces those of competitors.

Several writers have proposed that psychopathy represents an evolutionarily based cheating strategy that would have promoted reproductive success in ancestral environments (e.g., Beck & Freeman, 1990). However, although it might be expected that as cooperation in groups for mutual support became more adaptive, it should replace cheating as a heritable strategy, evolutionary theorists have proposed that genes for alternative strategies can survive through frequency-dependent selection (Buss, 1999). This means that the payoff for one strategy decreases as its frequency increases relative to the alternative strategy. For example, a cheating strategy is only effective when the majority are cooperators, and as the number of cheaters increases, so does the average cost to the cooperative group, which inflicts costs on "cheaters." The average payoff of a cheating strategy then decreases, maintaining the prevalence of cheaters at a small frequency in a predominantly cooperative population.

This selection theory is basic to Mealey's "integrated" evolutionary model of psychopathy (Mealey, 1995). "Sociopathy" is the product of evolutionary pressures leading to a life strategy of manipulative and predatory social interactions. Mealey surveys a wide range of evidence from genetics, developmental research, and theories such as those of Eysenck, Zuckerman, and Newman and concludes that there is a genotype for socially deviant behavior associated with temperamental and physiological differences that makes people less responsive to cues for socialization, and that is associated with deficits in the social emotions of shame, guilt, and love.

Sociopathy is held to be a normally distributed continuum manifest in many when environmental pressures encourage an antisocial strategy, but which takes two distinct, more extreme forms. In primary sociopathy, a small number of cheaters are selected for in every society, giving rise to a low, but stable proportion of psychopaths in all cultures through frequency-dependent selection in response to varying environmental circumstances, which fills an evolutionary niche. This is the outcome of genetically based individual differences in a single antisocial strategy and is unrelated to social background.

Secondary sociopaths are the product of individual differences in early developmental response to environmental conditions that give rise to a less extreme strategy involving the differential use of cooperative or deceptive social strategies. These individuals are less extreme on the continuum and not emotionally unresponsive. They are more the outcome of environmental conditions and less tied to genetic factors. Criminal behavior is one kind of cheating strategy related to factors affecting resource competition, and it entails the use of cheating strategies by individuals at a competitive disadvantage. This is reflected in two pathways to delinquency, unsocialized and socialized delinquency. Most upper-class sociopaths will be primary sociopaths. Secondary psychopaths are more likely to come from lower-class or disadvantaged groups.

Mealey's model is similar to several others, and Lykken (1995) considers her primary–secondary distinction to be in agreement with his own distinction between psychopathy and sociopathy. However, in integrating a broad range of theories, Mealey's retains some of their weaknesses. Critical commentaries noted that her assumptions that sociopathy represents cheating rather than violent competition, that physiological differences are necessarily genetic, and that socialization is mediated primarily through punishment are all largely untested. Similarly, there is consistent evidence for a genetic contribution to antisocial behavior (Lykken, 1995), but although one recent twin study found evidence for a genetic contribution to psychopathy as measured by self-report (Blonigen, Carlson, Krueger, & Patrick, 2003), there is as yet no comparable study using the PCL-R. Baldwin (1995) also pointed out that her concept of a continuum does not require two discrete classes, and that variations along a single genetic-environment continuum would be a more economic assumption. In an addendum, Mealey suggested that primary sociopathy is reflected in Factor 1 of the PCL-R and secondary sociopathy in Factor 2. However, because these are correlated factors, this suggestion is difficult to reconcile with a concept of distinct types.

Harris, Skilling, and Rice (2001) proposed a very similar model, but rather than two distinct types of psychopath, they suggest two different paths to chronic criminality. One is associated with developmental neuropathology and competitive disadvantage, the other being nonpathological. However, Harris et al. argued that the latter represents a taxon or discrete category.

CONCLUSIONS

It is perhaps easier to see the differences among the models described in this chapter than to see similarities. Although several focus on inadequate socialization, there are differences among them in how far they see this primarily as located in the inborn characteristics of the child and how far in the failures of the socializing environment. Several also construe psychopathy as a deficit but differ as to whether this is primarily affective or primarily cognitive. There are similarly differences in the extent to which the models emphasize a more reductionist, physiological level of analysis and explanation or a more molar psychological level. Although a convergence of the two is desirable, physiology and psychology refer to different phenomena and tend to represent different assumptions about causality and the nature of human personality. For example, Eysenck's neobehaviorist theory construes biological processes as causes of behavior but treats thought as an epiphenomenon. In contrast, Beck's cognitive theory assumes that beliefs and expectancies have causal agency, consistent with the view that cognitions are emergent properties of matter with the causal power to determine emotional and social behavior (Sperry, 1993). Again, accounts of psychopathy in terms of biologically based dispositions provide at best only partial explanations for the deviant acts of psychopaths. These acts require reference to reasons in the form of motives, intentions, and beliefs for a more complete causal explanation (see Blackburn, 1993, chap. 1, for a brief overview of philosophy of science issues in the explanation of crime).

Two points of similarity are, however, noteworthy. First, despite the claimed contentiousness of the debate over whether psychopathy is a discrete category or the extreme of a continuum, most theories explicitly adopt the latter view. Second, all theories reviewed here share the significant limitation that attempts to test them empirically have so far been carried out almost exclusively with adult male offenders or forensic psychiatric patients

Most also share the assumption that psychopaths are a homogeneous group, and that the central components of the particular model are necessary and sufficient to account for the range of characteristics of psychopathy described in the literature. Yet it seems unlikely that a single model will capture all these or encompass the more significant empirical findings that different models claim in support. Widiger and Lynam (1998; see also Lynam & Derefinko, Chapter 7, this volume) suggested that the diversity among the various models may be clarified by identifying the domain of personality in the FFM that each emphasizes, consistent with the different domains of functioning represented by the PCL-R. They argued, for example, that the low-fear model focuses on low neuroticism, deficient response modulation on low conscientiousness, and the Cleckley–Hare model on antagonism (low agreeableness). It is clear that models that rely on self-report measures in defining their central construct tend to correlate more with Factor 2 than with Factor 1 of the PCL-R. Whether this means that these models are more valid in accounting for the impulsive, antisocial features of psychopathy than for explaining the affective deficits held to be central in Cleckley's conceptualization or whether it reflects the constraints of method variance is one of the many issues that remain to be addressed.

REFERENCES

American Psychiatric Association. (1994). *Diagnostic and statistical manual of mental disorders* (4th ed.). Washington, DC: Author.

Andrews, D. A., & Wormith, J. S. (1989). Personality and crime: Knowledge destruction and construction in criminology. *Justice Quarterly, 6,* 289–309.

Arnett, P. A., Howland, E. W., Smith, S. S., & Newman, J. P. (1993). Autonomic responsivity during passive avoidance in incarcerated psychopaths. *Personality and Individual Differences, 14,* 173–184.

Arnett, P. A., Smith, S. S., & Newman, J. P. (1997). Approach and avoidance motivation in psychopathic criminal offenders during passive avoidance. *Journal of Personality and Social Psychology, 72,* 1413–1428.

Baldwin, J. D. (1995). Continua outperform dichotomies. *Behavioral and Brain Sciences, 18,* 543–544.

Bandura, A. (1986). *Social foundations of thought and action.* Englewood Cliffs, NJ: Prentice-Hall.

Beck, A. T. (1976). *Cognitive therapy and the emotional*

disorders. New York: International Universities Press.

Beck, A. T., & Freeman, A. (1990). *Cognitive therapy of personality disorders*. New York: Guilford Press.

Blackburn, R. (1978). Psychopathy, arousal, and the need for stimulation. In R. D. Hare & D. Schalling (Eds.), *Psychopathic behaviour: Approaches to research* (pp. 157–164). Chichester, UK: Wiley.

Blackburn, R. (1979). Cortical and autonomic arousal in primary and secondary psychopaths. *Psychophysiology, 16,* 143–150.

Blackburn, R. (1987). Two scales for the assessment of personality disorder in antisocial populations. *Personality and Individual Differences, 8,* 81–93.

Blackburn, R. (1993). *The psychology of criminal conduct: Theory, research and practice*. Chichester, UK: Wiley.

Blackburn, R. (1998). Psychopathy and personality disorder: Implications of interpersonal theory. In D. J. Cooke, A. E. Forth, & R. D. Hare (Eds.), *Psychopathy: Theory, research and implications for society* (pp. 269–301). Amsterdam: Kluwer.

Blackburn, R. (2005). Psychopathy as a construct of personality. In S. Strack (Ed.), *Handbook of personology and psychopathology* (pp. 271–291). New York: Wiley.

Blackburn, R., & Lee-Evans, J. M. (1985). Reactions of primary and secondary psychopaths to anger evoking situations. *British Journal of Clinical Psychology, 24,* 93–100.

Blonigen, D. M., Carlson, S. R., Krueger, R. F., & Patrick, C. J. (2003). A twin study of self-reported psychopathic personality traits. *Personality and Individual Differences, 35,* 179–197.

Bowlby, J. (1969). *Attachment and loss: Vol 1. Attachment*. New York: Basic Books.

Buss, D. M. (1999). Human nature and individual differences: The evolution of human personality. In L. A. Pervin & O. P. John (Eds.), *Handbook of personality theory and research* (2nd ed., pp. 31–56). New York: Guilford Press.

Carson, R. C. (1979). Personality and exchange in developing relationships. In R. L. Burgess & T. L. Huston (Eds.), *Social exchange in developing relationships* (pp. 247–269). New York: Academic Press.

Carver, C. S., & White, T. L. (1994). Behavioral inhibition, behavioral activation, and affective responses to impending reward and punishment: The BIS/BAS scales. *Journal of Personality and Social Psychology, 67,* 319–333.

Cleckley, H. (1982). *The mask of sanity* (6th ed.). St. Louis, MO: Mosby. (Original work published 1941)

Cloninger, C. R. (1987). A systematic method for the clinical description and classification of personality variants. *Archives of General Psychiatry, 44,* 573–588.

Day, R., & Wong, S. (1996). Anomalous perceptual asymmetries for negative emotional stimuli in the psychopath. *Journal of Abnormal Psychology, 105,* 648–652.

Depue, R. A., & Lenzenweger, M. F. (2001). A neurobehavioral dimensional model. In W. J. Livesley (Ed.), *Handbook of personality disorders: Theory, research, and treatment* (pp. 277–306). New York: Guilford Press.

Diaz, A., & Pickering, A. D. (1993). The relationship between Gray's and Eysenck's personality spaces. *Personality and Individual Differences, 15,* 297–305.

Doren, D. (1987). Gough's theory—The psychopath as deficient in role-playing abilities. In D. Doren, *Understanding and treating the psychopath* (pp. 14–21). New York: Wiley.

Eysenck, H. J. (1977). *Crime and personality* (3rd ed.). London: Paladin.

Eysenck, H. J. (1996). Personality and crime: Where are we now? *Psychology, Crime and Law, 2,* 143–152.

Eysenck, H. J., & Gudjonsson, G. H. (1989). *The causes and cures of criminality*. New York: Plenum Press.

Forth, A., & Tobin, F. (1995). Psychopathy and young offenders: Rates of childhood maltreatment. *Forum on Corrections Research, 7,* 20–22.

Fowles, D. C. (1980). The three arousal model: Implications of Gray's two-factor learning theory for heart rate, electrodermal activity, and psychopathy. *Psychophysiology, 17,* 87–104.

Fowles, D. C. (1987). Applications of a behavioral theory of motivation to the concepts of anxiety and impulsivity. *Journal of Research in Personality, 21,* 417–435.

Gibbs, J. C., & Schnell, S. V. (1985). Moral development "versus" socialization: A critique. *American Psychologist, 40,* 1071–1080.

Gorenstein, E. (1991). A cognitive perspective on antisocial personality. In P. A. Magaro (Ed.), *Cognitive bases of mental disorders* (pp. 100–133). Newbury Park, CA: Sage.

Gorenstein, E., & Newman, J. P. (1980). Disinhibitory psychopathology: A new perspective and a model for research. *Psychological Review, 87,* 301–315.

Gough, H. G. (1948). A sociological theory of personality. *American Journal of Sociology, 53,* 359–366.

Gough, H. G. (1994). Theory, development, and interpretation of the CPI Socialization scale. *Psychological Reports, 75,* 651–700.

Gray, J. A. (1970). The psychophysiological basis of introversion–exatraversion. *Behaviour Research and Therapy, 8,* 249–266.

Gray, J. A. (1981). A critique of Eysenck's theory of personality. In H. J. Eysenck (Ed.), *A model of personality* (pp. 246–276). New York: Springer-Verlag.

Gray, J. A. (1987). The neuropsychology of emotion and personality. In S. M. Stahl, S. D. Iverson, & E. C. Goodman (Eds.), *Cognitive neurochemistry* (pp. 171–190). Oxford, UK: Oxford University Press.

Hare, R. D. (1965). Acquisition and generalisation of a conditioned fear response in psychopathic and non-psychopathic criminals. *Journal of Psychology, 59,* 367–370.

Hare, R. D. (1970). *Psychopathy: Theory and research*. New York: Wiley.

Hare, R. D. (1979). Psychopathy and laterality of cerebral functioning. *Journal of Anormal Psychology, 88,* 605–610.

Hare, R. D. (1982). Psychopathy and the personality dimensions of psychoticism, extraversion and neuroticism. *Personality and Individual Differences, 3,* 35–42.

Hare, R. D. (1991). *The Hare Psychopathy Checklist—Revised.* Toronto, ON, Canada: Multi-Health Systems.

Hare, R. D. (1998). Psychopathy, affect, and behavior. In D. J. Cooke, A. E. Forth, & R. D. Hare (Eds.), *Psychopathy: Theory, research and implications for society* (pp. 105–137). Dordrecht, The Netherlands: Kluwer.

Hare, R. D., & Jutai, J. W. (1988). Psychopathy and cerebral asymmetry in semantic processing. *Personality and Individual Differences, 9,* 329–337.

Hare, R. D., & McPherson, L. M. (1984). Psychopathy and perceptual asymmetry during verbal dichotic listening. *Journal of Abnormal Psychology, 93,* 141–149.

Hare, R. D., & Quinn, M. (1971). Psychopathy and autonomic conditioning. *Journal of Abnormal Psychology, 77,* 223–235.

Hare, R. D., Williamson, S. E., & Harpur, T. J. (1988). Psychopathy and language. In T. E. Moffitt & S. A. Mednick (Eds.), *Biological contributions to crime causation* (pp. 68–92). Dordrecht, The Netherlands: Martinus Nijhoff.

Harpur, T. J., Hare, R. D., & Hakstian, A. R. (1989). Two-factor conceptualization of psychopathy: Construct validity and assessment implications. *Psychological Assessment, 1,* 6–17.

Harpur, T. J., Hart, S. D., & Hare, R. D. (2002). Personality of the psychopath. In P. T. Costa & T. A. Widiger (Eds.), *Personality disorders and the five-factor model of personality* (2nd ed., pp. 299–324). Washington, DC: American Psychological Association.

Harris, G. T., Skilling, T. A., & Rice, M. E. (2001). The construct of psychopathy. In M. Tonry (Ed.), *Crime and justice: An annual review of research* (Vol. 28, pp.197–263). Chicago: University of Chicago Press.

Hiatt, K. D., Lorenz, A. R., & Newman, J. P. (2002). Assessment of emotion and language processing in psychopathic offenders: Results from a dichotic listening task. *Personality and Individual Differences, 32,* 1255–1268.

Intrator, J., Hare, R. D., Stritzke, P., Brichtswein, K., Dorfman, D., Harpur, T. J., et al. (1997). A brain imaging (single photon emission computerized tomography) study of semantic and affective processing in psychopaths. *Biological Psychiatry, 42,* 96–103.

Johnson, J. G., Cohen, P., Brown, J., Smailes, E. M., & Bernstein, D. P. (1999). Childhood maltreatment increases risk for personality disorders during early adulthood. *Archives of General Psychiatry, 56,* 600–606.

Jones, A. (1969). Stimulus seeking behaviour. In J. P. Zubek (Ed.), *Sensory deprivation: Fifteen years of research* (pp. 57–81). New York: Appleton-Century-Croft.

Karpman, B. (1948). The myth of the psychopathic personality. *American Journal of Psychiatry, 104,* 523–534.

Kegan, R. (1986). The child behind the mask: Sociopathy as developmental delay. In W. H. Reid, D. Dorr, J. I. Walker, & J. W. Bonner (Eds.), *Unmasking the psychopath: Antisocial personality and related syndromes* (pp. 45–77). New York: Norton.

Kernberg, O. (1996). A psychoanalytic theory of personality disorders. In J. F. Clarkin & M. F. Lenenweger (Eds.), *Major theories of personality disorder* (pp. 106–140). New York: Guilford Press.

Kiesler, D. J. (1996). *Contemporary interpersonal theory and research: Personality, psychopathology, and psychotherapy.* New York: Wiley.

Klass, E. T. (1980). Cognitive appraisal of transgression among sociopaths and normals. *Cognitive Research and Therapy, 4,* 353–369.

Kohlberg, L. (1984). *The psychology of moral development.* New York: Harper & Row.

Kosson, D. S., & Newman, J. P. (1989). Socialisation and attentional deficits under focusing and divided attention conditions. *Journal of Personality and Social Psychology, 57,* 87–99.

Kosson, D. S., Smith, S. S., & Newman, J. P. (1990). Evaluation of the construct validity of psychopathy in black and white inmates: Three preliminary studies. *Journal of Abnormal Psychology, 99,* 250–259.

Kosson, D. S., Steuerwald, B. L., Forth, A. E., & Kirkhart, K. J. (1997). A new method for assessing the interpersonal behavior of psychopathic individuals: Preliminary validation studies. *Psychological Assessment, 9,* 89–101.

Lazarus, R. S. (1991). Cognition and motivation in emotion. *American Psychologist, 46,* 352–367.

Leary, T. (1957). *Interpersonal diagnosis of personality.* New York: Ronald Press.

Levenson, M. R. (1992). Rethinking psychopathy. *Theory and Psychology, 2,* 51–71.

Levenson, M. R., Kiehl, K. A., & Fitzpatrick, C. M. (1995). Assessing psychopathic attributes in a noninstitutionalised population. *Journal of Personality and Social Psychology, 68,* 151–158.

Luntz, B. K., & Widom, C. S. (1994). Antisocial personality disorder in abused children grown up. *American Journal of Psychiatry, 151,* 670–674.

Lykken, D. T. (1957). A study of anxiety in the sociopathic personality. *Journal of Abnormal and Social Psychology, 55,* 6–10.

Lykken, D. T. (1995). *The antisocial personalities.* Hillsdale, NJ: Erlbaum.

McCord, W. M., & McCord, J. (1964). *The psychopath: An essay on the criminal mind.* New York: Van Nostrand.

Mealey, L. (1995). The sociobiology of sociopathy: An integrated evolutionary model. *Behavioral and Brain Sciences, 18,* 523–599.

Meichenbaum, D. (1993). Changing conceptions of cognitive behavior modification: Retrospect and prospect. *Journal of Consulting and Clinical Psychology*, 61, 202–204.

Meloy, J. R., & Gacono, C. B. (1998). The internal world of the psychopath. In T. Millon, E. Simonsen, M. Birket-Smith, & R. D. Davis (Eds.), *Psychopathy: Antisocial, criminal, and violent behaviour* (pp. 95–109). New York: Guilford Press.

Millon, T., & Davis, R. (1996). *Disorders of personality: DSM-IV and beyond*. New York: Wiley.

Nass, M. L. (1966). The superego and moral development in the theories of Freud and Piaget. *Psychoanalytic Study of the Child*, 21, 51–68.

Newman, J. P. (1997). Conceptual models of the nervous system: Implications for antisocial behavior. In D. M. Stoff, J. Breiling, & J. D. Maser (Eds.), *Handbook of antisocial behavior* (pp. 324–326.). New York: Wiley.

Newman, J. P. (1998). Psychopathic behavior: An information processing perspective. In D. J. Cooke, A. E. Forth, & R. D. Hare (Eds.), *Psychopathy: Theory, research and implications for society* (pp. 81–104). Dordrecht, The Netherlands: Kluwer.

Newman, J. P., & Kosson, D. S. (1986). Passive avoidance learning in psychopathic and nonpsychopathic offenders. *Journal of Abnormal Psychology*, 95, 252–256.

Newman, J. P., Patterson, C. M., Howland, E. W., & Nichols, S. L. (1990). Passive avoidance in psychopaths: The effects of reward. *Personality and Individual Differences*, 11, 1101–1114.

Newman, J. P., Patterson, C. M., & Kosson, D. S. (1987). Response perseveration in psychopaths. *Journal of Abnormal Psychology*, 96, 145–148.

Newman, J. P., & Schmitt, W. A. (1998). Passive avoidance in psychopathic offenders: A replication and extension. *Journal of Abnormal Psychology*, 107, 527–532.

Newman, J. P., Schmitt, W. A., & Voss, W. D. (1997). The impact of motivationally neutral cues on psychopathic individuals: Assessing the generality of the response modulation hypothesis. *Journal of Abnormal Psychology*, 106, 563–575.

O'Kane, A., Fawcett, D., & Blackburn, R. (1996). Psychopathy and moral reasoning: Comparison of two classifications. *Personality and Individual Differences*, 20, 505–514.

Passingham, R. E. (1972). Crime and personality: A review of Eysenck's theory. In V. D. Nebylitsin & J. A. Gray (Eds.), *Biological bases of individual behavior* (pp. 342–371). New York: Academic Press.

Patrick, C. J. (1994). Emotion and psychopathy: Startling new insights. *Psychophysiology*, 31, 319–330.

Patterson, C. M., & Newman, J. P. (1993). Reflectivity and learning from aversive events: Towards a psychological mechanism for the syndromes of disinhibition. *Psychological Review*, 100, 716–736.

Pickering, A. D., & Gray, J. A. (1999). The neuroscience of personality. In L. A. Pervin & O. P. John (Eds.),

Handbook of personality: Theory and research (pp. 277–300). New York: Guilford Press.

Quay, H. C. (1965). Psychopathic personality as pathological stimulation seeking. *American Journal of Psychiatry*, 122, 180–183.

Quay, H. C. (1977). Psychopathic behavior: Reflections on its nature, origins, and treatment. In F. Weizmann & I. Uzigiris (Eds.), *The structuring of experience* (pp. 155–171). New York: Plenum Press.

Reed, C. F., & Cuadra, C. A. (1957). The role-taking hypothesis in delinquency. *Journal of Consulting Psychology*, 21, 386–390.

Rescorla, R. A. (1988). Pavlovian conditioning: It's not what you think it is. *American Psychologist*, 43, 151–160.

Schalling, D. (1978). Psychopathy-related variables and the psychophysiology of socialization. In R. D. Hare & D. Schalling (Eds.), *Psychopathic behaviour: Approaches to research* (pp. 85–106). Chichester, UK: Wiley.

Schmitt, W. A., & Newman, J. P. (1999). Are all psychopathic individuals low anxious? *Journal of Abnormal Psychology*, 108, 353–358.

Serin, R. C. (1991). Psychopathy and violence in criminals. *Journal of Interpersonal Violence*, 6, 423–431.

Skrzypek, G. J. (1969). Effect of perceptual isolation and arousal on anxiety, complexity preference, and novelty preference in psychopathic and neurotic delinquents. *Journal of Abnormal Psychology*, 74, 321–329.

Sperry, R. W. (1993). The impact and promise of the cognitive revolution. *American Psychologist*, 48, 878–875.

Tellegen, A. (1985). Structures of mood and personality and their relation to assessing anxiety, with an emphasis on self-report. In A. H. Tuma & J. D. Maser (Eds.), *Anxiety and anxiety disorders* (pp. 681–706). Hillsdale, NJ: Erlbaum.

Thornquist, M., & Zuckerman, M (1995). Psychopathy, passive avoidance learning and basic dimensions of personality. *Personality and Individual Differences*, 19, 525–534.

Trasler, G. B. (1978). Relations between psychopathy and persistent criminality. In R. D. Hare & D. Schalling (Eds.), *Psychopathic behavior: Approaches to research* (pp. 273–298). New York: Wiley.

Vaillant, G. E. (1975). Sociopathy as a human process: A viewpoint. *Archives of General Psychiatry*, 32, 178–183.

Verona, E., Patrick, C. J., & Joiner, T. E. (2001). Psychopathy, antisocial personality, and suicide risk. *Journal of Abnormal Psychology*, 110, 462–470.

Watson, D., & Clark, L. A. (1984). Negative affectivity: The disposition to experience aversive emotional states. *Psychological Bulletin*, 96, 465–490.

Watson, D., Clark, L. A., & Harkness, A. R. (1994). Structures of personality and their relevance to psychopathology. *Journal of Abnormal Psychology*, 103, 18–31.

Widiger, T. A., & Lynam, D. R. (1998). Psychopathy and the five-factor model of personality. In T. Millon, E. Simonsen, M. Birket-Smith, & R. D. Davis (Eds.), *Psychopathy: Antisocial, criminal, and violent behavior* (pp. 171–187). New York: Guilford Press.

Widom, C. S. (1976). Interpersonal and personal construct systems in psychopaths. *Journal of Consulting and Clinical Psychology, 44,* 614–623.

Wiggins, J. S., & Trapnell, P. D. (1996). A dyadic-interactional perspective on the five-factor model. In J. S. Wiggins (Ed.), *The five-factor model of personality; Theoretical perspectives* (pp. 88–162). New York: Guilford Press.

Williamson, S., Harpur, T. J., & Hare, R. D. (1991). Abnormal processing of affective words by psychopaths. *Psychophysiology, 28,* 260–273.

Zuckerman, M. (1991). *Psychobiology of personality.* Cambridge, UK: Cambridge University Press.

Zuckerman, M., & Cloninger, C. R. (1996). Relationships between Cloninger's, Zuckerman's, and Eysenck's dimensions of personality. *Personality and Individual Differences, 21,* 283–285.

Zuckerman, M., Kuhlman, D. M., & Camac, C. (1988). What lies beyond E and N?: Factor analyses of scales believed to measure basic dimensions of personality. *Journal of Personality and Social Psychology, 54,* 96–107.

Zuckerman, M., Kuhlman, D. M., Joireman, J., Teta, P., & Kraft, M. (1993). A comparison of three structural models for personality: The Big Three, the Big Five, and the Alternative Five. *Journal of Personality and Social Psychology, 65,* 757–768.

4

The PCL-R Assessment of Psychopathy

Development, Structural Properties, and New Directions

ROBERT D. HARE
CRAIG S. NEUMANN

In this chapter we review the impetus for, and the development of, the Hare Psychopathy Checklist—Revised (PCL-R; Hare, 1991, 2003), discuss its psychometric properties, examine recent research on its structural characteristics, and suggest several directions and paradigms for new research. Reference also is made to direct derivatives of the PCL-R (referred to here as the PCL scales): The Hare Psychopathy Checklist: Screening Version (PCL:SV; Hart, Cox, & Hare, 1995) and the Hare Psychopathy Checklist: Youth Version (PCL:YV; Forth, Kosson, & Hare, 2003). These scales are described briefly below. Extensive discussions and reviews of the construct validity of these instruments are available in their respective manuals and elsewhere (e.g., this volume; Cooke, Forth, & Hare, 1998; Gacono, 2000).

INTRODUCTION TO THE PCL SCALES

Description

The PCL-R is a 20-item construct rating scale for use in research, clinical, and forensic settings. It uses a semistructured interview, file and collateral information, and specific scoring criteria to assess inferred personality traits and behaviors related to widely understood, traditional conceptions of psychopathy (see next section). The PCL-R yields dimensional scores but also may be used to classify individuals for research and clinical purposes. The items have been grouped statistically into several clusters, or factors. Several factor structures have been proposed, including the original two-factor structure (Hare, 1991), a three-factor model (Cooke, Michie, & Hart, Chapter 5, this volume), and a four-factor model (Hare, 2003). For reasons discussed in later sections, we believe that a four-factor model represents well the construct the PCL-R and its derivatives were designed to measure.

Each item in the PCL-R is scored on a 3-point scale (0, 1, 2) according to the extent to which the rater judges that it applies to a given individual. Total scores can range from 0 to 40, reflecting the degree to which the individual matches the prototypical psychopath. In North America a score of 30 typically is used as a cut score for the research on psychopathy. Other cut scores have been used, depending on the purpose of the assessments and the context in which they are used.

The PCL scales are widely used in basic and applied research, including the mental health and criminal justice systems. The qualifications for use of these instruments in clinical and forensic work are more stringent than those for research, for the simple reason that ratings of psychopathy have important implications for the individual and for society (Douglas, Vincent, & Edens, Chapter 27, this volume; Edens & Petrila, Chapter 29, this volume; Hare, 2003). It is not sufficient for users of the PCL scales to be familiar only with the contents of a manual. It is incumbent upon them to remain abreast of the current clinical and empirical literature on psychopathy, to have an understanding of the basic principles and limitations of psychological testing and interpretation, and to ensure that their assessments are conducted in accordance with appropriate professional and legal standards for psychological testing. They also must have enough clinical and forensic training and experience to use the PCL scales reliably and appropriately (American Educational Research Association, American Psychological Association, & National Council on Measurement in Education, 1999).

Properly used, the PCL scales provide a reliable and valid assessment of the clinical construct of psychopathy. Strictly speaking, that is all they do. They were not designed specifically to assess risk for antisocial or criminal activities or to determine treatment options. Nevertheless, the utility of the PCL scales for these and other applied purposes has been well established, in large part because the construct they measure plays a major role in understanding many of the problematic behaviors encountered by the criminal justice and mental health systems.

The generalizability of the PCL-R (as well as the PCL:SV and PCL:YV) makes it possible to assess psychopathy in a wide variety of contexts and in different racial, ethnic, cultural, and socioeconomic groups. Important provisos are that sufficient hard information is available to score the items, and that the user is able to take into account and evaluate, in an unbiased manner, cultural and other differences in which the features measured by the PCL scales might be expressed. Item response theory (IRT) is proving useful in this regard (cf. Sullivan & Kosson, Chapter 22, this volume).

Derivatives

PCL:SV

The PCL:SV is a 12-item version of the PCL-R that was developed for use in the MacArthur Risk Assessment study (Steadman et al., 2000). Like the PCL-R, each item is scored on a 3-point scale (0, 1, 2), with total scores that can range from 0 to 24. A cut point of 18 for a diagnosis of psychopathy has proven useful for research purposes. The PCL:SV is conceptually, psychometrically, and empirically related to the PCL-R (Cooke, Michie, Hart, & Hare, 1999; Hart et al., 1995), and exhibits the same factor structure (Hill, Neumann, & Rogers, 2004; Vitacco, Neumann, & Jackson, 2005). It is used as a screen for psychopathy in forensic populations or as a stand-alone instrument for research with forensic psychiatric populations and with noncriminals, including civil psychiatric patients. There is rapidly accumulating evidence for the construct validity of the PCL:SV, including its ability to predict aggression and violence in offenders and in both forensic and civil psychiatric patients (cf. Douglas et al., Chapter 27, this volume).

PCL:YV

The PCL:YV is 20-item age-appropriate modification of the PCL-R intended for use with adolescents. Like the PCL-R, each item is scored on a 3-point scale (0, 1, 2), with total scores that can range from 0 to 40. It appears to have much the same psychometric and predictive properties as its adult counterpart (see Forth et al., 2003, for review), as well as a four-factor structure. Because of its potential implications for adolescents, particularly young offenders, the PCL:SV is not used to diagnose psychopathy per se but, rather, to assess its adolescent precursors and features and to develop appropriate intervention strategies.

BACKGROUND

Clinical Tradition

Clinical tradition generally describes psychopathy as a combination of inferred personality traits and socially deviant behaviors (see Berrios, 1996; Blackburn, 1998; Cleckley, 1976; Coid, 1993; Doren, 1987; Hare,

1998; Hare & Cox, 1978; Hare & Schalling, 1978; Kernberg, 1984; McCord & McCord, 1964; Meloy, 1988; Millon, Simonson, & Birket-Smith, 1998; Pichot, 1978). McCord and McCord (1964), for example, viewed the psychopath as a selfish, impulsive, aggressive, and loveless individual who feels no guilt or remorse for behavior that is often appalling by most societal standards. Craft (1965) considered the psychopath to be an impulsive and aggressive individual who seriously lacks shame, remorse, or feeling for others. Buss (1966) described psychopathy as a personality disorder in which there is a fundamental incapacity for love or true friendship; a lack of insight, guilt, or shame; an inability to control impulses or to delay gratification; unreliability in fulfilling obligations; pathological lying; thrill seeking; poor judgment; disregard for societal conventions; and asocial and antisocial behavior. Karpman (1961) characterized the psychopath as a callous, two-dimensional person able to simulate emotions and affectional attachments when it is to his advantage to do so. Social and sexual relations with others are superficial but demanding and manipulative. Judgment is poor and behavior is often guided by impulse and current needs, with the result that he is frequently in trouble. Attempts to extricate himself often produce an intricate and contradictory web of blatant lies, coupled with theatrical and convincing explanations and promises. Kernberg (1984) referred to psychopathy as a form of malignant narcissism characterized by a combination of narcissistic personality, antisocial behavior, ego-syntonic aggression or sadism, and a paranoid orientation.

The clinical descriptions provided by Hervey Cleckley have been very influential in North American research. The characteristics considered by Cleckley (1941, 1976) to be typical of the psychopath were as follows: superficial charm and good intelligence; absence of delusions and other signs of irrational thinking; absence of nervousness or psychoneurotic manifestations; unreliability; untruthfulness or insincerity; lack of remorse or shame; inadequately motivated antisocial behavior; poor judgment and failure to learn from experience; pathologic egocentricity and incapacity for love; general poverty in major affective relations; specific loss of insight; unresponsiveness in general interpersonal relations; fantastic and uninviting behavior with drink and sometimes without; suicide rarely carried out; impersonal, trivial, and poorly integrated sex life; and failure to follow any life plan. This list contains a number of features that clearly are antisocial or socially disruptive in nature.

Role of Antisocial Behavior

Some commentators have suggested (incorrectly, in our view) that Cleckley and other influential clinicians defined psychopathy *solely* in terms of personality traits, without reference to antisocial behaviors. Furthermore, they argue that psychopathy *should* be defined in this way, that antisocial behaviors merely are "downstream" from, or manifestations of, core personality dispositions, and that these dispositions should be measured *without* reference to antisocial or socially deviant behaviors (e.g., Cooke, Michie, Hart, & Clarke, 2004). How this is to be done is unclear, given that many of the key personality traits considered most relevant to psychopathy are themselves inferred from behaviors that are antisocial, asocial, or otherwise harmful to others (see Hare, 2003). Until we have the science and technology to tap "directly" into relevant biopsychological processes we will have to rely on inference of these processes from behaviors, some of which are antisocial in nature. Further, the issue of what is upstream (core) and what is downstream (manifestation) is far from clear, as we discuss here and later in this chapter.

There are cogent arguments that an integral part of psychopathy is the emergence of an early and persistent pattern of antisocial behaviors, and that these behaviors are important in defining the condition (e.g., Harris & Rice, Chapter 28, this volume; Quinsey, Harris, Rice, & Cormier, 1998; Robins, 1966, 1978). Indeed, from an evolutionary psychology perspective (e.g., Harpending & Sobus, 1987; Harris, Rice, & Lalumiére, 2001; Lalumiére, Harris, Quinsey, & Rice, in press; MacMillan & Kofoed, 1984; Mealey, 1995), psychopathy is less a biopsychological defect than a heritable adaptive life strategy. In this view, the early emergence of antisocial behavior, including aggressive sexuality, is central to psychopathy (Harris & Rice, Chapter 28, this volume;

G. Harris, personal communication, July 30, 2004). Furthermore, this model helps to explain the psychophyisological, electrocortical, and functional imaging findings from cognitive/affective neuroscience (described throughout this volume; see also Hare, 2003) as normal (not pathological) concomitants of a particular adaptive life strategy.

DSM-III

With respect to the early emergence of antisocial behavior, it is relevant that the DSM-III (American Psychiatric Association, 1980) description and diagnostic criteria for antisocial personality disorder (APD) were "based on longitudinal studies of children whose antisocial behavior persisted into adult life" (p. 379). These studies were conducted and reported by Lee Robins (1966). Millon and colleagues (1998) had this to say about the study:

> What is noteworthy in these findings is the close correspondence they show to the behaviors specified as characteristic of psychopathic personalities 50 years earlier by Kraepelin. What made these data so historically important was that they comprised, in almost every detail, the diagnostic criteria promulgated in the DSM-III definition of antisocial personality disorder. . . . Despite the history of alternative models and theories available for consideration, the DSM-III Task Force voted to base its diagnostic guidelines on this single, albeit well-designed, follow-up study of delinquency cases referred to one child guidance clinic in a large western city. (pp. 20–21)

Robins is a sociologist, and her studies were reinforced by a belief that clinicians and researchers could not make reliable and valid inferences about psychological processes (Robins, 1978). This belief probably was cemented by a NATO Advanced Study Institute (ASI), directed by Hare and the late Daisy Schalling, and held in Les Arcs, France, in 1975. The 10-day ASI ostensibly was on psychopathy and was attended by some 80 prominent researchers, including Hans Eysenck, Charles Spielberger, Marvin Zuckerman, Ronald Blackburn, Samuel Guze, Sarnoff Mednick, Dan Olweus, Cathy Widom, Robert Cloninger, Irwin Sarason, and Lee Robins (see Hare & Schalling, 1978). Within days it became clear that few attendees were on the same diagnostic page

(see Hare, 1996) and that confusion reigned. It is quite possible that the seeds for the DSM-III (American Psychiatric Association, 1980) category APD were nurtured there. Robins certainly recognized that inferring psychological constructs and processes from behavior is "bread and butter" for psychologists and psychiatrists, but because they often were not very good at it she thought that it was "more parsimonious to stick to behavior and skip the inferences until such time as we have a way to validate them independently of behavior" (Robins, 1978, p. 256). The result is that the DSM strategy for operationalizing the construct of psychopathy may in fact have introduced a related, but not identical construct to the field, one that continues in DSM-IV (American Psychiatric Association, 1994).

Psychopathy and APD

In forensic populations the prevalence of APD is two or three times higher than the prevalence of psychopathy, as measured by the PCL-R. The result is an asymmetric association between the PCL-R and APD; most offenders with a high PCL-R score meet the criteria for APD, but most of those with APD do not have high PCL-R scores. In this respect, it is noteworthy that APD is strongly associated with PCL-R Factor 2 items but only weakly associated with Factor 1 items. Yet, DSM-IV states that antisocial personality disorder is also known as psychopathy, effectively equating two different constructs. About this unfortunate and untenable position, Rogers, Salekin, Sewell, and Cruise (2000) had this to say: "As noted by Hare (1998), DSM-IV does considerable disservice to diagnostic clarity in its equating of APD to psychopathy" (pp. 236–237). Extensive discussions of psychopathy and APD are available elsewhere (e.g., Hare, 1996; Hare & Hart, 1995; Rogers, Dion, & Lynett 1992; Rogers et al., 2000; Widiger et al., 1996). Parenthetically, Hare recalls a conversation with Lee Robins in which she suggested that antisocial behavior probably was more discriminating of psychopathy in the general population than in prison populations, where antisocial behavior is very common. As indicated in the section "Structure of Psychopathy," there is new evidence that she may be right.

ORIGINS OF THE PCL-R

The Les Arcs ASI brought into stark relief a fundamental problem in the study of psychopathy: the lack of a common metric for the disorder. Researchers used a variety of assessment and diagnostic procedures, most conceptually and empirically unrelated to one another. Because there was no reliable, valid, and generally acceptable method for the assessment of psychopathy, it was difficult or impossible to compare results from different researchers and studies. DSM-III attempted to rectify the situation by adopting clear and objective diagnostic criteria, heavily influenced by readily observed antisocial behaviors. The PCL-R began about the same time (see Hare, 1980) as an attempt to develop a common metric by combining personality traits and antisocial behaviors, in line with clinical tradition. Detailed descriptions of its evolution from a 22-item scale (Hare, 1980), referred to later as the Psychopathy Checklist (PCL), into the current 20-item PCL-R are available elsewhere (Hare, 1991, 2003). Only a brief account is given here.

The PCL

Around the time that the task force was preparing for DSM-III, Hare and his colleagues had undertaken to determine what specific diagnostic information they had actually used to separate psychopathic from nonpsychopathic offenders in their research investigations to that point (Hare, 1980). The immediate forerunner to the PCL was a global clinical procedure in which Hare and colleagues ordered prison inmates along a 7-point rating scale according to the extent to which their personality and behavior over a long period were deemed consistent with the clinical construct of psychopathy as reflected in the work of Cleckley (1941, 1976). The procedure required a thorough understanding of the clinical framework for these prototypicality ratings, as well as an ability to integrate extensive interview and case-history data into a single score. Under these conditions, the ratings were surprisingly reliable, but it was difficult for others to determine precisely what case facts entered into a particular rating. Consequently, there was a need for a more objective procedure—one in which the basis for assessment is explicit and compatible with the rich fund of clinical experience accumulated over the years. The problem was highlighted by the finding that various different procedures for the assessment of psychopathy failed to relate to one another in a meaningful way (Hare, 1985a).

Work on the development of a new assessment procedure began in 1978 with psychometric analyses of the Cleckley criteria, followed by a listing of the traits and behaviors explicitly or implicitly used in making global ratings of psychopathy. Many of the more than 100 items that resulted were redundant or would have been difficult to score; these items were eliminated. Preliminary scoring criteria were worked out for the remaining items. Each was scored by two experienced investigators from interview and file information, using a 3-point ordinal scale: 0 indicated that the characteristic definitely was not present or did not apply, 1 indicated some uncertainty about whether or not it applied, and 2 indicated that it definitely was present or applied. A series of statistical analyses was then carried out to determine which items had the best psychometric properties and best discriminated between prison inmates with low and high (7-point) global ratings of psychopathy. Twenty-two items were retained, and a mimeographed manual (Hare & Frazelle, 1980) was made available to other investigators. Some of the items involved complex behaviors and traits and, in most cases, required judgment and clinical inference. Nevertheless, initial analyses indicated that the items generally had acceptable interrater reliabilities (Hare, 1980). The total scores, which could range from 0 to 44, were very reliable; the correlation between two independent sets of scores obtained from 143 prison inmates was .93, and Cronbach's coefficient alpha was .88. The total scores were also highly correlated ($r = .83$) with global ratings of psychopathy. Subsequent research with prison inmates confirmed the reliability and validity of this set of 22 items (now named the PCL, but initially referred to as a Research Scale for the Assessment of Psychopathy).

THE PCL-R

1985 Draft Version

Experience with the PCL, as well as feedback from other users, suggested that several improvements could be made without compromising the original intent of the exercise. Two items were deleted, reducing the list to 20. Item 22 ("Drug or alcohol abuse not direct cause of antisocial behavior") was dropped because it was sometimes difficult to score. Item 2 ("Previous diagnosis as psychopath or similar") was deleted because it relied on diagnoses of uncertain meaning and reliability, and because it provided little useful information. Item 6 ("Irresponsible behavior as a parent") was too specific; it was changed to "Irresponsibility" in general, and the scoring procedure was modified to take this into account. The titles of 10 other items were changed slightly without altering the nature of the trait or behavior being rated. The item descriptions and scoring procedures were described in more detail than they had been in the PCL, and some difficulties and apparent inconsistencies in the scoring criteria were removed. The procedure for dealing with inadequate information was changed. With the PCL, a score of 1 was assigned if there was insufficient evidence to score an item with confidence, whereas now the item was omitted and the total score prorated. The scoring instructions for the PCL included some examples of the sorts of behaviors that would qualify for scores of 0, 1, and 2. After some deliberation and pretesting Hare decided to provide only a prototypical description of the item (with the exception of items 9, 17–20) and to assign a score of 0, 1, or 2 on the basis of the extent to which an individual's personality or behavior fit the item description. These revisions of the PCL formed the basis for a draft version of the PCL-R (Hare, 1985b), widely circulated to researchers.

1991 Edition

Soon after the manual for the draft PCL-R found its way into circulation, further minor modifications were made to the item descriptions and scoring criteria. These changes amounted to little more than fine-tuning designed to clarify the scoring criteria and to make it easier for other investigators to use them. Care was taken to ensure that the changes did not have any effect on the actual scores assigned to an item. As a result, the draft and the 1991 published edition of the instrument, now referred to as the Hare PCL-R, were substantively the same and yielded identical results. All the data ob-

tained using the draft manual for the PCL-R were directly applicable to the 1991 version. Table 4.1 lists the PCL-R items.

The 1991 manual contained psychometric data for 1,192 male offenders (M = 23.6, SD = 7.9) and 440 male forensic psychiatric patients (M = 20.6, SD = 7.8). Reliabilities of the items were generally respectable, and internal consistency was high, with Cronbach's alpha coefficients of .87 for the offenders and .85 for the forensic psychiatric patients. Interrater reliability also was high: the intraclass correlation (ICC) for a single rating was .83 for the offenders and .86 for the patients, while the ICC for two ratings averaged was .91 for the offenders and .93 for the patients. The standard error of measurement, the standard deviation of observed scores if the true score is held constant, was estimated at 3.25 for both offenders and patients. Evidence for the validity of the PCL-R is extensive, as reflected in several hundred published studies since its inception.

Exploratory factor analyses (EFAs) of the data sets described in the 1991 edition yielded two correlated factors (see Table 4.1). Factor 1 (Items 1, 2, 4, 5, 6, 7, 8, 16) has been described as Interpersonal/Affective and Factor 2 (Items 3, 9, 10, 12, 13, 14, 15,

TABLE 4.1. PCL-R Items

1. Glibness/superficial charm[a]
2. Grandiose sense of self-worth[a]
3. Need for stimulation/proneness to boredom[b]
4. Pathological lying[a]
5. Conning/manipulative[a]
6. Lack of remorse or guilt[a]
7. Shallow affect[a]
8. Callous/lack of empathy[a]
9. Parasitic lifestyle[b]
10. Poor behavioral controls[b]
11. Promiscuous sexual behavior
12. Early behavior problems[b]
13. Lack of realistic, long-term goals[b]
14. Impulsivity[b]
15. Irresponsibility[b]
16. Failure to accept responsibility for own actions[a]
17. Many short-term marital relationships
18. Juvenile delinquency[b]
19. Revocation of conditional release[b]
20. Criminal versatility[c]

Note. From Hare (1991). Copyright 1991 by R. D. Hare and Multi-Health Systems. Reprinted by permission.
[a] Original Factor 1 items.
[b] Original Factor 2 items.
[c] Added to Factor 2 in the 2nd edition (Hare, 2003).

18, 19) as Social Deviance, although other labels have also been used by different investigators. Items 11 and 17 did not load on either factor. There have been many replications of this two-factor model of psychopathy and it has played an important role in helping us to understand the disorder.

Recent analyses indicate that other models may fit the data better. For example, factor analyses of a selected subset of 13 items (Cooke & Michie, 2001; Cooke et al., Chapter 5, this volume) suggested that the PCL-R measures a superordinate construct underpinned by six testlets and three correlated clusters of items, or factors, that reflect, respectively, the interpersonal (four items), affective (four items), and behavioral/lifestyle (five items) features of psychopathy. The first two factors represent a simple split of the original PCL-R Factor 1 into two parts (Items 1, 2, 4, 5; Items 6, 7, 8, 16). The third factor consists of five of the nine items in the original PCL-R Factor 2 (Items 3, 9, 13, 14, 15). The 13 items in this three-factor model were described as forming the "core" of psychopathy, while the remaining seven "orphaned" items were at first (but since changed; see Cooke et al., 2004) considered to form a unidimensional construct (antisocial behavior) that appeared to reflect antisocial manifestations of the core factors (D. J. Cooke, personal communication, August 8, 2001).

The three-factor model (see Cooke et al., Chapter 5, this volume), though appealing in some respects, is incomplete and, in our view, the procedures used to select the items and to conduct the analyses do not stand up to careful scrutiny. Arbitrary, subjective criteria were used to reduce the PCL-R item set from 20 items down to 13 (e.g., some items that displayed low-to-poor factor loadings in an initial EFA were retained, whereas others that showed low-to-good loadings were eliminated. The testlet (item grouping) strategy that was employed in deriving the three-factor model raises concerns about overfitting (i.e., 10 factors were invoked to model the covariance of 13 items; cf. Skeem, Mulvey, & Grisso, 2003). Related to this, some of the residual error terms for standardized estimates in the model were listed as zero, probably as a function of lower bound errors (i.e., the EQS software used for modeling fitting estimated negative residual

error variances in some instances, and these were arbitrarily set to zero; see Bentler, 1995, for an extended discussion of this issue). These and other limitations of the three-factor model are described in detail elsewhere (Hare, 2003; Vitacco et al., 2005). Our position, articulated below in the section titled "Structure of the Psychopathy," is that a four-factor model encompassing Interpersonal, Affective, Lifestyle, Antisocial facets of psychopathy is more defensible not only for the PCL-R but for its derivatives, the PCL:SV and the PCL:YV.[1]

The PCL-R 2nd Edition (2003)

The 2nd edition of the PCL-R manual was published in 2003. There were no compelling grounds for making substantive revisions to the PCL-R items. Fine-tuning of the scoring criteria for several items might have made them a bit easier to apply in some contexts but at the risk of introducing subtle, though potentially important, changes in the meaning of PCL-R scores. For this reason, and also to maintain continuity with the large research and clinical literature on the PCL-R that has developed in the past decade, new items were not introduced and the scoring criteria for individual items remained unchanged from the first edition. This is a conservative strategy, but one that is consistent with recent recommendations for determining the need for revisions to a psychological test or instrument (Knowles & Condon, 2000; Silverstein & Nelson, 2000; Strauss, Spreen, & Hunter, 2000).

Changes from the 1st Edition

The 2nd edition differs from the 1991 manual in several respects. The major difference is the large amount of data now available for establishing comparison tables and descriptive statistics for selected groups, and for addressing issues of item characteristics, reliability, validity, generalizability, and factor structure. Since the appearance of the PCL-R in 1991 there has been a dramatic surge in published theory and research on psychopathy, and many new articles featuring the PCL-R, as well as the PCL:SV and the PCL:YV, appear every year, adding to the hundreds of articles, scores of chapters, reviews, and books currently available (see www.hare.org for an up-to-date reference list). Not all users of these instruments are familiar with this burgeoning literature. In many cases, it seems that clinicians who produce psychological reports for the criminal justice system or who testify in court rely primarily on material published in the 1991 manual. As a result, it is not uncommon for a prosecuting or defense attorney to argue that the PCL-R is not applicable to a particular group or context because the relevant information is not contained in the manual. The PCL-R: 2nd Edition helps to correct this problem, but it is the responsibility of users to keep abreast of the research literature, particularly as it applies to minority and legal issues (see Sullivan & Kosson, Chapter 22; Edens & Petrila, Chapter 29, this volume).

Included in the 2nd edition are descriptive and validation data for use of the PCL-R with male and female offenders, substance abusers, sex offenders, African American offenders, and forensic psychiatric patients, as well as with offenders in several other countries. Because of these additions, the 2nd edition is three times as large as the first edition (222 vs. 77 pages).

Descriptive Statistics

The descriptive statistics in the 2nd edition are based on large pooled samples of North American male offenders, male forensic psychiatric patients, and female offenders, all assessed from interview and file information (standard procedure), as well as a large sample of male offenders and a smaller sample of male forensic psychiatric patients assessed from only file reviews (no interviews). Statistics also are provided for 1,117 male offenders from England (standard assessments) and 615 male offenders and forensic psychiatric patients from Sweden (file reviews only). Table 4.2 presents a summary of the means, standard deviations, and reliability indices for each of the North American data sets; values are provided for total and factor scores.

The distributions are approximately normal for the female offenders, slightly negatively skewed for the male offenders and male forensic psychiatric patients and slightly positively skewed for the file reviews (see Hare, 2003). The largest difference among data sets is the relatively low scores of offenders assessed from only file reviews.

TABLE 4.2. Descriptive PCL-R Statistics for Pooled Samples in the 2nd Edition

	Standard			File reviews	
	Male offenders	Male forensic patients	Female offenders	Male offenders	Male forensic patients
N	5,408	1,246	1,218	2,622	402
Total					
Mean	22.1	21.5	19.0	16.5	17.4
SD	7.9	6.9	7.5	8.3	9.3
Factor 1: Interpersonal					
Mean	3.6	3.1	3.3	2.5	2.0
SD	2.2	2.1	2.2	2.3	2.4
Factor 2: Affective					
Mean	4.8	4.9	4.1	4.2	4.7
SD	2.1	2.1	2.3	2.3	2.6
Factor 3: Lifestyle					
Mean	5.8	6.1	5.8	4.5	5.7
SD	2.6	2.2	2.5	3.0	3.4
Factor 4: Antisocial					
Mean	5.7	5.9	4.3	4.1	4.1
SD	2.8	2.6	2.5	2.8	2.8

Note. Factors 1 and 2 consist of four items each. Factors 3 and 4 consist of five items each. In the 2 × 4 hierarchical model (Hare, 2003) the factors described here are referred to as facets. See Note 1. Complete details are provided in Hare (2003).

The use of file reviews alone is a nonstandard procedure but one that is used by researchers who are unable to conduct interviews with offenders or patients. In some cases, the file reviews are part of postdictive or retrospective analyses designed to identify variables related to behaviors or events that occurred before or after the compilation of archival data. The advantages of such analyses are that a great deal of useful information can be gathered in a short time, and that it is not necessary to wait years to find out if a variable "predicts" a particular behavior or event (e.g., recidivism). A disadvantage, at least with respect to PCL-R assessments, is that without an interview there may not be sufficient information to adequately score the items that tap interpersonal and affective features. The rater then must rely solely on what others have recorded in the files. IRT analyses (see below) indicated that when standard assessments were used, Factors 1 and 2 provided more information about the latent trait of psychopathy than did Factors 3 and 4. However, this was not the case with file reviews: Factors 1 and 2 carried about the same amount of information as did Factors 3 and 4. These differences between ratings based on file reviews alone and those based on the standard (interview + file review) procedure may be due to differences in the samples used, the amount of information available, and/or the way in which the information is scored. To firmly establish the basis of differences, we need large-scale studies in which offenders and patients are scored, independently, from file reviews and from use of the standard procedure.

The PCL-R scores of the 1,117 English male offenders described in the 2nd edition were representative of the population of Her Majesty's Prison (HMP) Service. The scores were normally distributed, with a mean of 17.2 and a standard deviation of 7.3. The Swedish data were from 265 male offenders and 350 male forensic psychiatric patients and were based on file reviews. The mean PCL-R score was 21.2 ($SD = 9.1$) for the offenders, and 19.5 ($SD = 8.0$) for the forensic patients.

The 2nd edition of the manual also contains descriptive statistics for sex offenders, for substance-dependent patients, and for African American and Caucasian offenders, male and female.

Reliability of Scores

Like its predecessor, the 2nd edition provides strong evidence for the reliability of the PCL-R items and scores. Table 4.3 provides a summary of the reliability indices for total and factor scores for each data set. Internal consistency is generally high (alpha, mean interitem correlation), as is interrater reliability for single ratings (ICC_1) and for the average of two ratings (ICC_2). For the pooled standard assessment data sets, ICC_1 and ICC_2 values for the total score were .87 and .93, respectively. For the pooled file review data sets, alpha was .87 and the mean interitem correlation was .25

The reliabilities of the English and Swedish PCL-R scores were much the same as those of the North American scores. For the English sample, coefficient alpha was .79, ICC_1 was .89, and ICC_2 was .94. For the pooled Swedish samples, pooled coefficient alpha was .81. ICCs were not available for these data.

Standard Error of Measurement

The standard error of measurement is a joint function of the standard deviation and the reliability of measurement. The more reliable the measure and the smaller the standard deviation, the smaller the standard error of measurement, defined as the standard deviation of observed scores if the true score is held constant. In the 1991 edition of the PCL-R the estimated standard error of measurement was 3.25 for total scores. Because of the gradual increase in the reliability of PCL-R assessments as more and more researchers began to use the instrument, the standard error of measurement for the 2nd edition decreased to approximately 3.0 for a single rating and 2.0 for averaged ratings.

For the English sample, the standard error of measurement was the same as that for North American offenders: 3.0 for a single rating and 2.0 for averaged ratings. The standard error of measurement for the Swedish sample was calculated from coefficient alpha, and was approximately 3.0.

A MULTIGROUP IRT ANALYSIS OF THE PCL-R

Because of its demonstrated importance in the criminal justice system, the PCL-R has been subjected to unusually intense scrutiny

TABLE 4.3. PCL-R Reliabilities for Pooled Samples in the 2nd Edition

	Standard			File reviews	
	Male offenders	Male forensic patients	Female offenders	Male offenders	Male forensic patients
Total score					
ICC$_1$	.86	.88	.94	—	—
ICC$_2$	.92	.93	.97	—	—
Alpha	.85	.81	.82	.87	.89
Mean interitem r	.23	.19	.19	.25	.28
Factor 1: Interpersonal					
ICC$_1$	.71	.80	.84	—	—
ICC$_2$	.83	.89	.91	—	—
Alpha	.71	.74	.69	.71	.77
Mean interitem r	.40	.42	.36	.39	.46
Mean interitem r	.40	.72	.36	.40	.46
Factor 3: Lifestyle					
ICC$_1$	.75	.76	.87	—	—
ICC$_2$	.86	.86	.93	—	—
Alpha	.67	.65	.64	.80	.83
Mean interitem r	.31	.29	.28	.45	.50
Factor 4: Antisocial					
ICC$_1$	.84	.88	.89	—	—
ICC$_2$	.91	.93	.94	—	—
Alpha	.64	.61	.60	.70	.73
Mean interitem r	.27	.23	.25	.32	.35

Note. Factors 1 and 2 consist of four items each. Factors 3 and 4 consist of five items each. In the 2 × 4 hierarchical model (Hare, 2003) the factors described here are referred to as facets. See Note 1. Complete details are provided in Hare (2003). ICC$_1$ and ICC$_2$, interrater reliability for single ratings and for the average of two ratings, respectively.

and critical analysis, both conceptual and statistical. Although it has fared very well on both fronts, like all psychological instruments its generalizability requires continual evaluation. One goal has been to determine the extent to which the PCL-R score metric has scalar equivalence, a condition that holds where test scores represent the same level of a construct (e.g., psychopathy) across diverse populations.

The application of IRT to psychopathy as measured by the PCL-R and the PCL:SV is described in detail elsewhere (Bolt, Hare, Vitale, & Newman, 2004; Cooke et al., Chapter 5, this volume[2]; Cooke & Michie, 1997; Cooke et al., 1999). Briefly, IRT models provide a mathematical expression of the relationship between a score on an individual item and the underlying construct or latent trait, theta (θ), often standardized to have a mean of 0 and a standard deviation of 1. For PCL-R items a graded response model (GRM) characterizes each item according to three parameters: a, an indication of the discriminating value of the item with respect to θ; b_1, the threshold or level of θ at which a

score of "1" becomes more probable than a score of 0; and b_2, the threshold or level of θ at which a score of 2 becomes more probable than a score of 1. IRT also provides estimates of the amount of information provided by a test and its items, and the precision of estimates at various levels of the trait. When comparing groups for scalar equivalence, IRT provides information on group differences in the trait-item score relationship. When a difference occurs the item is said to exhibit *differential item functioning* (DIF). IRT also provides information about the scalar equivalence of total test scores, depicted by test characteristic curves (TCCs).

The results and discussions presented in this section are based on the published version of the IRT analyses of the 2nd edition North American data sets by Bolt and colleagues (2004), to which the reader is referred. The total number of offenders and forensic psychiatric patients was 8,938. The samples in these analyses included 3,847 male offenders, 1,219 female offenders, and 1,246 male forensic psychiatric patients—all assessed with the standard PCL-R procedure (interview plus file information)—plus 2,626 male offenders assessed from file reviews. These large samples permitted assessment of DIFs with considerably more power than was available in previous IRT studies of the PCL-R (Cooke & Michie, 1997, 1999).

Unidimensionality of the PCL-R

IRT analyses typically assume unidimensionality, with only one latent dimension underpinning the data. Although the factor structure of the PCL-R is under debate, all models obtain correlated factors, implying the strong influence of a single underlying factor, psychopathy. Several criteria were used to test this assumption: the eigenvalues of the reduced polychoric correlation matrix; the fit of a single-factor model to the polychoric correlation matrix; and the general factor saturation (GFS) index. The ratio of the first to second eigenvalues of the reduced polychoric correlation matrix was 5.6:1 for male offenders, 3.4:1 for female offenders, 3.7:1 for male forensic psychiatric patients, and 3.9:1 for male offenders rated from file reviews. Similar values were obtained by Cooke and Michie (1997) in their analysis of the 1991 PCL-R data set. These results indicate the presence of a dominant first factor but also are indicative of some multidimensionality in the data. Nevertheless, a single-factor model, using the weighted least-squares estimation, fit the data well for all four data sets, based on several fit indices: the minimum-fit-function chi-square test, the comparative fit index (CFI), the Tucker–Lewis index (TLI), and the root-mean-square error of approximation index (RMSEA). The CFI, TLI, and RSMEA were, respectively, .94, .93, and .065 for male offenders, .91, .90, and .084 for male forensic psychiatric patients, .92, .91, and .074 for female offenders, and .95, .95, and .077 for male offenders rated from file reviews. For each group, a single dimension was relatively successful in accounting for the interitem polychoric correlations.

The GFS index represents the proportion of the total variance that can be accounted for by the single underlying factor, with values above .50 indicative of sufficient unidimensionality for IRT. To estimate the GFS, the two-factor, four-facet model of the PCL-R described in Hare (2003) was fit, but with the addition of a third-order factor to account for the correlation between the two second-order factors. The GFS estimate was .56 for female offenders, .59 for male forensic psychiatric patients, .59 for male offenders rated from file reviews, and .71 for male offenders. The values for the male offenders are similar to the GFS estimate of .77 obtained by Cooke and Michie (2001) in their analysis of the 1991 PCL-R data set, and to the GFS estimate of .74 obtained by Cooke and colleagues (2001) for both white and African American offenders. The higher values for the male offenders may be due to the fact that the selection of items for the PCL was based on work with male offenders assessed from interviews and file reviews. Bolt and colleagues (2004) also allowed the two items excluded from the two-factor, four-facet model (promiscuous sexual behavior, many short-term marital relationships) to load on the general factor. The GFS estimates remained the same, indicating that all 20 PCL-R items measure a single underlying factor, sufficient for IRT analyses of the data.

Multigroup Graded Response Model

Differential Item Functioning

Separate DIF analyses were conducted on each data set, using the male offenders as a reference. DIF tests were performed with all three GRM item parameters (a, b_1, b_2). Detailed results of these and other analyses are reported by Bolt and colleagues (2004). Briefly, for the female offenders and the male forensic psychiatric patients, the items that showed DIF with respect to the reference group tended to come from Factor 2, whereas for the offenders rated from file reviews the items that showed DIF tended to come from Factor 1. These findings are discussed later. Items that did not show DIF were used as anchors for a multigroup GRM analysis.

In the multigroup GRM the item parameters of all four groups were estimated simultaneously. The analysis allows for separate GRM estimates for each group but uses anchor items to connect the estimates of the groups to a common latent metric. Table 4.4 presents the results. Items in bold were left unconstrained in the multigroup model because they displayed DIF. Items not in bold

TABLE 4.4. Graded Response Model Item Parameter Estimates, Multigroup Analysis

Item	Male off			Fem off			Psych			File		
	a	b_1	b_2	a	b_1	b_2	a	b_1	b_2	a	b_1	b_2
1	1.19	−0.65	1.46	1.19	−0.65	1.46	1.03	−0.01	2.01	1.18	−0.27	1.33
2	1.20	−0.71	1.24	1.20	−0.71	1.24	1.06	−0.21	1.76	1.27	−0.70	0.76
3	1.30	−1.43	0.24	1.30	−1.43	0.24	1.30	−1.43	0.24	1.30	−1.43	0.24
4	1.26	−1.07	1.13	1.26	−1.07	1.13	1.26	−1.07	1.13	1.21	−0.54	1.02
5	1.41	−0.90	0.77	0.89	−1.63	0.39	1.41	−0.90	0.77	1.20	−1.50	−0.05
6	1.58	−1.83	−0.18	1.58	−1.83	−0.18	1.58	−1.83	−0.18	1.58	−2.32	−0.89
7	1.23	−0.95	1.04	1.23	−0.95	1.04	1.04	−1.90	0.72	0.79	−0.72	1.43
8	1.84	−1.18	0.47	1.84	−1.18	0.47	1.84	−1.18	0.47	1.48	−1.64	−0.26
9	0.96	−1.71	1.14	0.64	−2.43	0.55	0.96	−1.71	1.14	1.05	−1.21	0.65
10	1.02	−1.63	0.20	0.87	−1.10	0.55	1.08	−2.43	−0.20	1.02	−1.63	0.20
11	0.92	−1.29	0.41	0.84	−0.85	0.29	0.54	−1.59	0.42	0.68	−1.74	−0.28
12	1.16	−0.42	0.82	0.94	0.16	1.59	0.97	−1.07	0.35	1.16	−0.42	0.82
13	1.03	−1.47	0.44	0.94	−1.26	0.61	1.00	−1.50	0.99	1.03	−1.47	0.44
14	1.11	−2.02	0.32	1.07	−1.87	−0.03	1.24	−2.72	−0.29	1.22	−2.06	−0.20
15	1.15	−2.19	0.10	0.82	−2.97	−0.55	1.15	−2.19	0.10	1.15	−2.19	0.10
16	0.98	−1.95	0.21	0.98	−1.95	0.21	0.98	−1.95	0.21	1.16	−2.44	−0.85
17	0.65	0.05	1.76	0.30	−0.51	3.01	0.22	3.71	7.77	0.33	3.67	6.24
18	0.91	−1.00	0.28	0.89	0.03	1.58	0.91	−1.00	0.28	0.91	−1.00	0.28
19	0.67	−2.37	−1.12	0.37	−3.04	−0.88	0.51	−2.20	−0.43	0.73	−1.39	−0.24
20	0.85	−1.56	0.24	0.69	−1.32	0.84	0.85	−1.56	0.24	0.63	−0.93	0.64

Note. From Bolt, Hare, Vitale, and Newman (2004). Copyright 2004 by the American Psychological Association. Reprinted by permission. **Boldface** implies different item parameter values in the corresponding group according to the differential item functioning analysis. Male off, male criminal offenders; Fem off, female criminal offenders; Psych, male forensic psychiatric patients; File, male criminal offenders scored only from file review. The a parameter is an estimate of the discriminating value of the item with respect to θ. The b_1 and b_2 parameters indicate, respectively, the threshold or level of θ at which a score of 1 becomes more probable than a score of 0, and the threshold or level of θ at which a score of 2 becomes more probable than a score of 1.

are anchor items. For each group, Factor 1 items had higher discrimination estimates (larger a) than did Factor 2. Factor 1 items also discriminated at higher levels of the trait (larger b values) than did Factor 2 in all groups except the group assessed with file reviews. That is, for all but the file reviews a higher "level" of psychopathy is required for the manifestation of Factor 1 traits and behaviors than for the manifestation of Factor 2 traits and behaviors. These results are consistent with those reported by Cooke and Michie's (1997) IRT analysis of the PCL-R scores from 10 North American samples of male offenders, 8 of whom were from the "normative" samples described in the 1991 PCL-R manual. In each case there was considerable variation in the a parameter, indicating that some items were more discriminating than others of the underlying trait, θ. There also was considerable variation in b parameters, indicating that items discriminated at different levels of the underlying trait. Cooke and Michie concluded, as do we, that the PCL-R is a good measure of psy-

chopathy because all items contribute to the estimate of θ and because different items function efficiently at different levels of the trait.

Eight items (seven from Factor 1) did not show DIF in the female offenders (i.e., the items performed the same as in male offenders). Ten items (five from Factor 1) did not show DIF in the male forensic psychiatric patients. Six items (all from Factor 2) did not show DIF in the offenders assessed with file reviews. It is apparent that Factor 1 (interpersonal/affective) items tended to perform in much the same way as the reference group for groups assessed with the standard PCL-R procedure (interview plus file review), whereas it was Factor 2 items that performed the same for the file-review procedures. The causes of DIF for Factor 1 items scored from file reviews were generally more difficult to interpret than were those for the standard procedure. It is possible that the file-review sample differed from the reference group in ways other than the method of scoring (note that there was not random assignment to the

PCL-R scoring conditions). Factor 1 items may be relatively difficult to assess without the information provided by an interview. However, Bolt and colleagues (2004) noted that these items did not display DIF in a consistent direction. Relative to the samples assessed with the standard procedure, it appeared that file reviews were associated with some Factor 1 item scores that were overestimated (Items 5, 6, 8, 16) and some that were underestimated (Items 1, 2, 4, 7). In this respect, it is interesting that the items that were overestimated had the highest mean scores in the male offender reference group, while those that were underestimated had the lowest scores in the reference group. Most raters are familiar with the mean scores for items scored with the standard procedure. Thus, one explanation for the finding that some Factor 1 items show DIF in one direction and others in the opposite direction may be that in the absence of information needed to score Factor 1 items, raters rely heavily on the known marginal base rates for these items.

Test Characteristic Curves

A TCC plots the expected PCL-R score as a function of the latent trait of psychopathy. With male offenders as the reference group, and using a common latent trait metric, Bolt and colleagues (2004) compared TCCs for each of the four data sets described earlier. A chi-square test based on the differential functioning of items and tests (DFIT) procedure (Flowers, Oshima, & Raju, 1999) indicated that the TCC for the male offenders (reference group) differed significantly from the TCC for the female offenders and for the male forensic psychiatric patients ($p < .01$ in each case), but not from the TCC for file reviews. However, the TCCs were very similar for all groups, particularly in the midrange of the trait, with only small differences at the lower and upper levels of the trait (see Bolt et al., Figure 3). This suggests that in midrange a given PCL-R score may represent much the same level of psychopathy in male offenders, male forensic psychiatric patients, female offenders, and male offenders assessed from file reviews. Exceptions occurred at relatively low PCL-R scores, where the level of psychopathy (relative to male offenders) appeared to be slightly overestimated in the

other groups, and at higher PCL-R scores where the level of psychopathy appeared to be slightly underestimated, in each case by only 1 or 2 points.

Bolt and colleagues (2004) also compared TCCs for each of the four PCL-R facet scores across the four participant samples. The largest difference was for Facet 4 (Antisocial), in which female offenders received lower scores than did male offenders (see Bolt et al., Figure 3). This suggests that for female offenders a relatively high level of psychopathy is required for the manifestation of antisocial traits. The other difference of note occurred for Facet 2 (Affective), with file reviews having higher scores than the reference group. This suggests that for file reviews, a relatively low level of psychopathy is required for manifestation of affective features, for reasons that are not yet clear.

Information Functions

IRT can be used to estimate the amount of information provided by a test and its items, and to determine the precision of estimates at various levels of the trait. Cooke and Michie (1997) computed the information functions for each PCL-R item, each factor, and the whole test. The maximum amount of information carried by the whole test and by Factor 1 centered near the middle of the distribution, a level of θ where the estimates are based on the largest number of cases.

Bolt and colleagues (2004) computed information functions for PCL-R Total and Facet scores for each of the four groups described previously, based on a common latent trait metric. The information functions for Total scores appeared very similar to one another, although slightly more information was provided by the PCL-R for male offenders than for the other groups (see Bolt et al., Figure 4). The maximum amount of information was near the middle of the trait ($\theta = 0$), with the point of maximum information somewhat lower for file reviews. For standard assessments (interview plus file), Factor 1 (Facets 1 and 2) provided more information than did Factor 2 (Facets 3 and 4), especially at higher levels of the trait. With file reviews, however, Factors 1 and 2 provided much the same amount of information. At higher levels of the latent trait, the file reviews provided less information than did the other groups, primarily because of Facet 2 (Affective) and to a lesser extent, Facet 1 (Interpersonal). This is not surprising, because the Interpersonal/Affective items, which function most effectively at high levels of the trait, may be more difficult to measure with file reviews. With female offenders, the least information was provided by Facet 3 (Lifestyle) and Facet 4 (Antisocial). The items in these facets are less prevalent among female offenders than among male offenders and are less discriminating of psychopathy, as indicated by their *a* parameters.

A Multigroup IRT Analysis of English PCL-R Data

On the basis of their IRT analyses, Cooke and Michie (1997) argued that four of the PCL-R Factor 2 items (10, 12, 18, 19) and three items that did not load on either factor (11, 17, 20) could be excluded from the instrument because they were less discriminating of psychopathy and provided less information, than Factor 1 items. Cooke and Michie (2001) also asserted that these items were not part of the factor structure of the PCL-R or the PCL:SV. However, as noted earlier, the criteria that Cooke and Michie used to exclude items were arbitrary and subjective, and in particular, their decision to omit antisocial behavior items from the PCL-R ignores a sizable literature attesting to the importance of such behaviors to the construct of psychopathy. Here we present IRT analyses of data from English male prisoners that illustrate the importance of Factor 2 items in assessing psychopathy (see Bolt & Hare, 2004; Hare, 2003, Appendix A). The two English samples were provided by HMP Service and consisted of a representative sample of 669 inmates drawn from seven prisons and from a national database of new admissions to HMP Service, and a sample of 448 inmates from cognitive skills programs at six HMP Service prisons. The two samples (B-1 and B-2, respectively, in the 2nd edition) were pooled to form a sample of 1,117 offenders.

Analyses similar to those described above for the North American data sets were conducted on the pooled English sample. In these analyses, a multigroup GRM was fitted to the item response data from the North American male offenders and English male offenders. This model resulted in a common latent trait metric against which the two groups could be compared concurrently, with the North American male offenders as the reference group.

Differential Item Functioning

Ten items functioned the same in North American and English offenders (did not show DIF) and served as anchor items for comparing the two groups. Of the 10 items that did not did not show DIF, one was from the Interpersonal factor (Item 5), four were from the Affective factor (Items 6, 7, 8, 16), two were from the Lifestyle factor (Items 3, 14), two were from the Antisocial factor (Items 10, 12), plus Item 17, which did not load on any factor. Unlike the North American data, the Lifestyle and Antisocial factors were about as discriminating of the trait of psychopathy as were the Interpersonal and Affective factors. Items 18–20 were particularly discriminating of the trait of psychopathy among English offenders, much more so than among North American offenders. Ironically, these three items were among the seven items that Cooke and Michie (2001) considered not to be an integral part of the psychopathy trait.

Test Characteristic Curves

Figure 4.1 presents plots of the TCC relating the expected PCL-R score to the level of the underlying trait of psychopathy in North American and English offenders. The curves are very similar, particularly at middle and higher levels. Scores below about 25 may slightly overestimate the level of the trait among English offenders, but higher scores appear to have much the same meaning with respect to the latent trait of psychopathy for English and North American male offenders. To put it another way, a score of 30 reflects about the same level of psychopathy in both groups of offenders.

Information Functions

The information functions for PCL-R Total and factor scores based on the common latent trait metric are described in Appendix B of the 2nd edition (Hare, 2003). Unlike the North American data, in which the Interper-

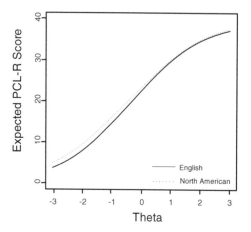

FIGURE 4.1. Test characteristic functions for North American and English male offenders relating the expected PCL-R score to the level of the latent trait, theta. Based on a multigroup analysis (Bolt & Hare, 2004; Hare, 2003).

sonal and Antisocial factors carried more information than did the Lifestyle and Antisocial factors, the English data indicate that the latter two carried as much information as did the former other two factors.

It appears that the presence of impulsive lifestyle and antisocial features are more informative of psychopathy in English male offenders than in North American offenders. One possibility is that the English sample contained many more "minor" criminals from jails and low-security facilities than did the North American sample. Note that the distribution of the English scores was normal, with a mean of 17.2 (*SD* = 7.3), whereas the distribution of the North American scores was negatively skewed (more scores at the upper end of the distribution than at the lower end), with a mean of 22.1 (*SD* = 7.9). Antisocial items may be more discriminating of psychopathy in groups with a relatively low prevalence of psychopathic features. We provide some empirical support for this possibility in a later section.

Some Implications of IRT Analyses

Detailed discussions of the value of IRT in understanding the construct of psychopathy are available elsewhere (Bolt et al., 2004: Cooke et al., Chapter 5, this volume), and only some general comments are provided here.

The multigroup analyses described earlier indicate that a significant proportion of the PCL-R items showed DIF in each of the groups that were compared with the male offender reference group. However, the specific items with DIF were not the same in each comparison group, suggesting that proposals to eliminate or modify items of the PCL-R on the basis of data from circumscribed samples are premature. Our findings indicate that the task of retaining or developing items that show little or no DIF across various populations, groups, and settings is likely to be a formidable one. Furthermore, the amount of DIF in a given item was relatively small in practical terms, though statistically significant because of the power to detect small differences in DIF associated with the very large sample sizes used (Ankenmann, Witt, & Dunbar, 1999). In many cases, DIF items in a particular comparison group canceled one another out, with the result that the total PCL-R scores showed scalar equivalence with the reference group. A similar effect was observed by Cooke and colleagues (2001) in their analyses of African American and white offenders. Bolt and colleagues (2004) commented that "the fact that PCL-R generally performs similarly in terms of both expected scores and information for the comparison groups is encouraging. The differences observed with respect to the test characteristic curves do not appear to require the use of different cut scores in identifying individuals with psychopathy" (p. 166).

The same reasoning also applies to the English data. That is, a PCL-R score of 30, typically used for a research diagnosis of psychopathy, appears to have about the same meaning with respect to level of psychopathy in North American male offenders, female offenders, male forensic psychiatric patients, male offenders assessed from file reviews, and English male offenders. Concerning the latter, the conclusions are at odds with those reached by Cooke and Michie (1999), who used IRT analyses to argue that a cut score of 25 in Scottish male offenders reflects the same level of the latent construct of psychopathy as does a score of 30 in North American male offenders. A similar cut score was proposed for English offenders (D. Cooke, personal communication, April 26, 2000). However, the Cooke and Michie sample was relatively small ($N = 246$) and the common latent trait metric was estimated from only three anchor items (4, Pathological lying; 12, Early behavior problems; 20, Criminal versatility), two of which (12 and 20) were antisocial items that Cooke and Michie (2001) later concluded were not part of the construct of psychopathy. This suggests that the common latent trait in their study was more related to antisociality than to psychopathy.

Bolt and colleagues (2004) urged caution in the use of IRT analyses to establish scalar equivalence, for several reasons. First, there are different procedures for the selection of anchor items that comprise the basis for scaling of the latent trait metric. In this regard, Bolt et al. noted that the PCL-R items that function the same across race (Cooke et al., 2001) and across the comparison groups described earlier tended to come from Factor 1, allowing researchers to specify, a priori, the items that should be unbiased. It may be useful, therefore, to consider Factor 1 items as anchors for future analyses (Bolt et al., 2004), or at least as supplementary to whatever other procedure is used to select anchors.

A second reason for caution is that traditional IRT analyses ignore rater effects. "For example, it is conceivable that raters may develop a sophisticated understanding of the contingencies among items and apply those in largely the same way across groups, with less regard for whether those same contingencies should be applied in the same way for all comparison groups" (Bolt et al., 2004, p. 167).

It also is important to realize that IRT analyses are concerned exclusively with the internal performance of items in a scale, and the extent to which they are used in the same way in different groups. The point is illustrated by the PCL-R assessments based entirely on file reviews. Although there was scalar equivalence between this group and the reference group of male offenders, the mean score for the file reviews was considerably lower than that of the reference group. This raises the possibility that the offenders scored from file reviews differed in some important ways from those scored with the standard procedure. It also is possible that there was a more systematic bias in scoring offenders from file reviews, one that is not effectively studied with IRT. These issues indicate that IRT analyses are not by themselves sufficient for interpreting the meaning of equivalent test characteristic curves. External validation is necessary (e.g., cognitive, affective, biological, and behavioral correlates) before we can conclude with confidence that the PCL-R measures an identical construct on the same score metric in different contexts and populations.

STRUCTURE OF PSYCHOPATHY

Fundamentally important to the study of any psychological construct is the clear delineation of its underlying dimensionality. Not only is this necessary for proper interpretation of scores on a measure (e.g., verbal vs. visual intelligence), but the different dimensions of a construct may correlate differentially with critical external variables (Reise, 1999). For instance, Neumann and colleagues (Salekin, Neumann, Leistico, & Zalot, 2004; Vitacco et al., 2005) have recently shown that interpersonal features of psychopathy are positively associated with intelligence whereas impulsive behavioral features are negatively associated with intelligence. Similar findings have been reported between the interpersonal and behavioral–antisocial features of psychopathy, respectively, and serotonin levels (Dolan & Anderson, 2003). Findings of differential relations between the psychopathy factors and various external correlates highlight the multidimensional nature of this construct and the likelihood of multiple causal determinants in its manifestation. Therefore, precise and comprehensive elucidation of its dimensionality is essential.

Given that psychopathy involves disturbances in personality functioning, it is helpful to consider how prominent investigators have conceptualized the dimensions of normative personality (see also Lynam & Derefinko, Chapter 7, this volume). For Allport (1961), personality consisted of "the dynamic organization within the individual of those psychophysical systems that determined his characteristic behavior and thought" (p. 28). While this definition has served well as a starting point for understanding personality, there is considerable debate as to what constitute the essential domains of personality (Heatherton & Nichols,

1994). As noted by Costa and Widiger (2002, p. 5), "Personality traits are often defined as enduring dimensions of individual differences in tendencies to show consistent patterns of thoughts, feelings, and actions." Helson and Stewart (1994) suggested that motives, attitudes, and adaptations are important components of personality viewed from a longitudinal perspective. Zuckerman (1991) proposed that human personality traits are based on inherited variations in certain biological structures, but he also emphasized that personality traits involve purposive direction of behavior including sociability and antisocial tendencies. Trull and Durrett (2005) have also discussed the evidence for a dissocial domain of personality functioning. Cloninger (1998), in line with a long tradition, discussed two major domains of personality: temperament and character. The former involves automatic associative responses to basic emotional stimuli, and the latter involves self-awareness concepts that influence voluntary intentions and attitudes. Finally, Caspi, Roberts, and Shiner (2005) discuss how broad traits such as extraversion may represent the most general dimensions of individual differences, but lower-order traits such as sociability (and, conversely, antisociality) may provide better prediction of behavioral outcomes.

With respect to psychopathy, the broad domains of conscientiousness and constraint may be applicable. Caspi and colleagues (2005) indicate that this personality domain includes at least six lower-order traits including self-control (vs. impulsivity) and responsibility (vs. irresponsibility). Similarly, individuals low on the broad trait of agreeableness may manifest a lower-order personality trait of aggressivity. Taken together, it is reasonable to posit that major dimensions of personality reflect not only traits, but characteristic adaptations to the environment as well. In the case of psychopathic personality, such adaptations are likely to be fundamentally related to undercontrolled or externalizing pathology (Blonigen, Hicks, Krueger, Patrick, & Iacono, 2005; Patrick, Hicks, Krueger, & Lang, 2005), in conjunction with interpersonal, affective, and impulsive traits (Vitacco, Rogers, Neumann, Harrison, & Vincent, in press). Thus, each of these personality domains (traits and adaptations) may be necessary in the conceptualization of psychopathic personality.

This broad view of personality is consistent with recent evidence from evolutionary psychology (Harris & Rice, Chapter 28, this volume) indicating that psychopathy may be conceptualized as a heritable adaptive life strategy in which a central figure is the early emergence of antisocial behavior, including aggressive sexuality. The position that major dimensions of personality reflect trait dispositions and characteristic adaptations to the environment (Zuckerman, 1991) also is consistent with twin studies on the heritability of antisocial behavior (Slutske, 2001) and on the trait and action features of psychopathy (Blonigen et al., 2005; Blonigen, Carlson, Krueger, & Patrick, 2003; Viding, Blair, Moffitt, & Plomin, 2005). Thus, we would argue that PCL-R items reflecting poor behavioral controls and severe, versatile, antisocial tendencies are necessary in the conceptualization and measurement of psychopathy. Furthermore, there is evidence (Blonigen et al., 2005) that impulsive–antisocial components of psychopathology show significant genetic overlap with the externalizing psychopathy domain. These results are consistent with early theoretical and empirical research indicating that impulsive (Berrios, 1996) and antisocial (Robins, 1966) dispositions are important features of psychopathic personality. In terms of recent research, youth studies indicate that poor childhood behavioral controls are significant predictors of subsequent externalizing psychopathology (Caspi, Henry, McGee, Moffitt, & Silva, 1995) and adult psychopathy (Lynam & Gudonis, 2005). Moreover, childhood antisocial tendencies are significant predictors of the longitudinal stability of other psychopathic traits (Frick, Kimonis, Dandreaux, & Farell, 2003; Frick & Marsee, Chapter 18, this volume; Lynam & Derefinko, Chapter 7, this volume; Lynam & Gudonis, 2005).

Rather than eliminating externalizing pathology, such as antisocial tendencies, from the construct of psychopathy, we argue that both basic research on normal personality and studies on psychopathy support the position that characteristic adaptations, reflecting undercontrolled or externalizing antisocial tendencies, are important components of the psychopathy construct.

Taken together, it is reasonable to posit that major dimensions of personality reflect not only trait dispositions but characteristic adaptations to the environment as well. This broad view of personality is helpful for understanding prior and current factor-analytic research aimed at describing the dimensions or facets of the psychopathy construct.

Latent-Variable Analyses of the PCL Instruments

As discussed in detail elsewhere (Neumann, Kosson, & Salekin, in press), both early (e.g., Hare, 1980; Harpur, Hakstian, & Hare, 1988; Raine, 1985) and more recent exploratory factor-analytic research (e.g., Cooke & Michie, 2001; Templeman & Wong, 1994) with adults has revealed that between two to five factors can be extracted from measures of psychopathy. Within each factor solution, the results indicate that critical dimensions of psychopathy involve disturbances in interpersonal and affective traits, as well as behavioral dysregulation and antisocial tendencies. Similar results have been found for adolescent samples (Forth et al., 2003). This pattern of findings is entirely consistent with the broad notion of personality discussed previously in that both specific traits (e.g., interpersonal superficiality) and adaptations to the environment (e.g., criminal versatility) are necessary for a comprehensive representation of the dimensions that underlie psychopathic personality.

While EFA research on the dimensions of psychopathy has been helpful, this EFA-based research also has certain limitations (Neumann et al., in press). In particular, interpretation of this literature is hampered by the indeterminacy of factor solutions and factor structure invariance, and by the fact that skew, kurtosis, and the ordinal nature of the PCL items have not been adequately dealt with. In contrast, confirmatory factor analysis (CFA), which relies on advances in model-based measurement theory (Embretson, 1996; Embretson & Hershberger, 1999), is a powerful statistical method for modeling theoretical constructs and the relations among constructs (Bentler, 1980; Dunn, Everitt, & Pickels, 1993; Hoyle, 1995; MacCallum & Austin, 2000).

A strength of CFA is that this multivariate approach allows investigators to examine whether sets of observed or manifest variables (MVs) are valid indicators of specific hypothetical constructs or latent variables (LVs). A specific LV (e.g., deficient affect) is hypothesized to account for the correlations among a specific set of MVs (e.g., PCL-R items 6, 7, 8, & 16). Thus the essence of CFA involves covariance structure analysis (Dunn et al., 1993). The value of LV CFA models is that they represent the common factor variance in a set of MVs separately from their unique/error variance (Bentler, 1980, 1995). Therefore, these models can be used to evaluate the intercorrelations between factors (e.g., dimensions of psychopathy) in a less biased manner (Hoyle, 1995). Moreover, structural equation modeling programs such as EQS (Bentler, 1995) and Mplus (Muthen & Muthen, 2001) provide methods for handling skew, kurtosis, and categorical or ordinal items. These latter benefits are particularly important given that clinical data are often highly non-normal and based on ordinal rating scales, as is true for the PCL instruments. Failure to account for these issues is likely to result in biased parameter estimates (e.g., factor loadings) and underestimation of model fit (Neumann et al., in press; West, Finch, & Curran, 1995). Finally, an additional advantage of the Mplus statistical routine is that it generates item threshold values when the items are binary or ordinal variables. Threshold parameters provide information on the difficulty or extremity of each item (Reise, 1999). In the case of the PCL instruments, item threshold parameters allow investigators to identify which items tend to be endorsed at high levels of the psychopathy latent trait.

In conducting CFA, investigators must specify *a priori* models with precise variable-to-factor and factor-to-factor relations, which are then tested via strict model fit criteria (Bentler, 1995; Hoyle, 1995). Incremental (or relative) fit indices such as the TLI (also known as the non-normed fit index [NNFI]) and the CFI test how well a hypothesized model fits relative to a null (unstructured) model. Absolute indices such as the standardized root mean square (SRMR) and RMSEA test how well a hypothesized model reproduces the observed covariance matrix (Hu & Bentler, 1995). Incremental indices close to .95 along with SRMR and RMSEA values close to .08 and .06, respectively, suggest excellent model fit (Hu & Bentler, 1999). Finally, it is possible to conduct multiple group CFA to unambiguously determine factor structure invariance by constraining various parameters (e.g., factor loadings and correlations) to be the same across groups and then statistically testing the viability of such constraints (Bentler, 1995).

Latent variable structural equation modeling (SEM) has become "social and behavior science's most successful methodology" for testing psychological theories with nonexperimental data (Barnes, Murray, Patton, Bentler, & Anderson, 2000, p. 102). For instance, clinical researchers have been able to use LV CFA, which is a special case of SEM, to further our conceptualization of major mental disorders. In three separate population-based studies (Krueger, 1999; Krueger, Caspi, Moffitt, & Silva, 1998; Vollebergh et al., 2001), investigators have advanced our understanding of the underlying structure of common mental disorders using the SEM approach. Critical in each of these studies to achieving good model fit was employment of methods to adequately handle the dichotomous nature of DSM disorder variables. Most important, these studies show that broad continuous latent variable dimensions (internalizing and externalizing disorders) can be used to explain the prominent comorbidity among individuals with mental disorders despite the claim that the DSM is a categorical system. Thus, it is reasonable to propose that psychopathy can be understood in terms of continuous latent variable dimensions as well, rather than as a discrete disease or disorder category.

A Four-Factor Model of Psychopathy

Consonant with the EFA research on psychopathy cited previously, Hare (2003) recently proposed that four latent variable dimensions are needed to represent the construct of psychopathy: an Interpersonal factor (PCL-R/YV items, 1, 2, 4, 5; PCL:SV items, 1, 2, 3), an Affective factor (PCL-R/YV items, 6, 7, 8, 16; PCL:SV items, 3, 4, 6), a behavioral Lifestyle factor (PCL-R/YV items, 3, 9, 13, 14, 15; PCL:SV items, 7, 9, 10), and an Antisocial factor (PCL-R/YV items, 10, 12, 18, 19, 20; PCL:SV items, 8, 11, 12). Recent CFA studies have revealed good support for a four-factor model for the PCL-R (Neumann et al., in press; Vitacco et al., in press), the PCL:SV (Hill et al., 2004; Vitacco et al., 2005), and the PCL:YV (Forth

et al., 2003; Kosson, Neumann, Forth, & Hare, 2004; Salekin, Neumann, Leistico, DiCicco, & Duros, 2004). Interestingly, these CFA studies are consistent with recent large-sample taxometric analyses of the PCL-R which suggest that all four factors reflect continuous latent variable dimensions of psychopathy (Guay, Ruscio, Knight, & Hare, 2004). Similarly, a recent large-sample multidimensional scaling (MDS) analysis indicated that the PCL-R could be described by two broad dimensions and by four more specific dimensions, all in accordance with the CFAs of the PCL-R (Bishopp & Hare, 2004).

New Evidence for the Four-Factor Model of Psychopathy

For the current chapter we present new findings in support of the four-factor model of psychopathy using large samples of individuals who were assessed with either the PCL-R, PCL:YV, or the PCL:SV. All CFA analyses were conducted with Mplus (Muthen & Muthen, 2001) unless stated otherwise, items were treated as ordinal variables, and a robust weighted least-squares parameter estimation procedure was used. We believe that these methodological approaches are appropriate to use when conducting CFA on the PCL instruments (cf. Neumann et al., in press). The samples for the analyses presented here, all from North America, included 5,964 adult offenders (17% female) assessed with the PCL-R (Hare, 2003), 1,631 adolescents (11% female) assessed with the PCL:YV (Forth et al., 2003), and 514 participants (61% female) from a community sample assessed with the PCL:SV as part of the MacArthur Risk Assessment Study (Monahan & Steadman, 1994). Only cases with complete data for all PCL items were used for these analyses. The purpose of these analyses was to evaluate the generalizability of the four-factor model across distinctive samples, consisting of adults, adolescents, and general community participants.

Males and females were combined within each of the separate samples (adult, adolescent, community) to facilitate comparison of the four-factor model across samples. Before collapsing gender subsamples, we first tested whether each subsample had equivalent covariance matrices by constraining the variances/covariances to be equal across gender groups, and then examining model fit indices to assess how well the constrained model could reproduce the observed covariance matrices for male and female subsamples (cf. Dunn et al., 1993). The covariance equivalence analyses revealed that the males and females had very similar covariance matrices for both the adult offender (TLI = .96, RMSEA = .01) and adolescents (TLI = .95, RMSEA = .03) samples. The covariance equivalence model was also able to reproduce the observed covariance matrices for the males and females in the community sample with adequate precision (RMSEA = .08). This provided a foundation for combining males and females within each participant sample in the four-factor model analyses.

First, we tested fit of the four-factor model separately for the adult offender and adolescent samples. Fit was good for both the adult (TLI = .94, RMSEA = .07, SRMR = .05) and adolescent (TLI = .97, RMSEA = .07, SRMR = .05) samples. Figures 4.2 and 4.3 display the standardized parameter estimates for these two samples, in which the PCL-R and PCL:YV, respectively, were used. Viewed "side by side" the four-factor model parame-

ters for adult and adolescent samples look very similar, except for some slight, and perhaps theoretically meaningful, differences.

To facilitate comparison of parameter profiles across the adult offender and adolescent samples, Figure 4.4 depicts PCL-R and PCL:YV item (b_2) threshold parameters (Panel A), and item factor loadings (Panel B) for each sample. In Figure 4.4, items are ordered by their factor designation. As in IRT, the factor loadings reflect how well an item can discriminate individuals on the latent psychopathy trait. In contrast, larger threshold values signify items that are likely to be assigned higher ratings for individuals who score higher on the latent trait (Reise, 1999). Note that only b_2 threshold parameters are provided here.

Generally, the overlap in profiles for factor loadings and item thresholds suggests that the PCL-R and PCL:YV items work similarly when used for discriminating and precisely rating both adults and adolescents with psychopathic features. In particular, the Affective factor on average yielded the largest factor loadings, and the Interpersonal factor on average yielded the largest threshold values for both samples. Notably, there were items

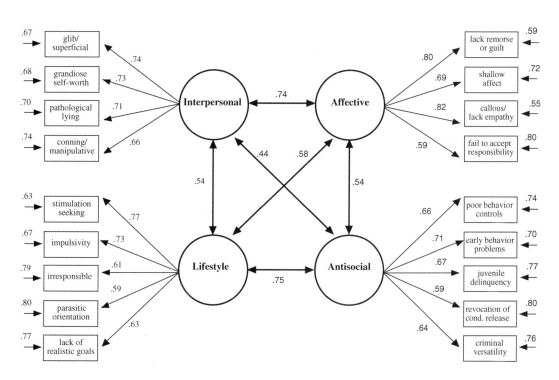

FIGURE 4.2. PCL-R four-factor model of psychopathy.

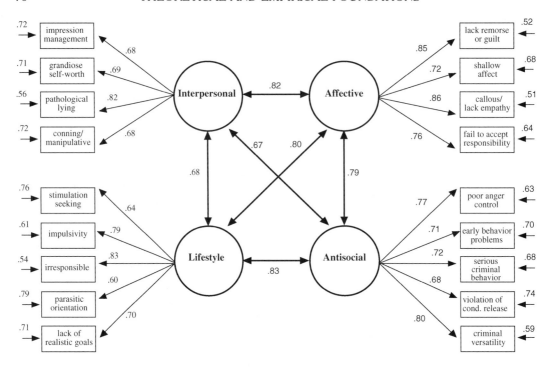

FIGURE 4.3. PCL:YV Four-factor model of psychopathy.

from the Interpersonal (2, 4), Affective (7), Lifestyle (9, 13), and Antisocial (12) factors that displayed good discrimination and threshold parameters across both samples. Nonetheless, we believe that the PCL–R and PCL:YV are good measures of psychopathy because *all items* contribute to the estimate of the latent psychopathy trait; however, different items function efficiently at different levels of the trait.

There are also some interesting differences in the parameter profiles between the adult offender and adolescent samples. One of the most interesting comparative features in the figures and graphs for the four-factor model is that the antisocial items tend to have larger factor loadings and in some cases higher threshold values for the adolescents, compared to the adults. Indeed, the mean factor loading for the Antisocial factor is .74 for adolescents and .65 for adults. Also notable is the fact that items 19 and 20 have larger threshold values for the adolescents, whereas items 12 and 18 have higher threshold values for the adults. Thus, prominent antisocial acts tend to be endorsed (or rated) at high levels of psychopathy in adolescents, but early behavior problems and juvenile antiso-

cial behavior are endorsed at high levels of psychopathy in adults. Finally, the factor correlations between the Antisocial factor and the other psychopathy factors are stronger for the adolescents. Collectively, the findings suggest that antisocial behavior is a slightly more prominent feature of psychopathy in adolescence than in adulthood. However, *early* manifestations of externalizing and antisocial behavior represent critical indicators of psychopathy in adults.

Clearly, one reason for the difference in the salience of antisocial behavior between the adults and the adolescents is that the former sample consisted entirely of incarcerated offenders, whereas less than half of the adolescents were offenders (see Forth et al., 2003). However, another reason may relate to the significance of antisocial behavior (e.g., criminal versatility) in a younger sample. As suggested by other authors (Harris & Rice, Chapter 28, this volume; Quinsey et al., 1998; Robins, 1966, 1978), the early emergence of antisocial behavior is prominent in the development of psychopathic personality. Consistent with this second interpretation, the PCL-R antisocial items reflecting early behavior problems (#12) and

Panel A

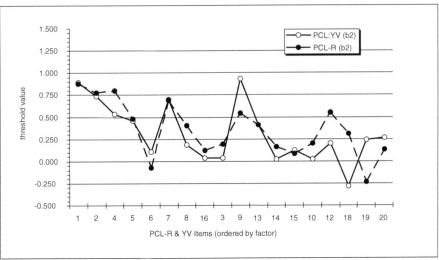

Panel B

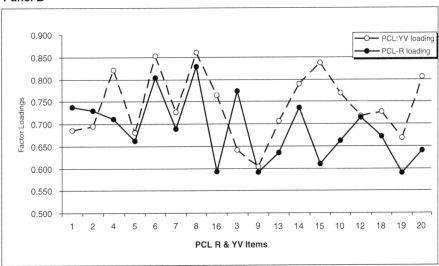

FIGURE 4.4. PCL-R and PCL:YV item threshold (b_2) parameters (Panel A) and factor loadings (Panel B).

juvenile delinquency (#18) had the largest factor loadings and threshold parameters among the antisocial items in the adult offenders.

As discussed previously, Lee Robins (1966, 1978) suggested some time ago that antisocial behavior was likely to be a more discriminating psychopathic trait in the general population than in prison populations. To test this proposal, we evaluated the four-factor model in the large sample of community participants from the MacArthur Risk Assessment study, which was administered the PCL:SV. Fit statistics for the model were excellent (TLI = .98, RMSEA = .04, SRMR = .05), indicating that the four-factor model can easily be extended to a general population sample. Figure 4.5 displays the standardized parameter estimates for the four-factor PCL:SV model. Clearly, the items on

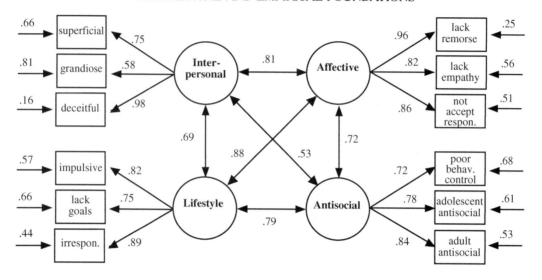

FIGURE 4.5. PCL:SV four-factor model of psychopathy: MacArthur community sample.

the Antisocial factor have substantial factor loadings, highlighting the critical nature of antisocial behavior as indicators of the psychopathy construct. Also, consistent with the previously presented results, as well as other research with forensic and clinical populations, the Affective factor has on average the strongest set of factor loadings, signifying the importance of shallow, callous affect in psychopathic personality.

Finally, we compared results for the MacArthur community sample to those for a large forensic/psychiatric sample. Figure 4.6 displays the item (b_2) threshold values for the current MacArthur data alongside those reported by Cooke and colleagues (1999) from an IRT analysis of the PCL:SV standardization data. The community sam-

ple participants have much higher threshold values, as would be expected, suggesting that higher overall levels of psychopathy need to be present in individuals from the general population before receiving a rating of 2 on any particular PCL:SV item. Also, consistent with previous research, the items for the Interpersonal and Affective factors tend to have the highest threshold values. However, it is also apparent that antisocial items reflecting poor behavioral controls and adolescent antisocial behavior have relatively high threshold values. Taken together, the modeling results for the adult offender, adolescent, and adult community samples provide solid evidence for the inclusion of antisocial behavior in the assessment of psychopathy.

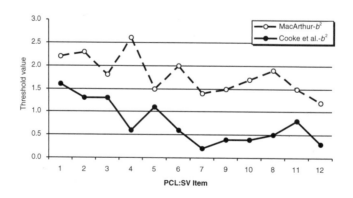

FIGURE 4.6. PCL:SV item threshold (b_2) parameters.

Criterion-Related Validity Evidence
for the Four-Factor Model of Psychopathy

In addition to its substantive and structural validity, evidence for the criterion-related validity of the four-factor model has recently been reported. Two studies by Neumann and colleagues that used the PCL:SV found that the four-factor model, compared to the three-factor model, accounted for greater variance in maximum security patients' aggression at 6-month follow up (Hill et. al., 2004) and in psychiatric patients' community violence at 10-week follow-up (Vitacco et al., 2005). Each of these studies found that, in addition to the antisocial factor, other psychopathy factors were also significant predictors. In another study that dealt with adolescent offenders, Salekin and colleagues (2004) found that a higher-order four-factor model was the only significant predictor of violent offenses, above and beyond a disruptive behavior factor and an Axis I symptoms factor. Thus, current findings suggest that the four-factor model has good external validity and, in the two PCL:SV studies, displays incremental validity over the three-factor model in predicting important external correlates of psychopathy.

Alternative Form
of the Four-Factor Model: Dealing
with Small-*N* and Non-Normal Data

The aforementioned results for the four-factor model have the benefit of being grounded in strong statistical methodology (large sample sizes, reduced skew/kurtosis, and appropriate treatment of ordinal data). However, most clinical and forensic studies do not have the good fortune of large samples ($N \geq 250$) and normally distributed data. Nonetheless, as sample size goes down, so does the veracity of the parameter estimates, particularly with non-normal data (West et al., 1995). Thus, Bentler (1995) suggests that the ratio of subjects-to-free parameters may go as low as 5:1 with normally distributed data but believes that a 10:1 ratio would be better in other circumstances. This recommendation means that evaluation of an 18-item four-factor model with 42 free parameters should have a sample size between 210 and 420.

Given the ordinal (and usually non-normal) nature of the items on the PCL instruments, as well as sample size concerns, an appropriate strategy is to reexpress the items of the PCL-R to form item composites or "parcels" (cf. West et al., 1995). This approach involves summing or taking the mean of different items indexing the same facet (or subdimension) of a construct to obtain variables that more closely approximate a normal distribution than the original items (Bagozzi & Heatherton, 1994; Little, Cunningham, Shahar, & Widaman, 2002). The use of item-based parcels rather than all single items as indicators for LVs has been established in applications of structural equation modeling (Greenbaum & Dedrick, 1998; Little et al., 2002; Marsh, 1994).

The use of parcels, versus single items, as indicators of LVs in a structural model is advantageous because parcels are more reliable and valid indicators of LVs, have higher communalities, provide more efficient (low variability) parameter estimates, and reduce the number of parameters that have to be estimated, thus improving the subjects: free-parameters ratio for samples of a given size (Bagozzi & Heatherton, 1994; Little et al., 2002; West et al., 1995).

Note that parcels (i.e., sums or means of item groupings) are quite different from testlets (i.e., items set to load on particular first-order factors), even though each may have similar purposes (e.g., controlling for systematic specific or error variance). The most obvious difference is that parceling items results in a different covariance matrix to be modeled, compared to the same item set that is not parceled. For example, suppose someone wanted to test a two-factor model based on a measure that has 20 items. To create a two-factor parcel model, one could take pairs of items from the 20 items to form 10 parcels and then load 5 parcels onto one (first-order) common factor and the remaining 5 parcels set to load onto the second (first-order) common factor. This 10-"item" parcel model has 55 data points to be modeled (i.e., variances/covariances = $10 \times 11/2 = 55$), is estimating 21 free parameters (10 factor loadings, 10 error variances, and 1 factor correlation), and, thus, has 34 degrees of freedom. Conversely, a 20-item testlet model could be created which uses 10 testlets (with two items each serving as indicators for one of the respective testlets—i.e., first-order factors) and then have 5 testlets loading onto one (second-order) common factor, and the remaining 5 testlets set to load onto the second (second-order) common factor. This 20-item testlet model has 210 data points to be modeled ($20 \times 21/2$), is estimating 41 free parameters (10 first-order factor loadings [given that one loading/testlet must be set to unity], 20 error variances, 10 second-order factor loadings and 1 second-order factor correlation), and thus, has 169 degrees of freedom. Conceptually, each model may be similar, but statistically they are completely different.

The Four-Factor Parcel Model

In related research, we have reported good fit for the four-factor parcel model using incarcerated males from two studies of adolescent offenders (Forth et al., 2003; Kosson et al., 2004), as well as adult male offenders from another study cited earlier (Neumann et al., in press). Here, we present results for the four-factor parcel model using the large sample of male and female adult offenders ($N = 5964$) described earlier in the section entitled "New Evidence for the Four-Factor Model of Psychopathy." Eight parcels were created from the 18 PCL-R items of the four-factor model by computing the mean of the following item pairs or item triplets: (a) 1 and 2, (b) 4 and 5, (c) 7 and 8, (d) 6 and 16, (e) 3, 14, and 15, (f) 9 and 13, (g) 10 and 12, and, finally, (h) 18, 19, and 20. The foregoing item groupings are based primarily on IRT analyses of the PCL-R discussed by Cooke and Michie (2001) which identified local dependence (or specific variance) shared by certain item pairs or triplets, and secondarily on each item's conceptual relatedness to other items. Each item correlated on average .82 with its respective parcel. Two parcels were designated as indicators for each of the four factors in the model: Interpersonal (parcels a, b), Affective (c, d), Lifestyle (e, f), or Antisocial (g, h). The model is depicted in Figure 4.7. As recommended by Little and colleagues (2002), the loadings for each parcel associated with a given factor were constrained to be equal to avoid underidentification of each factor within the model. Because the parcels are continuous variables, robust maximum likelihood parameter estimation was used via EQS. The results indicated good fit for the four-factor parcel model (robust CFI = .95, RMSEA = .07, SRMR = .04). Figure 4.7 shows the standardized parameter estimates for this model, which are generally similar to those for the item-based four-factor model.

Finally, measures vary in terms of unwanted sources of systematic error variance (e.g., rating bias, and social desirability), which can result in a misspecified model (e.g., spurious factors). Parcels have been shown to cancel out random and systematic error variance by aggregating across such errors (Little et al., 2002) and thus may aid in dealing with such nuisance variance at the item level for PCL ratings of males versus females. Although good fit for the four-factor PCL-R item-based model discussed above with the females and males combined provides some support for similar factor structures across gender, this result is not a definitive test of factor structure invariance. Therefore, we used the four-factor PCL-R parcel model to provide such a test. In this multiple group CFA, the two samples consisted of the male and female adult offenders. The factor loadings and factor correlations were constrained to be equal across the two groups. The results indicated good fit (CFI = .95, RMSEA = .04, SRMR = .05), demonstrating that there is invariance of factor structure across the male and female offenders, at least at the level of parcels.

Implications of the Structural Equation Modeling Results

The four-factor model provides a statistically viable model for representing the dimensions of PCL-R psychopathy, with distinct advantages. In contrast to the three-factor model, it incorporates most of the items of the PCL-R (i.e., 18 of 20), and it allows one to test whether the Interpersonal, Affective, or Lifestyle factors exhibit incremental validity, above and beyond the Antisocial factor, in predicting important external criteria. The four-factor parcel model may be particularly useful in such research, because it has a good subject: parameter ratio. That is, the eight-"item" parcel model estimates 22 free parameters (eight factor loadings, eight error variances, and six factor correlations), which

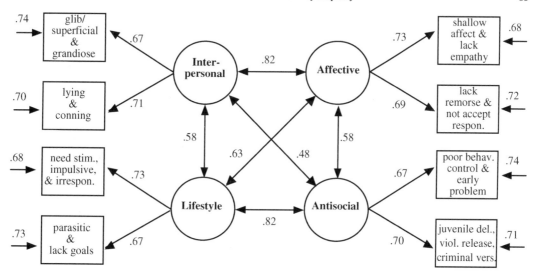

FIGURE 4.7. PCL-R four-factor parcel model.

(assuming normally distributed parcels) could be efficiently estimated with a sample size of 110. Thus, the four-factor parcel might be helpful when additional factors (e.g., symptoms of psychopathology and parental style) are included for testing more complex models without having to substantially increase sample size. Another valuable direction for future research with the four-factor model will be to investigate whether certain facets of psychopathy may serve as developmental antecedents to others. For example, Cooke and colleagues (2004) speculate on the basis of structural analyses of the PCL-R items that antisocial behavior and relationship instability represent *consequences* of more basic Interpersonal, Affective, and Lifestyle facets of psychopathy. However, structural equation modeling of cross-sectional data *cannot* be used to infer causality; longitudinal investigations are required to do this, and we look forward to studies of this kind (see Neumann, Vitacco, & Hare, 2005, for a detailed critique of Cooke et al., 2004). Another important direction for future research lies in behavioral and molecular genetic bases of psychopathy and its facets (see Waldman & Rhee, Chapter 11; and MacDonald & Iacono, Chapter 19, this volume). For example, recent twin studies of children (Viding et al., 2005), adolescents (Larrson, Andershed, & Lichtentein, in press), and adults (Blonigen et al., 2003,

2005) clearly indicate that both the interpersonal–affective and the lifestyle–antisocial features of psychopathy have significant heritabilities. Research along these lines will be facilitated by the recent evidence for the dimensionality of psychopathy and its factors (Guay & Knight, 2003; Guay, Ruscio, Knight, & Hare, 2005; Marcus, John, & Edens, 2004), and by the view that psychopathy can be described and understood from the perspective of general personality theory. Concerning the latter, Lynam (2002) and Widiger and Lynam (1998) have mapped out in detail the association between each of the PCL-R items and the domains and facets of the five-factor model of personality (FFM; Costa & McCrae, 1992). They view psychopathic personality as a maladaptive variant of common personality traits (many of which are antisocial in nature). This view of psychopathy is consistent with a recent study in which multidimensional scaling (MDS) was used to unfold the dimensions that underlie the PCL-R (Bishopp & Hare, 2005). Viding and colleagues (in press) reported that the callous–unemotional traits associated with psychopathy have high heritability, particularly when associated with antisocial behaviors. Similarly, a twin study of adults by Blonigen and colleagues (2003) found that the personality traits associated with psychopathy were under "significant genetic influence" (p. 179).

Finally, there is a host of other latent variable approaches (e.g., multilevel, growth, MIMIC, and mixture models) that can be used to address other issues in the psychopathy area, such as treatment outcome, change in psychopathic traits over time, the effects of background variables on the expression of psychopathy, and alternative manifestations (subtypes) of psychopathy.

CONCLUSIONS

Early theorists such as Pinel (1801) and Pritchard (1835) employed the terms "manie sans delire" and "moral insanity" to describe individuals with no apparent psychopathology who eschewed basic social norms and engaged repeatedly in antisocial behavior. Cleckley (1941), based on his practice with mainly noncriminal psychiatric patients, developed a list of traits describing the psychopathic personality, which included both personality characteristics (e.g., poverty in affective relationships and incapacity for love), and behavioral criteria (e.g., inadequately motivated antisocial behavior) as fundamental indicators for the psychopathy construct. The aforementioned structural equation modeling results provide good empirical support for the clinical insights of these early investigators.

Collectively, there is a clear theme that runs through the modeling results that may aid in understanding of the psychopathy construct: the juxtaposition of affective interpersonal traits with *antisocial behavior*. Most human behavior is typified by genuine interpersonal relationships, authentic emotional expressions, controlled and responsible lifestyles, and, of course, law-abiding behavior. With respect to the current results, our conclusion is that the construct of psychopathy reflects the covariation of the four psychopathy factors, and not simply one of the factors in isolation, or in superordinate relation to the others. For example, conning and manipulative interpersonal behavior displayed by a gambler during a poker game would not constitute psychopathy. Similarly, a surgeon operating in a cold and unempathic manner would not signify psychopathy. Instead, deceitful interpersonal behavior, deficient affect, and behavioral dysregulation in the context of violating critical social contracts, be they moral or legal, represent the manifestation of psychopathy proper. Thus, the antisocial items are critical for understanding psychopathy.

As such, we do not agree with suggestions that antisocial behavior is a nuisance variable or that psychiatric diagnosis will be hampered by including it in the construct (Cooke et al., 2004). Rather, we believe that antisociality is a characteristic feature that helps to differentiate psychopathy from other psychiatric syndromes. For example, individuals with histrionic personality disorder are flamboyant, insincere, and shallow (Serin & Marshall, 2003). Individuals with schizoid personality disorders have persistently shallow affect, and persons with attention-deficit/hyperactivity disorder or substance abuse display behavioral dysregulation. However, none of these mental disorders runs the risk of being confused with psychopathy because none has antisociality as a characteristic feature. Furthermore, consonant with DSM-IV field trial results for APD (Widiger et al., 1996), the analyses reported in this chapter indicate that antisocial tendencies are especially important indicators of psychopathy in nonincarcerated, community samples.

In line with recent calls for a dimensional perspective in understanding mental disorders (cf. Widiger & Coker, 2003), and with population-based modeling studies that highlight the importance of antisocial behavior in our conceptualization of such disorders, we propose that four dimensions can be used for understanding the construct of psychopathy (cf. Bishopp & Hare, 2004). Research aimed at elucidating the unique aspects and covariation of these four dimensions of psychopathy will be helpful and consistent with a venerable clinical tradition that has defined psychopathy in terms of interpersonal, affective, and impulsive–irresponsible traits combined with socially deviant behaviors.

NOTES

1. Recent exploratory and confirmatory factor analyses support the viability of the original two-factor model for the PCL-R, with the addition of *Criminal Versatility* to Factor 2

(Hare, 2003). The pattern of correlations among the four factors described in this chapter also implies the presence of two broad factors, suggesting a hierarchical model of psychopathy that consists of two broad and four narrow factors. This 2×4 model, described by Hare (2003), refers to the four narrow factors as *facets*. The model allows users of the PCL-R to determine the level of descriptive analysis to be used. For convenience and consistency we retain the term *factor* for the dimensions described in this chapter.

2. Cooke, Michie, and Hart would not provide us with a copy of their chapter for this volume before its publication. However, we assume the content of their chapter is consistent with their prior published work.

REFERENCES

Allport, G. W. (1961). *Pattern and growth in personality*. New York: Holt, Rinehart & Winston.

American Educational Research Association, American Psychological Association, & National Council on Measurement in Education. (1999). *Standards for educational and psychological testing*. Washington, DC: American Educational Research Association.

American Psychiatric Association. (1980). *Diagnostic and statistical manual of mental disorders* (3rd ed.). Washington, DC: Author.

American Psychiatric Association. (1994). *Diagnostic and statistical manual of mental disorders* (4th ed.). Washington, DC: Author.

Ankenmann, R. D., Witt, E. A., & Dunbar, S. B. (1999). An investigation of the power of the likelihood ratio goodness-of-fit statistic in detecting differential item functioning. *Journal of Educational Measurement, 36*, 277–300.

Bagozzi, R. P., & Heatherton, T. F. (1994). A general approach to representing multifaceted personality constructs: Application to state self-esteem. *Structural Equation Modeling, 1*, 35–67.

Barnes, G. E., Murray, R. P., Patton, D., Bentler, P. M., & Anderson, R. E. (2000). *The addiction prone personality: Longitudinal research in the social sciences*. New York: Plenum Press.

Bentler, P. M. (1980). Multivariate analysis with latent variables: Causal modeling. *Annual Review of Psychology, 31*, 419–456.

Bentler, P. M. (1995). *EQS structural equations program manual*. CA: Multivariate Software.

Berrios, G. E. (1996). *The history of mental symptoms: Descriptive psychopathology since the nineteenth century*. Cambridge, UK: Cambridge University Press.

Bishopp, D., & Hare, R. D. (2005). *A multidimensional scaling analysis of the PCL-R*. Manuscript under review.

Blackburn, R. (1998). Psychopathy and personality disorder: Implications of interpersonal theory. In D. J. Cooke, A. E. Forth, & R. D. Hare (Eds.), *Psychopathy: Theory, research, and Implications for society* (pp. 269–301). Dordrecht, The Netherlands: Kluwer.

Blonigen, D. M., Carlson, S. R., Kreuger, R. F., & Patrick, C. J. (2003). A twin study of self-reported psychopathic personality traits. *Personality and Individual Differences, 35*, 179–197.

Blonigen, D. M., Hicks, B. M., Krueger, R. F., Patrick, C. J., & Iacono, W. (2005). Psychopathic personality traits: Heritability and genetic overlap with internalizing and externalizing psychopathology. *Psychological Medicine, 35*, 1–12.

Bolt, D., & Hare R. D. (2004). *An IRT analysis of the Hare PCL-R in an English prison population*. Manuscript in preparation.

Bolt, D., Hare, R. D., Vitale, J., & Newman, J. P. (2004). A multigroup item response theory analysis of the Hare Psychopathy Checklist—Revised. *Psychological Assessment, 16*, 155–168

Buss, A. H. (1966). *Psychopathology*. New York: Wiley.

Caspi, A., Henry, B., McGee, R. O., Moffitt, T. E., & Silva, P. A. (1995). Temperamental origins of child and adolescent behavior problems: From age 3 to age 15. *Child Development, 66*, 55–68.

Caspi, A., Roberts, B. W., & Shiner, R. L. (2005). Personality development: Stability and change. *Annual Review of Psychology, 56*, 453–484.

Cleckley, H. (1941). *The mask of sanity*. St. Louis, MO: Mosby.

Cleckley, H. (1976). *The mask of sanity* (5th ed.). St. Louis, MO: Mosby.

Cliff, N. (1983). Some cautions concerning the application of causal modeling. *Multivariate Behavioral Research, 18*, 115–126.

Cloninger, R. C. (1998). The genetics and psychobiology of the seven-factor model of personality. In K. R. Silk (Ed.), *Biology of personality disorders* (pp. 63–92). Washington, DC: American Psychiatric Press.

Coid, J. (1993). Current concepts and classifications of psychopathic disorder. In P. Tyrer & G. Stein (Eds.), *Personality disorder reviewed* (pp. 113–164). London: Royal College of Psychiatrists, Gaskell Press.

Cooke, D. J., Forth, A. E., & Hare, R. D. (Eds.). (1998). *Psychopathy: Theory, research, and implications for society*. Dordrecht, The Netherlands: Kluwer.

Cooke, D. J., Kosson, D. S., & Michie, C. (2001). Psychopathy and ethnicity: Structural, item and test generalizability of the Psychopathy Checklist—Revised (PCL-R) in Caucasian and African-American participants. *Psychological Assessment, 13*, 531–542.

Cooke, D. J., & Michie, C. (1997). An item response theory analysis of the Hare Psychopathy Checklist—Revised. *Psychological Assessment, 9*, 3–14.

Cooke, D. J., & Michie, C. (1999). Psychopathy across cultures: North America and Scotland compared. *Journal of Abnormal Psychology, 108*, 58–68.

Cooke, D. J., & Michie, C. (2001). Refining the construct of psychopathy: Towards a hierarchical model. *Psychological Assessment, 13,* 171–188.

Cooke, D. J., Michie, C., Hart, S. D., & Clark, D. A. (2004). Reconstructing psychopathy: Clarifying the significance of antisocial behavior in the diagnosis of psychopathic personality disorder. *Journal of Personality Disorders, 18,* 337–356.

Cooke, D. J., Michie, C., Hart, S. D., & Hare, R. D. (1999). The functioning of the Clinical Version of the Psychopathy Checklist: An item response theory analysis. *Psychological Assessment, 11,* 3–13.

Costa, P. T., & McCrae, R. R. (1992). The five-factor model of personality and its relevance to personality disorders. *Journal of Personality Disorders, 6,* 343–359.

Costa, P. T., & Widiger, T. A. (2002). *Personality disorder and the five-factor model of personality* (2nd ed.). Washington, DC: American Psychological Association.

Craft, M. J. (1965). *Ten studies into psychopathic personality.* Bristol, UK: John Wright.

Dolan M. C., & Anderson, I. M. (2003). The relationship between serotonergic function and the Psychopathy Checklist: Screening Version. *Journal of psychopharmacology, 17,* 216–222.

Doren, D. M. (1987). *Understanding and treating the psychopath.* New York: Wiley.

Dunn, G., Everitt, B., & Pickels, A. (1993). *Modeling covariance structures using EQS.* New York: Chapman & Hall.

Edens, J. F. (2001). Misuses of the Hare Psychopathy Checklist—Revised in court: Two case examples. *Journal of Interpersonal Violence, 16,* 1082–1094.

Embretson, S. E. (1996). The new rules of measurement. *Psychological Assessment, 8,* 341–349.

Embretson, S. E., & Hershberger, S. L. (1999). *The new rules of measurement: What every psychologist and educator should know.* Mahwah, NJ: Erlbaum.

Flowers, C. P., Oshima, T. C., & Raju, N. S. (1999). A description and demonstration of the polytomous–DFIT framework. *Applied Psychological Measurement, 23,* 309–326.

Forth, A. E., Kosson, D. S., & Hare, R. D. (2003). *The Psychopathy Checklist: Youth Version manual.* Toronto, ON, Canada: Multi-Health Systems.

Frick, P. J., Kimonis, E. R., Dandreaux, D. M., & Farrell, J. M. (2003). The 4 years of stability of psychopathic traits in non-referred youth. *Behavioral Sciences and the Law, 21,* 1–24.

Gacono, C. B. (Ed.). (2000). *The clinical and forensic assessment of psychopathy: A practitioner's guide.* Mahwah, NJ: Erlbaum.

Greenbaum, P. E., & Dedrick, R. F. (1998). Hierarchical confirmatory factor analysis of the Child Behavior Checklist/4-18. *Psychological Assessment, 10,* 149–155.

Guay, J. P., & Knight, R. A. (2003, July). *Assessing the underlying structure of psychopathy factors using taxometrics.* Poster session presented at the Developmental and Neuroscience Perspectives on Psychopathy conference, Madison, WI.

Guay, J. P., Ruscio, J. Knight, R. A., & Hare, R. D. (2005). *A taxometric analysis of the latent structure of psychopathy: Evidence for dimensionality.* Manuscript submitted for publication.

Hare, R. D. (1980). A research scale for the assessment of psychopathy in criminal populations. *Personality and Individual Differences, 1,* 111–119.

Hare, R. D. (1985a). Comparison of the procedures for the assessment of psychopathy. *Journal of Consulting and Clinical Psychology, 53,* 7–16.

Hare, R. D. (1985b). *The Psychopathy Checklist.* Unpublished manuscript, University of British Columbia, Vancouver, BC, Canada.

Hare, R. D. (1991). *The Hare Psychopathy Checklist— Revised.* Toronto, ON, Canada: Multi-Health Systems.

Hare, R. D. (1996). Psychopathy and antisocial personality disorder: A case of diagnostic confusion. *Psychiatric Times, 13,* 39–40.

Hare, R. D. (1998). Psychopaths and their nature: Implications for the mental health and criminal justice systems. In T. Millon, E. Simonson, M. Burket-Smith, & R. Davis (Eds.), *Psychopathy: Antisocial, criminal, and violent behavior* (pp. 188–212). New York: Guilford Press.

Hare, R. D. (2003). *The Hare Psychopathy Checklist— Revised, 2nd edition.* Toronto, ON, Canada: Multi-Health Systems.

Hare, R. D., & Cox, D. N. (1978). Clinical and empirical conceptions of psychopathy, and the selection of subjects for research. In R. D. Hare & D. Schalling (Eds.), *Psychopathic behavior: Approaches to research* (pp. 1–21). Chichester, UK: Wiley.

Hare, R. D., & Frazelle, J. (1980). *Some preliminary notes on the use of a research scale for the assessment of psychopathy in criminal populations.* Unpublished manuscript, University of British Columbia, Vancouver, BC, Canada.

Hare, R. D., & Hart, S. D. (1995). Commentary on antisocial personality disorder: The DSM-IV field trial. In W. J. Livesley (Ed.), *The DSM-IV personality disorders* (pp. 127–134). New York: Guilford Press.

Hare, R. D., & Schalling, D. (Eds.). (1978). *Psychopathic behaviour: Approaches to research.* Chichester, UK: Wiley.

Harpending, H. C., & Sobus, J. (1987). Sociopathy as an adaptation. *Ethology and Sociobiology, 3,* 63S–72S.

Harpur, T. J., Hakstian, A. R., & Hare, R. D. (1988). Factor structure of the Psychopathy Checklist. *Journal of Consulting and Clinical Psychology, 56,* 741–747.

Harris, G. T., Rice, M. E., & Lalumière, M. (2001). Criminal violence: The roles of psychopathy, neurodevelopmental insults and antisocial parenting. *Criminal Justice and Behavior, 28,* 402–426.

Hart, S., Cox, D., & Hare, R. D. (1995). *Manual for the Psychopathy Checklist: Screening Version (PCL:SV).* Toronto, ON, Canada: Multi-Health Systems.

Heatherton, T. F., & Nichols, P. A. (1994). Conceptual issues in assessing whether personality can change. In T. F. Heatherton & J. L. Weinberger (Eds.), *Can personality change?* (pp. 3–18). Washington, DC: American Psychological Association.

Helson, R., & Stewart, A. (1994). Personality change in adulthood. In T. F. Heatherton & J. L. Weinberger (Eds.), *Can personality change?* (pp. 201–226). Washington, DC: American Psychological Association.

Hill, C., Neumann, C. S., & Rogers, R. (2004). Confirmatory Factor Analysis of the Psychopathy Checklist: Screening Version (PCL:SV) in Offenders with Axis I Disorders. *Psychological Assessment, 16*, 90–95.

Hoyle, R. H. (1995). *Structural equation modeling: Concepts, issues and applications.* Thousand Oaks: Sage.

Hu, L., & Bentler, P. M. (1995). Evaluating model fit. In R. H. Hoyle (Ed.), *Structural equation modeling: Issues, concepts, and applications* (pp. 76–99). Newbury Park, CA: Sage.

Hu, L., & Bentler, P. M. (1999). Cut-score criteria for fit indexes in covariance structure analysis: Conventional criteria versus new alternatives. *Structural Equation Modeling, 6*, 1–55.

Karpman, B. (1961). The structure of neurosis: With special differentials between neurosis, psychosis, homosexuality, alcoholism, psychopathy, and criminality. *Archives of Criminal Psychodynamics, 4*, 599–646.

Kernberg, O. T. (1984). *Severe personality disorders: Psychotherapeutic strategies.* New Haven, CT: Yale University Press.

Knowles, E. S., & Condon, C. A. (2000). Does the rose still smell as sweet? Item variability across test forms and revisions. *Psychological Assessment, 12*, 245–252.

Kosson, D., Neumann, C. S., Forth, A., & Hare, R. (2004). *Factor structure of the Hare Psychopathy Checklist: Youth Version in incarcerated adolescents.* Manuscript submitted for publication.

Krueger, R. F. (1999). The structure of common mental disorders. *Archives of General Psychiatry, 56*, 921–926.

Krueger, R. F., Caspi, A., Moffitt, T. E., & Silva, P.A. (1998). The structure and stability of common mental disorders (DSM-III-R): A longitudinal-epidemiological study. *Journal of Abnormal Psychology, 107*, 216–227.

Lalumière, M. L., Harris, G. T., Quinsey, V. L., & Rice, M. E. (in press). *The causes of rape: Understanding individual differences in the male propensity for sexual aggression.* Washington, DC: American Psychological Association.

Larsson, H., Andershed, H., & Lichtenstein, P. (in press). A genetic factor explains most of the variation in the psychopathic personality. *Journal of Abnormal Psychology.*

Little, T. D., Cunningham, W. A., Shahar, G., &

Widaman, K. F. (2002). To parcel or not to parcel: Exploring the questions, weighting the merits. *Structural Equation Modeling, 9*, 151–173.

Lynam, D. R. (2002). Psychopathy from the perspective of the five-factor model of personality. In P. T. Costa & T. A. Widiger (Eds.), *Personality disorder and the five-factor model of personality* (2nd ed., pp. 325–348). Washington, DC: American Psychological Association.

Lynam, D. R., & Gudonis, L. (2005). The development of psychopathy. *Annual Review of Clinical Psychology, 1*, 381–407.

MacCallum, R. C., & Austin, J. (2000). Applications of structural equation modeling in psychological research. *Annual Review of Psychology, 51*, 201–226.

MacMillan, J., & Kofoed, L. (1984). Sociobiology and antisocial personality. *Journal of Nervous and Mental Disease, 172*, 701–706.

Marcus, D. K., John, S. L., & Edens, J. F. (2004). A taxometric analysis of psychopathic personality. *Journal of Abnormal Psychology, 113*, 626–635.

Marsh, H. W. (1994). Using the National Longitudinal Study of 1988 to evaluate theoretical models of self-concept: The Self Description Questionnaire. *Journal of Educational Measurement, 21*, 153–217.

McCord, W., & McCord, J. (1964). *The psychopath: An essay on the criminal mind.* Princeton, NJ: Van Nostrand.

Mealey, L. (1995). The sociobiology of sociopathy: An integrated evolutionary model. *Behavioral and Brain Sciences, 18*, 523–599.

Meloy, J. R. (1988). *The psychopathic mind: Origins, dynamics, and treatments.* Northvale, NJ: Jason Aronson.

Millon, T., Simonson, E., & Birket-Smith, (1998). Historical conceptions of psychopathy in the United States and Europe. In T. Millon, E. Simonson, M. Birket-Smith, & R. D. Davis (Eds.), *Psychopathy: Antisocial, criminal, and violent behavior* (pp. 3–31). New York: Guilford Press.

Monahan, J., & Steadman, H. J. (1994). *Violence and mental disorder: Developments in risk assessment.* Chicago: University of Chicago Press.

Mulaik, S. A. (2002). Commentary on Meehl and Waller's (2002) path analysis and verisimilitude. *Psychological Methods, 7*, 316–322.

Muthen, L. K., & Muthen, B. O. (2001). *Mplus user's guide* (2nd ed.). Los Angeles, CA: Muthen & Muthen.

Neumann, C. S., Kosson, D., & Salekin, R. T. (in press). Exploratory and confirmatory factor analysis of the psychopathy construct: Methodological and conceptual issues. In H. Hervé & J. Yuille (Eds.), *Psychopathy: Theory, research, and social implications.* New York: Erlbaum.

Neumann, C. S., Vitacco, M. J., & Hare, R. D. (2005). *Re-construing the reconstruction of psychopathy: A reply to Cooke, Michie, Hart, & Clark.* Manuscript under review.

Patrick, C. J., Hicks, B. M., Krueger, R. F., & Lang, A.

R. (2005). Relations between psychopathy facets and externalizing psychopathology in a criminal offender sample. *Journal of Personality Disorders, 19,* 339–356.

Pichot, P. (1978). Psychopathic behaviour: A historical overview. In R. D. Hare & D. Schalling (Eds.). *Psychopathic behaviour: Approaches to research* (pp. 55–70). Chichester, UK: Wiley.

Pinel, P. (1801). *Traite medico-philosophique sur l'alientation mentale.* Paris: Caille et Ravier.

Pritchard, J. C. (1835). *A treatise on Insanity.* New York: Hafner.

Quinsey, V. L., Harris, G. T., Rice, M. E., & Cormier, C. (1998). *Violent offenders: Appraising and managing risk.* Washington, DC: American Psychological Association.

Raine, A. (1985). A psychometric assessment of Hare's checklist for psychopathy on an English prison population. *British Journal of Clinical Psychology, 24,* 247–258.

Reise, S. P. (1999). Personality measurement issues viewed through the eyes of IRT. In S. E. Embretson & S. L. Hershberger (Eds.), *The new rules of measurement* (pp. 219–242). Mahwah, NJ: Erlbaum.

Robins, L. N. (1966). *Deviant children grown up.* Baltimore: Williams & Wilkins.

Robins, L. N. (1978). Aetiological implications in studies of childhood histories relating to antisocial personality. In R. D. Hare & D. Schalling (Eds.), *Psychopathic behavior: Approaches to research* (pp. 255–271). Chichester, UK: Wiley.

Rogers, R., Dion, K. L., & Lynett, E. (1992). Diagnostic validity of antisocial personality disorder: A prototypical analysis. *Law and Human Behavior, 16,* 677–689.

Rogers, R., Salekin, R. T., Sewell, K. W., & Cruise, K. R. (2000). Prototypical analysis of antisocial personality disorder: A study of inmate samples. *Criminal Justice and Behavior, 27,* 234–255.

Salekin, R. T., Neumann, C. S., Leistico, A. R., DiCicco, T. M. & Duros, R, L. (2004). Construct validity of psychopathy in a youth offender sample: Taking a closer look at psychopathy's potential importance over disruptive behavior disorders. *Journal of Abnormal Psychology, 113,* 416–427.

Salekin, R. T., Neumann, C. S., Leistico, A. R., & Zalot, A. A. (2004). Psychopathy in youth and intelligence: An investigation of Cleckley's hypothesis. *Journal of Clinical Child and Adolescent Psychology, 33,* 731–742.

Silverstein, M. L., & Nelson, L. D. (2000). Clinical and research implications of revising psychological tests. *Psychological Assessment, 12,* 298–303.

Skeem, J. L., Mulvey, E. P., & Grisso, T. (2003). Applicability of traditional and revised models of psychopathy to the Psychopathy Checklist: Screening Version. *Psychological Assessment, 15,* 41–55.

Slutske, W. S. (2001). The genetics of antisocial behavior. *Current Psychiatry Reports, 3,* 158–162.

Steadman, H. J., Silver, E., Monahan, J. Appelbaum, P. S., Robbins, P. C., Mulvey, E. P., et al. (2000). A classification tree approach to the development of actuarial violence risk assessment tools. *Law and Human Behavior, 24,* 83–100.

Strauss, E., Spreen, O., & Hunter, M. (2000). Implications of test revisions for research. *Psychological Assessment, 12,* 237–244.

Templeman, R., & Wong, S. (1994). Determining the factor structure of the psychopathy checklist: A converging approach. *Multivariate Experimental Clinical Research, 10,* 157–166.

Trull, T. J., & Durrett, C. A. (2005). Categorical and dimensional models of personality disorder. *Annual Review of Clinical Psychology, 1,* 355–380.

Viding, E., Blair, R. J. R., Moffitt, T. E., & Plomin, R. (2005). Evidence for substantial genetic risk for psychopathy in 7-year olds. *Journal of Child Psychology and Psychiatry, 46,* 592–597.

Vitacco, M. J., Neumann, C. S., & Jackson, R. (2005). Testing a four-factor model of psychopathy and its association with ethnicity, gender, intelligence, and violence. *Journal of Consulting and Clinical Psychology, 73,* 466–478.

Vitacco, M. J., Rogers, R., Neumann, C. S., Harrison, K., & Vincent, G. (in press). A comparison of factor models on the PCL-R with mentally disordered offenders: The development of a four-factor model. *Criminal Justice and Behavior.*

Vollebergh, W. A., Iedema, J., Bijl, R. V., de Graaf, R., Smit, F., & Ormel, J. (2001). The structure and stability of common mental disorders: The NEMESIS study. *Archives of General Psychiatry, 5,* 597–603.

West, S. G., Finch, J. F., & Curran, P. J. (1995). Structural equation modeling with nonnormal variables: Problems and remedies. In R. H. Hoyle (Ed.), *Structural equation modeling: Concepts, issues and applications* (pp. 56–75). Thousand Oaks, CA: Sage.

Widiger, T. A., Cadoret, R., Hare, R. D., Robins, L., Rutherford, M., Zanarini, M., et al. (1996). DSM-IV antisocial personality disorder field trial. *Journal of Abnormal Psychology, 105,* 3–16.

Widiger, T. A., & Coker, L. A. (2003). Mental disorders as discrete clinical conditions: dimensional versus categorical classification. In M. Hersen & S. M. Turner (Eds.), *Adult psychopathology and diagnosis* (pp. 3–35). Hoboken, NJ: Wiley.

Widiger, T. A., & Lynam, D. R. (1998). Psychopathy and the five-factor model of personality. In T. Millon, E. Simonson, M. Birket-Smith, & R. D. Davis (Eds.), *Psychopathy: Antisocial, criminal, and violent behavior* (pp. 171–187). New York: Guilford Press.

Zuckerman, M. (1991). *Psychobiology of personality.* New York: Cambridge University Press

II

ISSUES IN CONCEPTUALIZATION AND ASSESSMENT

5

Facets of Clinical Psychopathy

Toward Clearer Measurement

DAVID J. COOKE
CHRISTINE MICHIE
STEPHEN D. HART

> The wicked in his pride does persecute the poor . . . the wicked through the pride of his countenance, will not seek after God . . . his ways are always grievous . . . he has said in his heart, I shall not be moved for I *shall* never *be* in adversity. His mouth is full of cursing and deceit and fraud: under his tongue *is* mischief and vanity. He sitteth in the lurking places of the villages: in the secret places doth he murder the innocent.
>
> —PSALM 10:2–8, King James VI version

The constellation of personality characteristics that today is labeled "psychopathy" has long been recognized, both across time and across cultures. The psalmist identified key features central to contemporary accounts of the disorder: wickedness or immoral behavior, pride, vanity, grievousness, a sense of invulnerability, deceitfulness, manipulation, and extreme violence. Other historical sources, including the Icelandic Sagas, identified a similar pattern (Hoyersten, 2001). The pattern has been recognized in many societies: Murphy (1976) in her classic anthropological study argued that members of two preindustrial societies, the Inuit of North West Alaska and the Yoruba tribe of Nigeria, could distinguish this disorder from other forms of mental disorder and had specific terms for the disorder: *kulangeta* and *aranakan*, respectively.

Although thought to be more prevalent in men, psychopathy has long been described in women. From Greek mythology to contemporary cinema (e.g., Medea, Salome, Manon Lescaut), *les femmes fatales* harmed others by being seductive, manipulative, cruel, egocentric, callous, affectionless and unfaithful. Using their sensuality and sexuality, they controlled and dominated others (Forouzan & Cooke, 2004).

The clinical description of this disorder can be traced back to the case studies of Pinel and Pritchard (Berrios, 1996), their primary contribution being the understanding that mental disorder can exist even when reasoning is intact. These and other influential alienists described mental disorders characterized by a disturbance of emotion or volition, which they gave names such as *manie sans délire, monomanie, moral insanity,* and *folie lucide* (Millon, 1981). The motivation for describing these disorders was forensic: To ensure that their testimony would be relevant, the alienists of the 19th century had to extend their expertise beyond the realm of "total insanity." Even 200 years ago it was argued that a mental disorder whose symptomatology includes antisocial behavior is a moral judgment or tautology that is open to abuse in forensic settings (Berrios, 1996). The first half of the 20th century saw a narrowing of the concept of psychopathy to refer to personality disorder in general. Little consensus existed about the specific forms of personality disorder and the nosology that should be applied; nonetheless, a consensus emerged that an important cluster of symptoms related to aggression, impulsivity, and antisocial behavior (Berrios, 1996). Henderson described the "predominantly aggressive psychopath"; Kahn, the "impulsive," "weak," and "sexual" psychopath; Schneider, the "labile," "explosive," and "wicked" psychopath (Berrios, 1996).

The second half of the last century saw a further narrowing of the construct of psychopathy, to a disorder defined by specific interpersonal, affective, and behavioral features. Rich clinical descriptions—such as those of Arieti (1963), Cleckley (1976), and McCord and McCord (1964)—have provided a framework for describing these individuals. There is broad agreement that interpersonally, psychopathic individuals are dominant, forceful, arrogant, and deceptive; affectively, they lack appropriate emotional responses, with any emotional responses being limited and short-lived; behaviorally, they are impulsive and lack planfulness. Current work suggests that clinicians experienced with this group of patients have a more sophisticated view of the disorder, adding further domains including problems of self, attachment, and cognitive processes (e.g., Cooke, 2004).

The Psychopathy Checklist—Revised (PCL-R) was developed to operationalize a particular conceptualization of psychopathy, namely, that of Hervey Cleckley: "the 'Cleckley psychopath' is the clinical basis for the PCL and the PCL-R" (Hare, 1991, p. 2). However, it is important to note that the PCL-R—and other tests derived from it, such as the Screening Version (PCL:SV; Hart, Cox, & Hare, 1995) and the Youth Version (PCL:YV; Forth, Kosson, & Hare, 2003) of the PCL-R—include some clinical features not considered by Cleckley and exclude others to which Cleckley did refer (Blackburn, in press; Forouzan & Cooke, 2004).

There are two broad approaches to the exploration of a clinical construct and its facets, the "bottom up" and the "top down." In the realm of personality disorder, the bottom-up approach (e.g., Clark, 1992, Livesley, Jackson, & Schroeder, 1992) entails selecting a large number of traits that provide a broad and systematic representation of the domain of interest. Data are then subjected to structural analyses that provide information about the lower- and higher-order dimensions underlying the disorder. The top-down approach is perhaps more efficient in that a restricted number of traits are selected for study based on an established conceptualization of a disorder; however, this has the limitation that any resulting model can only be as good as the original conceptualization. If the original concept is based on experience in only a limited number of subjects or settings, as was the case with Cleckley's concept, then there is a significant danger of both construct underrepresentation and the inclusion of "surplus construct irrelevancies," that is, traits that are irrelevant to the target construct (Cook & Campbell, 1979; Lillienfeld, 1994; Shadish, 1999). The PCL-R thus suffers from the fundamental limitation inherent in any psychological test developed using a top-down approach to the measurement of a construct: If the conceptualization on which the test is based missed key features or included irrelevant features of the disorder, then it will provide a biased measure of the latent construct (Cook & Campbell, 1979; Pedhazur & Schmelkin, 1991; Shadish, Cook, & Campbell, 1999).

There can be little doubt that the development and application of the PCL-R has made a crucial contribution to research in this area. Using the PCL-R, psychopathy has been assessed in a standardized manner by numerous investigators, in a wide range of settings, and in both laboratory and applied research contexts (Cooke, Forth, & Hare, 1998). This has led to a body of research findings that can be contrasted and even cumulated across studies. Yet, after almost two decades of use, it is perhaps time to stand back and consider what has been learned about the limitations of the PCL-R as a psychological test. In doing so, we can start to develop new measures of psychopathy, thereby avoiding the dangers inherent in mono-operation bias, also known as monomeasure bias (Pedhazur & Schmelkin, 1991; Smith, Fischer, & Fister, 2003). Reviewing the psychometric properties of the PCL-R, identifying important limitations of the test, and clarifying what is known about the construct of psychopathy are the purposes of this chapter.

EXPLORING THE FACETS OF PSYCHOPATHY WITH MODERN PSYCHOMETRIC APPROACHES

Modern psychometric procedures can be used to answer many questions alluded to, or implied, in the brief review of the preclinical and clinical literatures. These questions include the following:

1. Do the symptoms of psychopathy form a coherent syndrome?
2. Is antisocial behavior a primary or secondary symptom of psychopathy?
3. Which symptoms of psychopathy are most diagnostic?
4. Does the diagnostic efficiency of symptoms of psychopathy vary according to the severity of the disorder?
5. Is the expression of psychopathic symptomatology affected by culture, race, gender, and the presence of other mental disorders, such as schizophrenia or mental retardation?
6. Can the precision of measurement of psychopathic symptoms be improved by using different definitions of the disorder?
7. How well can clinicians distinguish the intensity of psychopathic symptoms?

The first two questions can be explored using confirmatory factor analysis (CFA) and structural equation modeling (SEM), and the remainder can be explored using item response theory (IRT) methods.

We start by looking at the overall structure of the disorder. We then consider the individual symptoms of the disorder and how they are best measured. We finish by considering the special challenges that confront us when we try to assess change in facets of this disorder.

DO THE SYMPTOMS OF PSYCHOPATHY FORM A COHERENT CONSTRUCT?

The construct of psychopathy has not been without its critics: Toch (1998) argued that the term was a form of negative countertransference, whereas Calvaldino (1998) suggested it was "a moralism masquerading as medical science" (p. 5). The process of validating a psychopathological construct is never complete (Shadish et al., 1999). The success of validation must be judged by a range of criteria, including evidence of reliable assessment, evidence of convergent and divergent validity, evidence of predictive utility, evidence of a diathesis, and, finally, evidence for associations with basic abnormalities of a psychological or biological nature (Blashfield & Draguns, 1976; Eysenck, 1970; Kendell, 1989; Robins & Guze, 1970). Fundamentally, however, these forms of validation can only stand if there is firm support for the existence of a coherent syndrome (i.e., a cluster of symptoms that occur together and that is distinct from other clusters of symptoms).

Obtaining greater understanding of the structural properties of a disorder can yield many advantages (Watson, Clark, & Harkness, 1994). First, it can serve as a starting point for the identification of fundamental psychological structures or processes. Watson and colleagues (1994) argued, for example, that structural research on intelligence tests revealed distinct verbal and spatial factors, with subsequent research indicating that these factors measured separate neuropsychological subsystems. Second, explication of the structure of a disorder can clarify measurement; failure to group items into unidimensional constructs may result in a lack of clarity in the nomological net linking constructs to other variables. For example, Verona, Patrick, and Joiner (2001) clarified Cleckley's view that psychopaths are relatively immune from suicide by demonstrating that although such behavior was associated with chronic antisocial deviance features of the disorder, it was not associated with affective or interpersonal features of the disorder. Third, an appreciation of structure can improve scales, by providing direction on where new variables should be added to improve construct representation, or removed to reduce construct-irrelevant variance (Lilienfeld, 1994). For example, it has been argued elsewhere (Cooke & Michie, 2001) that the measurement of psychopathy could potentially be improved by the addition of items to measure features implicated in other descriptions of psychopathy—for example, emotional coldness, incapacity for love, egocentricity, fearlessness, and absence of anxiety (e.g., Harris, Rice, & Quinsey, 1994; Poythress, Edens, & Lilienfeld, 1999)—and by the removal of items that are essentially counts of antisocial acts (Blackburn, 1992; Cooke, Michie, Hart, & Clark, 2004; see later).

The very diversity of the characteristics attributed to psychopathy challenges the *prima facie* notion that the construct of psychopathy is a coherent syndrome: The empirical evidence reflects this. Hare (1980) made an early attempt to evaluate the structure of psychopathy by carrying out a principal component analysis of the 16 criteria for psychopathy described by Cleckley (1976) and extracted five components. Raine (1985) used oblique factor analysis and extracted seven factors. With the publication of the original PCL-R manual (Hare, 1991), the lack of clarity about the structure of the disorder remained. The manual contained, implicitly or explicitly, three putative models: a three-facet model, a two-factor model, and a hierarchical model. Hare (1991), following the clinical tradition, identified and specified three distinct domains—the interpersonal, affective and behavioral—thought to underpin the expression of psychopathy. At other points in the manual he implied a hierarchical structure: "There is heuristic value in viewing psychopathy as a higher-order construct composed of two correlated factors, one reflecting the personality traits widely considered to be descriptive of this syndrome, and the other reflecting socially deviant behaviors. Together, the factors provide a useful description of the syndrome" (Hare, 1991, p. 37).

For a number of years, a two-factor model of the PCL-R (Hare et al., 1990; see also Harpur, Hakstian, & Hare, 1988) was widely accepted by investigators in the field. In this model, PCL-R items were considered to be underpinned by two distinct but correlated factors: the affective and interpersonal items formed a factor termed "the selfish, callous, and remorseless use of others" and the behavioral items formed a factor termed "the chronically unstable and antisocial lifestyle; social deviance" factor (Hare, 1991, p. 76). However, the two-factor model can be questioned on various statistical grounds. For example, the development of the model was overreliant on congruence coefficients. These coefficients are used to assess the similarity among factors across samples; however, their utility has been called into question (e.g., Van de Vijver & Leung, 1997). The major function of factor analysis is to demonstrate that the variation in scores can be summarized in terms of a few major dimensions, that is, by a simple structure; examination of factor loading plots indicated that a simple structure based on two factors was not present in PCL-R data.

Also, at a conceptual level, Lilienfeld (1994) posed the critical question, "What is psychopathy?" (p. 28), arguing that accounts of the two-factor model do not make it clear whether the two factors are distinct forms of psychopathy or whether the first factor is the core of the disorder. Other authors have shared this concern (e.g., Widiger & Lynam, 1998). This concern is perhaps based on a misinterpretation of the model. The two-factor model (like the three-factor model, described later) is inherently hierarchical in that the factors can be considered to underpin a higher-order construct; that is, they can be regarded as distinct facets of a superordinate construct in the way that verbal and performance intelligence underpins general intelligence.

In earlier work, we reviewed difficulties with the two-factor model. Using both IRT and CFA methods, we established that 13 of the 20 PCL-R items are conceptually distinct and psychometrically nonredundant (Cooke & Michie, 2001). There is no good psychometric evidence that the remaining seven items measure the construct of psychopathy (Cooke et al., 2004; also see later). We developed a *hierarchical* structure with good fit in which the superordinate trait, psychopathy, was underpinned by three highly correlated symptom facets. We called these factors Arrogant and Deceitful Interpersonal Style, Deficient Affective Experience, and Impulsive and Irresponsible Behavioral Style. The first factor was specified by *Glibness/superficial* charm, Grandiose sense of self worth, Pathological Lying, and Conning/manipulative; the second factor by Lack of remorse or guilt, Shallow affect, Callous/lack of empathy, and Failure to accept responsibility for own actions; and the third factor by Need for stimulation/proneness to boredom, Irresponsibility, Impulsivity, Parasitic lifestyle, and Lack of realistic, long-term goals.

There are perhaps three points to emphasize regarding this three-factor model. First, the structure is hierarchical, with a superordinate construct that was sufficiently unidimensional to be regarded as a coherent psychopathological construct or syndrome (Cooke & Michie, 2001, Zinbarg, Barlow, & Brown, 1997). Second, the three facets can be regarded as having reliable general variance as a consequence of the influence of the broad construct shared with the other facets, but in addition, there was reliable specific variance unique to each particular facet. The value of refining the broad construct into specific facets has advantages in that the specificity between aspects of the disorder and external variables may be clearer (e.g., Dolan & Anderson, 2003; Hall, Benning, & Patrick, 2004; Raine, Lencz, Bihrle, LaCasse, & Colletti, 2000; Soderstrom et al., 2002). Third, the model encompasses only 13 of the 20 PCL-R items. The excluded items primarily reflect antisocial behavior rather than core traits. Some personality theorists distinguish between basic tendencies and characteristic adaptations, the former being core personality traits and the latter being overt manifestations (McCrae & Costa, 1995). Although this distinction is clearly one of degree rather than one of kind, Lilienfeld (1998) has argued that the items associated with Hare's original Factor One (e.g., Shallow affect, Grandiose sense of self-worth) are basic tendencies whereas those associated with Hare's original Factor Two (e.g., Poor behavioral controls, Revocation of conditional release) are characteristic adaptations.

The failure of the other items to coalesce into a coherent syndrome raises important theoretical questions—questions that can be traced back to the alienists of the 19th century—about the relationship between antisocial behavior and psychopathy: It is to this issue that we return shortly.

The factor structure replicated well in data from the United Kingdom as well as in ratings based on the PCL:SV (Hart et al., 1995) and the various criterion sets used in the DSM-IV Antisocial Personality Disorder Field Trial (Widiger et al., 1996). This model has since been replicated in independent samples of adults and adolescents in North America, the United Kingdom, and continental Europe (Cooke, Kosson, & Michie, 2001; Cooke, Michie, Hart, & Clark, 2005a, 2005b) and by independent investigators (e.g., Andershed, Kerr, Stattin, & Levander, 2002; Johansson, Andershed, Kerr, & Levander, 2002; Skeem, Mulvey, & Grisso, 2003; Vincent, 2002; Warren et al., 2003).

In his recent revision of the PCL-R manual, Hare (2003) rejected the three-factor model and proposed an alternative, two-factor/four-facet hierarchical model. Unfortunately, the manual does not specify the details of the model or provide sufficient information to permit a full evaluation of it, and there are no other publications that might shed light on the issue. Based on the brief description in the PCL-R manual we have several concerns about the statistical viability of the four-facet model.[1] First, Hare (2003) claims a two-factor solution fits the data but does not provide fit statistics, relying solely on an examination of a factor-loading plot (Hare, 2003, Figure 7.2). However, no simple structure is evident in the plot: the factor loadings do not cluster around the factors but, rather, form an arc between the two axes. We tested the four-facet model presented in schematic form in Figure 7.3 of the new manual (Hare, 2003), a hierarchical one in which the three factors of Cooke and Michie (2001) were supplemented with a fourth comprising five items related to criminality (Poor behavioral controls, Early behavior problems, Juvenile delinquency, Revocation of conditional release, and Criminal versatility). Using large data sets from the United Kingdom, Europe, and North America we demonstrated not only that this model failed to achieve, or approach, acceptable levels of fit but that it was also substantially poorer in fit than the three-factor solution (Cooke, Michie, Hart, & Clark, 2005a, 2005b).

A recent study by Hill, Neumann, and Rogers (2004) highlighted a problem emerging in the field, namely, the failure to distinguish between hierarchical and nonhierarchical models. The primary function of factor analysis in this context is to demonstrate that symptoms cluster to form a coherent syndrome. Such a model postulates a higher-order construct, psychopathy, which is underpinned by distinct but related symptom facets. In other words, the various expressions of the disorder can be construed as a consequence of the general variance "produced" by a broad construct that is shared with the lower-order facets. In addition, there may be reliable specific variance unique to each particular facet. This type of hierarchical model parallels models of intelligence in which general intelligence underpins more specific aspects including verbal and performance intelligence.

To claim that psychopathy is a coherent syndrome it is therefore necessary to think hierarchically. Only two- and three-factor models are inherently hierarchical insofar as correlated factor models are mathematically equivalent to models that include a superordinate factor overarching subordinate factors. With four or more factors, the equivalence of hierarchical and correlated factor models no longer pertains. This is because the number of parameters in the hierarchical model is less than that in the correlated factor model. As a result, the correlated model is less parsimonious, because fewer constraints are applied than within the hierarchical model. The apparent fit of the correlated (i.e., less constrained) model will thus appear to be better. It is therefore necessary to test a four-factor hierarchical model against a four-correlated-factor model and be aware of the differences in interpretation.

Specifically, the distinction between these two models has conceptual importance. As noted earlier, the hierarchical model implies some general latent trait underpinned by distinct facets of the disorder; the four-factor correlated model could reflect merely an array of related but conceptually distinct domains that are not unified by an overarching latent trait. The following example is offered to illustrate this point.

Psychopathy has been observed to be associated with body building, tattoos, steroid use, and body piercing (e.g., Post, 1968), at least in adult male prisoners in North America. If these items were included in the PCL-R, it is plausible that a "Body enhancement" factor would emerge. It does not make conceptual sense to assume that body building

and tattoos are primary symptoms of psychopathy, given that the frequency of these activities clearly is influenced by norms that vary across cultures and across time within cultures. These activities are characteristic adaptations rather than basic tendencies. If "Body enhancement" is not a core feature of the disorder, then a hierarchical model would fit poorly, but a correlated factor model could fit the data well.

We have chosen this perhaps extreme example for didactic purposes. However, this argument is equally true for the inclusion of items that are essentially counts of antisocial behaviors in the model. The findings of Hill, Neumann, and Rogers (2004) indicate only that the three factors identified by Cooke and Michie (2001) are correlated with antisocial behavior; their data do not demonstrate that antisocial behavior is a distinct facet of a coherent superordinate psychopathy construct. We will now turn to consider the association between psychopathy and antisocial behavior in detail.

IS ANTISOCIAL BEHAVIOR A PRIMARY OR SECONDARY SYMPTOM OF THE DISORDER?

The link between psychopathy and antisocial behavior is formalized in the diagnostic criteria of nosological systems such as the *ICD-10 Classification of Mental and Behavioural Disorders* (ICD-10; World Health Organization, 1992) and the fourth edition of *Diagnostic and Statistical Manual of Mental Disorders* (DSM-IV; American Psychiatric Association, 1994). Yet, the nature of the association between psychopathy and antisocial behavior is unclear. Is antisocial behavior a *symptom* of psychopathy or is it simply a *consequence*? A symptom generally is considered to be a direct manifestation of a disease process or disorder, and therefore it plays an important role in assessment and diagnosis. In contrast, a consequence—also referred to as a secondary symptom or sequela—is indirectly associated with a disease. A consequence may be a marker or predictor of the disease but is likely to have low sensitivity or specificity. This could be the result of equifinality, in that the same consequences may result from several different diseases or disorders.

Theoretical Support
for the Consequence Hypothesis

There are at least four theoretical arguments supporting the view that antisocial behavior is a consequence (i.e., an effect), rather than a symptom, of psychopathy; we term this the "consequence hypothesis." First, classical clinical descriptions of psychopathy (e.g., Arieti, 1963; Gough, 1948; Karpman, 1961; McCord & McCord, 1964) do not include antisocial behavior as a central feature or symptom of the disorder. As the McCords argued, "Much of psychology's confusion over the psychopath can be traced to a basic mistake: equating deviant behavior with the psychopathic personality. . . . Deviant behavior, then, is an inadequate criterion of psychopathy. [A]ny adequate study of the psychopath must look beyond asociality" (McCord & McCord, 1964, p. 8). Both Schneider (1950) and Cleckley (1976) indicated that many psychopaths have no history of antisocial behavior. Schneider explicitly stated that antisocial behavior is secondary to personality pathology. Diagnostic criteria for psychopathy that appear to overfocus on antisocial behavior have been heavily criticized (Hare, 1991; Millon, 1981; Rogers & Dion, 1991).

Second, there are rational reasons to argue that psychopathy may play a causal role in regard to antisocial behavior: "the personality features that are encompassed under psychopathy seem likely to result in and drive antisocial behavior" (McDermott et al., 2000, p. 185). For example, interpersonal symptoms of psychopathy, such as grandiosity, predispose individuals with the disorder to engage in sadistic criminal acts, motivated by a desire to control, demean, or humiliate a victim; affective deficits, such as lack of empathy and anxiety, result in a failure to inhibit antisocial (and especially violent) thoughts and urges; and impulsivity increases the likelihood of engaging in criminal acts without considering their consequences (e.g., Baumeister, Smart, & Boden, 1996; Blackburn, 1993, 1998; Blair, Jones, Clark, & Smith, 1995; Fowles & Missel, 1994; Hare, Cooke, & Hart, 1999; Hart, 1998; Kernberg, 1998; Malamuth & Brown, 1994; Meloy, 1988; Serin, 1991).

Third, antisocial and socially deviant behavior can be considered to be qualitatively different from other symptoms of psychopathy insofar as they reflect specific acts rather than general personality traits. Blackburn (1988) emphasized that to define or diagnose personality disorder in terms of both traits and acts is to mix criteria from distinct conceptual domains (see also Widiger & Lynam, 1998). In a similar vein, Lilienfeld (1994) criticized diagnostic criteria for psychopathy (e.g., PCL-R criteria) that conflated both "basic tendencies" (traits) and "characteristic adaptations" (acts).

Fourth, theoretical views of crime and violence suggest that antisocial behavior results from the influence of a wide range of biological, psychological, and social factors (e.g., Gottfredson & Hirschi, 1990). In general theories of crime, psychopathic personality disorder is only one of many important causal factors. Other mental disorders that have been linked to antisocial behavior include psychotic disorders, mental retardation, substance use and dependence, and other personality disorders.

Recently, we endeavored to examine the link between the three-factor hierarchical model of psychopathy and the seven PCL-R items that did not aggregate into the coherent latent trait we call psychopathy in large sets of North American, U.K., and Continental European data (Cooke et al., 2004). We first examined the structure of these seven PCL-R items. Using PCL-R ratings from a sample of 1,316 British prisoners, we carried out exploratory factor analysis and extracted two factors. The first, which we interpreted as *Criminal Behavior*, was marked by *Juvenile Delinquency* (Item 18), *Revocation of conditional release* (Item 19), and *Criminal versatility* (Item 20); the second, which we interpreted as *Relationship lability*, was marked by *Promiscuous sexual behavior* (Item 11) and *Many short-term marital relationships* (Item 17). CFA indicated that good fit could be achieved (Cooke et al., 2004).

We then examined how these dimensions related to the three-factor model of psychopathy. Are they additional factors that parallel the interpersonal, affective, and behavioral factors identified previously (Cooke & Michie, 2001), or are they better conceptualized as consequences of the disorder? We used SEM methods to examine these questions. SEM has two major advantages over traditional correlational methods (Hull,

Lehn, & Tedlie, 1991). First, it allows the estimation of the unique effects of one symptom factor controlling for the other symptom factors. Second, it estimates and controls for measurement error: Thus, the relative importance of symptom factors can be compared directly, without concern that the effects are attenuated by differential measurement reliability.

As a first step, we generated a five-factor hierarchical model in which *Criminal behavior* and *Relationship lability* were considered to be facets additional to those in the three-factor model. The fit of this model was unacceptable using standard criteria, and also was substantially poorer than that achieved by the three-factor model. Put simply, adding items related to antisocial behavior actually degraded the measurement of psychopathy. The second step was to develop and evaluate a causal model. We started model building

by selecting a 50% random sample of our U.K. data in order to build the model on one subsample and cross-validate it on the second subsample.

In the absence of any specific *a priori* hypothesis, the initial model was parameterized on the broad hypothesis that *Criminal behavior* and *Relationship lability* were, in part, the product of the three factors; the model contained all paths between the three factors and the presumed consequences. We then simplified this model by excluding nonsignificant paths; the fit of the model remained adequate but more parsimonious. To improve the comprehensiveness of the model we tried to include the remaining two PCL-R items, *Poor behavioral controls* and *Early behavioral problems*. The first of these items could not be fitted to the model, but the second could. This final model (depicted in Figure 5.1) was cross-validated on the other

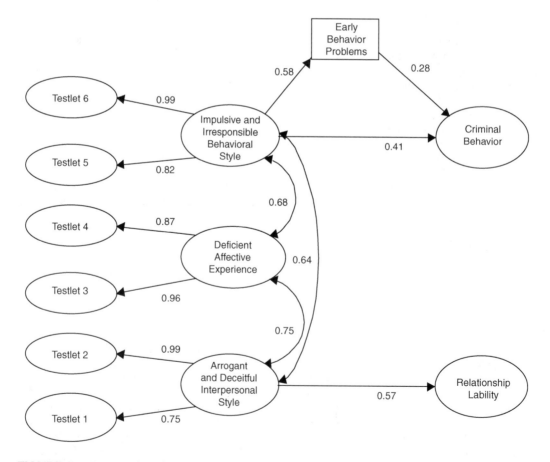

FIGURE 5.1. Structural model of three-factor model of psychopathy and its links to relationship lability and antisocial behavior: Standardized estimates from complete U.K. sample.

random subsample of the U.K. data, and then in large samples from continental Europe and from Canada. This cross-validation process demonstrated the robustness and cross-cultural stability of this model.

In the final model, the *Arrogant and Deceitful Interpersonal Style* facet of psychopathy was linked strongly to *Relationship lability*. The *Impulsive and Irresponsible Behavioral Style* facet was linked to *Criminal behavior* both directly, and also indirectly, through *Early behavioral problems*. These findings challenge current conceptualizations of psychopathy as operationalized by the PCL-R and suggest that the domain tapped by the PCL-R items is too broad, embracing both the disorder and certain consequences of the disorder. We conclude that the PCL-R construct of psychopathy has drifted from the traditional conceptualizations of the disorder (e.g., Cleckley, 1976; Karpman, 1961; McCord & McCord, 1964; Schneider, 1950), and that it may be time to correct this course. It may be time to "reconstruct" psychopathy by reducing or eliminating reliance on criteria that are overly saturated with antisocial and socially deviant behavior, thus putting personality back at the heart of this personality disorder.

Having considered the complex structure of the disorder of psychopathy as operationalized using the PCL-R, we now explore several other important conceptual and measurement issues raised in the initial discussion. To do this, we rely on a different analytic approach, namely, item response theory. We therefore preface our discussion of conceptual issues with a brief account of IRT.

ITEM RESPONSE THEORY: "THE NEW PSYCHOMETRICS"

Measurement of psychological characteristics is indirect: An individual's level of a psychological characteristic (e.g., intelligence, depression, or psychopathy) cannot be observed directly but has to be inferred from observable behavior, such as responses to test items or verbal accounts of symptoms. In the language of test theory, a person's standing on the unobservable latent trait (e.g., intelligence) is inferred from manifest variables (e.g., scores on tests of abstract reasoning; Waller, Thompson, & Wenk, 2000).

IRT methods provide a comprehensive description of the performance of individual items with an understanding of the performance of tests, or facets of tests, being achieved by a bottom-up approach. Item characteristic curves (ICCs) provide graphical representation of key item qualities. Three hypothetical ICCs are presented in Figure 5.2 for purposes of illustration. On the horizontal axis is the level of the hypothetical trait, while on the vertical axis is the probability of a positive response on the item. Curves A and B are parallel—they are equally steep—and thus are equally good at discriminating between low and high levels of the latent trait. Although they are equally discriminating, they discriminate at different levels of the trait: Item B discriminates at a higher level of the trait compared with Item A. Item C differs from the other curves in that it has a lower slope and therefore it is less discriminating.

A concrete example may assist the illustration. The Vocabulary subtest of the Wechsler Adult Intelligence Scale—Revised (WAIS-III; Wechsler, 1997) requires the participant to define progressively more difficult words. If an IRT analysis was carried out on the Vocabulary subtest then a latent trait measuring general vocabulary skills should emerge. The ICC for simple words such as *"Ship"* or *"Breakfast"* might be represented by Curve A, whereas more complex words such as *"Matchless"* or *"Tirade"* might be represented by Curve B—a curve which becomes positive at higher levels of the trait. Curve C may represent a word that is a specialist term used in a particular trade, profession, or hobby; for example, most sailors could define the term "Burgee" (a type of flag used to indicate apparent wind direction) whereas nonsailors might not be familiar with the term. The ability to define *Burgee* is not a good indicator of general vocabulary skill; it is merely an indicator of particular interests or experience. It is through the examination of curves of this type that IRT analyses can assist in the development and refining of scales. If an item has an ICC curve like that depicted in Curve C, then this item could be eliminated from the test because it does not provide useful information about the latent trait of interest.

By focusing at the individual item level we can gain greater understanding of the key

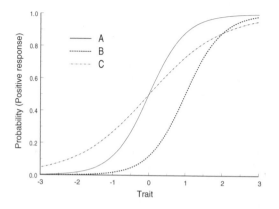

FIGURE 5.2. Hypothetical item characteristic curves.

features of the disorder and also gain understanding of how to improve our approach to measurement. In the next section we examine what IRT methods tell us about which symptoms are most diagnostic, which symptoms raters can make fine distinctions about, whether detailed symptom descriptions enhance or detract from symptom ratings, and how we can clarify item definitions to ensure item independence.

UNDERSTANDING ITEM PERFORMANCE: IMPORTANCE FOR MEASUREMENT AND CONCEPTUALIZATION

Which Symptoms Are Most Diagnostic?

The items in the PCL-R are weighted equally (i.e., unit-weighted), based on the assumption that all items—and the symptoms or features they reflect—are equally diagnostic. IRT analysis can demonstrate whether this assumption is unwarranted, thereby resulting in loss of measurement precision (Cooke & Michie, 1997; Cooke et al., 1998, 2001, 2005a, 2005b).

Examination of PCL-R items in a variety of samples has revealed that items vary considerably in their slopes, and thus in their usefulness as measures of the underlying trait (Cooke & Michie, 1997). PCL-R items such as *Promiscuous sexual behavior, Poor behavioral controls,* and *Criminal versatility,* have shallow slopes, whereas items such as *Callous/lack of empathy, Lack of remorse or*

guilt, and *Grandiosity* have steep slopes. The latter items are much more useful in the measurement of psychopathy than the former. Adding poor or irrelevant items to a test can degrade measurement: Less can be more (Smith et al., 2003). Thus to improve our measurement of the facets of psychopathy it is important to include only items that discriminate well. In addition, from the perspective of theory, this approach assists in identifying the core features of the disorder (i.e., those that are most diagnostic).

Do Different Symptoms Reflect Different Severities of Disorder?

In a series of IRT analyses, we have demonstrated that the PCL-R items reflect different levels of severity of the disorder; some tend to be present at low levels of severity, whereas others tend to be present only at high levels (Cooke & Michie, 1997, 1999; Cooke et al., 2004; Cooke, Michie, Hart, & Hare, 1999). Broadly speaking, the symptoms related to the Impulsive and Irresponsible Behavioral Style factor are most diagnostic at low levels of psychopathy; symptoms related to Deficient Affective Experience are diagnostic at moderate levels; and symptoms related to the Arrogant and Deceitful Interpersonal Factor are diagnostic at high levels of the trait. This ordering suggests that if patients present with features such as grandiosity and superficial charm, then they are very likely also to have symptoms such as shallow emotions and the poor impulse control; however, many patients with symptoms such as poor impulse control will not exhibit interpersonal or affective symptoms of psychopathy. This finding allows the rational selection of symptoms for different purposes. For example, if the goal is to make a categorical diagnosis of psychopathy, then the emphasis should be on the assessment of symptoms that discriminate around the diagnostic cutoff on the latent trait; but if the goal is to assess the severity of the disorder in dimensional terms, then the emphasis should be on assessing symptoms that reflect the entire range of the latent trait. From the perspective of theory, understanding which symptoms discriminate at different levels of the trait assists in identifying the conceptual core of the disorder.

Can Raters Distinguish Different Degrees of a Symptom?

ICCs can also be used to understand how well raters distinguish different levels of a symptom. The PCL-R and related tests use a simple three-point scheme for coding items: 0 = *Does not apply*, 1 = *Applies to some extent* or *Mixed evidence*, and 2 = *Definitely applies*. Analysis of PCL-R data has revealed that the coding of some items is essentially binary; raters appear to distinguish between the presence and the absence of a symptom. For other symptoms, the distinctions between codes of 1 and 2 appear to be more meaningful (Hart, Cooke, & Douglas, 2001).

Figure 5.3 plots the ICC for the item *Callous/Lack of empathy* estimated on approximately 2,000 PCL-R ratings from North America (Cooke & Michie, 1997). The left-hand curve plots the probability of a "0" rating on this item at different points of the underlying trait, the middle curve plots the probability of receiving a "1" rating, and the right-hand curve the probability of a "2" rating. The curves are steep, demonstrating that this item is a good indicator of the underlying trait. But in addition, it is clear that raters can distinguish validly among the three response options. This is in distinct contrast to the pattern for the item *Irresponsibility* (see Figure 5.4), where raters are only able to make essentially binary decisions. It remains an empirical question whether raters can dis-

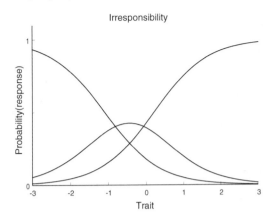

FIGURE 5.4. Item characteristic curves for Irresponsibility.

tinguish finer graduations in some symptoms of psychopathy as compared with others. However, clearer definitions of categories may assist measurement and clearer definitions of symptoms may assist raters to make finer distinctions.

Are Short Item Definitions Sufficient?

The definitions of PCL-R items are complex, some running to several hundred words. In the development of the PCL:SV (Hart et al., 1995) and the Psychopathy Criterion Set (PCS; Widiger et al., 1996), great efforts were made to simplify the definitions. Direct comparisons of the PCL-R and PCL:SV ratings in the standardization sample of the PCL-R revealed that even with simpler definitions, the level of discrimination achieved with the simpler PCL:SV definitions was equivalent, and in some cases even superior, to that obtained with the more complex definitions (Cooke et al., 1999). It is possible that the longer definitions result in cognitive overload, making it difficult for raters to integrate the information required.

This leads to a related question: Are broad or narrow definitions of symptoms preferable? Once again IRT methods can provide an answer. IRT methods allow the computation of information functions; these functions estimate the precision of measurement; the more information an item provides the better is the estimate of the level of psychopathy expressed by an individual. It is possible to plot

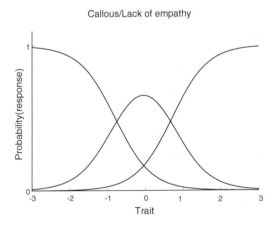

FIGURE 5.3. Item characteristic curves for Callous/lack of empathy.

information functions across the latent trait and these plots can be used to determine which item, facet, or test of a construct yields the most precise measurement. The higher the information function the greater the precision of measurement at that point on the latent trait. These plots can therefore be used to determine where precision is best; for example, if a cutoff score is being applied then ideally precision ought to be maximal around this cutoff score.

To illustrate this, we consider results from the DSM-IV Antisocial Personality Disorder Field Trial. In the Field Trial, three sets of diagnostic criteria were compared: DSM-III-R criteria for antisocial personality disorder, ICD-10 dissocial personality disorder, and a PCS based on simplified PCL:SV ratings. Both the PCS and the DSM-III-R criterion sets had an item that measured impulsivity. Examination of Figure 5.5 indicates that the PCS item provided more information and, therefore, greater precision of measurement than did the DSM-III-R item. This is perhaps not surprising. The DSM-III-R definition of impulsivity is rather specific, seeking a narrow subset of examples of impulsive behavior, specifically: "Fails to plan ahead, or is impulsive, as indicated by one or both of the following: a) traveling from place to place without a prearranged job or clear goal for the period of travel or clear idea about when the travel will terminate; b) lack of a fixed address for a month or more" (p. 345). In contrast, the PCS definition seeks a broader range of examples: "The individual

does things on the spur of the moment, without adequately considering the consequences of his behavior; frequently changes employment, sexual partners, or residence; frequently engages in risky and exciting activities." These IRT analyses suggested that broad descriptions of broad symptoms may work better.

Can the Distinction among Symptoms Be Ensured?

A difficulty with the definitions of PCL-R items is that they are not sufficiently independent of one another; rather, subsets of items are locally dependent, forming what are known as testlets (Chen & Thissen, 1997). Testlets occur when items are more highly associated than can explained by their relationship with the underlying latent trait; thus, a pair of items that form a testlet can be construed as being somewhere between one and two items. Indeed, in a study of PCL-R ratings for more than 2,000 participants, all items except *Poor behavioral controls* formed testlets with other items (Cooke & Michie, 2001). Examples of item pairs that formed testlets included (1) *Shallow affect* and *Callous/lack of empathy*; and (2) *Early behavioral problems* and *Juvenile delinquency*. The items *Need for stimulation/proneness to boredom, Impulsivity,* and *Irresponsibility* formed a three-item testlet. Testlets can emerge for a variety of reasons but the most common reason in a rating scale is the overlap of content in item definitions. PCL-R item definitions are replete with overlapping definitions. For example, item 6 ("lack of remorse") makes reference to both an inability to recognize the seriousness of actions that cause damage or difficulty to others and a tendency to blame such action on external factors (e.g., other people, situational influences). The latter criterion overlaps clearly with item 16 ("failure to accept responsibility for own actions"), which focuses on rationalization and externalization of blame.

The presence of testlets in a scale indicates potential problems. First, it suggests that the structure underpinning the data is more complex and the assumption that a unidimensional trait is underpinning the test may be invalid. Second, it suggests that estimates of the information provided by the test may

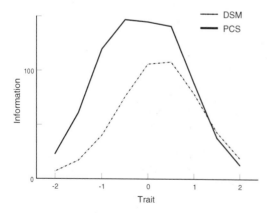

FIGURE 5.5. Item information functions for two definitions of "impulsivity."

be inaccurate, specifically, that they may be inflated: The test appears to be more accurate than is actually the case. Third, the presence of testlets indicates that the test does not allow clinicians to distinguish adequately among conceptually distinct symptoms (Chen & Thissen, 1997).

In summary, this review of previous analyses of measures of psychopathy, including the PCL-R, PCL:SV, PCS, and DSM-III-R criteria, has identified several key issues relevant for those wishing to build on what has been learned so far concerning the measurement of the facets of psychopathy and who wish to develop new approaches to its measurement. First, there are at least three key domains of symptoms to consider, the interpersonal, the affective, and the behavioral. However, this formulation should be treated with caution because it may be a consequence of a top-down approach to the conceptualization of the disorder: That is, an approach based on a single conceptualization (i.e., Cleckley, 1976). Broader sampling of key symptoms may identify more domains or subdomains. As noted previously, current work suggests that additional domains are required to provide a comprehensive description of psychopathy. Second, certain types of symptoms are more useful than others for measuring the psychopathy construct and at indexing severity of the disorder. Accordingly, we encourage research efforts directed toward identifying symptoms that add measurement precision at the moderate to high range of psychopathy. Third, simplifying item definitions, limiting the overlap across item definitions, being more flexible in the response formats used, and providing raters with more sophisticated guidance regarding response coding for individual items should increase measurement precision.

CONCLUSION

In conclusion, historical accounts and clinical descriptions have provided clear evidence for the complex multifaceted nature of psychopathy. The development of the PCL-R has provided a useful procedure for increasing our understanding of this disorder; however, we must be alert to the danger that mono-operation bias may lead us into a conceptual cul-de-sac. As the prefatory quote

from the Psalms illustrates, psychopathy is a venerable construct—it is not here today and gone tomorrow. Thus, it is important to build on what has been learned in the last decade so that both the measurement and the conceptualization of this important disorder can be enhanced through a greater understanding of the facets that compose it.

NOTE

1. Regrettably our request for the full details of the model was declined.

REFERENCES

American Psychiatric Association. (1994). *Diagnostic and statistical manual of mental disorders* (4th ed.). Washington, DC: Author.

Andershed, H., Kerr, M., Stattin, H., & Levander, S., (2002). Understanding the abnormal by studying the normal. *Acta Psychiatrica Scandanavica, 106*, 75–80.

Arieti, S. (1963). Psychopathic personality: Some views on its psychopathology and psychodynamics. *Comprehensive Psychiatry, 4*, 301–312.

Baumeister, R. F., Smart, L., & Boden, J. M. (1996). Relation of threatened egotism to violence and aggression: The dark side of self-esteem. *Psychological Review, 103*, 5–33.

Berrios, G. E. (1996). *The history of mental symptoms: Descriptive psychopathology since the nineteenth century*. Cambridge, UK: Cambridge University Press.

Blackburn, R. (1988). On moral judgments and personality disorders: the myth of psychopathic personality revisited. *British Journal of Psychiatry, 153*, 505–512.

Blackburn, R. (1992). Criminal behaviour, personality disorder, and mental illness: the origins of confusion. *Criminal Behaviour and Mental Health, 2*, 66–77.

Blackburn, R. (1993). *The psychology of criminal conduct: Theory, research and practice*. Chichester, UK: Wiley.

Blackburn, R. (1998). Psychopathy and personality disorder: implications of interpersonal theory. In D. J. Cooke, A. E. Forth, & R. D. Hare (Eds.), *Psychopathy: Theory, research and implications for society* (pp. 269–301). Dordrecht, The Netherlands: Kluwer.

Blackburn, R. (in press). Conceptualizing psychopathy. In S. Strack (Ed.), *Handbook of personology and psychopathology*. New York: Wiley.

Blair, R., Jones, L., Clark, F., & Smith, M. (1995). Is the psychopath morally insane? *Personality and Individual Differences, 19*, 741–752.

Blashfield, R. K., & Draguns, J. G. (1976). Evaluative

criteria for psychiatric classification. *Journal of Abnormal Psychology, 85,* 140–150.

Calvadino, P. (1998). Death to the psychopath. *Journal of Forensic Psychiatry, 9,* 5–8.

Chen, W. H., & Thissen, D. (1997). Local dependence indices for item pairs using item response theory. *Journal of Educational and Behavioral Statistics, 22,* 265–289.

Clark, L. A. (1992). Resolving taxonomic issues in personality disorders: the value of large scale analyses of symptom data. *Journal of Personality Disorders, 6,* 360–376.

Cleckley, H. (1976). *The mask of sanity* (5th ed.). St Louis, MO: Mosby.

Cook, T. D., & Campbell, D. T. (1979). *Quasi-experimentation, design and analysis issues for field settings.* Chicago: Rand McNally.

Cooke, D. J. (2004, March 22–24). *Measuring psychopathy: Things that I have learned so far.* Keynote Address at the 13th annual Conference of the Division of Forensic Psychology, University of Leicester.

Cooke, D. J., Forth, A., & Hare, R. D. (1998). *Psychopathy: theory, research and implications for society.* Dordrecht, The Netherlands: Kluwer.

Cooke, D. J., Kosson, D. S., & Michie, C. (2001). Psychopathy and ethnicity: Structural, item and test generalizability of the Psychopathy Checklist—Revised (PCL-R) in Caucasian and African-American participants. *Psychological Assessment, 13,* 531–542.

Cooke, D. J., & Michie, C. (1997). An item response theory evaluation of Hare's Psychopathy Checklist. *Psychological Assessment, 9,* 2–13.

Cooke, D. J., & Michie, C. (1999). Psychopathy across cultures: North America and Scotland compared. *Journal of Abnormal Psychology, 108,* 55–68.

Cooke, D. J., & Michie, C. (2001). Refining the construct of psychopathy: Towards a hierarchical model. *Psychological Assessment, 13,* 171–188.

Cooke, D. J., Michie, C., Hart, S. D., & Clark, D. (2004). Reconstructing psychopathy: Clarifying the significance of antisocial and socially deviant behavior in the diagnosis of psychopathic personality disorder. *Journal of Personality Disorders, 18,* 337–357.

Cooke, D. J., Michie, C., Hart, S. D., & Clark, D. (2005a). Assessing psychopathy in the United Kingdom: Concerns about cross-cultural generalisability. *British Journal of Psychiatry, 186,* 339–345.

Cooke, D. J., Michie, C., Hart, S. D., & Clark, D. (2005b). Searching for the pan-cultural core of psychopathic personality disorder: Continental Europe and North American compared. *Personality and Individual Differences, 39,* 283–295.

Cooke, D. J., Michie, C., Hart, S. D., & Hare, R. D. (1999). The functioning of the Screening Version of the Psychopathy Checklist—Revised: An item response theory analysis. *Psychological Assessment, 11,* 3–13.

Dolan, M., & Anderson, I. M. (2003). The relationship between serotonergic function and the psychopathy checklist: Screening version. *Journal of Psychopharmacology, 17,* 211–217.

Eysenck, H. J. (1970). The classification of depressive illness. *British Journal of Psychiatry, 117,* 241–250.

Forouzan, E., & Cooke, D. J. (2004). *Figuring out la femme fatale: Conceptual and assessment issues concerning psychopathy in females.* Manuscript under review.

Forth, A. E., Kosson, D. S., & Hare, R. D. (2003). *The Psychopathy Checklist: Youth Version manual.* Toronto, ON, Canada: Multi-Health Systems.

Fowles, D. C., & Missel, K. A. (1994). Electrodermal hyporeactivity, motivation, and psychopathy: Theoretical issues. In D. C. Fowles, P. Sutker, & S. H. Goodman (Eds.), *Special focus on psychopathy and antisocial personality disorder: A developmental perspective* (pp. 263–283). New York: Springer.

Gottfredson, M. R., & Hirschi, T. (1990). *A general theory of crime.* Stanford, CA: Stanford University Press.

Gough, H. G. (1948). A sociological theory of psychopathy. *American Journal of Sociology, 53,* 359–366.

Hall, J., Benning, S. D., & Patrick, C. J. (2004). Criterion-related validity of the three-factor model of psychopathy: Personality, behavior, and adaptive functioning. *Assessment, 11,* 4–16.

Hare, R. D. (1980). A research scale for the assessment of psychopathy in criminal populations. *Personality and Individual Differences, 1,* 111–119.

Hare, R. D. (1991). *Manual for the Hare Psychopathy Checklist—Revised.* Toronto, ON, Canada: Multi-Health Systems.

Hare, R. D. (2003). *Manual for the Hare Psychopathy Checklist—Revised* (2nd ed.). Toronto, ON, Canada: Multi-Health Systems.

Hare, R. D., Cooke, D. J., & Hart, S. D. (1999). Psychopathy and sadistic personality disorder. In T. Millon, P. H. Blaney, & R. D. Davies (Eds.), *Oxford textbook of psychopathology* (pp. 555–584). Oxford, UK: Oxford University Press.

Hare, R. D., Harpur, T. J., Hakstian, A. R., Forth, A. E., Hart, S. D., & Newman, J. P. (1990). The Revised Psychopathy Checklist: Reliability and factor structure. *Psychological Assessment: A Journal of Consulting and Clinical Psychology, 2,* 238–341.

Harpur, T. J., Hakstian, A., & Hare, R. D. (1988). Factor structure of the Psychopathy Checklist. *Journal of Consulting and Clinical Psychology, 56,* 741–747.

Harris, G. T., Rice, M. E., & Quinsey, V. L. (1994). Psychopathy as a taxon: Evidence that psychopaths are a discrete class. *Journal of Consulting and Clinical Psychology, 62,* 387–397.

Hart, S. D. (1998). Psychopathy and risk for violence. In D. J. Cooke, A. E. Forth, & R. D. Hare (Eds.), *Psychopathy: Theory, research and implications for society* (pp. 355–374). Utrecht, The Netherlands: Kluwer.

Hart, S. D., Cooke, D. J., & Douglas, K. (2001, November 28–31). *Advanced workshop on the PCL-R.* Paper presented at the international conference on "Violence risk assessment and management: Bringing science and practice closer together," Sundsvall, Sweden.

Hart, S. D., Cox, D. N., & Hare, R. D. (1995). *The Hare Psychopathy Checklist: Screening Version* (1st ed.). Toronto, ON, Canada: Multi-Health Systems.

Hill, C. D., Neumann, C. S., & Rogers, R. (2004). Confirmatory factor analysis of the Psychopathy Checklist: Screening version in offenders with Axis I disorders. *Psychological Assessment, 16,* 90–95.

Hoyersten, J. G. (2001). The Icelandic Sagas and the idea of personality and deviant personalities in the Middle Ages. *History of Psychiatry,* 199–212.

Hull, J. G., Lehn, D. A., & Tedlie, J. C. (1991). A general approach to testing multifaceted personality constructs. *Journal of Personality and Social Psychology, 61,* 932–945.

Karpman, B. (1961). The structure of neuroses: With special differentials between neurosis, psychosis, homosexuality, alcoholism, psychopathy and criminality. *Archives of Criminal Psychodynamics, 4,* 599–646.

Kendell, R. E. (1989). Clinical validity. *Psychological Medicine, 19,* 45–55.

Kernberg, O. F. (1998). The psychotherapeutic management of psychopathic, narcissistic, and paranoid transferences. In T. Millon, E. Simonsen, M. Birket-Smith, & R. D. Davis (Eds.), *Psychopathy: antisocial, criminal and violent behavior* (pp. 372–392). New York: Guilford Press.

Lilienfeld, S. O. (1994). Conceptual problems in the assessment of psychopathy. *Clinical Psychology Review, 14,* 17–38.

Lilienfeld, S. O. (1998). Methodological advances and developments in the assessment of psychopathy. *Behaviour Research and Therapy, 36,* 99–125.

Livesley, W. J., Jackson, D. N., & Schroeder, M. (1992). Factorial structure of traits delineating personality disorders in clinical and general population samples. *Journal of Abnormal Psychology, 101,* 432–440.

Malamuth, N., & Brown, A. J. (1994). Sexually aggressive men's perceptions of women's communications: Testing three explanations. *Journal of Personality and Social Psychology, 67,* 699–712.

McCord, W., & McCord, J. (1964). *The psychopath: An essay on the criminal mind.* Princeton, NJ: Van Nostrand.

McCrae, R. R., & Costa, P. T. (1995). Trait explanations in personality psychology. *European Journal of Personality, 9,* 231–252.

McDermott, P. A., Alterman, A. I., Cacciola, J. S., Rutherford, M. J., Newman, J. P., & Mulholland, E. M. (2000). Generality of Psychopathy Checklist—Revised factors over prisoners and substance-dependent patients. *Journal of Consulting and Clinical Psychology, 68,* 181–186.

Meloy, J. R. (1988). *The psychopathic mind: Origins, dynamics, and treatments.* Northvale, NJ: Jason Aronson.

Millon, T. (1981). *Disorders of personality.* New York: Wiley.

Murphy, J. M. (1976). Psychiatric labeling in cross-cultural perspective: Similar kinds of disturbed behavior appear to be labeled abnormal in diverse cultures. *Science, 191,* 1019–1028.

Post, R. S. (1968). The relationship of tattoos to personality disorder. *Journal of Criminal Law, Criminology and Police Science, 59,* 516–524s.

Poythress, N. G., Edens, J. F., & Lilienfeld, S. O. (1999). Criterion related validity of the psychopathic personality inventory in a prison sample. *Psychological Assessment, 10,* 426–430.

Pedhazur, E. J., & Schmelkin, L. P. (1991). *Measurement, design, and analysis: An integrated approach.* Hillsdale, NJ: Erlbaum.

Raine, A., Lencz, T., Bihrle, S., LaCasse, L., & Colletti, P. (2000). Reduced prefrontal gray matter volume and reduced autonomic activity in antisocial personality disorder. *Archives of General Psychiatry, 57,* 119–127.

Robins, E., & Guze, S. B. (1970). Establishment of diagnostic validity in psychiatric illness: Its application to schizophrenia. *American Journal of Psychiatry, 126,* 983–987.

Rogers, R., & Dion, K. L. (1991). Rethinking the DSM-III-R diagnosis of antisocial personality disorder. *Bulletin of the American Academy of Psychiatry and Law, 19,* 21–31.

Schneider, K. (1950). *Psychopathic personalities.* London: Cassell.

Serin, R. C. (1991). Psychopathy and violence in criminals. *Journal of Interpersonal Violence, 6,* 423–431.

Shadish, W. R., Cook, T. D., & Campbell, D. T. (1999). *Experimental and quasi-experimental designs for generalized causal inference.* Boston: Houghton Mifflin.

Skeem, J. L., Mulvey, E. P., & Grisso, T. (2003). Applicability of the traditional and revised models of psychopathy to the Psychopathy Checklist: Screening Version (PCL:SV). *Psychological Assessment, 15,* 41–55.

Smith, G. T., Fischer, S., & Fister, S. (2003). Incremental validity principles in test construction. *Psychological Assessment, 15,* 467–477.

Soderstrom, H., Hultin, L., Tullberg, M., Wikkelso, C., Ekholm, S., & Forsman, A. (2002). Reduced frontotemporal perfusion in psychopathic personality. *Psychiatry Research Neuroimaging, 114,* 81–94.

Toch, H. (1998). Psychopathy or antisocial personality in forensic settings. In T. Millon, E. Simonsen, M. Birket-Smith, & R. D. Davies (Eds.), *Psychopathy, antisocial, criminal and violent behavior* (pp. 144–158). New York: Guilford Press.

Van de Vijver, F. J., & Leung, K. (1997). *Methods and data analysis for cross-cultural research.* Thousand Oaks, CA: Sage.

Verona, E., Patrick, C. J., & Joiner, T. E. (2001). Psychopathy, antisocial personality, and suicide risk. *Journal of Abnormal Psychology, 110,* 462–470.

Vincent, G. M. (2002). *The legitimacy of psychopathy assessments in young offenders: Contributions of item response theory* Unpublished doctoral thesis, Simon Fraser University, Burnaby, BC, Canada.

Vincent, G. M., & Hart, S. D. (2002). Psychopathy in childhood and adolescence: Implications for the assessment and management of multi-problem youths. In R. R. Corrado, R. Roesch, S. D. Hart, & J. K. Gierowski (Eds.), *Multi-problem violent youth* (pp. 150–163). Amsterdam: IOS Press.

Waller, N. G., Thompson, J. S., & Wenk, E. (2000). Using IRT to separate measurement bias from true group difference on homogenous *and* heterogeneous scales: An illustration with the MMPI. *Psychological Methods, 5,* 125–146.

Warren, J., Burnette, M., South, S. C., Chauhan, R. B., Friend, R., & Van Patten, I. (2003). Psychopathy in women: structural thinking and comorbidity. *International Journal of Law and Psychiatry, 372,* 1–21.

Watson, D., Clark, L. A., & Harkness, A. R. (1994). Structures of personality and their relevance to psychopathology. *Journal of Abnormal Psychology, 103,* 18–31.

Wechsler, D. (1997). *Wechsler Adult Intelligence Scale—Third edition.* San Antonio, TX: Psychological Corporation.

Widiger, T. A., Cadoret, R., Hare, R. D., Robins, L. N., Rutherford, M. J., Zanarini, M., et al. (1996). DSM-IV antisocial personality disorder field trial. *Journal of Abnormal Psychology, 105,* 3–16.

Widiger, T. A. E., & Lynam, D. R. (1998). Psychopathy and the five-factor model of personality. In T. Millon, E. Simonsen, M. Birket-Smith, & R. D. Davies (Eds.), *Psychopathy: Antisocial, criminal and violent behavior* (pp. 171–187). New York: Guilford Press.

World Health Organization. (1992). *The ICD-10 classification of mental and behavioural disorders: Clinical descriptions and diagnostic guidelines.* Geneva: Author.

Zinbarg, R. E., Barlow, D. H., & Brown, T. A. (1997). Hierarchical structure and general factor saturation of the anxiety sensitivity index: Evidence and implications. *Psychological Assessment, 9,* 277–284.

6

The Self-Report Assessment of Psychopathy

Problems, Pitfalls, and Promises

SCOTT O. LILIENFELD
KATHERINE A. FOWLER

The idea of detecting psychopaths by asking them about themselves surely strikes many readers as paradoxical. After all, why would one attempt to identify a condition marked by dishonesty by asking individuals to respond honestly to questions regarding this condition? To many, the enterprise seems pointless, doomed utterly to failure. Yet the self-report assessment of psychopathy has a lengthy, albeit checkered, history. Moreover, despite lingering controversies and serious setbacks over the past few decades, it appears to be experiencing a renaissance. Notwithstanding a host of potential pitfalls (Lilienfeld, 1994, 1998), the use of questionnaires to detect psychopathy may prove considerably more fruitful than once believed.

GOALS OF THE CHAPTER

In this chapter, we review the conceptual and methodological challenges confronting the assessment of psychopathy by means of self-report. We begin by examining the advantages and disadvantages of self-report measures in the assessment of psychopathy and dispelling several widespread misconceptions regarding the use of self-report mea-

sures to assess psychopathy. We next discuss long-standing problems that plague the questionnaire assessment of psychopathy and revisit the shortcomings of older, but still commonly administered, self-report measures that purportedly assess psychopathy. We then survey the contemporary status of self-report psychopathy measures with an emphasis on their psychometric properties, research and clinical uses, and limitations. We conclude with a clarion call for further research on several undeservedly neglected topics concerning the self-report assessment of psychopathy.

ADVANTAGES OF SELF-REPORT MEASURES IN THE ASSESSMENT OF PSYCHOPATHY

The Self as Observer

As the great American psychologist Gordon Allport observed, the self is in a privileged position with respect to its own mental status. For Allport (1961), the self is the "warm, central, private region of our life" (p. 110). As a consequence, self-report measures may be of particular utility in the assessment of subjective emotional states and traits. With respect to psychopathy, the relative *absence* of such states and traits, such as guilt, empathy, fear, and feelings of intimacy toward others, is probably most diagnostically relevant. Nevertheless, psychopaths may experience certain emotions, such as alienation and anger, more frequently than do nonpsychopaths.

Moreover, self-reports of personality converge with reports from others. Self-ratings of personality traits tend to concur moderately with ratings of personality traits by knowledgeable observers (r = .30 to .50), with agreement typically being higher for more observable traits (e.g., extraversion) than for less unobservable traits (e.g., neuroticism) (Kendrick & Funder, 1988). Nevertheless, the substantial amount of nonshared variance between self and observer ratings of personality introduces the possibility that each information source possesses incremental validity (Meehl, 1959; Sechrest, 1963) above and beyond the other for predicting psychologically important variables. For example, self-reports may be especially useful for detecting affects and enduring affective dispositions (see Grove & Tellegen, 1991), although this possibility has received surprisingly scant research attention.

Economy

A second and more self-evident advantage of using self-reports to detect psychopathy is economy. Self-report measures tend to be brief and easy to complete, and they require minimal training on the part of test administrators. In this respect, they stand in sharp contrast to the Psychopathy Checklist—Revised (PCL-R; Hare, 1991), a lengthy (e.g., 90-minute) semistructured interview for psychopathy that requires access to file information and extensive interviewing training. As discussed in several chapters in this book, the PCL-R has increasingly come to be regarded as the "gold standard" in psychopathy research (e.g., Fulero, 1995), although it should be recalled that genuine gold standards are probably unattainable in the domain of personality and psychopathology (Cronbach & Meehl, 1955; Faraone & Tsuang, 1994). Because the PCL-R is time- and labor-intensive, research on psychopathy in institutional settings has often been difficult to conduct (Lilienfeld, 1994). Moreover, because the PCL-R requires access to

corroborative information, much research on psychopathy in noninstitutional (e.g., college and community) settings has similarly run afoul of logistical roadblocks.

Assessment of Response Styles

A third and often unappreciated advantage of self-report measures is that they can assess response styles systematically (Widiger & Frances, 1987). In this respect, they are advantageous in comparison with interviews, virtually none of which (the PCL-R included) contain well-constructed and carefully normed response-style indicators. Certain response styles, such as positive impression management and malingering, may be particularly problematic among psychopaths (Hart, Hare, & Harpur, 1992; Lilienfeld, 1994). Although such response styles may adversely affect the validity of psychopaths' self-reports, questionnaires can help to detect such response styles by means of validity scales (see Paulhus, 1991, for a review).

Reliability

Finally, it perhaps goes without saying that interrater reliability is not even a consideration for self-report measures, because these measures are completed by respondents and do not require "judgment calls" by interviewers or other observers. It is worth noting that many of the core features of psychopathy, such as lack of empathy and guiltlessness, require considerable clinical inference on the part of observers and therefore are unlikely to achieve anywhere near perfect interrater reliability. Because validity is limited by the square root of reliability (Meehl, 1986), the subjectivity inherent to interview-based measures will, *ceteris paribus*, constrain their validity.

Summary

In summary, self-report measures possess several advantages in the assessment of psychopathy. They may yield useful information regarding the absence of affective states and traits, they are economical and easily administered, and they permit the systematic detection of response styles that may be especially problematic among psychopaths, namely, positive impression management and malingering. In addition, the validity of self-report measures is not constrained by low interrater reliability. Nevertheless, as seen in the following section, it is unclear whether these advantages outweigh several potential disadvantages.

DISADVANTAGES OF SELF-REPORT MEASURES IN THE ASSESSMENT OF PSYCHOPATHY

Dishonesty

The first disadvantage of using self-reports to detect psychopathy is obvious: Psychopaths lie frequently. Moreover, psychopaths' notorious dishonesty is not limited to situations in which they can obtain tangible benefits. Instead, psychopaths frequently lie for the sheer fun of it, a phenomenon that Ekman (1985) termed "duping delight." Psychopaths also lie with impunity and with minimal guilt or anxiety. As Cleckley (1941/ 1988) noted:

> The psychopath shows a remarkable disregard for truth and is to be trusted no more in his accounts of the past than in his promises for the future of his statement of present intentions. . . . Typically he is at ease and unpretentious in making a serious promise or in (falsely) exculpating himself from accusations, whether grave or trivial. (p. 341)

Although such lying on questionnaires may sometimes be detected by response style indicators, many of these indicators, such as the Lie scale of the Minnesota Multiphasic Personality Inventory, second edition (MMPI-2), tend to be insensitive to subtle or sophisticated forms of impression management (Greene, 2000; Kroger & Turnbull, 1975; Vincent, Linsz, & Greene, 1966).

Making matters worse, the nature of psychopaths' lying may depend largely on situational demands and therefore cannot be readily predicted without knowledge of contextual variables. That is, if psychopaths are placed in a situation in which crafting a positive impression is desirable (e.g., applying for a job) they may attempt to make themselves look good, whereas if they are placed in a situation in which crafting a negative impression is desirable (e.g., being evaluated for an insanity plea) they may attempt to make themselves look bad.

In some cases, psychopaths' prevarication on self-report measures reaches remarkable proportions. Hare (1985) described such a case:

> To take what admittedly is an extreme example, 1 inmate (a classic psychopath by any criterion) confided (and we were able to verify) that he had his own MMPI manual, a set of scoring keys, and several books on the clinical interpretation of the MMPI. As a result, he was able to produce a given type of profile on demand, not only for himself but also for other inmates. For the latter, he operated his own consulting service, advising inmates on how they should respond to certain types of items in order to obtain the "appropriate" MMPI profile. (pp. 15–16)

Although we suspect that such cases are rare, it seems likely that psychopaths who are motivated to create a specific impression on questionnaires will exhibit scant compunction about acquiring the information needed to do so.

Lack of Insight

Second, psychopaths often lack insight into the nature and extent of their psychological problems. In his discussion of psychopaths' "specific loss of insight," Cleckley (1941/ 1988) went so far as to conjecture that

> in the sense of realistic evaluation, the psychopath lacks insight more consistently than some schizophrenic patients. He has absolutely no capacity to see himself as others see him. It is perhaps more accurate to say that he has no ability to know how others feel when they see him or to experience subjectively anything comparable about the situation. (p. 350)

The glaring inability—or at least failure—of many psychopaths to perceive themselves as others perceive them may limit the usefulness of certain self-report items, especially those that require at least a modicum of accurate knowledge regarding the impact of their behavior on others.

As a consequence, observers may be superior to psychopathic individuals when reporting on certain overt behaviors and their consequences. Grove and Tellegen (1991) argued that observer reports may be especially useful for detecting "blind spots" among individuals with ego-syntonic personality disorders, that is, personality disorders that are consistent with the self-concept. Psychopathy, which is marked by a striking absence of awareness into the impact of one's actions on others, is in many respects the quintessential ego-syntonic personality disorder.

One can conceptualize the potential disadvantages and advantages of self-report measures of psychopathy and related conditions by means of the *Johari window* (named, curiously enough, after the first names of its developers Joseph Luft and Harry Ingham) which schematically represents the four major "regions" of personality as perceived by both self and observers (Luft, 1969; see Figure 6.1). This window consists of four cells: the region of personality known to both self and others (the "open" quadrant), the region of personality known to the self but not others (the "hidden" quadrant), the region of personality known to others but not the self (the "blind" quadrant), and finally, and perhaps most interesting, the region of personality known to neither self nor others (the "unknown" quadrant). Observer reports are potentially of particular utility in assessing the blind quadrant, where others can report on attributes that psychopaths are either unable or unwilling to report.

Semantic Aphasia

Third, it may be inherently problematic to ask individuals who have never experienced an emotion (or who have experienced only weak variants of this emotion) to report on its absence. As George Kelly (1955) observed, a full understanding of a dimension requires an appreciation of both of its poles. For example, the experience of "cold" has

no subjective meaning unless one has experienced heat. Similarly, asking psychopaths to report on the absence of guilt may be fruitless given that they have had scant experience with its presence.

Taking this argument a step further, Cleckley (1941/1988; see also Hare, 1993) speculated that the core deficit in psychopathy is analogous to the brain syndrome of "semantic aphasia," a condition that ostensibly leads them to mislabel affective experiences. According to Cleckley (1941/1988), "just as meaning and the adequate sense of things as a whole are lost with semantic aphasia in the circumscribed field of speech although the technical mimicry of language remains intact, so in most psychopaths the purposiveness and the significance of all life-striving and of all subjective experience are affected without obvious damage to the outer appearance or superficial reactions of the personality" (p. 383). Cleckley therefore viewed psychopathy as akin to color-blindness. Just as color-blind individuals often learn to refer to apples as red and leaves as green because they are aware of the verbal labels attached to natural objects, psychopaths may erroneously learn to label certain emotions as "guilt" or "fear" even though they have never experienced them. For example, they may learn to refer to "guilt" when they experience negative affect after committing an antisocial act and receiving punishment for it, even though they are actually experiencing regret (displeasure upon getting caught) rather than remorse. From this perspective, psychopaths' reporting of many emotions may be inaccurate but not insincere.

Saturation with Negative Emotionality

Fourth, many self-report measures of psychopathology are heavily saturated with Negative Emotionality (NE), a pervasive higher-order personality dimension reflecting a disposition to experience negative affects of many kinds, including anxiety, irritability, hostility, and mistrust. Indeed, one of the great challenges in constructing self-report measures of psychopathology is to develop questionnaires that are not saturated with NE (Finney, 1985; Tellegen, 1985). The substantial saturation of many self-report

	known to self	not known to self
known to others	OPEN	BLIND
not known to others	HIDDEN	UNKNOWN

FIGURE 6.1. The Johari window conceptualizes personality as a multilayered construct, with quadrants representing combinations of self and other awareness (Luft, 1969).

psychopathology measures with NE reduces their discriminant validity, because NE courses through many psychiatric conditions, including mood disorders, anxiety disorders, psychotic disorders, eating disorders, and somatoform disorders (Watson & Clark, 1984). Although one might expect measures of psychopathy to be largely independent of NE, many measures designed to detect psychopathy, such as the MMPI-2 Psychopathic deviate (Pd) scale, are substantially contaminated by NE (Lilienfeld, 1994). This is especially true of self-report measures that assess the antisocial lifestyle and impulsive behaviors associated with psychopathy (e.g., Harpur, Hare, & Hakstian, 1989).

Summary

In summary, there are several reasons to be skeptical regarding the use of self-report measures in the assessment of psychopathy. Psychopaths lie frequently, and their dishonesty may extend to responses on psychological tests. Psychopaths also lack insight into the nature and extent of their psychological problems. Moreover, because they have not experienced certain affective states (e.g., guilt and empathy) they may be unable to report accurately on their absence. In addition, many self-report measures designed to assess psychopathy are heavily saturated with NE, reducing their discriminant validity for distinguishing psychopathy from a motley assortment of other conditions marked by antisocial behavior.

The problems highlighted in this section have led some authors to conclude that self-report measures may be inherently ill-suited for assessing psychopathy. For example, Edens, Hart, Johnson, Johnson, and Olver (2000) contended that the use of questionnaires to detect psychopathy may be an example of a "method-mode mismatch" (see Haynes, Richard, & Kubany, 1995) resulting from the use of a method, in this case, self-report, that is not optimal for the assessment of a construct, in this case psychopathy. As we argue later in the chapter, method-mode mismatch remains a viable hypothesis for the less than stellar psychometric showing of some self-report measures of psychopathy, but alternative hypotheses have yet to be excluded.

MISCONCEPTIONS AND MISUNDERSTANDINGS REGARDING THE SELF-REPORT ASSESSMENT OF PSYCHOPATHY

Although several of the disadvantages of self-report psychopathy measures raise important questions regarding their validity, we would be remiss not to address three misconceptions that have found their way into the psychopathy literature. These misconceptions have led to misunderstandings regarding the potential uses and misuses of questionnaires for detecting psychopathy and have led some authors to prematurely discount the potential value of self-reports in the assessment of this condition.

The Requirement of Veridical Responding

The first misconception regarding self-report measures is that their validity hinges on the assumption of veridical responding (Lilienfeld, 1994). This misconception has led some to question whether self-reports can be useful in the assessment of psychopathy given that psychopaths' dishonesty and lack of insight presumably lead to inaccurate responding. But as Meehl (1945) noted, the responses to self-report items can be conceptualized as interesting samples of verbal behavior in their own right. These responses may or may not be factually accurate, but they can offer diagnostically helpful information regarding respondents' apperceptions of themselves and the world.

For example, consider the item, "I often get blamed for things that aren't my fault," which appears on the Psychopathic Personality Inventory (PPI; Lilienfeld & Andrews, 1996), a self-report measure of psychopathy discussed later. A "true" response to this item is a valid indicator of psychopathy, even though it is unlikely to be factually accurate. After all, most psychopaths are probably not blamed nearly enough for things that go wrong in their lives, and those things that do go wrong are typically their fault! Nevertheless, this item provides useful information regarding psychopaths' well-known propensity to externalize blame (Hare, 1991) and to perceive others as malevolent (Millon, 1981). Similarly, the item "I can read people like a book," which appears on the Self-

Report Psychopathy Scale (see Hare, 1985), is a valid indicator of the narcissism associated with psychopathy, although it is not at all clear that psychopathic individuals' interpersonal perception skills are better than those of nonpsychopathic individuals. In fact, the admittedly limited research literature on this question suggests that they are probably not (Morgan, 2000; Stevens, Charman, & Blair, 2001).

Propensity toward Positive Impression Management

A second misconception is that psychopaths consistently engage in positive impression management on self-report measures. In fact, self-report measures of psychopathy tend to be slightly or moderately *negatively* correlated with indices of social desirability and positive impression management (e.g., Hare, 1982; Lilienfeld & Andrews, 1996; Ray & Ray, 1982). Although perhaps puzzling, this finding is understandable given that psychopathic individuals' behaviors and personality traits tend to be socially undesirable. Moreover, one might conjecture that psychopaths possess a different conception of what is socially undesirable compared with the average person; for example, they may perceive as "normal" antisocial behaviors that others perceive as undesirable. This negative correlation suggests that psychopaths often report accurately on the presence of socially devalued characteristics, such as antisocial behaviors, recklessness, hostility, and poor impulse control (Lilienfeld, 1994). It should also be borne in mind that response style measures, such as self-report lie scales, are not entirely independent of trait variance (Paulhus, 1991; Piedmont, McCrae, Reimann, & Angleitner, 2000). As a consequence, extreme (either high or low) scores on these scales are probably heterogeneous in origin, as they reflect genuine variance relevant to personality and psychopathology on the part of most respondents in addition to conscious dissimulation on the part of others.

Aptitude for Malingering

A third misconception is that psychopaths are particularly skilled at manipulating their responses to self-report measures. So, this reasoning goes, their responses are even more untrustworthy than those of nonpsychopathic dissimulators. Nevertheless, there is no evidence supporting this claim and at least some preliminary evidence against it. Edens, Buffington, and Tomicic (2000) asked 143 college students to take the PPI, which as noted earlier is a self-report measure of psychopathy, under two conditions: honestly and with instructions to malinger psychosis. They found that PPI scores were not significantly related to malingering success, as measured by scores on a malingering index containing "bogus" symptoms of psychosis. Nevertheless, PPI scores were significantly and positively correlated with willingness to malinger, as well as self-perceived ability to malinger a mental disorder. Therefore, although psychopaths may be more inclined than nonpsychopaths to malinger on psychological tests when it is in their best interests (Rogers et al., 2002), there is no evidence that they are especially adept at doing so (see Poythress, Edens, & Watkins, 2002, for similar conclusions using a correlational design).

LONG-STANDING EMPIRICAL PROBLEMS IN THE SELF-REPORT ASSESSMENT OF PSYCHOPATHY

Until fairly recently, the self-report assessment of psychopathy was regarded by many as a deeply troubled endeavor (e.g., Hare, 1985; Hart et al., 1992), perhaps even a hopeless morass. In particular, this field was bedeviled by three major empirical problems. As we will see, these problems persist even to the present day, although there has been promising progress toward their resolution.

Low Correlations among Psychopathy Questionnaires

First, the results of several early studies indicated that questionnaires designed to assess psychopathy were weakly or at best negligibly intercorrelated. Such findings suggest that these measures assess only slightly overlapping aspects of the same construct, and that putatively comparable measures of psychopathy are by no means interchangeable.

For example, Hundleby and Ross (1977) administered the Activity Preference Questionnaire (Lykken, Tellegen, & Katzenmeyer, 1973), a measure of fearfulness found previously to distinguish psychopaths from nonpsychopaths (Lykken, 1957; see also Lilienfeld & Andrews, 1996), the Eysenck Personality Inventory (Eysenck & Eysenck, 1964), the MMPI (Hathaway & McKinley, 1940), the Sensation-Seeking Scale (SSS; Zuckerman, Kolin, Price, & Zoob, 1964), and the Personal Opinion Study (Quay & Parsons, 1971) to 397 male adult prison inmates. They found low intercorrelations among these self-report measures. In addition, they found that no general factor corresponding to psychopathy emerged in lower-order factor analyses. Nevertheless, other work has demonstrated that several of the questionnaires they administered, such as Eysenck's extraversion scale and numerous MMPI scales, are only peripherally relevant to psychopathy. Moreover, Hundleby and Ross did not conduct a higher-order factor analysis to determine whether a higher-order psychopathy dimension would emerge from their lower-order factors. Given that Cleckley (1941/1988), Hare (1991), and other authors have argued that psychopathy comprises a variety of personality traits, there is no reason to expect a single psychopathy factor to emerge at the lower-order level.

More compelling evidence comes from a study by Hare (1985), who administered a number of self-report measures, including the MMPI Pd scale and Hypomania (Ma) scales, Gough's (1960) California Psychological Inventory (CPI) Socialization (So) scale (see also Kosson, Steuerwald, Newman, & Widom, 1994), which is often scored in reverse as a measure of psychopathy, and the Self-Report Psychopathy (SRP) scale, to 274 male adult prison inmates. In addition, trained raters completed a number of clinical–behavioral assessments, including the Psychopathy Checklist and a measure of the DSM-III (American Psychiatric Association, 1980) criteria for antisocial personality disorder (APD). Like Hundleby and Ross, Hare found low or at best moderate correlations among the self-report measures, with the absolute value of the correlations ranging from .14 to .53. Moreover, some measures previously viewed as virtually interchangeable shared little variance; for example, the MMPI Pd scale and So scale were correlated only $r = -.34$.

Widom and Newman (1985) reported somewhat more promising results. They recruited 40 participants from the Bloomington, Indiana, community using a newspaper advertisement that featured many of the Cleckley (1941/1988) characteristics of psychopathy framed in socially desirable language. For example, part of the advertisement requested "adventurous, carefree people who've led exciting impulsive lives" (p. 58). Widom and Newman administered a variety of self-report (including the MMPI Pd scale and Gough's So scale) and interview (including the Robins's, 1966, criteria for sociopathy and the Research Diagnostic Criteria [RDC] for APD) measures relevant to psychopathy and antisocial behavior. The absolute values of these correlations were higher than reported by Hare (1985), and ranged from $r = .43$ to .89. Moreover, in contrast to Hare, the MMPI Pd scale and So scale were correlated $r = -.78$. The reason for the discrepancy across studies is unclear; they are not attributable to differences in variance because the variances of the Pd and So scales in Hare's study were actually larger than in Widom and Newman's study. Nevertheless, Widom and Newman found that the correlations between the MMPI Pd scale and other measures were below $r = .5$.

The Role of Method Covariance

Although the correlations among self-report measures of psychopathy are often low or modest, even these correlations may partly reflect method variance arising from the shared use of a self-report format.

In the study mentioned in the previous section, Hare (1985) conducted a principal components analysis of the self-report and clinical–behavioral measures administered to prison inmates. This analysis yielded a two-component solution that accounted for 71.5% of the variance among measures. Distressingly, these two components appeared to reflect method variance rather than content variance. Specifically, the first component was marked by high loadings on the clinical–behavioral measures, whereas the second component was marked by high loadings on the self-report measures. The content of the scales appeared to exert little impact on the pattern of intercorrelations. For example, even though the PCL and

DSM-III criteria for APD ostensibly assess different constructs (psychopathy versus APD, respectively; see Hare, 1991; Lilienfeld, 1994), they loaded more highly with each other than with self-report measures ostensibly assessing the same construct.

Widom and Newman (1985) reported roughly comparable results in the study reported in the previous section. Specifically, they found that the absolute value of the correlation between the MMPI Pd Scale and CPI So scale, was high (as noted above, $r = -.78$) as was the correlation between Robins's (1966) criteria for sociopathy and the RDC criteria for APD ($r = .89$). In contrast, the absolute values of correlations between these two sets of measures (questionnaires and interviews, respectively) were lower, ranging from $r = .43$ to .57. Although Widom and Newman did not test the differences in correlations against each other, we performed such tests and found that, with the exception of the correlation between the Robins criteria and So scale (absolute $r = .67$), the cross-method correlations were significantly ($p < .05$) lower than the within-method correlations. These findings again suggest the possibility of method covariance between both self-report measures and interview measures, although one cannot exclude the rival hypothesis that assessment mode (i.e., self-report vs. interview) was confounded with substantive content (e.g., item coverage of the core affective and interpersonal features psychopathy versus the antisocial and impulsive lifestyle sometimes associated with psychopathy).

Nonspecific Measures of Behavioral Deviance

Another shortcoming of many self-report psychopathy measures is that they appear primarily to be nonspecific measures of behavioral deviance, that is, global antisocial and criminal behavior, rather than measures of the core affective and interpersonal features of psychopathy, such as guiltlessness, callousness, lovelessness, and egocentricity.

In one of the first studies to address this issue, Harpur and colleagues (1989) examined the correlations of the two major PCL factors with several self-report indices relevant to psychopathy, including the MMPI Pd and Ma scales, the So scale, the Eysenck Personality Questionnaire Psychoticism scale (Eysenck & Eysenck, 1975), the SSS, and the SRP. The correlations of these questionnaires with PCL Factor II, which assesses an antisocial and impulsive lifestyle, were moderately high and were generally in the $r = .3$ to .5 range. In contrast, the correlations of these questionnaires with PCL Factor I, which assesses the core affective and interpersonal features of psychopathy, were negligible to low, and were generally in the $r = .05$ to .15 range. Perhaps most surprisingly, two of the most frequently administered self-report measures of psychopathy (Hare & Cox, 1978), the MMPI Pd scale and the So scale, correlated with PCL Factor I at only $r = .05$ and $-.06$, respectively (this latter correlation, albeit minimal, is in the expected direction, as lower So scores are ostensibly related to higher psychopathy).

Of all major self-report measures examined by Harpur and colleagues (1989), the two that fared "best" were the SRP and the addition of the MMPI Pd and Ma scales, both of which correlated only $r = .18$ with the PCL Factor I (see also Gynther, Altman, & Warbin, 1973, who found that psychiatric inpatients with the MMPI Pd-Ma codetype reported significantly *more* guilt feelings than other inpatients, perhaps reflecting the heavy saturation of this codetype with NE, and Hare & Cox, 1978, who reported that the MMPI Pd-Ma codetype did not distinguish between inmates with high and low global ratings of psychopathy). Harpur et al.'s findings suggest that several widely used self-report measures of psychopathy, including the MMPI Pd scale, are largely unrelated to the core personality features of this condition (see also Hawk & Peterson, 1973; Lovering & Douglas, 2004). Instead, these measures appear to be markers of behavioral deviance, which do not distinguish psychopathy from a variety of other conditions often associated with antisocial and criminal behavior (see Lykken, 1995, for a discussion).

Several investigators have reported similar results for other self-report measures that ostensibly assess psychopathy or closely allied constructs. In a sample of 119 male prison inmates, Hart, Forth, and Hare (1991) found that Scales 6A (Antisocial) and 6B (Aggressive/Sadistic) of the Millon Clinical Multiaxial Inventory—II (MCMI-II; Millon,

1987) were more highly correlated with Factor II of ($r = .51$ and $.34$, respectively) than with Factor I ($r = .24$ and $.28$), respectively, of the PCL-R. With the exception of the correlation between Scale 6A and Factor I, all of these correlations were statistically significant. Hart et al. did not report partial correlations examining the associations between Scales 6A and 6B with each PCL-R factor controlling for the influence of the other factor. Nevertheless, their findings indicate that the two MCMI-II scales ostensibly most relevant to psychopathy are only weakly related to the core interpersonal and affective features of this condition.

In an investigation of 46 forensic psychiatric inpatients, Edens, Hart, and colleagues (2000) found that the Antisocial (ANT) scale of the Personality Assessment Inventory (PAI; Morey, 1991) correlated moderately ($r = .44$) with Factor I of the Psychopathy Checklist: Screening Version (PCL:SV; Hart, Cox, & Hare, 1995), although the correlation with Factor II was somewhat higher ($r = .56$). Nevertheless, after controlling statistically for scores on the other PCL:SV factor, the ANT scale was nonsignificantly correlated with Factor I ($r = .07$) but significantly correlated with Factor II ($r = .39$). These findings suggest that the ANT scale is moderately related to Factor I traits, although this association is largely attributable to the overlap between Factors I and II. A second investigation by Edens, Hart, and colleagues yielded even less promising findings for the PAI ANT scale. In a sample of 55 sex offenders, they found that the ANT scale was nonsignificantly correlated ($r = .07$) with PCL-R Factor I, but moderately related to PCL-R Factor II ($r = .53$). After controlling for the influence of the other factor, the correlation with Factor I became negative ($r = -.17$) whereas the correlation with Factor II remained virtually identical ($r = .54$) (see Lovering & Douglas, 2004, for similar findings).

Summary

The self-report assessment of psychopathy has been plagued by three enduring empirical problems. Questionnaires designed to assess psychopathy and cognate constructs frequently exhibit low or modest intercorrelations, indicating that they are not fungible indices of the same construct. In addition, the correlations among psychopathy questionnaires may be inflated by shared method variance arising from the use of a self-report format, although the extent to which this format is confounded with substantive content (e.g., relative emphasis on the core affective and interpersonal features of psychopathy vs. antisocial behaviors) is unclear. It is worth noting, however, that the problem of method covariance is not unique to self-report measures and may be equally problematic for interview-based measures of psychopathy. Finally, most commonly used self-report indices of psychopathy, including the MMPI Pd scale, CPI So scale, MCMI-II Antisocial scale, and PAI Antisocial scale, are related preferentially to Factor II rather to than Factor I of the PCL and its variants, suggesting that they are measures of nonspecific behavioral deviance rather than of the core interpersonal and affective features of psychopathy (e.g., guiltlessness and callousness) delineated by Cleckley (1941/1988) and others.

PROMISING NEW SELF-REPORT MEASURES OF PSYCHOPATHY

The shortcomings of extant psychopathy questionnaires have led several investigators to develop new self-report measures in the hopes of remedying these problems. As we will see, the extent to which these investigators have been successful remains a matter of debate.

In this section, we review the psychometric status, strengths, and weaknesses of three recently developed self-report measures of psychopathy, the Levenson Primary and Secondary Psychopathy scales (Levenson, Kiehl, & Fitzpatrick, 1995), the SRP (see Hare, 1985) and its revisions, the SRP-II and SRP-III, and the PPI (Lilienfeld, 1990; Lilienfeld & Widows, 2005). We have elected to focus on these three measures because (1) they were designed at least in part to remedy the shortcomings of previously developed psychopathy measures (e.g., the MMPI Pd scale), (2) they were designed to be measures of psychopathy *per se* as opposed to generalized behavioral deviance (cf. the MMPI-2 Antisocial Practices scale; Butcher, Graham, Williams, & Ben-Porath, 1990; Lilienfeld,

1996), and (3) they have been examined in a number of published studies.

We have elected not to examine self-report measures of psychopathy in children given that (1) the status of the childhood psychopathy construct is highly controversial (Edens, Skeem, Cruise, & Kauffman, 2001; Johnstone & Cooke, 2004; see also Salekin, Chapter 20, this volume), and (2) the evidence regarding the psychometric properties of self-report measures of childhood psychopathy is highly preliminary (see Poythress et al., 2004). We have also elected not to examine self-report measures of adult psychopathy and related constructs that are inadequately researched, such as the MMPI-based Sociopathy scale (Spielberger, Kling, & O'Hagan, 1978), the Psychopathic State Inventory (Haertzen, Martin, Ross, & Niedert, 1980), Levenson's Psychopathy Scale (Levenson, 1990), the Social Psychopathy Scale (Edelmann & Vivian, 1988; Smith, 1985), or the Antisocial Personality Questionnaire (Blackburn & Fawcett, 1999).

Levenson Primary and Secondary Psychopathy Scales

Construction

The Levenson Primary and Secondary Psychopathy scales (LPSP) were developed by Levenson and colleagues (1995) to detect self-reported psychopathic features in noninstitutional samples. They consist of 26 items in a 1–4 Likert-type format. The Primary and Secondary scales of the LPSP were rationally constructed to provide indices of PCL-R Factors I and II, respectively. As predicted, Levenson et al.'s exploratory factor analyses revealed a two-factor structure that appeared to parallel the two factors of the PCL-R.

Following from the classic writings of Karpman (1948), Levenson and colleagues hypothesized that PCL-R Factor I is primarily a marker of "primary" (Cleckley) psychopathy, whereas PCL-R Factor II is primarily a marker of "secondary" psychopathy. The latter, which can be thought of as "pseudopsychopathy," is presumably a heterogeneous mélange of conditions (Lykken, 1995) characterized largely by elevated neuroticism and impulsivity, as well as intact interpersonal relationships and loyalty toward others. Therefore, Levenson and colleagues reasoned, the LPSP Primary and Secondary Psychopathy scales can be differentiated on the basis of trait anxiety, with high scorers on the former scale being low in trait anxiety and high scorers on the latter scale being high in trait anxiety. A representative item from the Primary Psychopathy Scale is "Looking out for myself is my top priority," whereas a representative item from the Secondary Psychopathy Scale is "I am often bored."

Psychometric Properties

In an investigation of 487 undergraduates, Levenson and colleagues (1995) reported that the LPSP Primary Psychopathy Scale exhibited adequate internal consistency (Cronbach's alpha = .82), although the internal consistency of the Secondary Psychopathy scale was marginal (Cronbach's alpha = .63). Moreover, these two scales were moderately correlated ($r = .40$). The interpretation of this correlation is unclear. On the one hand, this correlation may support the convergent validity of the LPSP Primary and Secondary Psychopathy scales if one assumes that each scale is a lower-order marker of a higher-order psychopathy dimension. On the other hand, this correlation may call into question the discriminant validity of the LPSP Primary and Secondary Psychopathy scales given that Karpman (1948) regarded primary and secondary psychopathy to be etiologically distinct, perhaps even negatively correlated, conditions. Levenson and colleagues found that males scored significantly higher than females on both scales, although only the difference for Primary Psychopathy was marked in magnitude. This difference is consistent with previous findings that males tend to be higher in psychopathy than females (Lykken, 1995).

Levenson and colleagues (1995) further reported that both scales were positively and significantly correlated with a self-report measure of trait anxiety, although the correlation with the Primary Psychopathy Scale was weak ($r = .09$). The absence of a substantial negative correlation between the Primary Psychopathy Scale and trait anxiety calls into question this scale's construct validity, as Levenson and colleagues predicted that primary psychopaths should be low in trait anxiety (see McHoskey, Worzel, & Szyarto, 1998, for similar findings).

Both scales were significantly and positively correlated with a measure of antisocial behavior, although this finding is difficult to interpret because Levenson et al. included (reverse-scored) prosocial behaviors (e.g., volunteerism) along with criminal and irresponsible actions in this measure. Some authors, such as Lykken (1982, 1995), maintain that antisocial and prosocial behaviors may be positively, not negatively, correlated, as both types of behaviors may stem from a shared underlying disposition (e.g., fearlessness) (see Krueger, Hicks, & McGue, 2001, for evidence that antisocial behavior and altruism are largely orthogonal).

Finally, Levenson and colleagues (1995) found that both LPSP psychopathy scales were positively correlated with the Boredom Susceptibility and Disinhibition subscales of the SSS (Zuckerman, 1989) but were essentially uncorrelated with the SSS Experience Seeking and Thrill-and-Adventure-Seeking subscales. These findings are broadly supportive of the construct validity of the LPSP given the centrality of risk taking to the psychopathy construct (see also McHoskey et al., 1998).

Lynam, Whiteside, and Jones (1999) examined the psychometric properties of the LPSP in two undergraduate samples. In the first study, Lynam and colleagues administered the LPSP, a self-report measure of delinquency and substance use, the Big Five Inventory (BFI; John & Srivastava, 1999), a measure of the five-factor model of personality, to 1,154 college students. Confirmatory factor analyses suggested that a two-factor solution for the LPSP was appropriate, as suggested by Levenson and colleagues (1995). Moreover, both LPSP scales were reasonably internally consistent, although the internal consistency for the Secondary Psychopathy Scale was again somewhat lower (Cronbach's alpha = .68) than that of the Primary Psychopathy Scale (Cronbach's alpha = .84). Again, the two scales were moderately correlated (r = .43).

Lynam and colleagues reported that both LPSP scales were positively correlated with measures of antisocial behavior, alcohol use, and drug use, with most correlations in the r = .20 to .30 range. Nevertheless, the Primary and Secondary scales failed to demonstrate clear discriminant validity for these external criteria, as the correlations for the Primary scales were, contrary to expectation, approximately as high—and in some cases nonsignificantly higher—than the correlations for the Secondary scales (the lone exception was for variety of drug use over the past year, which was significantly more highly correlated with the Secondary than with the Primary Scale). The relations of the LPSP to the BFI scales were generally supportive of the LPSP's construct validity. The LPSP Primary Scale was primarily related (negatively) to Agreeableness (see also McHoskey et al., 1998, for findings linking the Primary Scale to Machiavellianism, which is associated with low agreeableness), whereas the LPSP Secondary Scale was related to Agreeableness (negatively), Conscientiousness (negatively), and Neuroticism (positively). The lattermost correlation is consistent with the view that secondary psychopathy is associated with elevated anxiety (Karpman, 1948). In contrast, the correlation of the LPSP Primary Scale with Neuroticism was negative and significant, albeit negligible (r = −.05), again raising questions concerning the construct validity of this scale as a marker of primary psychopathy.

In a second study, Lynam and colleagues examined the relation of the LPSP to two laboratory measures of response modulation, the go–no-go task and the Q task (see Hiatt & Newman, Chapter 17, this volume), in 70 male prisoners. Because Newman and his colleagues (e.g., Newman & Kosson, 1986) consider deficits in response modulation to lie at the core of psychopathy, this study provides an informative test of the LPSP's construct validity. Lynam and colleagues also administered the SRP-II, a self-report psychopathy measure to be discussed shortly, as an additional indicator of convergent validity.

Lynam and colleagues found that LPSP scales were significantly (or in the case of the Secondary Scale, marginally significantly) related to passive avoidance (commission) errors on the go–no-go task and marginally significantly related to (low) response interference on the Q task. The absolute values of the correlations ranged from r = .18 to .23, and there was no significant difference in the correlates of the two LPSP scales. Both the Primary (r = .66) and Secondary (r = .42) scales were moderately to highly correlated with the SRP-II. In contrast to some findings (e.g., Hare, 1985) using earlier psychopathy measures, this finding suggests adequate convergent validity for at least some self-report psychopathy measures.

Brinkley, Schmitt, Smith, and Newman (2001) provided further evidence for the construct validity of the LPSP. They examined its factor structure, as well as its relations with a self-report index of alcohol use, performance on a go–no-go task, and the PCL-R and its two factors, in 270 Caucasian and 279 African American prisoners. Although confirmatory factor analyses suggested that a two-factor model was optimal, factor invariance analyses revealed that the pattern of item loadings differed somewhat for the two racial groups. As in previous analyses, the two LPSP scales were moderately internally consistent, with slightly lower internal consistency for the Secondary Scale.

In both Caucasian and African American samples, the LPSP Secondary Scale, but not the Primary Scale, was significantly correlated with alcohol use. In addition, analyses for the combined sample revealed that total LPSP scores were related to the number of passive avoidance errors on the go–no-go task. Analyses for the separate LPSP scales on the go–no-go task were not reported.

Moreover, in both Caucasian and African American samples, the LPSP Primary Scale displayed a clear pattern of convergent and discriminant validity with the two PCL-R factors, whereas the LPSP Secondary Scale did not. Specifically, the Primary Scale was more highly correlated with PCL-R Factor 1 (r's = .30 in both Caucasians and African Americans), than with Factor 2 (r's = .19 and .08 in Caucasians and African Americans, respectively), whereas the Secondary Scale correlated about equally with PCL-R Factor 2 (r's = .45 and .26 in Caucasians and African Americans, respectively) as with PCL-R Factor 1 (r's = .37 and .28 in Caucasians and African Americans, respectively).

Notably, several other investigators have reported that the LPSP Primary Scale lacks discriminant validity. In a sample of 661 participants drawn from prison and substance abuse settings, Lilienfeld, Skeem, and Poythress (2004) reported that the LPSP Primary Scale was much more highly correlated (r = .62) with the Factor 2 scale of the PPI (Lilienfeld, 1990; see section on "Psychopathic Personality Inventory") than with the

Factor I scale of the PPI (r = .16). Moreover, they found that the Primary Scale was as highly correlated (r = .52) with a self-report measure of DSM-IV APD symptoms as was the Secondary scale (r = .53). Wilson, Frick, and Clements (1999) and Lilienfeld and Hess (2001) similarly found that the LPSP Primary Scale was more highly correlated with Factor 2 self-report psychopathy measures (e.g., PPI Factor 2) than with Factor 1 measures. Finally, in a sample of 125 undergraduates, McHoskey and colleagues (1998) reported that the LPSP Primary and Secondary scales were about equally correlated with a self-report measure of antisocial actions (r's = .46 and .47, respectively).

Summary

The LPSP and its component scales appear to hold promise as self-report measures of psychopathy. For example, the LPSP exhibits a two-factor structure similar to the PCL-R, offering support for its factorial validity (Guilford, 1946) as a measure of the major component traits underpinning psychopathy. In addition, the LPSP demonstrates theoretically meaningful relations with self-report measures of sensation seeking and antisocial behavior, as well as with laboratory measures of response modulation. In particular, LPSP scores have been linked to passive avoidance errors, which are often regarded as indicators of a core deficit in psychopathy (Lykken, 1995). Nevertheless, the construct validity of the LPSP Primary Scale is problematic. In several studies, this scale has been found to be more highly related to measures of secondary psychopathy and antisocial behaviors than to measures of the core affective and interpersonal features of psychopathy.

Self-Report Psychopathy Scale

Construction

The Self-Report Psychopathy Scale was constructed by Hare and his colleagues (see Hare, 1985) using a combination of rational, empirical, and internal consistency approaches. Hare initially identified 75 items that distinguished high from low PCL scorers. This preliminary item pool was refined by selecting 29 items that showed high correlations with the PCL total score. Nevertheless, the original version of the SRP correlated only modestly with the PCL (Hare, 1985) and did not provide adequate content coverage of several traits traditionally considered central to psychopathy, including superficial charm, callousness, and dishonesty.

The SRP was revised using item analytic techniques to increase its correlation with the PCL (now the PCL-R) and to provide more comprehensive content coverage of the core personality traits of psychopathy (Hare, Hemphill, & Paulhus, 2002). Like the PCL-R, this revised measure, the SRP-II, contains two factors, with the first factor assessing primarily the core interpersonal and affective features of psychopathy and the second factor assessing primarily an antisocial and impulsive lifestyle. SRP-II items include "I can read people like a book" (Factor I) and "I have often done something dangerous just for the thrill of it" (Factor II).

Psychometric Properties

There has been less published research on the reliability and validity of the SRP and SRP-II than on the LPSP. In a prison sample, Hare (1985) found that the SRP was internally consistent (Cronbach's alpha = .80) and that it correlated $r = .26$ with the MMPI Pd scale, $r = -.53$ with the CPI So scale, $r = .35$ with clinician ratings of the DSM-III criteria for APD, and $r = .38$ with the PCL. The fact that the SRP correlated almost as highly with a measure of APD as with a measure of psychopathy (the PCL) raises concerns about its construct validity, in particular its discriminant validity from generalized behavioral deviance (although it is worth noting that PCL and PCL-R total scores also correlate quite highly with measures of APD; see Hare, 1991). Nevertheless, these concerns may have been remedied with the development of the SRP-II.

In the DSM-IV field trials, Widiger and colleagues (1996) administered the SRP-II, along with various measures of psychopathy and APD, to over 400 males recruited from various clinical (prison, psychiatric) sites. Across these samples, the SRP-II correlated at an average of $r = .35$ with DSM-III-R diagnoses of APD and at an average of $r = .38$ with a 10-item abbreviated version of the PCL-R (see Zagon & Jackson, 1994). Although the approximately equal correlation of the SRP-II with DSM-III-R APD and with PCL-R psychopathy may again raise concerns regarding its discriminant validity, the 10-item version of the PCL-R may not have provided adequate content coverage of psychopathy to afford a stringent test of the SRP-II's capacity to distinguish psychopathy from APD.

In an undergraduate sample, Lilienfeld and Penna (2001) reported that that although the SRP-II total score was internally consistent (Cronbach's alpha = .91), the internal consistency of SRP-II Factor 1 was marginal (Cronbach's alpha = .59). The internal consistency of SRP-II Factor 2 was adequate (Cronbach's alpha = .72).

In another sample of undergraduates, Zagon and Jackson (1994) reported that the SRP-II correlated significantly and moderately ($r = .62$) with a self-report measure of narcissism, the Narcissistic Personality Inventory (NPI; Raskin & Hall, 1979). This correlation is consistent with the grandiosity and egocentricity traditionally considered central to psychopathy (Cleckley, 19411988; Hare, 1991). In addition, the SRP-II correlated significantly and negatively ($r = -.30$ in both cases) with a self-report measure of trait anxiety, the trait form of the State–Trait Anxiety Inventory (Spielberger, Gorsuch, Lushene, Vagg, & Jacobs, 1983) and a self-report measure of empathy, the Interpersonal Reactivity Index (Davis, 1983). Again, both correlations are consistent with classic clinical descriptions of psychopathy, although the relation between psychopathy and trait anxiety is controversial (Schmitt & Newman, 1999; but see Frick, Lilienfeld, Ellis, Loney, & Silverthorn, 1999; Frick et al., 2000; Harpur et al., 1989; Verona, Patrick, & Joiner, 2001). Moreover, all these correlations were comparable in males and females. Trait anxiety was selectively related to SRP-II Factor I, whereas narcissism and empathy were related to both SRP-II factors. Zagon and Jackson found that the two SRP-II factors were significantly but moderately correlated ($r = .37$), roughly paralleling findings for the two factors of the PCL-R (Hare, 1991). Finally, Zagon and Jackson reported that males scored significantly higher than females on both the SRP total score and its component factors.

Other investigators have reported high correlations between the SRP-II and alternative self-report measures of psychopathy. For example, Lilienfeld and Andrews (1996) reported high correlations of $r = .91$ and $r =$

.62 between the PPI and SRP-II in two undergraduate samples. Lilienfeld (1996) reported that the SRP-II correlated $r = .27$ and $r = .52$ with MMPI-2 Pd and Antisocial Practices (ASP) content scale, respectively, in undergraduates. The discrepancy between these two correlations is consistent with data indicating that the MMPI-2 ASP content scale appears to be more closely related to the Cleckley features of psychopathy than the MMPI-2 Pd scale (Lilienfeld, 1996, 1999).

Overall, these findings suggest that previous concerns regarding low correlations among self-report measures of psychopathy (e.g., Hundleby & Ross, 1977) are no longer warranted. Although the reason for the superior showing of most recently developed psychopathy measures is unclear, the superior content coverage of psychopathic personality traits (e.g., guiltlessness, callousness, and narcissism) by these measures is a prime candidate. Whereas many earlier measures (e.g., the MMPI Pd scale and the CPI *So* scale) contained few items assessing psychopathic personality traits, the SRP-II and other recently developed measures were explicitly constructed with such traits in mind.

Williams, Nathanson, and Paulhus (2002) conducted an oblique (oblimin) factor analysis of an abbreviated 31-item version of the SRP-II in an undergraduate sample. They found both two- (Cold Affect and Antisocial Behavior) and three-factor (Deficient Affect, Interpersonal Callousness, and Antisocial Behavior) solutions to be interpretable, although they did not test the model fit of these two solutions against each other. Moreover, because they used an abbreviated version of the SRP-II, the extent to which their findings apply to the full SRP-II is unclear. Williams and colleagues found that the SRP-II total score correlated significantly at $r = .38$ with self-reported delinquency (including violent crime, cheating, and bullying), even after three SRP-II items tapping delinquent acts were removed from computation of the total score. Moreover, in the two-factor solution, the antisocial lifestyle factor was the only significant predictor of delinquency; in the three-factor solution, both the interpersonal callousness and antisocial lifestyle factors were significantly (and about equally) correlated with delinquency.

Paulhus and Williams (2002) examined the correlates of the SRP-III, a revised version of the SRP-II, in a sample of 245 undergraduates. They found that the internal consistency (Cronbach's alpha) of the SRP-III was .79. In terms of convergent validity, they reported that that the SRP-III correlated significantly with the NPI ($r = .50$) and with a questionnaire measure of Machiavellianism, the MACH-IV ($r = .31$) (Christie & Geis, 1970). The former finding replicates that of Zagon and Jackson (1994). Paulhus and Williams also reported significant correlations between the SRP-III and all five dimensions of the five-factor model as measured by the BFI (John & Srivastava, 1999). Specifically, they found that the SRP-III was correlated positively with extraversion and openness to experience (r's = .34 and .24, respectively) and negatively with agreeableness, conscientiousness, and neuroticism (r's = −.25, −.24, and −.34, respectively). These correlations are broadly consistent with that reported for the PCL-R:SV (Hart & Hare, 1994), although some previous investigators (e.g., Harpur, Hart, & Hare, 1993) have reported that the PCL is associated primarily with agreeableness and conscientiousness rather than with the other dimensions of the five-factor model. Finally, Paulhus and Williams found that SRP-III scores were slightly but significantly related ($r = .14$) to participants' propensity to overestimate their intelligence (as ascertained by the discrepancy between estimated and actual IQ), but they were not significantly related to a measure of "overclaiming" (which measured participants' claimed familiarity with various nonexistent persons, events, and objects).

Summary

The SRP and its offspring have shown promising internal consistency and construct validity in various samples, although questions remain regarding the internal consistency of SRP-II Factor II. The SRP total score correlates highly with other self-report measures relevant to psychopathy, including the PPI and MMPI-2 APD content scale, and exhibits meaningful convergent relations with self-report measures of traits ostensibly related to psychopathy, including narcissism, empathy, (reversed) agreeableness, and (reversed) conscientiousness. Nevertheless, the discriminant validity of the SRP from generalized antisocial behavior requires clarification, although this potential shortcoming appears to be less of an issue for the SRP-II than for the LPSP. In addition, there is little published research on the differential correlates of the two SRP factors or the relation between the SRP and laboratory measures that ostensibly tap the core deficits of psychopathy, such as passive-avoidance tasks or psychophysiological measures of sensitivity to threat cues (see Lykken, 1995).

Psychopathic Personality Inventory

Construction

The Psychopathic Personality Inventory was developed by Lilienfeld (1990) to detect psychopathic traits in noncriminal (e.g., student) samples. It consists of 187 items in a 4-point Likert-type format. In addition to eight subscales that assess lower-order facets of psychopathy, the PPI yields a total score representing global psychopathy. The PPI also contains validity scales intended to detect three response styles that are potentially problematic among psychopaths, namely positive impression management (the Unlikely Virtues Scale), malingering (the Deviant Responding Scale), and careless or random responding (the Deviant Responding Scale).

Using an exploratory approach to test construction (Loevinger, 1957; Tellegen & Waller, in press), Lilienfeld (1990) cast a broad net by identifying a large number of characteristics deemed by diverse authors as potentially relevant to psychopathy (e.g., Albert, Brigante, & Chase, 1959; Gray & Hutchinson, 1964; Hare, 1991). He then wrote items to assess these characteristics and submitted responses to these items to successive factor analyses in undergraduate samples. Based on the results of each factor analysis, Lilienfeld revised both scales and items. Test construction proceeded across three rounds of factor analysis involving 1,156 participants.

Factor analyses of the PPI item pool yielded eight replicable factors: Machiavellian Egocentricity (a ruthless willingness to manipulate and take advantage of others; e.g., "I sometimes try to get others to bend the rules for me if I can't change them any other way"), Social Potency (interpersonal impact and skill at influencing others; e.g.,

"Even when others are upset with me, I can usually win them over with my charm"), Fearlessness (a willingness to take physical risks and an absence of anticipatory anxiety; e.g., "Making a parachute jump would really frighten me," keyed in the false direction), Coldheartedness (callousness, guiltlessness, and absence of empathy; e.g., "I have had 'crushes' on people that were so intense that they were painful," keyed in the false direction), Impulsive Nonconformity (a flagrant disregard for tradition; e.g., "I sometimes question authority figures 'just for the hell of it' "), Blame Externalization (a tendency to attribute responsibility for one's mistakes to others; e.g., "When I'm in a group of people who do something wrong, somehow it seems like I'm usually the one who ends up getting blamed"), Carefree Nonplanfulness (an insouciant attitude toward the future; e.g., "I weigh the pros and cons of major decisions carefully before making them," keyed in the false direction), and Stress Immunity (sangfroid and absence of tension in anxiety-provoking situations; e.g., "I can remain calm in situations that would make many other people panic").

The PPI has recently been revised to lower its reading level and to eliminate psychometrically problematic or culturally specific items (Lilienfeld & Widows, 2005). Nevertheless, there is no published research on the revised PPI (now the PPI-R) as of this writing.

Psychometric Properties

Lilienfeld and Andrews (1996; see also Lilienfeld, 1990) examined the reliability and construct validity of the PPI in four undergraduate samples. They reported that the PPI was internally consistent (Cronbach's alphas ranged from .90 to .93), as were its subscales (Cronbach's alphas ranged from .70 to .90, with 75% of the alpha coefficients in the .80–.90 range). In addition, they reported that the PPI total score displayed a test–retest reliability of $r = .95$ over a mean 26-day interval. Test–retest reliabilities of the PPI subscales ranged from $r = .82$ to .94 (see Chapman, Gremore, & Farmer, 2003, for comparable data on the PPI's internal consistency and test–retest reliability). Lilienfeld and Andrews also reported that the PPI subscales did not exhibit uniform positive manifold. Specifically, although most of the subscales were positively correlated, some (e.g., Blame Externalization and Stress Immunity) were either slightly or moderately negatively correlated (see also Chapman et al., 2003). This finding calls into question the claim that the PPI subscales assess a unitary construct. Lilienfeld and Andrews also found that PPI total scores were significantly higher in males than females; moreover, this difference was large in magnitude (Cohen's $d = .97$). Scores on six PPI subscales, namely Machiavellian Egocentricity (Cohen's $d = .53$), Fearlessness (Cohen's $d = .79$), Coldheartedness (Cohens' $d = .73$), Impulsive Nonconformity (Cohen's $d = .52$), Blame Externalization (Cohen's $d = .19$), and Stress Immunity (Cohen's $d = .74$) were also significantly higher in males than females.

Lilienfeld and Andrews (1996) further reported that the PPI displayed convergent and discriminant validity with self-report measures of psychopathy and antisocial behavior, including the CPI *So* scale ($r = -.59$), MMPI-2 ASP content scale ($r = .56$ and $.58$ in two samples), and the Personality Diagnostic Questionnaire—Revised APD scale ($r = .58$ and $r = .43$ in two samples), as well as with theoretically relevant self-report scales from the Multidimensional Personality Questionnaire (MPQ; Tellegen, 1982), including Social Potency ($r = .39$), Aggression ($r = .38$), Harmavoidance ($r = -.55$), Control vs. Impulsiveness ($r = -.27$), and Traditionalism ($r = -.20$). In addition, the PPI displayed convergent validity with a measure of peer rated Cleckley psychopathy ($r = .45$), interview-rated Cleckley psychopathy ($r = .60$), and with APD ($r = .59$) and Narcissistic Personality Disorder ($r = .35$) as measured by the Structured Clinical Interview for DSM-III-R (Spitzer, Williams, & Gibbon, 1987).

The finding that the PPI assesses APD at least as much as, if not more than, psychopathy raises concerns regarding its discriminant validity from generalized antisocial behavior. Nevertheless, the PPI displayed discriminant validity (low and nonsignificant correlations) from measures of several constructs that are conceptually unrelated to psychopathy, including the Perceptual Aberration Scale (Chapman, Chapman, & Raulin, 1976), the Schizoidia Scale (Golden & Meehl, 1979), the General Behavior Inventory (GBI) Depression Scale (Depue et al.,

1981), and the PDQ-R Schizotypal and Schizoid scales (see also Salekin, Trobst, & Krioukova, 2001, for evidence that the correlates of PPI are largely specific to features of Cluster B [dramatic, emotional] disorders). These findings suggest that the PPI is largely unrelated to measures of depression and schizophrenia spectrum conditions.

Finally, Lilienfeld and Andrews (1996) used hierarchical multiple regression techniques to examine the incremental validity of the PPI above and beyond other self-report measures of psychopathy and antisocial behavior. They used both peer-rated and interviewer-rated Cleckley psychopathy as dependent measures. In both cases, the MMPI-2 Pd scale, MMPI-2 ASP content scale, PDQ-R ASPD scale, and MMPI Antisocial Personality Scale (Morey, Blashfield, Webb, & Jewell, 1988) were entered on the first step, followed by the PPI total score on the second step. For peer-rated Cleckley psychopathy, the addition of the PPI increased prediction by 10% of the variance ($p < .01$), while for interviewer-rated Cleckley psychopathy, the addition of the PPI increased prediction by 38% of the variance ($p < .001$). These analyses demonstrate that the PPI contains meaningful variance not shared with several self-report measures of psychopathy and antisocial behavior.

Although the PPI was designed for noncriminal samples, several investigators have examined its correlates in prisoners. In a sample of 100 male inmates, Sandoval and colleagues (2000) found that the PPI correlated $r = -.45$ with the Questionnaire Measure of Emotional Empathy (Mehrabian & Epstein, 1972) and $r = .60$ with the Buss and Perry (1992) Aggression Questionnaire. Both correlations are consistent with the clinical portrait of psychopaths as callous and as having low frustration tolerance (Hare, 1991). Contrary to prediction, the PPI was not significantly (negatively) correlated with the Protestant Ethic Scale (Mirels & Garrett, 1971), a measure of work ethic attitudes.

In a sample of 60 male inmates, Edens, Poythress, and Watkins (2001) found that the PPI exhibited a theoretically meaningful pattern of relations with the scales of the PAI (Morey, 1991). For example, the PPI correlated significantly with the PAI Antisocial ($r = .68$), Aggression ($r = .57$), Dominance ($r =$

.38), and Borderline ($r = .39$) scales. The lattermost correlation is difficult to interpret given that the relation between psychopathy and borderline personality disorder (BPD) is unclear (see Lilienfeld & Andrews, 1996, for similar results) and that BPD appears to be etiologically heterogeneous (Akiskal et al., 1985). Moreover, Edens and colleagues found that the PPI correlated significantly with physical ($r = .26$) and nonaggressive ($r = .37$) disciplinary infractions, although the correlation ($r = .19$) with verbal disciplinary infractions only approached significance ($p = .08$; see Edens, Poythress, & Lilienfeld, 1999, for additional data on the PPI and disciplinary infractions).

Poythress, Edens, and Lilienfeld (1998) examined the relation between the PPI and the PCL-R in 50 male inmates. They found that the PPI and PCL-R correlated at $r = .54$, suggesting a moderately high association between self-report and interview-based measures of psychopathy. Perhaps more important, the PPI correlated $r = .54$ with PCL-R Factor 1 and $r = .40$ with PCL-R Factor 2, suggesting that the PPI may be the first self-report measure of psychopathy to be associated substantially with the core interpersonal and affective features of psychopathy (but see Skeem & Lilienfeld, 2004, who found a more modest $r = .31$ correlation between the PPI and PCL-R Factor I, and a significantly higher correlation of $r = .48$ with PCL-R Factor II). Moreover, partial correlation analyses between the PPI and each PCL-R factor controlling for the variance shared with the other PCL-R factor revealed that the PPI was selectively associated with PCL-R Factor I (partial $r = .40$, $p < .01$) rather than with PCL-R Factor II (partial $r = .14$, ns). Finally, Machiavellian Egocentricity was the best PPI subscale correlate ($r = .57$) of the PCL-R total score, although Social Potency, Coldheartedness, and Impulsive Nonconformity were also significant PCL-R correlates.

Chapman and colleagues (2003) examined the psychometric properties of the PPI in 153 female inmates. They found that the PPI total score correlated $r = -.60$ with the CPI *So* scale and $r = .81$ with the PAI ANT scale. The latter correlation, although providing evidence for the PPI's convergent validity, may raise questions regarding its discriminant validity given that the PAI ANT scale is largely a measure of antisocial behavior

rather than the core personality traits of psychopathy (Edens, Hart, et al., 2000). Chapman and colleagues also reported that PPI total scores in their sample did not differ significantly from those obtained from female undergraduates in a previous study (Hamburger, Lilienfeld, & Hogben, 1996). This finding raises concerns regarding the PPI's criterion-related validity, although differences in age, education, social class, and other potential covariates between the two samples render this finding difficult to interpret.

Although Lilienfeld (1990) initially conceptualized the PPI as consisting of eight lower-order factors and a total score, factor analyses by Benning, Patrick, Hicks, Blonigen, and Krueger (2003) demonstrated that the PPI conforms to a two-factor structure conceptually related to that of PCL-R. In these factor analyses, Social Potency, Fearlessness, and Stress Immunity loaded on Factor 1, whereas Machiavellian Egocentricity, Impulsive Nonconformity, Blame Externalization, and Carefree Nonplanfulness loaded on Factor 2. Interestingly, Coldheartedness, which assesses many of the deficits traditionally regarded as central to psychopathy, particularly guiltlessness and lovelessness (McCord & McCord, 1964), did not load substantially on either factor. In sharp contrast to the two PCL-R factors, which are moderately correlated, the two PPI factors are essentially orthogonal. Therefore, PPI-assessed psychopathy does not comprise a classic psychopathological syndrome, that is, a condition marked by covarying signs and symptoms (see Kazdin, 1983; Lilienfeld, Waldman, & Israel, 1994).

The two PPI factors exhibit strikingly divergent, in some cases even directly opposite, correlates. For example, in a sample of 353 adult community males, Benning and colleagues (2004) found that PPI Factor 1 was positively correlated with educational level, high school class rank, and adult antisocial behavior. In contrast, PPI Factor 2 was negatively correlated with educational achievement, income, and verbal intelligence, and age of first substance use, and positively correlated with both child and adult antisocial behaviors. In addition, PPI Factor 1 was primarily associated (positively) with MPQ scales assessing Positive Emotionality, such as Well Being, and secondarily associated (negatively) with MPQ scales assessing Negative Emotionality, such as Stress Reaction. In contrast, PPI Factor 2 was moderately to highly associated (positively) with MPQ scales assessing Negative Emotionality, particularly Alienation and Aggression and (negatively) with MPQ scales assessing Constraint, particularly Control versus Impulsiveness. Benning and colleagues suggested that PPI Factor 1 may reflect emotional resilience (see also Block, 1965, for a discussion of "ego resilience"), whereas PPI Factor 2 may reflect a broad predisposition toward externalizing behavior. This possibility is consistent with preliminary analyses from prison and substance samples indicating that although PPI Factor 2 is positively associated with suicide ideation and attempts, PPI Factor 1 is negatively associated with such variables (Douglas, Lilienfeld, & Poythress, 2004). Thus, some features of psychopathy, especially those linked to high interpersonal influence and low anticipatory anxiety, may exert a protective influence against suicidal thinking and behavior.

Finally, Skeem and Lilienfeld (2004) found that, in contrast to the LPSP Primary and Secondary Psychopathy scales, the two PPI factors displayed a relatively clear convergent/discriminant pattern of relations with other measures. For example, PPI Factor 1 was more highly correlated with PCL-R Factor 1 than with PCL-R Factor 2 (although this difference did not reach significance), and vice versa for PPI Factor 2. In addition, PPI Factor 1 was virtually unrelated to self-reported features of DSM-IV APD ($r = .06$) whereas PPI Factor 2 was highly related to these features ($r = .61$).

Summary

The PPI holds considerable potential as a self-report measure of psychopathy. Both its total score and its subscales are internally consistent and stable over time. The PPI total score displays good convergent and discriminant validity with self-report, interview, and observer-rated measures of psychopathy, antisocial behavior, DSM personality disorders, and normal-range personality traits. In addition, the PPI correlates moderately to highly with PCL-R Factor 1, suggesting that it assesses at least some of the core affective and interpersonal deficits of psychopathy. Never-theless, the PPI also correlates moderately to highly with PCL-R Factor 2, indicating that it is not selective to these deficits. Finally, the PPI's two factors appear to exhibit promising convergent and discriminant validity with measures of psychopathy and antisocial behavior, as well as strikingly different demographic and personality correlates.

Nevertheless, important questions regarding the PPI's validity remain. Scant published research has examined the PPI's relation to laboratory indices relevant to psychopathy (e.g., go–no-go tasks, fear-potentiated startle, neuropsychological measures of prefrontal lobe dysfunction, neuroimaging findings) (see Lilienfeld, Hess, & Rowland, 1996, for an exception). Such evidence is needed to fill out the still sketchy nomological network linking the PPI to measures of psychobiological deficits ostensibly underpinning psychopathy. More evidence is also required to demonstrate that the PPI distinguishes individuals in prison versus nonprison samples, as the limited evidence on this issue is not supportive of the PPI's criterion-related validity (Chapman et al., 2003). Finally, the presence of negative correlations among some PPI subscales and the virtual orthogonality of the two PPI factors suggest that the PPI does not assess a unitary construct. As we discuss in the next section, it is unclear whether this finding calls into question the PPI's structural validity (see Loevinger, 1957) or whether it points toward the need to rethink the construct of psychopathy.

DISCUSSION AND FUTURE DIRECTIONS

The past 10–15 years have witnessed significant advances in the self-report assessment of psychopathy. Previous pessimistic conclusions regarding the low correlations among self-report psychopathy measures (e.g., Hundleby & Ross, 1977) must now be revised in light of new evidence. It seems likely that these earlier conclusions were largely a consequence of the suboptimal content validity of many widely used "psychopathy" measures, including the MMPI Pd scale and CPI So scale, as few of these measures provided adequate coverage of the Cleckley (1941/1988) criteria for psychopathy. The convergent associations among the LPSP, SRP, and PPI have proven considerably more promising than those of earlier measures, as have their convergent validities with measures of normal-range personality traits and DSM-IV personality disorder features. In addition, the PPI correlates moderately to highly with PCL-R Factor I (Poythress et al., 1998), suggesting that at least some self-report psychopathy measures adequately assess the core interpersonal and affective features of psychopathy. Hence, claims that self-report measures are intrinsically unsuited for the assessment of psychopathy are difficult to sustain in light of recent evidence.

At the same time, the past 10–15 years of research on the self-report assessment of psychopathy has raised significant questions concerning (1) the potential limitations of self-reports measures in the assessment of psychopathy and (2) the nature of the psychopathy construct itself. We address both of these questions in turn.

Potential Limitations of Self-Report Psychopathy Measures

Given psychopaths' well-known propensities toward dissimulation, it seems clear that self-report measures should rarely, if ever, be used by themselves to assess psychopathy in clinical settings (see Shadish, Cook, & Campbell, 2001, for a discussion of "mono-method bias"). In such settings, self-report measures should typically be supplemented with corroborative information, including file data and observer ratings. Presumably, such corroborative information can often provide incremental validity above and beyond self-reports, especially in settings in which the motivation to create either a positive or negative impression on questionnaires is high.

Nevertheless, there is surprisingly little research bearing on the question of whether other modes of assessment confer incremental validity above and beyond self-reports in the assessment of psychopathy. In the only published study to our knowledge to address this issue, Edens and colleagues (1999) found that both the PPI and PCL-R correlated significantly with disciplinary infractions among inmates, although neither measure afforded significant incremental validity

above and beyond the other for this quasi-criterion. This finding suggests that the PPI and PCL-R may tap largely overlapping (and therefore redundant) regions of the criterion space, at least as far as institutional misbehavior is concerned. Nevertheless, the low correlations of both measures with institutional infractions (most r's were in the .20–.30 range) render this study a less than optimal test of incremental validity. In evaluating future research on the incremental validity of self-report measures above and beyond interview measures, and vice versa, investigators will need to accord careful consideration to the issue of criterion contamination. For example, we would expect the PPI to possess incremental validity above and beyond the PCL-R for self-report measures of antisocial behavior, and vice versa for file-based measures of antisocial behavior. If so, these findings could be difficult to interpret, as they may reflect merely a largely tautological association between measures that assess overlapping content.

In addition, researchers should examine the relative incremental validity of self-reports and observer ratings of psychopathy while bearing in mind both the hidden and blind quadrants of the Johari window (Luft, 1969). In the hidden quadrant, self-reports may be especially useful for detecting ego-dystonic affective traits common in psychopaths, such as chronic feelings of alienation, frustration, and boredom. In contrast, in the blind quadrant, observer reports may be especially useful for detecting ego-syntonic emotional affective traits common in psychopaths, such as chronic feelings of ethical superiority or contempt toward others. Such traits may be important "blind spots" (Grove & Tellegen, 1991) that are readily missed by self-report measures of psychopathy.

Observer reports may also provide incremental validity in detecting the *absence* of certain long-standing emotional dispositions, such as guilt, warmth, love, and empathy. After all, it may be inherently paradoxical to ask psychopathic individuals to report on the absence of emotions they have rarely, if ever, experienced. To adapt terminology from Gestalt psychology, the absence of such emotions may not be noticed by psychopathic individuals as "ground" because they have never experienced their presence as "figure." As noted earlier, Kelly (1955) argued that one must experience both poles of a construct to derive meaning from it (see Kelly's, 1955, discussion of the "dichotomy corollary"). As a consequence, in Kelly's terms psychopaths may have no (or at best poorly developed) "personal constructs" of guilt, warmth, love, and empathy. Moreover, according to Kelly, empathy stems from the capacity to construe others' construct systems (or in modern parlance, from what might be termed "theory of mind"; Premack & Woodruff, 1978). Because psychopaths presumably possess absent or poorly developed personal construct systems for guilt and similar emotions, they may be understandably bewildered by others' reactions to their callous behaviors. Psychopaths' lack of personal construct systems for such emotions may explain their striking "absence of insight" (Cleckley, 1941/1988).

Observers, in contrast, may accurately infer the absence of such emotions from certain highly diagnostic behaviors, such as cruel behaviors toward people or animals or a chronic lack of fidelity in romantic relationships. If so, observer reports may exhibit especially marked incremental validity above and beyond self-reports for the "cold" and "calculating" behaviors traditionally viewed as prototypical for psychopathy.

The "Kelly paradox" may explain why many self-report measures of psychopathy correlate weakly or at best moderately with PCL-R Factor I traits. It may also explain why the PPI Coldheartedness subscale, which assesses a lack of guilt, empathy, love, and other interpersonal emotions, loads negligibly on both PPI factors (Benning et al., 2003) and correlates negligibly with most other PPI subscales (Chapman et al., 2003; Lilienfeld & Andrews, 1996).

Still, we should not reflexively assume that the modest or negligible correlations between most self-report psychopathy measures and PCL-R Factor I represent a shortcoming of the former rather than of the latter. Indeed, it is equally plausible that neither the interview component of the PCL-R—which is, after all, scored on the basis of self-report combined with clinical judgment—nor the file component of the PCL-R adequately assesses the absence of guilt and other interpersonal emotions (see Hall, Benning, & Patrick, 2004, for evidence that

in contrast to the "interpersonal" and "behavioral" factors derived from a three-factor solution of the PCL-R, the "affective factor" of the PCL-R correlates minimally with variables in the domains of personality, intelligence, and adaptive functioning). It would be premature to exclude the hypothesis that certain self-report measures of psychopathy actually provide better measures of such interpersonal emotions than do the PCL-R, in part because they contain many questions assessing these traits and thereby capitalize on the Spearman–Brown formula (see Epstein, 1979, for a discussion of the principle of aggregation in personality assessment). An important direction for future research will be to compare the incremental validity of PCL-R Factor I and self-report instruments, such as the PPI Coldheartedness subscale, to predict performance on laboratory tasks that ostensibly tap psychopaths' affective deficits, such as lexical decision-making tasks using emotional and nonemotional words (e.g., Lorenz & Newman, 2002; Williamson, Harpur, & Hare, 1991).

The Nature of the Psychopathy Construct

The finding that the PPI's two factors are essentially orthogonal (e.g., Benning et al., 2003) invites two very different interpretations. The first is that this finding suggests a fundamental problem with the PPI's construct validity, stemming from inadequate construct conceptualization, inadequate test construction, or the aforementioned Kelly paradox, which may produce a "method–mode mismatch" (Edens, Buffington, & Tomick, 2000; see also Haynes et al., 1995) between the self-report mode of assessment and certain constructs of interest (e.g., guiltlessness and callousness).

The second and more intriguing possibility is that this finding may suggest the need for a reconceptualization of the psychopathy construct itself. Rather than a classical syndrome, which as noted earlier consists of a constellation of covarying signs and symptoms (Kazdin, 1983), psychopathy may instead be a maladaptive *configuration* of at least two (PPI Factors 1 and 2), and possibly three (PPI Factors 1, 2, and Coldheartedness), largely independent dimensions (Lilienfeld & Andrews, 1996; see also Benning et al., 2003, Grove & Tellegen,

1991). Patrick (in press) has referred to these alternative conceptualizations of psychopathy as "unitary" process and "dual process" models, respectively.

The dual-process view of psychopathy is consistent with interpersonal models of personality, which imply that certain traits, which need not be positively correlated, combine to produce configurations associated with malignant interpersonal consequences. As an example, take passive–aggressive personalities. In many interpersonal circumplex models of personality, passivity and aggressiveness are essentially or entirely orthogonal dimensions (e.g., Wiggins, 1982). Yet when passivity and aggressiveness are both present, they combine to create a potent—and highly noxious—interpersonal style that cannot be predicted from either dimension alone. In the case of psychopathy, individuals who are *both* guiltless and callous on the one hand *and* risk taking and irresponsible on the other may be especially untrustworthy in interpersonal interactions, because such individuals may be especially prone to acting on their malevolent intentions. More speculatively, such individuals may be especially likely to activate evolutionarily selected algorithms tuned to cheater detection (Cosmides & Tooby, 1992).

In the industrial–organizational psychology literature, the distinction between *multifaceted* traits and *compound* traits (Hough & Schneider, 1995; Smith, Fischer, & Fister, 2003) is helpful in this regard. Whereas multifaceted traits "consist of narrower facets that covary because of the causal influence of the higher order . . . trait" (Smith et al., 2003, p. 471), compound traits are emergent composites of separable, often unrelated, lower-order traits (see also Lykken, Bouchard, McGue, & Tellegen, 1992, for a discussion of "emergenesis"). Whereas virtually all psychopathy measures, including the PCL-R and most self-report indexes, implicitly or explicitly treat psychopathy as a multifaceted trait, findings on the PPI's factor structure suggest that psychopathy might best be regarded as a compound trait. This possibility is consistent with preliminary twin data indicating that the PPI and several of its subscales may contain substantial nonadditive genetic variance stemming from dominance (interactions among alleles within genes), epistasis (interactions among

genes), or both (Blonigen, Carlson, Krueger, & Patrick, 2003), although these data require replication with larger samples.

If so, this heretical view of psychopathy may call for alternative models of scoring and interpreting self-report psychopathy measures. Specifically, investigators would do well to examine configural (multiplicative or interactive) models of scoring the PPI and perhaps other self-report psychopathy measures instead of, or at least in addition to, more traditional linear (additive) models that rely on merely summing scores on lower-order psychopathy dimensions. Although configural models of personality assessment have rarely fared well in head-to-head comparisons with linear models (Goldberg, 1965; Pritchard, 1977), this negative outcome may be largely a consequence of the weak theoretical underpinnings of most configural models. Most of these models have been exploratory and largely devoid of a compelling theoretical rationale. The situation may be different in the case of psychopathy, because the conceptualization of psychopathy as a compound trait accords well with the rich literature on interpersonal models of personality and personality disorders. Moreover, in their laboratory studies Newman and colleagues (see Hiatt & Newman, Chapter 17, this volume) have similarly embraced a dual-process view of psychopathy. Specifically, they have often found that the response modulation deficits ostensibly underpinning psychopathy are limited to individuals with both elevated PCL-R scores and low trait anxiety, but neither attribute alone.

This alternative conception of psychopathy also calls for investigation of the reason(s) for the marked discrepancy between the PPI, on the one hand, and PCL-R, LPSP, and SRP, on the other, in the correlation between their two underlying factors. As noted earlier, this discrepancy could point to a fundamental defect in the PPI's construct validity. Alternatively, this discrepancy could point to overlooked psychometric shortcomings, such as method covariance, in the other psychopathy measures. For example, when scoring the PCL-R, interviewers frequently use file information to inform their scoring of both Factors I and II. Moreover, their clinical impressions regarding Factor II characteristics (e.g., antisocial behaviors) may "spill over" to influence their ratings of Factor I characteristics. Such spillover may at times be warranted, as in the case of a PCL-R interviewer who rates a participant high on both "Callous/Lack of Empathy" and "Poor Behavioral Controls" for committing sadistic and uncontrolled violence against people and household pets. Nevertheless, such spillover may also introduce method covariance arising from halo effects (Landy, Vance, Barnes-Farrell, & Steele, 1980), logical errors (Guilford, 1954), and other response style artifacts. Such possibilities merit empirical investigation.

CONCLUDING THOUGHTS

To paraphrase Mark Twain, rumors of the death of self-report measures of psychopathy have been greatly exaggerated. Recent findings demonstrate that the self-report assessment of psychopathy is alive and well. At the same time, the often perplexing literature we have reviewed raises at least as many questions as answers. Nevertheless, there is ample reason to be optimistic, because these unresolved questions may suggest answers to more fundamental questions regarding the conceptualization and etiology of psychopathy.

REFERENCES

Akiskal, H. S., Chen, S. E., Davis, G. C., Puzantian, V. R., Kashgarian, M., & Bolinger, J. M. (1985). Borderline: An adjective in search of a noun. *Journal of Clinical Psychiatry*, 46, 41–48.

Albert, R. S., Brigante, T. R., & Chase, M. (1959). The psychopathic personality: A content analysis of the concept. *Journal of General Psychology*, 60, 17–28.

Allport, G. (1961). *Pattern and growth in personality*. New York: Holt, Reinhart, & Winston.

American Psychiatric Association. (1980). *Diagnostic and statistical manual of mental disorders* (3rd ed.). Washington, DC: Author.

Benning, S. D., Patrick, C. J., Hicks, B. M., Blonigen, D. M., & Krueger, R. F. (2003). Factor structure of the Psychopathic Personality Inventory: Validity and implications for clinical assessment. *Psychological Assessment*, 15, 340–350.

Blackburn, R., & Fawcett, D. (1999). The antisocial personality questionnaire: An inventory for assessing personality deviation in offender populations. European *Journal of Psychological Assessment*, 15, 14–24.

Block, J. (1965). *The challenge of response sets*. New York: Appleton-Century-Crofts.

Blonigen, D. M., Carlson, S. R., Krueger, R. F., & Patrick, C. J. (2003). A twin study of self-reported psychopathic personality traits. *Personality and Individual Differences*, 35, 179–197.

Brinkley, C. A., Schmitt, W. A., Smith, S. S., & Newman, J. P. (2001). Construct validation of a self-report psychopathy scale: Does Levenson's self-report psychopathy scale measure the same constructs as Hare's psychopathy checklist-revised? *Personality and Individual Differences*, 31, 1021–1038.

Buss, A. H., & Perry, M. (1992). The aggression questionnaire. *Journal of Personality and Social Psychology*, 63, 452–459.

Butcher, J. N., Graham, J. R., Williams, C. L., & Ben-Porath, Y. (1990). *Development and use of the MMPI-2 content scales*. Minneapolis: University of Minnesota Press.

Chapman, A. L., Gremore, T. M., & Farmer, R. F. (2003). Psychometric analysis of the Psychopathic Personality Inventory (PPI) with female inmates. *Journal of Personality Assessment*, 80, 164–172.

Chapman, L. J., Chapman, J. P., & Raulin, M. L. (1976). Body-image aberration in schizophrenia. *Journal of Abnormal Psychology*, 87, 374–382.

Christie, R., & Geis, F. L. (1970). *Studies in Machiavellianism*. London: Academic Press.

Cleckley, H. (1988). *The mask of sanity*. St. Louis, MO: Mosby. (Original work published 1941)

Cosmides, L., & Tooby, J. (1992). Cognitive adaptations for social exchange. In J. Barkow, L. Cosmides, & J. Tooby (Eds.), *The adapted mind: Evolutionary psychology and the generation of culture* (pp. 163–228). New York: Oxford University Press.

Cronbach, L. J., & Meehl, P. E. (1955). Construct validity in psychological tests. *Psychological Bulletin*, 52, 281–302.

Davis, M. H. (1983). Measuring individual differences in empathy: Evidence for a multidimensional approach. *Journal of Personality and Social Psychology*, 44, 113–126.

Depue, R. A., Slater, J. F., Wolfstetter-Kausch, H., Klein, D., Goplerud, E., & Farr, D. (1981). A behavioral paradigm for identifying persons at risk for bipolar depressive disorder: A conceptual framework and five validation studies. *Journal of Abnormal Psychology*, 90, 57–68.

Douglas, K. S., Lilienfeld, S. O., & Poythress, N. G. (2004). *Psychopathy and suicide*. Paper presented at the annual meeting of the American Psychology–Law Society, Scottsdale, AZ.

Edelmann, R. J., & Vivian, S. E. (1988). Further analysis of the social psychopathy scale. *Personality and Individual Differences*, 9, 581–587.

Edens, J. F., Buffington, J. K., & Tomicic, T. L. (2000). An investigation of the relationship between psychopathic traits and malingering on the Psychopathic Personality Inventory. *Assessment*, 7, 281–296.

Edens, J. F., Hart, S. D., Johnson, D. W., Johnson, J. K.,

& Olver, M. E. (2000). Use of the personality assessment inventory to assess psychopathy in offender populations. *Psychological Assessment*, *12*, 132–139.

Edens, J. F., Poythress, N. G., & Lilienfeld, S. O. (1999). Identifying inmates at risk for disciplinary infractions: A comparison of two measures of psychopathy. *Behavioral Sciences and the Law*, *17*, 435–443.

Edens, J. F., Poythress, N. G., & Watkins, M. M. (2001). Further validation of the psychopathic personality inventory among offenders: Personality and behavioral correlates. *Journal of Personality Disorders*, *15*, 403–415.

Edens, J. F., Skeem, J. L., Cruise, K. R., & Cauffman, E. (2001). Assessment of "juvenile psychopathy" and its association with violence: A critical review. *Behavioral Sciences and the Law*, *19*, 53–80.

Ekman, P. (1985). *Telling lies*. New York: Norton.

Epstein, S. (1979). The stability of behavior: I. On predicting more of the people more of the time. *Journal of Personality and Social Psychology*, *37*, 1097–1126.

Eysenck, H. J., & Eysenck, S. B. G. (1964). *Manual of the Eysenck Personality Inventory*. London: University of London Press.

Eysenck, S. B. G., & Eysenck, H. J. (1975). *Manual of the Eysenck Personality Questionnaire*. London: University of London Press.

Faraone, S. V., & Tsuang, M. T. (1994). Measuring diagnostic accuracy in the absence of a "gold standard." *American Journal of Psychiatry*, *151*, 650–657.

Finney, J. C. (1985). Anxiety: Its measurement by objective personality tests and self-report. In A. H. Tuma & J. D. Maser (Eds.), *Anxiety and the anxiety disorders* (pp. 645–673). Hillsdale, NJ: Erlbaum.

Frick, P. J., Lilienfeld, S. O., Edens, J. F., Poythress, N. G., Ellis, M., & McBurnett, K. (2000). The association between anxiety and antisocial behavior. *Primary Psychiatry*, *7*, 52–57.

Frick, P. J., Lilienfeld, S. O., Ellis, M., Loney, B., & Silverthorn, P. (1999). The association between anxiety and psychopathy dimensions in children. *Journal of Abnormal Child Psychology*, *27*, 383–392.

Fulero, S. (1995). Review of the Hare Psychopathy Checklist—Revised. In J. C. Conoley, J. C. Impara, & L. L. Murphy (Eds.), *Twelfth mental measurements yearbook* (pp. 453–454). Lincoln, NE: Buros Institute.

Goldberg, L. R. (1965). Diagnosticians vs. diagnostic signs: The diagnosis of psychosis vs. neurosis from the MMPI. *Psychological Monographs*, *79*(9, Whole No. 602), 29.

Golden, R. R., & Meehl, P. E. (1979). Detection of the schizoid taxon with MMPI indicators. *Journal of Abnormal Psychology*, *88*, 217–233.

Gough, H. G. (1960). Theory and method of socialization. *Journal of Consulting and Clinical Psychology*, *24*, 23–30.

Gray, K. G., & Hutchinson, H. C. (1964). The psychopathic personality: A survey of Canadian psychiatrists' opinions. *Canadian Psychiatric Association Journal*, *9*, 452–461.

Greene, R. L. (2000). *The MMPI-2: An interpretive manual* (2nd ed.). Boston: Allyn & Bacon.

Grove, W. M., & Tellegen, A. (1991). Problems in the classification of personality disorders. *Journal of Personality Disorders*, *5*, 31–42.

Guilford, J. P. (1946). New standards for test evaluation. *Educational and Psychological Measurement*, *6*, 427–438.

Guilford, J. P. (1954). *Psychometric methods*. New York: McGraw Hill.

Gynther, M. D., Altman, H., & Warbin, R. W. (1973). Behavioral correlates for the Minnesota Multiphasic Personality Inventory 4–9, 9–4 code types: A case of the emperor's new clothes? *Journal of Consulting and Clinical Psychology*, *40*, 259–263.

Haertzen, C. A., Martin, W. R., Ross, F. E., & Neidert, G. L. (1980). Psychopathic states inventory (PSI): Development of a short test for measuring psychopathic states. *International Journal of the Addictions*, *15*, 137–146.

Hall, J. R., Benning, S. D., & Patrick, C. J. (2004). Criterion-related validity of the three-factor model of psychopathy: Personality, behavior, and adaptive functioning. *Assessment*, *11*, 4–16.

Hamburger, M. E., Lilienfeld, S. O., & Hogben, M. (1996). Psychopathy, gender, and gender roles: Implications for antisocial and histrionic personality disorders. *Journal of Personality Disorders*, *10*, 41–55.

Hare, R. D. (1982). Psychopathy and the personality dimensions of psychoticism, extraversion, and neuroticism. *Personality and Individual Differences*, *3*, 35–42.

Hare, R. D. (1985). A comparison of procedures for the assessment of psychopathy. *Journal of Consulting and Clinical Psychology*, *53*, 7–16.

Hare, R. D. (1991). *The Hare Psychopathy Checklist—Revised*. Toronto, ON, Canada: Multi-Health Systems.

Hare, R. D. (1993). *Without conscience: The disturbing world of the psychopaths among us*. New York: Pocket Books.

Hare, R. D., & Cox, D. N. (1978). Clinical and empirical conceptions of psychopathy, and the selection of subjects for research. In R. D. Hare & D. Schalling (Eds.), *Psychopathic behaviour: Approaches to research* (pp. 1–21). Chichester, UK: Wiley.

Hare, R. D., Hemphill, J. F., & Paulhus, D. (2002). *The Self-Report Psychopathy Scale—II (SRP-II)*. Manuscript in preparation.

Harpur, T. J., Hare, R. D., & Hakstian, A. R. (1989). Two-factor conceptualization of psychopathy: Construct validity and assessment implications. *Psychological Assessment*, *1*, 6–17.

Harpur, T. J., Hart, S. D., & Hare, R. D. (1993). Personality of the psychopath. In P. A. Costa & T. A. Widiger (Eds.), *Personality disorders and the five-factor model* (pp. 149–173). Washington, DC: American Psychological Association.

Hart, S. D., Cox, D. N., & Hare, R. D. (1995). *Manual for the Psychopathy Checklist: Screening Version (PCL:SV)*. Toronto, ON, Canada: Multi-Health Systems.

Hart, S. D., Forth, A. E., & Hare, R. D. (1991). The MCMI-II and psychopathy. *Journal of Personality Disorders, 5*, 318–327.

Hart, S. D., & Hare, R. D. (1994). Psychopathy and the Big Five: Correlations between observers' ratings of normal and pathological personality. *Journal of Personality Disorders, 8*, 32–40.

Hart, S. D., Hare, R. D., & Harpur, T. J. (1992). The Psychopathy Checklist: Overview for researchers and clinicians. In J. Rosen & P. McReynolds (Eds.), *Advances in psychological assessment* (Vol. 7, pp. 103–130). New York: Plenum Press.

Hathaway, S. R., & McKinley, J. C. (1940). A multiphasic personality schedule (Minnesota): I. Construction of the schedule. *Journal of Psychology, 10*, 249–254.

Hawk, S. S., & Peterson, R. A. (1973). Do MMPI psychopathic deviancy scores reflect psychopathic deviancy or just deviancy? *Journal of Personality Assessment, 38*, 362–368.

Haynes, S. N., Richards, D. C. S., & Kubany, E. S. (1995). Content validity in psychological assessment: A functional approach to concepts and methods. *Psychological Assessment, 7*, 238–247.

Hough, L. M., & Schneider, R. J. (1995). Personality traits, taxonomies, and applications in organizations. In K. R. Murphy (Ed.), *Individuals and behavior in organizations* (pp. 31–88). San Francisco: Jossey-Bass.

Hundleby, J. D., & Ross, B. E. (1977). A comparison of questionnaire measures of psychopathy. *Journal of Consulting and Clinical Psychology, 45*, 702–703.

John, O. P., & Srivastava, S. (1999). The Big Five trait taxonomy: History, measurement, and theoretical perspectives. In L. A. Pervin & O. P. John (Eds.), *Handbook of personality: Theory and research* (2nd ed., pp. 102–138). New York: Guilford Press.

Johnstone, L., & Cooke, D. J. (2004). Psychopathic-like traits in childhood: Conceptual and measurement concerns. *Behavioral Sciences and the Law, 22*, 103–125.

Karpman, B. (1948). The myth of psychopathic personality. *American Journal of Psychiatry, 103*, 523–534.

Kazdin, A. E. (1983). Psychiatric diagnosis, dimensions of dysfunction, and child behavior therapy. *Behavior Therapy, 14*, 73–99.

Kelly, G. A. (1955). *The psychology of personal constructs* (Vols. 1 & 2). New York: Norton.

Kendrick, D., & Funder, D. (1988). Profiting from controversy: Lessons from the person–situation debate. *American Psychologist, 43*, 23–34.

Kosson, D. S., Steuerwald, B. L., Newman, J. P., & Widom, C. S. (1994). The relation between socialization and antisocial behavior, substance use, and family conflict in college students. *Journal of Personality Assessment, 63*, 473–488.

Kroger, R. O., & Turnbull, W. (1975). Invalidity of validity scales: The case of the MMPI. *Journal of Consulting and Clinical Psychology, 43*, 48–55.

Krueger, R. F., Hicks, B. M., & McGue, M. (2001). Altruism and antisocial behavior: Independent tendencies, unique personality correlates, distinct etiologies. *Psychological Science, 12*, 397–402.

Landy, F. J., Vance, R. J., Barnes-Farrell, J. L., & Steele, J. W. (1980). Statistical control of halo error in performance ratings. *Journal of Applied Psychology, 65*, 501–506.

Levenson, M. (1990). Risk taking and personality. *Journal of Personality and Social Psychology, 58*, 1073–1081.

Levenson, M. R., Kiehl, K. A., & Fitzpatrick, C. M. (1995). Assessing psychopathic attributes in a noninstitutionalized population. *Journal of Personality and Social Psychology, 68*(1), 151–158.

Lilienfeld, S. O. (1990). *Development and preliminary validation of a self-report measure of psychopathic personality*. Doctoral dissertation, University of Minnesota, Minneapolis.

Lilienfeld, S. O. (1994). Conceptual problems in the assessment of psychopathy. *Clinical Psychology Review, 14*, 17–38.

Lilienfeld, S. O. (1996). The MMPI-2 Antisocial Practices content scale: Construct validity and comparison with the Psychopathic Deviate scale. *Psychological Assessment, 8*, 281–293.

Lilienfeld, S. O. (1998). Methodological advances and developments in the assessment of psychopathy. *Behaviour Research and Therapy, 36*, 99–125.

Lilienfeld, S. O. (1999). The relation of the MMPI-2 Pd Harris–Lingoes subscales to psychopathy, psychopathy facets, and antisocial behavior: Implications for clinical practice. *Journal of Clinical Psychology, 55*, 241–255.

Lilienfeld, S. O., & Andrews, B. P. (1996). Development and preliminary validation of a self report measure of psychopathic personality traits in noncriminal populations. *Journal of Personality Assessment, 66*, 488–524.

Lilienfeld, S. O., & Hess, T. (2001). Psychopathic personality traits and somatization: Sex differences and the mediating role of negative emotionality. *Journal of Psychopathology and Behavioral Assessment, 23*, 11–24.

Lilienfeld, S. O., Hess, T., & Rowland, C. (1996). Psychopathic personality traits and temporal perspective: A test of the short time horizon hypothesis. *Journal of Psychopathology and Behavioral Assessment, 18*, 285–314.

Lilienfeld, S. O., & Penna, S. (2001). Anxiety sensitivity: Relations to psychopathy, DSM-IV personality disorders, and personality traits. *Journal of Anxiety Disorders, 15*, 367–393.

Lilienfeld, S. O., Skeem, J. L., & Poythress, N. G. (2004, March). *Psychometric properties of self-report psychopathy measures*. Paper presented at the annual meeting of the American Psychology–Law Society, Scottsdale, AZ.

Lilienfeld, S. O., Waldman, I. D., & Israel, A. C. (1994). A critical note on the use of the term and concept of "comorbidity" in psychopathology research. *Clinical Psychology: Science and Practice, 1,* 71–83.

Lilienfeld, S. O., & Widows, M. (2005). *Manual for the Psychopathic Personality Inventory—Revised (PPI-R).* Manuscript in preparation.

Loevinger, J. (1957). Objective tests as instruments of psychological theory. *Psychological Reports, 9,* 635–694.

Lorenz, A., & Newman, J. P. (2002). Do emotion and information processing deficiencies found in Caucasian psychopaths generalize to Africa-American psychopaths? *Personality and Individual Differences, 32,* 1077–1086.

Lovering, A., & Douglas, K. S. (2004, March). *Comparative analysis of multiple self-report measures' association with the construct of psychopathy among criminal offenders.* Poster presented at the annual meeting of the American Psychology–Law Society, Scottsdale, AZ.

Luft, J. (1969). *Of human interaction.* Palo Alto, CA: National Press.

Lykken, D. T. (1957). A study of anxiety in the sociopathic personality. *Journal of Abnormal and Social Psychology, 55,* 6–10.

Lykken, D. T. (1982, March). Fearlessness: Its carefree charms and deadly risks. *Psychology Today, 16,* 20–28.

Lykken, D. T. (1995). *The antisocial personalities.* Mahwah, NJ: Erlbaum.

Lykken, D. T., Bouchard, T. J., McGue, M., & Tellegen, A. (1992). Emergenesis: Genetic traits that may not run in families. *American Psychologist, 47,* 1565–1577.

Lykken, D. T., Tellegen, A., & Katzenmeyer, C. (1973). *Manual for the Activity Preference Questionnaire.* Minneapolis: University of Minnesota Press.

Lynam, D. R., Whiteside, S., & Jones, S. (1999). Self-reported psychopathy: A validation study. *Journal of Personality Assessment, 73,* 110–132.

McCord, W., & McCord, J. (1964). *The psychopath: An essay on the criminal mind.* Princeton, NJ: Van Nostrand.

McHoskey, J. W., Worzel, W., & Szyarto, C. (1998). Machiavellianism and psychopathy. *Journal of Personality and Social Psychology, 74,* 192–210.

Meehl, P. E. (1945). The dynamics of "structured" personality tests. *Journal of Clinical Psychology, 1,* 296–303.

Meehl, P. E. (1959). Some ruminations on the validation of clinical procedures. *Canadian Journal of Psychology, 13,* 102–128.

Meehl, P. E. (1986). Diagnostic taxa as open concepts: Meta-theoretical and statistical questions about the reliability and construct validity in the grand strategy of nosological questions. In T. Millon & G. L. Klerman (Eds.), *Contemporary directions in psychopathology: Toward the DSM-IV* (pp. 215–231). New York: Guilford Press.

Mehrabian, A., & Epstein, N. (1972). A measure of emotional empathy. *Journal of Personality, 40,* 525–543.

Millon, T. (1981). *Disorders of personality, DSM-III: Axis II.* New York: Wiley.

Millon, T. (1987). *Millon Clinical Multiaxial Inventory—II: Manual for the MCMI-II.* Minneapolis, MN: National Computer Systems

Mirels, H. I., & Garrett, J. B. (1971). The Protestant ethic as a personality variable. *Journal of Consulting and Clinical Psychology, 36,* 40–44.

Morey, L. (1991). *Personality Assessment Inventory: Professional Manual.* Tampa, FL: Psychological Assessment Resources.

Morey, L. C., Blashfield, R. K., Webb, W. W., & Jewell, J. (1988). MMPI scales for DSM-III personality disorders: A preliminary validation study. *Journal of Clinical Psychology, 44,* 47–50.

Morgan, A. B. (2000). *The relation of social information processing to psychopathic personality traits.* Unpublished master's thesis, Emory University, Atlanta, GA.

Newman, J. P., & Kosson, D. S. (1986). Passive avoidance learning in psychopathic and nonpsychopathic offenders. *Journal of Abnormal Psychology, 95,* 252–256.

Patrick, C. J. (in press). Getting to the heart of psychopathy. In H. Herve & J. C. Yuille (Eds.), *Psychopathy: Theory, research, and social implications.* Mahwah, NJ: Erlbaum.

Paulhus, D. L. (1991). Measurement and control of response bias. In J. P. Robinson & P. R. Shaver (Eds.), *Measures of personality and social psychological attitudes* (pp. 17–59). San Diego, CA: Academic Press.

Paulhus, D. L., & Williams, K. M. (2002). The dark triad of personality: Narcissism, Machiavellianism, and psychopathy. *Journal of Research in Personality, 36,* 556–563.

Piedmont, R. L., McCrae, R. R., Riemann, R., & Angleitner, A. (2000). On the invalidity of validity scales: Evidence from self-reports and observer ratings in volunteer samples. *Journal of Personality and Social Psychology, 78,* 582–593.

Poythress, N. G., Edens, J. F., & Lilienfeld, S. O. (1998). Criterion-related validity of the Psychopathic Personality Inventory in a prison sample. *Psychological Assessment, 10,* 426–430.

Poythress, N. G., Edens, J. F., & Watkins, M. M. (2002). The relationship between psychopathic personality features and malingering symptoms of major mental illness. *Law and Human Behavior, 25,* 567–582.

Premack, D., & Woodruff, G. (1978). Does the chimpanzee have a theory of mind? *Behavioral and Brain Sciences, 1,* 515–526

Pritchard, D. A. (1977). Linear versus configural statistical prediction. *Journal of Consulting and Clinical Psychology, 45,* 559–563.

Quay, H. C., & Parsons, L. B. (1971). *The differential behavioral classification of the juvenile offender.* Laboratory report, Philadelphia.

Raskin, R. R., & Hall, C. S. (1979). Narcissistic Personality Inventory. *Psychological Reports, 45,* 590.

Ray, J. J., & Ray, J. A. B. (1982). Some apparent advantages of sub-clinical psychopathy. *Journal of Social Psychology, 117,* 135–142.

Robins, L. R. (1966). *Deviant children grown up.* Baltimore: Williams & Wilkins.

Rogers, R., Vitacco, M. J., Jackson, R. L., Martin, M., Collins, M., & Sewell, K. W. (2002). Faking psychopathy: An examination of response styles with antisocial youth. *Journal of Personality Assessment, 78,* 31–46.

Salekin, R. T., Trobst, K. K., & Krioukova, M. (2001). Construct validity of psychopathy in a community sample: A nomological net approach. *Journal of Personality Disorders, 15,* 425–441.

Sandoval, A. R., Hancock, D., Poythress, N., Edens, J. F., & Lilienfeld, S. (2000). Construct validity of the Psychopathic Personality Inventory in a correctional sample. *Journal of Personality Assessment, 74,* 262–281.

Schmitt, W. A., & Newman, J. P. (1999). Are all psychopathic individuals low-anxious? *Journal of Abnormal Psychology, 108,* 353–358.

Sechrest, L. (1963). Incremental validity: A recommendation. *Educational and Psychological Measurement, 23,* 153–158.

Shadish, W. R., Cook, T. D., & Campbell, D. T. (2001). *Experimental and quasi-experimental designs for generalized causal inference.* Boston: Houghton Mifflin.

Skeem, J., & Lilienfeld, S. O. (2004). *Psychometric properties of self-report psychopathy measures.* Paper presented at the annual meeting of the American Psychology–Law Society, Scottsdale, AZ.

Smith, G. T., Fischer, S., & Fister, S. M. (2003). Incremental validity principles in test construction. *Psychological Assessment, 15,* 467–477.

Smith, R. J. (1985). The concept and measurement of social psychopathy. *Journal of Research in Personality, 19,* 219–231.

Spielberger, C. D., Gorsuch, R. L., Lushene, R. E., Vagg, P. R., & Jacobs, G. A. (1983). *Manual for the State–Trait Anxiety Inventory.* Palo Alto, CA: Consulting Psychologists Press.

Spielberger, C. D., Kling, J. K., & O'Hagan, S. E. (1978). Dimensions of psychopathic personality: Antisocial behavior and anxiety. In R. D. Hare & D. Schalling (Eds.), *Psychopathic behaviour: Approaches to research* (pp. 23–46). Chichester, UK: Wiley.

Spitzer, R. L., Williams, J. B. W., & Gibbon, M. (1987). *Structured clinical interview for DSM-III-R Axis II (SCID-II).* Washington, DC: American Psychiatric Association Press.

Stevens, D., Charman, T., & Blair, R. J. (2001). Recognition of emotion in facial expressions and vocal tones in children with psychopathic tendencies. *Journal of Genetic Psychology, 162,* 201–211.

Tellegen, A. (1982). *Manual for the Multidimensional Personality Questionnaire.* Unpublished manuscript, University of Minnesota. (Original work published 1978)

Tellegen, A. (1985). Structure of mood and personality and their relevance to assessing anxiety, with an emphasis on self-report. In A. H. Tuma & J. D. Maser (Eds.), *Anxiety and the anxiety disorders* (pp. 681–706). Hillsdale, NJ: Erlbaum.

Tellegen, A., & Waller, N. (in press). Exploring personality through test construction: Development of the Multidimensional Personality Questionnaire. In S. R. Briggs, & J. M. Cheek (Eds.), *Personality measures: Development and evaluation* (Vol. I). Greenwich, CT: JAI Press.

Verona, E., Patrick, C. J., & Joiner, T. E. (2001). Psychopathy, antisocial personality, and suicide risk. *Journal of Abnormal Psychology, 110,* 462–470.

Vincent, N. M. P., Linsz, N. L., & Greene, M. I. (1966). The L scale of the MMPI as an index of falsification. *Journal of Clinical Psychology, 22,* 214–215.

Widiger, T. A, Cadoret, R., Hare, R., Robins, L., Rutherford, M., Zanarini, M., et al. (1996). DSM-IV antisocial personality disorder field trial. *Journal of Abnormal Psychology, 105,* 3–16.

Widiger, T. A., & Frances, A. (1987). Interviews and inventories for measurement of personality disorders. *Clinical Psychology Review, 7,* 49–75.

Widom, C. S., & Newman, J. P. (1985). Characteristics of noninstitutionalized psychopaths. In J. Gunn & D. Farrington (Eds.), *Current research in forensic psychiatry and psychology* (Vol. 2, pp. 57–80). New York: Wiley.

Wiggins, J. S. (1982). Circumplex models of interpersonal behavior in clinical psychology. In P. C. Kendall & J. M. Butcher (Eds.), *Handbook of research methods in clinical psychology* (pp. 183–221). New York: Wiley.

Williams, K., Nathanson, C., & Paulhus, D. (2002). *Factor structure of the self-report psychopathy scale: Two and three factor solutions.* Paper presented at the annual meeting of the Canadian Psychological Association, Vancouver, BC, Canada.

Williamson, S. E., Harpur, T. J., & Hare, R. D. (1991). Abnormal processing of affective words by psychopaths. *Psychophysiology, 28,* 260–273.

Wilson, D. L., Frick, P. J., & Clements, C. B.(1999). Gender, somatization, and psychopathic traits in a college sample. *Journal of Psychopathology and Behavioral Assessment, 21,* 221–235.

Zagon, I., & Jackson, H. (1994). Construct validity of a psychopathy measure. *Personality and Individual Differences, 17,* 125–135.

Zuckerman, M. (1989). Personality in the third dimension: A psychobiological approach. *Personality and Individual Differences, 10,* 391–418.

Zuckerman, M., Kolin, E. A., Price, L., & Zoob, I. (1964). Development of a Sensation-Seeking Scale. *Journal of Consulting Psychology, 28,* 477–482.

7

Psychopathy and Personality

DONALD R. LYNAM
KAREN J. DEREFINKO

In 1937, Allport offered one of the first systematic definitions of personality: "personality is the dynamic organization within the individual of those psychophysical systems that determine his unique adjustment to the environment" (p. 48). Since that time, dozens of other similar definitions have appeared. Our preferred definition is a simple one: Personality refers to an individual's characteristic patterns of thinking, feeling, and acting. All these definitions share several features. First, personality is internal; it resides within the individual. Second, personality is manifested broadly; it has cognitive, affective, interpersonal, and behavioral components. Third, personality accounts for stable behavior patterns across time and situations. Using this definition, psychopathy can be understood as a particular personality pattern.

The idea of psychopathy as a personality configuration is not new. Cleckley's (1976) seminal description of psychopaths is a study in personality. By looking across the lives of certain individuals, Cleckley deduced their consistent patterns of behavior (i.e., their personalities). Cleckley's list of 16 diagnostic criteria for psychopathy is replete with personality traits. Nine of his diagnostic criteria are fairly standard personality descriptors: interpersonally charming, (absence of) nervousness, unreliability, insincerity, (lack of) shame, poor judgment, egocentricity, affec-

tively impoverished, and interpersonally unresponsive. Five of the remaining seven characteristics reference "enduring patterns" of behavior and can therefore be considered to be assessing personality: inadequately motivated antisocial behavior, fantastic and uninviting behavior with drink and sometime without, suicide rarely carried out, an impersonal sex life, and failure to follow any life plan.

The emphasis on personality is also found in Hare's operationalization of psychopathy, the 20-item Hare Psychopathy Checklist—Revised (PCL-R; Hare, 1991). In the PCL-R, 13 of the 20 items assessed represent standard personality descriptors: glibness, grandiosity, need for stimulation, untruthfulness, manipulativeness, lack of guilt, shallow affect, callousness, poor behavioral control, lack of planning, impulsivity, irresponsibility, and failure to accept responsibility. At least four of the remaining seven reference enduring behavior patterns: parasitic lifestyle, promiscuous sexual behavior, many short-term marital relations, and criminal versatility.

This chapter does not argue that psychopathy is related to personality. That is already demonstrated and widely accepted. Instead, this chapter presents evidence that psychopathy *is* personality. That is, a basic premise of this chapter is that psychopathy can be understood as a particular constellation of basic personality traits available in a variety of structural models of personality. By "structural," we refer to models from basic research in personality that use multiple dimensions, domains, or superfactors to organize the array of personality traits according to their interrelations (Wiggins & Pincus, 1992). These models of personality share fundamental assumptions that traits are the basic building blocks of personality, there are a finite number of basic traits, and traits provide comprehensive coverage of human personality. There are several benefits to using such models. First, these models were developed in research efforts to identify and organize the primary building blocks of personality. Traits from these models, then, are based more in the science of personality and less in the minds of psychopathy observers and theorists. Second, because these models were identified in basic science efforts and not in efforts to predict specific criteria, problems with predictor-criterion overlap are minimized. Third, each of these models has been widely used and well validated in various kinds of research. Thus, these models are very well grounded. Fourth, these models have been used to study issues in personality, including genetics, development, and neurobiology. As such, these models have much to offer the study of psychopathy.

In the pages that follow, we argue that psychopathy is best understood as a configuration of traits from a general, structural model of personality. First, we present several similar descriptions of psychopathy in terms of structural personality models generated by different methods. Second, we provide evidence that psychopathy can be assessed using such structural models. Third, we examine how the use of structural models of personality resolves lingering issues in the field of psychopathy. Finally, we discuss unresolved issues and potential future directions.

Using models of general personality functioning to understand psychopathy is consistent with research on personality psychopathology. There has been increasing concern regarding the validity of the categorical model underlying personality disorders. Critics of this categorical model have pointed to the model's failure to adequately differentiate abnormal from normal functioning and one type of disordered functioning from another (see Widiger & Clark, 2000). In response, authors have suggested that a dimensional model of personality disorders might be more useful (see Widiger & Frances, 2002). In the last 15 years alone, there have been over 50 studies looking at the relations between just the five-factor model of personality and personality disorders (Widiger & Costa, 2002). There are more studies using different dimensional models. In general, the results from these studies support the thesis that personality disorders can be understood from this perspective.

STRUCTURAL MODELS OF PERSONALITY

Since its inception, the field of personality research has been concerned with identifying the basic traits that represent the building blocks of personality. This research has developed and tested structural models of personality. The present study examines the relations between psychopathy and three widely used personality models: the five-factor model (FFM; McCrae & Costa, 1990), the Psychoticism–Extraversion–Neuroticism (PEN) model (Eysenck, 1977), and Tellegen's (1985) three-factor model (T-3). These models differ from each other in terms of the number and composition of the primary personality dimensions and in terms of how they were derived. The FFM is based on a lexical hypothesis which posits that the traits most important to human interaction, communication, and survival have been encoded in the natural language as single words (Allport, 1937). Based on this hypothesis, researchers have factor-analyzed trait terms taken from dictionaries in order to identify the major dimensions of personality. In contrast, Eysenck attempted to tie his personality domains to biological factors such as arousal level, testosterone, and the sympathetic nervous system. Finally, Tellegen developed his model and instrument through an iterative, exploratory approach to test construction that originally began as an effort to "explore personality characteristics that might be related to individual differences in hypnotic susceptibility" (Tellegen &

Waller, in press, p. 12) Despite these differences, there is a great deal of overlap between the models. Importantly, all three models have received sufficient study to warrant confidence in their reliability and validity.

Five-Factor Model

Table 7.1 lists the structural models reviewed in this study. The FFM was derived from studies of the English language to identify the domains of personality functioning most important in describing the personality traits of oneself and other persons (Digman, 1990; John & Srivastava, 1999; Wiggins & Pincus, 1992). This lexical research emphasized five broad domains, identified as Extraversion (E), Agreeableness (A), Conscientiousness (C), Neuroticism (N), and Openness (O) (John & Srivastava, 1999). E assesses an individual's proneness to positive emotions and sociability. A is concerned with an individual's interpersonal relationships and strategies; people high in A tend to be trusting, straightforward, and empathic whereas those who score low tend to be manipulative, arrogant, and unconcerned about others. C relates to the *"control of impulses,"* as well as to the ability to plan, organize, and complete behavioral tasks. The domain of N assesses emotional adjustment and stability. The domain of O refers to an individual's interest in culture and to the preference for new activities and emotions. Each of these five broad domains can be further divided into underlying facets or components. Costa and McCrae (1995a) have proposed six facets within each domain on the basis of their research with the NEO Personality Inventory—Revised (NEO PI-R; Costa & McCrae, 1992). For example, they parse the domain of Agreeableness (vs. Antagonism) into more specific facets of trust (vs. suspicion), straightforwardness (vs. deception), altruism (vs. exploitation), compliance (vs. aggression), modesty (vs. arrogance), and tender-mindedness (vs. tough-mindedness). We should note that because the psychopath is characterized by the negative pole of this dimension, we often speak of the psychopath as being high in Antagonism rather than low in Agreeableness.

Eysenck's PEN Model

Another enduring model is Eysenck's PEN, which includes Neuroticism (N), Extraversion (E), and Psychoticism (P) (Eysenck & Eysenck, 1970). These factors were origi-

TABLE 7.1. Personality Models and Dimensions

Model	Definitions
Five-factor model	
Neuroticism	Emotional stability and adjustment versus instability and maladjustment
Extraversion	Sociability and agency
Openness to Experience	Interest and willingness to try or consider new activities, ideas, beliefs; intellectual curiosity
Agreeableness	Interpersonal strategies: Agreeableness versus Antagonism
Conscientiousness	Ability to control impulses, carry out plans and tasks, organizational skills, follow one's internal moral code
Eysenck's PEN model	
Psychoticism	Egocentricity, interpersonal coldness and disconnectedness, lack of empathy, and impulsiveness
Extraversion	Sociability and agency
Neuroticism	Emotional stability and adjustment versus instability and maladjustment
Tellegen's three-factor model	
Positive Emotionality	Sociability, tendency to experience positive emotions, assertiveness, achievement orientation
Negative Emotionality	Tendency to experience negative emotions; one's ability to handle stress
Constraint	Ability to control impulses, avoid dangerous situations, and endorse traditional values and standards

nally derived from factor analyses of questionnaire items. Subsequently, Eysenck proposed that these factors were underlain by distinct biological systems. N, which measures emotional stability and adjustment, is believed to be related to the sympathetic nervous system and its activation threshold. E, which measures traits related to sociability and agency, is believed to be related to cortical arousal. Finally, Eysenck argued that P, which assesses egocentricity, (lack of) interpersonal warmth and connectedness, (lack of) empathy, and impulsiveness, is related to testosterone levels. This dimension was originally viewed as an underlying genotypic predisposition to schizophrenia.

Tellegen's Three-Factor Model

Tellegen's model posits three basic dimensions, each marked by a set of primary trait scales. Positive Emotionality refers to the tendency of individuals to be positively engaged with others and the world around them; it is marked by scales labeled wellbeing, social potency, social closeness, and achievement. Negative Emotionality reflects an individual's tendency to experience negative emotions (e.g., fear, anxiety, and anger) and his or her tendency to break down under stress; it is marked by subscales labeled "aggression," "alienation," and "stress reaction." Finally, Constraint assesses an individual's ability to control impulses, act deliberately, avoid potentially dangerous situations, and endorse traditional values and standards; it is marked by subscales labeled "traditionalism," "harm avoidance," and "control."

As noted earlier, there is good evidence for the validity of all of the models. For example, empirical support for the construct validity of the FFM is extensive, at both the domain and the facet levels, including convergent and discriminant validation across self, peer, and spouse ratings (Costa & McCrae, 1988), temporal stability across 7–10 years (Costa & McCrae, 1994), cross-cultural replication (De Raad, Perugini, Hrebickova, & Szarota, 1998), and heritability (Jang, McCrae, Angleitner, Reimann, & Livesley, 1998). The dimensions of Eysenck's PEN model have been replicated

cross-culturally in over 35 different countries (see Eysenck, 1990), show high temporal stability (Conley, 1985) and substantial genetic involvement (Eaves, Eysenck, & Martin, 1989), and are related to biological variables (Eysenck, 1990). Similar support exists for Tellegen's model; its structure has been replicated across raters (Harkness, Tellegen, & Waller, 1995) and countries (e.g., Almagor, Tellegen, & Waller, 1995), and it shows high heritabilities (Bouchard, Lykken, McGue, Segal, & Tellegen, 1990) and relations to biological variables (Depue, 1996).

Consensus Big Four

Readers may wonder how each model can be so well validated. The answer lies in recognizing that there is substantial agreement across the models in terms of the traits that are represented. The models all contain explicit representations of the "big two"—Extraversion (Positive Emotionality) and Neuroticism (Negative Emotionality). In addition, the FFM and Tellegen both contain dimensions related to control of impulses and orientation to convention—Conscientiousness and Constraint (C). Eysenck's model contains C, although it is not associated uniquely with a single factor: Empirical work suggests that Eysenck's Psychoticism dimension can be considered a blend of low C and low Agreeableness (Costa & McCrae, 1995b). All models also contain representations of Agreeableness (A). In Eysenck's model it is a component of the Psychoticism dimension. In Tellegen's model, it is represented on both the Negative Emotionality (aggression) and Positive Emotionality (social potency) dimensions (Church, 1994). Thus, these structural models are far from discrepant with one another. In fact, Watson, Clark, and Harkness (1994) have argued that "the Big Three and Big Five models define a common 'Big Four' space in which (a) two traits are equivalent (Neuroticism and Extraversion), (b) the third Big Three dimension (Constraint or Psychoticism) represents some combination of two Big Five factors (Conscientiousness and Agreeableness), and (c) the final Big Five trait (Openness, or imagination) is excluded "(p. 24). They go on to label the Big Four as Neuroticism (or negative emotionality), Extraversion (or Positive Emotionality), Conscientiousness (or Constraint), and Agreeableness.

PERSONALITY DESCRIPTIONS OF PSYCHOPATHY

The first step in coming to understand psychopathy as a specific personality configuration is determining what that specific configuration is. In what follows, we present the results of three approaches to generating a basic personality profile for psychopathy. In the first approach, we examine the empirical relations between each of the structural models and psychopathy through a meta-analytic framework. In the second approach, we discuss a translation of a psychopathy instrument into the language of a particular structural model, the FFM. In the third approach, we examine the personality profiles of psychopathy generated by experts. At this point, it is important to note that the latter profiles are couched almost entirely in terms of a single structural model, the FFM, simply because most of the work has been done using this model. We do not wish to imply that other structural models might not also be used to generate useful personality profiles of psychopathy.

Empirical Relations between Structural Models of Personality and Psychopathy

A number of studies have examined the empirical relations between psychopathy and various structural models of personality. Rather than rely on one or two of these studies to provide *the* empirical profile, we chose to combine studies and look at the composite profiles that emerged. There are two good reasons for taking this approach. First, we did not wish to allow our own biases and predispositions to influence which studies were reported. By including all relevant studies, we attempt to avoid claims of subjectivity and "cherry picking" of findings. Second, results of any individual study are constrained by the sample and the measures employed. Results of an aggregate of studies provide a more generalized profile. For both these reasons, we chose to conduct a meta-analysis of studies that examined one of the structural models and psychopathy.

Meta-Analytic Method

We conducted a comprehensive search for empirical research regarding the relations between the aforementioned structural models of personality and psychopathy. To do so we used PsychINFO (1963–2000). The personality-related terms included in the search were "psychoticism," "extraversion," "neuroticism," "Eysenck," "negative emotionality," "positive emotionality," "constraint," "Tellegen," "neuroticism," "extraversion," "openness," "agreeableness," "conscientious," and "five-factor model." These terms were crossed with psychopathy. Only studies using most components of a full structural model were included. Studies that reported relevant relations using several different samples were treated as independent samples and each was included in the meta-analysis. In studies in which multiple psychopathy assessments were conducted, results were averaged across method. Psychopathy was defined broadly and included ratings and self-reports.

We identified 20 studies that assessed both one of the major structural models of personality and psychopathy, variously defined. Six studies examined the relation to the PEN model (af Klinteberg, Humble, & Schalling, 1992; Andersen, Sestoft, Lillebaek, Mortensen, & Kramp, 1999; Harpur, Hare, & Hakstian, 1989; Harpur, Hart, & Hare, 2002; Shine & Hobson, 1997; Thornquist & Zuckerman, 1995); three studies (two in the same report) studied the relation with Tellegen's model (Lilienfeld & Andrews, 1996; Verona, Joiner, & Patrick, 2001); 11 studies (published in nine articles) yielded effect sizes between the FFM and psychopathy (Harpur et al., 1989, 2002; Hicklin & Widiger, in press; Lynam, 2002; Lynam et al., in press; Lynam, Whiteside, & Jones, 1999; Paulhus & Williams, 2002; Salekin et al., in press; Skeem, Miller, Mulvey, Tiemann, & Monahan, in press). In three studies that used the interpersonal circumplex, we transformed coefficients for dominance and love dimensions into effect sizes for Extraversion (E) and Agreeableness (A) from the FFM,[1] because dominance and love define the same two-dimensional space as E and A (McCrae & Costa, 1989); that is, dominance and love can be considered as 45-

degree rotations of E and A. Two studies were not included in this analysis because they examined the relation between structural models of personality and psychopathy using only the subfactors of psychopathy and not the total score (i.e., Benning, Patrick, Hicks, Blonigen, & Krueger, 2003; McHoskey, Worzel, & Szyarto, 1998).

Of the studies, 12 used the PCL-R to assess psychopathy, two used Lilienfeld's Psychopathic Personality Inventory (PPI; Lilienfeld & Andrews, 1996), two used Lynam's (1997) Childhood Psychopathy Scale (CPS), one used Hare's Self-Report Psychopathy (SRP) scale, two used Levenson's Self-Report Psychopathy (LSRP; Levenson, Kiehl, & Fitzpatrick, 1995) scale, and one used three different assessments. Eleven studies used incarcerated samples; five used student samples; four used community samples. Three studies, all with the FFM, were conducted in adolescent populations; the other studies were conducted in young to middle-age adult samples. Twelve of the effect sizes came from male only samples; eight

effect sizes came from samples that were at least 40% female.

Five-Factor Model

Table 7.2 provides a summary of the results. Each of the domains was significantly related to psychopathy although they differed in the strength of those relations. Neuroticism (N), Extraversion (E), and Openness (O) were all weakly related to psychopathy, whereas Agreeableness (A) and Conscientiousness (C) were strongly related. The weighted mean effect size for N is .16 with a 95% confidence interval ranging from .13 to .20. The weighted mean effect size for E was −.05 with a 95% confidence interval ranging from −.09 to −.02. The weighted mean effect size for O was −.09 with a 95% confidence interval ranging from −.14 to −.07. For A, the weighted effect size was −.52 with a 95% confidence interval of −.54 to −.50. For C, the weighted average effect size was −.38 with a 95% confidence interval ranging from −.41 to −.35.

TABLE 7.2. Results of Meta-Analysis on the Relations of Structural Models of Personality to Psychopathy

	Unweighted mean effect size	Weighted mean effect size	95% CI	No. of studies	Total N	Range of effect sizes
Five-factor model						
Neuroticism	.15	.16***	.13 to .20	10	3277	−.34 to .50
Extraversion	−.03	−.05*	−.09 to −.02	11	3457	−.25 to .34
Openness	−.09	−.10***	−.14 to −.07	9	3071	−.33 to .24
Agreeableness	−.51	−.52***	−.54 to −.50	11	3457	−.26 to −.65
Conscientiousness	−.39	−.38***	−.41 to −.35	10	3277	−.12 to −.64
Eysenck's PEN model						
Psychoticism	.25	.25***	.18 to .32	5	735	.14 to .33
Extraversion	.05	.07*	.00 to .14	6	824	−.20 to .13
Neuroticism	.12	.15***	.09 to .22	6	824	−.08 to .36
Tellegen's three-factor model						
Positive Emotionality	.13	.10*	.00 to .20	3	379	.14 to .33
Negative Emotionality	.30	.27***	.17 to .36	3	379	.22 to .35
Constraint	−.41	−.35***	−.44 to −.36	3	379	−.50 to −.24
Consensus Big Four						
Neuroticism	.13	.14***	.11 to .17	19	4480	−.34 to .50
Extraversion	.00	−.03*	−.05 to .00	20	4660	−.25 to .34
Agreeableness	−.42	−.49***	−.51 to −.47	19	4155	−.14 to −.65
Conscientiousness	−.36	−.37***	−.40 to −.35	18	3975	−.12 to −.64

Note. CI, confidence interval
*$p \leq .05$; **$p \leq .01$; ***$p \leq .001$.

Eysenck's PEN Model

The effect size for each higher-order factor was significantly different from zero, although there were significant differences in the sizes of the relations. The weighted mean effect size for Psychoticism was .25 with a 95% confidence interval of .18 to .32. The weighted mean effect size for Extraversion was .07 with a 95% confidence interval of .00 to .14; it should be noted this is in the direction opposite to that found for FFM Extraversion. The weighted mean effect size for Neuroticism was .15 with a 95% confidence interval of .09 to .22.

Tellegen's Three-Factor Model

There was a small, positive relation of .10 between Positive Emotionality and psychopathy with a 95% confidence interval ranging from 0 to .20. This positive relation is due almost entirely to the social potency subscale which had a weighted effect size of .27 compared to weighted effect sizes of −.02, −.06, and .03 for well-being, social closeness, and agency respectively. There was a moderate to large negative correlation of −.35 between Constraint and psychopathy with a 95% confidence interval ranging from −.44 to −.36. Negative Emotionality (NE) also bore a moderate, but positive relation, to psychopathy with a weighted effect size of .27 and a 95% confidence interval ranging from .17 to .36. However, the subscales within NE were differentially related to psychopathy; the aggression subscale was moderately to strongly related to psychopathy with a weighted effect size of .36, whereas the other two scales were much more weakly correlated with psychopathy (effect size =.10 and .17).

Consensus Big Four

Because of the similarities between various personality models, it is possible to provide effect sizes for the Consensus Big Four of Neuroticism/Negative Affect (N), Extraversion/ Positive Affect (E), Agreeableness (A), and Conscientiousness/Constraint (C). In order to construct the Big Four, it was necessary to decide which effect sizes to use, as the models of both Tellegen and Eysenck include only three of the four factors. In the case of

the PEN model, several studies have shown that P can be understood as a blend of FFM A and C (Costa & McCrae, 1995b). Thus, effect sizes for P were used as indices of A and C, although each was weighted by only half of the number of participants. Joint factor analyses of Tellegen's Multidimensional Personality Questionnaire (MPQ) and Costa and McCrae's NEO-PI-R (Church, 1994) suggest that A is represented in the MPQ dimensions of Negative Emotionality and Positive Emotionality in the form of aggression and social potency, respectively; that the stress reaction subscale of the MPQ is the best indicator of N; and that E is best approximated by well-being and social closeness. In summary, effect sizes for N came from FFM N, Eysenck's N, and MPQ stress reaction. Effect sizes for E came from FFM E, Eysenck's E, and the average of MPQ well-being and social closeness. Effect sizes for A came from FFM A, Psychoticism (reversed), and the average of MPQ aggression (reversed) and social potency (reversed). Effect sizes for C came from FFM C, Eysenck's P (reversed), and Constraint.

Results appear in Table 7.2. The weighted effect size for E is significantly different from zero but minuscule. N bears a small, positive relation to psychopathy with a weighted effect size of .14 and a 95% confidence interval ranging from .11 to .17. The effect for C is moderate to large and negative with weighted effect size of −.36 and a 95% confidence interval of −.38 to −.33. Finally, the relation between A and psychopathy is large and negative with a weighted average effect size of −.47 and a 95% confidence interval ranging from −.49 to −.44.

Based on these descriptions, the psychopathic individual is interpersonally antagonistic (low A). At the facet level, he is suspicious (low in trust), deceptive (low in straightforwardness), exploitive, aggressive, arrogant, and tough-minded. This individual has trouble controlling his impulses and endorses nontraditional values and standards (low C). Running somewhat counter to Cleckley's original description is a tendency for the psychopathic individual to experience negative emotions (e.g., anger and cravings-related distress), although this relation is weaker than the relations to A and C. There is little evidence that the psychopathic individual is high or low in Extraversion.

Translation of the PCL-R

A second approach to generating a personality profile of psychopathy based on a structural model of personality is to translate the criteria for psychopathy into the language of one or more structural models. Widiger and Lynam (1998) argued that all the core features of psychopathy operationalized in Hare's (1991) PCL-R have an explicit representation within one or more facets of the FFM. Table 7.3 provides a translation by Widiger and Lynam (1998) of the PCL-R

items into the facets of the FFM. Several aspects of this translation are worth noting.

First, facets of Agreeableness (A) and Conscientiousness (C) pervade the translation; facets from A appear in 14 of the PCL-R items, while facets of C appear in 13 of the items. For example, the PCL-R item of pathological lying is a direct expression of low straightforwardness (a facet of A). Cleckley (1976) stated that "the psychopath shows a remarkable disregard for truth and is to be trusted no more in his accounts of the past than in his promises for the future or his

TABLE 7.3. "Translation" of the PCL-R into the Language of the FFM

PCL-R item	FFM facets (domains)
Factor 1	
1. Glibness/superficial charm	Low self-consciousness (N–)
2. Grandiose sense of self-worth	Low modesty (A–)
4. Pathological lying	Low straightforwardness (A–)
5. Conning/ manipulative	Low straightforwardness, low altruism, low tender-mindedness (A–)
6. Lack of remorse or guilt	Low tender-mindedness (A–)
7. Shallow affect	Low warmth, low positive emotionality (E–), low altruism, low tender-mindedness (A–)
8. Callous/ lack of empathy	Low tender-mindedness (A–)
16. Failure to accept responsibility	Low straightforwardness, low tender-mindedness (A–), low dutifulness (C–)
Factor 2	
3. Need for stimulation	High excitement-seeking (E+), low self-discipline (C–)
9. Parasitic lifestyle	Low straightforwardness, low altruism, low modesty, low tender-mindedness (A–), low achievement striving, low self-discipline (C–)
10. Poor behavioral controls	High angry hostility (N+), low compliance (A–), low deliberation (C–)
12. Early behavior problems	Low straightforwardness, low altruism, low compliance (A–), low self-discipline, low deliberation (C–)
13. Lack of realistic, long-term goals	Low achievement striving, low self-discipline (C–)
14. Impulsivity	High impulsiveness (N+), low deliberation (C–)
15. Irresponsibility	Low competence, low dutifulness (C–)
18. Juvenile delinquency	Low straightforwardness, low altruism, low compliance, low modesty, low tender-mindedness (A–), low dutifulness, low self-discipline, low deliberation (C–)
19. Revocation of conditional release	Low straightforwardness, low altruism, low compliance, low modesty, low tender-mindedness (A–), low competence, low dutifulness, low self-discipline, low deliberation (C–)
Neither Factor 1 nor 2	
11. Promiscuous sexual behavior	Low straightforwardness, low altruism, low compliance, low modesty, low tender-mindedness (A–), low dutifulness, low self-discipline, low deliberation (C–)
17. Many short marital relationships	Low dutifulness (C–)
20. Criminal versatility	Low straightforwardness, low altruism, low compliance, low modesty, low tender-mindedness (A–), low dutifulness, low self-discipline, low deliberation (C–)

Note. Based on Widiger and Lynam (1998).

statements of present intentions" (p. 207). The lowest levels of FFM straightforwardness include being dishonest, cunning, misleading, deceptive, manipulative, shifty, and crooked. Similarly, the PCL-R item assessing responsibility is a direct expression of low dutifulness. As Cleckley (1976) noted, "Although the psychopath is likely to give an early impression of being a thoroughly reliable person, it will soon be found that on many occasions he shows no sense of responsibility whatsoever" (p. 206). Persons who are extremely low in dutifulness will be irresponsible, undependable, and unreliable.

It is also important to note that although facets of Agreeableness and Conscientiousness are the most widely represented, facets from Extraversion (E) and Neuroticism (N) are also included in the translation; in fact, both poles (low and high) of E and N are represented. For example, glibness and superficial charm, the tendency to be smooth, charming, slick, and verbally facile (Hare, 1991), are essentially the absence of self-consciousness, a facet of N (Costa & McCrae, 1992). The average person is characterized by a degree of self-consciousness and will be, to some extent, sensitive to ridicule, prone to embarrassment, socially anxious, or insecure (Costa & McCrae, 1992). On the other hand, the psychopath, is at the lowest levels of self-consciousness: "more than the average person, he is likely to seem free from social or emotional impediments, from the minor distortions, peculiarities, and awkwardness so common even among the successful" (Cleckley, 1976, p. 205). In terms of high N, the PCL-R item regarding poor behavioral controls, the tendency to become angry and aggressive over trivialities (Hare, 1991) is clearly related to the angry hostility facet of N—"the tendency to experience anger and related states such as frustration and bitterness" (Costa & McCrae, 1992, p. 16).

The final aspect to note about the translation is that although many PCL-R traits are well represented by single FFM facets (e.g., glibness, grandiosity, and lack of remorse) or multiple facets from the same domain (e.g., conning and irresponsibility), other PCL-R traits are represented by combinations of facets from different domains. This blending of facets from different domains may, at first, be difficult to understand given research documenting the distinctiveness of each domain

from the others. Such blending, however, makes sense in the present cases. The degree to which the PCL-R items map onto single FFM domains is, in part, a function of the degree to which the item represents an explicit personality trait rather than a behavior. For example, at least five of the seven PCL-R items translated as combinations of facets from Agreeableness and Conscientiousness reference antisocial behavior (i.e., promiscuous sexual behavior, early behavior problems, juvenile delinquency, revocation of conditional release, and criminal versatility). However, the blended translations offered for these items are quite consistent with what is known about the personality correlates of crime (Miller & Lynam, 2001). For the remaining PCL-R items the necessity to blend FFM domains was due primarily to either fuzziness in the PCL-R item itself (i.e., shallow affect) or to the placement of related facets, primarily those dealing with impulsivity (see Whiteside & Lynam, 2001), on different domains within the FFM itself.

Expert Descriptions

A third approach to arriving at a personality description of the psychopathic individual is to invite psychopathy experts to describe the personalities of prototypical psychopaths in the language of one or more structural models. From such ratings, prototypical descriptions of the psychopathic individual can be generated by averaging across experts. Such descriptions are useful as they bring out in stark contrast the aspects on which experts agree and blunt the idiosyncratic elements of each description. For example, if the experts all agree that the psychopath is low on a given facet, then the aggregate profile will include low values of that trait. If, however, only one or two experts believe that the psychopath is low in that trait, then that trait will appear to be about average in the aggregate.

FFM Expert Ratings

In the first expert study (Miller, Lynam, Widiger, & Leukefeld, 2001), researchers wrote to 21 nationally known psychopathy researchers and asked each to "rate the prototytpical, classic Cleckley psychopath" on each of 30 bipolar scales which corresponded to the 30 facets of the FFM. For example, to assess the facet of straightforwardness (a facet of Agreeableness), experts were asked "to what extent is the male [or female] psychopath honest, genuine, and sincere versus deceptive and manipulative?" Response choices ranged from 1 (extremely low) to 5 (extremely high). Experts were asked to rate a prototypical male and female psychopath; however, because results were similar across ratings, we present only results for the prototypical male psychopath. Sixteen experts returned the ratings. Table 7.4 gives the experts' mean rating on each of the facets as well as the standard deviations and ranges. As detailed in Miller and colleagues (2001), there was remarkable agreement in the descriptions of the prototypic psychopath, validating the approach itself.

What does the prototypical psychopath look like? Taking any facet with a mean score lower than 2 (low) or higher than 4 (high) as characteristic, the profile is similar to the one provided by Widiger and Lynam (1998). As with that profile, the psychopath is low in all facets of Agreeableness, three facets of Conscientiousness (dutifulness, self-discipline, and deliberation), self-consciousness (Neuroticism), and warmth (Extraversion), and high in impulsiveness (N) and excitement seeking (E). In addition, unconstrained by the definition inherent in the PCL-R, the experts indicated that the psychopath is low in anxiety (N), depression (N), vulnerability (N), trust (A), and openness to feelings (Openness), but high on assertiveness (E), openness to actions (O), and, perhaps surprisingly, competence (C). With the possible exception of psychopaths being characterized as high in competence, the additional traits included by our experts make good sense. Despite not being explicitly assessed by the PCL-R, low anxiety, a facet of N, is considered by some a cardinal characteristic of psychopathy (Lykken, 1995). Similarly, the trust (vs. suspiciousness) facet of A, which contrasts a disposition to believe that others are honest and well-intentioned with the tendency to be cynical and to assume that others may be dishonest or dangerous (Costa & McCrae, 1992), makes sense in a description of the prototypical psychopath. It is also easy to see why the psychopath would be characterized as low scoring on the two additional facets of N, depression and vulnera-

TABLE 7.4. Expert-Generated FFM Psychopathy Prototype

Domain and Facet	Mean	SD	Range
Neuroticism			
Anxiety	1.4s7	0.52	1–2
Angry hostility	**3.87**	0.64	3–5
Depression	1.40	0.51	1–2
Self-consciousness	1.07	0.26	1–2
Impulsiveness	**4.53**	0.74	3–5
Vulnerability	1.47	0.52	1–2
Extraversion			
Warmth	1.73	1.10	1–5
Gregariousness	3.67	0.62	3–5
Assertiveness	**4.47**	0.52	4–5
Activity	3.67	0.98	2–5
Excitement seeking	**4.73**	0.46	4–5
Positive emotions	2.53	0.92	1–4
Agreeableness			
Trust	1.73	0.80	1–3
Straightforwardness	1.13	0.35	1–2
Altruism	1.33	0.62	1–3
Compliance	1.33	0.49	1–2
Modesty	1.00	0.00	1–1
Tendermindedness	1.27	0.46	1–2
Conscientiousness			
Competence	**4.20**	1.00	1–5
Order	2.60	0.51	2–3
Dutifulness	1.20	0.78	1–4
Achievement striving	3.07	1.20	1–5
Self-discipline	1.87	0.83	1–4
Deliberation	1.60	1.10	1–4
Openness to Experience			
Fantasy	3.07	0.88	2–4
Aesthetics	2.33	0.62	1–3
Feelings	1.80	0.86	1–4
Actions	**4.27**	0.59	3–5
Ideas	3.53	1.10	1–5
Values	2.87	0.99	1–4

Note. Items were rated on a scale of 1 (extremely low) to 5 (extremely high). Characteristic items defined as less than or equal to 2, or greater than or equal to 4, appear as underlined (low) or **boldfaced** (high) values. From Miller, Lynam, Widiger, and Leukefeld (2001). Copyright 2001 by Blackwell Publishing. Reprinted by permission.

bility. In addition, the elevation on assertiveness makes sense given the description of high scorers as "dominant, forceful, and socially ascendant" (Costa & McCrae, 1992, p. 17).

The most difficult aspect of the experts' rating to understand is the characterization of the psychopath as high in competence. This issue is resolved, however, by noting that NEO-PI-R assessed competence is, in part, a self-assessment of efficacy. Costa and McCrae (1992) acknowledge that "of all the C[onscientiousness] facet scales, competence is most highly associated with self-esteem" (p. 18). There is, therefore, an interesting dissociation among the facets of C in psychopathic individuals; they see themselves as competent, but their life histories belie them.

Besides competence, three other facets (i.e., angry hostility, low positive emotions, and low achievement striving) that Widiger and Lynam identified within the PCL-R were not conceived as essential to psychopathy by the expert raters. All three were rated as being neither high nor low. The rating for angry hostility, however, almost surpassed our somewhat arbitrary criterion for being considered prototypical (i.e., $m = 3.87$ rather than ≥ 4). Ratings for positive emotions and achievement striving were among the most disagreed upon; both had standard deviations above 0.90, and the standard deviation for achievement striving was the highest of any item. Finally, low positive emotion was represented only by the most troublesome PCL-R item—shallow affect.

Expert Ratings on the Common Language Q-Sort

A second expert study (see Lynam, 2002) revealed that the impressive agreement between the expert raters and the FFM translation of the PCL-R was not due to constraining the raters to the 30 facets of the FFM. Similar results were obtained by having psychopathy experts rate the prototypical fledgling psychopath (Lynam, 2002) using the 100 items of the Common Language Version (CLQ; Caspi et al., 1992) of the California Child Q-set (CCQ; Block & Block, 1980). The CCQ does not represent any one theoretical viewpoint; instead, it reflects a general language for describing variations in children's personalities.

As in the previous study, psychopathy experts were contacted and asked to provide descriptions of the fledgling psychopath using the CLQ. Eight of 14 experts returned their Q-sorts of the fledgling psychopath, which were then used to construct a prototype by averaging across raters for each of the 100 items. Agreement among the returned Q-sorts was again excellent.

The 10 items most characteristic and the 10 items most uncharacteristic of the fledgling psychopath are provided in Table 7.5, along with how each item maps onto the FFM (John, Caspi, Robins, Moffitt, & Stouthamer-Loeber, 1994; Robins John, & Caspi, 1994). From this mapping, it can be seen that the prototype obtained from the Q-sort is quite similar to that obtained using the FFM. Ten of the defining items are relatively clear indicators of a single dimension; of these, five were indicators of low Agreeableness (A), three were indicators of low Conscientiousness (C), and two were indicators of low Neuroticism (N). The remaining 10 items were interstitial items that assessed both low A and low C. In sum, the psychopath, described using the atheoretical Q-sort, is extremely low in A, extremely low in C, and somewhat low in N.

Expert Ratings on the California Adult Q-Set

Reise and Oliver (1994) used a similar procedure to generate a profile of psychopathy using the California Adult Q-Set (Block, 1961). These authors had seven psychologists, five with clinical experience and two with training in personality assessment, use the CAQ to describe the psychopath. Again there was generally good agreement among judges. The authors developed a prototype by aggregating the ratings and provided the 13 most characteristic and 13 least characteristic descriptors. Mapping these characteristics onto the FFM (McCrae, Costa, & Busch, 1986), 22 of the 26 items assess low Agreeableness (A), low Conscientiousness (C), or a blend of more than one factor including A or C. The remaining four items assess low Neuroticism (N), low Openness (O), high Extraversion, and a blend of high N and high O.

A General Summary

The three methods to generating a psychopathy profile yield similar results. Across methods, the largest, most robust descriptor of psychopathy was low Agreeableness or high interpersonal antagonism. The psychopathic individual is egocentric, distrustful, aggressive, and unconcerned about others. Low Conscientiousness/Constraint was also very strongly and consistently related to psychop-

TABLE 7.5. Common Language Q-Sort Items Uncharacteristic and Characteristic of the Fledgling Psychopath

CLQ item	Mean	SD	Range	FFM scale
Uncharacteristic items				
76. He can be trusted; he's reliable and dependable.	1.3	0.46	1–2	C+
15. He shows concern about what's right and what's wrong.	1.9	0.99	1–4	A+, C+
62. He is obedient and does what he is told.	1.9	0.83	1–3	A+, C+
99. He thinks about his actions and behavior; he uses his head before doing or saying something.	1.9	0.83	1–3	C+
9. He makes good and close friendships with other people.	2.0	0.76	1–3	A+
67. He plans things ahead; he thinks before he does something; he "looks before he leaps."	2.0	0.93	1–3	C+
23. He is nervous and fearful.	2.3	0.89	1–3	N+
77. He feels unworthy; he has a low opinion of himself.	2.4	1.19	1–4	N+
2. He is considerate and thoughtful of other people.	2.5	1.60	1–5	A+
3. He is a warm person and responds with kindness to other people.	2.5	1.07	2–5	A+
Characteristic items				
11. He tries to blame other people for things he has done.	9.0	0.00	9–9	A–, C–
22. He tries to get others to do what he wants by playing up to them. He acts charming in order to get his way.	8.5	0.76	7–9	A–
65. When he wants something, he wants it right away. He has a hard time waiting for things he wants and likes.	8.5	0.53	8–9	A–, C–
20. He tries to take advantage of other people.	8.4	0.74	7–9	A–, C–
13. He tries to see how much he can get away with. He usually pushes limits and tries to stretch the rules.	8.3	0.71	7–9	A–, C–
21. He tries to be the center of attention.	8.0	1.07	6–9	A–, C–
85. He is aggressive.	8.0	0.76	7–9	A–, C–
10. His friendships don(t last long; he changes friends a lot.	7.6	1.69	4–9	A–, C–
91. His emotions don(t seem to fit the situation.	7.6	0.92	6–9	A–, C–
93. He's bossy and likes to dominate other people.	7.6	0.74	6–8	A–

Note. Each item is rated from 1 (extremely uncharacteristic) to 9 (extremely characteristic). A, C, and N denote the FFM domain (Agreeableness, Conscientiousness, and Neuroticism) and the sign indicates whether the item assesses the low (–) or high (+) pole of the domain. From Lynam (2002). Copyright 2002 by the American Psychological Association. Reprinted by permission.

athy. The psychopathic individual has trouble controlling his impulses and endorses nontraditional values and standards. Less consistent were the results for Neuroticism (N) and Extraversion (E), perhaps due to facets of these dimensions relating differentially to psychopathy. For example, expert ratings and the PCL-R translation both suggest that the psychopathic individual can be described as high in some elements of N (i.e., angry hostility and impulsiveness/urgency) but low in others (i.e., self-consciousness). These distinctions may get lost when one moves to the domain or higher-order factor level where N demonstrates a small, positive correlation with psychopathy in the meta-analyses. The case may be similar for E. Expert raters and the PCL-R translation agree that psycho-

pathic individuals are low in some elements of E (i.e., warmth and positive emotions) but high in others (i.e., excitement seeking). Again, these distinctions are lost at the domain level where E demonstrates a small, negative relation with psychopathy.

USING STRUCTURAL MODELS OF PERSONALITY TO ASSESS PSYCHOPATHY

Demonstrating that there is general agreement within and across approaches to defining psychopathy in terms of structural models of personality is only one step in showing that psychopathy can be described in terms of a particular constellation of basic traits. A second step lies in showing that psychopathy can be assessed using structural models of personality. To this end, Miller and Lynam and colleagues have conducted several studies (Miller & Lynam, 2003; Miller et al., 2001). Each study involves using the expert-generated FFM prototype to assess psychopathy among individuals, accomplished by computing the similarity of an individual's NEO-PI-R profile to the psychopathy prototype. The resultant number, the psychopathy resemblance index (PRI), serves as a measure of psychopathy in future analyses. Individuals who are more similar to the prototype are deemed more psychopathic.

In the first study, Miller and colleagues (2001) examined the relations between the PRI and antisocial behavior, substance use, and psychopathology in a community sample of 481 young men and women. These authors found that individuals high in psychopathy assessed using the FFM "looked like" psychopathic individuals assessed using other means (e.g., the PCL-R). These individuals scored high on a self-report inventory of psychopathy. They reported an earlier age at onset of delinquency, a greater variety of criminal offenses, and earlier and greater drug use. In addition, they reported more symptoms of antisocial personality and substance abuse and dependence. Importantly, these individuals were relatively immune to symptoms of internalizing disorders.

In a second study with college students, Miller and Lynam (2003) examined the relations between FFM psychopathy and antisocial behavior, aggression, risky sex, drug use, and laboratory measures of constructs relevant to psychopathy. Again, individuals identified as more psychopathic based on their resemblance to the psychopathy prototype "looked like" psychopaths identified using explicit psychopathy measures. Psychopathic students reported higher rates of substance use, riskier sexual behavior, and a greater variety of criminal acts. In terms of aggression, individuals high in psychopathy were more relationally, reactively, and proactively aggressive; in fact, psychopathy was more strongly related to proactive than reactive aggression, replicating previous work using incarcerated, PCL-R defined psychopaths (Cornell et al., 1996). Performance on the laboratory tasks was also in line with previous research. Psychopathic individuals

behaved more aggressively in an aggression task, were less willing to delay gratification in a discounting task, and generated more aggressive responses and were more likely to choose to enact an aggressive response in a social information-processing task.

RESOLUTION OF ISSUES IN THE AREA OF PSYCHOPATHY

The application of structural models of personality provides several clarifications of findings in the field. Specifically, the FFM clarifies (1) the PCL-R factor structure, (2) the patterns of comorbidity, (3) the litany of psychopathic deficits, and (4) the concept of successful psychopathy. In the next section, we describe these contributions.

The Two-Factor Structure of the PCL-R

There has long been an interest in subtyping psychopaths or breaking psychopathy into its constituent elements (see Poythress & Skeem, Chapter 9, and Cooke, Michie, & Hart, Chapter 5, this volume). Some attempts have been theoretical (e.g., Karpman, 1948; Lykken, 1995), whereas others have been empirical (Benning et al., 2003; Cooke & Michie, 2001; Harpur, Hakstian, & Hare, 1988; Harpur, Hare, & Hakstian, 1989). Most empirical attempts have involved factor analyses of psychopathy instruments, particularly the PCL-R. Original work argued for a two-factor structure (Harpur et al., 1988, 1989), whereas more recent work by Cooke and Michie (2001) has suggested that a three-factor model is more parsimonious. The most recent version of the manual for the Hare Psychopathy Checklist—Revised (Hare, 2003) retains the original two-factor solution but offers an alternative four-factor conceptualization (cf. Hare & Neumann, Chapter 4, this volume). Because most previous research, including research on self-report instruments, has examined a two-factor solution, we examine how a structural personality model can be used to understand the nature of the factors.

The interpretation of the two factors up to this point has been unclear and confusing; see Table 7.3 for the composition of the two factors. One interpretation, dropped in more recent writings, is that the two factors are primarily method factors. A second interpretation is that the first factor represents "a constellation of interpersonal and affective traits commonly considered to be fundamental to the construct of psychopathy," whereas the second reflects a "chronically unstable, antisocial, and socially deviant lifestyle" (Hare, 1991, p. 38). Although this interpretation is more substantive than the previous one, it has several shortcomings. It raises and leaves unanswered the question of what is psychopathy. The personality/behavior dichotomy into which this interpretation frequently slips is simplistic, overlooking the fact that Factor 2 includes several personality dimensions such as impulsivity, irresponsibility, and sensation seeking (Rogers & Bagby, 1994).

We offer two ways to understand the factor structure using personality models. The first is based on the translation of the PCL-R provided in Table 7.3. The items on Factor 1 are almost all indicators of low Agreeableness (A). Five of the eight items are mapped only onto low A, and two of the remaining three map onto low A and one other domain. Only the item assessing glibness fails to assess A. In contrast, Factor 2 items assess both low A and low Conscientiousness (C) with minimal representations of high Neuroticism and high Extraversion. This interpretation provides a substantive rather than methodological interpretation of the factors, acknowledges the presence of "personality" in both factors of the PCL-R, and does not suggest that one element is more central to psychopathy than another. In addition, this interpretation accounts for the strong correlation between factors (Hare, 1991); the factors are correlated because both include low A.

A second way to examine the structural makeup of the two factors is empirically, by looking across studies that have examined the correlations between structural models of personality and the two psychopathy dimensions. Because there are too few studies to conduct separate meta-analyses for each structural model, we focus on the Consensus Big Four. Seven studies provided eight effect sizes separately for two psychopathy factors (Benning et al., 2003; Harpur et al., 1989; Lynam, 2002; Lynam et al., in press; Lynam, Whiteside, & Jones, 1999; Shine & Hobson, 1997; Skeem et al., in press). Five of these studies used the FFM, two used Eysenck's PEN, and one used Tellegen's MPQ. In terms of psychopathy, four used the PCL-R, one used the LSRP, two used the CPS, and one used Lilienfeld's PPI. Six of the studies used adults and two used adolescents.

As can be seen from Table 7.6, results from the meta-analysis were consistent with the results obtained from the PCL-R translation. Neuroticism is uncorrelated with Factor 1 but moderately positively correlated with Factor 2 with a weighted effect size of .34 and a 95% confidence interval ranging from .31 to .37.[2] Similarly, Extraversion is uncorrelated with Factor 1 but weakly negatively correlated with Factor 2 with a weighted effect size of −.12 and a 95% confidence interval ranging from −.15 to −.09. Agreeableness is equally strongly negatively correlated with both Factor 1 and Factor 2 with a weighted effect size of −.43. Finally,

TABLE 7.6. Relations among the Consensus Big Four and Two Psychopathy Factors

	Unweighted mean effect size	Weighted mean effect size	95% CI	No. of studies	Total N	Range of effect sizes
Factor 1						
Neuroticism	−.01	.01	−.02 to .04	8	3301	−.41 to .34
Extraversion	.03	.00	−.03 to .03	8	3301	−.15 to .34
Agreeableness	−.39	−.46***	−.48 to −.43	8	3169	−.07 to −.65
Conscientiousness	−.22	−.22***	−.25 to −.19	8	3169	−.03 to −.44
Factor 2						
Neuroticism	.35	.34***	.31 to −.37	8	3301	.10 to .57
Extraversion	−.11	−.12***	−.15 to −.09	8	3301	−.31 to .03
Agreeableness	−.43	−.44***	−.46 to −.41	8	3169	−.21 to −.58
Conscientiousness	−.46	−.45***	−.48 to −.43	8	3169	−.02 to −.70

Conscientiousness is significantly, negatively, and weakly related to Factor 1 with a weighted effect size of –.21 and a 95% confidence interval ranging from –.25 to –.18. Alternatively, C is strongly, negatively related to Factor 2 with a weighted effect size of –.44 and a 95% confidence interval ranging from –.47 to –.42.

Thus, the two factors are similar in their assessments of low Agreeableness (A) but divergent in their relations to other dimensions. Factor 1 provides a fairly straightforward assessment of low A and some degree of low Conscientiousness (C), whereas Factor 2 strongly assesses both low A and low C with aspects of high Neuroticism and low Extraversion also included. On this account, the two factors are relatively highly correlated because of the overlap with low A but are divergent because the factors differentially assess the remaining three dimensions.

A recent study by Lynam and colleagues (in press) explicitly tested the idea that Agreeableness (A) is responsible for the overlap of F1 and F2. These authors examined the relations between psychopathy assessed using the Childhood Psychopathy Scale and the Big Five in two separate cohorts of the Pittsburgh Youth Study. Cohort 1 consisted of 405 12- to 13-year-old boys, and cohort 2 consisted of 435 17-year-old boys. Psychopathy and personality were assessed using mother-reports in both cohorts; additionally, boys reported on their own personalities in cohort 2. In an effort to explicitly test how much of the overlap between Factor 1 and Factor 2 is accounted for by A, Lynam and colleagues performed a series of hierarchical regression analyses. In cohort 1, two regression analyses were conducted. First, scores on F1 were regressed onto score for F2 at step one, with squared semipartial correlation providing an index of the degree of overlap. At step 2, A was entered; the squared semipartial correlation for F2 at this step provides an index of overlap after removing the overlap attributable to A. This analysis was repeated reversing the roles of Factors 1 and 2, and in cohort 2 for both mother- and self-reported personality. In all instances, the inclusion of A significantly reduced the overlap between the factors. In cohort 1 using mother-reports, the variance contributed by F2 in predicting F1 was reduced by 57% with the inclusion of A; the variance contributed by F1 in predicting F2 was reduced by 50%. In cohort 2 using mother-reports, the corresponding percentages were 68% and 65%; the percentages using self-reports of personality were 58% and 62%.

Explaining Comorbidity

Structural models of personality can also explain the comorbidity of psychopathy with other personality disorders (PDs) described in the fourth edition of the *Diagnostic and Statistical Manual of Mental Disorders* (DSM-IV; American Psychiatric Association, 1994; see Widiger, Chapter 8, this volume). Although high comorbidity presents a challenge to the validity of a categorical approach, it is easily accommodated within a dimensional model that views "categories" as configurations of basic dimensions of personality (Widiger & Frances, 2002). From this view, the apparent comorbidity among PDs is understood as the co-occurrence of diagnoses that have overlapping constellations of personality traits. Lynam and Widiger (2001) recently demonstrated how comorbidity can be understood as the sharing of FFM facets across PDs. Using expert-generated PD prototypes, these authors showed how the actual comorbidities among the DSM PDs can be predicted on the basis of FFM facet overlap alone. The argument is similar for psychopathy. More similar FFM profiles are predicted to have higher comorbidity. Antisocial personality disorder (APD) has an FFM profile that consists of low Agreeableness (A), low Conscientiousness (C), and somewhat high Neuroticism (N); see Table 7.7.[3] On the one hand, a strong positive correlation between psychopathy and APD would be expected because both prototypes include low A and low C; on the other hand, divergence would be expected given the differing relations to N, with psychopathy being associated primarily with low N and APD with somewhat higher N. Likewise, one expects an inverse relation between psychopathy and dependent personality disorder (DEP) given the divergence of these disorders on A, with psychopathy characterized by very low A and DEP characterized by high A (Lynam & Widiger, 2001).

To illustrate the effectiveness of the FFM in understanding the comorbidity between psychopathy and the other PDs, following

TABLE 7.7. FFM Profiles for Psychopathy and Three DSM-IV Personality Disorders

Domain and facet	Psychopathy	Antisocial	Dependent	Paranoid
Neuroticism				
Anxiousness	1.47	1.82	4.32	3.60
Angry hostility	3.87	4.14	2.42	4.00
Depressiveness	1.40	2.45	3.63	3.30
Self-consciousness	1.07	1.36	4.16	3.30
Impulsiveness	4.53	4.73	2.32	2.90
Vulnerability	1.47	2.27	4.32	3.60
Extraversion				
Warmth	1.73	2.14	3.84	1.30
Gregariousness	3.67	3.32	3.26	1.70
Assertiveness	4.47	4.23	1.32	2.90
Activity	3.67	4.00	2.26	2.90
Excitement seeking	4.73	4.64	2.26	2.20
Positive emotions	2.53	2.86	2.53	2.20
Openness				
Fantasy	3.07	2.82	3.05	2.90
Aesthetics	2.33	2.36	2.89	2.20
Feelings	1.80	2.27	3.74	2.40
Actions	4.27	4.23	2.21	2.00
Ideas	3.53	2.91	2.84	3.50
Values	2.87	3.00	2.89	1.90
Agreeableness				
Trust	1.73	1.45	4.26	1.00
Straightforwardness	1.13	1.41	3.11	2.00
Altruism	1.33	1.41	3.95	1.90
Compliance	1.33	1.77	4.68	1.40
Modesty	1.00	1.68	4.26	2.40
Tendermindedness	1.27	1.27	3.89	1.80
Conscientiousness				
Competence	4.20	2.09	2.58	3.30
Order	2.60	2.41	2.89	3.70
Dutifulness	1.20	1.41	3.79	3.40
Achievement striving	3.07	2.09	2.47	3.00
Self-discipline	1.87	1.81	2.84	3.50
Deliberation	1.60	1.64	3.00	3.80
Correlation with Psychopathy Profile		0.88	−0.84	0.10

Lynam and Widiger (2001), we generated the correlations between the FFM profiles for psychopathy and the other PDs. This was accomplished by treating facets as cases and PDs as variables. This provided a comorbidity estimate for psychopathy with each PD. These expected comorbidities are presented in the first column of Table 7.8.

Next, we meta-analyzed studies that included correlations between psychopathy and various personality disorders to generate an observed set of correlations. These studies examined the relations among the PCL-R

and the DSM-III criteria (Blackburn & Coid, 1998; Hart & Hare, 1989), the DSM-IV criteria (Reiss, Grubin, & Meux, 1999), the Millon Clinical Multiaxial Inventory–II (Hart, Forth, & Hare, 1991), the Personality Diagnostic Questionnaire, Revised (Shine & Hobson, 1997) and between the Psychopathy Q-Sort (PQS; Reise & Oliver, 1994) and the Morey Minnesota Multiphasic Personality Inventory (MMPI) Personality Disorder scales (Reise & Wink, 1995). Results are provided in the second and third column of Table 7.8. Finally, we compared, via a sec-

TABLE 7.8. Relations between Psychopathy and DSM-IV PDs Based on Facet Overlap and Empirical Studies

		Meta–analysis of empirical correlations		
	Facet overlap	Weighted observed *r*	95% CI	Range of *rs*
Paranoid	.10	.36	.28 to .43	.13 to .56
Schizoid	−.42	−.08	−.15 to 0	−.22 to .13
Schizotypal	−.25	.09	0 to .17	−.11 to .46
Antisocial	.88	.58	.53 to .63	.31 to .85
Borderline	.41	.33	.25 to .41	.13 to .60
Histrionic	.54	.25	.17 to .32	.14 to .44
Narcissistic	.85	.34	.27 to .40	.21 to .46
Avoidant	−.72	−.06	−.14 to .02	−.30 to .23
Dependent	−.84	−.16	−.26 to −.07	−.27 to .17
Obsessive–compulsive	−.36	−.07	−.17 to .03	−.20 to .28
Similarity to FFM correlations		.92		

Note. The "Facet overlap" column refers to the correlations between the FFM psychopathy prototype and the FFM personality disorder prototypes from Lynam and Widiger (2001). The "Weighted observed *r*" column represents the weighted mean effect size from six studies examining the correlations between psychopathy and other personality disorders (Blackburn & Coid, 1998; Hart et al., 1991; Hart & Hare, 1989; Reise & Wink, 1995; Reiss et al., 1999; Shine & Hobson, 1997). The number of studies including each personality ranged from 4 to 6; the number of participants for each disorder ranged from 409 to 673. "Similarity to FFM correlations" was calculated as a second–order correlation by correlating the entries in the "Facet overlap" column with those in the "Weighted *r*" column.

ond-order correlation, the correlations in column one to the correlations in column 2 to see how similar the results were. The correlations between psychopathy and other PDs expected based merely on facet overlap correspond extremely well to the correlations observed empirically, *r* = .92.

Alternative Models of "Psychopathic Deficits"

Much of the research in psychopathy has been oriented toward identifying and characterizing *the* core problem/deficit underlying psychopathy. Many candidate deficits have been proposed and are actively being studied; unfortunately, these various deficits are not easily subsumed under a single construct. That is, there does not appear to be *a* single etiological mechanism. This state of affairs is exactly what is expected if psychopathy were a constellation of personality traits from a general model of personality. How could a single deficit or deviation underlie low Agreeableness, low Conscientiousness, and low and high Neuroticism and Extraversion? Understood from a personality perspective, the variety of psychopathic deficits is due to the fact that different researchers are focused on different elements of the personality profile. For example, Patrick, Bradley, and Lang

(1993) have emphasized an emotional hyporeactivity as assessed by a fear-potentiated startle response. Patrick (1994) has specifically related this deficit to the broad domain of negative affectivity (neuroticism): "The observed absence of startle potentiation in psychopaths (Patrick et al., 1993) may reflect a temperamental deficit in the capacity for negative affect" (p. 325).

Lykken (1995) has also proposed a theory for psychopathy that is linked to general personality/temperament. He has suggested that the etiology of "primary" psychopathy may be constitutionally low levels of fear. In support of this hypothesis, Lykken (1995) cited data suggesting that psychopathic individuals demonstrate lower skin conductance (SC) when faced with negative stimuli and are more likely than controls to indicate a preference for risky rather than boring activities on the Activities Preference Questionnaire (APQ). Although neither the SC nor the APQ is a pure measure of Neuroticism, they are related (Watson & Clark, 1992).

In contrast to the emphasis on Neuroticism within the models of Lykken (1995) and Patrick (1994), the response modulation model of Newman (1998) may place more emphasis on low Conscientiousness/Constraint (C). According to Newman, the psychopath has a deficit in the ability to suspend a dominant response in order to assimilate feedback from the environment. Most recently, Newman (1998) has placed more emphasis on the role of shifting attention from the organization and implementation of behavior to its evaluation. In either case, the pathology would be expected to relate to low C, which is concerned with impulse control. For example, the FFM contains two facets of C that seem particularly relevant—deliberation and discipline. Persons low in discipline are impaired in their "ability to begin tasks and carry them through to completion despite boredom and other distractions," and persons low in deliberation are "hasty and often speak or act without considering the consequences" (Costa & McCrae, 1992, p. 18). The description of the attentional deficit by Newman is clearly more specific than the description of discipline and deliberation by Costa and McCrae (1992), but "a lack of prospective reflection or, in other words, a lack of planful thought and sound judgment" (Patterson & Newman, 1993, p. 722) is likely to be related in meaningful ways to deficits in deliberation and discipline present in persons who are low in C.

Successful Psychopathy

The FFM also brings clarity to the variety of conceptions of "successful" psychopathy. Hare (1993) has written that "many psychopaths never go to prison or any other facility. They appear to function reasonably well—as lawyers, doctors, psychiatrists, academics, mercenaries, police officers, cult leaders, military personnel, business people, writers, artists, entertainers, and so forth . . . " (p. 113). He indicated that if he could not study psychopathy in prisons, his next choice would "be a place like the Vancouver Stock Exchange" (p. 119). In contrast, Lykken's "successful" psychopath is the hero: "the hero and the psychopath are twigs from the same branch. Both are relatively fearless. . . . Had Chuck Yeager had slightly different parents (not necessarily bad parents, just more ordinary ones), he might have become a con man or a Gary Gilmore" (Lykken, 1982, p. 22).

These are two very different conceptualizations of successful psychopathy. An understanding of psychopathy as a collection of traits from a general model of personality, however, suggests that all versions of the suc-

cessful psychopath target only a subset of the traits in the psychopathic profile. The individuals Hare described are clearly deceptive, exploitive, arrogant, and callous (i.e., extremely low in Agreeableness). However, these individuals have frequently obtained advanced degrees and moved far in their fields; they seem to lack other important characteristics possessed by the prototypical psychopath such as unreliability, aimlessness, and poor impulse control (i.e., low Conscientiousness/Constraint). Similarly, Lykken's description focuses on only a subset of the traits involved in psychopathy, namely, the traits associated with low Neuroticism. Lykken neglects the fact that Yeager lacks the low A (i.e., deceptiveness, exploitativeness, aggressiveness, arrogance, and callousness) and low C (i.e., unreliability, aimlessness, negligence, and carelessness) that Gilmore possessed. In short, Yeager may share some characteristics with Gilmore (i.e., low fear, high excitement seeking, and high openness to actions), but there are more elements to prototypical psychopathy than these. Such an understanding of successful psychopathy is consistent with Cleckley's (1976) original descriptions of "incomplete manifestations or suggestions of the disorder" (p. 188).

FUTURE DIRECTIONS AND HYPOTHESES

We believe that there are a number of implications and future directions implied by understanding psychopathy as a collection of traits from a structural model of personality. These implications and directions are wide-ranging and include some suggestions for current practices and directions for future research on psychopathy as personality.

Implications for Current Practices

We believe that the current analysis of psychopathy as personality has implications for current practices. Specifically, we believe, first, that progress in understanding psychopathy can be advanced by studying its specific elements, with reference to one or more structural models of personality. Second, the current analysis suggests that researchers stop looking for a single psychopathic deficit. These researchers may be better served by looking for which traits are associated with which kinds of problems. Third, we believe that researchers may benefit by moving away from the traditional extreme groups designs (contrasting those who are very high in psychopathy against those who are very low) used in most psychopathy research. Such designs can be powerful and efficient but may make it difficult to study the contributions that individual traits make; those who are high in psychopathy have virtually all of the traits, whereas those who are low have very few, if any.

Future Research

Extensions of Current Research

There seems to be enough support and potential utility to continue studying psychopathy from the perspective of one or more dimensional models of personality. Replication and extension of the current findings across different measures, settings, and samples would be helpful. The inclusion of additional measures of psychopathy would be useful; there are various derivatives of the Hare Psychopathy Checklist available for use in different settings and with different populations as well as several well-validated self-report instruments that might be used. Future research would also be well served by using additional methods for assessing personality. Previous research has relied primarily on self-reports of personality, but these have shortcomings, depending as they do on individuals' ability and willingness to accurately report (but see Lilienfeld & Fowler, Chapter 6, this volume). In terms of the FFM, a rating form of the NEO-PI-R exists, as does a Structural Interview for the Five Factor Model (SIFFM; Trull & Widiger, 1997). Research showing that these approaches yield results similar to self-reports would be quite compelling. Future research might also look to employ samples of differing ages. Current research shows that psychopathy can be assessed relatively early in development; more research in adolescence (Lynam et al., in press; Salekin, Leistico, Trobst, & Schrum, in press) would be helpful as would research in older adults. In general, we agree with Robins (1978): "the more the populations studied differ, the wider the historical eras

they span, the more the details of the methods vary, the more convincing becomes that replication" (p. 611).

We would also like to see more research examining the utility of assessing psychopathy with structural models of personality and testing key hypotheses from this account. If psychopathy can be understood as a collection of traits from a structural model of personality, then it should be possible to use such a model to reliably and validly assess psychopathy. Although some initial work has been done, much work remains. Both studies by Miller and Lynam (2003; Miller et al., 2001) used young adult samples drawn from community or undergraduate populations. It would be useful to examine this issue in incarcerated populations using additional structural models.

New Hypotheses

In terms of moving beyond replication, there are several hypotheses that fall out of the present account. There is research supporting the two-factor reconceptualization of the PCL-R and the account of comorbidity provided by structural models, but there is little research examining the idea that different psychopathic deficits line up along the lines of the personality dimensions from the structural models. There is also little research on the issue of successful psychopathy. Both ideas are amenable to empirical test in a variety of settings.

The present account also generates several additional hypotheses, some of which make predictions in directions opposite to those expected based on understanding psychopathy as a categorical entity. For example, a categorical, deficit-driven model seems to predict a single genetic influence on psychopathy, whereas the dimensional model allows for multiple, additive genetic effects. Given that all the major dimensions in the structural models of personality have strong genetic components, one would expect to see these same effects apparent in the genetics of psychopathy. Using multivariate behavior genetics, one could ask whether the genes underlying the dimensions of personality are the same or different as the genes underlying psychopathy.

An additional prediction concerns sex differences. Although there was not enough research on psychopathy and personality in women to allow discussion in this chapter (for a review of existing research on psychopathy in women, see Verona & Vitale, Chapter 21, this volume), there is enough research to conclude that women are generally less psychopathic than men (e.g., Vitale, Smith, Brinkley, & Newman, 2002). These sex differences are entirely consistent with the present perspective which suggests that sex differences in levels of psychopathy should mirror sex differences in the personality traits comprising psychopathy. Gender differences in personality traits relevant to psychopathy have been well documented (Costa, Terracciano, & McCrae, 2001). Women score higher (almost one-third of a standard deviation higher) on all facets of Agreeableness, higher on all facets of Neuroticism except for angry hostility, and higher on some facets of Extraversion (e.g., warmth and positive emotions) but lower on others (e.g., assertiveness and excitement seeking). In fact, the pattern of sex differences closely mirrors the expert-generated FFM psychopathy prototype. The current model predicts that sex differences in psychopathy should disappear when sex differences in personality are taken into account.

In sum, we have offered an account of psychopathy as a collection of basic personality traits. Extant evidence supports this account. The specific traits involved are well delineated; the same personality profile emerges across methods. This profile can be used to assess psychopathy. Understanding psychopathy as personality in this way resolves a number of issues in the field. Perhaps more important, understanding psychopathy from this perspective generates a variety of new hypotheses and directions for research.

ACKNOWLEDGMENT

The writing of this chapter was supported in part by Grant No. MH60104 from the National Institute of Mental Health.

NOTES

1. Specifically, the effect size for E was computed as: cosine(45)*dominance + cosine(45)*love. The effect size for A was computed as: cosine(45)*love – cosine(45)*dominance.

2. However, several studies have noted a cooperative suppressor effect between the two factors and trait anxiety, such that Factor 1 bears a negative relation to anxiety once the variance shared with Factor 2 is removed (e.g., Frick, Lilienfeld, Ellis, Loney, & Silverthorn, 1999; Verona, Joiner, & Patrick, 2001).

3. It should be noted that the correspondence between the FFM profiles for psychopathy and APD is quite high. We believe this is due to two influences. First, many of our APD experts likely thought of the psychopath when rating the personality of the individual with APD. Second and relatedly, we did not restrict the experts to the facets that are included in the DSM APD criteria. When such a restriction is applied (see Widiger, Trull, Clarkin, Sanderson, & Costa, 2002), the correspondence between these FFM profiles should decrease. In fact, the correlation between the psychopathy prototype and Widiger et al. APD prototype is .60.

REFERENCES

Studies followed by an asterisk were included in the meta-analysis on personality and psychopathy. Those followed by two asterisks were also included in the meta-analysis on personality and psychopathy factors.

af Klinteberg, B., Humble, K., & Schalling, D. (1992). Personality and psychopathy of males with a history of early criminal behavior. *European Journal of Personality*, 6, 245–266.*

Allport, G. W. (1937). *Personality: A psychological interpretation*. New York: Holt

Almagor, M., Tellegen, A., & Waller, N. (1995). The big seven model: A cross-cultural replication and further exploration of the basic dimensions of natural language trait descriptors. *Journal of Personality and Social Psychology*, 69, 300–307.

American Psychiatric Association. (1994). *Diagnostic and statistical manual of mental disorders* (4th ed.). Washington, DC: Author.

Andersen, H. S., Sestoft, D., Lillebaek, T., Mortensen, E. L., & Kramp, P. (1999). Psychopathy and psychopathological profiles in prisoners on remand. *Acta Psychiatrica Scandinavia*, 99, 33–39.*

Benning, S. D., Patrick, C. J., Hicks, B. M., Blonigen, D. M., & Kreuger, R. F. (2003). Factor structure of the Psychopathic Personality Inventory: Validity and implications for clinical assessment. *Psychological Assessment*, 15, 340–350.**

Blackburn, R., & Coid, J. W. (1998). Psychopathy and the dimensions of personality disorder in violent offenders. *Personality and Individual Differences*, 25, 129–145.

Block, J. (1961). *The Q-sort method in personality as-*

sessment and psychiatric research. Springfield, IL: Thomas.

Block, J. H., & Block, J. (1980). *The California Child Q-Set.* Palo Alto, CA: Consulting Psychologists Press.

Bouchard, T. J., Lykken, D. T., McGue, M., Segal, N. L., & Tellegen, A. (1990). Sources of human psychological differences: The Minnesota Study of Twins Reared Apart. *Science, 250,* 223–228.

Caspi, A., Block, J., Block, J. H., Klopp, B., Lynam, D., Moffitt, T. E., & Stouthamer-Loeber, M. (1992). A "common language" version of the California Child Q-Set (CCQ) for personality assessment. *Psychological Assessment, 4,* 512–523.

Church, T. A. (1994). Relating the Tellegen and five factor models of personality structure. *Journal of Personality and Social Psychology, 67,* 898–909.

Cleckley, H. (1976). *The mask of sanity* (5th ed.). St. Louis, MO: Mosby.

Cooke, D. J., & Michie, C. (2001). Refining the construct of psychopathy: Towards a hierarchical model. *Psychological Assessment, 13,* 171–188.

Cornell, D. G., Warren, J., Hawk, G., Stafford, E., Oram, G., & Pine, D. (1996). Psychopathy in instrumental and reactive violent offenders. *Journal of Consulting and Clinical Psychology, 64,* 783–790.

Costa, P. T., & McCrae, R. R. (1988). Personality in adulthood: A six-year longitudinal of self-reports and spouse ratings on the NEO Personality Inventory. *Journal of Personality and Social Psychology, 54,* 853–863.

Costa, P. T., & McCrae, R. R. (1992). *Revised NEO Personality Inventory (NEO-PI-R) and NEO Five-Factor Inventory (NEO-FFI) Professional Manual.* Odessa, FL: Psychological Assessment Resources.

Costa, P. T., & McCrae, R. R. (1994). Set like plaster? Evidence for the stability of adult personality. In T. Heatherton & J. L. Weinberger (Eds.), *Can personality change?* (pp. 21–40). Washington, DC: American Psychological Association.

Costa, P. T., & McCrae, R. R. (1995a). Domains and facets: Hierarchical personality assessment using the revised NEO personality inventory. *Journal of Personality Assessment, 64,* 21–50.

Costa, P. T., & McCrae, R. R. (1995b). Primary traits of Eysenck's P-E-N model: Three- and five-factor solutions. *Journal of Personality and Social Psychology, 69,* 308–317.

Costa, P. T., Terracciano, A. & McCrae, R. R. (2001). Gender differences in personality traits across cultures: Robust and surprising findings. *Journal of Personality and Social Psychology, 81,* 322–331.

Depue, R. A. (1996). A neurobiological framework for the structure of personality and emotion: Implications for personality disorders. In J. F. Clarkin & M. F. Lenzenweger (Eds.), *Major theories of personality disorder* (pp. 347–390). New York: Guilford Press.

De Raad, B., Perugini, M., Hrebickova, M., & Szarota, P. (1998). Lingua franca of personality: Taxonomies and structures based on the psycholexical approach. *Journal of Cross-Cultural Psychology, 29,* 212–232.

Digman, J. (1990). Personality structure: Emergence of the five factor model. *Annual Review of Psychology, 41,* 417–440.

Eaves, L. J., Eysenck, H. J., & Martin, N. G. (1989). *Genes, culture, and personality: An empirical approach.* London: Academic Press.

Eysenck, H. J. (1977). *Crime and personality.* London: Routledge & Kegan Paul.

Eysenck, H. J. (1990). Biological dimensions of personality. In L. A. Pervin & O. P. John (Eds.), *Handbook of personality: Theory and research* (2nd ed., pp. 102–138). New York: Guilford Press.

Eysenck, S. G., & Eysenck, H. J. (1970). Crime and personality: An empirical study of the three-factor theory. *British Journal of Criminology, 10,* 225–239.

Frick, P. J., Lilienfeld, S. O., Ellis, M., Loney, B., & Silverthorn, P. (1999). The association between anxiety and psychopathy dimensions in children. *Journal of Abnormal Child Psychology, 27,* 383–392.

Haapsalo, J., & Pulkkinen, L. (1992). The psychopathy checklist and non-violent offender groups. *Criminal Behaviour and Mental Health, 2,* 315–328.*

Hare, R. D. (1991). *The Hare Psychopathy Checklist—Revised.* Toronto, ON, Canada: Multi-Health Systems.

Hare, R. D. (2003). *The Hare Psychopathy Checklist—Revised* (2nd ed.). Toronto, ON, Canada: Multi-Health Systems.

Harkness, A. R., Tellegen, A., & Waller, N. (1995). Differential convergence of self-report and informant data for Multidimensional Personality Questionnaire traits: Implications for the construct of Negative Emotionality. *Journal of Personality Assessment, 64,* 185–204.

Harpur, T. J., Hakstian, A. R., & Hare, R. D. (1988). Factor structure of the Psychopathy Checklist. *Journal of Consulting and Clinical Psychology, 56,* 741–747.

Harpur, T. J., Hare, R. D., & Hakstian, A. R. (1989). Two-factor conceptualization of psychopathy: Construct validity and assessment implications. *Psychological Assessment, 1,* 6–17.**

Harpur, T. J., Hart, S. D., & Hare, R. D. (2002). Personality of the psychopath. In P. T. Costa & T. A. Widiger (Eds.), *Personality disorders and the five-factor model of personality* (2nd ed., pp. 299–324). Washington, DC: American Psychological Association.*

Hart, S. D., Forth, A. E., & Hare, R. D. (1991). The MCMI-II and psychopathy. *Journal of Personality Disorders, 5,* 318–327.

Hart, S. D., & Hare, R. D. (1989). Discriminant validity of the Psychopathy Checklist in a forensic psychiatric population. *Psychological Assessment, 1,* 211–218.

Hicklin, J., & Widiger, T. A. (in press). Similarities and differences among antisocial and psychopathic self-report inventories from the perspective of general personality functioning. *European Journal of Psychology.**

Jang, K., McCrae, R. R., Angleitner, A., Riemann, R., & Livesley, W. J. (1998). Heritability of facet-level traits in a cross-cultural twin sample: Support for a hierarchical model of personality. *Journal of Personality and Social Psychology, 74,* 1556–1565.

John, O. P., Caspi, A., Robins, R. W., Moffitt, T. E., & Stouthamer-Loeber, M. (1994). The "Little Five": Exploring the nomological network of the Five-Factor Model of personality in adolescent boys. *Child Development, 65,* 160–178.

John, O. P., & Srivastava, S. (1999). The Big Five trait taxonomy: History, measurement, and theoretical perspectives. In L. A. Pervin & O. P. John (Eds.), *Handbook of personality. Theory and research* (2nd ed., pp. 102–138). New York: Guilford Press.

Karpman, B. (1948). The myth of the psychopathic personality. *American Journal of Psychiatry, 104,* 523–534.

Levenson, M. R., Kiehl, K. A., & Fitzpatrick, C. M. (1995). Assessing psychopathic attributes in a noninstitutional population. *Journal of Personality and Social Psychology, 68,* 151–158.

Lilienfeld, S. O., & Andrews, B. P. (1996). Development and preliminary validation of a self-report measure of psychopathic personality traits in noncriminal populations. *Journal of Personality Assessment, 66,* 488–524.*

Lykken, D. T. (1982, September). Fearlessness. *Psychology Today,* pp. 6–10.

Lykken, D. T. (1995). *The antisocial personalities.* Hillsdale, NJ: Erlbaum.

Lynam, D. R. (1997). Childhood psychopathy: Capturing the fledgling psychopath in a nomological net. *Journal of Abnormal Psychology, 106,* 425–438.

Lynam, D. R. (2002). Psychopathy from the perspective of the five factor model. In P. T. Costa & T. A. Widiger (Eds.), *Personality disorders and the five-factor model of personality* (2nd ed., pp. 325–350). Washington, DC: American Psychological Association.**

Lynam, D. R., Caspi, A., Moffitt, T. E., Raine, A., Loeber, R., & Stouthamer-Loeber, M. (in press). Adolescent psychopathy and the Big Five: Results from two samples. *Journal of Abnormal Child Psychology.**

Lynam, D. R., Whiteside, S., & Jones, S. (1999). Self-reported psychopathy: A validation study. *Journal of Personality Assessment, 73,* 110–132.**

Lynam, D. R., & Widiger, T. A. (2001). Using the Five Factor Model to represent the DSM-IV personality disorders: An expert consensus approach. *Journal of Abnormal Psychology, 110,* 401–412.

McCrae, R. R., & Costa, P. T., Jr. (1989). The structure of interpersonal traits: Wiggins's circumplex and the Five-Factor Model. *Journal of Personality and Social Psychology, 56,* 586–595.

McCrae, R. R., & Costa, P. T. (1990). *Personality in adulthood.* New York: Guilford Press.

McCrae, R. R., Costa, P. T., & Busch, C. M. (1986). Evaluating comprehensiveness in personality systems: The California Q-Set and the five-factor model. *Journal of Personality, 54,* 430–446.

McHoskey, J. W., Worzel, W., & Szyarto, C. (1998). Machiavellianism and psychopathy. *Journal of Personality and Social Psychology, 74,* 192–210.

Miller, J. D., & Lynam, D. R. (2001). Structural models of personality and their relation to antisocial behavior: A meta-analytic review. *Criminology, 39,* 765–792.

Miller, J. D., & Lynam, D. R. (2003). Psychopathy and the Five Factor Model of personality: A replication and extension. *Journal of Personality Assessment, 81,* 168–178.

Miller, J. D., Lynam, D. R., Widiger, T. A., & Leukefeld, C. (2001). Personality disorders as extreme variants of common personality dimensions: Can the Five-Factor Model adequately represent psychopathy? *Journal of Personality, 69,* 253–276.

Newman, J. P. (1998). Psychopathy: An information processing perspective. In D. J. Cooke, A. E. Forth, & R. D. Hare (Eds.), *Psychopathy: Theory, research, and implications for society* (pp. 81–104). London: Kluwer.

Patrick, C. J. (1994). Emotion and psychopathy: Startling new insights. *Psychophysiology, 31,* 319–330.

Patrick, C. J., Bradley, M. M., & Lang, P. J. (1993). Emotion in the criminal psychopath: Startle reflex modulation. *Journal of Abnormal Psychology, 102,* 82–92.

Patterson, M. C., & Newman, J. P. (1993). Reflectivity and learning from aversive events: Toward a psychological mechanism for the syndromes of disinhibition. *Psychological Review, 100,* 76–736.

Paulhus, D. L., & Williams, K. M. (2002). The dark triad of personality: Narcissism, machaivellianism, and psychopathy. *Journal of Research in Personality, 36,* 556–563.*

Reiss, D., Grubin, D., & Meux, C. (1999). Institutional performance of male "psychopaths" in a high-security hospital. *Journal of Forensic Psychiatry, 10,* 290–299.

Reise, S. P., & Oliver, C. J. (1994). Development of a California Q-Set indicator of primary psychopathy. *Journal of Personality Assessment, 62,* 130–144.

Reise, S. P., & Wink, P. (1995). Psychological implications of the Psychopathy Q-Sort. *Journal of Personality Assessment, 65*(2), 300–312.

Robins, L. (1978). Sturdy childhood predictors of adult antisocial behavior: Replications from longitudinal studies. *Psychological Medicine, 8,* 611–622.

Robins, R. W., John, O. P., & Caspi, A. (1994). Major dimensions of personality in early adolescence: The Big Five and beyond. In C. F. Halverson, G. A. Kohnstamm, & R. P. Martin (Eds.), *The developing structure of temperament and personality from infancy to adulthood* (pp. 267–291). Hillsdale, NJ: Erlbaum.

Salekin, R. T., Leistico, A. R., Trobst, K. K., & Schrum,

C. L. (in press). Adolescent psychopathy and the interpersonal circumplex: Expanding evidence of a nomological net. *Journal of Abnormal Child Psychology.**

Shine, J., & Hobson, J. (1997). Construct validity of the Hare Psychopathy Checklist, Revised, on a UK prison population. *Journal of Forensic Psychiatry, 8,* 546–561.***

Skeem, J. L., Miller, J. D., Mulvey, E., Tiemann, J., & Monahan, J. (in press). Personality traits and violence among psychiatric patients. *Journal of Consulting and Clinical Psychology.***

Tellegen, A. (1985). Structures of mood and personality and their relevance to assessing anxiety with an emphasis on self-report. In A. H. Tuma & J. D. Maser (Eds.), *Anxiety and the anxiety disorders* (pp. 681–706). Hillsdale, NJ: Erlbaum.

Tellegen, A., & Walker, N. G. (in press). Exploring personality through test construction: Development of the Multidimensional Personality Questionnaire. In S. R. Briggs & M. Cheek (Eds.), *Personality measures: Development and evaluation* (Vol. 1). Greenwich, CT: JAI Press.

Thornquist, M. H., & Zuckerman, M. (1995). Psychopathy, passive-avoidance learning and basic dimensions of personality. *Personality and Individual Differences, 19,* 525–534.*

Trull, T. J., & Widiger, T. A. (1997). *Structured Interview for the Five Factor Model of Personality.* Odessa, FL: Psychological Assessment Resources.

Verona, E., Joiner, T. E., & Patrick, C. J. (2001). Psychopathy, antisocial personality, and suicide risk. *Journal of Abnormal Psychology, 110,* 462–470.*

Vitale, J. E., Smith, S. S., Brinkley, C. A., & Newman, J. P. (2002). The reliability and validity of the Psychopathy Checklist—Revised in a sample of female offenders. *Criminal Justice and Behavior, 29,* 202–231.

Watson, D., & Clark, L. A. (1992). Affects separable and inseparable: On the hierarchical arrangement of the negative affects. *Journal of Personality and Social Psychology, 62,* 489–505.

Watson, D., Clark, L. A., & Harkness, A. R. (1994). Structures of personality and their relevance to psychopathology. *Journal of Abnormal Psychology, 103,* 18–31.

Whiteside, S. P., & Lynam, D. R. (2001). The Five Factor Model and impulsivity: Using a structural model of personality to understand impulsivity. *Personality and Individual Differences, 30,* 669–689.

Widiger, T. A., & Clark, L. A. (2000). Toward DSM-V and the classification of psychopathology. *Psychological Bulletin, 126,* 946–963.

Widiger, T. A. & Costa, P. T. (2002). Five-factor model personality disorder research. In P. T. Costa & T. A. Widiger (Eds.), *Personality disorders and the five-factor model of personality* (2nd ed., pp. 59–88). Washington, DC: American Psychological Association.

Widiger, T. A., & Frances, A. J. (2002). Towards a dimensional model for the personality disorders. In P. T. Costa & T. A. Widiger (Eds.), *Personality disorders and the five-factor model of personality* (2nd ed., (pp. 23–44). Washington, DC: American Psychological Association.

Widiger, T. A., & Lynam, D. R. (1998). Psychopathy and the five-factor model of personality. In T. Millon, E. Simonsen, M. Birket-Smith, & R. D. Davis (Eds.), *Psychopathy: Antisocial. criminal, and violent behaviors* (pp. 171–187). New York: Guilford Press.

Widiger, T. A., Trull, T. J., Clarkin, J. F., Sanderson, C., & Costa, P. T. (2002). A description of the DSM-IV personality disorders with the five-factor model of personality. In P. T. Costa & T. A. Widiger (Eds.), *Personality disorders and the five-factor model of personality* (2nd ed., pp. 89–102). Washington, DC: American Psychological Association.

Wiggins, J. S., & Pincus, A. L. (1992). Personality: Structure and assessment. *Annual Review of Psychology, 43,* 473–504.

8

Psychopathy and DSM-IV Psychopathology

THOMAS A. WIDIGER

The purpose of this chapter is to consider the relationship of psychopathy with disorders included within the American Psychiatric Association's (2000) *Diagnostic and Statistical Manual of Mental Disorders* (DSM-IV-TR). The co-occurrence of one disorder, such as psychopathy, with another disorder is often described as comorbidity (i.e., the comorbid presence of two disorders). The term "comorbidity" made its first appearance in the title or abstract of a psychiatric journal in the early 1980s (Lilienfeld, Waldman, & Israel, 1994), but "with meteoric speed, 'comorbidity' has emerged as the single most important concept for psychiatric research and practice" (Lewinsohn, 1990, p. ii).

The term "comorbidity" refers to the co-occurrence of independent disorders, each with presumably its own, separate etiology, pathology, and treatment implications (Feinstein, 1970). Diagnostic comorbidity is important in part because it is a pervasive phenomenon. It is a rare psychiatric patient who meets diagnostic criteria for just one mental disorder (Clark, Watson, & Reynolds, 1995; Lilienfeld et al., 1994; Mineka, Watson, & Clark, 1998). Diagnostic comorbidity is also important because it is evident that the etiology, course, treatment, and outcome of a disorder are influenced heavily by the presence of comorbid conditions. And, finally, comorbidity is also important be-

cause the nature and extent of its occurrence are problematic to the conceptualization of mental disorders as distinct clinical conditions (Lilienfeld et al., 1994; Widiger & Clark, 2000). "The greatest challenge that the extensive comorbidity data pose to the current nosological system concerns the validity of the diagnostic categories themselves—do these disorders constitute distinct clinical entities?" (Mineka et al., 1998, p. 380). Diagnostic co-occurrence can reflect simply overlapping diagnostic criterion sets, an artifact of a setting in which the data were obtained, or the presence of a common, underlying pathology (Frances, Widiger, & Fyer, 1990). This chapter illustrates these possible interpretations of the apparent comorbidity of psychopathy with other conditions with respect to the comorbidity of psychopathy with personality disorders and Axis I mental disorders.

PERSONALITY DISORDERS

A number of studies have explored the comorbidity and covariation of psychopathy with the American Psychiatric Association (2000) personality disorders. The two personality disorders with which psychopathy has been consistently reported to covary have been the antisocial and the narcissistic. Each is discussed in turn.

Antisocial Personality Disorder

There has been a considerable amount of research on the diagnostic co-occurrence of psychopathy with antisocial personality disorder (APD) (Chapman, Gremore, & Farmer, 2003; Edens, Poythress, & Watkins, 2001; Hare, 1996, 2003; Lilienfeld & Andrews, 1996; Salekin, Rogers, & Sewell, 1997). This research has generally suggested that most cases of psychopathy diagnosed within prison or other forensic settings will meet the DSM-IV criteria for APD, but perhaps as few as only half of the cases of APD will meet criteria for psychopathy (Hare, 1996, 2003; Widiger, Corbitt, & Millon, 1992). Much has been written on the differences between psychopathy, as diagnosed with the Hare Psychopathy Checklist—Revised (PCL-R; Hare, 2003) and the American Psychiatric Association (1980, 2000) APD criterion sets (Hare, Hart, & Harpur, 1991; Lilienfeld, 1994; Rogers, Salekin, Sewell, & Cruise, 2000; Widiger et al., 1992). However, it is perhaps equally important to acknowledge their similarities, overlap, and correspondence.

The description of APD within the second edition of the American Psychiatric Association's (1968) DSM resembled reasonably well the description of psychopathy provided by Cleckley (1941). However, the DSM-II criterion sets were being applied so unreliably in research and clinical practice that the validity of most of the diagnoses within the manual was highly questionable (Spitzer, Endicott, & Robins, 1975). The authors of DSM-III therefore turned to the more specific and explicit criterion sets developed for research purposes by Feighner and colleagues (1972) and Spitzer, Endicott, and Robins (1978). The only personality disorder included within these research criterion sets was APD, due in large part to the seminal work of Robins (1966).

Robins (1966) conducted a systematic follow-up study of 524 children who had been seen 30 years previously at a child guidance clinic for juvenile delinquents. Robins used 19 criteria for her diagnosis of "sociopathy." She preferred the term "sociopathy" over the DSM-I (American Psychiatric Association, 1952) antisocial diagnosis "because it resembles the older term 'psychopathic personality'" (p. 79). Thus, it was her intention to identify persons who would be considered to

be psychopathic, as diagnosed by Cleckley. "It is hoped that Cleckley is correct that despite the difficulties in terminology and definition, there is broad agreement on which kinds of patients are psychopaths" (Robins, 1966, p. 79). Robins included in her study items to assess lack of guilt, remorse, and shame, but these were not successful in differentiating the sociopath from other clinical groups, due in part to difficulties in assessing them reliably. These aspects of psychopathy were therefore not included in the subsequent revisions of her criterion set by Feighner and colleagues (1972), Spitzer and colleagues (1978), and DSM-III (American Psychiatric Association, 1980).

The DSM-III criterion set for APD proved to be quite successful in obtaining adequate levels of reliability. In contrast, it was notably difficult to construct behaviorally specific criterion sets for the complex and broad behavior patterns that constituted the other personality disorders (Widiger & Trull, 1987). As acknowledged by the authors of DSM-III-R, "for some disorders, . . . particularly the Personality Disorders, the criteria require much more inference on the part of the observer" (American Psychiatric Association, 1987, p. xxiii). APD was considered to be an exception to this difficulty, due in large part to the experiences and efforts of Robins (1966), Feighner and colleagues (1972), and Spitzer and colleagues (1978). Indeed, APD has been the only personality disorder to be diagnosed reliably in general clinical practice (Mellsop, Varghese, Joshua, & Hicks, 1982; Spitzer, Forman, & Nee, 1979). Nevertheless, the APD criterion set also received considerable criticism, suggesting to many that validity had been sacrificed for reliability (Frances, 1980; Hare, 1983; Millon, 1981) due to its failure to include all the features of psychopathy identified by Cleckley (1941), such as glib charm, low anxiousness, arrogance, lack of remorse, and lack of empathy. The authors of the DSM-III-R APD criterion set responded in part to these criticisms by adding lack of remorse as a criterion (Widiger, Frances, Spitzer, & Williams, 1988). Neither the DSM-IV nor the PCL-R criterion set has included low anxiousness (Cleckley, 1941).

The impression that the DSM-IV APD criterion set provides an inadequate representation of psychopathy is suggested in part by its differential correlation with the two commonly identified factors of the PCL-R (Lilienfeld, 1994). PCL-R psychopathy is often differentiated with respect to two correlated factors (Hare et al., 1990; Harpur, Hare, & Hakstian, 1989). The first factor describes a "selfish, callous, and remorseless use of others" (Hare, 1991, p. 38) and the second factor a "chronically unstable and antisocial lifestyle" (p. 31). The eight items in Factor 1 describe "a constellation of interpersonal and affective traits commonly considered to be fundamental to the construct of psychopathy" (Hare, 2003, p. 79). Whereas Factor 1 is said to describe the core features of psychopathy, Factor 2 is at times said to refer simply to "social deviance" (Hare, 2003, p. 79).

Many studies have indicated that the APD criterion set correlates more highly with Factor 2 than with Factor 1 (e.g., Hart & Hare, 1989; Shine & Hobson, 1997), suggesting perhaps that the APD criterion set is not identifying the core, personality features of psychopathy and is identifying instead simply the tendency to be aimless, impulsive, irresponsible, delinquent, or criminal (Hare, 1996). "Research that uses a DSM diagnosis of [APD] taps the social deviance component of psychopathy but misses much of the personality component, whereas each component is measured by the PCL-R" (Hare, 2003, p. 92). Nevertheless, it should be noted that PCL-R items that are central to Factor 1 are included within the DSM-IV criterion set for APD; specifically, conning/manipulative and pathological lying (represented by the DSM-IV deceitfulness criterion) and lack of remorse or guilt and failure to accept responsibility (represented by DSM-IV lack of remorse criterion). In addition, in most of the studies in which the APD criterion set has correlated more highly with Factor 2 than Factor 1, the APD criterion set has correlated significantly with Factor 1. Studies have reported that the association between PCL-R Factor 1 and the APD criterion set is negligible after the variance shared by the two factors is removed, whereas the reverse is not true (e.g., Verona, Patrick, & Joiner, 2001). This does suggest that there is unique variance in PCL-R Factor 1 that is not entirely accounted for by the APD criterion set. On the other hand, these analyses do not necessarily suggest that the APD crite-

rion set does not include a significant proportion of Factor 1 variance. Much of the variance shared by Factors 1 and 2 could perhaps represent core, fundamental traits of psychopathy. In any case, it is evident that the PCL-R does include additional traits of psychopathy that are not included within APD (i.e., glib charm, lack of empathy, shallow affect, and arrogance) and it is possible that the unique variance in Factor 1 not accounted for by the APD criterion represent these features.

The APD criterion set might itself be differentiated into subfactors that distinguish between a callous exploitation of others and an impulsive disinhibition (Livesley & Schroeder, 1991; Morey, 1988). Skilling, Harris, Rice, and Quinsey (2002) recently demonstrated in two samples of male offenders "that when the PCL-R (whether scored from file alone or from file and interview) and DSM APD criteria are each scored as continuous measures the association between them is extremely high" (p. 34). They concluded that "persistently antisocial individuals not only exhibit such APD characteristics as antisocial behavior beginning early in life, but (with extremely high likelihood) also exhibit psychopathic glibness, superficiality, failure to take responsibility, shallow affect, and so on" (p. 35). If appropriate cutoff scores are used and adequate consideration is given to measurement error, "individuals would be categorized nearly identically by the two approaches" (pp. 34–35).

In sum, the DSM-IV APD and PCL-R psychopathy criterion sets do not appear to be identifying different disorders. The two respective criterion sets are instead quite similar albeit alternative efforts at identifying the same personality disorder (Hare et al., 1991; Millon et al., 1996). This does not suggest, however, that the inclusion within the PCL-R of glib charm, arrogant self-appraisal, lack of empathy, and shallow affect do not contribute to a more thorough and at times valid assessment of the disorder. In fact, it is acknowledged in DSM-IV that the PCL-R items not included within the criterion set for APD will at times improve the validity of the assessment of APD: "Lack of empathy, inflated self-appraisal, and superficial charm are features that have been commonly included in traditional conceptions of psychopathy that may be particularly distinguishing of the disorder and more predictive of recidivism in prison or forensic settings where criminal, delinquent, or aggressive acts are likely to be non-specific" (American Psychiatric Association, 2000, p. 703).

On the other hand, it is possible that much of the differences between the two criterion sets could reflect the fact that most of this research has been conducted within prison settings. The DSM-IV criteria for APD does place relatively more emphasis on delinquent, criminal, and irresponsible behaviors than the PCL-R criterion set for psychopathy, and antisocial, criminal behaviors are of course endemic within a prison setting, contributing to the higher prevalence rate of APD within this setting. It would be of interest for future research to explore the diagnostic co-occurrence of APD and psychopathy within settings or populations that might be characterized by high rates of glib charm, exploitation, manipulation, shallow affect, and confident self-presentation, coupled with relatively low rates of overt criminal, reckless, and delinquent activity. It is possible that in such settings (e.g., perhaps the professions of sales, law, or politics) the rate of APD might be lower than the rate of PCL-R psychopathy and the specificity of criminal, delinquent, and irresponsible behaviors for the diagnosis of PCL-R psychopathy might improve.

For example, the DSM-IV field trial compared the co-occurrence of psychopathy and APD across different settings (Widiger et al., 1996). Number of arrests and convictions correlated significantly with both APD and psychopathy in the drug–homelessness clinic, the methadone maintenance clinic, and the psychiatric inpatient hospital but not with either APD or psychopathy within the prison setting. Items that were unique to the PCL-R (e.g., lacks empathy, inflated and arrogant self-appraisal, and glib, superficial charm) correlated more highly with interviewers' ratings of APD and psychopathy within the prison setting but not within the clinical settings. The PCL-R items that were most predictive of clinician's impressions of psychopathy within a drug treatment and homelessness site included adult antisocial behavior. Within a psychiatric inpatient site, the most predictive items were adult antisocial behavior and early behavior problems, along with glib, superficial charm. In contrast, the most predictive items within the prison site were inflated, arrogant self-appraisal, lack of empathy, irresponsibility, deceitfulness, and glib, superficial charm.

The relationship of APD to criminality is much lower outside prison settings. On the basis of the National Institute of Mental Health (NIMH) Epidemiological Catchmant Area (ECA) data, Robins, Tipp, and Pryzbeck (1991) reported that only 47% of those who met the APD criteria had a significant arrest record (total $N = 628$). "Rather than criminality, the adult symptoms that typify the antisocial personality are job troubles (found in 94%), violence (found in 85%), multiple moving traffic offenses (found in 72%), and severe marital difficulties (desertion, multiple separations or divorces, multiple infidelities, found in 67%)" (p. 260). The occurrence of a significant arrest record was not predictive of an APD diagnosis. Only 37% of those with multiple nontraffic arrests (40% for males) met the APD criteria.

Criminality

The relationship of criminality to psychopathy warrants particular consideration. There are many studies on the comorbidity of psychopathy and criminal behavior (Coid, 2002; Dolan & Doyce, 2000; Hare, Cooke, & Hart, 1999; Hart & Hare, 1997; Hemphill, Hare, & Wong, 1998; Salekin, Rogers, & Sewell, 1996). "The clinical concept of psychopathy is linked inextricably to criminal behavior, and in particular to criminal violence" (Hart, 1998, p. 355). Psychopathy is a diagnostic concept that was developed in large part to help understand or explain criminal behavior (Blackburn, 1993; Hare, 1996). Many studies have indicated that the construct of psychopathy has been successful in identifying a particularly callous, dangerous, and remorseless subset of criminals who repeatedly engage in particularly heinous, brutal, and exploitative acts (Salekin et al., 1996; Serin, 1991). Psychopathic persons begin their criminal careers earlier, commit a greater variety of offenses, and offend at higher rates (Hart & Hare, 1997). PCL-R scores are associated with higher rates of violent crime and with a higher risk of criminal recidivism (Salekin et al., 1996). The PCL-R often provides incremental validity in the prediction of violence, recidivism, and institutional misbehavior over standard actuarial risk scales based on other demographic and historical variables (Hart, 1998). In sum, the construct of psychopathy does appear to be an important moderating variable in the understanding of a particular subset of physically abusive and violent males, including the sexually assaultive, sexually abusive, pedophilic, and serial murdering (Dorr, 1998; Hare, 2003; Hare et al., 1999; Stone, 1998).

"In psychopaths . . . it seems that certain symptoms (e.g., impulsivity, grandiosity, lack of empathy) both increase the likelihood that affected individuals will consider engaging in criminal conduct and decrease the likelihood that the decision to act will be inhibited" (Hart & Hare, 1997, p. 31). It perhaps takes little imagination to understand how such personality traits as lack of empathy, arrogance, and callousness, along with disinhibitory impulsivity, would provide a disposition toward, or at least risk for, engaging in criminal, exploitative, and even violent behavior. On the other hand, it might be equally difficult to consider persons with such dispositions not engaging in criminal behavior. Criminality and psychopathy are not the same constructs. Glib charm, callousness, arrogance, shallow affect, deceitfulness, and lack of empathy do not necessarily involve or imply criminal behavior (Hare, 1991, 1998) and "only a small minority of those who engage in criminal conduct are psychopaths" (Hart & Hare, 1997, p. 22). Nevertheless, it is also true that the existing research on psychopathy has usually conjoined criminality and psychopathy with respect to both the sampling of subjects and the assessment of the construct.

There have been few studies of psychopaths, as assessed by the PCL-R, who lack a history of criminal behavior (Gustafson & Ritzer, 1995). In fact, the vast majority of PCL-R studies have been conducted within prison or other forensic settings (Hare, 1991, 1996, 1998, 2003) and, as discussed further below, PCL-R assessments rely substantially on this criminal behavior to assess psychopathic personality traits. Commonly cited efforts to conduct studies of noncriminal (successful) psychopaths have often failed to identify persons who lacked criminal behavior. For example, Widom (1977) lamented that "we have no knowledge of the extent to which psychopathy remains undetected in the general population or even whether the concept is a meaningful one outside the prison or psychiatric hospital" (p. 675). She therefore placed advertisements in a Boston counterculture newspaper seeking "adventurous carefree people who've led exciting impulsive lives" (p. 675). Seventy-three persons responded and 28–30 subjects participated in a series of tests and interviews. However, the psychopaths she identified were not appreciably different from those who would be sampled from a clinical setting. Sixty-one percent reported some form of psychiatric experience, 46% had been in outpatient treatment, 21% had been an inpatient, and 29% had a history of suicide attempts. Most important, 74% had been arrested and 50% had been incarcerated.

"The contribution of personality characteristics to antisocial behaviour is an empirical question that can only be answered if the two are identified independently" (Blackburn, 1988, p. 507). Many of the PCL-R items refer explicitly to criminal behavior, notably the childhood items concerned with early behavior problems and juvenile delinquency, and the adult items concerned with revocation of conditional release and criminal versatility. Their inclusion within the criterion set complicates studies of the comorbidity and contribution of psychopathy to criminal behavior. These four items (along with others) were in fact excluded from the reformulation of psychopathy by Cooke and Michie (2001) in part to define the construct independently from criminal behavior.

However, the exclusion of the four PCL-R items concerned explicitly with criminal history would not ensure that the assessment is in fact independent of criminal behavior. Many of the remaining PCL-R items are still heavily dependent on or at least informed by criminal behavior. PCL-R assessments are often based largely on the review of a person's criminal record (Hare, 1991, 1998, 2003). The PCL-R was "designed for use with adult male prison inmates and forensic psychiatric patients" (Hart & Hare, 1997, p. 23) and it is their criminal record that often provides the basis for the assessment of the core, fundamental traits of psychopathy. For example, lack of empathy or callousness can be inferred on the basis of the commission of particularly brutal, heinous acts of violence or criminal exploitation or the person's attitude toward a victim's suffering. Lack of empathy could alternatively be assessed on the basis of the manner in which a person describes people who have been victimized by other perpetrators, but it is not clear how the core features have in fact been assessed in much of the existing psychopathy studies. PCL-R assessments have not generally included an explicit set of questions that must be administered to each respondent, and there is often no record of the basis on which items have been assessed. It is quite possible, perhaps even likely, that the assessment of many of the core features of psychopathy have been assessed on the basis of a prisoner's antisocial, criminal behaviors. In fact, it is unclear whether psychopathy, as diagnosed by the PCL-R, could even be assessed in the absence of a criminal history, given its reliance on the collateral (institutional, prison record) information for its assessment. An alternative approach would be to use instruments that do not appear to rely so heavily on criminal history for their assessment (e.g., Levenson, Kiehl, & Fitzpatrick, 1995; Lilienfeld & Andrews, 1996; Morey, 1991), although it is also possible that a respondent's answers to self-report inventory items that do not refer explicitly to criminal behavior could still have relied heavily on the respondent's criminal history as a basis for affirmative responses.

It will be informative for future studies on the relationship of psychopathy to criminal behavior to dismantle the construct in order to isolate and identify which particular components, items, or facets of psychopathy are in fact predicting the occurrence of the violent, heinous, or repetitive criminal behaviors. The construct of psychopathy, as assessed by the PCL-R, is heterogeneous in its coverage of maladaptive personality traits (Brinkley, Newman, Widiger, & Lynam, 2004). The two factors commonly identified within the PCL-R have been helpful in distinguishing between two broad components of psychopathy (e.g., McDermott et al., 2000; Patrick, Bradley, & Lang, 1993; Patrick, Cuthbert, & Lang, 1994). It is possible that the substantial variance shared by the two factors represents the core features of the disorder, but it is also possible that the shared variance represents method variance due to the use of criminal records to assess the affective and interpersonal traits. The person-

ality traits that are involved in the second factor of the PCL-R should be further articulated (Lilienfeld, 1994; Lynam, 2002). Cooke and Michie (2001) suggest that further distinctions can be obtained through an alternative three-factor model, and others have suggested that each of the two factors should themselves be differentiated into two more specific components (Hill, Neumann, & Rogers, in press; Vitacco, Rogers, Neumann, Harrison, & Vincent, in press). Further differentiation could also be provided by the dismantling of psychopathy in terms of more general models of personality functioning (e.g., Benning, Patrick, Hicks, Blonigen, & Krueger, 2003; Blackburn, 1998; Livesley, 1998; Widiger & Lynam, 1998). For example, Benning and colleagues (2003) and Verona and colleagues (2001) dismantle PCL-R psychopathy in terms of the Multidimensional Personality Questionnaire (MPQ; Tellegen, 2000) traits of well-being, social potency, stress reaction, alienation, aggression, control, and harm avoidance. Lynam (2002) describes psychopathy in terms of the five-factor model of general personality functioning, including neuroticism facets associated with low anxiousness, feelings of invulnerability, and angry hostility; antagonism facets that represent callousness (i.e., tough-mindedness), deceitfulness, and exploitation; conscientiousness facets of low deliberation, low self-discipline, and low dutifulness; and extraversion facets of excitement seeking and assertiveness.

Narcissistic Personality Disorder

An additional personality disorder with which psychopathy is often reported to be comorbid is the narcissistic personality disorder (Blackburn, Logan, Donnelly, & Renwick, 2003; Gustafson & Ritzer, 1995; Morey & Jones, 1998; Paulhus & Williams, 2002; Salekin, Trobst, & Krioukova, 2001). Narcissistic personality disorder often loads on the first factor of psychopathy (Harpur et al., 1989), along with APD, but, in contrast to APD, tends not to load as highly on the second factor (Hare et al., 1991; Hart, Forth, & Hare, 1991; Hart & Hare, 1998). Morey (1988) cluster analyzed all of the DSM-III-R personality disorder diagnostic criteria and found that the APD criterion set split into two independent clusters. One cluster appeared to be defined largely by aggressive behaviors, the other combined with items from the narcissistic personality disorder. "This [latter] cluster was named psychopathic, because the inclusion of the exploitative narcissistic personality features and the removal of the overtly aggressive antisocial aspects creates a syndrome reminiscent of the older psychopathic concept" (Morey, 1988, p. 319).

Narcissistic personality disorder has a theoretical and clinical literature that is quite independent of PCL-R studies of psychopathy (Cooper, 1998; Gunderson, Ronningstam, & Smith, 1991; Hare, 1991, 1998; Kernbeg, 1970). Nevertheless, psychodynamic views of narcissism do suggest common features (Gacono, Meloy, & Berg, 1992; Kernberg, 1998; Perry & Cooper, 1989). Antisocial and psychopathic tendencies are conceptualized as being on a continuum with narcissism, with both involving a motivation to dominate, humiliate, and manipulate others. As noted by Stone (1993), "all commentators on psychopathy . . . allude to the attribute of (pathological) narcissism—whether under the rubric of egocentricity, self-indulgence, or some similar term" (p. 292). He went so far as to suggest that "all psychopathic persons are at the same time narcissistic persons" (Stone, 1993, p. 292). Kernberg (1970) has similarly stated that "the antisocial personality may be considered a subgroup of the narcissistic personality" (p. 51). Hart and Hare (1998) generally agree that there is a close correspondence between psychopathy and narcissism but suggest instead that "psychopathy can be viewed as a higher-order construct with two distinct, albeit related facets, one of which is very similar to the clinical concept of narcissism" (p. 429).

Some of the features of DSM-IV narcissistic personality disorder are explicitly suggestive of psychopathy, notably a grandiose sense of self-importance and arrogant, haughty behaviors (comparable to psychopathic arrogant self-appraisal), lack of empathy and being unwilling to recognize or identify with the feelings and needs of others (closely related to psychopathic lack of empathy), and interpersonal exploitation (corresponding to psychopathic manipulativeness, deceitfulness, and antisocial behaviors). It has even been intimated that narcissistic personality disorder is closer to the

Cleckley's conceptualization of psychopathy than APD (Hare et al., 1991; Harpur et al., 1989; Harpur, Hart, & Hare, 2002).

Consideration was given in the development of the DSM-IV criteria for APD to include the components of PCL-R psychopathy that are not already contained within the APD criterion set; notably glib charm, arrogance, and lack of empathy (Widiger et al., 1992). The DSM-IV APD field trial focused specifically on this proposal (Widiger et al., 1996). However, one concern was that these features are also central to the diagnosis of narcissistic personality disorder and their inclusion within the criterion set for APD would increase markedly their diagnostic co-occurrence and undermine their differential diagnosis (Widiger & Corbitt, 1995). The authors of the DSM-IV criterion set for narcissistic personality disorder (Gunderson et al., 1991) considered the personality disorders to be qualitatively distinct conditions, as do many theorists of psychopathy. Those who support this categorical perspective argue that the criterion sets should increase the ability of clinicians to differentiate among these distinct disorders rather than complicate this effort by increasing criterion set overlap (Gunderson, 1992). "The high comorbidity of narcissistic personality disorder with other personality disorders makes differential diagnosis essential" (Ronningstam, 1999, p. 681).

The final decision for DSM-IV was to at least acknowledge that glib charm, arrogance, and lack of empathy are included within other conceptualizations of APD and that their inclusion within the criterion set would likely increase the validity of the assessment of APD within prison and other forensic settings (American Psychiatric Association, 2000). To help differentiate the narcissistic and antisocial personality disorders, it has been suggested that "narcissists are usually more grandiose, while APD patients are exploitative, have a superficial value system, and are involved in recurrent antisocial activities" (Ronningstam, 1999, p. 681). It is also suggested that "exploitiveness in antisocial patients is probably more likely to be consciously and actively related to materialistic or sexual gain, while exploitive behavior in narcissistic patients is more passive, serving to enhance self-image by attaining praise or power" (Ronningstam,

1999, p. 681). Kernberg (1998) suggests "the way to differentiate . . . narcissistic personality disorder from an antisocial personality disorder proper is the absence in the latter of the capacity for feeling guilt and remorse" (pp. 42–43). Narcissistic persons will feel guilty and remorseful when confronted with the negative effects of their exploitative use of others, whereas antisocial persons will not. These speculations are compelling and have perhaps been beneficial in clinical practice, but they have not yet been empirically evaluated.

Dimensional Model of Personality Disorder

A compelling rejoinder to the concerns over differential diagnosis is questioning "the assumption that these two disorders should be largely independent" (Hare & Hart, 1995, p. 132). Hare and Hart suggested that the categorical assumption is perhaps illusory, or at least equally problematic for all the existing personality disorder diagnoses. "The diagnostic approach used [in DSM-IV] represents the categorical perspective that Personality Disorders are qualitatively distinct clinical syndromes" (American Psychiatric Association, 2000, p. 689). DSM-IV provides diagnostic criterion sets to help guide a clinician toward the correct diagnosis and a section devoted to differential diagnosis that indicates "how to differentiate [the] disorder from other disorders that have similar presenting characteristics" (American Psychiatric Association, 2000, p. 10). The intention is to help the clinician determine which particular disorder is present, the selection of which would, ideally, indicate the presence of a specific pathology that will explain the occurrence of the symptoms and suggest a specific treatment that would ameliorate the patient's suffering (Frances, First, & Pincus, 1995).

It is evident, however, that DSM-IV routinely fails in the goal of guiding the clinician to the presence of one specific personality disorder. Despite the efforts of the authors of various editions of the diagnostic manual, diagnostic co-occurrence continues to be problematic (Bornstein, 1998; Lilienfeld et al., 1994). Widiger and Trull (1998) provided co-occurrence rates for the DSM-III-R personality disorder diagnoses obtained for the construction of the DSM-IV criterion sets

from unpublished data provided by six research sites. "If one takes a rate of 33.3% as indicating problematic co-occurrence (i.e., at least a third of the persons meet the criteria for another personality disorder), then there is problematic co-occurrence for each personality disorder" (Widiger & Trull, 1998, p. 362).

Kernberg (1998) does in fact consider the antisocial and narcissistic personality disorders to lie along a common continuum of psychopathology. "Pathological narcissism constitutes a dimension within the field of personality disorders that includes—in order of progressive severity—narcissistic personality disorder, malignant narcissism syndrome, and antisocial personality disorder" (Kernberg, 1998, p. 47). Hare and Hart (1995) suggested that the authors of the DSM-IV criterion sets should have abandoned the effort to maintain the illusory diagnostic boundaries and put the criterion sets for all the personality disorders, along with the PCL-R, "into one large pot, to determine whether natural factors or clusters of items would emerge" (p. 133). Such research has since been conducted (Clark & Livesley, 2002). Hare and Hart speculated that "it is quite possible, even likely, that we would have ended up with a reliable combination of items from several criteria sets—a combination that would have looked a lot like the PCL-R" (p. 133), but this has not in fact been the typical result of these analyses. Instead, this research has consistently identified four broad personality factors.

For example, Livesley, Jang, and Vernon (1998) compared the phenotypical and genetic structure of a comprehensive set of personality disorder symptoms in samples of 656 patients with personality disorder, 939 general community participants, and 686 twin pairs. Principal components analysis yielded four broad dimensions (identified by Livesley as emotional dysregulation, dissocial behavior, inhibitedness, and compulsivity) that were replicated across all three samples. Multivariate genetic analyses also yielded the same four factors. The dissocial behavior factor would correlate highly with PCL-R psychopathy, but it is not equivalent to psychopathy (Livesley, 1998). It is defined by such scales as rejection, suspiciousness, conduct problems, interpersonal disesteem, passive oppositionality, and narcissism. Some of these components are included within PCL-R psychopathy (e.g., conduct problems, narcissism, and interpersonal disesteem) but some are not (e.g., suspiciousness). In addition, other components of PCL-R psychopathy are not included within this domain (e.g., impulsivity, need for stimulation, and irresponsibility).

Livesley and colleagues (1998) also noted the remarkable consistency of the four broad domains of personality disorder with four of the five broad domains consistently identified in studies of the five-factor model (FFM) of general personality functioning (Widiger & Costa, 2002). Emotional dysregulation corresponds closely to FFM Neuroticism, dissocial behavior to FFM Antagonism, inhibitedness to FFM Introversion, and compulsivity to FFM Conscientiousness. Livesley and colleagues concluded that "the higher-order traits of personality disorder strongly resemble dimensions of normal personality" (p. 941). Indeed, joint factor analyses of measures of the general personality functioning and comprehensive representations of personality disorder symptoms have consistently confirmed a common underlying structure (Cannon, Turkheimer, & Oltmanns, 2003; Clark & Livesley, 2002; Krueger & Tacket, 2003; Larstone, Jang, Livesley, Vernon, & Wolf, 2002; O'Connor & Dyce, 1998; Watson, Clark, & Harkness, 1994). It is "striking that an extensive history of research to develop a dimensional model of normal personality functioning that has been confined to community populations is so closely congruent with a model that was derived from an analysis confined to personality disorder symptoms" (Widiger, 1998a, p. 865).

It is now acknowledged in DSM-IV that "an alternative perspective to the categorical approach is the dimensional perspective that personality disorders represent maladaptive variants of personality traits that merge imperceptibly into normality and into one another" (American Psychiatric Association, 2000, p. 689). The categorical diagnoses of psychopathy, APD, and narcissistic personality disorder can be understood from the perspective of a dimensional model of general personality functioning, but in doing so they no longer retain their identity as qualitatively distinct conditions. More specifically, psychopathy from the perspective of the FFM includes primarily facets of the personality

domain of antagonism (manipulative, deceptive, exploitative, aggressive, callous, lacking remorse, and ruthless) and the domain of low constraint (rashness, negligence, hedonism, immorality, undependability, & irresponsibility). Prototypic cases of psychopathy would also include facets of low emotional dysregulation, such as low anxiousness, low self-consciousness, glib charm, and fearlessness, as well as other facets of neuroticism and extraversion (Brinkley et al., 2004; Lynam, 2002; Widiger, 1998b; Widiger & Lynam, 1998). Empirical support for this alternative conceptualization of psychopathy is provided by Miller, Lynam, Widiger, and Leukefeld (2001) and Miller and Lynam (2003).

AXIS I DISORDERS

There has been a considerable amount of research on the comorbidity of psychopathy with Axis I disorders, running the gamut from mild anxiety disorders to schizophrenia (Cloninger, Bayon, & Przybeck, 1997; Dahl, 1998; Hare, 2003; Knop, Jensen, & Mortensen, 1998; Sutker & Allain, 2001). This review is confined largely to the anxiety and substance use disorders.

Anxiety Disorders

The relationship of psychopathy to anxiety disorders has been controversial (Frick, Lilienfeld, Elllis, Loney, & Silverthorn, 1999; Schmitt & Newman, 1999). Cleckley (1941) included within his original criteria for psychopathy an "absence of 'nervousness' or psychoneurotic manifestations" (p. 206). Rather than be troubled by the presence of anxiety disorders it was suggested that "it is highly typical for [psychopaths] not only to escape the abnormal anxiety and tension . . . but also to show a relative immunity from such anxiety and worry as might be judged normal or appropriate" (Cleckley, 1941, p. 206). Miller and colleagues (2001) surveyed 15 psychopathy researchers, asking them to describe the prototypic psychopath in terms of the domains and facets of the FFM description of general personality functioning. Their description included very low levels of anxiousness, inconsistent with the PCL-R assessment of psychopathy but consistent with the earlier description of this disorder by Cleckley (1941). In stark contrast, it is stated in DSM-IV that "individuals with this disorder [APD] may also experience dysphoria, including complaints of tension, inability to tolerate boredom, and depressed mood" (American Psychiatric Association, 2000, p. 702). It is noted more specifically that "they may have associated anxiety disorders [and] depressive disorders" (American Psychiatric Association, 2000, p. 702).

The suggestion in DSM-IV that APD is associated with anxiety disorders can be attributed in part to the confinement of many of the APD studies to clinical populations (Lilienfeld, 1994). Anxiousness is common among persons in treatment for mental disorders. However, increased prevalence rates of panic disorder, agoraphobia, social phobia, and obsessive–compulsive personality have also been reported among persons diagnosed with APD in the NIMH (Robins et al., 1991) and Edmonton (Swanson, Bland, & Newman, 1994) epidemiological community studies. Dahl (1998) suggested that "these findings clearly demonstrate that Cleckley (1941) was wrong when he stated that psychopaths did not show manifest anxiety" (p. 298).

An association of APD with anxiety disorders could reflect in part the use of DSM-IV criteria for APD in the epidemiological studies rather than the PCL-R criterion set, although the PCL-R does not itself include low anxiousness within its criterion set (Hare, 1980, 2003). The callous–unemotional traits of psychopathy have at times correlated negatively with measures of anxiousness (e.g., Harpur et al., 1989), but psychopathic persons will report clinically high levels of anxiousness (Schmitt & Newman, 1999). Some researchers have therefore recommended including low anxiousness, along with meeting a diagnostic threshold on the PCL-R, to identify persons with psychopathy (Brinkley et al., 2004; Lykken, 1995; Newman, 1998; Rogers, 1995; Salekin, Rogers, & Machin, 2001; Schmitt & Newman, 1999). This is to some extent consistent with the suggestion to make a distinction between primary and secondary psychopathy (Blackburn, 1998). Primary psychopaths would have low levels of anxiousness, whereas secondary psychopaths would have high levels of anxiousness. For example, the Levenson Self-Report Psy-chopathy (LSRP; Levenson et al., 1995) scale distinguishes between primary and secondary psychopaths, with the latter characterized in part by high levels of anxiousness.

It may also be useful to distinguish between fearfulness and anxiousness (Lilienfeld, 1994). Fearfulness and anxiousness can appear to be quite similar constructs, but they may in fact be different. Fearfulness involves a sensitivity to cues or signs of impending danger, whereas anxiousness is distress associated with the perception that impending danger is imminent or inevitable (Frick et al., 1999; Watson & Clark, 1984) . The opposite of fearfulness would perhaps be a fearlessness that some suggest is in fact central to the construct of psychopathy (Lykken, 1995). Persons who are high in fearlessness engage in substantial risk taking, and may then often experience anxiousness secondary to their producing and encountering highly stressful events (Frick et al., 1999; Lilienfeld, 1994). The assessment of fearlessness has often used measures of thrill seeking, sensation seeking, and adventure seeking that generally load on the broad personality domain of constraint rather than a negative affectivity domain that would include anxiousness. However, it is not entirely clear whether the thrill-seeking behavior is best understood as reflecting fearlessness, an impulsive disinhibition, or both.

Another approach to this issue is statistical. Researchers have demonstrated that callous–unemotional traits of psychopathy will correlate negatively with anxiousness when variance that can be accounted for by the impulsive, deviant, or antisocial lifestyle factor is removed (e.g., Frick et al., 1999; Verona et al., 2001). For example, Frick and colleagues (1999) reported that callous–unemotional traits of psychopathy (e.g., lack of guilt or empathy and shallow affect) did not correlate with fearlessness (i.e., thrill and adventure seeking) or with anxiousness in a sample of clinic children. However, after controlling for the variance accounted for by conduct disorder symptoms, these traits correlated positively with fearlessness (thrill and adventure seeking) and negatively with anxiousness. Verona and colleagues (2001) similarly reported in a sample of adult male inmates that the affective–interpersonal traits of psychopathy (i.e., Factor 1) correlated negatively with anxiousness (i.e., stress reaction) when the variance accounted for by the second factor of psychopathy was removed. These findings could suggest that the variance that is unique to the Factor 1 traits is in fact correlated negatively with anxiousness, consistent with the original theory of Cleckley (1941). Nevertheless, it might still be important to recognize that lack of guilt, lack of empathy, glib charm, deceitfulness, and other components of the affective–interpersonal traits of psychopathy traits will often fail to correlate negatively with anxiousness. They may do so after variance that can be accounted for by other features of psychopathy are removed, but it is also possible that these findings might say more about the variance that has been removed than the affective–interpersonal traits themselves (Cohen & Cohen, 1983).

Substance Use Disorders

Psychopathy has been consistently related to substance use, gambling, "and other disorders of impulse control" (American Psychiatric Association, 2000, p. 704). In the ECA study, 84% of persons diagnosed with APD reported at least some form of substance use disorder (Robins et al., 1991). Approximately one-third of opioid users are often diagnosed with APD (Alterman et al., 1998; Ball, Tennen, Poling, Kranzler, & Rounsaville, 1997). Morgenstern, Langenbucher, Labouvie, and Miller (1997) reported a relatively high rate of APD among women undergoing treatment for alcohol and drug disorders. APD has been shown to provide a significant risk for dyscontrolled drug and alcohol usage in a variety of comorbidity studies (Grant et al., 2004; Kessler & Walters, 2002; Skodol, Oldham, & Gallaher, 1999). Smith and Newman (1990) reported that 93% of a sample of incarcerated psychopaths met criteria for alcohol dependence or abuse (26% for opioid dependence or abuse).

However, this comorbidity has also been somewhat controversial, as it has been suggested that it could reflect, at least in part, overlapping diagnostic criterion sets (Verheul, van den Brink, & Hartgers, 1995). For example, many of the behaviors that would count toward a diagnosis of APD can be due, at least in part, to a history of dyscontrolled drug usage, such as thefts, deception, conning, poor work history, and

recklessness. In each of the recent revisions of the American Psychiatric Association DSM, it has been suggested that an exclusion criterion be added to APD to disallow the diagnosis when the behaviors involved substance usage (Widiger & Corbitt, 1995). This exclusion criterion has not been added though because differentiation of APD and substance dependence is facilitated by the requirement in DSM-IV for evidence of a conduct disorder. The presence of a conduct disorder prior to the age of 15 will often date the onset of APD prior to the onset of a substance-related disorder, making it unlikely that the adult antisocial acts involving substance-related behavior are secondary to an adult substance-related disorder. The PCL-R includes two similar diagnostic criteria (i.e., early behavior problems and juvenile delinquency), but, in contrast to DSM-IV, the PCL-R does not require the childhood antecedents for the diagnosis of psychopathy.

Differentiation of APD and substance use disorder is more complicated if the onset and course of the substance usage are congruent with the onset and course of the APD behaviors (Widiger, Verheul, & van den Brink, 1999). However, if both have been evident prior to the age of 15 and evident thereafter consistently into adulthood, then it might then be clinically meaningless to differentiate them. Both disorders would likely be present. Persons with APD can develop a substance dependence, and a substance dependence can contribute to the development of APD (Sher & Trull, 1994). In such cases, it might be useful to recognize that both warrant recognition and treatment.

APD, psychopathy, and substance-related disorders may also share a common underlying psychopathology (Krueger, 2002; Markon, Krueger, Bouchard, & Gottesman, 2002; Sher & Trull, 1994; Watson et al., 1994). Many twin studies have suggested a common genetic contribution to antisocial and substance use disorders (Sher & Slutske, 2003). Krueger and colleagues (2002) explored this hypothesis in a sample of 1,048 17-year-old twins. "Our analyses indicated that co-occurrence among alcohol dependence, drug dependence, conduct disorder, adolescent antisocial behavior, and a disinhibitory personality style assessed in late adolescence can be traced to a highly heritable externalizing factor" (Krueger et al.,

2002, p. 419). The association between PCL-R psychopathy and substance abuse does appear to be accounted for largely by Factor 2 of psychopathy (Reardon, Lang, & Patrick, 2002; Smith & Newman, 1990). This disinhibitory temperament could be the basis for both the irresponsibility, impulsivity, undependability, and negligence of APD, as well as the harmful, reckless, and dyscontrolled drug usage.

CONCLUSIONS

Psychopathy, particularly as assessed with the PCL-R, has established itself as an important clinical construct, especially within forensic, prison settings. The ability of the PCL-R to predict future violence, substance use, and recidivism clearly has implications for making important forensic decisions related to sentencing, conditional release, and institutional placement (Brinkley et al., 2004). Of particular importance for future research, however, will be to dismantle the PCL-R and the construct of psychopathy to isolate its particular facets or components that are contributing to its predictive validity. This effort could take the form of the dismantling of psychopathy in terms of more general models of personality functioning (e.g., Benning et al., 2003; Clark & Livesley, 2002; Widiger & Lynam, 1998) or through the use of assessment instruments that do not rely on criminal history for their assessment and that provide subscales for different components of psychopathy (e.g., Lilienfeld & Andrews, 1996; Morey, 1991). It will also be useful for future research to be conducted in populations of persons for whom moderate to high levels of psychopathy are likely to be found in the absence of overt criminal behavior.

REFERENCES

Alterman, A. I., McDermott, P. A., Cacciola, J. S., Rutherford, M. J., Boardman, C. R., McKay, J. R., & Cook, T. G. (1998). A typology of antisociality in methadone patients. *Journal of Abnormal Psychology, 107,* 412–422.

American Psychiatric Association. (1952). *Diagnostic and statistical manual of mental disorders.* Washington, DC: Author.

American Psychiatric Association. (1968). *Diagnostic and statistical manual of mental disorders* (2nd ed.). Washington, DC: Author.

American Psychiatric Association. (1980). *Diagnostic and statistical manual of mental disorders* (3rd ed.). Washington, DC: American Psychiatric Association.

American Psychiatric Association. (1987). *Diagnostic and statistical manual of mental disorders* (3rd ed., rev). Washington, DC: Author.

American Psychiatric Association. (2000). *Diagnostic and statistical manual of mental disorders* (4th ed., text rev.). Washington, DC: Author.

Ball, S. A., Tennen, H., Poling, J. C., Kranzler, H. R. A., & Rounsaville, B. J. (1997). Personality, temperament, character dimensions and the DSM-IV personality disorders in substance abusers. *Journal of Abnormal Psychology, 106,* 545–553.

Benning, S. D., Patrick, C. J., Hicks, B. M., Blonigen, D. M., & Krueger, R. F. (2003). Factor structure of the Psychopathy Personality Inventory: Validity and implications for clinical assessment. *Psychological Assessment, 15,* 340–350.

Blackburn, R. (1988). On moral judgements and personality disorders: The myth of psychopathic personality revisited. *British Journal of Psychiatry, 153,* 505–512.

Blackburn, R. (1993). *The psychology of criminal conduct: Theory, research and practice.* Chichester, UK: Wiley.

Blackburn, R. (1998). Psychopathy and the contribution of personality to violence. In T. Millon & E. Simonsen (Eds.), *Psychopathy: antisocial, criminal, and violent behavior* (pp. 50–68). New York: Guilford Press.

Blackburn, R., Logan, C., Donnelly, J., & Renwick, S. (2003). Personality disorders, psychopathy, and other mental disorders: Co-morbidity among patients at English and Scottish high-security hospitals. *Journal of Forensic Psychiatry and Psychology, 14,* 111–137.

Bornstein, R. F. (1998). Reconceptualizing personality disorder diagnosis in the DSM-V: The discriminant validity challenge. *Clinical Psychology: Science and Practice, 5,* 333–343.

Brinkley, C. A., Newman, J. P., Widiger, T. A., & Lynam, D. R. (2004). Two approaches to parsing the heterogeneity of psychopathy. *Clinical Psychology: Science and Practice, 11,* 69–94.

Cannon, T., Turkheimer, E., & Oltmanns, T. F. (2003). Factorial structure of pathological personality as evaluated by peers. *Journal of Abnormal Psychology, 112,* 81–91.

Chapman, A. L., Gremore, T. M., & Farmer, R. F. (2003). Psychometric analysis of the Psychopathic Personality Inventory (PPI) with female inmates. *Journal of Personality Assessment, 80,* 164–172.

Clark, L. A., & Livesley, W. J. (2002). Two approaches to identifying the dimensions of personality disorder: Convergence on the five-factor model. In P. T. Costa & T. A. Widiger (Eds.), *Personality disorders and the five-factor model of personality* (2nd ed., pp. 161–

176). Washington, DC: American Psychological Association.

Clark, L. A., Watson, D., & Reynolds, S. (1995). Diagnosis and classification of psychopathology: Challenges to the current system and future directions. *Annual Review of Psychology, 46,* 121–153.

Cleckley, H. (1941). *The mask of sanity.* St. Louis, MO: Mosby.

Cloninger, C. R., Bayon, C., & Przybeck, T. R. (1997). Epidemiology and Axis I comorbidity of antisocial personality. In D. M. Stoff, J. Breiling, & J. D. Maser (Eds.), *Handbook of antisocial behavior* (pp. 12–21). New York: Wiley.

Cohen, J., & Cohen, P. (1983). *Applied multiple regression for the behavioral sciences* (2nd ed.). Hillsdale, NJ: Erlbaum.

Coid, J. (2002). Personality disorders in prisoners and their motivation for dangerous and disruptive behaviour. *Criminal Behaviour and Mental Health, 12,* 209–226.

Cooke, D. J., & Michie, C. (2001). Refining the construct of psychopathy: Towards a hierarchical model. *Psychological Assessment, 13,* 171–188.

Cooper, A. M. (1998). Further developments in the clinical diagnosis of narcissistic personality disorder. In E. F. Ronningstam (Ed.), *Disorders of narcissism: Diagnostic, clinical, and empirical implications* (pp. 53–74). Washington, DC: American Psychiatric Press.

Dahl, A. A. (1998). Psychopathy and psychiatric comorbidity. In T. Millon, E. Simonsen, M. Birket-Smith, & R. D. Davis (Eds.), *Psychopathy: Antisocial, criminal, and violent behaviors* (pp. 292–303). New York: Guilford Press.

Dolan, M., & Doyle, M. (2000). Violence risk prediction: Clinical and actuarial measures and the role of the Psychopathy Checklist. *British Journal of Psychiatry, 177,* 303–311.

Dorr, D. (1998). Psychopathy in the pedophile. In T. Millon, E. Simonsen, M. Birket-Smith, & R. D. Davis (Eds.), *Psychopathy: Antisocial, criminal, and violent behaviors* (pp. 304–320). New York: Guilford Press.

Edens, J. F., Poythress, N. G., & Watkins, M. M. (2001). Further validation of the Psychopathic Personality Inventory among offenders: Personality and behavioral correlates. *Journal of Personality Disorders, 15*(5), 403–415.

Feighner, J. P., Robins, E., Guze, S. B., Woodruff, R. A., Winokur, G., & Munoz, R. (1972). Diagnostic criteria for use in psychiatric research. *Archives of General Psychiatry, 26,* 57–63.

Feinstein, A. R. (1970). The pre-therapeutic classification of co-morbidity in chronic disease. *Journal of Chronic Diseases, 23,* 455–468.

Frances, A. J. (1980). The DSM-III personality disorders section: A commentary. *American Journal of Psychiatry, 137,* 1050–1054.

Frances, A. J., First, M. B., & Pincus, H. A. (1995). *DSM-IV guidebook.* Washington, DC: American Psychiatric Press.

Frances, A., Widiger, T. A., & Fyer, M. R. (1990). The influence of classification methods on comorbidity.

In J. D. Maser & C. R. Cloninger (Eds.), *Comorbidity of mood and anxiety disorders* (pp. 41–60). Washington, DC: American Psychiatric Press.

Frick, P. J., Lilienfeld, S. O., Ellis, M., Loney, B., & Silverthorn, P. (1999). The association between anxiety and psychopathy dimensions in children. *Journal of Abnormal Child Psychology, 27,* 383–392.

Gaconoa, C. B., Meloy, J. R., & Berg, J. L. (1992). Object relations, defensive operations, and affective states in narcissistic, antisocial, and borderline personality disorder. *Journal of Personality Assessment, 59,* 32–49.

Grant, B. F., Stinson, F. S., Dawson, D. A., Chou, S. P., Ruan, W. J., & Pickering, R. P. (2004). Co-occurrence of 12-month alcohol and drug use disorders and personality disorders in the United States. Results from the National Epidemiologic Survey on Alcohol and Related Conditions. *Archives of General Psychiatry, 61,* 361–368.

Gunderson, J. G. (1992). Diagnostic controversies. In A. Tasman & M. B. Riba (Eds.), *Review of psychiatry* (Vol. 11, pp. 9–24). Washington, DC: American Psychiatric Press.

Gunderson, J. G., Ronningstam, E., & Smith, L. (1991). Narcissistic personality disorder: A review of data on DSM-III-R descriptions. *Journal of Personality Disorders, 5,* 167–177.

Gustafson, S. B., & Ritzer, D. R. (1995). The dark side of normal: A psychopathy-linked pattern called aberrant self-promotion. *European Journal of Personality, 9,* 147–183.

Hare, R. D. (1980). A research scale for the assessment of psychopathy in criminal populations. *Personality and Individual Differences, 1,* 111–117.

Hare, R. D. (1983). Diagnosis of antisocial personality disorder in two prison populations. *American Journal of Psychiatry, 140,* 887–890.

Hare, R. D. (1991). *The Hare Psychopathy Checklist-Revised manual.* North Tonawanda, NY: Multi-Health Systems.

Hare, R. D. (1996). Psychopathy: A clinical construct whose time has come. *Criminal Justice and Behavior, 23,* 25–54.

Hare, R. D. (1998). Psychopathy, affect, and behavior. In D. J. Cooke, A. E. Forth, & R. D. Hare (Eds.), *Psychopathy: theory, research, and implications for society* (pp. 104–137). Dordrecht, The Netherlands: Kluwer.

Hare, R. D. (2003). *Hare Psychopathy Checklist—Revised (PCL-R). Technical manual.* North Tonawanda, NY: Multi-Health Systems.

Hare, R. D., Cooke, D. J., & Hart, S. D. (1999). Psychopathy and sadistic personality disorder. In T. Millon, P. H. Blaney, & R. D. Davies (Eds.), *Oxford textbook of psychopathology* (pp. 555–584). Oxford, UK: Oxford University Press.

Hare, R. D., Harpur, T. J., Hakstian, A. R., Forth, A. E., Hart, S. D., & Newman, J. P. (1990). The revised Psychopathy Checklist: Reliability and factor structure. *Psychological Assessment, 2,* 338–341.

Hare, R. D., & Hart, S. D. (1995). Commentary on antisocial personality disorder: The DSM-IV field trial. In W. J. Livesley (Ed.), *The DSM-IV personality disorders* (pp. 127–134). New York: Guilford Press.

Hare, R. D., Hart, S. D., & Harpur, T. J. (1991). Psychopathy and the DSM-IV criteria for antisocial personality disorder. *Journal of Abnormal Psychology, 100*, 391–398.

Harpur, T. J., Hare, R. D., & Hakstian, A. R. (1989). Two-factor conceptualization of psychopathy: Construct validity and assessment implications. *Psychological Assessment, 2*, 338–341.

Harpur, T. J., Hart, S. D., & Hare, R. D. (2002). Personality of the psychopath. In P. T. Costa & T. A. Widiger (Eds.), *Personality disorders and the five factor model of personality* (2nd ed., pp. 299–324). Washington, DC: American Psychological Association.

Hart, S. D. (1998). Psychopathy and risk for violence. In D. J. Cooke, A. E. Forth, & R. D. Hare (Eds.), *Psychopathy: Theory, research, and implications for society* (pp. 355–373). Dordrecht, The Netherlands: Kluwer.

Hart, S. D., Forth, A. E., & Hare, R. D. (1991). The MCMI-II and psychopathy. *Journal of Personality Disorders, 5*, 318–327.

Hart, S. D., & Hare, R. D. (1989). Discriminant validity of the Psychopathy Checklist in a forensic psychiatric population. *Psychological Assessment, 1*, 211–218.

Hart, S. D., & Hare, R. D. (1997). Psychopathy: assessment and association with criminal conduct. In D. M. Stoff, J. Maser, & J. Breiling (Eds.), *Handbook of antisocial behavior* (pp. 22–35). New York: Wiley.

Hart, S. D., & Hare, R. D. (1998). Association between psychopathy and narcissism: theoretical reviews and empirical evidence. In E. F. Ronningstam (Ed.), *Disorders of narcissism. Diagnostic, clinical, and empirical implications* (pp. 415–436). Washington, DC: American Psychiatric Press.

Hemphill, J. F., Hare, R. D., & Wong, S. (1998). Psychopathy and recidivism: A review. *Legal and Criminological Psychology, 3*, 139–170.

Hill, C. D., Neumann, C. S., & Rogers, R. (in press). Confirmatory factor analysis of the Psychopathy Checklist: Screening Version (PCL:SV) in offenders with Axis I disorders. *Psychological Assessment.*

Kernberg, O. F. (1970). Factors in the treatment of narcissistic personalities. *Journal of the American Psychoanalytic Association, 18*, 51–85.

Kernberg, O. F. (1998). Pathological narcissism and narcissistic personality disorder: Theoretical background and diagnostic classification. In E.F. Ronningstam (Ed.), *Disorders of narcissism. Diagnostic, clinical, and empirical implications* (pp. 29–52). Washington, DC: American Psychiatric Press.

Kessler, R. C., & Walters, E. E. (2002). The National Comorbidity Survey. In M. T. Tsuang & M. Tohen (Eds.), *Textbook in psychiatric epidemiology* (2nd ed., pp. 343–362). New York: Wiley.

Knop, J., Jensen, P., & Mortensen, E. L. (1998). Comorbidity of alcoholism and psychopathy. In T. Millon, E. Simonsen, M. Birket-Smith, & R. D.

Davis (Eds.), *Psychopathy: Antisocial, criminal, and violent behaviors* (pp. 321–331). New York: Guilford Press.

Krueger, R. F. (2002). Personality from a realist's perspective: personality traits, criminal behaviors, and the externalizing spectrum. *Journal of Research in Personality, 36*, 564–572.

Krueger, R. F., Hicks, B. M., Patrick, C. J., Carlson, S. R., Iacono, W. G., & McGue, M. (2002). Etiologic connections among substance dependence, antisocial behavior, and personality: Modeling the externalizing spectrum. *Journal of Abnormal Psychology, 111*, 411–424.

Krueger, R. F., & Tackett, J. L. (2003). Personality and psychopathology: Working toward the bigger picture. *Journal of Personality Disorders, 17*, 109–128.

Larstone, R. M., Jang, K. L., Livesley, W. J., Vernon, P. A., & Wolf, H. (2002). The relationship between Eysenck's P-E-N model of personality, the five factor model of personality, and traits delineating personality dysfunction. *Personality and Individual Differences, 33*, 25–37.

Levenson, M. R., Kiehl, K. A., & Fitzpatrick, C. M. (1995). Assessing psychopathic attributes in a noninstitutionalized population. *Journal of Personality and Social Psychology, 68*, 151–158.

Lewinsohn, P. M. (1990). Forward. In J. D. Maser & C. R. Cloninger (Eds.), *Comorbidity of mood and anxiety disorders* (p. ii). Washington, DC: American Psychiatric Press.

Lilienfeld, S. O. (1994). Conceptual problems in the assessment of psychopathy. *Clinical Psychology Review, 14*, 17–38.

Lilienfeld, S. O., & Andrews, B. P. (1996). Development and preliminary validation of a self-report measure of psychopathic personality traits in noncriminal populations. *Journal of Personality Assessment, 66*, 488–524.

Lilienfeld, S. O., Waldman, I. D., & Israel, A. C. (1994). A critical examination of the use of the term "comorbidity" in psychopathology research. *Clinical Psychology: Science and Practice, 1*, 71–83.

Livesley, W. J. (1998). The phenotypic and genotypic structure of psychopathic traits. In D. J. Cooke, A. E. Forth, & R. D. Hare (Eds.), *Psychopathy: Theory, research, and implications for society* (pp. 69–80). London: Kluwer.

Livesley, W. J., Jang, K. L., & Vernon, P. A. (1998). Phenotypic and genetic structure of traits delineating personality disorder. *Archives of General Psychiatry, 55*, 941–948.

Livesley, W. J., & Schroeder, M. (1991). Dimensions of personality disorder: The DSM-III-R cluster B diagnoses. *Journal of Nervous and Mental Disease, 179*, 320–328.

Lykken, D. T. (1995). *The antisocial personalities.* Hillsdale, NJ: Erlbaum.

Lynam, D. R. (2002). Psychopathy from the perspective of the five-factor model of personality. In P. T. Costa & T. A. Widiger (Eds.), *Personality disorders from the perspective of the five-factor model* (2nd ed., pp. 325–348). Washington, DC: American Psychological Association.

Markon, K. E., Krueger, R. F., Bouchard, T. J., & Gottesman, I. (2002). Normal and abnormal personality traits: Evidence for genetic and environmental relationships in the Minnesota Study of Twins Reared Apart. *Journal of Personality, 70,* 661–693.

McDermott, P. A., Alterman, A. I., Cacciola, J. S., Rutherford, M. J., Newman, J. P., & Mulholland, E. M. (2000). Generality of Psychopathy Checklist—Revised factors over prisoners and substance-dependent patients. *Journal of Consulting and Clinical Psychology, 68,* 181–186.

Mellsop, G., Varghese, F. T. N., Joshua, S., & Hicks, A. (1982). Reliability of Axis II of DSM-III. *American Journal of Psychiatry, 139,* 1360–1361.

Miller, J. D., & Lynam, D. R. (2003). Psychopathy and the five-factor model of personality: A replication and extension. *Journal of Personality Assessment, 81,* 168–178.

Miller, J. D., Lynam, D. R., Widiger, T. A., & Leukefeld, C. (2001). Personality disorders as extreme variants of common personality dimensions: Can the Five-Factor Model adequately represent psychopathy? *Journal of Personality, 69,* 253–276.

Millon, T. (1981). *Disorders of personality: DSM-III: Axis II.* New York: Wiley.

Millon, T., Davis, R. D., Millon, C. M., Wenger, A. W., Van Zuilen, M. H., Fuchs, M., & Millon, R. B. (1996). *Disorders of personality: DSM-IV and beyond.* New York: Wiley.

Mineka, S., Watson, D., & Clark, L. E. A. (1998). Comorbidity of anxiety and unipolar mood disorders. *Annual Review of Psychology, 49,* 377–412.

Morey, L. C. (1988). The categorical representation of personality disorder: A cluster analysis of DSM-III-R personality features. *Journal of Abnormal Psychology, 97,* 314–321.

Morey, L. C. (1991). *The Personality Assessment Inventory professional manual.* Odessa, FL: Psychological Assessment Resources.

Morey, L. C., & Jones, J. K. (1998). Empirical studies of the construct validity of narcissistic personality disorder. In E. F. Ronningstam (Ed.), *Disorders of narcissism: Diagnostic, clinical, and empirical implications* (pp. 351–373). Washington, DC: American Psychiatric Press.

Morgenstern, J., Langenbucher, J., Labouvie, E., & Miller, K. J. (1997). The comorbidity of alcoholism and personality disorders in a clinical population: Prevalence rates and relation to alcohol typology variables. *Journal of Abnormal Psychology, 106,* 74–84.

Newman, J. P. (1998). Psychopathy: An information processing perspective. In D. J. Cooke, A. E. Forth, & R. D. Hare (Eds.), *Psychopathy: Theory, research, and implications for society* (pp. 81–104). London: Kluwer.

O'Connor, B. P., & Dyce, J. A. (1998). A test of models of personality disorder configuration. *Journal of Abnormal Psychology, 107,* 3–16.

Patrick, C. J., Bradley, M. M., & Lang, P. J. (1993). Emotion in the criminal psychopath: Startle reflex modulation. *Journal of Abnormal Psychology, 102,* 82–92.

Patrick, C. J., Cuthbert, B. N., & Lang, P. J. (1994). Emotion in the criminal psychopath: Fear image processing. *Journal of Abnormal Psychology, 103,* 523–534.

Paulhus, D. L., & Williams, K. M. (2002). The dark triad of personality: Narcissism, machiavellianism, and psychopathy. *Journal of Research in Personality, 36,* 556–563.

Perry, J. C., & Cooper, A. (1989). An empirical study of defense mechanisms: I. Clinical interview and life vignette ratings. *Archives of General Psychiatry, 46,* 444–452.

Reardon, M. L., Lang, A. R., & Patrick, C. J. (2002). An evaluation of relations among antisocial behavior, psychopathic traits, and alcohol problems in incarcerated men. *Alcoholism: Clinical and Experimental Research, 26,* 1188–1197.

Robins, L. N. (1966). *Deviant children grown up.* Baltimore: Williams & Wilkins.

Robins, L. N., Tipp, J., & Przybeck, T. (1991). Antisocial personality. In L. N. Robins & D. A. Regier (Eds.), *Psychiatric disorders in America* (pp. 258–290). New York: Free Press.

Rogers, R. (1995). *Diagnostic and structured interviewing: A handbook for psychologists.* Odessa, FL: Psychological Assessment Resources.

Rogers, R., Salekin, R. T., Sewell, K. W., & Cruise, K. R. (2000). Prototypical analysis of antisocial personality disorder: A study of inmate samples. *Criminal Justice and Behavior, 27,* 234–255.

Ronningstam, E. (1999). Narcissistic personality disorder. In T. Millon, P. H. Blaney, & R. D. Davis (Eds.), *Oxford textbook of psychopathology* (pp. 674–693). New York: Oxford University Press.

Salekin, R. T., Rogers, R., & Machin, D. (2001). Psychopathy in youth: Pursuing diagnostic clarity. *Journal of Youth and Adolescence, 30,* 173–195.

Salekin, R. T., Rogers, R., & Sewell, K. W. (1996). A review and meta-analysis of the Psychopathy Checklist and Psychopathy Checklist—Revised: Predictive validity of dangerousness. *Clinical Psychology: Science and Practice, 3,* 203–215.

Salekin, R., Trobst, K. K., & Krioukova, M. (2001). Construct validity of psychopathy in community sample: A nomological net approach. *Journal of Personality Disorders, 15,* 425–441.

Schmitt, W. A., & Newman, J. P. (1999). Are all psychopathic individuals low-anxious? *Journal of Abnormal Psychology, 108,* 353–358.

Serin, R. C. (1991). Psychopathy and violence in criminals. *Journal of Interpersonal Violence, 6,* 423–431.

Sher, K. J., & Slutske, W. S. (2003). Disorders of impulse control. In G. Stricker & T. A. Widiger (Eds.), *Handbook of psychology: Clinical psychology* (Vol. 8., pp. 195–228). New York: Wiley.

Sher K. J., & Trull, T. J. (1994). Personality and disinhibitory psychopathology: Alcoholism and antisocial personality disorder. *Journal of Abnormal Psychology, 103,* 92–102.

Shine, J., & Hobson, J. (1997). Construct validity of the Hare Psychopathy Checklist, Revised, in a UK prison population. *Journal of Forensic Psychiatry, 8,* 546–561.

Skilling, T. A., Harris, G. T., Rice, M. E., & Quinsey, V. L. (2002). Identifying persistently antisocial offenders using the Hare Psychopathy Checklist and DSM antisocial personality disorder criteria. *Psychological Assessment, 14,* 27–38.

Skodol, A. E., Oldham, J. M., & Gallaher, P. E. (1999). Axis II comorbidity of substance use disorders among patients referred for treatment of personality disorders. *American Journal of Psychiatry, 156,* 733–738.

Smith, S. S., & Newman, J. P. (1990). Alcohol and drug abuse-dependence disorders in psychopathic and nonpsychopathic criminal offenders. *Journal of Abnormal Psychology, 99,* 430–439.

Spitzer, R. L., Endicott, J., & Robins E. (1975). Clinical criteria for psychiatric diagnosis and DSM-III. *American Journal of Psychiatry, 132,* 1187–1192.

Spitzer, R. L., Endicott, J., & Robins, E. (1978). Research diagnostic criteria. Rationale and reliability. *Archives of General Psychiatry, 35,* 773–782.

Spitzer, R. L., Forman, J. B. W., & Nee, J. (1979). DSM-III field trials: I. Initial interrater diagnostic reliability. *American Journal of Psychiatry, 136,* 815–817.

Stone, M. (1993). *Abnormalities of personality. Within and beyond the realm of treatment.* New York: Norton.

Stone, M. (1998). Sadistic personality in murderers. In T. Millon, E. Simonsen, M. Birket-Smith, & R. D. Davis (Eds.), *Psychopathy: Antisocial, criminal, and violent behaviors* (pp. 346–355). New York: Guilford Press.

Sutker, P. B., & Allain, A. N. (2001). Antisocial personality disorder. In P. B. Sutker & H. E. Adams (Eds.), *Comprehensive handbook of psychopathology* (3rd ed., pp. 445–490). New York: Plenum Press.

Swanson, M. C., Bland, R. C., & Newman, S. C. (1994). Antisocial personality disorders. *Acta Psychiatrica Scandinavica, 89*(Suppl. 376), 63–70.

Tellegen, A. (2000). *Manual of the Multidimensional Personality Questionnaire.* Minneapolis: University of Minnesota Press.

Verheul, R., van den Brink, W., & Hartgers, C. (1995). Prevalence of personality disorders among alcoholics and drug addicts: An overview. *European Addiction Research, 1,* 166–177.

Verona, E., Patrick, C. J., & Joiner, T. E. (2001). Psychopathy, antisocial personality, and suicide risk. *Journal of Abnormal Psychology, 110,* 462–470.

Vitacco, M. J., Rogers, R, Neumann, C. S., Harrison, K., & Vincent, G. (in press). A comparison of factor models on the PCL-R with mentally disordered offenders: The development of a four-factor model. *Criminal Justice and Behavior.*

Watson, D., & Clark, L. A. (1984). Negative affectivity: The disposition to experience aversive emotional states. *Psychological Bulletin, 98,* 219–235.

Watson, D., Clark, L. A., & Harkness, A. R. (1994). Structures of personality and their relevance to psychopathology. *Journal of Abnormal Psychology, 103,* 18–31.

Widiger, T. A. (1998a). Four out of five ain't bad. *Archives of General Psychiatry, 55,* 865–866.

Widiger, T. A. (1998b). Psychopathy and normal personality. In D. J. Cooke, A. E. Forth, & R. D. Hare (Eds.), *Psychopathy: Theory, research and implications for society* (pp. 47–68). Dordrecht, The Netherlands: Kluwer.

Widiger, T. A., Cadoret, R., Hare, R., Robins, L., Rutherford, M., Zanarini, M., et al. (1996). DSM-IV antisocial personality disorder field trial. *Journal of Abnormal Psychology, 105,* 3–16.

Widiger, T. A., & Clark, L. A. (2000). Toward DSM-V and the classification of psychopathology. *Psychological Bulletin, 126,* 946–963.

Widiger, T. A., & Corbitt, E. M. (1995). Antisocial personality disorder in DSM-IV. In W. J. Livesley (Ed.), *The DSM-IV personality disorders* (pp. 103–126). New York: Guilford Press.

Widiger, T., Corbitt, E., & Millon, T. (1992). Antisocial personality disorder. In A. Tasman & M. Riba (Eds.), *Review of psychiatry* (Vol. 11, pp. 63–79). Washington, DC: American Psychiatric Press.

Widiger, T. A., & Costa, P. T. (2002). Five factor model personality disorder research. In P. T. Costa & T. A. Widiger (Eds.), *Personality disorders and the five factor model of personality* (2nd ed., pp. 59–87). Washington, DC: American Psychological Association.

Widiger, T., Frances, A., Spitzer, R., & Williams, J. (1988). The DSM-III-R personality disorders: An overview. *American Journal of Psychiatry, 145,* 786–795.

Widiger, T. A., & Lynam, D. R. (1998). Psychopathy from the perspective of the five-factor model of personality. In T. Millon, E. Simonsen, M. Birket-Smith, & R. D. Davis (Eds.), *Psychopathy: Antisocial, criminal, and violent behaviors* (pp. 171–187). New York: Guilford Press.

Widiger, T., & Trull, T. (1987). Behavioral indicators, hypothetical constructs, and personality disorders. *Journal of Personality Disorders, 1,* 82–87.

Widiger, T. A., & Trull, T. J. (1998). Performance characteristics of the DSM-III-R personality disorder criteria sets. In T. A. Widiger, A. J. Frances, H. A. Pincus, R. Ross, M. B. First, W. W. Davis, & M. Klein (Eds.), *DSM-IV sourcebook* (Vol. 4., pp. 357–373). Washington, DC: American Psychiatric Association.

Widiger, T. A., Verheul, R., & van den Brink, W. (1999). Personality and psychopathology. In L. Pervin & O. John (Eds.), *Handbook of personality: Theory and research* (2nd ed., pp. 347–366). New York: Guilford Press.

Widom, C. S. (1977). A methodology for studying noninstitutionalized psychopaths. *Journal of Consulting and Clinical Psychology, 45,* 674–683.

9

Disaggregating Psychopathy

Where and How to Look for Subtypes

NORMAN G. POYTHRESS
JENNIFER L. SKEEM

In this chapter we consider the issue of subtypes[1] of psychopathy. Although there have been many efforts to classify criminal offenders into different subtypes (e.g., Bohn, Carbonell, & Megargee, 1995; Toch & Adams, 1994; Van Voorhis, 1994), there have been few efforts to identify subtypes of psychopathy (see Blackburn, 1975). Contemporary conceptualizations of psychopathy date to Cleckley's (1941/1976) influential characterization of what has come to be called the *primary* psychopath. For the next half century, this conceptualization drove most psychopathy research. Cleckley's contemporary, psychiatrist Benjamin Karpman (1941), proposed a subtype (*secondary* psychopath) that was constitutionally different from, but phenotypically similar to Cleckley's psychopath. Nevertheless, little conceptual or empirical work regarding subtypes of psychopathy occurred during this period.

Several developments have rekindled interest in the search for psychopathy subtypes. One was the publication of Hare's Psychopathy Checklist—Revised (PCL-R; Hare, 1991), which provided researchers with a reliable and valid measure of criminal psychopathy. The PCL-R comprises two correlated factors[2] that reliably fractionate in different directions with respect to a number of criterion measures relevant to theoretical subtypes (see Hicks, Markon, Patrick, & Krueger, 2004). A second is the theoretical work of Fowles (1980) and Gray (1987), whose disaggregation of the neuropsychological response system into behavioral activation system (BAS) and behavioral inhibition (BIS) components accommodates the early work of Lykken (1957) and others to provide a framework for exploring subtypes of psychopathy in terms of etiologies associated with unique temperamental underpinnings (see Lykken, 1995).

Third, the field has experienced rejuvenated interest in noncriminal psychopathy. As Raine (1988) noted, Cleckley's original description of the syndrome derived from his clinical work with nonoffenders, and only one of Cleckley's criteria ("inadequately motivated antisocial behaviour") related to criminality, and then only in an indirect fashion. Consistent with Hare's (1993) assertion that psychopaths are "to be found everywhere—in business, the home, the professions, the military, the arts, the entertainment industry, the news media, academe, and the blue-collar world" (p. 115), investigators are receptive to notions of "successful" or subclinical subtypes of psychopathy that may be identified in community samples. This, in turn, has encouraged the development of psychopathy measures for use with nonclinical samples (e.g., Levenson, Kiehl, & Fitzpatrick, 1995; Lilienfeld & Andrews, 1996), and efforts to define psychopathy in terms of extreme variations on basic personality dimensions (e.g., Miller, Lynam, Widiger, & Leukefeld, 2001; Reise & Oliver, 1994) rather than as a categorical entity.

In the first part of this chapter we review historical conceptions of psychopathy subtypes from Karpman's (1941, 1946) early work to the contemporary writings of Lykken (1995) and draw from our own work (Skeem, Poythress, Edens, Lilienfeld, & Cale, 2003) and recent empirical findings to suggest the best candidate domains for identifying these theoretical subtypes in future research. In the second part, we focus on contemporary research strategies for uncovering subtypes, which chiefly emphasize cluster analysis, and review findings from selected studies. Given space limitations, we do not review relevant studies of children (e.g., Christian, Frick, Hill, Tyler, & Frazer, 1997) or adolescents (e.g., Andershed, Kerr, Statin, & Levander, 2002). Readers are referred to these referenced articles and other chapters in this book (see Salekin, Chapter 20, this volume) for further information on these topics.

CONCEPTIONS OF PSYCHOPATHY SUBTYPES AND PROMISING DOMAINS FOR IDENTIFICATION (WHERE TO LOOK)

Primary and Secondary Psychopathy

Key Theories

Karpman. Benjamin Karpman's (1941) seminal distinction between *primary* and *secondary* psychopathy set the template for much subsequent work on psychopathy subtypes. Like Cleckley's (1941/1976) work, Karpman's was based on clinical observation. According to Karpman's theory, primary and secondary subtypes generally are phenotypically similar: They cheat, con, and swindle others, "*seemingly* have no feeling or regard for others," and often manifest antisocial behavior (Karpman, 1948a, p. 457, emphasis added). However, primary psychopaths' symptoms reflect an affective[3] *deficit*

that is constitutional, whereas secondary psychopaths' symptoms reflect an affective *disturbance* based on early psychosocial learning. The secondary psychopaths' hostility can be understood as an emotional adaptation to such factors as parental rejection and abuse. Unlike the primary psychopath, who possesses the "instinctive emotional organization of a subhuman animal" (Karpman, 1948b, p. 533), the secondary psychopath occasionally manifests such "higher human emotions" as empathy or a wish for acceptance (Karpman, 1941). Indeed, the secondary psychopath suffers from an underlying anxiety, depression, or character neurosis.

In addition to these core etiological and affective differences, Karpman believed that primary and secondary psychopaths differed in their impulsivity and amenability to treatment: "the primary psychopath often acts purposefully and directly to maximize his gain or excitement, whereas the secondary psychopath typically acts out of such emotions as hatred and revenge, often in reaction to circumstances that exacerbate his or her neurotic conflict" (Skeem, Poythress, et al., 2003, p. 520; see Karpman, 1948b, 1955). Furthermore, given their capacity for "moral training," Karpman (1948b) viewed secondary, but not primary, psychopaths as amenable to psychotherapy.

Lykken. David Lykken (1995; see also Lewis, 1991) built on Karpman's theory by linking it with Gray's (1987; Gray & McNaughton, 1996) biological model of personality. The two central components of Gray's model are the BIS, which regulates responsiveness to aversive stimuli and is associated with the experience of negative affect (including anxiety), and the BAS, which regulates appetitive motivation and is associated with the experience of positive affect (and impulsivity). Deficits in these systems may indicate distinct constitutional abnormalities that underlie primary and secondary psychopathy. The primary psychopath may possess an underactive BIS: He or she fails to experience anticipatory anxiety that causes most people to inhibit activity that will not be rewarded (Fowles, 1980; Fowles & Missel, 1994). In contrast, the secondary psychopath may possess an overactive BAS: "He is likely to show poor passive avoidance in the real world when . . . confronted with incentives that attract him strongly enough to overcome his fear. . . . It is his overactive BAS that pushes him into stressful situations" (Lykken, 1995, pp. 160–161). This conceptualization is consistent with Karpman's view that secondary (but not primary) psychopaths experience negative affect and behave quite impulsively.[4] Lykken (1995), however, posits that both primary and secondary psychopathy reflect two extreme temperaments, or constitutional abnormalities. Lykken recommended that the term "sociopath" be reserved for individuals who appear phenotypically psychopathic due to environmental stressors (e.g., inadequate socialization).

Porter. Like Karpman, Stephen Porter (1996) postulated that primary psychopathy chiefly reflects a congenital affective deficit whereas secondary psychopathy chiefly reflects an acquired, environmentally based affective disturbance. According to Porter, however, secondary psychopathy is more *dissociative* than neurotic: A specific environmental insult (extreme physical or sexual abuse, or abandonment) leads to disillusionment and interferes with this individual's ability to form (or if formed, to sustain) significant interpersonal attachments based on positive affect. Although "born with" the capacity for "empathic responding" and positive attachments with others, this individual copes with trauma by dissociating, "turning off," or "deactivating" his or her emotions. Thus, the individual *acquires* features of psychopathy (i.e., shallow affect) and develops a lifestyle centered on self-promotion and self-interest.

Based on a sample of 521 prison inmates and substance abuse treatment residents, Skeem and Poythress (2004) explored Porter's hypothesis using standardized self-report measures and a cross-sectional design. Specifically, they tested whether dissociative symptoms mediated the relationship between child abuse and PCL-R psychopathy (particularly its affective features). Standard regression-based analyses (Baron & Kenny, 1986) indicated that child abuse related positively and directly to psychopathy (PCL-R Total), and that dissociative symptoms partially mediated this relationship. Among factors of psychopathy as specified

in Cooke and Michie's (2001) three-factor model, child abuse was positively and directly associated with the behavioral features of psychopathy (impulsive and irresponsible behavioral style), and this association was partially mediated by dissociative experiences. Child abuse was unrelated to the interpersonal features of psychopathy (arrogant and deceitful interpersonal style). More relevant to Porter's theory were complex findings relating child abuse to the Affective features of psychopathy (deficient affective experience). For this facet of the psychopathy construct, a negative *direct* association was obtained, but a *positive* indirect effect was present via the mediating role of dissociative features.

Although these results are largely consistent with Porter's theory, further research is necessary to draw firm conclusions regarding dissociation as a pathogenic mechanism for secondary psychopathy. In this study all effects were small and child abuse was measured based on retrospective self-report, which introduces the potential for recall and reporting biases. Moreover, no correction was made for measurement error. Future analyses based on structural equation modeling techniques may clarify the relations among these constructs by attempting to control for the unreliability of their measures (which would serve to attenuate any relationships) and for potential method bias (which would serve to exaggerate some relationships, e.g., the relation between the self-report measures of dissociation and child abuse).

Blackburn. Unlike other theories of psychopathy subtypes, Blackburn's (1975, 1999) conceptualization combines empirical results with interpersonal theory. This conceptualization began as an investigation of Megargee's typology of violent offenders, which consisted of over- and undercontrolled types (see Blackburn, 1998). On the basis of cluster analyses of Minnesota Multiphasic Personality Inventory (MMPI) profiles of forensic patients treated in maximum-security hospitals, Blackburn (1968, 1971) identified a fourfold typology of mentally disordered offenders, two of which were labeled "primary" and "secondary" psychopaths. This typology has been replicated in the United Kingdom with various offender populations using Blackburn's (1982) MMPI-based Special Hospitals Assessment of Personality and Socialization (SHAPS; see Blackburn, 1975, 1998, 1999; Blackburn & Coid, 1999). The SHAPS assesses "Belligerence" (impulsive aggression/psychopathy vs. control) and "Withdrawal" (withdrawal vs. sociability) (Blackburn, 1999) and correlates moderately with overall scores on the PCL-R.[5]

According to Blackburn (1998), the chief distinction between primary and secondary psychopaths lies in their degree of withdrawal. Both subtypes share extreme traits of Belligerence (aggressive, hostile, impulsive). However, the primary psychopath is extraverted, confident, dominant, and low to average in anxiety, whereas the secondary psychopath is emotionally disturbed, socially anxious, withdrawn, moody, more submissive, and low in self-esteem (Blackburn, 1985, 1998). These subtypes differ in theoretically coherent ways across a diverse array of variables separate from those used to define them, including: aggression, symptoms and personality disorder diagnoses, self-reported physiological arousal (e.g., sweating; heart racing) in response to provoking hypothetical scenarios, and interpersonal behavior, as rated by self and others (for a review, see Blackburn, 1998).

Morrison and Gilbert (2001) used Blackburn's (1999) Antisocial Personality Questionnaire to classify 50 mentally disordered offenders into primary, secondary, and nonpsychopathic groups. All offenders completed self-report measures of social rank, internalized shame, and anger. Relative to primary psychopaths, secondary psychopaths perceived themselves as possessing significantly lower social rank, greater shame-proneness, and greater general angriness. These differences in self- and social evaluative processes are in keeping with the core dimension of withdrawal–sociability on which Blackburn distinguishes psychopathy subtypes. More generally, Blackburn's distinction between primary and secondary psychopathy is consistent with the results of other typological research conducted with prisoners, mentally disordered offenders, "difficult" psychiatric patients, and male batterers (for a review, see Skeem et al., 2004).

Promising Domains of Inquiry

In our view, there are three promising domains of inquiry for identifying primary and secondary subtypes of psychopathy, as conceptualized by Karpman, Lykken, Porter, and Blackburn. These domains are etiological (etiology and "mechanism markers"), trait-based (psychopathic trait constellations; anxiety or negative affectivity), and behavioral (suicidal and violent behavior).

Etiological. Given that most of these theories distinguish between phenotypically similar variants of psychopathy that chiefly are genetically based (primary) or environmentally based (secondary), etiology will be a crucial domain of inquiry in future research. Current research on the etiology of psychopathy (as currently operationalized) is in its infancy. Most research merely identifies risk factors for psychopathy, treating psychopathy as a homogeneous entity (for a review, see Skeem, Poythress, et al., 2003). In future research, variants of psychopathy should be examined with behavior genetic designs (e.g., twin and adoption studies) that can separate etiological influences on psychopathic traits into specific sources of variance (see Plomin, Ashbury, & Dunn, 2001). In this regard, Krueger and colleagues (2002) employed structural equation modeling to twin study data ($N = 1,048$) to estimate genetic, shared environmental, and nonshared environmental etiological contributions to both a general latent "externalizing" factor representing the shared variance among various disinhibitory disorders and personality traits, and the unique part of each individual phenotype (i.e., conduct disorder, adult antisocial behavior, alcohol dependence, drug dependence, and unconstrained personality). A similar approach could be applied to delineate, for example, etiological influences underlying broad ("general psychopathy") and specific ("distinct facets") elements of the psychopathy construct.

Although etiological research is in its infancy, primary and secondary subtypes may also be distinguished by two groups of "mechanism" markers. First, as noted earlier, Lykken (1995) posits that psychopathy subtypes can be distinguished based on nervous system structures represented by the BIS (underactive in primary psychopathy) and the BAS (overactive in secondary psychopathy). Similar theories (e.g., Gottman, 2001) suggest that these subtypes can be distinguished based on their degree of physiological arousal during provoking situations (hypoarousal-primary; hyperarousal-secondary). Self-report (e.g., Carver & White, 1994; Torrubia, Avila, Molto, & Caseras, 2001), or performance-based, laboratory measures (see Gottman, 2001) of these mechanisms or their markers might be used to disaggregate individuals with phenotypically similar psychopathy profiles. For example, in a study that employed self-report measures of BIS, BAS, and psychopathy with students, results indicated that primary psychopathy is inversely associated with BIS, whereas secondary psychopathy is positively associated with BIS and BAS (McHoskey, Worzel, & Szyarto, 1998).

Second, as noted earlier, some theories posit that primary psychopathy is distinguished by a (heritable) affective deficit, whereas secondary psychopathy is marked by an (acquired) affective disturbance. To investigate this promising domain for identifying psychopathy subtypes, one could apply laboratory measures of affective processing (e.g., Christianson et al., 1996; Patrick, Bradley, & Lang, 1993; Williamson, Harpur, & Hare, 1991) or emotional skills (see Mayer, Salovey, & Caruso, 2000) to determine whether psychopathy factor scores or subgroups fractionate in a theoretically coherent manner.[6]

Trait-Based. Two groups of trait constellations may distinguish between primary and secondary psychopathy. The first group is psychopathic traits. Most measures of psychopathy distill groups of traits across which primary and secondary subtypes might differ.[7] For example, Factor 1 of the PCL-R captures the interpersonal and affective core of psychopathy, whereas Factor 2 largely reflects impulsive and socially deviant behavior.[8] These clusters of interpersonal, affective, and behavioral psychopathic traits hold promise for distinguishing subtypes of psychopathy (see below, Part 2, Strategy 1).[9] Given the aforementioned theories, one might expect primary psychopaths to manifest traits strongly suggestive of an *affective* deficit (i.e., more emotional detachment and

a relative elevation on F1), whereas secondary psychopaths might display more pronounced impulsivity and hostile, deviant *behavior* (i.e., relative elevation on F2). Some evidence suggests that deficits on etiological markers (e.g., indices of affective processing) correlate more strongly with Factor 1 than Factor 2 (Harpur, Hare, & Hakstian, 1989; Patrick, Zempolich, & Levenston, 1997). In fact, there is substantial evidence that Factors 1 and 2 relate to a range of external variables in a manner that is consistent with theories of primary and secondary psychopathy (see Benning et al., 2003).

Second, trait anxiety, neuroticism, or negative affectivity may also assist in discriminating between primary and secondary subtypes. Although Cleckley (1964) asserted that psychopathy is characterized by a lack of anxiety, Karpman (1941; see also Lykken, 1957) suggested that only primary psychopaths lack anxiety (and other "higher human emotions"), whereas secondary psychopaths experience intense anxiety associated with underlying conflict and character neurosis. In keeping with this notion, Kosson and Newman (1995) have identified "high anxious" and "low anxious" individuals with high PCL-R psychopathy scores (see also Andersen, Sestoft, Lillebaek, Mortensen, & Kramp, 1999; Kosson, Smith, & Newman, 1990; Schmitt & Newman, 1999). These high-anxious and low-anxious psychopaths have been shown to differ in their emotional responsiveness (an etiological marker for psychopathy variants) and information processing (e.g., Fagan & Lira, 1980; Goldman, Lindner, Dinitz, & Allen, 1971; Kosson & Newman, 1995). Moreover, measures of anxiety appear inversely associated with psychopathy scales that assess emotional detachment and positively associated with those that assess social deviance (Frick, Lilienfeld, Edens, Poythress, & McBurnett, 2000; Hare, 1991; Verona, Patrick, & Joiner, 2001).

Suicidal and Violent Behavior. In addition to etiological and trait domains, behavioral domains may also aid in differentiating primary and secondary subtypes. First, suicide-related behavior (O'Carroll et al., 1996) may distinguish between primary and secondary subtypes. Primary psychopaths typically are viewed as emotionally stable individuals at distinctly low risk for suicide. Indeed, Cleckley's (1941/1976) diagnostic criteria for psychopathy included "suicide rarely carried out." However, to the extent that secondary psychopaths are anxious, dysphoric, hostile, impulsive, and withdrawn, they may be at high risk for suicide and suicide-related behavior. In keeping with this notion, several studies indicate that suicidal tendencies (attempts and/or ideation) are preferentially associated with PCL-R Factor 2 (or analogous factors of other psychopathy measures) and, at least partially mediated by trait dimensions of negative emotionality and low constraint (Douglas, Lilienfeld, & Poythress, 2004; Verona et al., 2001).

Primary and secondary psychopaths also may be differentiated based on the nature of their violent behavior. Given their emotional detachment and underactive BIS, primary psychopaths may be less prone to *reactive* violence but more likely to employ *instrumental* violence to obtain some extrinsic goal (see Cornell et al., 1996; Porter & Woodworth, Chapter 24, this volume; Stafford & Cornell, 2003; Williamson, Hare, & Wong, 1987). In contrast, due to their overactive BAS, secondary psychopaths may be more prone to relatively frequent, *reactive* violence:

> The loss (or potential loss) of reward (e.g., dissolution of a valued interpersonal relationship) or self-esteem is more likely to result in anger that provokes immediate violence in individuals whose characterological features include impulsivity, poor behavior controls, and (theoretically) a type of covert narcissism that is less stable in the face of challenge or insult and is associated with underlying feelings of insecurity and vulnerability. (Skeem, Poythress, et al., 2003, p. 537; citations omitted)

The results of a study by Hart and Dempster (1997) are partially in keeping with this hypothesis. Ratings of offenders' crime scenarios revealed that PCL-R Factor 1 scores were positively associated with ratings of instrumentality, goal-directedness, and planning but negatively associated with intoxication and co-combatant provocation. In contrast, Factor 2 was negatively associated with ratings of planning and positively associated with intoxication.

Psychopathy Subtypes with Distinctive Traits of Other Disorders

Key Theories

Theories of primary and secondary psychopathy focus on how individuals with phenotypically similar symptoms differ etiologically. An additional set of theories focuses on describing phenotypical differences among individuals with psychopathic traits by referencing comorbid traits and features of other personality disorders. This approach focuses on recurring patterns of overlap between psychopathic and other traits (Murphy & Vess, 2003), or psychodynamic personality organization (Meloy & Gacono, 1992, 1993; Millon & Davis, 1998).

Based on clinical observations at a forensic hospital, Murphy and Vess (2003) asserted that four subtypes of psychopathy can be distinguished, based on prominent comorbid features of other "dramatic, erratic" Cluster B personality disorders. The *sadistic* subtype is distinguished by assaultiveness and pleasure derived from the suffering of others; the *narcissistic* subtype by features of grandiosity, entitlement, and callous disregard for others; the *antisocial* subtype by impulsivity, stimulation seeking, and socially deviant behavior; and the *borderline* subtype by affective instability and self-destruction. The authors muse about whether these subtypes might be placed on a continuum anchored by the aggressive *sadistic* and unstable *borderline* types. Given the authors' description of the subtypes, however, one might conceptualize the subtypes as organized by correlated trait dimensions rather than a single trait dimension.

Millon and Davis (1998) and Meloy and Gacono (1992, 1993) propose subtypes of psychopathy using a similar approach, but they do so from a psychodynamic perspective. Because these theories may be relatively difficult to operationalize and evaluate empirically using strategies like those proposed below, we note them only briefly here. Of Millon and Davis's 10 proposed subtypes of psychopathy, the "malevolent," "covetous," and "unprincipled"[10] are similar to Murphy and Vess's (2003) sadistic, narcissistic, and antisocial subtypes. Meloy and Gacono (1992, 1993) present two case studies: one of a *borderline* psychopath similar to that of

Murphy and Vess, and another of a *psychotic* psychopath. The psychotic psychopath bears some resemblance to Karpman's (1948b, 1955) occasional description of secondary psychopathy as underpinned by psychosis and Kallman's (1938) recognition of "schizoid psychopaths," who manifest traits of both psychopathy and subclinical features of schizophrenia. According to this view, psychopathy may share some common affective deficit with schizophrenia spectrum disorders (Raine, 1986; see also Eysenck & Eysenck, 1975).

Promising Domains of Inquiry: Cluster B Traits

These theories and relevant data suggest that traits of borderline personality disorder and narcissism may distinguish among particular subtypes of psychopathy (see Skeem, Poythress, et al., 2003, for a detailed review). They may also distinguish between primary and secondary psychopathy. Blackburn (1996) described secondary psychopaths as "predominantly borderline personalities" (p. 19) (see also Blackburn, 1998; Blackburn & Coid, 1999; Hart & Hare, 1989). For these individuals, disturbed emotional capacities may often manifest in hostile reactivity that interferes with stable relationships and adaptive functioning. Indeed, there is some evidence that borderline personality disorder is more strongly associated with PCL-R Factor 2 than the emotional detachment of Factor 1 (e.g., Hart & Hare, 1989; Rutherford, Alterman, Cacciola, & McKay, 1997; Salekin, Rogers, & Sewell, 1997; Shine & Hobson, 1997).

Raine (1992) found a "subgroup" of offenders with mid-high range scores on the PCL-R who manifested "borderline–schizotypal" personality characteristics. These characteristics were most strongly related to PCL-R (Factor 2) items that referenced an impulsive, unstable lifestyle. Notably, the self-report measures of schizotypal personality used in this study included features that overlap quite clearly with borderline traits (i.e., hypersensitivity and social withdrawal, subclinical perceptual aberrations), and clinical ratings of borderline and schizotypal personality were strongly correlated ($r = .57$). Thus, this finding appears more in keeping with the notion of a psychopathy subtype with borderline traits that occasionally shows psychotic-like experiences, than with the notion that psychosis per se (i.e., hallucinations, delusions, formal thought disorder) is an intrinsic feature of the subtype.

Some of the theories reviewed earlier suggest that there may be a "narcissistic" subtype of psychopathy. Narcissism may mark either a unique subtype of psychopathy (e.g., Millon & Davis, 1998) or primary psychopathy per se. In keeping with the latter possibility, Hare (1991; see also Hart & Hare, 1989) found that narcissistic personality disorder was more strongly associated with PCL-R Factor 1 than with Factor 2. Similar findings have been reported using self-report measures of psychopathy (Blackburn, 1998; Blackburn & Coid, 1999; McHoskey et al., 1998).

Although primary psychopaths may be "narcissistic" in the obvious sense of the term, secondary psychopaths may possess a less obvious constellation of narcissistic traits. Empirical work by Wink (1991) distinguishes *overt* and *covert* forms of narcissism. Primary psychopaths may manifest overt narcissism, or "grandiosity–exhibitionism," whereas secondary psychopaths manifest covert narcissism, or "vulnerability–sensitivity." In keeping with Blackburn's distinction between subtypes, primary psychopaths may be characterized by dominance and obvious arrogance, whereas secondary psychopaths manifest a lack of self-confidence. Unhappy with their subordinate status, secondary psychopaths may be viewed as defensive, bitter, and sensitive to ego threat. Behavioral rating systems that capture the extent to which interpersonal interactions are dominant/controlling or hostile/submissive (e.g., Benjamin, 1974) may aid in distinguishing between primary and secondary psychopaths.

STRATEGIES FOR IDENTIFYING SUBTYPES (HOW TO FIND THEM)

Whereas research on the nature of psychopathy has relied primarily on variable-centered approaches, a person-centered approach—primarily cluster analysis—has been the method of choice among investigators attempting to identify subtypes. However, investigations have differed considerably in their strategies regarding samples, clustering variables, and criterion measures used to validate the emergent clusters. As employed to date, these strategies involve explicit or implicit assumptions about the critical defining features of psychopathy, as reflected in the choices of samples and measures that investigators have employed.

Strategy 1: Clustering the PCL-R Profiles of Identified "Psychopaths"

Description and Exemplar of Strategy 1

Given that popular research measures of psychopathy distill trait constellations into factors or facets that could fit theories specifying phenotypical differences among primary and secondary subtypes, one research strategy involves selecting a sample of identified "psychopaths" according to some *a priori* criterion and attempting to identify subtypes based exclusively on the configurations of these factors or facets. Exemplary of this approach is the unpublished work of Hervé and colleagues. Hervé, Ling, and Hare (2000) selected the protocols of 202 federal inmates who scored above 27 on the PCL-R.[11] These protocols were used to compute scores on the three PCL-R facets (Interpersonal, Affective, and Lifestyle) delineated by Cooke and Michie (2001). Various clustering algorithms were used to identify relatively homogeneous groups of inmates. The authors reported that a four-cluster solution best fit the data and replicated across clustering methods. This solution also replicated across psychopathy models, as a similar four-cluster solution was identified when the authors added a fourth facet (Antisocial) that Hare (2003) recently added to Cooke and Michie's (2001) model (Hervé & Hare, 2004). This solution also reportedly replicated across other offender/forensic psychiatric samples (Hervé & Hare, 2002). Figure 9.1 shows the profiles of these four groups.

The cluster labels appear to be based strictly on profile shape and elevation. The designation of *prototypical* psychopath was given to the group that was (relatively) higher across the board on all psychopathy facet scores. Hervé and colleagues (2000) surmised that the *manipulative* psychopaths, higher on interpersonal but lower on lifestyle, might be "talkers" especially prone to crimes involving fraud and deception, whereas the *macho* psychopaths, lacking the glibness and charm required for confidence games (i.e., relatively lower on the interper-

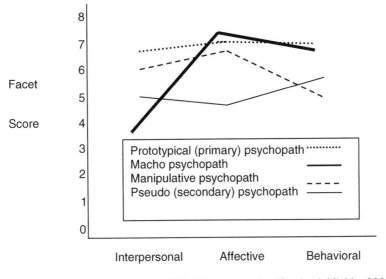

FIGURE 9.1. Psychopathy subtypes defined by PCL-R facet profiles. Adapted with permission of the authors from Hervé, Ling, and Hare (2000).

sonal factor), might manipulate others more through force and intimidation (e.g., robberies and assaults). The fourth group, with the lowest affective facet score and second lowest scores on the other two facets, were initially described as *sociopaths* (Hervé, Ling, & Hare, 2000); this group was later labeled the *pseudo-* (or secondary) psychopath (Hervé & Hare, 2002, 2004).

Recently, Hervé and Hare (2004) examined the relation between group membership and past types of crimes committed by participants. Their findings suggested that *pseudo* and *prototypical* psychopaths have a greater number of past offenses than the other two groups; *pseudo* and *macho* psychopaths have more anger-related past offenses (arson, vandalism, threats) than the other two groups; *manipulative* psychopaths have the fewest past offenses, least serious interpersonal violence, and greatest "fraud for needs" (but not "fraud for money") offenses, and *macho* psychopaths have the greatest number of drug offenses. These findings provided only mixed support for the authors' *a priori* hypotheses. For example, *manipulative* psychopaths were relatively prone to con and deceive in some circumstances (fraud for needs, but not money), but there was little evidence that *macho* psychopaths were particularly likely to force and intimidate (through serious interpersonal violence).

The field awaits further evidence regarding the construct validity of the identified clusters and whether identifying subtypes (in part) on the basis of criminal *modus operandi* can be accommodated into a viable theoretical framework. This validation strategy may be vulnerable to problems of criterion contamination because prior criminality and style of influencing/ manipulating others are factors considered in scoring the PCL-R items, from which the clustering factors are derived. To validate identified subgroups of psychopathy, one must determine whether those subgroups differ on *external* variables that were not tapped in the original clustering solution. Without such external validation, it is unclear whether the groups identified are valid and meaningful.

It will also be interested to see whether and how the *pseudo* group compares with the *prototypical* group on relevant criterion measures. Hervé and Hare (2004) found that

pseudo psychopaths engaged in as much or more antisocial and violent behavior as *prototypic* psychopaths. This is in keeping with the foregoing discussion of primary and secondary psychopathy, as is the putative *pseudo* group's relatively higher elevation on the lifestyle factor (compared to their scores on affective and interpersonal factors). However, a perusal of Figure 1 suggests that the overall difference between these two groups may be mainly in terms of profile elevation. In the absence of evidence that these groups differ systematically on important external variables, a viable alternative interpretation is that *both* clusters are primary psychopaths that differ merely in the degree of saturation or severity of their features. As described in the next section, Alterman and colleagues (1998) found that, of three cluster groups evidencing psychopathic features,[12] peculiarly high PCL-R scores did not distinguish the group that appeared most like primary psychopaths in terms of scores on criterion measures.

Evaluation of Strategy 1

Regarding this general strategy for identifying subtypes, the selection of only individuals who meet an *a priori* criterion for being psychopaths caters to the view of psychopathy as a taxon, or discrete class of individuals who differ from others not in degree, but in *kind*. In the absence of clear evidence that psychopathy is a taxon, information about meaningful subtypes may be lost by excluding those subjects who do not meet a putative cutscore to be regarded "psychopaths." It may be the case that (at least minor) variations in elevation may be less important than profile configuration for identifying a particular subtype, and that important information is lost by excluding individuals with slightly lower elevations but otherwise similar profiles. That said, however, starting with relatively higher scorers on a psychopathy measure seems an appropriate strategy for *initial* explorations of possible subtypes.

Other problems may result from restricting the array of clustering variables to psychopathy factor scores. First, in some studies the PCL-R factors have been so highly correlated that investigators have found them to be of limited use in distinguishing subtypes (e.g., Alterman et al., 1998). Second, because similar psychopathy phenotypes may arise from different etiologies, individuals with the same (or very similar) configuration of factor scores may differ in ways that are obscured by the exclusion of clustering variables related to etiology. Other clustering strategies may be less vulnerable to these potential problems.

Strategy 2: Clustering Using Psychopathic Features *and* Other Variables

Description and Exemplar of Strategy 2

If important features that define subtypes of psychopathy are not well represented in existing psychopathy measures, then one alternative is to expand the array of clustering variables to include measures of these features. The study by Alterman and his colleagues (1998) illustrates this general approach, although their objective was to discriminate subtypes of antisociality rather than psychopathy per se. Because these investigators judged that no single measure adequately captured all the features relevant to antisociality, they used multiple clustering variables, including measures of (1) conduct disorder, (2) adult antisocial behavior, (3) the Socialization scale from the California Psychological Inventory, and (4) PCL-R scores.[13] Cluster analyses of these variables in a sample of 252 males in a methadone maintenance program yielded six stable and replicable subtypes, three of which (Types 1, 2, and 5) had relatively high PCL-R elevations.[14] Types 1 and 2 had highly similar scores on all clustering variables except conduct disorder symptoms (higher for Type 1), whereas Type 5 was similar to Types 1 and 2 on PCL-R elevation only and lower on the other variables.

Alterman and colleagues (1998) also used an extensive array of external validation measures that yielded interesting comparisons among these three groups. Both Type 1 and Type 2 obtained scores on external correlates that are consistent with clinical characterizations of *secondary* psychopath, including serious involvement in criminality and substance abuse, higher levels of negative emotionality (anxiety and depression), moderately high guilt, and high levels of hostility. Type 5, in contrast, shared only the feature of significant criminality with the other

psychopathic types. In keeping with features of *primary* psychopathy, Type 5 showed less substance abuse involvement, less negative emotionality and hostility, and the lowest level of guilt of all subtypes.

Enhancement of Strategy 2

To enhance the ability of Strategy 2 to identify psychopathy subtypes, one might focus more specifically on psychopathy and apply a theoretical approach for deriving and validating subtypes.[15] For example, one might use Lykken's (1995) classification of psychopathy subtypes as a blueprint for investigation. Lykken suggested that primary psychopathy, secondary psychopathy, and (phenotypically similar) sociopathy differ in their basic etiology. Indications of low BIS, high BAS, and inadequate socializing resources, respectively, might distinguish exemplars of these subtypes. Based on this principle, investigators could cluster individuals not only on their psychopathy traits but also on "mechanism markers" (e.g., behavioral activation and inhibition) and socializing influences (e.g., childhood maltreatment).

Some variations in the configurations of psychopathy traits might be anticipated. Comparatively higher scores in the affective domain might be expected with primary psychopathy, whereas secondary psychopathy might result in a relative elevation on impulsive and deviant lifestyle indicators. Given this theory-driven strategy, investigators would determine whether these trait configurations varied in a coherent manner with hypothesized etiological factors. Such a pattern would permit investigators to identify groups of individuals representative of theoretical subtypes. If such groups were identified, they could be systematically validated by determining whether they differed as expected on measures of criterion variables (e.g., low vs. high anxiety, suicidality, or type of violence).

Strategy 3: Clustering Psychopathic Individuals on General Personality Indicators

A third strategy, exemplified in the work of Hicks and colleagues (2004), is to use a psychopathy measure only for purposes of selecting a sample of psychopathic individuals. Facets of the psychopathy measure itself are not used to identify subtypes; rather, clustering techniques are applied to indices of general personality traits to disaggregate the sample into relatively homogeneous subgroups, an approach that "rests on the assumption that personality disorders can be conceptualized as distinct configurations of extreme scores on normative personality traits" (Hicks et al., 2004, p. 277; Widiger & Lynam, 1998).

Using the PCL-R as a screening measure, Hicks et al. identified 96 male prison inmates with PCL-R Total scores ≥ 30. Scores on the brief form of the Multidimensional Personality Questionnaire (MPQ:BF, Patrick, Curtin, & Tellegen, 2002) were used as clustering variables to identify homogeneous clusters among these 96 male prisoners. The MPQ-BF was developed using data from a large community sample (675 males and 675 females), and yields scores on 11 primary trait scales that assess a range of distinct personality constructs. Trait scales include Social Potency, Social Closeness, Stress Reaction, Alienation, Aggression, Harm Avoidance, and Traditionalism (among others). These scales load on four superordinate factors: Agentic Positive Emotionality (PEM-A), Communal Positive Emotionality (PEM-C), Negative Emotionality (NEM), and Constraint (CON).

Hicks et al. reviewed the literature on different patterns of external correlates for PCL-R Factor 1 and Factor 2 and noted that these patterns of correlations[16] parallel the putative characteristics that distinguish primary and secondary psychopaths. Briefly, PCL-R Factor 2 is positively associated with measures of anxiety, neuroticism, negative emotionality, impulsivity, anger–aggression, substance abuse/dependence, and history of suicide attempt—a pattern consistent with a characterization of secondary psychopathy. In contrast, investigators have found that, consistent with a characterization of primary psychopathy, PCL-R Factor 1 is negatively associated with anxiety, neuroticism, and negative emotionality, whereas it is unrelated to impulsivity and anger or aggression, as well as substance use problems and suicide attempts.

Examination of these associations led

Hicks et al. to hypothesize that two distinct subgroups would emerge from the cluster analysis of MPQ:BF scores, one cluster low in anxiety, with personality features similar to those attributed to primary psychopaths, and a second cluster characterized by high anxiety, impulsivity, and aggression. As revealed in the profiles shown in Figure 9.2, the results from model-based clustering[17] confirmed this hypothesis.[18]

For one group ($N = 30$) the most extreme score was in the negative direction on the Stress Reaction scale; thus, this group was labeled Emotionally Stable psychopaths. For the second group ($N = 66$), the most extreme score was an elevation on the Aggression scale, thus these inmates were labeled Aggressive psychopaths. For the Emotionally Stable group, the average deviation from the normative T score mean (= 50) for the 11 MPQ:BF traits was 3.71. Significant deviations from MPQ community normative means were obtained for six MPQ traits and one higher-order personality dimension. Greater deviation from MPQ norms was observed in the Aggressive psychopaths' scores; for the 11 MPQ:BF traits, their average deviation from a T score mean of 50 was 6.61. Significant deviations from MPQ normative means were obtained for nine MPQ traits and three higher order personality dimensions.[19]

Interpreting the MPQ:BF score configurations, Hicks and colleagues (2004) concluded that the Emotionally Stable group reasonably supports the *primary* psychopathy construct. In addition to low anxiety (reflected in low Stress Reaction), Emotionally Stable psychopaths described themselves as socially dominant (high PEM-A) and relatively fearless (low on Harm Avoidance), although not impulsive (high on Control) individuals. In contrast, trait characteristics of the Aggressive group included aggressiveness (high Aggression), difficulty establishing or maintaining relationships with others (high Alienation, low PEM-C), and greater likelihood of impulsive behavior and reactive hostility toward others (high Stress Reaction, low Constraint)—all features associated with *secondary* psychopathy. Group differences on other self-report criterion measures were consistent with these interpretations. Specifically, Aggressive psychopaths

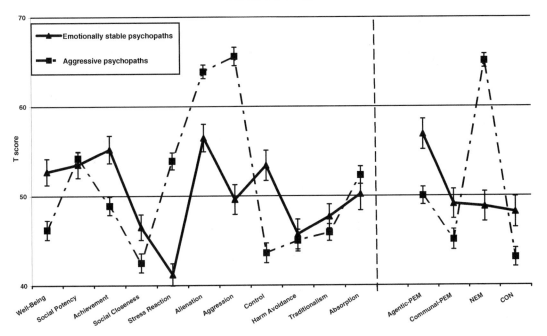

FIGURE 9.2. Two empirically derived subtypes of psychopathy. Adapted with permission from Hicks et al. (2004).

reported significantly more childhood and adult fights, higher scores on an alcohol abuse inventory, lower socialization scores, and higher trait anxiety than did Emotionally Stable psychopaths.

The importance of this strategy is highlighted by the fact that these empirically derived psychopathy subtypes were phenotypically similar in terms of PCL-R features. The clusters did not differ on PCL-R Total or Factor 1 scores, although the Aggressive group did score slightly (and significantly) higher on Factor 2. Thus, although the methodology employed by Hicks and colleagues appears, like Strategy 1, to cater to a conceptualization of psychopathy as a taxon, it avoids other potential problems with Strategy 1 related to clustering exclusively on the basis of psychopathy factor or facet scores. This study demonstrates that PCL-R diagnosed psychopaths can be disaggregated into theoretically meaningful subgroups despite extensive phenotypic similarity, and that the investigation of the psychopathy construct (including its subtypes) may be furthered in the larger domain of general personality constructs.

Strategy 4: Psychopathy Prototypes based on General Personality Constructs

Description and Exemplar of Strategy 4

The aforementioned strategies all involve, in some fashion, scores on some measure of psychopathy as a starting point for the identification of discrete subtypes. The first two strategies include measures of psychopathy facets as clustering variables; the third strategy uses measures of psychopathy only to identify a sample of psychopathic individuals that is then disaggregated by clustering on indices of a general personality inventory. A fourth potential strategy does not involve the use of explicit measures of psychopathy but, like the third strategy, employs broad measures of general personality. Briefly, this strategy involves the use of psychopathy experts to define the quintessential psychopath using the specific items or facets of a general personality measure. The resulting profile can then be used as a criterion against which to compare the profiles of individuals of interest. The work of Lynam and colleagues (Brinkley, Newman, Widiger, & Lynam,

2004; Lynam, 2002; Miller et al., 2001; Widiger & Lynam, 1998) (see also Lynam & Derefinko, Chapter 7, this volume) best illustrates this strategy.[20]

Miller and colleagues (2001) developed a prototypical profile based on expert ratings of the five-factor model (FFM: McCrae & Costa, 1990, 2003) of normal personality, whose broad domains of normal personality include Neuroticism (or negative affectivity), Extraversion (or positive affectivity), Openness to experience (or unconventionality), Agreeableness (vs. Antagonism), and Conscientiousness (vs. low constraint). Each of these five domains includes six facets that represent conceptually distinct aspects of the domain. A panel of 16 psychopathy experts provided ratings from 1 (extremely uncharacteristic of psychopaths) to 5 (extremely characteristic of psychopaths) for each of the 30 FFM facets. The mean scores across experts resulted in a prototype that was low in all facets of Agreeableness, some facets of Conscientiousness (e.g., Self-Discipline and Deliberation), Warmth (a facet of Extraversion) and Openness to Feelings. The psychopath was described as high on a single facet of Neuroticism (i.e., Impulsivity), high on Extraversion (Assertiveness, Excitement Seeking), and, unexpectedly, high in Conscientiousness (Competence).

Miller and colleagues (2001) used this prototypical profile to develop a psychopathy resemblance index (PRI), which is a Q-correlation between an individual's own FFM scores and those of the psychopathy prototype. Based on a sample of 481 community residents, these authors provided preliminary evidence for the validity of the PRI, which was moderately correlated (r = .52) with Total scores on Levenson's Self-Report Psychopathy (LSRP; Levenson et al., 1995) scale. The authors also found evidence of convergent and discriminant validity with measures of a variety of internalizing and externalizing disorders.

High congruence between measures of psychopathy and indices of general personality traits have also been demonstrated with methods other than expert prototype matching. The congruence of the Impulsivity and Withdrawal dimensions of Blackburn's (1999) Antisocial Personality Questionnaire (APQ) with the higher-order latent factors of

the NEO Five Factor Inventory (Costa & McCrae, 1992) has been demonstrated using structural equation modeling (Blackburn, Renwick, Donnelly, & Logan, 2004). Similarly, Benning and colleagues (2003) have shown that the factor scores of Lilienfeld and Andrews's (1996) Psychopathic Personality Inventory (PPI) can be predicted well using scores from Tellegen's MPQ. Thus, it may be possible to compute, for individuals, psychopathy resemblance indicators for the APQ and PPI using prototypical profiles derived from these measures.

Enhancement and Evaluation of Strategy 4

With respect to identifying subtypes of psychopathy on the basis of prototypes, there are at least two directions investigators might pursue. One approach would be to identify a group of participants as likely "psychopathic" on the basis of high(er) resemblance indices, and then use clustering methods to further sort these individuals into more homogeneous groups. Widiger and Lynam (1998) reviewed literature related to primary theories of psychopathy. They suggested that variations among FFM configurations, all of which have a high PRI, might distinguish among individuals with (1) fearless temperament (i.e., relatively lower Neuroticism) (2) cognitive deficits (e.g., Patterson & Newman, 1993) that result in lack of planning and impaired judgment (i.e., relatively lower Conscientiousness), or (3) socially acquired information-processing deficits, such as hostile attributions (e.g., Dodge, 1993), as reflected in relatively higher Antagonism. These particular personality variations appear, at least descriptively, similar to Lykken's (1995) primary psychopath (low behavioral inhibition), secondary psychopath (impulsive pursuit of awards), and sociopath (environmentally acquired psychopathic features), respectively.

A second approach would be to have psychopathy experts provide different sets of prototype ratings for different theoretical subtypes (e.g., primary vs. secondary psychopathy). This would permit the computation of a resemblance index (Q-correlation) for a given individual with each prototype, with assignments of individuals to groups representing theoretically different subtypes on the basis of differences between correlations.

This strategy avoids some problems in the selection of measures in psychopathy research. Hare's PCL-R is not appropriate for research with nonforensic samples, whereas the evidence for the validity of some other psychopathy measures (e.g., LSRP and PPI) with forensic and clinical samples is (presently) limited. Well-normed general personality measures offer standardized criteria against which to compare the performance of individuals from a wide variety of populations. "Psychopathy" measures may still have a role in such studies, perhaps as criterion measures for validating prototypes rather than as a basis for sample selection or as primary clustering variables. This strategy is compatible with that of Hicks and colleagues, discussed earlier, in which psychopathy can be represented dimensionally as "a collection of personality traits rather than a homogeneous, qualitatively distinct condition . . . on a continuum with normal personality functioning, with different pathologies reflecting the different facets of personality that are involved" (Widiger & Lynam, 1998, p. 185).

General Comments on Clustering Strategies

As the foregoing discussion reveals, in choosing a strategy for identifying subtypes of psychopathy, investigators must make several decisions, some of which are associated with important underlying assumptions. In this section, we briefly review five important decisions, including choice of sample, analytic technique, variables, and validation framework.

First, one must decide what population to study. Ideally, one would study a representative sample of community residents to capture the nature, prevalence, and full range of psychopathy subtypes. Given practical constraints, however, investigators typically study psychopathy in referred populations (e.g., correctional offenders, substance abuse patients, and psychiatric patients), thereby risking underinclusiveness. Most efforts to date to study psychopathy in adult community samples have been limited to highly select groups such as students (e.g., Lilienfeld & Andrews, 1996; Lynam, Whiteside, & Jones, 1999) or members of twin registries (e.g., Benning et al., 2003; Blonigen, Carlson, Krueger, & Patrick, 2003), or have utilized recruitment strategies that attract substantial numbers of criminal offenders who, perhaps only for the moment, are not incarcerated (e.g., Belmore & Quinsey, 1994; Widom, 1977).

When choosing a sample, one must consider how mental health and criminal justice systems "sort" individuals to estimate whether the referred population will include the subtypes of interest. For example, "charismatic psychopaths" (Lykken, 1995) may be such accomplished confidence artists that they are unlikely to be present in any referred sample. Consistent with this hypothesis, Hervé and Hare (2004) found a very low base rate (7%) of manipulative psychopaths in a recent sample of offenders. On the other hand, secondary psychopaths ("neurotic," "dissociative," or "borderline") may be abundant in psychiatric samples.

In addition to choosing the population from which to sample, the investigator often determines the selection criteria for study inclusion. As in some of the studies reviewed previously, some investigators have searched for subtypes using only those individuals who surpass the conventional PCL-R threshold (Total score ≥30) for diagnosing psychopathy. Although this is a defensible strategy for investigations of individuals with the most extreme manifestations, particularly at this early stage in the search for valid subtypes, it is an approach that is problematic on a number of counts. First, it caters to the notion that psychopathy is a taxon and, as noted later, the limited evidence currently available cuts against this notion. Empirically, there is evidence that individuals with mid-to-high range scores on the PCL-R often experience comorbid anxiety (Schmitt & Newman, 1999), psychopathology (Andersen et al., 1999), and Cluster B-like traits (Raine, 1992). To the extent that these individuals are secondary psychopaths, excluding them from analyses is a crucial omission that probably will go undetected.

This strategy is also hostile to the notion of the "successful" or "subclinical" psychopath, the individual who may have substantial psychopathic traits but sufficient skills or protective features to avoid the behavioral excesses that result in incarceration. The PCL-R is applicable only to corrections and forensic populations for whom ample file information is available, and thus it cannot be used to study psychopathy in community samples.[21] Other developing measures of psychopathy (see Lilienfeld & Fowler, Chapter 6, this volume) may offer greater flexibility in the study of psychopathy.

A third decision is whether to use categorical or dimensional analytic techniques. Cluster analyses, for example, assume that subtypes are discrete categories; inverse or "Q" factor analysis (see Banks & Phillip, 1965) assumes that variants may be placed along dimensions. An investigator could find discrete groups or continuous dimensions, based solely on the technique applied. Ideally, then, investigators will choose a technique based on a defensible theory about whether subtypes or variants represent categories, or dimensions (see later).

Fourth, one must choose variables for analysis that will best distinguish among putative subtypes. The best guide for choosing variables is a carefully articulated hypothesis about the subtypes of psychopathy that will be found in the population of interest. Such a hypothesis will go far both in identifying variables that maximally differentiate among the hypothesized subtypes and in interpreting the results of analyses. An articulated hypothesis also makes the investigators' assumptions about subtypes and their distinct features transparent, allowing others to determine whether a subtype of interest had an opportunity to be identified (in that failure to include at least one dimension that differentiates the subtype from others ensures that it will not).

Finally, an investigator must decide how to validate the subtypes of psychopathic individuals identified. This involves determining whether the groups or dimensions of individuals identified relate in a theoretically coherent manner to variables that were not used to derive them. The choice of validation variables may set up an "easy" or a "stringent" test and involves assumptions about the nomological network in which each subtype is embedded. For example, one might determine whether secondary psychopaths respond to treatment more readily than primary psychopaths. A more stringent test would be to determine whether Porter's dissociative secondary psychopath and Blackburn's withdrawn/borderline psychopath were uniquely responsive to exposure therapy (see Foa, Hearst-Ikeda, & Perry, 1995) and dialectical behavior therapy (Linehan, 1993), respectively. The more specific the prediction, the more credible the identified subtype.

SUMMARY AND CLOSING COMMENTS

The notion of subtypes of psychopathy has a rich history over the past half century, dating at least to the work of Karpman (1941, 1946) and more recently to the work of Blackburn (1975) and Lykken (1995). Focusing mainly on the *primary* versus *secondary* psychopathy distinction and related theoretical issues, we have suggested some promising domains and strategies for identifying subtypes of psychopathy and reviewed some studies that illustrate select strategies in contemporary subtype research.

The field has just begun systematically and empirically to investigate subtypes of psychopathy. Research lags far behind clinical and theoretical musings about the potentially wide array of subtypes (Lykken, 1995; Millon & Davis, 1988) but promises to refine our understanding of the psychopathy construct. For example, subtyping research may shed some light on the debate about psychopathy as a categorical versus dimensional entity. Although psychopathy often is discussed predominantly in categorical terms, the evidence to date offers little support for taxonicity (see Marcus, Edens, & Lilienfeld, 2004; Marcus, John, & Edens, 2004). In fact, the most favorable evidence for taxonicity (Harris, Rice, & Quinsey, 1994) is limited to a subset of PCL-R features that some have recommended for exclusion from the construct (Cooke & Michie, 2001; Skeem, Mulvey, & Grisso, 2003).

This debate about the categorical versus dimensional nature of psychopathy bears on a central question in subtyping research. If subtypes are found, will all of them be "psychopaths"? This is a particularly salient question in the context of studies that seek to identify "subclinical" or "successful" psychopaths in community and other noncorrectional samples. Although clustering algorithms will identify groups of relatively similar individuals in a given sample, they provide no guidance on the propriety of assigning particular labels to the emergent groups. Instead, these groups must be interpreted based on testable and sound theories. Simply put, important decisions will have to be made about when to assign the label of "psychopath" to a group, lest we be finding psychopaths under every stone.

The question is also an important one with respect to more traditional samples in psychopathy research. In offender and forensic populations, scores of 30 or higher on Hare's PCL-R provide a heuristic for classifying individuals as "psychopaths." One possible outcome of subtyping studies is that groups may emerge containing individuals who are phenotypically similar on explicit measures of psychopathic features (i.e., similar PCL-R patterns and elevations) but etiologically heterogeneous. To the degree that one or more clusters were distinguished by unique environmental etiological factors, the results would support Lykken's (1995) proposal for distinguishing the latter group of (phenotypical) psychopaths as "sociopaths." Alternatively, one or more clusters may have psychopathy scores that fall beneath the traditional PCL-R threshold for diagnosing psychopathy but who are indistinguishable from clusters with higher PCL-R scores, in terms of etiological patterns and performance on criterion measures. It also is possible that some clusters may be identified primarily by features associated with a psychopathy taxon, whereas others are identified by features associated with a (dimensional) psychopathy trait (see Waller, Putnam, & Carlson, 1996; Waller & Ross, 1977; cf. Watson, 2003, for such findings in studies of the dissociation construct).

Each of these scenarios gives rise to questions about the wisdom and utility of using the same construct to capture heterogeneous groups of individuals. Given this array of possible outcomes, at the end of the day subtyping research may offer some direction to the field regarding Lilienfeld's (1994) troubling question: "What is psychopathy?" (p. 28).

ACKNOWLEDGMENT

Preparation of this chapter was supported in part by Grant No. R01 MH63783-01A1 (Personality Features in Social Deviancy) from the National Institute of Mental Health.

NOTES

1. Throughout this chapter, we use the term "subtype" to refer to primary, secondary, and other potential forms of psychopathy. Although this term suggests that these forms of psychopathy are discrete categories, we make no assumption that this is the case. As noted later, forms of psychopathy may be construed as subtypes or variants, depending on whether the construct is dimensional or taxonic.

2. Although three-factor (Cooke & Michie, 2001) and four-factor (Hare, 2003) models have recently been proposed, overwhelmingly the research to date has employed the two-factor conceptualization.

3. Although Karpman (1948a) labeled this as absent, versus disturbed, "conscience" in primary and secondary psychopaths, respectively, the essence of his discussion focuses on emotional capacities.

4. "[P]aradoxical as it may seem, the true [primary] psychopath is in a sense the least impulsive of them all. . . . Rather than being hasty, the psychopath often coolly and deliberately plans his actions . . . there is no hotheadedness here at all of the type we are accustomed to seeing in neurotics and psychotics" (Karpman, 1948b, pp. 527–528).

5. Blackburn's operationalization of psychopathy overlaps (but is not synonymous) with the PCL-R operationalization. Only roughly 50% of SHAPS-classified primary psychopaths exceed the PCL-R threshold for a diagnosis of psychopathy, compared with roughly 15% of SHAPS-classified secondary psychopaths and 8% of SHAPS-classified nonpsychopaths (Blackburn, 1999). In contrast with many theoretical conceptualizations of secondary psychopathy, then, Blackburn's (1999) secondary psychopathy may share few phenotypical characteristics with primary psychopathy. Nevertheless, he contends that "Cleckley psychopaths [can] be divided according to high and low trait anxiety . . . whatever the appropriate term, this is a clinically distinct and deviant group which seems to be prevalent among offenders" (p. 95).

6. However, even if psychopathy subtypes were found to be differentiable on psychophysio-

logical and laboratory measures of these mechanisms, it would be premature to draw inferences about etiology, given that the heritability of such laboratory response measures is unclear (Skeem, Poythress, et al., 2003).

7. Implications are not restricted to investigating primary and secondary psychopathy. For example, Lykken (1995) described an attractive, charming, "charismatic psychopath," who was particularly adept at conning and manipulating others. This variant of psychopathy would be expected to have substantially higher *interpersonal* features of psychopathy than other groups.

8. Somewhat analogous two-factor structures have been identified in Levenson's Self-Report Psychopathy Scale (LSRP; Levenson, et al., 1995) and Lilienfeld and Andrews's (1996) Psychopathic Personality Inventory (PPI; see Benning, Patrick, Hicks, Blonigen & Krueger, 2003).

9. Recently proposed three-factor (Cooke & Michie, 2001; Skeem, Mulvey, & Grisso, 2003) and 4-facet (Hare, 2003) structures for the PCL-R may permit a more differentiated examination of patterns of psychopathic features; in these models, traditional Factor 1 affective and interpersonal features are divided into separate factors or facets). Studies reporting the differential correlates of the three-factor model are just beginning to appear in the literature (Hall, Benning, & Patrick, 2004).

10. Millon and Davis's other variants are: risk-taking, spineless, explosive, abrasive, tyrannical, disingenuous, and malignant.

11. Total scores had to be 27.5 or higher, which is within 1 standard error of measurement of the traditionally recommended score of 30 for "diagnosing" psychopathy.

12. However, that absolute level of PCL-R elevation for subjects in the Alterman et al. (1998) study was lower than that of Hervé et al. (2000). Thus, sample differences may explain this finding.

13. As noted previously, these investigators found that entering PCL-R factor scores separately as clustering variables did not help discriminate subgroups; therefore they added F1 and F2 scores to form a single index based on 17 items.

14. The mean 17-item PCL-R scores for Types 1, 2, and 5 were 20.7, 23.1, and 20.4, respectively. Prorated to 20 items, these mean scores are 24.4, 27.2, and 24.0.

15. Investigators seeking to identify subtypes within a psychodynamic framework (e.g., Meloy, 1988; Millon & Davis, 1998) might propose radically different indicators than those suggested here to supplement psychopathy factor scores as clustering variables, or different criterion variables to validate emergent clusters.

16. Because of the positive correlation between F1 and F2 (usually about .5), and cooperative suppression effects between these factors, partial correlations have proven especially useful in revealing the unique associations of PCL-R factors with external correlates (e.g., Patrick, 1994; Verona et al., 2001). See Fowles and Dindo, Chapter 2, this volume.

17. The chief advantage of model-based clustering, compared to conventional cluster-analytic methods, is that it employs a statistical, goodness-of-fit criterion for deciding among alternative cluster solutions. See Banfield and Raftery (1993).

18. Scores were scaled to T scores (mean = 50, $SD = 10$) based on data for the MPQ normative sample (1,350 community residents).

19. In comparison to a control group of prisoners (PCL-R Total ≤ 20), significant differences were observed on only 1 of 11 MPQ traits (lower Stress Reaction) for the Emotionally Stable group, whereas significant differences were found on 10 of 11 MPQ traits (all except Absorption) for the Aggressive group. Thus, in comparison to both the MPQ normative sample and nonpsychopathic inmates, the Emotionally Stable group appears to present a more convincing "mask of sanity" with respect to general personality features.

20. The interested reader is referred to similar work in this area by Reise and colleagues (Reise & Oliver, 1994; Reise & Wink, 1995), who have used expert sortings of the California Q-Set to develop a psychopathy prototype.

21. Even the Psychopathy Checklist: Screening Version (PCL:SV; Hart, Cox, & Hare, 1995), designed for use with nonoffender samples, requires collateral information that may not regularly be available for many community samples.

REFERENCES

Alterman, A. I., McDermott, P. A., Cacciola, J. S., Boardman, C. R., McKay, J. R., & Cook, T. G. (1998). A typology of antisociality in methadone patients. *Journal of Abnormal Psychology, 107,* 412–422.

Andershed, H., Kerr, M., Stattin, H., & Levander, S. (2002). Psychopathic traits in non-referred youths: Initial test of a new assessment tool. In E. Blaauw & L. Sheridan (Eds.), *Psychopaths: Current interna-*

tional perspectives (pp. 131–158). The Hague, The Netherlands: Elsevier.

Andersen, H. Sestoft, D., Lillebaek, T., Mortensen, E. L., & Kramp, P. (1999). Psychopathy and psychopathological profiles in prisoners on remand. *Acta Psychiatrica Scandinavica, 99,* 33–39.

Banfield, J. D., & Raftery, A. E. (1993). Model-based Gaussian and non-Gaussian clustering. *Biometrics, 49,* 803–821.

Banks, A. S., & Phillip, G. (1965). Grouping political systems: Q-Factor analysis of "A Cross-Polity Survey." *American Behavioral Scientist, 9,* 3–6.

Baron, R., & Kenny, D. (1986). The moderator–mediator variable distinction in social psychological research: Conceptual, strategic, and statistical considerations. *Journal of Personality and Social Psychology, 51,* 1173–1182.

Belmore, M. F., & Quinsey, V. (1994). Correlates of psychopathy in a noninstitutional sample. *Journal of Interpersonal Violence, 9,* 339–349.

Benjamin, L. (1974). Structural analysis of social behavior. *Psychological Review, 81,* 392–425.

Benning, S. D., Patrick, C. J., Hicks, B. M., Blonigen, D. M., & Krueger, R. F. (2003). Factor structure of the Psychopathic Personality Inventory: Validity and Implications for clinical assessment. *Psychological Assessment, 15,* 340–350.

Blackburn, R. (1968). Personality in relation to extreme aggression in psychiatric offenders. *British Journal of Psychiatry, 114,* 821–828.

Blackburn, R. (1971). Personality types among abnormal homicides. *British Journal of Criminology, 11,* 14–31.

Blackburn, R. (1975). An empirical classification of psychopathic personality. *British Journal of Psychiatry, 127,* 456–460.

Blackburn, R. (1982). *The special hospitals assessment of personality and socialisation (SHAPS).* Unpublished manuscript, University of Liverpool.

Blackburn, R. (1985). Psychological approaches to problems of aggression and violence. In E. Karas (Ed.), *Current issues in clinical psychology* (Vol. 2, pp. 239–250). New York: Plenum Press.

Blackburn, R. (1996). Psychopathy and personality disorder: implications of interpersonal theory. *Issues in Criminological and Legal Psychology, 24,* 18–23.

Blackburn, R. (1998). Psychopathy and the contribution of personality to violence. In T. Millon, E. Simonsen, M. Birket-Smith, & R. D. Davis (Eds.), *Psychopathy: Antisocial, criminal, and violent behavior* (pp. 50–67). New York: Guilford Press.

Blackburn, R. (1999). Personality assessment in violent offenders: The development of the Antisocial Personality Questionnaire. *Psychologica Belgica, 39,* 87–111.

Blackburn, R., & Coid, J. (1999). Empirical clusters of DSM-III personality disorders in violent offenders. *Journal of Personality Disorders, 13,* 18–34.

Blackburn, R., Renwick, S. J. D., Donnelly, J. P., & Logan C. (2004). Big Five or Big Two? Superordinate

factors in the NEO Five Factor Inventory and the Antisocial Personality Questionnaire. *Personality and Individual Differences, 37,* 957–970.

Blonigen, D. M., Carlson, S. R., Krueger, R. F., & Patrick, C. J. (2003). A twin study of self-reported psychopathic personality traits. *Personality and Individual Differences, 35,* 179–197.

Bohn, M., Carbonell, J., & Megargee, E. (1995). The applicability and utility of the MMPI-based offender classification system in a correctional mental health unit. *Criminal Behaviour and Mental Health, 5,* 14–33.

Brinkley, C. A., Newman, J. P., Widiger, T. A., & Lynam, D. R. (2004). Two approaches to parsing the heterogeneity of psychopathy. *Clinical Psychology: Science and Practice, 11,* 69–94.

Carver, C. S., & White, T. L. (1994). Behavioral inhibition, behavioral activation, and affective responses to impending reward and punishment: The BIS/BAS scales. *Journal of Personality and Social Psychology, 67,* 319–333.

Christian, R. E., Frick, P. J., Hill, N. L., Tyler, L., & Frazer, D. R. (1997). Psychopathy and conduct problems in children: II. Implications for subtyping children with conduct problems. *Journal of the American Academy of Child and Adolescent Psychiatry, 36,* 233–241.

Christianson, S., Forth, A. E., Hare, R. D., Strachan, C., Lidberg, L., & Thorell, L. (1996). Remembering details of emotional events: A comparison between psychopathic and non-psychopathic offenders. *Personality and Individual Differences, 20,* 437–443.

Cleckley, H. (1964). *The mask of sanity* (2nd ed.). St. Louis, MO: Mosby.

Cleckley, H. (1976). *The mask of sanity.* St. Louis, MO: Mosby. (Original work published 1941)

Cooke, D. J., & Michie, C. (2001). Refining the construct of psychopathy: Towards a hierarchical model. *Psychological Assessment, 13,* 171–188.

Cornell, D. G., Warren, J., Hawk, G., Stafford, E., Oram, G., & Pine, D. (1996). Psychopathy in instrumental and reactive violent offenders. *Journal of Consulting and Clinical Psychology, 64,* 783–790.

Costa, P. T., & McCrae, R. R. (1992). *Revised NEO Personality Inventory and Neo Five Factor professional manual.* Odessa, FL: Psychological Assessment Resources.

Dodge, K. A. (1993). Social-cognitive mechanisms in the development of conduct disorder and depression. *Annual Review of Psychology, 44,* 559–584.

Douglas, K., Lilienfeld, S. O., & Poythress, N. G. (2004, March). Psychopathy and suicide. In N. G. Poythress (Chair), *Contemporary issues in psychopathy research.* Symposium presented at the biennial conference of the American Psychology–Law Society, Scottsdale, AZ.

Eysenck H., & Eysenck, S. (1976). *Psychoticism as a dimension of personality.* London: Hodder & Stoughton.

Fagan, T., & Lira, F. (1980). The primary and secondary

sociopathic personality: Differences in frequency and severity of antisocial behaviors. *Journal of Abnormal Psychology, 89,* 493–496.

Foa, E. B., Hearst-Ikeda, D. E., & Perry, K. J. (1995). Evaluation of a brief cognitive-behavioral program for the prevention of chronic PTSD in recent assault victims. *Journal of Consulting and Clinical Psychology, 63,* 948–955.

Fowles, D. (1980). The three arousal model: Implications for Gray's two-factor learning theory for heart rate, electrodermal activity, and psychopathy. *Psychophysiology, 17,* 87–104.

Fowles, D., & Missel, K. (1994). Electrodermal hyporeactivity, motivation, and psychopathy: Theoretical issues. In D. Fowles, P. Sutker, & S. Goodman (Eds.), *Special focus on psychopathy and antisocial personality disorder: A developmental perspective* (pp. 263–283). New York: Springer.

Frick, P. J., Lilienfeld, S. O., Edens, J. F., Poythress, N. G., & McBurnett, K. (2000). The association between anxiety and antisocial behavior. *Primary Psychiatry, 7,* 52–57.

Goldman, H., Lindner, L., Dinitz, S., & Allen, H. (1971). The simple sociopath: Physiologic and sociologic characteristics. *Biological Psychiatry, 3,* 77–83.

Gottman, J. M. (2001). Crime, hostility, wife battering, and the heart: On the Meehan et al. (2001) failure to replicate the Gottman et al. (1995) typology. *Journal of Family Psychology, 15*(3), 409–414.

Gray, J. (1987). *The psychology of fear and stress* (2nd ed.). Cambridge, UK: Cambridge University Press.

Gray, J., & McNaughton, N. (1996). The neuropsychology of anxiety: reprise. In D. Hope & C. Izard (Eds.), *Nebraska symposium on motivation, 1995: Perspectives on anxiety, panic, and fear* (pp. 61–134). Lincoln: University of Nebraska Press.

Hall, J. R., Benning, S. D., & Patrick, C. J. (2004). Criterion-related validity of the three-factor model of psychopathy: Personality, behavioral, and adaptive functioning. *Assessment, 11,* 4–16.

Hare, R. D. (1991). *The Hare Psychopathy Checklist—Revised.* Toronto, ON, Canada: Multi-Health Systems.

Hare, R. D. (1993). *Without conscience: the disturbing world of the psychopaths among us.* New York: Pocket Books.

Hare, R. D. (2003). *The Hare Psychopathy Checklist—Revised* (2nd ed.). Toronto, ON, Canada: Multi-Health Systems.

Harpur, T. J., Hare, R. D., & Hakstian, A. R. (1989). Two-factor conceptualization of psychopathy: Construct validity and assessment implications. *Psychological Assessment, 1,* 6–17.

Harris, G. T., Rice, M. E., & Quinsey, V. L. (1994). Psychopathy as a taxon: Evidence that psychopaths are a discrete class. *Journal of Consulting and Clinical Psychology, 62,* 387–397.

Hart, S. D., Cox, D. N., & Hare, R. D. (1995). The *Hare PCL:SV: Psychopathy Checklist Screening Version.* Toronto, ON, Canada: Multi-Health Systems.

Hart, S., & Dempster, R. (1997). Impulsivity and psychopathy. In C. Webster & M. Jackson (Eds.), *Impulsivity: Theory, assessment and treatment* (pp. 212–232). New York: Guilford Press.

Hart, S. D., & Hare, R. D. (1989). Discriminant validity of the Psychopathy Checklist in a forensic psychiatric population. *Psychological Assessment, 1,* 211–218.

Hervé, H. F., & Hare, R. D. (2002, March). *Criminal psychopathy and its subtypes: Reliability and generalizability.* Paper presented at the biennial conference of the American Psychology–Law Society, Austin, TX.

Hervé, H. F., & Hare, R. D. (2004, March). *Psychopathic subtypes and their crimes: A validation study.* Paper presented at the annual conference of the American Psychology–Law Society, Scottsdale, AZ.

Hervé, H. F., Ling, J. Y. H., & Hare, R. D. (2000, March). *Criminal psychopathy and its subtypes.* Paper presented at the biennial conference of the American Psychology–Law Society, New Orleans, LA.

Hicks, B. M., Markon, K. E., Patrick, C. J., & Krueger, R. F. (2004). Identifying psychopathy subtypes based on personality structure. *Psychological Assessment, 16,* 276–288.

Kallman, F. J. (1938). *The genetics of schizophrenia.* New York: Locust Valley.

Karpman, B. (1941). On the need for separating psychopathy into two distinct clinical types: Symptomatic and idiopathic. *Journal of Criminology and Psychopathology, 3,* 112–137.

Karpman, B. (1946). Psychopathy in the scheme of human typology. *Journal of Nervous and Mental Disease, 103,* 276–288.

Karpman, B. (1948a). Conscience in the psychopath: Another version. *American Journal of Orthopsychiatry, 18,* 455–491.

Karpman, B. (1948b). The myth of the psychopathic personality. *American Journal of Psychiatry, 104,* 523–534.

Karpman, B. (1955). Criminal psychodynamics: A platform. *Archives of Criminal Psychodynamics, 1,* 3–100.

Kosson, D., & Newman, J. (1995). An evaluation of Mealey's hypotheses based on Psychopathy Checklist—Identified groups. *Behavioral and Brain Sciences, 18,* 562–563.

Kosson, D., Smith, S., & Newman, J. (1990). Evaluating the construct validity of psychopathy in Black and White male inmates: Three preliminary studies. *Journal of Abnormal Psychology, 99,* 250–259.

Krueger, R. F., Hicks, B. M., Patrick, C. J., Carlson, S. R., Iacono, W. G., & McGue, M. (2002). Etiologic connections among substance dependence, antisocial behavior, and personality: Modeling the externalizing spectrum. *Journal of Abnormal Psychology, 111,* 411–424.

Levenson, M. R., Kiehl, K. A., & Fitzpatrick, C. M. (1995). Assessing psychopathic attributes in a noninstitutionalized population. *Journal of Personality and Social Psychology, 68,* 151–158.

Lewis, C. (1991). Neurochemical mechanisms of chronic antisocial behavior (psychopathy). *Journal of Nervous and Mental Disease, 179,* 720–727.

Lilienfeld, S. O. (1994). Conceptual problems in the assessment of psychopathy. *Clinical Psychology Review, 14,* 17–38.

Lilienfeld, S. O., & Andrews, B. P. (1996). Development and preliminary validation of a self-report measure of psychopathic personality traits in non-criminal populations. *Journal of Personality Assessment, 66,* 488–524.

Linehan, M. M. (1993). *Cognitive behavioral treatment of borderline personality disorder.* New York: Guilford Press

Lykken, D. (1957). A study of anxiety in the sociopathic personality. *Journal of Abnormal Psychology, 55,* 6–10.

Lykken, D. (1995). *The antisocial personalities.* Hillsdale, NJ: Erlbaum.

Lynam, D. R. (2002). Psychopathy from the perspective of the five-factor model of personality. In P. T. Costa & T. A. Widiger (Eds.), *Personality disorders and the five-factor model of personality* (2nd ed., pp. 325–350). Washington, DC: American Psychological Association.

Lynam, D. R., Whiteside, S., & Jones, S. (1999). Self-reported psychopathy: A validation study. *Journal of Personality Assessment, 73,* 110–132.

Marcus, D. K., Edens, J. F., & Lilienfeld, S. O. (2004, March). Is psychopathy a taxon? In N. G. Poythress (Chair), *Contemporary issues in psychopathy research* Symposium presented at the biennial conference of the American Psychology–Law Society, Scottsdale, AZ.

Marcus, D. K., John, S. L., & Edens, J. F. (2004). A taxometric analysis of psychopathic personality. *Journal of Abnormal Psychology, 113,* 626–635.

Mayer, J., Salovey, P., & Caruso, D. (2000). Models of emotional intelligence. In R. J. Sternberg (Ed.), *Handbook of intelligence* (pp. 396–420). New York: Cambridge University Press.

McCrae, R. R., & Costa, P. T. (1990). *Personality in adulthood.* New York: Guilford Press.

McCrae, R. R., & Costa, P. T. (2003). *Personality in adulthood* (2nd ed.). New York: Guilford Press.

McHoskey, J., Worzel, W., & Szyarto, C. (1998). Machiavellianism and psychopathy. *Journal of Personality and Social Psychology, 74,* 192–210.

Meloy, J. R. (1988). *The psychopathic mind: Origins, dynamics, and treatment.* Northvale, NJ: Jason Aronson.

Meloy, J. R., & Gacono, C. (1992). A psychotic (sexual) psychopath: "I just had a violent thought . . . ". *Journal of Personality Assessment, 58,* 480–493.

Meloy, J., & Gacono, C. (1993). A borderline psychopath: "I was basically maladjusted . . . " *Journal of Personality Assessment, 58,* 358–373.

Miller, D. J., Lynam, D. R., Widiger, T. A., & Leukefeld, C. (2001). Personality disorders as extreme variants of common personality dimensions: Can the five-factor model adequately represent psychopathy? *Journal of Personality, 69,* 253–276.

Millon, T., & Davis, R. D. (1998). Ten subtypes of psychopathy. In T. Millon, E. Simonsen, M. Birket-Smith, & R. D. Davis (Eds.), *Psychopathy: Antisocial criminal, and violent behavior* (pp. 161–170). New York: Guilford Press.

Morrison, D., & Gilbert, P. (2001). Social rank, shame and anger in primary and secondary psychopaths. *Journal of Forensic Psychiatry, 12,* 330–356.

Murphy, C., & Vess, J. (2003). Subtypes of psychopathy: Proposed differences between narcissistic, borderline, sadistic, and antisocial psychopaths. *Psychiatric Quarterly, 74,* 11–29.

O'Carroll, P. W., Berman, A. L., Maris, R. W., Moscicki, E. K., Tanney, B. L., & Silverman M. M. (1996). Beyond the Tower of Babel: A nomenclature for suicidology. *Suicide and Life-Threatening Behavior, 26,* 237–252.

Patrick, C. J. (1994). Emotion and psychopathy: Startling new insights. *Psychophysiology, 31,* 319–330.

Patrick, C. J, Bradley, M., & Lang, P. (1993). Emotion in the criminal psychopath: Startle reflex modulation. *Journal of Abnormal Psychology, 102,* 82–92.

Patrick, C. J., Curtin, J. J., & Tellegen, A. (2002). Development and validation of a brief form of the Multidimensional Personality Questionnaire. *Psychological Assessment, 14,* 150–163.

Patrick, C. J, Zempolich, K., & Levenston, G. (1997). Emotionality and violent behavior in psychopaths: A biosocial analysis. In A. Raine (Ed.), *Biosocial bases of violence* (pp. 145–161). New York: Plenum Press.

Patterson, M. C., & Newman, J. P. (1993). Reflectivity and learning from aversive events: Toward a psychological mechanism for the syndromes of disinhibition. *Psychological Review, 100,* 716–736.

Plomin, R., Ashbury, K., & Dunn, J. (2001). Why are children in the same family so different? Nonshared environment a decade later. *Canadian Journal of Psychiatry in Review, 46,* 225–233.

Porter, S. (1996). Without conscience or without active conscience? The etiology of psychopathy revisited. *Aggression and Violent Behavior, 1,* 179–189.

Raine, A. (1986). Psychopathy, schizoid personality and borderline/schizotypal personality disorders. *Personality and Individual Differences, 13,* 717–721.

Raine, A. (1988). Psychopathy: A single or dual concept? *Personality and Individual Differences, 9,* 825–827.

Raine, A. (1992). Schizotypal and borderline features in psychopathic criminals. *Personality and Individual Differences, 13,* 717–722.

Reise, S. P., & Oliver, C. J. (1994). Development of a California Q-set indicator of primary psychopathy. *Journal of Personality Assessment, 62,* 130–144.

Reise, S. P., & Wink, P. (1995). Psychological implications of the Psychopathy Q-sort. *Journal of Personality Assessment, 65,* 300–312.

Rutherford, M., Alterman, A., Cacciola, J., & McKay, J. (1997). Validity of the Psychopathy Checklist—Revised in male methadone patients. *Drug and Alcohol Dependence, 44,* 143–149.

Salekin, R. T., Rogers, R., & Sewell, K. W. (1997). Construct validity of psychopathy in a female offender sample: A multitrait–multimethod evaluation. *Journal of Abnormal Psychology, 106,* 576–585.

Schmitt, W., & Newman, J. (1999). Are all psychopathic individuals low-anxious? *Journal of Abnormal Psychology, 108,* 353–358.

Shine, J., & Hobson, J. (1997). Construct validity of the Hare Psychopathy Checklist, Revised on a UK prison population. *Journal of Forensic Psychiatry, 8,* 546–561.

Skeem, J., Mulvey, E., Appelbaum, A., Banks, S., Grisso, T., Silver, E., & Robbins, P. (2004). Identifying subtypes of civil psychiatric patients at high risk for violence. *Criminal Justice and Behavior, 31,* 392–437.

Skeem, J. L., Mulvey, E. P., & Grisso, T. (2003). Applicability of traditional and revised models of psychopathy to the Psychopathy Checklist:Screening Version. *Psychological Assessment, 15,* 41–55.

Skeem, J., & Poythress, N. (2004, March). Porter's secondary psychopath. In N. Poythress (Chair), *Contemporary issues in psychopathy research.* Symposium at the American Psychology–Law Society's Annual Conference, Scottsdale, AZ.

Skeem, J. L., Poythress, N. G., Edens, J. F., Lilienfeld, S. O., & Cale, E. M. (2003). Psychopathic personality or personalities? Exploring potential variants of psychopathy and their implications for risk assessment. *Aggression and Violent Behavior, 8,* 513–546.

Stafford, E., & Cornell, D. G. (2003). Psychopathy scores predict adolescent inpatient aggression. *Assessment, 10,* 102–112.

Toch, H., & Adams, K. (1994). *The disturbed violent offender* (2nd ed.). Washington, DC: American Psychological Association.

Torrubia, R., Avila, C., Molto, J., & Caseras, X. (2001). The Sensitivity to Punishment and Sensitivity to Reward Questionnaire (SPSRQ) as a measure of Gray's anxiety and impulsivity dimensions. *Personality and Individual Differences, 31,* 837–862.

Van Voorhis, P. (1994). *Psychological classification of the adult male prison inmate.* New York: State University of New York Press.

Verona, E., Patrick, C. J., & Joiner, T. E. (2001). Psychopathy, antisocial personality, and suicide risk. *Journal of Abnormal Psychology, 110,* 462–470.

Waller, N. G., Putnam, F. W., & Carlson, E. B. (1996). Types of dissociation and dissociative types: A taxometric analysis of dissociative experiences. *Psychological Methods, 1,* 300–321.

Waller, N. G., & Ross, C. A. (1997). The prevalence and biometric structure of pathological dissociation in the general population: Taxometric and behavior genetic findings. *Journal of Abnormal Psychology, 106,* 499–510.

Watson, D. (2003). Investigating the construct validity of the dissociative taxon: Stability analyses of normal and pathological dissociation. *Journal of Abnormal Psychology, 112,* 298–305.

Widiger, T. A., & Lynam, D. R. (1998). Psychopathy and the five-factor model of personality. In T. Millon, E. Simonsen, M. Birket-Smith, & R. Davis (Eds.), *Psychopathy: Antisocial, criminal, and violent behavior* (pp. 171–187). New York: Guilford Press.

Widom, C. (1977). A methodology for studying noninstitutionalized psychopaths. *Journal of Consulting and Clinical Psychology, 45,* 674–683.

Williamson, S., Hare, R. D., & Wong, S. (1987). Violence: criminal psychopaths and their victims. *Canadian Journal of Behavioral Science, 19,* 454–462.

Williamson, S., Harpur, T., & Hare, R. (1991). Abnormal processing of affective words by psychopaths. *Psychophysiology, 28,* 260–273.

Wink, P. (1991). Two faces of narcissism. *Journal of Personality and Social Psychology, 61,* 590–597.

10

Perspectives on the Conceptualization of Psychopathy

Toward an Integration

ROBERT F. KRUEGER

The purpose of this chapter is to outline some potential new possibilities for the conceptualization of psychopathy, with an eye toward integrating various perspectives presented in this section of the *Handbook of Psychopathy*. In particular, I suggest that an integrative perspective is a tractable and desirable goal in psychopathy research, and I emphasize the utility of integrating the results from various statistical approaches in striving toward an optimal, empirically based model of psychopathy. A first step in this endeavor is to summarize the ways in which psychopathy is currently conceptualized, as reflected in the other contributions to this section of the *Handbook of Psychopathy*.

CONCEPTUALIZING PSYCHOPATHY: A DIVERSITY OF APPROACHES

The excellent collection of other chapters in this section of the *Handbook of Psychopathy* provides an unusually rich snapshot of current thinking about the nature of psychopathy and its assessment. Widiger (Chapter 8, this volume) tackles the issue of psychopathy as it intersects with psychopathological con-

structs in the current DSM-IV (American Psychiatric Association, 1994) nomenclature. The conceptualization of psychopathy that emerges is multifaceted, in the sense that Widiger views psychopathy—especially the construct identified by the Psychopathy Checklist—Revised (PCL-R; Hare, 1991, 2003)—as intersecting with multiple DSM-IV constructs (e.g., both antisocial and narcissistic personality disorders), rather than mapping on to a specific DSM-IV construct in a 1:1 fashion. Widiger calls for a "dismantling" of psychopathy, in an attempt to identify which features are contributing to particular aspects of the validity of psychopathy. The conceptualization that emerges is one in which psychopathy may be better understood as a configuration of multiple personality traits and specific behavioral tendencies, as opposed to a unitary categorical entity. Also of note is Widiger's call for a better understanding of psychopathy in nonforensic settings, a call compatible with the conceptualization of psychopathy in personality trait terms. A potentially provocative implication of this perspective could be that the "whole" of psychopathy might consist of little more than the individual predictive validities of its constituent parts. For example,

Widiger implies that some of the utility of the psychopathy construct in predicting criminal behavior might be traced to ways in which PCL-R ratings rely on criminal behavior.

Lynam and Derefinko's (Chapter 7, this volume) conceptualization of psychopathy is also in terms of personality traits; indeed, they write that "psychopathy *is* personality" (emphasis theirs). In particular, these authors assert that structural models of dimensional personality traits provide a useful conceptual framework for understanding psychopathic personality. Moreover, these authors point out how major structural models of personality define a common higher-order factor space and differ primarily on how they parse that space. When this approach is taken, the psychopath is primarily characterized as "interpersonally antagonistic" and as having "trouble controlling his impulses" and endorsing "nontraditional values and standards"—that is, a blend of low agreeableness and low conscientiousness (using the terms associated with these factors in the five-factor model of personality [FFM]; McCrae & Costa, 1990). Allowing for some differences in the details, this personality profile also results from the translation of specific PCL-R items into the facet-level language of the FFM, and from expert descriptions of psychopathy using the FFM facets and Q-sort ratings.

Interestingly, as these authors note, some cardinal features of "primary" psychopathy (such as a lack of anticipatory anxiety; Lykken, 1995) are not well captured by low agreeableness and low conscientiousness and have complex relations with other domains within models of the higher-order structure of personality, such as the FFM. For example, the combination of low "self-consciousness" and high "angry hostility" entails having distinct facets of the higher-order domain of neuroticism scored in different directions, such that a summary profile of the psychopath in terms of the broader neuroticism domain could be misleading (see Lynam & Derefinko, Chapter 7, this volume, Table 7.3). Lynam and Derefinko echo Widiger's call for research on specific elements within psychopathy, and call for movement away from the idea that psychopathy is a single "coherent entity" associated with a single core deficit.

David Cooke and his colleagues have been pioneers in applying sophisticated modern psychometric methods to problems in the measurement and conceptualization of psychopathy. In their contribution to this volume, Cooke, Michie, and Hart (Chapter 5, this volume) review the conceptualization of psychopathy that has emerged from these efforts. Cooke and his colleagues focus on their three-factor model, consisting of factors they label Arrogant and Deceitful Interpersonal Style, Deficient Affective Experience, and Impulsive and Irresponsible Behavioral Style. In addition, they conceptualize antisocial and socially deviant behavior as a consequence of psychopathy, as opposed to a core symptom of psychopathy. Finally, they show how item response theory methods can point us toward further refinements in the conceptualization and measurement of psychopathy.

Poythress and Skeem (Chapter 9) tackle the challenging area of psychopathy subtypes. They provide a review of existing work on subtyping psychopathy, which tends to converge on a distinction between primary and secondary psychopathy, with the former linked more to deficiencies in the experience of anxiety and the latter linked more to impulsivity and negative affect. In addition, they review various decisions and strategies that are inherent in the subtyping effort. They describe empirical research in this area as lagging behind theoretical thinking regarding psychopathy subtypes. Accordingly, their chapter emphasizes the importance of pulling together various approaches under a more unified framework, a topic we return to later.

Lilienfeld and Fowler (Chapter 6, this volume) focus on assessment of psychopathy by self-report. They note that self-reports of personality disorder constructs such as psychopathy have a variety of conceptual strengths and weaknesses, but, nevertheless, some of the putative weaknesses of self-report psychopathy assessment have been overstated or misunderstood. Answers to self-report items need not be veridical to have construct validity (e.g., a psychopath's propensity for self-aggrandizement could lead to factually inaccurate but psychologically telling descriptions of the self). Moreover, self-report psychopathy indices are negatively correlated with social desirability, suggesting that psychopaths have little compunction about reporting on their socially unacceptable traits.

BRINGING CONCEPTUALIZATIONS TOGETHER: EXTERNALIZING, NEUROTICISM, AND PSYCHOPATHY

One thing that seems particularly striking about the chapters in this section of the *Handbook of Psychopathy* is their relative diversity. Some of this diversity can be traced to the distinct foci of different chapters (e.g., subtyping vs. self-report assessment), but even keeping this in mind, it is very challenging to provide a succinct answer to the question, "What is psychopathy?" based on the diversity of approaches and views represented by the leaders in the field. Can we work toward integrating these approaches and views?

Working toward integrating these approaches and views could provide a useful organizing framework for psychopathy research and also help in linking psychopathy research with other areas of inquiry in personality and psychopathology. For example, various conceptual models in psychopathy research likely have distinct signatures in relevant data. Identifying the optimal model for aspects of a domain such as psychopathy thereby offers a compelling way to link conceptual ideas with empirical data. To take one prominent issue as an example, if some aspects of psychopathy form a discrete latent class in nature (or a "taxon"), qualitatively distinct from normality, this situation should have a specific "signature" in pertinent data (cf. Harris, Rice, & Quinsey, 1994; Skilling, Harris, Rice, & Quinsey, 2002; Skilling, Quinsey, & Craig, 2001). The key is to identify this signature, as well as the signatures of other situations that might occur in nature (e.g., psychopathy is a configuration of personality traits that blend imperceptibly into normality), and then to determine which model provides a better account of the data.

The challenge inherent in attempting to integrate various perspectives involves placing different conceptualizations and their associated models on a level playing field, so they can be compared in a direct fashion. Along these lines, the state of psychopathy research is not unlike the state of other areas of psychopathology research in the sense that a number of sophisticated models have been fit to pertinent data, but integrating the results from different studies is a challenge because it is not always clear how to directly compare the results generated by fitting different models. To name a few prominent models in order to provide specific examples, psychopathy data have been fit by factor-analytic models (e.g., Cooke & Michie, 2001), by taxometric models (e.g., Harris et al., 1994; Skilling et al., 2001, 2002), by mixture models (e.g., Hicks, Markon, Patrick, Krueger, & Newman, 2004), by cluster analysis (e.g., unpublished work by Hervé and colleagues, as described by Poythress & Skeem, Chapter 9, this volume), and by item response theory models (which can be conceptualized as one-dimensional factor models for categorical observed variables; see, e.g., Cooke & Michie, 1997).

Each of these models can be informative by itself. For example, recognizing the existence of subfactors of the PCL-R has been influential and useful in informing the search for neurophysiological systems undergirding psychopathy (Patrick, in press). Nevertheless, by fitting each model individually, deeper conceptual issues at the intersection of the models remain unresolved. Specifically, a collection of results from each of these approaches still leaves open the question of which of the various models embodied in these approaches is the most optimal model for conceptualizing the phenomena associated with the psychopathy construct. As described by Poythress and Skeem (Chapter 9, this volume), "an investigator could find discrete groups or continuous dimensions, based solely on the technique applied" (p. 186). Similarly, one could add that various investigators could arrive at various conceptualizations depending on their particular vantage point, embodied, for example, in how they assess psychopathic qualities and the sorts of models they consider for their data. This situation seems to calls for viewing research on psychopathy from a broad perspective.

The Externalizing Spectrum vis-à-vis Psychopathy

Rather than being focused on a specific clinical disorder, such as psychopathy, much of my own research has been aimed at understanding broader factors that might be help-ful in understanding patterns of comorbidity among common forms of adult psychopath-ology, as described in official nosological sys-tems such as the ICD and DSM (for a recent review, see Krueger & Tackett, 2003). One consistent finding from this program of re-search is that antisocial behavior disorders such as conduct disorder and antisocial per-sonality disorder, substance dependence, and personality characteristics related to impul-sivity and aggression are sufficiently interre-lated that they can be conceptualized as elements within a coherent "externalizing spectrum" of personality and psychopathol-ogy. Of particular importance, the spectrum shows coherence at an etiological level, as the aforementioned disorders and traits form a unitary genetic factor in multivariate be-havioral genetic research published by multi-ple research groups, including our own (see Kendler, Prescott, Myers, & Neale, 2003; Krueger et al., 2002; Young, Stallings, Cor-ley, Krauter, & Hewitt, 2000). In the popula-tion at large, the etiology of externalizing disorders and traits appears mostly genetic, and mostly in common. This suggests that psychopathology research might focus most profitably on what these disorders and traits have in common, rather than studying these disorders and traits in relative isolation, a common but potentially misleading strategy.

Nevertheless, it is also important to em-phasize the role of the environment in the externalizing spectrum, as the unified genetic etiological contributions to the externalizing spectrum are importantly shaped by the en-vironment. Environmental forces play a key role in shaping the underlying genetic risk both by differentiating among externalizing phenomena and determining the severity of expression (see e.g., Krueger et al., 2002), as well as by constraining or enhancing genetic variation in the population (a form of gene × environment interaction). For example, Dick, Rose, Viken, Kaprio, and Koskenvuo (2001) found that socioregional environ-ment moderated the extent of genetic var-iation in alcohol use. Similarly, specific environmental factors (e.g., childhood mal-treatment) appear to interact with genotype in the prediction of antisocial behavior (Caspi et al., 2002).

The externalizing spectrum is broader than psychopathy per se. Nevertheless, the spectrum does appear to be related to psy-chopathy as defined by the PCL-R. Externalizing phenomena are correlated with PCL-R scores, in particular, the antiso-cial behavior factor of the PCL-R (using the classical two-factor PCL-R model; see Pat-rick, Hicks, Krueger, & Lang, 2005; Smith & Newman, 1990). Thus, PCL-R defined psychopathy is linked with the externalizing spectrum, both conceptually and empirically. In particular, the antisocial behavior features of psychopathy appear to be manifestations or indicators of a broad but coherent domain of human individual differences. This per-spective is somewhat different from other perspectives on the relationship between psy-chopathy and antisocial behavior. From this perspective, antisocial behavior is not a con-sequence of core psychopathy traits. It is also not a symptom of psychopathy. Rather, it is an indicator of a different (externalizing) do-main that intersects with psychopathy as de-fined by the PCL-R.

This connection is important because psy-chopathy research per se has mostly been con-fined to forensic settings. Widiger (Chapter 8, this volume) states this situation succinctly: "Psychopathy, particularly as assessed with the PCL-R, has established itself as an impor-tant clinical construct, especially within fo-rensic, prison settings" (p. 167). The connec-tion between the externalizing spectrum and psychopathy helps to connect psychopathy re-search with broader issues in the classification of psychopathology, with individual differ-ences in the population at large, and with re-search on the genetic and environmental bases of psychopathology. In sum, the antisocial behavior aspects of psychopathy research may be well conceived as elements within the externalizing spectrum.

Psychopathy, Externalizing, and the Vexing Role of Neuroticism

One perpetually vexing issue in psychopathy research pertains to "the rest" of psychopa-thy, i.e., the aspects of psychopathy beyond impulsive-antisocial deviance. Complex is-sues related to these phenomena arise in vari-ous forms in each of the chapters in this sec-tion of the *Handbook*. For example, Cooke and colleagues (Chapter 5, this volume) re-gard antisocial behavior as a "consequence" of psychopathy, not a core part of the syndrome. Another key example arises in Chapter 7 by Lynam and Derefinko. As they write, "Despite not being explicitly assessed by the PCL-R, low anxiety, a facet of N [neuroticism], is considered by some a cardinal characteristic of psychopathy (Lykken, 1995) (p. 142)." Of course, Lykken's (1995) account was not novel, as he drew on the classical description of psychopathy provided by Cleckley (1941/1976), which included "absence of 'nervousness' " as a core feature.

In spite of the putative role of low anxiety in psychopathy, the account of psychopathy from the FFM perspective is of the psychopath as disagreeable (−A) and unconscientious (−C), with neuroticism (N) showing inconsistent associations with psychopathy. The association of the psychopathy construct embodied by the PCL-R with two putatively separate domains of the FFM (−A and −C) may at first seem somewhat surprising, in the sense that the domains of the FFM are often conceptualized as entirely independent (orthogonal). Nevertheless, it is important to keep in mind that the domains of the FFM are often arrived at via orthogonal rotation of factors, such that the factors are forced to be independent. When correlations between A and C are freely estimated, these domains do appear to be nontrivially correlated (see meta-analytic analyses of the relevant literature provided by Digman, 1997, and Markon, Krueger, & Watson, 2005). Indeed, the other personality trait models considered by Lynam and Derefinko (Eysenck's Psychoticism–Extraversion–Neuroticism [PEN] model and Tellegen's three-factor model of the Multidimensional Personality Questionnaire) model the correlation between disagreeableness and unconsciousness via higher order constructs of psychoticism and the lack of constraint, respectively.

Markon and colleagues (2005) integrate these observations in a joint hierarchical model of normal and abnormal personality in which the FFM domains lie at a lower level of the personality hierarchy than the big three domains. In the Markon and colleagues model, the construct combining low agreeableness and low conscientiousness is labeled "disinhibition." Table 7.3 (Lynam & Derefinko, Chapter 7, this volume) is informative in terms of linking disinhibition and PCL-R defined psychopathy. Note that in Table 7.3, Factor 1 of the PCL-R is linked primarily to a lack of agreeableness in the FFM, and Factor 2 of the PCL-R is linked primarily to a lack of conscientiousness. Inasmuch as Factors 1 (−A) and 2 (−C) are correlated, and PCL-R defined psychopathy is what Factors 1 and 2 have in common, PCL-R defined psychopathy aligns well with the higher-order construct of disinhibition (i.e., the confluence of −A and −C.

Indeed, this vector at the juncture of −A and −C appears to be at the core of the externalizing spectrum. Consider, for example, the joint factor analysis of personality scales from the Multidimensional Personality Questionnaire (MPQ; Tellegen, 1985) and criminal behavior presented in Krueger (2002). In this analysis, criminal behavior per se and the trait of aggression marked the higher end of a dimension that was anchored on the lower end by traditionalism, harm avoidance, social closeness, and control over one's impulses. This dimension can be conceptualized as the main vector linking phenomena in the externalizing spectrum; that is, disinhibition appears to be the source of the spectrum's phenotypical and genetic coherence, and, in FFM terms, the vector intermediate between −C and −A.

But What about Neuroticism?

Returning to the role of neuroticism (N) in psychopathy, in every structural model of personality considered by Lynam and Derefinko, a tendency to be worried, anxious, and on edge is located in a different part of the factor space from the part of the space pertaining to externalizing (i.e., unconscientious and disagreeable tendencies). Moreover, the PCL-R does not assess this dimension explicitly. Consider Cooke and colleagues' (Chapter 5, this volume) three-factor model of PCL-R psychopathy. Although Deficient Affective Experience is considered a core aspect of the syndrome, the PCL-R items that tap this pertain to −A (e.g., callous/lack of empathy) rather than −N (which is not measured directly by the PCL-R). So how can we resolve the role of low anxiety (-N) in psychopathy?

The answer may lie in assessing low anxiety explicitly in the context of assessing psychopathic personality traits and examining the nature of the resulting joint factor space. For example, the Psychopathic Personality

Inventory (PPI; Lilienfeld & Andrews, 1996) contains scales that capture both the externalizing and low anxiety aspects of the psychopathy construct. When the scales of the PPI are factor-analyzed, two major higher-order factors result, one marked primarily by "stress immunity," the other marked primarily by "Machiavellian egocentricity" (a tendency to be aggressive and self-centered—i.e., disagreeable) and "Impulsive nonconformity" (unconscientiousness).

These two factors also appear to be uncorrelated (Benning, Patrick, Hicks, Blonigen, & Krueger, 2003). This may seem a surprising finding, given that the PPI is intended to measure the putatively single domain of "psychopathy" (Lilienfeld & Fowler, Chapter 6, this volume). Nevertheless, it makes sense in the context of structural models of personality such as the FFM, and it makes sense in the context of the emerging view, running throughout the contributions in this section of the handbook, that psychopathy is not a "single entity" but, rather, that the phenomena captured by the idea of "psychopathy" are aspects of personality. As noted earlier, in the FFM, the domain pertaining to low anxiety (a lack of neuroticism) is separate from the domains pertaining to externalizing tendencies (disagreeableness and a lack of conscientiousness). Thus, the factor structure of the PPI makes sense in the context of the factor structure of personality in general. That is, as posited in the FFM, individual differences in anxiety proneness (neuroticism) pertain to a different domain when contrasted with individual differences in disagreeableness and conscientiousness.

In short, all the characteristics historically associated with the construct of "psychopathy" cannot be accommodated within a single domain of human variation. As suggested by Widiger (Chapter 8, this volume), this situation calls for "dismantling" psychopathy. That is, it may be more accurate to conceptualize "psychopathy" as the psychopathological implications of personality traits that undergird various pathways to behavior described in the clinical literature as "psychopathic." Because these personality traits are located in different parts of the structure of personality, there is no single pathway to psychopathy, and, hence, it is unlikely that there is a single psychopathic deficit underlying a unitary "psychopathic syndrome" (cf. Lynam & Derefinko, Chapter 7, this volume). Hence, a unified perspective on psychopathy may actually be best achieved by recognizing multiple pathways to behavior historically labeled "psychopathic." As noted earlier, at least two separate processes can be identified by integrating various perspectives on psychopathy: a process involving deficient anxiety and a process involving aggressive impulsivity (cf. Fowles & Dindo, Chapter 2, this volume; Patrick, in press).

INTEGRATIVE QUANTITATIVE MODELING

Recognizing the possibility of distinct psychopathic processes helps in integrating various perspectives but leaves a parallel conceptual puzzle unanswered. As emphasized in particular in Chapter 9 (Poythress & Skeem), this puzzle pertains to the issue of how psychopathic processes are distributed. Are these processes distributed as continuous dimensions of variation, or do they give rise to discrete psychopathic categories? Some novel methodological perspectives on this issue have developed in the course of our work on the externalizing spectrum.

The externalizing spectrum is conceptualized in dimensional terms, in the sense that disorders within the spectrum are viewed as blending into each other, as well as into more "normal" realms of human variation, in a graded, continuous fashion. Nevertheless, this conceptualization remains a hypothesis until it encounters empirical data. The challenge, then, is to determine how to map this hypothesis, as well as rival hypotheses, onto the same data. For example, a relevant rival hypothesis could be that disorders within the spectrum constitute relatively distinct classes of psychopathology that cannot be meaningfully linked by a unifying continuum of variation.

We recently undertook research designed to compare these conceptualizations directly (Krueger, Markon, Patrick, & Iacono, in press). Specifically, we were interested in patterns of comorbidity among DSM-defined externalizing syndromes assessed in adults—that is, conduct disorder (CD), adult antisocial behavior (AAB), alcohol dependence (AD), marijuana dependence (MD), and drug dependence (DD). These disorders were assessed via in-person interviews with adult parents of adolescent twins who participated in the Minnesota Twin-Family Study (N = 2,835). Because the study began before the publication of DSM-IV (American Psychiatric Association, 1994), the diagnoses were made using DSM-III-R (American Psychiatric Association, 1987) criteria. AAB comprised criterion C (adult) symptoms of antisocial personality disorder (APD); the threshold for the diagnosis was four symptoms, consistent with criterion C of the APD diagnosis in DSM-III-R. That is, we separated APD into its two constituent parts (CD and AAB) for the purposes of this analysis.

With these data in hand, we sought to evaluate the fit of distinct models of patterns of comorbidity among the five externalizing diagnoses. Were the data more compatible with a model in which the diagnoses were conceptualized as elements along a continuum of variation, or were the data better fit by a model in which the diagnoses were conceptualized as forming distinct latent classes? The initial challenge in this research, therefore, was to identify relevant statistical models that map onto these conceptual models, and to figure out how to compare these models in a direct fashion.

One way to approach this issue is via taxometric methods (see, e.g., Waller & Meehl, 1998). However, taxometric methods have a notable shortcoming in that they do not directly parameterize the model that constitutes the alternative to the taxonic hypothesis. That is, if the taxonic hypothesis is rejected, one is left without an explicit, quantitative model of the latent structure of the domain. This serves to illustrate a point raised earlier: By fitting specific models individually, deeper conceptual issues at the intersection of various models remain unresolved.

We therefore sought to identify statistical models that map onto different conceptualizations of the comorbidity among externalizing disorders, and to determine how to compare the fit of those models in a direct fashion. The model that maps onto the hypothesis of continuity can be termed a "latent trait model" (LTM; see Heinen, 1996). Models under the LTM rubric are often called item response theory (IRT), but we prefer to use LTM because (1) the models are

not limited to analysis of item responses and (2) "theory" is typically used to refer to conceptual ideas about a domain, as opposed to the statistical formalisms that seem to us better captured by the term "model."

The latent trait model can be contrasted with the latent class model (LCM), which represents the alternative to the continuity hypothesis. The difference between the models can be understood as follows: in the LCM, elements within a domain (in this case, DSM-defined mental disorders in the externalizing spectrum) are understood as indicators of membership in a series of discrete and mutually exclusive groups. For example, it could be the case that persons with AD are an entirely separate group from persons with AAB, such that the diagnoses cannot be meaningfully arrayed along a dimension. In contrast, in a unidimensional LTM, elements within a domain are understood as indicators of a single dimension of variation. For example, it could be the case that persons with AAB are likely to have AD, in a probabilistic sense. If this were the case, then it should be possible to array AAB and AD along a dimension encompassing tendencies toward externalizing behavior, such that AAB represents a more "severe" manifestation of those tendencies than AD.

We fit a series of both LCMs and LTMs to our data: LCMs positing two to five distinct classes to explain the comorbidity among the externalizing disorders, discrete LTMs positing latent traits with two to five values, and an LTM positing a normal underlying latent distribution. Compared with the other models we fit, the model that provided the most optimal fit to the data was the LTM positing a normal underlying latent distribution. The clear implication is that the comorbidity among the various disorders within this spectrum can be understood as a function of an underlying, continuous "externalizing" disposition.

In addition, when we turned to interpret the parameter estimates from the best-fitting LTM, we found that the diagnoses were arrayed along the underlying externalizing continuum in a way that made conceptual sense. For example, AD was the least severe substance dependence diagnosis, followed by MD, with DD being the most severe. This makes sense if one thinks about the general externalizing tendency in terms of continuously increasing risk for continuously more abnormal or socially prohibited behaviors, with the more licit substances acting as a "gateway" to the more illicit substances. In addition, CD and AAB differed in their correlation with this underlying externalizing dimension, with variation in AAB being more closely linked to variation along the externalizing continuum (in the parlance of LTMs, AAB was more discriminating than CD). This also makes sense, as the etiology of CD is complex, with some cases representing developmentally limited expressions of antisocial behavior (Moffitt, 1993). As revealed by the LTM, CD is not as indicative of the extent of adult externalizing problems, when compared with AAB, which is more indicative of overall externalizing problems in adulthood.

Because the approach we employed in this research is embedded in a general latent variable modeling framework, it can also be extended in a number of directions in future research. For example, the approach is directly amenable to modeling distributions other than the normal distribution; in addition to fitting a normal distribution LTM, one could also fit a model positing a specific nonnormal distribution (e.g., the Poisson). Along these same lines, the discrete LTM is essentially an exploratory model of the distribution of the latent trait. That is, with a sufficient number of latent trait values freely estimated, one is using the data to empirically approximate the distribution of the latent trait. This opens up a number of new possibilities for conceptualizing the processes underlying psychopathology. For example, those processes could be continuous but non-normally distributed, and this possibility can be evaluated empirically in a latent variable modeling framework.

This work is relevant to psychopathy research per se for a number of specific reasons. Inasmuch as the externalizing spectrum appears to be continuous in nature when it is modeled using DSM-defined diagnoses, this work suggests that the antisocial variant of psychopathy is likely continuous as well. This issue has also been approached using taxometric methods, although the picture emerging from taxometric studies is unclear, with some studies presenting evidence of the continuity of psychopathy using taxometrics, and others presenting evidence for dis-

continuity in this domain on the basis of taxometric analyses (see Poythress & Skeem, Chapter 9, this volume). In addition, the approaches we employed in modeling the externalizing spectrum could be employed in modeling psychopathy data per se. Related approaches (IRT) have been ably employed by Cooke and his colleagues in modeling PCL-R data and refining our understanding of that instrument. Nevertheless, without fitting both LCMs and LTMs (IRT models) to the data, one cannot directly evaluate the empirical evidence for discontinuous versus continuous conceptualizations of a domain. This is not a criticism of Cooke and colleagues' work, which has been groundbreaking in terms of increasing the level of psychometric sophistication in psychopathy research. Rather, it is a suggestion regarding some potential new directions made possible by pairing an integrative perspective on statistical modeling with a recognition that various perspectives on psychopathy might be integrated by recognizing that psychopathy is not a single thing.

For example, it is not entirely clear what one might predict regarding the discrete versus continuous nature of the low anxiety variant of psychopathy, a variant distinct from the antisocial variant (indeed, uncorrelated when psychopathy is assessed by the PPI, and conceptually uncorrelated when viewed in the context of, for example, the FFM, as described earlier). Trait anxiety, and the higher-order domain of human variation in which it is embedded (neuroticism or negative emotionality), is likely a continuous domain. Nevertheless, the psychopathological implications of low anxiety might themselves be discontinuous, resulting in a discontinuity, or perhaps non-normality, in the latent distribution of the confluence of deficient anxiety and its psychopathological implications. One might therefore speculate that pure "primary psychopathy," characterized by an essential absence of anxiety, could constitute a relatively distinct group of persons because the impact of declining anxiety on social behavior accelerates as anxiety declines. Put differently, it is one thing to be relatively less anxious than most people but perhaps quite another thing to be entirely lacking in the capacity for appropriate anxious arousal. Thus, one could imagine a nonlinear regression of trait anxiety on the tendency to violate societal norms, such that the conjunction of a basic lack of anxiety with norm violation represents a rather distinct group of persons. Or, it may be that the combination of low anxiety and norm violation is best modeled by a non-normal latent distribution. The point is that these possibilities are not unreasonable, and they can be evaluated empirically via new developments in latent variable modeling.

CONCLUSIONS

The development and application of more integrative approaches to modeling data should be helpful in furthering our understanding of psychopathy, in particular if such work is paired with recognition of the multiple psychopathological processes that appear to be linked to the concept of "psychopathy." In addition to the integrative potential provided by developments in statistical modeling, many authors in this section of the *Handbook* note that an integrative perspective will require a broad approach to assessing psychopathy in multiple populations.

The psychopathy literature has been very fortunate to have a reliable and valid measure of its core construct for going on 25 years in the form of the PCL and its various versions, extensions, and adaptations (Hare, 1980, 1991, 2003). Nevertheless, no single instrument can be expected to fulfill all the assessment needs of an area of research. As Cooke and colleagues (Chapter 5, this volume) note, "after almost two decades of use, it is perhaps time to stand back and consider what has been learned about the limitations of the PCL-R as a psychological test. In doing so, we can start to develop new measures of psychopathy, thereby avoiding the dangers inherent in mono-operation bias" (pp. 92–93). One could also add that many ideas about psychopathy cannot be readily evaluated in forensic settings. For example, the distribution of psychopathic personality processes cannot be readily evaluated in forensic settings, owing to the complex factors that lead to incarceration and that render incarcerated samples unrepresentative of the population at large. Broader sampling could provide important new insights into the details of psychopathic phenomena. For example, Cooke et al. note that impulsive and irresponsible behavioral style items of the PCL-R are more diagnostic at lower levels of PCL-R psychopathy, whereas arrogant and deceitful interpersonal style items are more diagnostic at the higher end. In theory, this arrangement could be linked to the ways in which these indicators function in a prison population, where impulsivity and irresponsibility are relatively common, and might not function in this manner in the population at large. Such a possibility can be evaluated only by sampling from a broader, nonforensic population.

A broad perspective on psychopathy is needed, as has been called for throughout this section of the *Handbook*. Novel assessment and novel sampling from nonforensic populations, combined with novel statistical modeling, have the potential to result in a more integrated perspective on psychopathy.

REFERENCES

American Psychiatric Association. (1987). *Diagnostic and statistical manual of mental disorders* (3rd ed., rev). Washington, DC: Author.

American Psychiatric Association. (1994). *Diagnostic and statistical manual of mental disorders* (4th ed.). Washington, DC: Author.

Benning, S. D., Patrick, C. J., Hicks, B. M., Blonigen, D. M., & Krueger, R. F. (2003). Factor structure of the psychopathic personality inventory: Validity and implications for clinical assessment. *Psychological Assessment, 15,* 340–350.

Caspi, A., McClay, J., Moffitt, T. E., Mill, J., Martin, J., Craig, I. W., et al. (2002). Role of genotype in the cycle of violence in maltreated children. *Science, 297,* 851.

Cleckley, H. (1941/1976). *The mask of sanity.* St. Louis, MO: Mosby. (Original work published 1941)

Cooke, D. J., & Michie, C. (1997). An Item Response Theory evaluation of Hare's Psychopathy Checklist. *Psychological Assessment, 9,* 2–13.

Cooke, D. J., & Michie, C. (2001). Refining the construct of psychopathy: Towards a hierarchical model. *Psychological Assessment, 13,* 171–188.

Dick, D. M., Rose, R. J., Viken, R. J., Kaprio, J., & Koskenvuo, M. (2001). Exploring gene-environment interactions: Socioregional moderation of alcohol use. *Journal of Abnormal Psychology, 110,* 625–632.

Digman, J. M. (1997). Higher-order factors of the Big Five. *Journal of Personality and Social Psychology, 73,* 1246–1256.

Hare, R. D. (1980). A research scale for the assessment of psychopathy in criminal populations. *Personality and Individual Differences, 1,* 111–119.

Hare, R. D. (1991). *Manual for the Hare Psychopathy Checklist—Revised* (1st ed.). Toronto, ON, Canada: Multi-Health Systems.

Hare, R. D. (2003). *Manual for the Hare Psychopathy Checklist—Revised* (2nd ed.). Toronto, ON, Canada: Multi-Health Systems.

Harris, G. T., Rice, M. E., & Quinsey, V. L. (1994). Psychopathy as a taxon: Evidence that psychopaths are a discrete class. *Journal of Consulting and Clinical Psychology, 62,* 387–397.

Heinen, T. (1996). *Latent class and discrete latent trait models: Similarities and differences.* Thousand Oaks, CA: Sage.

Hicks, B. M., Markon, K. E., Patrick, C. J., Krueger, R. F., & Newman, J. (2004). Identifying psychopathy subtypes based on personality structure. *Psychological Assessment, 16,* 276–288.

Kendler, K. S., Prescott, C. A., Myers, J., & Neale, M. C. (2003). The structure of genetic and environmental risk factors for common psychiatric and substance use disorders in men and women. *Archives of General Psychiatry, 60,* 929–937.

Krueger, R. F. (2002). Personality from a realist's perspective: Personality traits, criminal behaviors, and the externalizing spectrum. *Journal of Research in Personality, 36,* 564–572.

Krueger, R. F., Hicks, B. M., Patrick, C. J., Carlson, S. R., Iacono, W. G., & McGue, M. (2002). Etiologic connections among substance dependence, antisocial behavior, and personality: Modeling the externalizing spectrum. *Journal of Abnormal Psychology, 111,* 411–424.

Krueger, R. F., Markon, K. E., Patrick, C. J., & Iacono, W. G. (in press). Externalizing psychopathology in adulthood: A dimensional-spectrum conceptualization and its implications for DSM-V. *Journal of Abnormal Psychology.*

Krueger, R. F., & Tackett, J. L. (2003). Personality and psychopathology: Working toward the bigger picture. *Journal of Personality Disorders, 17,* 109–128.

Lilienfeld, S. O., & Andrews, B. P. (1996). Development and preliminary validation of a self report measure of psychopathic personality traits in noncriminal populations. *Journal of Personality Assessment, 66,* 488–524.

Lykken, D. T. (1995). *The antisocial personalities.* Hillsdale, NJ: Erlbaum.

Markon, K. E., Krueger, R. F., & Watson, D. (2005). Delineating the structure of normal and abnormal personality: An integrative hierarchical approach. *Journal of Personality and Social Psychology, 88,* 139–157.

McCrae, R. R., & Costa, P. T. (1990). *Personality in adulthood.* New York: Guilford Press.

Moffitt, T. E. (1993). Adolescent-limited and life-course-persistent antisocial behavior: A developmental taxonomy. *Psychological Review, 100,* 674–701.

Patrick, C. J. (in press). Getting to the heart of psychopathy. In H. Herve & J. C. Yuille (Eds.), *Psychopathy: Theory, research, and social implications.* Hillsdale, NJ: Erlbaum.

Patrick, C. J., Hicks, B. M., Krueger, R. F., & Lang, A. R. (2005). Relations between psychopathy facets and externalizing in a criminal offender sample. *Journal of Personality Disorders, 19,* 339–356.

Skilling, T. A., Harris, G. T., Rice, M. E., & Quinsey, V. L. (2002). Identifying persistently antisocial offenders using the Hare psychopathy checklist and DSM antisocial personality disorder criteria. *Psychological Assessment, 14,* 27–38.

Skilling, T. A., Quinsey, V. L., & Craig, W. M. (2001). Serious antisocial behavior in boys: Evidence of an underlying taxon. *Criminal Justice and Behavior, 28,* 450–470.

Smith, S. S., & Newman, J. P. (1990). Alcohol and drug abuse–dependence disorders in psychopathic and nonpsychopathic criminal offenders. *Journal of Abnormal Psychology, 99,* 430–439.

Tellegen, A. (1985). Structure of mood and personality and their relevance to assessing anxiety, with an emphasis on self-report. In A. H. Tuma & J. D. Maser (Eds.), *Anxiety and the anxiety disorders* (pp. 681–706). Hillsdale, NJ: Erlbaum.

Waller, N. G., & Meehl, P. E. (1998). *Multivariate taxometric procedures: Distinguishing types from continua.* Thousand Oaks, CA: Sage.

Young, S. E., Stallings, M. C., Corley, R. P., Krauter, K. S., & Hewitt, J. K. (2000). Genetic and environmental influences on behavioral disinhibition. *American Journal of Medical Genetics (Neuropsychiatric Genetics), 96,* 684–695.

III

ETIOLOGICAL MECHANISMS

11

Genetic and Environmental Influences on Psychopathy and Antisocial Behavior

IRWIN D. WALDMAN
SOO HYUN RHEE

There are many research approaches to illuminating and understanding the etiology of disorders or traits, such as psychopathy and antisocial behavior. Behavior genetic designs have the advantage of disentangling genetic and environmental influences, the effects of nature and nurture, and characterizing their relative magnitudes as an important first step in explaining etiology, to be followed by the search for specific candidate genes and environmental risk factors. Although it is not possible to disentangle genetic from environmental influences in family studies because these are confounded in nuclear families, twin and adoption studies have the unique ability to disentangle genetic and environmental influences and to estimate the magnitude of both simultaneously. In this chapter, we summarize the literature on genetic and environmental influences on psychopathy and antisocial behavior. After a brief review of important concepts and methods underlying behavior genetic designs, we present the results of a recent meta-analysis of twin and adoption studies of antisocial behavior (Rhee & Waldman, 2002) followed by a summary of the small but burgeoning recent behavior genetic literature on psychopathy. We conclude with some future directions for research on the genetic and environmental influences underlying psychopathy and antisocial behavior. These include the selection of relevant candidate genes and environmental risk factors as specific etiological mechanisms and the use of endophenotypes to help find genes for psychopathy and antisocial behavior and explain the biopsychological mechanisms underlying their effects.

Although more than 100 twin and adoption studies of antisocial behavior have been published, it is difficult to draw clear conclusions regarding the magnitude of genetic and environmental influences on antisocial behavior given the current literature. The main reason for this difficulty is the considerable heterogeneity of the results in this area of research, with published estimates of heritability (i.e., the magnitude of genetic influences) ranging from very low (e.g., .00; Plomin, Foch, & Rowe, 1981) to very high (e.g., .71; Slutske et al., 1997). Various hypotheses have been proposed to explain this heterogeneity in results across studies, including differences in the age of the sample (e.g., Cloninger & Gottesman, 1987), the age of onset of antisocial behavior (e.g., Moffitt, 1993), and the measurement of antisocial behavior (e.g., Plomin, Nitz, & Rowe, 1990).

Given such hypotheses, we examined the possible moderating effects of three study characteristics (i.e., the operationalization of antisocial behavior, assessment method, and zygosity determination method) and two participant characteristics (i.e., the age and sex of the participants) on the magnitude of genetic and environmental influences on antisocial behavior. These study and participant characteristics were chosen because clarifying the moderating effects of these characteristics will improve our understanding of the etiology of antisocial behavior. Examining these moderators has the potential to clarify issues regarding the degree of heterogeneity in the etiology of antisocial behavior (i.e., examination of the operationalization of antisocial behavior, age of the participants, and sex of the participants), the development of antisocial behavior (i.e., examination of the age of the participants), and the effects of potential methodological confounders (i.e., examination of the assessment method and zygosity determination method) on the results. We conducted a meta-analysis of 51 twin and adoption studies in order to provide a clearer and more comprehensive picture of the magnitude of genetic and environmental influences on antisocial behavior, and to test several alternative hypotheses regarding moderating variables that may explain the heterogeneity in the magnitude of these influences on antisocial behavior.

THE META-ANALYSIS

Hypothesis 1: Operationalization as a Moderator

The operationalizations of antisocial behavior can be divided into three major categories (Plomin et al., 1990). First, antisocial behavior has been examined in terms of psychiatric diagnoses, such as antisocial personality disorder (APD) and conduct disorder (CD). Second, antisocial behavior has been operationalized in terms of the violation of legal or social norms (i.e., as criminality and delinquency). Third, antisocial behavior has been operationalized as aggressive behavior. In addition to these definitions, several researchers have examined an omnibus operationalization that includes both aggression and delinquency items, such as the externalizing scale from the Child Behavior Checklist (Achenbach & Edelbrock, 1983).

Past reviews have focused on only one operationalization (e.g., aggression in Miles & Carey, 1997) or reviewed the results of studies separately by operationalization (e.g., Plomin et al., 1990). Thus, we tested whether the magnitude of genetic and environmental influences on antisocial behavior varies with the operationalization of antisocial behavior.

As mentioned previously, studies that used *Diagnostic and Statistical Manual of Mental Disorders* (DSM; American Psychiatric Association, 1994) criteria to assess APD or CD were included in the "diagnosis" category of operationalization. It was not as clear whether studies examining psychopathy should also be included in this category, as some researchers emphasize the difference between the DSM criteria and the traditional concept of psychopathy, noting that the DSM criteria for APD focus on antisocial behavior whereas the traditional concept of psychopathy focuses on affective–interpersonal traits (e.g., Hare, Hart, & Harpur, 1991; Hare, 2003). Given evidence that psychopathy measures and DSM criteria are related (e.g., Cooney, Kadden, & Litt, 1990; Taylor, McGue, Iacono, & Lukken, 2000), psychopathy measures were included as an operationalization of diagnosis. Nonetheless, given the concern that psychopathy and APD are not synonymous (e.g., Hare et al., 1991), the meta-analysis was repeated after excluding studies examining psychopathy to assess the impact of such studies on the results. We also conducted a separate meta-analysis of behavior genetic studies of psychopathy alone for purposes of comparison. Table 11.1 presents the characteristics of these nine behavior genetic studies of psychopathy.

Hypothesis 2: Assessment Method as a Moderator

Antisocial behavior has been assessed via self-report, report by others (i.e., parent or teacher report), objective measures (i.e., aggression toward a Bobo doll; Plomin et al., 1981), official records of criminality, and reactions to aggressive material (e.g., whether or not one finds aggressive humor to be funny; Wilson, Rust, & Kasriel, 1977).

Several studies have shown that assessment method can influence the results of

TABLE 11.1. Effect Sizes for Twin and Adoption Studies of Psychopathy

Study	Measure	Zygosity determination	Age (mean)	Sex	N	Relationship	Effect size
Texas Adoption Study: Loehlin et al. (1987)	MMPI Pd	N/A	N/A	Both-m Both-fm	81 81	a-bf a-bm	.12 .07
Minnesota Twins Reared Apart Study: DiLalla et al. (1996)	MMPI Pd	Blood grouping	40.4 45.1	Both-both	66 54	MZ ra DZ ra	.62 .14
Minnesota Twin Study (1960s—high school sample): Gottesman (1963, as cited in Gottesman & Goldsmith, 1994)	MMPI Pd	Blood grouping	16.0	Both-both	34 34	MZ DZ	.57 .18
Boston Twin Study (adolescents): Gottesman (1965, as cited in Gottesman, 1994)	MMPI Pd	Blood grouping	16.0	Both-both	80 68	MZ DZ	.46 .25
National Merit Scholarship Twin Study: Loehlin & Nichols (1976)	CPI So	Questionnaire	18.0	m-m fm-fm	202 124 288 193	MZ DZ MZ DZ	.52 .15 .55 .48
Norwegian Twin Study (psychiatric sample): Torgersen et al. (1993)	SCID-II Unreliable Scale	Not reported	Not reported	Both-both	24 28	MZ DZ	.22 .20
Indiana Twin Study: Brandon and Rose (1995, personal communication)	MMPI Pd	Blood grouping/questionnaire	20.4	Both-both	289 228	MZ DZ	.48 .27
Minnesota Twin Registry: Blonigen et al. (2003)	PPI	Blood grouping/questionnaire	~38.5	m-m	89 47	MZ DZ	.46 −.26
Minnesota Twin Family Study: Taylor et al. (2003)	MTI	Blood grouping/questionnaire/ ponderal index/cephalic index/ fingerprint ridge count/	11.0 17.0	m-m m-m	128 58 142 70	MZ DZ MZ DZ	.42 .16 .40 .17
Minnesota Twin Family Study: Taylor et al. (2000)[a]	CPI So	Blood grouping/questionnaire/ ponderal index/cephalic index/ fingerprint ridge count/	17.0	m-m fm-fm	145 77 107 52	MZ DZ MZ DZ	.51 .29 .60 .38

Note. Information within the parentheses indicates whether the data were obtained from personal communication or another publication. m, male; fm, female; both, both male and female; a-bf, adoptee-biological father; a-bm, adoptee-biological mother; MZ, MZ twin pairs; DZ, DZ twin pairs; MZ ra, MZ twin pairs reared apart; DZ ra, DZ twin pairs reared apart; MMPI Pd, Minnesota Multiphasic Personality Inventory Psychopathic Deviate Scale; CPI So, California Psychological Inventory Socialization Scale; SCID-II, Structural Clinical Interview for DSM-III-R Personality Disorders; MTI, Minnesota Temperament Inventory (the average correlation for the Antisocial and Detachment scales is presented); PPI, Psychopathic Personality Inventory.
[a] Study not included in the meta-analysis given the overlap in twin sample with that in Taylor et al. (2003).

behavior genetic studies. McCartney, Harris, and Bernieri (1990) compared parent and self-reports of sociability and found that parent reports resulted in higher correlations than seif-reports in monozygotic (MZ) twins but resulted in lower correlations than self-reports in dizygotic (DZ) twins. They also found that for activity–impulsivity, parent reports resulted in higher correlations than self-reports in both MZ and DZ twins. In contrast, Miles and Carey (1997) found that behavior genetic studies of aggression using parent reports resulted in a lower heritability estimate when compared with those using self-reports.

Researchers studying temperament have found that parent reports tend to yield DZ correlations that are very low or even negative. This may be the result of parents exaggerating the differences between their DZ twins, which has been described as a rater contrast effect (Loehlin, 1992a). One example of such a finding emerged from the MacArthur Longitudinal Twin Study (Emde et al., 1992). No resemblance of DZ twins on measures of behavioral inhibition and shyness was found using parent reports, but significant DZ resemblance was found using observational measures of the same constructs. Plomin's (1981) review of twin studies examining personality concluded that objectively assessed behavior yielded lower heritabilities than self-reports and parent reports. Similarly, Miles and Carey's (1997) meta-analysis of behavior genetic studies of aggression concluded that two studies using an objective method found little evidence of genetic influences on aggression, in contrast to studies using self-report or parent report. We thus tested whether assessment method is a moderator of the magnitude of genetic and environmental influences on antisocial behavior.

Hypothesis 3: Zygosity Determination Method as a Moderator

We also tested whether zygosity determination method is a moderator of genetic and environmental influences on individual differences in antisocial behavior. Zygosity determination methods used in twin studies of antisocial behavior include blood grouping, questionnaires, and a combination of the two methods. The inaccuracy of blood

grouping in determining the zygosity of twin pairs is less than 1% (e.g., Smith & Penrose, 1955). Questionnaire methods of determining zygosity, which involve asking about the physical similarity of the twin pairs, have been found to agree highly with zygosity diagnosis by blood grouping and DNA markers. For example, Kasriel and Eaves (1976) found that if all twin pairs who agree that they were confused in childhood and are alike in appearance are determined to be MZ, only 3.9% of the sample would be diagnosed incorrectly, while Rietveld and colleagues (2000) found that agreement between zygosity determined by the questionnaire method and zygosity determined by DNA markers and blood typing was around 93%.

Although all zygosity determination methods used in behavior genetic studies of antisocial behavior have been shown to be valid, the estimates of the magnitude of genetic and environmental influences may be affected by the zygosity determination method. McCartney and colleagues (1990) predicted that studies that used blood grouping would have higher effect sizes for MZ twins and lower effect sizes for DZ twins because use of blood grouping in zygosity determination would purify the MZ and DZ samples. They found that studies using blood grouping did have higher effect sizes for MZ twins, but that the zygosity determination method did not moderate effect sizes for DZ twins. In the present review, studies using blood groupings, questionnaires, and a combination of the two methods (i.e., studies using the questionnaire method for the whole sample and the blood grouping method for a subset of the sample) were compared.

Hypothesis 4: Age as a Moderator

In the present meta-analysis, we used participants' age as a moderator, comparing results for children (below age 13), adolescents (ages 13–18), and adults (above age 18). Age was tested as a moderator of the magnitude of genetic and environmental influences on antisocial behavior for two reasons. First, in the behavior genetics literature, there is a general finding for a variety of traits that as age increases, the magnitude of genetic and nonshared environmental influences increases, whereas the magnitude of shared environmental influences decreases (Loehlin, 1992a; Plomin, 1986). One example of such a finding is Matheny's (1989) longitudinal study of temperament. Over 12 to 30 months of age, MZ twins became more concordant than DZ twins for age-to-age changes in temperament measures of emotional tone, fearfulness, and approach. In Miles and Carey's (1997) meta-analysis of behavior genetic studies examining aggression, the magnitude of shared environmental influences decreased and the magnitude of genetic influences increased from childhood to adulthood.

Second, age was examined because of the potential to test an interesting alternative hypothesis regarding the development of antisocial behavior. DiLalla and Gottesman (1989) and Moffitt (1993) have suggested that antisocial individuals can be divided into a smaller group whose antisocial behavior is persistent throughout the life course and influenced predominantly by genetic influences, and a larger group whose antisocial behavior is limited to adolescence and influenced predominantly by environmental influences. If their hypothesis is correct, the relative magnitude of genetic influences on antisocial behavior should be lower in adolescence than in childhood or adulthood.

Hypothesis 5: Sex as a Moderator

No matter how antisocial behavior is operationalized or assessed, it is more prevalent in males than females (e.g., Hyde, 1984; Wilson & Herrnstein, 1985). Given this sex difference in prevalence, it is important to consider whether the magnitude of genetic and environmental influences differs in males and females. Past literature reviews (e.g., Widom & Ames, 1988) have suggested that the magnitude of genetic and environmental influences on antisocial behavior is equal for the two sexes, whereas Miles and Carey (1997) found that the magnitude of genetic influences on aggression was slightly higher for males than for females.

Confounding among Moderators

Antisocial behavior is operationalized and assessed differently for children, adolescents, and adults (e.g., CD assessed via parent report in children versus APD assessed via self-report in adults). Also, certain operationalizations of antisocial behavior are most frequently or readily assessed using certain methods (e.g., criminality via official records). Therefore, age of the participants, operationalization, and assessment method may be highly correlated across studies of antisocial behavior. Such confounding among moderators can make the interpretation of results difficult in two ways. First, if two confounded moderators are both found to be significant, it is possible that the second moderator is significant only because it covaries with the first. Fortunately, this problem can be assessed in the present meta-analysis by testing the significance of a particular moderator after other moderators are controlled for statistically. Second, if one level of a moderator is completely confounded with a level of another moderator (e.g., all studies examining criminality being assessed by records) it is impossible to determine whether the results reflect the first or second moderator. Although we cannot resolve this problem in the present review, it can be addressed in future research by diversifying the pairings among operationalization, assessment method, and age (e.g., more studies of criminality using a variety of assessment methods, rather than official records alone). We conducted tests of moderators in the meta-analysis that address this confounding in order to provide a guide to fruitful directions for future behavior genetic studies of antisocial behavior.

Search Strategy

We began our search for twin and adoption studies of antisocial behavior by examining the PsycInfo and Medline databases. Appendix 11.1 shows the search terms used in this process. The references from the research studies and review papers found through this method were examined for any additional studies that might have been missed or published before the databases were established. Also, information about relevant unpublished manuscripts or manuscripts in press was obtained by examining pertinent review papers and the abstracts of the 1995, 1996, 1997, and 1998 Behavior Genetics Association meetings and searching the Dissertations Abstracts and ERIC databases. Authors of 14 manuscripts provided unpublished data; 4 of these manuscripts were published subsequently.

One hundred forty-one twin and adoption studies examining antisocial behavior were identified. After excluding unsuitable studies according to the criteria described later (i.e., construct validity, inability to calculate tetrachoric or intraclass correlations, and assessment of related disorders), 96 studies remained. After addressing the problem of nonindependence in these studies, 51 studies (i.e., 10 independent adoption samples and 42 independent twin samples, including two separate samples examined in Eley, Lichtenstein, & Stevenson, 1999) remained. Rhee and Waldman (2002) present the references for these studies.

Inclusion Criteria for Studies in the Meta-Analysis

Construct Validity

The validity of the measures used in the studies considered for the meta-analysis was an important issue in deciding whether to include or exclude a study. Only studies examining antisocial behavior were included, and those examining related constructs such as anger and hostility were excluded. A study was included if it was clearly evident that the study examined APD, CD, criminality, aggression, or antisocial behavior (an omnibus operationalization including both delinquency and aggression items). In addition, a study was included if there was empirical evidence that the measure of antisocial behavior used successfully discriminated between an antisocial group and a control group, or if the measure was significantly related to a more established operationalization of antisocial behavior. As stated previously, we also reanalyzed the data after excluding behavior genetic studies that examined psychopathy in order to ascertain the sensitivity of the results to the effect sizes from those studies.

Inability to Calculate Tetrachoric or Intraclass Correlations

The effect sizes used in this meta-analysis were the Pearson product–moment or intraclass correlations that were reported in the studies, or tetrachoric correlations estimated from the concordances or percentages reported in the studies. These effect sizes were analyzed using a model-fitting program (i.e., Mx; Neale, 1995) that estimates the magnitude of genetic and environmental influences. Studies were excluded if these effect sizes were not reported or if there was not enough information to calculate them.

Assessment of Related Disorders

In several studies, another variable related to antisocial behavior (e.g., alcoholism, somatization disorder, or other personality disorders) was studied in addition to antisocial behavior. For example, one adoption study (Schulsinger, 1972) examined the aggregate risk for psychopathy, criminality, alcoholism, drug abuse, or mental illness in adoptees of psychopathic biological parents and nonpsychopathic biological parents. This means that some adoptees who do not engage in antisocial behavior could have been counted as "affected" because of their problems with alcohol or drug abuse (i.e., variables outside the scope of this meta-analysis). Such studies were not included because the assessment of other disorders interfered with the assessment of antisocial behavior (e.g., alcoholism or drug abuse being counted as antisocial behavior).

Nonindependent Samples

In many studies considered for the present meta-analysis, data from the same sample were reported more than once. When authors published the same data in two different sources (e.g., Mednick, Gabrielli, & Hutchings, 1983, 1984), we only considered one of the studies for the meta-analysis. Other factors leading to nonindependent samples are more complicated. First, some authors of a single publication examined more than one dependent measure of antisocial behavior in their sample (e.g., Ghodsian-Carpey & Baker 1987). Second, several publications were a collection of follow-up data on the same sample (e.g., Cadoret, 1978; Cadoret, Troughton, O'Gorman, & Heywood, 1986). Third, several authors (in different publications) examined different dependent measures in the same sample (e.g., Grove et al., 1990; Tellegen et al., 1988). In model-fitting analyses, the sample size must be indicated. In cases in which the sample size was identical across the nonindependent samples, the average of the multiple effect sizes was used. If the sample size was not identical across the nonindependent samples, the effect size from the largest sample was used.

Determination of Effect Size

Some adoption and twin studies used a continuous variable to measure antisocial behavior and reported either Pearson product–moment or intraclass correlations. For these studies, the reported effect sizes were used. Other studies used a dichotomous variable to measure antisocial behavior and reported concordances, percentages, or a contingency table that included the number of twin pairs with both members affected, one member affected, and neither member affected. The information from the concordances or percentages was transformed into a contingency table, which was then used to estimate the tetrachoric correlation (i.e., the correlation between the latent continuous variables that are assumed to underlie the observed dichotomous variables). For these studies, the tetrachoric correlation was the effect size used in the meta-analysis.

Biometric Model-Fitting Analyses

In behavioral genetic analyses, alternative models containing different sets of causal influences are compared for their fit to the observed data (i.e., twin or familial correlations or covariances). These models posit that the etiology of antisocial behavior comprises different types of causal influences: additive genetic influences (A—genetic influences where alleles from different genetic loci are independent and "add up" to influence the liability for a trait), nonadditive genetic influences (D—genetic influences where alleles interact with each other to influence the liability for a trait, either at a single genetic locus or at difference loci), shared environmental influences (C—environmental influences that are experienced in common by family members that make them similar to one another), and nonshared environmental influences (E—environmental influences that are experienced uniquely by family members that make them different from one another). The magnitude of additive genetic influences,

nonadditive genetic influences, shared environmental influences, and nonshared environmental influences are represented by a^2, d^2, c^2, and e^2, respectively.

We included in the meta-analysis two types of adoption studies (1, parent–offspring studies comparing the correlation between adoptees and their adoptive parents and the correlation between adoptees and their biological parents; and 2, sibling adoption studies comparing the correlation between adoptive siblings and the correlation between biological siblings) and two types of twin studies (1, twin pairs reared together; and 2, twin pairs reared apart). The effect sizes from each study were entered in separate groups in the model-fitting program Mx (Neale, 1995). In the model-fitting program, the correlations between pairs of relatives are explained in terms of the components of variance that are shared between the relatives (A, C, or D). Nonshared environmental influences (i.e., E) do not explain any part of the correlation between relatives because, by definition, nonshared environmental influences are not shared between relatives. The correlation between different types of relatives is explained by different sets of influences and their appropriate weights, as shown in Appendix 11.2. These weights reflect the genetic or environmental similarity between pairs of relatives.

The analyses were performed in a series of steps. First, the analyses were conducted for all data appropriate for the meta-analysis, and five alternative models (the ACDE model, the ACE model, the AE model, the CE model, and the ADE model) were compared. The fit of each model was assessed using the χ^2 statistic and the Akaike Information Criterion (AIC), a fit index that reflects both the fit of the model as well as its parsimony (Loehlin, 1992b). Among competing models, that with the lowest AIC and the lowest χ^2 relative to its degrees of freedom is considered to be the best-fitting model.

It is not possible to estimate c^2 and d^2 simultaneously or to test an ACDE model with data only from twin pairs reared together because the estimation of c^2 and d^2 both rely on the same information (i.e., the difference between the MZ and DZ twin correlations). If certain other types of data, such as the correlations between adoptees and their adoptive and biological parents, also are included in the analyses, this additional source of information allows for the simultaneous estimation of c^2 and d^2, and the ACDE model can be tested. Therefore, it was only possible to test the ACDE model when analyzing all of the data included in the meta-analysis.

Second, we tested the moderating effects of operationalization (i.e., diagnoses, criminality, aggression, and antisocial behavior), assessment method (i.e., self-report, report by others, objective test, reaction to aggressive material, and records), zygosity determination method (i.e., blood typing, questionnaire, and a combination of the two), sex (i.e., male and female), and age (i.e., children, adolescents, and adults) by contrasting the fit of a model where the parameter estimates are constrained to be equal across levels of each moderator to the fit of a model where the parameter estimates are free to vary across levels of each moderator. If the fit of the two models is significantly different, this indicates the significance of the moderator. It is possible that a nonsignificant difference may be due to lack of power, especially if there is little variability in the levels of a moderator. It was not possible to test moderators within the context of the ACDE model because both twin and adoption studies were not always available across different types of studies representing different levels of a moderator.

Third, we tested whether operationalization, assessment method, and age each was a significant moderator after statistically controlling for the other moderators by testing whether estimating separate parameter estimates for studies at each level of *both* moderators resulted in a better fit than estimating separate parameter estimates for studies at each level of only one of the moderators. For example, when examining whether assessment method is a significant moderator after the effects of operationalization have been statistically controlled, two models are compared. In the first, less restrictive model, parameter estimates are allowed to vary across both the four operationalizations and the five assessment methods conjointly. This model is compared with a second, more restrictive model, in which parameter estimates are allowed to vary only across the four operationalizations. If the fit of the first model (i.e., with

both operationalization and assessment method as moderators) is significantly better than the fit of the second model (i.e., with only operationalization as a moderator), this indicates that assessment method is a significant moderator even after the effects of operationalization are statistically controlled.

META-ANALYSES OF ALL DATA

In this section, the number of "samples" refers to the number of independent studies in the analyses. The number of "groups" refers to the total number of independently analyzed units in the samples. For example, Slutske and colleagues (1997) and Torgersen, Skre, Onstad, Edvardsen, and Kringlen (1993) examined two independent samples, the Australian adult twins and the Norwegian twins. There are five groups (male–male MZ twin pairs, male–male DZ twin pairs, female–female MZ twin pairs, female–female DZ twin pairs, and male–female DZ twin pairs) in Slutske and colleagues, and two groups (MZ twin pairs and DZ twin pairs) in Torgersen and colleagues. Therefore, if data from Slutske and colleagues and Torgersen and colleagues are used in the analysis, it would comprise two samples and seven groups.

The results of analyses of the data from all the samples meeting the inclusion criteria (N = 52 samples; 149 groups; 55,525 pairs of participants) are presented in Table 11.2. As shown in the table, the full ACDE model fit best as compared with the other, more restrictive models. Excluding the studies that examined psychopathy did not alter the results, as parameter estimates did not differ after excluding these studies. We also present the meta-analytic results of psychopathy studies alone below.

Assessment of Potential Moderators

Table 11.3 shows the results of analyses examining operationalization, assessment method, zygosity determination method, sex, and age as moderators of the magnitude of genetic and environmental influences on antisocial behavior. The χ^2 difference between a model where the parameter estimates are constrained to be equal and a

TABLE 11.2. Standardized Parameter Estimates and Fit Statistics—Inclusion of All Data

	Parameter estimates				Fit statistics			
	a^2	c^2	e^2	d^2	χ^2	df	p	AIC
ACDE model	.32	.16	.43	.09	1394.46	146	< .001	1102.46
ACE model	.38	.18	.44	—	1420.38	147	< .001	1126.38
ADE model	.41	—	.42	.17	1590.58	147	< .001	1296.58
AE model	.55	—	.45	—	1707.89	148	< .001	1411.89
CE model	—	.45	.55	—	2364.90	148	< .001	2068.90
	Data from studies of psychopathy only							
ACE model	.49	.00	.51	—	45.77	19	< .001	7.77
ADE model	.40	—	.51	.09	45.16	19	< .001	7.16
AE model	.49	—	.51	—	45.77	20	< .001	5.77
CE model	—	.39	.61	—	116.17	20	< .001	76.17

TABLE 11.3. Standardized Parameter Estimates and Fit Statistics for the Best-Fitting Models: Test of Moderators

	Fit statistics			
	χ^2	df	p	AIC
Operationalization				
Parameters constrained to be equal	1406.50	139	< .001	1128.50
Parameters free to vary	1066.63	130	< .001	806.63
χ^2 difference test	339.87	9	< .001	321.87
Assessment method				
Parameters constrained to be equal	1361.73	139	< .001	1083.73
Parameters free to vary	530.47	128	< .001	274.47
χ^2 difference test	831.26	11	< .001	809.26
Zygosity determination method				
Parameters constrained to be equal	1305.79	110	< .001	1085.79
Parameters free to vary	945.65	104	< .001	737.65
χ^2 difference test	360.14	6	< .001	348.14
Age				
Parameters constrained to be equal	1351.30	133	< .001	1085.30
Parameters free to vary	1107.35	127	< .001	853.35
χ^2 difference test	243.95	6	< .001	231.95
Sex				
Parameters constrained to be equal	870.61	66	< .001	738.61
Parameters free to vary	869.07	63	< .001	743.07
χ^2 difference test	1.53	3	.68	–4.47

model where the parameter estimates are free to vary across the different levels of the moderator is shown for each moderator.

Operationalization

The χ^2 difference test was significant for operationalization, $\Delta\chi^2(9) = 339.87$, $p < .001$, indicating significant differences in the magnitude of genetic and environmental influences on diagnosis (14 samples; 40 groups; 11,681 pairs of participants), criminality (5 samples; 13 groups; 34,122 pairs of participants), aggression (14 samples; 40 groups; 4,408 pairs of participants), and antisocial behavior (15 samples; 48 groups; 4,365 pairs of participants). The ACE model was the best fitting model for diagnosis ($a^2 = .44$, $c^2 = .11$, $e^2 = .45$), aggression ($a^2 = .44$, $c^2 = .06$, $e^2 = .50$), and antisocial behavior ($a^2 = .47$, $c^2 = .22$, $e^2 = .31$), whereas the ADE model was the best-fitting model for criminality ($a^2 = .33$, $d^2 = .42$, $e^2 = .25$). Within the operationalization of diagnosis, significant differences were found between studies examining APD (8 samples; 17 groups; 5,019 pairs of participants) and CD (5 samples; 22 groups; 6560 pairs of participants). Although the magnitude of shared environmental influences (i.e., c^2) was similar, the heritability estimate (i.e., a^2) was higher in studies examining CD ($a^2 = .50$, $c^2 = .11$, $e^2 = .39$), whereas the magnitude of nonshared environmental influences (i.e., e^2) was higher in studies examining APD ($a^2 = .36$, $c^2 = .10$, $e^2 = .54$).

These results suggest that operationalization is a significant moderator of the magnitude of genetic and environmental influences on antisocial behavior, but the possible effects of confounding between operationalization and assessment method and between operationalization and age should be considered when interpreting these results. Parent report was more frequently used in studies examining antisocial behavior than in studies examining diagnosis or aggression, and there were more studies examining antisocial behavior in children and adolescents than in adults. Also, all the behavior genetic studies of criminality entailed the examination of adults using the assessment method of official records. The specific comparison between studies examining the diagnoses of APD and CD showed that the magnitude of genetic influences was higher for CD, whereas the magnitude of nonshared environmental influences was higher for APD. These results may be explained by age differences (APD being assessed in adulthood and CD being assessed in childhood) or differences in assessment method (self-report being used more often to assess APD and parent report being used more often to assess CD).

Assessment Method

The χ^2 difference test indicated that assessment method is a moderator of the magnitude of genetic and environmental influences on antisocial behavior, $\Delta\chi^2(11) = 831.26$, $p < .001$. Self-report (23 samples; 69 groups; 13,329 pairs of participants), report by others (14 samples; 51 groups; 6,851 pairs of participants), records (5 samples; 13 groups; 34,122 pairs of participants), reaction to stimuli (2 samples; 6 groups; 146 pairs of participants), and objective assessment (1 sample; 2 groups; 85 pairs of participants) were compared. The ACE model was the best fitting model for self-report ($a^2 = .39$, $c^2 = .06$, $e^2 = .55$) and report by others ($a^2 = .53$, $c^2 = .22$, $e^2 = .25$), whereas the AE model was the best fitting model for reaction to aggressive stimuli ($a^2 = .52$, $e^2 = .48$). All the studies using the assessment method of records were also studies examining criminality; hence, the ADE model was the best-fitting model ($a^2 = .33$, $d^2 = .42$, $e^2 = .25$). Model fitting could not be conducted for the assessment method of objective test because of lack of information (i.e., only one study used an objective test).

While our meta-analysis suggested that results vary across the different assessment methods, caution is recommended in interpreting these results, given that only one study (Plomin et al., 1981) used an objective test, and only two studies (Owen & Sines, 1970; Wilson et al., 1977) used reaction to aggressive material. Also, all the studies using the assessment method of records were studies examining the operationalization of criminality. When the assessment methods of self-report and report by others were compared, the magnitude of familial influences (a^2 and c^2) was higher for report by others than for self-report. These results differ slightly from the conclusions of Miles and Carey (1997), who found lower a^2 and higher c^2 estimates for parent reports than for self-reports of aggression. Again, the possibility of confounding between moderators should be considered. Studies using the assessment method of self-report were more likely to be those examining the operationalization of diagnosis in adults or adolescents, whereas studies using the assessment method of parent report were more likely to be those examining the operationalization of antisocial behavior in children.

Zygosity Determination Method

The χ^2 difference test also indicated that zygosity determination method is a significant moderator, as the magnitude of genetic and environmental influences differed significantly across studies using blood grouping (8 samples; 18 groups; 1,020 pairs of participants), a combination of blood grouping and the questionnaire method (15 samples; 55 groups; 27,631 pairs of participants), and the questionnaire method (11 samples; 39 groups; 8,249 pairs of participants), $\Delta\chi^2(6) = 360.14$, $p < .001$. The ADE model was the best-fitting model for studies using blood grouping ($a^2 = .14$, $d^2 = .33$, $e^2 = .53$), whereas the ACE model was the best-fitting model for studies using the questionnaire method ($a^2 = .43$, $c^2 = .27$, $e^2 = .30$) and a combination of the two methods ($a^2 = .39$, $c^2 = .11$, $e^2 = .50$). These parameter estimates are a bit difficult to interpret, however, given that studies using the most and least stringent methods of zygosity determination (i.e., blood grouping and questionnaire, respectively) yielded higher estimates of genetic influences than studies using a combination of the two methods.

Age

Age also was a significant moderator of the magnitude of genetic and environmental influences on antisocial behavior in children (15 samples; 54 groups; 7,807 pairs of participants), adolescents (11 samples; 31 groups; 2,868 pairs of participants), and adults (17 samples; 50 groups; 27,671 pairs of participants), $\Delta\chi^2(6) = 243.95$, $p < .001$.

The ACE model was the best-fitting model for children ($a^2 = .46$, $c^2 = .20$, $e^2 = .34$), adolescents ($a^2 = .43$, $c^2 = .16$, $e^2 = .41$), and adults ($a^2 = .41$, $c^2 = .09$, $e^2 = .50$). The magnitude of familial influences (a^2 and c^2) decreased with age, whereas the magnitude of nonfamilial influences (e^2) increased with age.

Although age was a significant moderator, these results should be interpreted with caution for three reasons. First, although many studies examined a wide age range, we had to use either the mean or the midpoint to represent this range, given that access to the raw data for each study was not possible. Second, age was simplified into a categorical variable (i.e., children, adolescents, and adults) in our meta-analysis, given the difficulties of including continuous moderators in model-fitting analyses. As age increased, the magnitude of familial influences (i.e., both a^2 and c^2) decreased. These findings for behavior genetic studies of antisocial behavior differ somewhat from the general finding in the behavior genetics literature (Loehlin, 1992a; Plomin, 1986) that a^2 and e^2 estimates increase and c^2 estimates decrease with increasing age. These findings also differ from Miles and Carey's (1997) conclusion that a^2 estimates increase and c^2 estimates decrease with age. Third, the confounding among moderators should again be considered in interpreting these results. The same pattern of results found for age was found for assessment method, with studies using report by others (viz., used more with children) yielding higher estimates of familial influences than those using self-report (viz., used more with adolescents and adults), as well as for operationalization, with studies examining antisocial behavior (viz., assessed more in children) yielding higher estimates of familial influences than those examining diagnosis (viz., assessed more in adults and adolescents).

Both DiLalla and Gottesman (1989) and Moffitt (1993) have suggested that in order to show conclusive evidence regarding their hypotheses, future studies of antisocial behavior should include longitudinal data of the same individuals. A good example of such a study is Jacobson, Neale, Prescott, and Kendler's (2001) longitudinal study, where they examined the antisocial behavior of 1,070 adult male–male twin pairs during adolescence and adulthood. Jacobson and colleagues tested the developmental taxonomy hypothesis by examining the heritability of antisocial behavior during adolescence in two different groups, individuals who were antisocial as adults versus those who were not. Heritability for antisocial behavior during adolescence was significantly higher for individuals who were antisocial as adults (h^2 = .38; c^2 = .10) compared to those who were not (h^2 = .00; c^2 = .35), providing support for the developmental taxonomy hypothesis.

Given that so few twin studies of antisocial behavior have examined age of onset or developmentally different subtypes of antisocial behavior, the present review cannot provide conclusive support for DiLalla and Gottesman's (1989) and Moffitt's (1993) hypothesis that there are genetic influences on continuous antisocial behavior but not on transitory antisocial behavior. If the magnitude of genetic influences had been lower in adolescence than in childhood or adulthood, however, the results of the meta-analysis would have been consistent with DiLalla and Gottesman's and Moffitt's hypothesis. The results were not consistent with this hypothesis, given that the magnitude of genetic influences was lower in both adolescence and adulthood than in childhood, but again the presence of confounding among the moderators needs to be considered. Unfortunately, it is difficult to interpret the results of analyses examining age as a moderator after statistically controlling for assessment method because only one study examining children used self-report and only two studies examining adolescents used parent report.

Sex

Analyses were limited to studies that examined antisocial behavior in both males (17 samples; 34 groups; 5,610 pairs of participants) and females (17 samples; 34 groups; 7,225 pairs of participants). Studies examining antisocial behavior in only one sex were excluded, given the fact that the studies examining antisocial behavior in only one sex varied a great deal in the operationalization examined (e.g., dishonorable discharge in males and aggression in females) and the assessment method used (e.g., official records

in males and parent report in females). The $\Delta\chi^2$ test of sex differences in the magnitude of genetic and environmental influences on antisocial behavior was not significant, $\Delta\chi^2(3) = 1.53$, $p = .68$. The ACE model was the best fitting model for both males (a^2 = .43, c^2 = .19, e^2 = .38) and females (a^2 = .41, c^2 = .20, e^2 = .39), such that the magnitude of genetic and environmental influences on antisocial behavior was virtually identical for males and females. This result is consistent with those of traditional literature reviews (e.g., Widom & Ames, 1988), which concluded that the magnitude of genetic and environmental influences on antisocial behavior in males and females is similar, and inconsistent with those of Miles and Carey (1997), who found higher heritability estimates for aggression in males.

Assessment of Confounding among Moderators

When there is confounding among moderators being tested in a meta-analysis, one concern is whether a particular variable appears to be a significant moderator only because it is confounded with another moderating variable. The possibility of confounding was assessed between the following pairs of moderators: operationalization and assessment method, age and operationalization, and age and assessment method. All analyses revealed a significant effect for each moderator even after the effects of the possible confounding moderator were controlled statistically. For example, the model estimating separate parameter estimates for each level of operationalization and each level of assessment method fit significantly better than the model estimating separate estimates for each level of operationalization only, $\Delta\chi^2(13)$ = 633.67, $p < .001$, and the model estimating separate estimates for each level of assessment method only, $\Delta\chi^2(12) = 112.56$, $p < .001$. Similarly, assessment method was a significant moderator after controlling for age, $\Delta\chi^2(7) = 676.28$, $p < .001$, operationalization was a significant moderator after controlling for age, $\Delta\chi^2(18) = 410.52$, $p < .001$, and age was a significant moderator after controlling for operationalization, $\Delta\chi^2(15) = 335.44$, $p < .001$, and after controlling for assessment method, $\Delta\chi^2(7) = 102.73$, $p < .001$. Thus, each moderator was found to be significant even after the other potentially confounding moderator was controlled for statistically.

Gender, Race–Ethnicity, and Socioeconomic Status

We found that gender was not a significant moderator of the magnitude of genetic and environmental influences on antisocial behavior (males—a^2 = .43, c^2 = .19, e^2 = .38; females—a^2 = .41, c^2 = .20, e^2 = .39). There is a possibility of an interaction between gender and age of onset in the etiology of antisocial behavior, however. Silverthorn and Frick (1999) noted that antisocial girls typically have an adolescent onset of antisocial behavior despite showing the characteristic features of the childhood-onset pathway and developing life-course-persistent antisocial behavior. Given this inconsistency, they proposed a delayed-onset pathway for girls that is analogous to the childhood-onset pathway in boys and suggested that there is no developmental pathway to antisocial behavior that is analogous to the adolescent pathway in boys. The study that would be needed to expose Silverthorn and Frick's hypothesis to risk of refutation is a longitudinal study examining the same individuals throughout the lifespan with reliable information collected on the age of onset of antisocial behavior. According to Silverthorn and Frick's hypothesis, age of onset should be a significant moderator of the heritability of antisocial behavior in males, with heritability being greater with earlier age of onset. In contrast, age of onset should not be a significant moderator of the heritability of antisocial behavior in females, given that for girls, adolescent onset of antisocial behavior does not necessarily indicate the adolescent-limited antisocial behavior that is primarily attributable to environmental influences.

We were unable to test any hypotheses regarding race–ethnicity or socioeconomic status because none of the studies included in the meta-analysis presented separate results for groups differing in these variables. In addition to examining race–ethnicity or socioeconomic status as a moderator of the etiology of antisocial behavior, interesting questions regarding the potential interaction between race–ethnicity or socioeconomic status and age of onset remain unanswered. A potential limitation of both twin and adoption studies is the generalizability of the findings given reduced diversity of race–ethnicity and socioeconomic status in twin and adoption samples. Volunteers in social science studies tend to be above average in socioeconomic status, and this limitation would pertain to twin and adoption studies just as it does for other studies. Also, the range of the adoptee's adoptive home environment is restricted, with adoptees having several advantages over children in the general population in family stability, educational opportunities, standards of health care, material living standards, and mother–child interactions (e.g., Fergusson, Lynskey, & Horwood, 1995).

SUMMARY OF META-ANALYSIS OF BEHAVIOR GENETIC STUDIES OF ANTISOCIAL BEHAVIOR

In the current meta-analysis, we found that there were moderate additive genetic (a^2 = .32), nonadditive genetic (d^2 = .09), shared environmental (c^2 =.16), and nonshared environmental influences (e^2 =.43) on antisocial behavior. All the potential moderators examined except for sex (i.e., operationalization, assessment method, zygosity determination method, and age) were found to account for significant differences in the genetic and environmental influences on antisocial behavior. It was often difficult to make conclusive statements about the moderator hypotheses examined in the present meta-analysis given concerns regarding the validity of the assessment methods and the confounding between assessment method and other potential moderators (viz., operationalization and age) in the literature. To make stronger conclusions regarding the hypotheses examined here, future studies should diversify the assessment methods used to measure antisocial behavior. Although there are several additional interesting distinctions in the operationalization of antisocial behavior (viz., violent vs. nonviolent crimes, delinquency vs. criminality, and relational vs. overt aggression), we were not able to conduct a quantitative review of these distinctions given that none or very few behavior genetic studies examined them.

META-ANALYSES AND RESULTS OF BEHAVIOR GENETIC STUDIES OF PSYCHOPATHY

In addition to the main meta-analysis of behavior genetic studies of antisocial behavior, and the tests of the various moderators of the considerable heterogeneity in the genetic and environmental influences therein, we conducted a follow-up meta-analysis of data from studies of psychopathy alone. Although deletion of the data from these samples did not alter the results of the main meta-analysis, it is possible that the results of the meta-analysis of the data from only these samples may yield somewhat different results. All the studies examined psychopathy via self-report and included seven samples of reared-together twins, one sample of reared-apart twins, and one adoption sample that provided correlations between adoptees and their biological parents. It is important to note that with only two exceptions (i.e., Blonigen, Carlson, Krueger, & Patrick, 2003; Taylor, Loney, Bobadilla, Iacono, & McGue, 2003), these studies examined the etiology of the antisocial deviance aspect of psychopathy, rather than the affective–interpersonal traits that are considered more germane to the construct of psychopathy. Given the small number of samples, and the presence of only one parent–offspring adoption sample, it was not possible to estimate the full ACDE model. As shown in the bottom of Table 11.2, the estimates of c^2 and d^2 were near zero or relatively small, and the fit of the ACE and ADE models were thus no better than that of the AE model, which was the best-fitting model. Additive genetic influences accounted for 49% of the variance and nonshared environmental influences accounted for the remaining 51% of the variance in self-reports of psychopathy. Additive genetic influences were clearly more important than shared environmental influences in explaining the familiality of psychopathy, as the CE model (which omits genetic influences) did not fit the data. The inclusion of a twin study (Taylor et al., 2000) that used self-reports on the California Psychological Inventory (CPI) Socialization scale to assess psychopathy yielded identical results.

Since the completion of our initial meta-analysis, several twin studies of psychopathic personality traits have been published and have yielded similar findings. In the first study, Taylor and colleagues (2003) estimated genetic and environmental influences on two subscales (Antisocial and Detachment) of the Minnesota Temperament Inventory (viz., MTI) in two twin cohorts, ages 16–18, from the Minnesota Twin Family Study (cohort 1: 142 MZ and 70 DZ twin pairs; cohort 2: 128 MZ and 58 DZ twin pairs). The MTI is a 19-item self-report measure designed to assess the classical features of psychopathy as described by Cleckley (1941). The Antisocial scale contains seven items that index impulsive, antisocial behaviors, whereas the Detachment scale contains six items that reflect the callous and unemotional interpersonal detachment that is often characteristic of psychopathy (Taylor et al., 2003). Both scales showed adequate internal consistency (i.e., $\alpha > .70$) and evidence for construct validity. For example, the Antisocial scale showed moderate correlations with symptoms of childhood oppositional defiant disorder (ODD) and CD and the adult antisocial behavior symptoms of APD, and these correlations were significantly greater than they were with the Detachment scale, which in turn was inversely correlated more strongly with a measure of Social Closeness (Loney, Taylor, Butler, & Iacono, 2002; Taylor et al., 2003). For both scales, it was possible to constrain the parameter estimates to be equal across cohorts and to thus fit the models to both cohorts simultaneously. The best-fitting model for both scales was the AE model, with additive genetic influences accounting for 39% and 42%, and nonshared environmental influences accounting for the remaining 61% and 58%, of the variance in the Antisocial and Detachment scales, respectively. There was no evidence for shared environmental influences on either of the scales. Additive genetic influences accounted for 53% and nonshared environmental influences accounted for the remaining 47% of the covariation between the two psychopathy-related traits. Approximately 55% of the genetic influences and 79% of the nonshared environmental influences on Detachment were shared in common with those that also influence the Antisocial scale. This indicates that whereas the vast majority of the nonshared environmental influences on Detachment are the same as those on Antisociality, just over half of the genetic influences on Detachment are the same as those on Antisociality, suggesting that many of the genetic influences are unique to each psychopathy trait.

A second recent twin study (Blonigen et al., 2003) used an adult male twin sample from Minnesota (165 MZ and 106 DZ twin pairs) to estimate genetic and environmental influences on the total score and 8 subscales from the Psychopathic Personality Inventory (PPI; Lilienfeld & Andrews, 1996; Lilienfeld & Fowler, Chapter 6, this volume). The PPI subscales include Machiavelian Egocentricity, Social Potency, Fearlessness, Coldheartedness, Impulsive Nonconformity, Blame Externalization, Carefree Nonplanfulness, and Stress Immunity. The best-fitting model for the etiology of each of the subscales included genetic and nonshared environmental influences, with no evidence for shared environmental influences on any of the subscales. The genetic influences appeared to be nonadditive for all of the subscales except for Social Potency and Blame Externalization, for which the genetic influences were additive. Genetic influences accounted for 29–56% of the variance in each of the PPI subscales.

In a third recent twin study, Viding, Blair, Moffitt, and Plomin (in press) examined genetic and environmental influences on antisocial behavior and on the callous–unemotional traits germane to psychopathy in children (see Salekin, Chapter 20, this volume), as well as the extent to which the genetic and environmental influences on antisocial behavior varied as a function of callous–unemotional trait levels, in a sample of 3,487 7-year-old twin pairs in the United Kingdom. The authors first selected probands based on extremely high scores on each of the dimensions, then estimated the genetic and environmental influences on extreme status on the antisocial behavior and callous–unemotional traits. There was moderate heritability ($h_g^2 = .67$) of extreme callous–unemotional group status, which in turn moderated the heritability of antisocial behavior. Specifically, extreme antisocial behavior group status was highly heritable ($h_g^2 = .81$) with no evidence for shared environmental influences when accompanied by extreme callous–unemotional group status, whereas extreme antisocial behavior group status was only modestly heritable ($h_g^2 = .30$) with similar levels of shared environmental influences ($c_g^2 = .34$) when not accompanied by extreme callous–unemotional group status. These results suggest that callous–unemotional psychopathic traits are moderately to highly heritable and may identify a subtype of antisocial behavior that is highly heritable even in childhood.

SUMMARY OF META-ANALYSIS AND RECENT BEHAVIOR GENETIC STUDIES OF PSYCHOPATHY

A meta-analysis of behavior genetic studies of psychopathy, as well as recent twin studies thereof, suggested that genetic influences on psychopathic traits are appreciable and may be nonadditive, with moderate nonshared environmental influences but no evidence for shared environmental influences across studies (in contrast to the meta-analytic results for the aforementioned behavior genetic studies of antisocial behavior). These studies raise the possibility that some of the genetic influences on the development of antisocial behavior may be mediated via psychopathic personality traits (e.g., Taylor et al., 2003), and raise the question as to what extent the heritability of psychopathic traits is coextensive with genetic influences on "normal range" personality traits such as negative and positive emotionality, and daring or constraint (Benning, Patrick, Blonigen, Hicks, & Iacono, 2005; Lahey & Waldman, 2003). Unfortunately, all but three of the behavior genetic studies of psychopathy reviewed previously examined the antisocial deviance component exclusively, rather than the affective–interpersonal features that are considered more central to the psychopathy construct. Important future directions for behavior genetic studies of psychopathy thus include further examination of the genetic and environmental influences underlying the affective–interpersonal components of psychopathy, whether the magnitude of these influences are similar to the magnitude of the genetic and environmental influences underlying the antisocial deviance component, and to what extent the same or different genetic and environmental influences underlie these two broad facets of psychopathy.

In addition to examining the interesting aforementioned distinctions in operationalization, future directions for behavior genetic studies of psychopathy and antisocial behavior include multivariate analyses of the magnitude of common or specific genetic and environmental influences on different operationalizations of antisocial behavior; further examination of the relations between psychopathic and "normal range" personality traits and antisocial behavior, of differing etiological influences on different facets of psychopathy, of genotype–environment interactions, and of specific environmental influences; and longitudinal studies on the effects of age of onset and developmentally different subtypes on the genetic and environmental influences underlying antisocial behavior.

FUTURE DIRECTIONS

The Design of Future Behavior Genetic Studies of Antisocial Behavior Given Confounding among Moderators

It was often difficult to make conclusive statements about the moderators examined in the present meta-analysis given concerns regarding the validity of the assessment method or confounding between assessment method and other moderators. When there is confounding between assessment method and other moderators, the magnitude of genetic and environmental influences may reflect the assessment method rather than the moderators of greater conceptual importance, such as operationalization or age. First, all studies that examined criminality used official records as an assessment method. Therefore, given the current evidence, it is not possible to distinguish whether the behavior genetic results for criminality reflect the operationalization of criminality per se or the assessment method of official records. Second, studies assessing aggression via parent and self-report found that genetic influences are important, but the one study (Plomin et al., 1981) that examined aggression using an objective test found no evidence for genetic influences. The objective test used by Plomin et al. has been validated against peer ratings and teacher ratings of aggression (Johnston, DeLuca, Murtaugh, & Diener, 1977), but the sample size in Plomin et al.'s study is small. Larger behavior genetic studies using different types

of validated, objective tests of aggression are necessary to resolve this question.

Third, no matter which operationalization was being examined (i.e., diagnosis, aggression, or antisocial behavior), the magnitude of familial influences (a^2 and c^2) was lower in studies using the assessment method of self-report than in studies using the assessment method of report by others. The only exception occurred in studies examining antisocial behavior, where the a^2 estimate was .47 for both report by others and self-report. These results suggest the possibility that the lower h^2 and c^2 estimates may be more a function of the assessment method of self-report than a function of any of the operationalizations that were examined. Two separate raters are involved in the assessment method of self-report (i.e., each member of a twin pair completes his or her own questionnaire), whereas the same person rates both of the twins or siblings when parent report is used. It is possible that this difference in the number of raters itself led to lower familial correlations and a lower estimate of the magnitude of familial influences in studies using self-report.

Fourth, the confounding between age and assessment method precluded our ability to test DiLalla and Gottesman's (1989) hypothesis regarding genetic influences on continuous versus transitory antisocial behavior. The assessment method of report by others was used only in children and adolescents, whereas the assessment method of self-report was used only in adolescents and adults. Given the fact that the pattern of results for age (i.e., familial influences decreasing and nonfamilial influences increasing as age increases) was identical to the pattern of results for assessment method (i.e., familial influences smaller and nonfamilial influences larger for self-report than for report by others) and that age and assessment method are confounded, it is impossible to conclude definitively whether age moderates the magnitude of genetic and environmental influences on antisocial behavior.

Both DiLalla and Gottesman (1989) and Moffitt (1993) have suggested that in order to show conclusive evidence regarding their hypotheses, future studies of antisocial behavior should include longitudinal data on the same individuals. The assessment methods used in future behavior genetic studies of antisocial behavior should be diversified given the common concerns regarding the validity of the assessment method. For example, a combination of official records and self-report should be used to assess criminality given the shortcomings of each assessment method. Larger behavior genetic studies using different types of validated, objective tests of aggression are needed. Most important, the limitations of the assessment method chosen for a behavior genetic study of antisocial behavior should be acknowledged and considered given the evidence that the assessment method can influence the results. If multiple assessment methods are used to assess antisocial behavior in a single twin study, multivariate behavior genetic models can be used to estimate the magnitude of genetic and environmental influences that are common to the latent construct being examined (i.e., antisocial behavior), as well as of genetic and environmental influences that are specific to each assessment method (e.g., Riemann, 1999).

Candidate Genes and Environments for Antisocial Behavior and Psychopathy

Broadly speaking, there are two general strategies for identifying genes that contribute to the etiology of a disorder or trait. The first is a genome scan, in which linkage is examined between a disorder or trait and evenly spaced DNA markers (e.g., approximately 10,000 base pairs apart) distributed across the entire genome (Haines, 1998). Evidence for linkage between any of these DNA markers and the trait or disorder of interest implicates a broad segment of the genome that may contain hundreds of genes, and lack of evidence for linkage can, in some cases, be used to exclude genomic segments. Subsequent fine-grained linkage analyses can then use a new set of more tightly grouped markers within the implicated genomic region to locate the functional mutation. Thus, genome scans may be thought of as exploratory searches for putative genes that contribute to the etiology of a disorder. The fact that major genes have been found for many medical diseases via genome scans is testament to the usefulness of this method. Unfortunately, the power of linkage analyses in genome scans is typically quite low, making it very difficult, if not impossible, to detect genes that account for less than ~15% of the

variance in a disorder. Given this, the promise for genome scans of complex traits remains largely unknown.

The second strategy for finding genes that contribute to the etiology of a disorder is the candidate gene approach. In many ways, candidate gene studies are polar opposites of genome scans. In contrast to the exploratory nature of genome scans, well-conducted candidate gene studies represent a targeted test of the role of specific genes in the etiology of a disorder as the location, function, and etiological relevance of candidate genes are most often known or strongly hypothesized *a priori*. Thus, an advantage of well-conducted candidate gene studies in comparison with genome scans is that positive findings are easily interpretable because one already knows the gene's location, function, and etiological relevance, even if the specific polymorphism(s) chosen for study in the candidate gene is not functional and the functional mutation(s) in the candidate gene is as yet unidentified. There are also disadvantages to the candidate gene approach given that only previously identified genes can be studied. Thus, one cannot find genes that one has not looked for or have yet to be discovered, and because there are relatively few strong candidate genes for psychiatric disorders, the same genes are examined as candidates for almost all psychiatric disorders, regardless of how disparate the disorders may be in terms of their symptomatology or conjectured pathophysiology.

In well-designed studies, however, knowledge regarding the biology of the disorder is used to select genes based on the known or hypothesized involvement of their gene product in the etiology of the trait or disorder (i.e., its pathophysiological function and etiological relevance). With respect to antisocial behavior and psychopathy, genes underlying various aspects of the dopaminergic and serotonergic neurotransmitter pathways may be conjectured based on several lines of converging evidence suggesting a role for these neurotransmitter systems in the etiology and pathophysiology of these traits and their relevant disorders. For example, there is considerable overlap between antisocial behavior and childhood ADHD (e.g., Lilienfeld & Waldman, 1990)—thus candidate genes for attention-deficit/hyperactivity disorder (ADHD) may also be relevant candidates for antisocial behavior and psychopathy. Several genes within the dopamine system appear to be risk factors for ADHD (see Waldman & Gizer, in press, for a recent review). Dopamine genes are plausible candidates for ADHD, given that the stimulant medications that are the most frequent and effective treatments for ADHD appear to act primarily by regulating dopamine levels in the brain (Seeman & Madras, 1998; Solanto, 1984), and also affect noradrenergic and serotonergic function (Solanto, 1998). In addition, "knockout" gene studies in mice, in which the behavioral effects of the deactivation of specific genes are examined, have further demonstrated the potential relevance of genes within these neurotransmitter systems. Results of such studies have markedly strengthened the consideration as candidate genes for ADHD of genes within the dopaminergic system, such as the dopamine transporter gene (*DAT1*; Giros, Jaber, Jones, Wightman, & Caron, 1996) and the dopamine receptor D3 and D4 genes (*DRD3* and *DRD4*; Accili et al., 1996; Dulawa, Grandy, Low, Paulus, & Geyer, 1999; Rubinstein et al., 1997), as well as genes within the serotonergic system, such as the serotonin 1β receptor gene (*HTR1β*; Saudou et al., 1994). Serotonergic genes also are plausible candidates for antisocial behavior and psychopathy, given the demonstrated relations between serotonergic function and aggression and violence (Berman, Kavoussi, & Coccaro, 1997).

Candidate genes for neurotransmitter systems may include (1) *precursor genes* that affect the rate at which neurotransmitters are produced from precursor amino acids (e.g., tyrosine hydroxylase for dopamine, tryptophan hydroxylase for serotonin); (2) *receptor genes* that are involved in receiving neurotransmitter signals (e.g., genes corresponding to the five dopamine receptors, *DRD1, D2, D3, D4,* and *D5,* and to the serotonin receptors, such as *HTR1β* and *HTR2A*); (3) *transporter genes* that are involved in the reuptake of neurotransmitters back into the presynaptic terminal (e.g., the dopamine and serotonin transporter genes, *DAT1* and *5HTT*); (4) *metabolite genes* that are involved in the metabolism or degradation of these neurotransmitters (e.g., the genes for catechol-O-methyl-transferase, *COMT*, and

for monoamine oxidase A and B [i.e., *MAOA* and *MAOB*]); and (5) genes that are responsible for the *conversion* of one neurotransmitter into another (e.g., dopamine beta-hydroxylase, or *DβH*, which converts dopamine into norepinephrine).

There are many environmental variables that have been posited as risk factors for antisocial behavior and psychopathy. Relevant environmental domains include pre- and perinatal influences, such as maternal smoking and drinking and obstetrical complications; parenting variables, such as warmth, control, harsh discipline, supervision and monitoring; family background variables, such as family poverty, size, disruption, divorce, and single- versus dual-parent status; sibling and peer influences, such as aggression and antisocial behavior, substance use or abuse, academic achievement and aspirations; and neighborhood characteristics, such as economic inequality, cohesion, crime rates, and collective efficacy. Unfortunately, it is difficult to interpret much of the literature on the relation between environmental variables and antisocial behavior and psychopathy because the environmental and genetic influences that potentially underlie such relations are confounded. For example, the relation between parental harsh discipline and children's antisocial behavior could be due to a direct environmental influence, to background environmental influences such as socioeconomic status, or to shared genetic influences, in which the same genes that underlie parents' tendencies to discipline harshly also underlie their children's antisocial behavior. Given these confounds, such specific candidate environmental influences on antisocial behavior can best be considered putative, and require examination in genetically informative designs to validate their mechanism of effect as truly environmental.

Fortunately, several authors have recently proposed behavior genetic designs and analyses that are well-suited to discriminating among these causal possibilities (e.g., D'Onofrio et al., 2003), and studies are beginning to investigate the relations of such environmental variables with antisocial behavior in such genetically informative designs and thus to move their status from the putative to the actual. A recent example is a study by Jaffe, Caspi, Moffitt, and Taylor

(2004) in which the environmental effects of physical maltreatment on children's antisocial behavior were assessed within the context of a twin study design. Although physical maltreatment was significantly and substantially related to their parents' antisocial behavior, and the heritability of their own antisocial behavior was appreciable (h^2 = .67), the environmental effects of physical maltreatment on children's antisocial behavior remained after controlling for the genetic influences on their antisocial behavior (which accounted for 56% of the physical maltreatment effect).

Researchers also are beginning to seriously entertain the possibility that candidate genes and candidate environments may not simply act in an additive manner in their influence on antisocial behavior and psychopathy. Developmental psychopathology researchers have long been intrigued by the prospect of gene–environment interaction, and many have contended that one cannot understand the development of psychopathology without the consideration of such processes. One recent, high-profile example of gene–environment interaction for psychopathology that has garnered considerable attention and interest showed that the risk for adolescent antisocial behavior and violence based on abuse during early childhood depended on alleles at the *MAOA* gene (Caspi et al., 2002). Notable features of this study were the careful measurement of both the psychopathology outcome and the environmental risk factor, as well as the use of functional mutations in the *MAOA* gene. It is important to recognize the symmetrical nature of such gene–environment interactions—that is, gene–environment interaction refers both to the moderation of the effects of environmental risk factors as a function of individuals' genotypes at a particular gene and to the moderation of individuals' genetic predispositions for a certain disorder as a function of the environmental facets to which they are exposed and experience. It would be fairly easy to test whether the effects of various of the candidate genes mentioned previously vary as a function of many of the aforementioned environmental risk factors for antisocial behavior and psychopathy. We expect that more studies of gene–environment interaction for antisocial behavior and psychopathy will emerge in the near future.

Endophenotypes for Antisocial Behavior and Psychopathy

Clearly there is a large gap between candidate genes and the manifest symptoms of disorders or traits such as antisocial behavior and psychopathy as typically assessed by interviews or rating scales. It is desirable from both a conceptual and empirical perspective to find valid and meaningful mediational or intervening constructs that may help to bridge this gap. The term "endophenotype" is often used to describe such constructs and the variables that are used to measure them. Endophenotypes were first described with respect to psychiatric disorders by Gottesman and Shields over 30 years ago in their application to the genetics of schizophrenia (Gottesman & Shields, 1972) as "internal phenotypes discoverable by a biochemical test or microscopic examination" (Gottesman & Gould, 2003, p. 637; Gottesman & Shields, 1972). More generally, endophenotypes refer to constructs that are thought to underlie psychiatric disorders or relevant traits and to be more directly influenced by the genes relevant to disorder than are the manifest symptoms. As such, they are closer to the immediate products of such genes (i.e., the proteins they code for) and are thought to be more strongly influenced by the genes that underlie them than the manifest symptoms that they in turn undergird. Endophenotypes also are thought to be "genetically simpler" in their etiology than are complex traits such as manifest disorders or their symptom dimensions (Gottesman & Gould, 2003). This means that the underlying structure of genetic influences on endophenotypes is simpler than that of complex disorders and traits in that there are fewer individual genes (or sets thereof) that contribute to their etiology.

A number of researchers have outlined criteria for evaluating the validity and utility of putative endophenotypes (e.g., Castellanos & Tannock, 2002; Doyle et al., 2005; Gottesman & Gould, 2003; Waldman, 2005). These include

1. The endophenotype is related to the disorder and its symptoms in the general population.
2. The endophenotype is heritable.
3. The endophenotype is expressed regardless of whether the disorder is present.

4. The endophenotype and disorder are associated within families (i.e., they "cosegregate").

5. In addition to the endophenotype occurring to a greater extent in family members with a disorder than in family members who are unaffected (viz., criteria 4), it also will occur at a higher rate in the unaffected relatives of family members with a disorder than in randomly selected individuals from the general population (given that the endophenotype reflects the inherited liability to a disorder).

In addition to these foregoing criteria, several other criteria are pertinent to the validity and utility of endophenotypes. First, it is important that the genetic influences that underlie the endophenotype also underlie the disorder or related trait and that at least some (but likely not all) of the genetic influences that underlie the disorder or related trait underlie the endophenotype. Note that this last criterion is asymmetrical in that a higher proportion of the genetic influences on the endophenotype will be shared in common with those on the disorder or related trait, rather than vice versa. This criterion follows from the notion mentioned above that endophenotypes are thought to be genetically simpler than are complex traits such as disorders, in the sense that fewer genes contribute a greater magnitude to their etiology (Gottesman & Gould, 2003). Second, measures of the endophenotype must show association and/or linkage with one (or more) of the candidate genes or genetic loci that underlie the disorder or related trait. Third, the endophenotype measure should *mediate* the association and/or linkage between the candidate gene or genetic locus and the disorder or related trait, meaning that the effects of a particular gene or locus on a disorder or trait are expressed—either in full or in part—through the endophenotype. The prerequisites for this causal scenario are that the candidate gene influences both the disorder or trait and the endophenotype and that the endophenotype in turn influences the disorder or related trait. Fourth, the endophenotype should show association and linkage with a candidate gene over and above the gene's relation with the disorder or related trait (i.e., the endophenotype should incrementally contribute to asso-

ciation with the candidate gene) and thus aid in the search for genes that underlie the etiology of disorders or related traits.

Several biological, psychophysiological, and psychological mechanisms may be plausible candidates as putative endophenotypes for antisocial behavior and psychopathy. Given that this topic is treated in detail in other chapters in this volume, we will discuss it only briefly herein. Putative biological endophenotypes may include serotonin and dopamine levels, given their aforementioned relations to antisocial behavior and psychopathy (Berman et al., 1997) and related disorders such as ADHD. Putative psychophysiological endophenotypes may include avoidance conditioning (Lykken, 1957) and startle reflex modulation (Patrick, 1994), given findings of deficits in such variables in psychopathic relative to nonpsychopathic individuals. Putative psychological endophenotypes may include hostile perceptual and attributional biases (Waldman, 1996) and executive function deficits (Morgan & Lilienfeld, 2000), given their demonstrated relations to aggression and antisocial behavior. Future studies examining the extent to which these variables meet the criteria outlined above are necessary for evaluating their validity and utility as putative endophenotypes for antisocial behavior and psychopathy. In addition, in the case of a syndrome like psychopathy that involves distinct phenotypic facets (Cooke & Michie, 2001; Hare, 2003; Harpur, Hakstian, & Hare, 1988; Taylor et al., 2003), it will be important to evaluate whether certain endophenotypes are associated more with some features than with others (e.g., affective–interpersonal features vs. antisocial deviance features).

ACKNOWLEDGMENTS

This work was supported in part by Grant No. DA-13956 from the National Institute on Drug Abuse and Grant No. MH-01818 from the National Institute of Mental Health. We thank the authors who made data from unpublished studies available through personal communication. We also thank Deborah Finkel, Jenae Neiderhiser, Wendy Slutske, and Edwin van den Oord for making the data from their studies available before their publication, and Scott O. Lilienfeld, Kim Wallen, and Terrie E. Moffitt for helpful comments on earlier versions of this chapter. Earlier versions of this chapter were presented at the meeting of the American Society of Criminology in 1996 and the meeting of the Behavior Genetics Association in 1997, and a more extensive version of the meta-analysis was published in *Psychological Bulletin* in 2002.

REFERENCES

Asterisks following references entries indicate behavior genetic studies of psychopathy.

Accili, D., Fishburn, C. S., Drago, J., Steiner, H., Lachowicz, J. E., Park, B. H., et al. (1996). A targeted mutation of the D3 dopamine receptor gene is associated with hyperactivity in mice. *Proceedings of the National Academy of Sciences, USA, 93*, 1945–1949.

Achenbach, T. M., & Edelbrock, C. S. (1983). *Manual for the Child Behavior Checklist and revised behavior profile*. Burlington: University of Vermont.

American Psychiatric Association. (1994). *Diagnostic and statistical manual of mental disorders* (4th ed.). Washington, DC: Author.

Benning, S. D., Patrick, C. J., Blonigen, D. M., Hicks, B. M., & Iacono, W. G. (2005). Estimating facets of psychopathy from normal personality traits: A step toward community-epidemiological investigations. *Assessment, 12*, 3–18.

Berman, M. E., Kavoussi, R. J., & Coccaro, E. F. (1997). Neurotransmitter correlates of human aggression. In D. M. Stoff, J. Breiling, & J. D. Masur (Eds.), *Handbook of antisocial behavior* (pp. 305–313). New York: Wiley.

Blonigen, D. M., Carlson, S. R., Krueger, R. F., & Patrick, C. J. (2003). A twin study of self-reported psychopathic personality traits. *Personality and Individual Differences, 35*, 179–197.*

Brandon, K., & Rose, R. J. (1995). A multivariate twin family study of the genetic and environmental structure of personality, beliefs, and alcohol use. *Behavior Genetics, 25*(3), 257.*

Cadoret, R. J. (1978). Psychopathology in adopted-away offspring of biologic parents with antisocial behavior. *Archives of General Psychiatry, 35*, 176–184.

Cadoret, R. J., Troughton, E., O'Gorman, T. W., & Heywood, E. (1986). An adoption study of genetic and environmental factors in drug abuse. *Archives of General Psychiatry, 43* (12), 1131–1136.

Caspi, A., Sugden, K., Moffitt, T. E., Taylor, A., Craig, I. W., Harrington, H., et al. (2003). Influence of life stress on depression: moderation by a polymorphism in the 5-HTT gene. *Science, 301*, 386–389.

Castellanos, F. X., & Tannock, R. (2002). Neuroscience of attention-deficit/hyperactivity disorder: The search for endophenotypes. *Nature Reviews Neuroscience, 3*, 617–628.

Cleckley, H. (1941). *The mask of sanity*. St. Louis, MO: Mosby.

Cloninger, C. R., & Gottesman, I. I. (1987). Genetic and environmental factors in antisocial behavior disorders. In S. A. Mednick, T. E. Moffitt, & S. A. Stack (Eds.), *The causes of crime: New biological approaches* (pp. 92–109). New York: Cambridge University Press.

Cooke, D. J., & Michie, C. (2001). Refining the construct of psychopathy: Towards a hierarchical model. *Psychological Assessment, 13*, 171–188.

Cooney, N. L., Kadden, R. M., & Litt, M. D. (1990). A comparison of methods for assessing sociopathy in male and female alcoholics. *Journal of Studies on Alcohol, 51*(1), 42–48.

DiLalla, D. L., Carey, G., Gottesman, I. I., & Bouchard, T. J. (1996). Heritability of MMPI personality indicators of psychopathology in twins reared apart. *Journal of Abnormal Psychology, 105*(4), 491–499.*

DiLalla, L. F., & Gottesman, I. I. (1989). Heterogeneity of causes for delinquency and criminality: Lifespan perspectives. *Development and Psychopathology, 1*(4), 339–349.

D'Onofrio, B. M., Turkheimer, E. N., Eaves, L. J. Corey, L. A., Berg, K., Solaas, M. H., & Emergy, R. E. (2003). The role of the Children of Twins design in elucidating causal relations between parent characteristics and child outcomes. *Journal of Child Psychology and Psychiatry, 44*, 1130–1144.

Doyle, A. E., Faraone, S. V., Seidman, L. J., Willcutt, E., Nigg, J. T., Waldman, I. D., et al. (2005). Are endophenotypes based on measures of executive functions useful for molecular genetic studies of ADHD? *Journal of Child Psychology and Psychiatry, 44*, 1130–1144.

Dulawa, S. C., Grandy, D. K., Low, M. J., Paulus, M. P., & Geyer, M. A. (1999). Dopamine D4 receptor-knock-out mice exhibit reduced exploration of novel stimuli. *Journal of Neuroscience, 19*, 9550–9556.

Eley, T. C., Lichtenstein, P., & Stevenson, J. (1999). Sex differences in the etiology of aggressive and non-aggressive antisocial behavior: Results from two twin studies. *Child Development, 70*(1), 155–168.

Emde, R. N., Plomin, R., Robinson, J. A., Corley, R., DeFries, J., Fulker, D. W., et al. (1992). Temperament, emotion, and cognition at fourteen months: The MacArthur longitudinal twin study. *Child Development, 63*, 1437–1455.

Fergusson, D. M., Lynskey, M., & Horwood, L. J. (1995). The adolescent outcomes of adoption: A 16-year longitudinal study. *Journal of Child Psychology and Psychiatry, 36*(4), 597–615.

Ghodsian-Carpey, J., & Baker, L. A. (1987). Genetic and environmental influences on aggression in 4- to 7-year-old twins. *Aggressive Behavior, 13*, 173–186.

Giros, B., Jaber, M., Jones, S. R., Wightman, R. M., & Caron, M. G. (1996). Hyperlocomotion and indifference to cocaine and amphetamine in mice lacking the dopamine transporter. *Nature, 379*, 606–612.

Gottesman, I. I. (1963). Heritability of personality: A demonstration. *Psychological Monographs, 77*(9, Whole No. 572).*

Gottesman, I. I. (1965). Personality and natural selection. In S. G. Vandenberg (Ed.), *Methods and goals in human behavior genetics* (pp. 63–80). New York: Academic Press.*

Gottesman, I. I., & Goldsmith, H. H. (1994). Developmental psychopathology of antisocial behavior: Inserting genes into is ontogenesis and epigenesist. In C. A. Nelson (Ed.), *Threats to optimal development: Integrating biological, psychological, and social risk factors* (pp. 69–104). Hillsdale, NJ: Erlbaum.

Gottesman, I. I., & Gould, T. D. (2003). The endophenotype concept in psychiatry: Etymology and strategic intentions. *American Journal of Psychiatry, 160,* 636–645.

Gottesman, I. I., & Shields, J. (1972). *Schizophrenia and genetics: A twin study vantage point.* New York: Academic Press.

Grove, W. M., Eckert, E. D., Heston, L., Bouchard, T. J., Segal, N., & Lykken, D. T. (1990). Heritability of substance abuse and antisocial behavior: A study of monozygotic twins reared apart. *Biological Psychiatry, 27,* 1293–1304.

Haines, J. L. (1998). Genomic screening. In J. L. Haines & M. A. Pericak-Vance (Eds.), *Approaches to gene mapping in complex human diseases* (pp. 243–252). New York: Wiley.

Hare, R. D. (2003). *Manual for the Hare Psychopathy Checklist—Revised* (2nd ed.). Toronto, ON, Canada: Multi-Health Systems.

Hare, R. D., Hart, S. D., & Harpur, T. A. (1991). Psychopathy and the DSM-IV criteria for antisocial personality disorder. *Journal of Abnormal Psychology, 100*(3), 391–398.

Harpur, T. J., Hakstian, A., & Hare, R. D. (1988). Factor structure of the Psychopathy Checklist. *Journal of Consulting and Clinical Psychology, 56,* 741–747.

Hyde, J. S. (1984). How large are gender differences in aggression? A developmental meta-analysis. *Developmental Psychology, 20,* 722–736.

Jacobson, K. C., Neale, M. C., Prescott, C. A., & Kendler, K. S. (2001). Behavioral genetic confirmation of a life-course perspective on antisocial behavior: Can we believe the results? [Abstract]. *Behavior Genetics, 31,* 456.

Jaffee, S. R., Caspi, A., Moffitt, T. E., & Taylor, A. (2004). Physical maltreatment victim to antisocial child: Evidence of an environmentally mediated process. *Journal of Abnormal Psychology, 113,* 44–55.

Johnston, A., DeLuca, D., Murtaugh, K., & Diener, E. (1977). Validation of a laboratory play measure of child aggression. *Child Development, 48,* 324–327.

Kasriel, J., & Eaves, L. (1976). The zygosity of twins: Further evidence on the agreement between diagnosis by blood groups and written questionnaires. *Journal of Biosocial Science, 8,* 263–266.

Lahey, B. B., & Waldman, I. D. (2003). A developmental propensity model of the origins of conduct problems during childhood and adolescence. In B. B. Lahey, T. E. Moffitt, & A. Caspi (Eds.), *Causes of conduct disorder and juvenile delinquency* (pp. 76–117). New York: Guilford Press.

Lilienfeld, S. O., & Andrews, B. P. (1996). Development and preliminary validation of a self report measure of psychopathic personality traits in noncriminal populations. *Journal of Personality Assessment, 66,* 488–524.

Lilienfeld, S. O., & Waldman, I. D. (1990). The relation between childhood Attention-Deficit Hyperactivity Disorder and adult antisocial behavior reexamined: The problem of heterogeneity. *Clinical Psychology Review, 10,* 699–725.

Loehlin, J. C. (1992a). *Genes and environment in personality development.* Newbury Park, CA: Sage.

Loehlin, J. C. (1992b). *Latent variable models: An introduction to factor, path, and structural analysis* (2nd ed.). Hillsdale, NJ: Erlbaum.

Loehlin, J. C., & Nichols, R. C. (1976). *Heredity, environment, and personality.* Austin: University of Texas Press.*

Loehlin, J. C., Willerman, L., & Horn, J. M. (1987). Personality resemblance in adoptive families: A 10-year follow-up. *Journal of Personality and Social Psychology, 53*(5), 961–969.*

Loney, B. R., Taylor, J., Butler, M., & Iacono, W. G. (2002). *The Minnesota Temperament Inventory: A psychometric study of adolescent self-reported psychopathy.* Unpublished manuscript.

Lykken, D. T. (1957). A study of anxiety in the sociopathic personality. *Journal of Abnormal and Social Psychology, 55,* 6–10.

Matheny, A. P. (1989). Children's behavioral inhibition over age and across situations: Genetic similarity for a trait during change. *Journal of Personality, 57*(2), 215–235.

McCartney, K., Harris, M. J., & Bernieri, F. (1990). Growing up and growing apart: A developmental meta-analysis of twin studies. *Psychological Bulletin, 107,* 226–237.

Mednick, S. A., Gabrielli, W. F., & Hutchings, B. (1983). Genetic influences in criminal behavior: Evidence from an adoption cohort. In K. T. Van Dusen & S. A. Mednick (Eds.), *Prospective studies of crime and delinquency* (pp. 39–56). Boston: Kluwer-Nijhof.

Mednick, S. A., Gabrielli, W. F., & Hutchings, B. (1984). Genetic influences in criminal convictions: Evidence from an adoption cohort. *Science, 224,* 891–894.

Miles, D. R., & Carey, G. (1997). Genetic and environmental architecture of human aggression. *Journal of Personality and Social Psychology, 72*(1), 207–217.

Moffitt, T. E. (1993). Adolescence-limited and life-course-persistent antisocial behavior: A developmental taxonomy. *Psychological Review, 100*(4), 674–701.

Morgan, A. B., & Lilienfeld, S. O. (2000). A meta-analytic review of the relation between antisocial behavior and neuropsychological measures of executive function. *Clinical Psychology Review, 20,* 113–156.

Neale, M. C. (1995). *Mx: Statistical modeling.* Richmond: Department of Psychiatry, Medical College of Virginia, Virginia Commonwealth University.

Owen, D., & Sines, J. O. (1970). Heritability of personality in children. *Behavior Genetics 1*, 235–248.

Patrick, C. J. (1994). Emotion and psychopathy: Startling new insights. *Psychophysiology, 31*, 319–330.

Plomin, R. (1981). Heredity and temperament: A comparison of twin data for self-report questionnaires, parental ratings, and objectively assessed behavior. In L. Gedda, P. Parisi, & W. E. Nance (Eds.), *Twin research 3: Intelligence, personality, and development* (pp. 269–278). New York: Liss.

Plomin, R. (1986). *Development, genetics, and psychology.* Hillsdale, NJ: Erlbaum.

Plomin, R., Foch, T. T., & Rowe, D. C. (1981). Bobo clown aggression in childhood: Environment, not genes. *Journal of Research in Personality 15*, 331–342.

Plomin, R., Nitz, K., & Rowe, D. C. (1990). Behavioral genetics and aggressive behavior in childhood. In M. Lewis & S. M. Miller (Eds.), *Handbook of developmental psychopathology* (pp. 119–133). New York: Plenum Press.

Rhee, S. H., & Waldman, I. D. (2002). Genetic and environmental influences on antisocial behavior: A meta-analysis of twin and adoption studies. *Psychological Bulletin, 128*(3), 490–529.

Riemann, R. (1999, July). *Multi-method measurement of personality: First results from the German observational study of adult twins.* Paper presented at the meeting of the Behavior Genetics Association, Vancouver, BC, Canada.

Rietveld, M. J., van Der Valk, J. C., Bongers, I. L., Stroet, T. M., Slagboom, P. E., & Boomsma, D. I. (2000). Zygosity diagnosis in young twins by parental report. *Twin Research, 3*, 134–141.

Rubinstein, M., Phillips, T. J., Bunzow, J. R., Falzone, T. L., Dziewczapolski, G., Zhang, G., et al. (1997). Mice lacking dopamine D4 receptors are supersensitive to ethanol, cocaine, and methamphetamine. *Cell, 90*, 991–1001.

Saudou, F., Amara, D. A., Dierich, A., LeMeur, M., Ramboz, S., Segu, L., et al. (1994). Enhanced aggressive behavior in mice lacking 5-HT1? receptor. *Science, 265*, 1875–1878.

Schulsinger, F. (1972). Psychopathy: Heredity and environment. *International Journal of Mental Health 1*, 190–206.

Seeman, P., & Madras, B. K. (1998). Anti-hyperactivity medication: methylphenidate and amphetamine. *Molecular Psychiatry, 3*, 386–396.

Silverthorn, P., & Frick, P. J. (1999). Developmental pathways to antisocial behavior: The delayed-onset pathway in girls. *Development and Psychopathology, 11*, 101–126.

Slutske, W. S., Heath, A. C., Dinwiddie, S. H., Madden, P. A. F., Bucholz, K. K., Dunne, M. P., et al. (1997).

Modeling genetic and environmental influences in the etiology of conduct disorder: A study of 2,682 adult twin pairs. *Journal of Abnormal Psychology, 106*(2), 266–279.

Smith, S. M., & Penrose, L. S. (1955). Monozygotic and dizygotic twin diagnosis. *Annals of Human Genetics, 19*, 273–289.

Solanto, M. V. (1984). Neuropharmacological basis of stimulant drug action in attention deficit disorder with hyperactivity: A review and synthesis. *Psychological Bulletin, 95*, 387–409.

Solanto, M. V. (1998). Neuropsychopharmacological mechanisms of stimulant drug action in attention-deficit hyperactivity disorder: A review and integration. *Behavioural Brain Research, 94*, 127–152.

Taylor, J., Loney, B. R., Bobadilla, L., Iacono, W. G., & McGue, M. (2003). Genetic and environmental influences on psychopathy trait dimensions in a community sample of male twins. *Journal of Abnormal Child Psychology, 31*, 633–645.*

Taylor, J., McGue, M., Iacono, W. G., & Lykken, D. T. (2000). A behavioral genetic analysis of the relationship between the socialization scale and self-reported delinquency. *Journal of Personality, 68*, 29–50.*

Tellegen, A., Lykken, D. T., Bouchard, T. J., Wilcox, K., Segal, N., & Rich, S. (1988). Personality similarity in twins reared apart and together. *Journal of Personality and Social Psychology, 54*, 1031–1039.

Torgersen, S. Skre, I., Onstad, S., Edvardsen, J., & Kringlen, E. (1993). The psychometric-genetic structure of DSM-III-R personality disorder criteria. *Journal of Personality Disorders, 7*, 196–213.*

Viding, E., Blair, J. R., Moffitt, T. E., & Plomin, R. (in press). Psychopathic syndrome indexes strong genetic risk for antisocial behavior in 7-year-olds. *Journal of Child Psychology and Psychiatry.*

Waldman, I. D. (1996). Aggressive children's hostile perceptual and response biases: The role of attention and impulsivity. *Child Development, 67*, 1015–1033.

Waldman, I. D. (2005). Statistical approaches to complex phenotypes: Evaluating neuropsychological endophenotypes for ADHD. *Biological Psychiatry, 57*, 1347–1356.

Waldman, I. D., & Gizer, I. (in press). The genetics of ADHD. *Clinical Psychology Review.*

Widom, C. S., & Ames, A. (1988). Biology and female crime. In T. E. Moffitt & S. A. Mednick (Eds.), *Biological contributions to crime causation* (pp. 308–331). Dordrecht, The Netherlands: Martinus Nijhoff.

Wilson, G. D., Rust, J., & Kasriel, J. (1977). Genetic and family origins of humor preferences: A twin study. *Psychological Reports, 41*(2), 659–660.

Wilson, J. Q., & Herrnstein, R. J. (1985). *Crime and human nature.* New York: Simon & Schuster.

APPENDIX 11.1. Terms Used in PsycInfo and Medline Searches

aggressive or		twin(s) or
aggression or		adoptee(s) or
antisocial or		adoptive or
conduct or		genetic or
psychopathy or		genetics or
sociopathy or		genes or
crime or		environmental or
criminal or	and	environment
criminality or		
delinquent or		
delinquency or		
behavior problem(s) or		
problem behavior(s)		

APPENDIX 11.2. Correlations for Adoption and Twin Relationships

Relationship	Correlation
Adoption studies	
Adoptee–adoptive parent	1*C
Adoptee–biological parent	.5*A
Biological child–biological parent	.5*A + 1*C
Adoptive siblings	1*C
Biological siblings	.5*A + 1*C + .25*D
Twin studies	
MZ twin pairs reared together	1*A + 1*C + 1*D
DZ twin pairs reared together	.5*A + 1*C + .25*D
MZ twin pairs reared apart	1*A + 1*D
DZ twin pairs reared apart	.5*A + .25*D

12

Family Background and Psychopathy

DAVID P. FARRINGTON

Psychopathy, at least as operationally defined by the family of Psychopathy Checklist (PCL) measures, is not a unitary construct. It includes explanatory elements such as low empathy, impulsiveness, and a cold, callous and conning personality, as well as behavioral elements such as antisocial and criminal conduct. To investigate the causal linkages between personality and behavior, it has been suggested that psychopathy should be operationally defined only by the personality trait elements of an arrogant and deceitful interpersonal style, deficient affective experience, and an impulsive and irresponsible lifestyle (Cooke, Michie, Hart, & Clark, 2004). However, because this proposal has not yet achieved widespread acceptance, and because most research on family factors has focused on the general syndrome of psychopathy, I concentrate in this chapter on adult psychopathy as operationally defined by total scores on PCL measures.

Few researchers focusing on adult psychopathy have tried to investigate family factors that might predict, influence, or cause it. In contrast, researchers interested in juvenile psychopathy have been more concerned with family factors (see Campbell, Porter, & Santor, 2004; Forth & Burke, 1998). The neglect of family factors in adult studies is surprising in light of the pioneering research by William and Joan McCord (1964), who argued that parental rejection, an antisocial parent, erratic discipline, and poor parental supervision all influenced the development of psychopathy. Similarly, despite the seminal work of Lee Robins (1966, 1979), "we have relatively few studies that have measured the effects of these [child and family] risks, prospectively measured, an adult personality disorder symptoms" (Cohen, 1996, p.126). The neglect of family factors by adult psychopathy researchers is even more surprising in light of the influential research of John Bowlby (1951), who argued that if a child suffered a prolonged period of maternal deprivation during the first 5 years of life, it would have irreversible negative effects, including causing the child to become a cold "affectionless character" and a delinquent. There are very few recent reviews of family factors in relation to psychopathy (e.g., McCord, 2001).

The main aim of this chapter is to review what is known about family background factors as predictors of psychopathy. The best method of establishing that a family factor predicts later psychopathy is to carry out a prospective longitudinal survey, and the emphasis in this chapter is on results obtained in such surveys (see Kalb, Farrington, & Loeber, 2001; Loeber & Farrington, 1997). They avoid retrospective bias (e.g., where the recollections of parents about their child-rearing methods are biased by the knowledge that their child has become a psychopath) and help in establishing causal order. Also, psychopaths emerge naturally from an initially nonpsychopathic population in community surveys, avoiding the problem of how to choose a control group of nonpsychopaths. If extreme groups (e.g., psychopaths vs. well-behaved nonoffenders) are compared, it will lead to an overestimate of the strength of relationships between explanatory variables and psychopathy. Retrospective case–control studies of psychopaths (cases) and nonpsychopathic offenders (controls) are problematic, because it is not clear that they will shed much light on the development of psychopathy in the general population. In investigating the causes of psychopathy, prospective probabilities (e.g., the proportion of poorly supervised children who become psychopaths) are more relevant than retrospective probabilities (e.g., the proportion of psychopaths who were poorly supervised by their parents).

Unfortunately, there are very few prospective longitudinal surveys that specifically investigate the development of psychopathy in adults. Consequently, much of this chapter reviews knowledge gained in longitudinal surveys of criminal behavior. Psychopathy is highly correlated with persistent, serious and violent offending. As Hart and Hare (1997) pointed out: "Many psychopaths engage in chronic criminal conduct and do so at a high rate, whereas only a small minority of those who engage in criminal conduct are psychopaths. This means that psychopaths are responsible for a disproportionate amount of crime in our society" (p. 22).

On the other hand, it should be pointed out that the two widely accepted components of psychopathy (Factor 1, measuring affective–interpersonal symptoms; Factor 2, measuring an antisocial lifestyle) are differentially related to chronic offending and antisocial personality disorder. The affective/interpersonal component is much less strongly associated, particularly when its overlap with the antisocial lifestyle component is controlled for (Verona, Patrick, & Joiner, 2001).

The vast majority of persistent or chronic offenders score high on measures of antisocial personality; for example, in the Cambridge Study—discussed later—Farrington (2000) found that 93% of adult chronic offenders (with five or more convictions after age 21) were among the most antisocial

quarter of men, in terms of features of antisocial personality disorder, at age 32. However, there are few prospective longitudinal studies of family factors as predictors of persistent or chronic offending. Generally, chronic offenders are more extreme than nonchronic offenders in their possession of early family risk factors (Farrington & West, 1993). Therefore, studies of family factors as predictors of offending are likely to underestimate the strength of these factors as predictors of chronic offending or psychopathy in community samples.

One of the reasons for the scarcity of prospective longitudinal studies specifically focusing on psychopathy in community samples is the fact that the PCL-R was largely designed to be used with male prisoners. However, the development of the PCL:SV (Forth, Brown, Hart, & Hare, 1996) made longitudinal studies of psychopathy more feasible. The PCL:SV takes less time to complete, its scores are highly correlated (.8) with PCL-R scores, and it measures the same underlying constructs (Cooke, Michie, Hart, & Hare, 1999). There is still the problem of the low prevalence of "psychopaths" in community samples, but it seems useful to regard psychopathy as a dimension rather than a category and to investigate the causes and development of people with high psychopathy scores.

THE CAMBRIDGE STUDY

This chapter presents results obtained in the Cambridge Study in Delinquent Development, which is a 40-year prospective longitudinal survey of the development of offending and antisocial behavior. In this survey, 411 London boys have been followed up from age 8 to age 48 (Farrington, 2003; Farrington et al., in press). Various individual, family, and socioeconomic risk factors were measured at ages 8–10, before any of the boys could be convicted. At age 48, 365 of the 394 men who were still alive were interviewed (93%). Of the 365 who completed a social interview, 304 (83%) also completed a medical interview including the Structured Clinical Interview for DSM-IV (SCID-II) and the PCL:SV. The SCID-II assessed a wide variety of Axis II personality disorders, including avoidant, dependent, obsessive–compulsive, paranoid, schizoid, histrionic, narcissistic, borderline, and antisocial. The PCL:SV was originally scored by Dr. Crystal Romilly and checked by Dr. Simone Ullrich. Conviction records were taken into account in scoring the PCL:SV. Scores on the 12-item PCL:SV ranged from 0 to 17 (of a possible maximum of 24), with a mean of 3.5 and a standard deviation of 3.8.

Up to age 48, 165 men (40%) were convicted out of 404 at risk (that is, excluding 7 men who emigrated permanently before age 21 and therefore could not be searched for convictions). Of the convicted men, 29 were defined as chronic offenders because they had 10 or more convictions. These chronic offenders (7% of the sample) accounted for 53% of all convictions.

When PCL:SV scores were compared with numbers of convictions, it was clear that there were qualitative differences between those scoring 10 or more on the PCL-SV and the remainder. Table 12.1 shows that 97% of the 33 men scoring 10 or more (11% of the sample) were convicted, compared with 55% of those scoring 3–9 and only 17% of those scoring 0–2. Nearly half (48%) of the men scoring 10 or more were chronic offenders, compared with 1% of the remainder. The vast majority of chronic offenders who completed the medical interview (16 of 20) scored 10 or more on the PCL:SV. The average number of convictions and average number of antisocial personality disorder criteria fulfilled on the SCID-II were also high for those scoring 10 or more on the PCL:SV.

As expected, the affective–interpersonal (Factor 1) and antisocial lifestyle (Factor 2) components of the PCL:SV were differentially related to convictions and antisocial personality disorder (APD) criteria on the SCID-II. The affective component correlated

.53 with the number of convictions, compared with .72 for the antisocial component and .71 for the total score. Two of the antisocial items directly reflect adolescent and adult antisocial behavior. The affective component correlated .58 with the APD score, compared with .81 for the antisocial component and .79 for the total score. The affective and antisocial components correlated .65.

In light of these results, it was decided to investigate early risk factors for:

1. The 33 men who scored 10 or more on the PCL:SV (11%)—termed the "most psychopathic" males—versus the remaining 271.
2. The 31 men who scored 4 or more on the affective–interpersonal component (10%), versus the remaining 273.
3. The 32 men who scored 7 or more on the antisocial lifestyle component (11%), versus the remaining 272.

Half of the high antisocial scorers (16) were also high affective scorers.

Of course, it must be admitted that even the "most psychopathic" males in this community sample would not necessarily be classified as clinical "psychopaths." According to the PCL:SV manual (Hart, Cox, & Hare, 1995), a "high" score in a community sample is 16 or above. Only two men at age 48 achieved this score, suggesting that few of the "most psychopathic" men suffered from a severe personality disorder. Nevertheless, based on the distribution of PCL:SV scores within this sample, it is correct to say that 33 males were the "most psychopathic" at age 48 according to this measure of psychopathy. There is no other longitudinal study that has related childhood risk factors to measures of psychopathy or antisocial personality 40 years later.

TABLE 12.1 Differences among PCL:SV Scores

PCL:SV score	No. of men	Mean APD	Mean convictions	% convicted	% chronic
0–2	162	0.2	0.2	17.4	0.0
3–5	74	1.1	1.5	52.7	1.4
6–9	35	2.1	3.3	60.0	8.6
10+	33	5.8	9.3	97.0	48.5

Note. APD, number of antisocial personality disorder criteria fulfilled on the SCID-II.

FAMILY FACTORS

Reviews of the literature confirm the importance of family factors as predictors of offending. Smith and Stern (1997) concluded:

> We know that children who grow up in homes characterized by lack of warmth and support, whose parents lack behavior management skills, and whose lives are characterized by conflict or maltreatment will more likely be delinquent, whereas a supportive family can protect children even in a very hostile and damaging external environment.... Parental monitoring or supervision is the aspect of family management that is most consistently related to delinquency. (pp. 383–384)

Lipsey and Derzon (1998) reviewed the predictors at ages 6–11 of serious or violent offending at ages 15–25. The best explanatory predictors (i.e., predictors not measuring some aspect of the child's antisocial behavior) were antisocial parents, male gender, low socioeconomic status of the family, and psychological factors such as daring, impulsiveness, and poor concentration. Other moderately strong predictors were minority race, poor parent–child relations (poor supervision, discipline, low parental involvement, low parental warmth), other family characteristics (parent stress, family size, parental discord), antisocial peers, low intelligence, and low school achievement. In contrast, abusive parents and broken homes were relatively weak predictors. It is clear that some family factors are at least as important in the prediction of serious and violent offending as are gender and race.

Reviewing these kinds of results reveals the bewildering variety of family constructs that have been studied, and also the variety of methods used to classify them into categories. In this chapter, family factors are grouped into seven categories: (1) childrearing problems (poor supervision, poor discipline, coldness and rejection, low parental involvement with the child); (2) abuse (physical or sexual) or neglect; (3) parental conflict and disrupted families; (4) large family size; (5) criminal or antisocial parents or siblings; (6) other characteristics of parents (young age, substance abuse, stress or depression, working mothers); and (7) socioeconomic factors such as low income and poor housing. These groupings are somewhat arbitrary and reflect the organization of topics of investigation within the field. For example, harsh discipline is usually studied along with poor supervision but, at the extreme, it could shade into physical abuse. Physical neglect is usually grouped with physical abuse but of course it usually coincides with emotional neglect (cold and rejecting parents). Extrafamilial factors (peer, school, and neighborhood) are discussed later, along with biopsychosocial interactions and protective factors. Finally, findings on family-based prevention are reviewed.

CHILDREARING PROBLEMS

Many different types of childrearing problems predict offending, as well as chronic offending (Farrington & West, 1993) and high antisocial personality scores (Farrington, 2000). The most important dimensions of childrearing are supervision or monitoring of children, discipline or parental reinforcement, warmth or coldness of emotional relationships, and parental involvement with children. Unlike family size, these constructs are difficult to measure with high reliability and validity, and there is some evidence that results differ according to methods of measurement. In their extensive review of parenting methods in relation to childhood antisocial behavior, Rothbaum and Weisz (1994) concluded that the strength of associations between parent and child measures was greater when parenting was measured by observation or interview than when it was measured using questionnaires.

Parental supervision refers to the degree of monitoring by parents of the child's activities, and their degree of watchfulness or vigilance. Of all these childrearing methods, poor parental supervision is usually the strongest and most replicable predictor of offending (Farrington & Loeber 1999; Smith & Stern, 1997), as well as chronic offending (Farrington & West, 1993) and high antisocial personality scores (Farrington, 2000). Many studies show that parents who do not know where their children are when they are out, and parents who let their children roam the streets unsupervised from an early age, tend to have delinquent children. For example, in the classic Cambridge–Somerville study in Boston, poor parental supervision in childhood was the best predictor of both violent and property crimes up to age 45 (McCord, 1979).

Parental discipline refers to how parents react to a child's behavior. It is clear that harsh or punitive discipline (involving physical punishment) predicts offending, as the review by Haapasalo and Pokela (1999) showed. In a follow-up study of nearly 700 Nottingham children, John and Elizabeth Newson (1989) found that physical punishment at ages 7 and 11 predicted later convictions; 40% of offenders had been smacked or beaten at age 11, compared with 14% of nonoffenders. Erratic or inconsistent discipline also predicts delinquency (West & Farrington, 1973). This can involve either erratic discipline by one parent, sometimes turning a blind eye to bad behavior and sometimes punishing it severely, or inconsistency between two parents, with one parent being tolerant or indulgent and the other being harshly punitive. Just as inappropriate methods of responding to bad behavior predict offending, low parental reinforcement (not praising) of good behavior is also a predictor (Farrington & Loeber, 1999).

Cold, rejecting parents tend to have delinquent children, as McCord (1979) found in the Cambridge–Somerville study in Boston. She also concluded that parental warmth could act as a protective factor against the effects of physical punishment (McCord, 1997). Whereas 51% of boys with cold physically punishing mothers were convicted in her study, only 21% of boys with warm physically punishing mothers were convicted—similar to the 23% of boys with warm nonpunitive mothers who were convicted. The father's warmth was also a protective factor against the father's physical punishment.

Low parental involvement in the child's activities predicts subsequent offending, as the Newsons found in their Nottingham survey (Lewis, Newson, & Newson, 1982). In the Cambridge Study, having a father who never joined in the boy's leisure activities doubled his risk of conviction (West & Farrington, 1973), and this was the most important predictor of persistence in offending after age 21 as opposed to desistance (Farrington & Hawkins, 1991). Similarly, poor parent–child communication predicted

offending in the Pittsburgh Youth Study (Farrington & Loeber, 1999), and low family cohesiveness was the most important predictor of violence in the Chicago Youth Development Study (Gorman-Smith, Tolan, Zelli, & Huesmann, 1996).

Marshall and Cooke (1999) compared psychopathic and nonpsychopathic prisoners in Scotland using the PCL-R and found that significantly more of the psychopathic prisoners had experienced parental indifference or neglect, poor parental supervision, and poor parental discipline. In the Cambridge Study, poor parental supervision, measured at age 8, significantly predicted high psychopathy scores at age 48 (actually based on information between ages 18 and 48). Table 12.2 shows that 24% of boys who were poorly supervised at age 8 (because their parents did not know where they were when they went out) had high psychopathy scores at age 48, compared with 8% of the remainder (odds ratio [OR] = 3.6, confidence interval 1.9–7.0, 2 = 3.22, p = .0006, one-tailed tests used in light of directional predictions). Generally, an OR of 2.0 or greater indicates a strong relationship (Cohen, 1996). Interestingly, poor parental supervision predicted high antisocial (Factor 2) scores (OR = 3.9) but not high affective (Factor 1) scores (OR = 1.9).

In contrast, harsh or erratic parental discipline at age 8 predicted both high affective component scores and high antisocial component scores; 19% of boys suffering harsh discipline at age 8 had high total scores at age 48, compared with 8% of the remainder (OR = 2.6, CI 1.4–4.8, z = 2.47, p = .007). Low paternal involvement with the boy (the father not joining in the boy's activities) was a strong predictor of high psychopathy scores (OR = 6.5) and it predicted high affective scores most (Table 12.2).

Most explanations of the link between childrearing methods and later offending focus on attachment or social learning theories. Attachment theory was inspired by the work of Bowlby (1951) and suggests that children who are not emotionally attached to warm, loving, and prosocial parents tend to become antisocial (Carlson & Sroufe, 1995). Social learning theories (e.g., Patterson, 1982, 1995) suggest that children's behavior depends on parental rewards and punishments and on the models of behavior that

TABLE 12.2. Early Predictors of Psychopathy at age 48

Risk factor at ages 8–11	% PCL:SV 10+			Affective OR	Antisocial OR
	No	Yes	OR		
Poor supervision	8	24	3.6*	1.9	3.9*
Harsh discipline	8	19	2.6*	2.3*	2.0*
Father uninvolved	4	23	6.5*	4.7*	2.7*
Physical neglect	8	34	5.9*	4.8*	5.2*
Disrupted family	7	25	4.3*	1.9*	4.6*
Large family size	7	22	3.5*	3.0*	3.8*
Convicted father	6	25	5.1*	4.4*	3.8*
Convicted mother	9	30	4.5*	3.2*	4.7*
Delinquent sibling	9	28	4.0*	3.6*	4.2*
Young mother	9	19	2.4*	1.4	2.6*
Depressed mother	8	18	2.7*	2.1*	3.3*
Low social class	8	22	3.1*	2.5*	2.8*
Low family income	7	25	4.6*	3.9*	3.6*
Poor housing	7	18	3.0*	1.7	2.9*
Unpopular	7	18	2.9*	2.9*	1.5
Delinquent school	7	24	3.9*	2.9*	2.7*
Low nonverbal IQ	8	18	2.4*	2.4*	1.9
Low verbal IQ	8	19	2.3*	3.5*	1.3
Low school track	7	19	3.0*	3.0*	2.1*
High daring	7	21	3.6*	2.0*	2.6*
Lacks concentration	8	23	3.6*	2.5*	2.8*
High impulsivity	8	18	2.4*	2.7*	1.9
Dishonest	7	22	4.1*	2.0	4.4*
Troublesome	8	23	3.4*	2.0*	2.7*

Note. The figures show the percentages of those without the risk factor (No) and with the risk factor (Yes) who scored 10+ on the PCL:SV. OR, odds ratio; Affective OR, OR for Factor 1; Antisocial OR, OR for Factor 2. Nonsignificant predictors: authoritarian parent, parental conflict, depressed father, low junior school attainment.
* $p < .05$, one-tailed.

parents provide. Children tend to become antisocial if parents do not respond consistently and contingently to their bad behavior and if parents themselves behave in an antisocial manner.

CHILD ABUSE AND NEGLECT

Children who are physically abused or neglected tend to become offenders later in life. The most famous study of this phenomenon was carried out by Widom (1989) in Indianapolis. She used court records to identify over 900 children who had been abused or neglected before age 11 and compared them with a control group matched on age, race, gender, elementary school class, and place of residence. A 20-year follow-up showed that the children who were abused or neglected were more likely to be arrested as juveniles and as adults than were the controls, and

they were more likely to be arrested for juvenile violence (Maxfield & Widom, 1996). Child sexual abuse and child physical abuse and neglect also predicted adult arrests for sex crimes (Widom & Ames, 1994). Most important, Luntz and Widom (1994) showed that child abuse predicted adult antisocial personality disorder, and Weiler and Widom (1996) found that child abuse predicted high PCL-R scores in adulthood, for males and females and African American and white children.

Similar results have been obtained in other studies. An extensive review by Malinosky-Rummell and Hansen (1993) confirmed that being physically abused as a child predicted later violent and nonviolent offending. For example, in the Cambridge–Somerville study in Boston, McCord (1983) found that about half of the abused or neglected boys were convicted for serious crimes, became alcoholics or mentally ill, or died before age 35.

In Stockholm, Lang, af Klinteberg, and Alm (2002) reported that boys who were abused or neglected at ages 11–14 tended to become violent and to have high PCL scores at age 36. Retrospective studies of offenders by Koivisto and Haapasalo (1996) in Finland and by Patrick, Zempolich, and Levenston (1997) in Florida found correlations between early child abuse and high PCL-R scores, but Marshall and Cooke (1999) in Scotland reported no difference in physical abuse histories between psychopathic and nonpsychopathic prisoners. In the Cambridge Study, physical neglect of the boy at age 8 predicted his high psychopathy scores 40 years later and also predicted high affective and antisocial component scores (Table 12.2).

Possible environmental causal mechanisms linking childhood victimization and later antisocial behavior were reviewed by Widom (1994). First, childhood victimization may have immediate but long-lasting consequences (e.g., shaking may cause brain injury). Second, childhood victimization may cause bodily changes (e.g., desensitization to pain) that encourage later violence. Third, child abuse may lead to impulsive or dissociative coping styles that, in turn, lead to poor problem-solving skills or poor school performance. Fourth, victimization may cause changes in self-esteem or in social information-processing patterns that encourage later violence. Fifth, child abuse may lead to changed family environments (e.g., being placed in foster care) that have deleterious effects. Sixth, juvenile justice practices may label victims, isolate them from prosocial peers, and encourage them to associate with delinquent peers.

PARENTAL CONFLICT AND DISRUPTED FAMILIES

Bowlby (1951) popularized the theory that broken homes cause delinquency. He argued that mother love in infancy and childhood was just as important for mental health as were vitamins and proteins for physical health. He thought that it was essential that a child should experience a warm, loving, and continuous relationship with a mother figure. If a child suffered a prolonged period of maternal deprivation during the first 5 years of life, it would have irreversible negative effects, including becoming a cold "affectionless character" and a criminal.

Most studies of broken homes have focused on the loss of the father rather than the mother, because the loss of a father is much more common. In general, it is found that children who are separated from a biological parent are more likely to offend than children from intact families. For example, in a birth cohort study of children born in Newcastle-upon-Tyne, Kolvin, Miller, Fleeting, and Kolvin (1988b) discovered that boys who experienced divorce or separation in their first 5 years of life had a doubled risk of conviction up to age 32 (53% as opposed to 28%).

McCord (1982) carried out an interesting study in Boston of the later serious offending (up to age 45) of boys from homes broken by loss of the biological father. She found that the prevalence of offending was high for boys from broken homes without affectionate mothers (62%) and for those from unbroken homes characterized by parental conflict (52%), irrespective of whether they had affectionate mothers. The prevalence of offending was low for those from unbroken homes without conflict (26%) and—importantly—equally low for boys from broken homes with affectionate mothers (22%). These results suggest that it might not be the broken home that is criminogenic but rather the parental conflict that often contributes to family breakdown. They also suggest that a loving mother might to some degree be able to compensate for the loss of a father.

A meta-analysis by Wells and Rankin (1991) showed that broken homes were more strongly related to delinquency when they were caused by parental separation or divorce rather than by death. In the Cambridge Study, coming from a disrupted family (separation from a parent before the 10th birthday for reasons other than death or hospitalization) predicted high antisocial personality scores at age 32 (Farrington, 2000) and high psychopathy scores at age 48 (Table 12.2). Coming from a disrupted family predicted the antisocial component of psychopathy but not the affective component. However, while the retrospective study by Koivisto and Haapasalo (1996) in Finland found a correlation between broken homes and high PCL-R scores, Patrick and colleagues (1997) in Florida reported that psychopathic prisoners were less likely than nonpsychopathic prisoners to come from single-parent homes.

Many studies show that parental conflict and interparental violence predict later antisocial behavior (see Buehler et al., 1997; Kolbo, Blakely, & Engleman, 1996). In the Christchurch Health and Development Study in New Zealand, children who witnessed violence between their parents were more likely to commit both violence and property offenses according to their self-reports (Fergusson & Horwood, 1998). The predictability of witnessing father-initiated violence held up after controlling for other risk factors such as parental criminality, parental substance abuse, parental physical punishment, a young mother, and low family income. Parental conflict also predicted offending in both the Cambridge and Pittsburgh studies (Farrington & Loeber, 1999). However, parental conflict at age 8 did not significantly predict later psychopathy scores at age 48 (Table 12.2), and Marshall and Cooke (1999) in Scotland found that psychopathic and nonpsychopathic prisoners were not quite significantly different on early parental discord.

Explanations of the relationship between disrupted families and later antisocial behavior fall into three major classes. Trauma theories suggest that the loss of a parent has a damaging effect on a child, most commonly because of the effect on attachment to the parent. Life-course theories focus on separation as a sequence of stressful experiences, and on the effects of multiple stressors such as parental conflict, parental loss, reduced economic circumstances, changes in parent figures, and poor child-rearing methods. Selection theories argue that disrupted families produce delinquent children because of preexisting differences from other families in risk factors such as parental conflict, criminal or antisocial parents, low family income, or poor child-rearing methods.

Hypotheses derived from the three theories were tested in the Cambridge Study (Juby & Farrington, 2001). While boys from broken homes (permanently disrupted families) were more delinquent than boys from intact homes; they were not more delinquent than boys from intact high conflict families. Overall, the most important factor was the postdisruption trajectory. Boys who remained with their mother after the separation had the same delinquency rate as boys from intact low-conflict families. Boys who remained with their father, with relatives, or with others (foster parents) had high offending rates. It was concluded that the results favored life-course theories rather than trauma or selection theories.

LARGE FAMILY SIZE

Large family size (a large number of children in the family) is a relatively strong and highly replicable predictor of offending (Ellis, 1988; Fischer, 1984). It was similarly important in the Cambridge and Pittsburgh studies, even though families were on average smaller in Pittsburgh in the 1990s than in London in the 1960s (Farrington & Loeber, 1999). In the Cambridge Study, if a boy had four or more siblings by his 10th birthday, his risk of being convicted as a juvenile was doubled (West & Farrington, 1973). Large family size was the most important independent predictor of convictions up to age 32 in a logistic regression analysis; 58% of boys from large families were convicted up to this age (Farrington, 1993). Large family size at the 10th birthday also predicted chronic offenders (Farrington & West, 1993), high antisocial personality scores at age 32 (Farrington, 2000), and high psychopathy scores at age 48 (Table 12.2).

There are many possible reasons why a large number of siblings might increase the risk of a child's delinquency. Generally, as the number of children in a family increases, the amount of parental attention that can be given to each child decreases. Also, as the number of children increases, the household tends to become more overcrowded, possibly leading to increases in frustration, irritation, and conflict. In the Cambridge Study, large family size did not predict delinquency for boys living in the least crowded conditions, with two or more rooms than there were children (West & Farrington, 1973). This suggests that household overcrowding might be an important factor mediating the association between large family size and offending.

CRIME RUNS IN FAMILIES

Generally, multimodal interventions are more effective than single-modality interventions (Wasserman & Miller, 1998). Multisystemic therapy (MST) is an important multiple-component family preservation program that was developed for chronic delinquents by Henggeler, Melton, Smith, Schoenwald, and Hanley (1993) in South Carolina. In this approach, the particular type of treatment is chosen according to the particular needs of the youth. Therefore, the nature of the treatment is different for each person. MST is delivered in the youth's home, school, and community settings. The treatment typically includes family intervention to promote the parent's ability to monitor and discipline the adolescent, peer intervention to encourage the choice of prosocial friends, and school intervention to enhance competence and school achievement

Similar results were obtained in the Pittsburgh Youth Study, a prospective longitudinal survey of Pittsburgh males ages 7–25. Arrests of fathers, mothers, brothers, sisters, uncles, aunts, grandfathers, and grandmothers all predicted the boy's own delinquency (Farrington, Jolliffe, Loeber, Stouthamer-Loeber, & Kalb, 2001). The most important relative was the father; arrests of the father predicted the boy's delinquency independently of all other arrested relatives. Only 8% of families accounted for 43% of arrested family members. There seems to be no longitudinal study specifically relating psychopathy of parents to psychopathy of children, but in Copenhagen Brennan, Mednick, and Mednick (1993) found that parental psychopathology (including psychopathy) significantly predicted violence by sons up to age 22. Also, Harris, Rice, and Lalumiere (2001) showed that antisociality in parents (identified on the basis of a composite measure incorporating parental criminality and alcoholism along with child abuse and neglect) was related to higher psychopathy in a sample of violent offenders drawn from a Canadian maximum security psychiatric hospital.

In the Cambridge Study, having a convicted parent or a delinquent older sibling by the 10th birthday were consistently among the best ages 8–10 predictors of the boy's later offending and antisocial behavior.

Apart from behavioral measures such as troublesomeness and daring, they were the strongest predictors of juvenile convictions (Farrington, 1992a) and chronic offending (Farrington & West, 1993). Having a convicted parent was the best predictor of high antisocial personality scores at age 32 (Farrington, 2000). Table 12.2 shows that having a convicted father, a convicted mother, or a delinquent sibling by the 10th birthday significantly predicted high psychopathy scores at age 48. Having a convicted father was a strong predictor of the most psychopathic males: 25% of males with a convicted father scored 10 or more on the PCL:SV, compared with 6% of the remainder (OR = 5.1, CI 2.7–9.7, z = 4.23, p < .0001).

Farrington and colleagues (2001) reviewed six possible explanations for why antisocial behavior was concentrated in families and transmitted from one generation to the next. First, there may be intergenerational continuities in exposure to multiple risk factors such as poverty, disrupted families, and living in deprived neighborhoods. Second, assortative mating (the tendency of antisocial females to choose antisocial males as partners) facilitates the intergenerational transmission of antisocial behavior. Third, family members may influence each other (e.g., older siblings may encourage younger ones to be antisocial). Fourth, the effect of an antisocial parent on a child's antisocial behavior may be mediated by environmental mechanisms such as poor parental supervision and inconsistent discipline. Fifth, intergenerational transmission may be mediated by genetic mechanisms. Sixth, there may be labeling and police bias against known criminal families.

OTHER PARENTAL FEATURES

Numerous other parental features predict antisocial behavior. For example, early childbearing or teenage pregnancy is a risk factor. Morash and Rucker (1989) analyzed results from four surveys in the United States and England (including the Cambridge Study) and found that teenage mothers tended to coincide with low-income families and tended to have welfare support and absent biological fathers. In addition they tended to use poor childrearing methods, and their children were often characterized by low school attainment and delinquency. However, the presence of the biological father mitigated many of these adverse factors and generally seemed to have a protective effect (see below). Similarly, a large-scale study in Washington State showed that children of teenage or unmarried mothers had a significantly increased risk of offending (Conseur, Rivara, Barnoski, & Emanuel, 1997). Boys born to unmarried mothers ages 17 or less showed an 11-fold increase in the risk of chronic offending compared with boys born to married mothers aged 20 or more.

In the Cambridge and Pittsburgh studies, the age of the mother at her first birth was only a moderate predictor of the boy's later delinquency (Farrington & Loeber, 1999). In the Cambridge Study, for example, 27% of sons of teenage mothers were convicted as juveniles, compared with 18% of the remainder. More detailed analyses in this study showed that teenage mothers who went on to have large numbers of children were especially likely to have convicted children (Nagin, Pogarsky, & Farrington, 1997). It was concluded that the results were concordant with a diminished resources theory: The offspring of adolescent mothers were more crime-prone because they lacked not only economic resources but also personal resources such as attention and supervision. Also, because juvenile delinquency is a predictor of causing an early pregnancy (Smith et al., 2000), the link between teenage parents and child delinquency may be a consequence of the link between teenage and criminal parents. Table 12.2 shows that the boys born to teenage mothers were significantly likely to have high PCL:SV scores at age 48. Teenage mothers also predicted high antisocial personality scores at age 32 (Farrington, 2000).

High parental stress and parental anxiety or depression also predicted delinquency in the Pittsburgh Youth Study (Loeber, Farrington, Stouthamer-Loeber, & van Kammen, 1998). In the Cambridge Study, having a mother who was anxious or depressed (according to psychiatric social worker ratings, a health questionnaire, or psychiatric records) predicted high antisocial personality scores at age 18 but not at age 32 (Farrington, 2000). However, having an anxious or depressed mother predicted high psychopathy scores at age 48 (Table 12.2).

Substance use by parents also predicts antisocial behavior by children, according to the findings of the Pittsburgh Youth Study (Loeber, Farrington, Stouthamer-Loeber, & van Kammen, 1998). Smoking by the mother during pregnancy is a particularly important risk factor. A large-scale follow-up of a general population cohort in Finland showed that maternal smoking during pregnancy doubled the risk of violent or persistent offending by male offspring, after controlling for other biopsychosocial risk factors (Rasanen et al., 1999). When maternal smoking was combined with a teenage mother, a single-parent family, and an unwanted pregnancy, the risk of offending increased 10-fold.

SOCIOECONOMIC FACTORS

In general, coming from a low-social-class family predicts later violence. For example, in the U.S. National Youth Survey, prevalence rates for self-reported assault and robbery were about twice as high among lower-class youth as among middle-class youth (Elliott, Huizinga, & Menard, 1989). In Project Metropolitan in Stockholm (Wikström, 1985) and in the Dunedin study in New Zealand (Henry, Caspi, Moffitt, & Silva, 1996), the socioeconomic status of a boy's family—based on the father's occupation—predicted his later violent crimes.

Low socioeconomic status is a less consistent predictor of offending. One source of variability relates to whether it is measured by income and housing or by occupational prestige. In the Cambridge Study, low family income and poor housing predicted official and self-reported, juvenile and adult offending, but low parental occupational prestige predicted only self-reported offending (Farrington, 1992a, 1992b). Also, low family income and low socioeconomic status (but not poor housing) significantly predicted chronic offending (Farrington & West, 1993) and high antisocial personality scores at age 32 (Farrington, 2000). Table 12.2 shows that low family income at age 8, low social class at ages 8–10 (based on occupational prestige), and poor housing at ages 8–10 all predicted high psychopathy scores at age 48. The strongest predictor was low family income. However, in their retrospective study, Patrick and colleagues (1997) found no significant relationship between socioeconomic status and PCL-R scores among prisoners.

PEER, SCHOOL, AND NEIGHBORHOOD FACTORS

It is well established that having delinquent friends is an important predictor of offending (Lipsey & Derzon, 1998). What is less clear is whether antisocial peers encourage and facilitate adolescent antisocial behavior, or whether it is merely the case that "birds of a feather flock together." Delinquents may have delinquent friends because of co-offending, which is particularly common under age 21 (Reiss & Farrington, 1991). However, Elliott and Menard (1996) in the U.S. National Youth Survey concluded that delinquent friends influenced an adolescent's own delinquency and that the reverse was also true: More delinquent adolescents were more likely to have delinquent friends. Delinquent friends were not measured until age 14 in the Cambridge Study, but chronic offenders significantly tended to have them (Farrington & West, 1993).

There is no doubt that highly aggressive children tend to be rejected by most of their peers (Coie, Dodge, & Kupersmidt, 1990). In the Oregon Youth Study, peer rejection at ages 9–10 significantly predicted adult antisocial behavior at ages 23–24 (Nelson & Dishion, 2004). In Stockholm, Freidenfelt and af Klinteberg (2003) found that unpopularity predicted high PCL scores among hyperactive boys but not among nonhyperactive boys. Low popularity at ages 8–10 was only a marginal predictor of adolescent aggression and teenage violence in the Cambridge Study (Farrington, 1989). It significantly predicted chronic offending (Farrington & West, 1993) but not high antisocial personality scores at age 32 (Farrington, 2000). Low popularity significantly predicted high affective and high total scores at age 48 (Table 12.2). Coie and Miller-Johnson (2001) found that it was the boys who were both aggressive and rejected by their classmates who became the self-reported and official offenders.

It is also well established that delinquents disproportionately attend high delinquency-rate schools, which have high levels of distrust between teachers and students, low commitment to the school by students, and unclear and inconsistently enforced rules (Graham, 1988). In the Cambridge Study, attending a high delinquency-rate school at age 11 significantly predicted a boy's own delinquency (Farrington, 1992a), as well as his chronic offending (Farrington & West, 1993) and high antisocial personality scores at age 32 (Farrington, 2000). Table 12.2 shows that attending a high delinquency-rate school also significantly predicted high psychopathy scores at age 48.

It is less clear how much the schools themselves influence antisocial behavior by their organization, climate, and practices, and how much the concentration of offenders in certain schools is mainly a function of their intakes. In the Cambridge Study, most of the variation between schools in their delinquency rates could be explained by differences in their intakes of troublesome boys at age 11 (Farrington, 1972). However, reviews of American research show that schools with clear, fair, and consistently enforced rules tend to have low rates of student misbehavior (Gottfredson, 2001; Herrenkohl, Hawkins, Chung, Hill, & Battin-Pearson, 2001).

Many studies show that boys living in urban areas are more violent than those living in rural ones. In the U.S. National Youth Survey, the prevalence of self-reported assault and robbery was considerably higher among urban youth (Elliott et al., 1989). Within urban areas, boys living in high-crime neighborhoods are more violent than those living in low-crime neighborhoods. In the Rochester Youth Development Study, living in a high-crime neighborhood significantly predicted self-reported violence (Thornberry, Huizinga, & Loeber, 1995). Similarly, in the Pittsburgh Youth Study, living in a bad neighborhood (either as rated by the mother, or based on census measures of poverty, unemployment, and female-headed households) significantly predicted official and reported violence (Farrington, 1998).

It is clear that offenders disproportionately live in inner-city areas characterized by physical deterioration, neighborhood disorganization, and high residential mobility

(Shaw & McKay, 1969). However, again, it is difficult to determine how much the areas themselves influence antisocial behavior and how much it is merely the case that antisocial people tend to live in deprived areas (because of their poverty or public housing allocation policies). Interestingly, both neighborhood researchers such as Gottfredson, McNeil, and Gottfredson (1991) and developmental researchers such as Rutter (1981) have concluded that neighborhoods have only indirect effects on antisocial behavior via their effects on individuals and families. However, Sampson, Raudenbush, and Earls (1997) argued that a low degree of "collective efficacy" in a neighborhood (a low degree of informal social control) caused high crime rates.

OTHER RISK FACTORS

Table 12.2 also shows the degree to which other well-known risk factors, measured at ages 8–10 in the Cambridge Study, predicted high psychopathy scores at age 48. Low nonverbal IQ, low verbal IQ, and low school track (but not low junior school attainment) predicted high psychopathy scores at age 48. Interestingly, these measures of intelligence and attainment predicted affective component scores (Factor 1) more strongly than antisocial component scores (Factor 2). High daring (taking many risks), poor concentration or restlessness, and high impulsivity on psychomotor tests all predicted the most psychopathic males. High dishonesty (rates by peers) and high troublesomeness (rated by peers and teachers) also significantly predicted high psychopathy scores at age 48. Daring, dishonesty, and troublesomeness were more strongly predictive of antisocial component scores, whereas high impulsivity was more strongly predictive of affective component scores. Overall, the best predictors of the most psychopathic males were having a convicted father or mother, physical neglect of the boy, low involvement of the father with the boy, low family income, and coming from a disrupted family.

Table 12.2 is only the starting point for analyzing the development and causes of adult psychopathy. More detailed multivariate research is needed to investigate how childhood risk factors predict juvenile conduct disorder and delinquency, and how later risk factors influence the continuity from juvenile to adult antisocial behavior and psychopathy. These more detailed analyses, which should also compare predictors of affective and antisocial component scores, are outside the scope of this review chapter.

BIOPSYCHOSOCIAL INTERACTIONS AND PROTECTIVE FACTORS

Risk factors have many different kinds of interaction effects—for example, between biological and psychosocial variables (see Farrington, 1997). However, the main distinction is between multiplicative effects, where the people with both types of risk factors have the worst outcomes, and protective effects, where in some way the "protective" end of one variable counteracts or nullifies the "risk" end of the other variable.

Multiplicative or additive effects are the most common. In general, the likelihood of an undesirable outcome such as psychopathy increases with the number of risk factors that a person possesses. For example, in the Cambridge Study Farrington (2000) found that the percentage of boys who were antisocial at age 32 increased from 13% of those with no risk factors at ages 8–10 to 61% of those with three or four risk factors at ages 8–10. Magnusson and Bergman (1988) found that many of the significant relationships between early risk factors and adult criminality and psychiatric illness disappeared when a small group of multiple-problem, multiple-risk-factor individuals were taken out of the analysis. Many of the findings regarding predictors of offending in general may be largely attributable to this small group of individuals, who are likely to be disproportionately chronic offenders and psychopaths.

Unfortunately, biopsychosocial interactions have not been studied specifically in relation to psychopathy, although they might be expected. For example, Lykken (1995) argued that people with a "hard-to-socialize temperament" would be at high risk of developing antisocial behavior in all childrearing environments, whereas people without this predisposing temperament would only develop antisocial behavior when exposed to poor childrearing. Wootton, Frick, Shelton, and Silverthorn (1995) tested this hypothesized interaction, using "callous–unemotional" as a measure of a "hard-to-socialize temperament" and poor supervision, inconsistent and harsh discipline, and low praise as measures of poor childrearing. As predicted, they found that the prevalence of conduct disorder/oppositional defiant disorder for callous–unemotional children was high at all levels of childrearing, whereas for other children it increased with the degree of dysfunctional parenting. This type of interaction effect was termed "suppressing–protective" by Farrington (1997) because the probability of a poor outcome is high except when both variables are favorable (here, with the combination of good childrearing and not callous–unemotional).

One of the earliest biopsychosocial interactions was reported by Wadsworth (1976) in the British National Survey of Health and Development. He found that a low pulse rate (resting heart rate) predicted violent and sexual offenses only among boys who had not experienced broken homes by age 4. Pulse rate was not predictive among boys from broken homes. This is again a "suppressing–protective" effect.

The most important research on biopsychosocial interactions has been carried out by Adrian Raine, Patricia Brennan, Sarnoff Mednick, and their colleagues (see, e.g., Raine, Brennan, Farrington, & Mednick, 1997). For example, in a Copenhagen longitudinal survey, Raine, Brennan, and Mednick (1994) found that children who had experienced both birth complications and early maternal rejection at age 12 months were particularly likely to be convicted of violent crimes by age 19. Using the same sample, Brennan and colleagues (1993) showed that children who had experienced both parental psychopathology (including psychopathy) and delivery complications were particularly likely to become violent offenders. These are multiplicative interaction effects.

As mentioned, most previous studies have reported multiplicative rather than protective effects. More research is needed to discover protective factors that might decrease the risk of psychopathy in people who are at risk. For example, in Hawaii, Werner and Smith (1982) studied children who possessed four or more risk factors for offending before age 2 but who nevertheless did not develop behavior problems during childhood or adolescence. They found that the major protective factors included being first-born, being active and affectionate during infancy, small family size, and receiving a large amount of attention from caretakers. In the Newcastle Thousand-Family Study, Kolvin, Miller, Fleeting, and Kolvin (1988a) investigated high-risk boys from deprived backgrounds who did not become delinquents. The major protective factors under age 5 were good mothering, good maternal health, an employed head of household, and being an oldest child. The key challenge is to discover family protective factors that counteract or nullify biological risk factors for psychopathy, and vice versa.

KEY METHODOLOGICAL ISSUES

It is difficult to determine what the precise causal mechanisms are that link family factors—such as parental criminality, young mothers, large family size, poor parental supervision, child abuse, or disrupted families—to later antisocial behavior or psychopathy. This is because these factors tend to be related not only to each other but also to other risk factors such as low family income, poor housing, impulsiveness, low IQ, and low school attainment. Just as it is hard to know what the key underlying family constructs are, it is equally hard to know what the key underlying constructs are in other domains of life. It is important to investigate what family factors predict psychopathy independently of other family factors, independently of genetic and biological factors, and independently of nonfamily factors (e.g., individual, peer, neighborhood, and socioeconomic).

It might be expected that family factors would have different effects on boys and girls, because there are well-documented gender differences in childrearing experiences. In particular, boys are more likely to receive physical punishment from parents (Lytton & Romney, 1991; Smith & Brooks-Gunn, 1997). However, in their extensive review of gender differences in antisocial behavior, Moffitt, Caspi, Rutter, and Silva (2001) concluded that boys were more antisocial essentially because they were exposed to more risk factors or a higher level of risk.

Family risk factors did not seem to have different effects on antisocial behavior for boys and girls.

Family factors may have different effects on African American and white children in the United States. It is clear that African American children are more likely to be physically punished, and that physical punishment is more related to antisocial behavior for white children than for African American children (see Deater-Deckard, Dodge, Bates, & Pettit, 1996; Kelley, Power, & Wimbush, 1992). In the Pittsburgh Youth Study, 21% of white boys who were physically punished (slapped or spanked) by their mothers were violent, compared with 8% of those not physically punished. In contrast, 32% of African American boys who were physically punished were violent, compared with 28% of those not physically punished (Farrington, Loeber, & Stouthamer-Loeber, 2003). It was suggested that physical punishment may have a different meaning in African American families. Specifically, in these families it may indicate warmth and concern for the child, whereas in white families it tended to be associated with a cold and rejecting parental attitude.

It is important to investigate sequential effects of risk factors on psychopathy. Several researchers have concluded that socioeconomic factors have an effect on offending through their effect on family factors (see Dodge, Pettit, & Bates, 1994; Larzelere & Patterson, 1990; Stern & Smith, 1995). In the Pittsburgh Youth Study, it was proposed that socioeconomic and neighborhood factors (e.g., poor housing) influenced family factors (e.g., poor supervision), which in turn influenced child factors (e.g., low guilt) which in turn influenced offending (Loeber et al., 1998, p. 10). There may also be sequential effects of some family factors on others (e.g., if young mothers tend to use poor childrearing methods: see Conger, Patterson, & Ge, 1995), or of family factors on other risk factors (e.g., if antisocial parents tend to have low incomes and live in poor neighborhoods).

Just as parental childrearing methods influence characteristics of children, so child characteristics may influence parenting, as Lytton (1990) suggested. For example, an antisocial child will provoke more punishment from a parent than a well-behaved child. In a longitudinal survey of children living in upper New York State, Cohen and Brook (1995) found that there were reciprocal influences between parental punishment and child behavior disorder.

FAMILY-BASED PREVENTION

Because family factors predict antisocial behavior, it is likely that family-based prevention can reduce antisocial behavior (see Farrington & Welsh, 2003). In the most famous intensive home visiting program implemented in Elmira (New York), Olds, Henderson, Chamberlin, and Tatelbaum (1986) randomly allocated 400 mothers to groups that received (1) home visits from nurses during pregnancy, (2) visits both during pregnancy and during the first 2 years of life, or (3) no visits (control group). Each visit lasted about 1¼ hours, and the mothers were visited on average every 2 weeks. The home visitors gave advice about prenatal and postnatal care of the child, about infant development, and about the importance of proper nutrition and avoiding smoking and drinking during pregnancy. Hence, this was a general parent education program.

The results of this experiment showed that the postnatal home visits caused a decrease in recorded child physical abuse and neglect during the first 2 years of life, especially by poor unmarried teenage mothers; 4% of visited versus 19% of nonvisited mothers within this category were guilty of child abuse or neglect. In a 15-year follow-up, the main focus was on lower-class unmarried mothers. Among these mothers, those who received prenatal and postnatal home visits had fewer arrests than those who received prenatal visits or no visits (Olds et al., 1997). Also, children of these mothers who received prenatal and/or postnatal home visits had less than half as many arrests as children of mothers who received no visits (Olds et al., 1998). Other studies (Kitzman et al., 1997; Stone, Bendell, & Field, 1988) also show that intensive home visiting can reduce later antisocial behavior of children.

One of the very few prevention experiments beginning in pregnancy and collecting outcome data on delinquency was the Syracuse (New York) Family Development Research Program of Lally, Mangione, and

Honig (1988). The researchers began with a sample of pregnant women (mostly poor African American single mothers) and gave them weekly help with childrearing, health, nutrition, and other problems. In addition, the children of these mothers received free full-time day care, designed to develop their intellectual abilities, up to age 5. This was not a randomized experiment, but a matched control group was chosen when the children were age 3. Ten years later, approximately 120 treated and control children were followed up to about age 15. Significantly fewer of the treated children (2% as opposed to 17%) had been referred to the juvenile court for delinquency offenses, and the treated girls showed better school attendance and school performance.

Perhaps the best-known method of parent training was developed by Patterson (1982) in Oregon. Parents were trained to notice what a child was doing, monitor behavior over long periods, clearly state house rules, make rewards and punishments contingent upon the child's behavior, and negotiate disagreements so that conflicts and crises did not escalate. This treatment program was shown to be effective in reducing child stealing and antisocial behavior over short periods in small-scale studies (Dishion, Patterson, & Kavanagh, 1992; Patterson, Chamberlain, & Reid, 1982; Patterson, Reid, & Dishion, 1992).

Webster-Stratton and Hammond (1997) evaluated the effectiveness of parent training and child skills training with about 100 Seattle children (average age 5) referred to a clinic because of conduct problems. The children and their parents were randomly allocated to groups receiving (1) parent training, (2) child skills training, (3) both parent and child training, or (4) no training (control group). The skills training aimed to foster prosocial behavior and interpersonal skills using video modeling, while the parent training involved weekly meetings between parents and therapists for 22–24 weeks. Parent reports and home observations showed that children in all three experimental conditions had fewer behavior problems than did control children, in both an immediate and a 1-year follow-up. There was little difference between the three experimental conditions, although the combined parent and child training condition produced the most signifi-

cant improvements in child behavior at the 1-year follow-up.

Scott, Spender, Doolan, Jacobs, and Aspland (2001) evaluated the Webster-Stratton parent training program in London, England. About 140 children ages 3–8 who were referred for antisocial behavior were allocated to receive parent training or to be in a control group. The program was successful. According to parent reports, the antisocial behavior of the experimental children decreased, while that of the control children did not change. Other studies also show that parent training is effective in reducing children's antisocial behavior (Kazdin, Siegel, & Bass, 1992; Strayhorn & Weidman, 1991).

Sanders, Markie-Dadds, Tully, and Bor (2000) in Brisbane, Australia, developed the Triple-P parenting program. This program can either be delivered to the whole community in primary prevention using the mass media or be used in secondary prevention with high-risk or clinic samples. Sanders and his colleagues evaluated the success of Triple-P with high-risk 3-year-olds by randomly allocating them either to receive Triple-P or to be in a control group. The Triple-P program involves teaching parents 17 child management strategies including talking with children, giving physical affection, praising, giving attention, setting a good example, setting rules, giving clear instructions, and using appropriate penalties for misbehavior ("time out," or sending the child to his or her room). The evaluation showed that the Triple-P program was successful in reducing children's antisocial behavior.

Another parenting intervention, termed "functional family therapy," was developed in Utah by Alexander and Parsons (1973; see also Alexander, Barton, Schiavo, & Parsons, 1976). This intervention aimed to modify patterns of family interaction by modeling, prompting, and reinforcement, in order to encourage clear communication between family members regarding requests and solutions and to minimize conflict. Essentially, all family members were trained to negotiate effectively, to set clear rules about privileges and responsibilities, and to use techniques of reciprocal reinforcement with each other. The program was evaluated by randomly allocating 86 delinquents to experimental or control conditions. The results showed that this technique halved the recidivism rate of delinquents in comparison with other approaches (client-centered or psychodynamic therapy). Its effectiveness with more serious offenders was confirmed in a replication study using matched groups (Barton, Alexander, Waldron, Turner, & Warburton, 1985).

In Oregon, Chamberlain and Reid (1998) evaluated treatment foster care (TFC), as an alternative to custody for delinquents. Custodial sentences for delinquents were thought to have undesirable effects especially because of the bad influence of delinquent peers. In TFC, families in the community were recruited and trained to provide a placement for delinquent youths. The TFC youths were closely supervised at home, in the community, and in the school, and their contacts with delinquent peers were thereby minimized. The foster parents provided a structured daily living environment with clear rules and limits, consistent discipline for rule violations, and one-to-one monitoring. The youths were encouraged to develop academic skills and desirable work habits. In the evaluation by Chamberlain and Reid (1998), 79 chronic male delinquents were randomly assigned to TFC or to regular group homes where they lived with other delinquents. A 1-year follow-up showed that the TFC boys had fewer criminal referrals and lower self-reported delinquency. Hence, this program seemed to be an effective treatment for chronic delinquency.

Generally, multimodal interventions are more effective than single-modality interventions (Wasserman & Miller, 1998). Multisystemic therapy (MST) is an important multiple-component family preservation program that was developed for chronic delinquents by Henggeler, Melton, Smith, Schoenwald, and Hanley (1993) in South Carolina. In this approach, the particular type of treatment is chosen according to the particular needs of the youth. Therefore, the nature of the treatment is different for each person. MST is delivered in the youth's home, school, and community settings. The treatment typically includes family intervention to promote the parent's ability to monitor and discipline the adolescent, peer intervention to encourage the choice of prosocial friends, and school intervention to enhance competence and school achievement.

Henggeler and colleagues (1993) evaluated this program by randomly assigning 84 serious delinquents (with an average age of 15) to receive either MST or the usual treatment (which mostly involved placing the juvenile outside home). The results showed that the MST group had fewer arrests and fewer self-reported crimes in a 1-year follow-up.

In another evaluation in Missouri, Borduin and colleagues (1995) randomly assigned 176 juvenile offenders (with an average age of 14) either to MST or to individual therapy focusing on personal, family, and academic issues. Four years later, only 29% of the MST offenders had been rearrested, compared with 74% of the individual therapy group. According to Aos, Phipps, Barnoski, and Lieb (2001), the benefit-to-cost ratio for MST is very high (28.3), largely because of the potential crime and criminal justice savings from targeting chronic juvenile offenders. Cohen (1998) calculated that the monetary cost to American society of a high-risk youth (taking account of juvenile and adult crimes, drug abuse, and school failure) was about $2 million.

Unfortunately, disappointing results were obtained in a large-scale independent evaluation of MST in Canada conducted by Leschied and Cunningham (2002). Over 400 youths who were either offenders or at risk of offending were randomly assigned to receive either MST or the usual services (typically probation supervision). Six months after treatment, 28% of the MST group had been reconvicted, compared with 31% of the control group, a nonsignificant difference. Therefore, it is unclear how effective MST is when it is implemented independently.

Although there are many evaluations suggesting that family-based prevention programs are effective, few have included a long-term follow-up and none have had an outcome measure of psychopathy. Future evaluations of early prevention programs should include long-term follow-ups and a wide range of outcome measures, including assessment of psychopathy.

CONCLUSIONS AND FUTURE DIRECTIONS

There has been too much emphasis on and reification of the PCL-R as a predictor of later crime and violence. More explanatory research is needed on psychopathy. More efforts should be made to integrate the personality constructs underlying psychopathy—an arrogant and deceitful interpersonal style, deficient affective experience, and an impulsive and irresponsible lifestyle—with larger systems of personality constructs (Lynam et al., in press; Widiger, 1998). More research is needed on the development of more unbiased, valid, and reliable instruments to measure psychopathy—preferably measures that are not contaminated by antisocial behavior and that do not rely on open-ended questions. It is important to supplement self-report data with other information (e.g., from case files).

The aim should be to develop and test causal models of psychopathy or of its constituent constructs such as low empathy and high impulsiveness. There is a great need to carry out prospective longitudinal surveys with high-risk community samples to investigate the development of psychopathy and the link between psychopathic parents and psychopathic children. In studying family factors, better measuring instruments are needed, with greater use of systematic observation of family interactions. More randomized experiments are needed to evaluate family-based interventions, with large samples and long-term follow-up periods, incorporating outcome measures of psychopathy. In principle, a great deal can be learned about causal effects of family factors from these experiments (Robins, 1992).

There is a pressing need for more research on independent, interactive, and sequential effects of family and other types of factors (e.g., biological and individual factors) on the development of psychopathy. Research should especially aim to identify protective effects, for example by studying family environments in which at-risk individuals (e.g., those with a biological risk factor) do not develop psychopathy. In addition, there should be more interplay between causal and intervention research. For example, the causal research could help to match types of interventions to types of people. Systematic reviews and meta-analyses should be carried out to assess the importance of both causal factors and intervention programs.

No one can doubt the importance of the construct of psychopathy, the need to develop better operational definitions of the underlying constructs, and the pressing need to advance knowledge about its development, explanation, prevention, and treatment. The time is ripe for Western countries to mount an ambitious coordinated program of research on psychopathy, focusing on international multidisciplinary collaboration and aiming to train a new generation of biopsychosocial researchers. Given the enormous social costs of psychopathy, the benefits of such a large-scale coordinated program of research should easily outweigh its costs. And, of course, a reduction in the number of psychopathic individuals and in the number of their victims would greatly increase the sum of human happiness.

ACKNOWLEDGMENTS

The ages 8–10 data collection of the Cambridge Study in Delinquent Development was funded by the Home Office and directed by Professor Donald West. The medical interview at age 48 was funded by the U.K. National Programme on Forensic Mental Health. The interview was conducted by Dr. Crystal Romilly under the supervision of Professor Jeremy Coid. The PCL:SV was scored by Dr. Crystal Romilly and Dr. Simone Ullrich. I am very grateful to Darrick Jolliffe for providing computerized age 48 data and to Professor David Cooke, Dr. Britt at Klinteberg, Professor Christopher Patrick, and Dr. Simone Ullrich for helpful comments on an earlier version of this chapter.

REFERENCES

Alexander, J. F., Barton, C., Schiavo, R. S., & Parsons, S. V. (1976). Systems-behavioral intervention with families of delinquents: Therapist characteristics, family behavior, and outcome. *Journal of Consulting and Clinical Psychology, 44,* 656–664.

Alexander, J. F., & Parsons, B. V. (1973). Short-term behavioral intervention with delinquent families: Impact on family process and recidivism. *Journal of Abnormal Psychology, 81,* 219–225.

Aos, S., Phipps, P., Barnoski, R. & Lieb, R. (2001). *The comparative costs and benefits of programs to reduce crime* (version 4.0). Olympia: Washington State Institute for Public Policy.

Barton, C., Alexander, J. F., Waldron, H., Turner, C. W., & Warburton, J. (1985). Generalizing treatment effects of functional family therapy: Three replications. *American Journal of Family Therapy, 13,* 16–26.

Borduin, C. M., Mann, B. J., Cone, L. T., Henggeler, S.

W., Fucci, B. R., Blaske, D. M., & Williams, R. A. (1995). Multisystemic treatment of serious juvenile offenders: Long-term prevention of criminality and violence. *Journal of Consulting and Clinical Psychology, 63*, 569–578.

Bowlby, J. (1951). *Maternal care and mental health.* Geneva, Switzerland: World Health Organization.

Brennan, P. A., Mednick, B. R., & Mednick, S. A. (1993). Parental psychopathology, congenital factors, and violence. In S. Hodgins (Ed.), *Mental disorder and crime* (pp. 244–261). Newbury Park, CA: Sage.

Buehler, C., Anthony, C., Krishnakumar, A., Stone, G., Gerard, J., & Pemberton, S. (1997). Interparental conflict and youth problem behaviors: A meta-analysis. *Journal of Child and Family Studies, 6*, 233–247.

Campbell, M. A., Porter, S., & Santor, D. (2004). Psychopathic traits in adolescent offenders: An evaluation of criminal history, clinical, and psychosocial correlates. *Behavioral Sciences and the Law, 22*, 23–47.

Carlson, E. A., & Sroufe, L. A. (1995). Contribution of attachment theory to developmental psychopathology. In D. Cicchetti & D. J. Cohen (Eds.), *Developmental psychopathology* (Vol. 1, pp. 581–617). New York: Wiley.

Chamberlain, P., & Reid, J. B. (1998). Comparison of two community alternatives to incarceration for chronic juvenile offenders. *Journal of Consulting and Clinical Psychology, 66*, 624–633.

Cohen, M. A. (1998). The monetary value of saving a high-risk youth. *Journal of Quantitative Criminology, 14*, 5–33.

Cohen, P. (1996). Childhood risks for young adult symptoms of personality disorder. *Multivariate Behavioral Research, 31*, 121–148.

Cohen, P., & Brook, J. S. (1995). The reciprocal influence of punishment and child behavior disorder. In J. McCord (Ed.), *Coercion and punishment in longterm perspectives* (pp. 154–164). Cambridge, UK: Cambridge University Press.

Coie, J. D., Dodge, K. A., & Kupersmidt, J. (1990). Peer group behavior and social status. In S. R. Asher & J. D. Coie (Eds.), *Peer rejection in childhood* (pp. 17–59). Cambridge, UK: Cambridge University Press.

Coie, J. D., & Miller-Johnson, S. (2001). Peer factors and interventions. In R. Loeber & D. P. Farrington (Eds.), *Child delinquents: Development, intervention, and service needs* (pp. 191–209). Thousand Oaks, CA: Sage.

Conger, R. D., Patterson, G. R., & Ge, X. (1995). It takes two to replicate: A mediational model for the impact of parents' stress on adolescent adjustment. *Child Development, 66*, 80–97.

Conseur, A., Rivara, F. P., Barnoski, R., & Emanuel, I. (1997). Maternal and perinatal risk factors for later delinquency. *Pediatrics, 99*, 785–790.

Cooke, D. J., Michie, C., Hart, S. D., & Clark, D. A. (2004). Reconstructing psychopathy: Clarifying the significance of antisocial and socially deviant behavior in the diagnosis of psychopathic personality disorder. *Journal of Personality Disorders, 18*, 337–357.

Cooke, D. J., Michie, C., Hart, S. D., & Hare, R. D. (1999). Evaluating the screening version of the Psychopathy Checklist—Revised (PCL-SV): An item response theory analysis. *Psychological Assessment, 11*, 3–13.

Deater-Deckard, K., Dodge, K. A., Bates, J. E., & Pettit, G. S. (1996). Physical discipline among African American and European American mothers: Links to children's externalizing behaviors. *Developmental Psychology, 32*, 1065–1072.

Dishion, T. J., Patterson, G. R., & Kavanagh, K. A. (1992). An experimental test of the coercion model: Linking theory, measurement and intervention. In J. McCord & R. Tremblay (Eds.), *Preventing antisocial behavior* (pp. 253–282). New York: Guilford Press.

Dodge, K. A., Pettit, G. S., & Bates, J. E. (1994). Socialization mediators of the relation between socioeconomic status and child conduct problems. *Child Development, 65*, 649–665.

Elliott, D. S., Huizinga, D., & Menard, S. (1989). *Multiple problem youth.* New York: Springer-Verlag.

Elliott, D. S., & Menard, S. (1996). Delinquent friends and delinquent behavior: Temporal and developmental patterns. In J. D. Hawkins (Ed.), *Delinquency and crime: Current theories* (pp. 28–67). Cambridge, UK: Cambridge University Press.

Ellis, L. (1988). The victimful–victimless crime distinction, and seven universal demographic correlates of victimful criminal behavior. *Personality and Individual Differences, 3*, 525–548.

Farrington, D. P. (1972). Delinquency begins at home. *New Society, 21*, 495–497.

Farrington, D. P. (1989). Early predictors of adolescent aggression and adult violence. *Violence and Victims, 4*, 79–100.

Farrington, D. P. (1992a). Explaining the beginning, progress, and ending of antisocial behavior from birth to adulthood. In J. McCord (Ed.), *Facts, frameworks and forecasts: Advances in criminological theory* (Vol. 3, pp. 253–286). New Brunswick, NJ: Transaction.

Farrington, D. P. (1992b). Juvenile delinquency. In J. C. Coleman (Ed.), *The school years* (2nd ed., pp. 123–163). London: Routledge.

Farrington, D. P. (1993). Childhood origins of teenage antisocial behaviour and adult social dysfunction. *Journal of the Royal Society of Medicine, 86*, 13–17.

Farrington, D. P. (1997). Key issues in studying the biosocial bases of violence. In A. Raine, P. A. Brennan, D. P. Farrington, & S. A. Mednick (Eds.), *Biosocial bases of violence* (pp. 293–300). New York: Plenum Press.

Farrington, D. P. (1998). Predictors, causes, and correlates of youth violence. In M. Tonry & M. H. Moore (Eds.), *Youth violence* (pp. 421–475). Chicago: University of Chicago Press.

Farrington, D. P. (2000). Psychosocial predictors of adult antisocial personality and adult convictions. *Behavioral Sciences and the Law, 18*, 605–622.

Farrington, D. P. (2003). Key results from the first 40 years of the Cambridge Study in Delinquent Development. In T. P. Thornberry & M. D. Krohn (Eds.), *Taking stock of delinquency* (pp. 137–183). New York: Kluwer/Plenum Press.

Farrington, D. P., Barnes, G., & Lambert, S. (1996). The concentration of offending in families. *Legal and Criminological Psychology, 1*, 47–63.

Farrington, D. P., Coid, J. W., Harnett, L., Jolliffe, D., Soteriou, N., Turner, R., & West, D. J. (in press). *The Cambridge Study in Delinquent Development: A prospective longitudinal survey from age 8 to age 48.* London: Home Office.

Farrington, D. P., & Hawkins, J. D. (1991). Predicting participation, early onset, and later persistence in officially recorded offending. *Criminal Behavior and Mental Health, 1*, 1–33.

Farrington, D. P., Jolliffe, D., Loeber, R., Stouthamer-Loeber, M., & Kalb, L. M. (2001). The concentration of offenders in families, and family criminality in the prediction of boys' delinquency. *Journal of Adolescence, 24*, 579–596.

Farrington, D. P., & Loeber, R. (1999). Transatlantic replicability of risk factors in the development of delinquency. In P. Cohen, C. Slomkowski, & L. N. Robins (Eds.), *Historical and geographical influences on psychopathology* (pp. 299–329). Mahwah, NJ: Erlbaum.

Farrington, D. P., Loeber, R., & Stouthamer-Loeber, M. (2003). How can the relationship between race and violence be explained? In D. F. Hawkins (Ed.), *Violent crime: Assessing race and ethnic differences* (pp. 213–237). Cambridge, UK: Cambridge University Press.

Farrington, D. P., & Welsh, B. C. (2003). Family-based prevention of offending: A meta-analysis. *Australian and New Zealand Journal of Criminology, 36*, 127–151.

Farrington, D. P., & West, D. J. (1993). Criminal, penal, and life histories of chronic offenders: Risk and protective factors and early identification. *Criminal Behavior and Mental Health, 3*, 492–523.

Fergusson, D. M., & Horwood, L. J. (1998). Exposure to interparental violence in childhood and psychosocial adjustment in young adulthood. *Child Abuse and Neglect, 22*, 339–357.

Fischer, D. G. (1984). Family size and delinquency. *Perceptual and Motor Skills, 58*, 527–534.

Forth, A. E., Brown, S. L., Hart, S. D., & Hare, R. D. (1996). The assessment of psychopathy in male and female noncriminals: Reliability and validity. *Personality and Individual Differences, 20*, 531–543.

Forth, A. E., & Burke, H. C. (1998). Psychopathy in adolescence: Assessment, violence, and developmental precursors. In D. J. Cooke, A. E. Forth, & R. D. Hare (Eds.), *Psychopathy: Theory, research, and implications for society* (pp. 205–229). Dordrecht, The Netherlands: Kluwer.

Freidenfelt, J., & af Klinteberg, B. (2003). Are negative social and psychological childhood characteristics of significant importance in the development of psychosocial functioning? *International Journal of Forensic Mental Health, 2*, 181–193.

Gorman-Smith, D., Tolan, P. H., Zelli, A., & Huesmann, L. R. (1996). The relation of family functioning to violence among inner-city minority youths. *Journal of Family Psychology, 10*, 115–129.

Gottfredson, D. C. (2001). *Schools and delinquency.* Cambridge, UK: Cambridge University Press.

Gottfredson, D. C., McNeil, R. J., & Gottfredson, G. D. (1991). Social area influences on delinquency: A multilevel analysis. *Journal of Research in Crime and Delinquency, 28*, 197–226.

Graham, J. (1988). *Schools, disruptive behaviour and delinquency.* London: Her Majesty's Stationery Office.

Haapasalo, J., & Pokela, E. (1999). Child-rearing and child abuse antecedents of criminality. *Aggression and Violent Behavior, 1*, 107–127.

Harris, G. T., Rice, M. E., & Lalumiere, M. (2001). Criminal violence: The roles of psychopathy, neurodevelopmental insults, and antisocial parenting. *Criminal Justice and Behavior, 28*, 402–426.

Hart, S. D., Cox, D. N., & Hare, R. D. (1995). *The Hare Psychopathy Checklist: Screening Version.* Toronto, ON, Canada: Multi-Health Systems.

Hart, S. D., & Hare, R. D. (1997). Psychopathy: Assessment and association with criminal conduct. In D. M. Stoff, J. Breiling, & J. D. Maser (Eds.), *Handbook of antisocial behavior* (pp. 22–35). New York: Wiley.

Henggeler, S. W., Melton, G. B., Smith, L. A., Schoenwald, S. K., & Hanley, J. H. (1993). Family preservation using multisystemic treatment: Long-term follow-up to a clinical trial with serious juvenile offenders. *Journal of Child and Family Studies, 2*, 283–293.

Henry, B., Caspi, A., Moffitt, T. E., & Silva, P. A. (1996). Temperamental and familial predictors of violent and nonviolent criminal convictions: Age 3 to age 18. *Developmental Psychology, 32*, 614–623.

Herrenkohl, T. I., Hawkins, J. D., Chung, I-J., Hill, K. G., & Battin-Pearson, S. (2001). School and community risk factors and interventions. In R. Loeber & D. P. Farrington (Eds.), *Child delinquents: Development, intervention, and service needs* (pp. 211–246). Thousand Oaks, CA: Sage.

Juby, H., & Farrington, D. P. (2001). Disentangling the link between disrupted families and delinquency. *British Journal of Criminology, 41*, 22–40.

Kalb, L. M., Farrington, D. P., & Loeber, R. (2001). Leading longitudinal studies on delinquency, substance use, sexual behavior, and mental health problems with childhood samples. In R. Loeber & D. P. Farrington (Eds.), *Child delinquents: Development, intervention, and service needs* (pp. 415–423). Thousand Oaks, CA: Sage.

Kazdin, A. E., Siegel, T. C., & Bass, D. (1992) Cognitive problem-solving skills training and parent management training in the treatment of antisocial behavior in children. *Journal of Consulting and Clinical Psychology, 60,* 733–747.

Kelley, M. L., Power, T. G., & Wimbush, D. D. (1992). Determinants of disciplinary practices in low-income black mothers. *Child Development, 63,* 573–582.

Kitzman, H., Olds, D. L., Henderson, C. R., Hanks, C., Cole, R., Tatelbaum, R., et al. (1997). Effect of prenatal and infancy home visitation by nurses on pregnancy outcomes, childhood injuries, and repeated childbearing: A randomized controlled trial. *Journal of the American Medical Association, 278,* 644–652.

Koivisto, H., & Haapasalo, J. (1996). Childhood maltreatment and adulthood psychopathy in light of file-based assessments among mental state examinees. *Studies on Crime and Crime Prevention, 5,* 91–104.

Kolbo, J. R., Blakely, E. H., & Engleman, D. (1996). Children who witness domestic violence: A review of empirical literature. *Journal of Interpersonal Violence, 11,* 281–293.

Kolvin, I., Miller, F. J. W., Fleeting, M., & Kolvin, P. A. (1988a). Risk/protective factors for offending with particular reference to deprivation. In M. Rutter (Ed.), *Studies of psychosocial risk* (pp. 77–95). Cambridge, UK: Cambridge University Press.

Kolvin, I., Miller, F. J. W., Fleeting, M., & Kolvin, P. A. (1988b). Social and parenting factors affecting criminal-offence rates: Findings from the Newcastle Thousand Family Study (1947–1980). *British Journal of Psychiatry, 152,* 80–90.

Lally, J. R., Mangione, P. L., & Honig, A. S. (1988). The Syracuse University Family Development Research Program: Long-range impact of an early intervention with low-income children and their families. In D. R. Powell (Ed.), *Parent education as early childhood intervention* (pp. 79–104). Norwood, NJ: Ablex.

Lang, S., af Klinteberg, B., & Alm, P-O. (2002) Adult psychopathy and violent behavior in males with early neglect and abuse. *Acta Psychiatrica Scandinavica, 106,* 93–100.

Larzelere, R. E., & Patterson, G. R. (1990). Parental management: Mediator of the effect of socioeconomic status on early delinquency. *Criminology, 28,* 301–324.

Leschied, A., & Cunningham A. (2002). *Seeking effective interventions for serious young offenders: Interim results of a four-year randomized study of multisystemic therapy in Ontario, Canada.* London, ON, Canada: London Family Court Clinic.

Lewis, C., Newson, E., & Newson, J. (1982). Father participation through childhood and its relationship with career aspirations and delinquency. In N. Beail & J. McGuire (Eds.), *Fathers: Psychological perspectives,* (pp. 174–193). London: Junction.

Lipsey, M. W., & Derzon, J. H. (1998). Predictors of violent or serious delinquency in adolescence and early adulthood: A synthesis of longitudinal research. In R. Loeber & D. P. Farrington (Eds.), *Serious and violent juvenile offenders: Risk factors and successful interventions* (pp. 86–105). Thousand Oaks, CA: Sage.

Loeber, R., & Farrington, D. P. (1997). Strategies and yields of longitudinal studies on antisocial behavior. In D. M. Stoff, J. Breiling, & J. D. Maser (Eds.), *Handbook of antisocial behavior* (pp. 125–139). New York: Wiley.

Loeber, R., Farrington, D. P., Stouthamer-Loeber, M., & van Kammen, W. B. (1998). *Antisocial behavior and mental health problems.* Mahwah, NJ: Erlbaum.

Luntz, B. K., & Widom, C. S. (1994). Antisocial personality disorder in abused and neglected children. *American Journal of Psychiatry, 151,* 670–674.

Lykken, D. T. (1995). *The antisocial personalities.* Hillsdale, NJ: Erlbaum.

Lynam, D. (1996). Early identification of chronic offenders: Who is the fledgling psychopath? *Psychological Bulletin, 120,* 209–234.

Lynam, D. R., Caspi, A., Moffitt, T. E., Raine, A., Loeber, R., & Stouthamer-Loeber, M. (in press). Adolescent psychopathy and the Big Five: Results from two samples. *Journal of Abnormal Child Psychology.*

Lytton, H. (1990). Child and parent effects in boys' conduct disorder: A reinterpretation. *Developmental Psychology, 26,* 683–697.

Lytton, H., & Romney, D. M. (1991). Parents' differential socialization of boys and girls: A meta-analysis. *Psychological Bulletin, 109,* 267–296.

Magnusson, D., & Bergman, L. R. (1988). Individual and variable-based approaches to longitudinal research on early risk factors. In M. Rutter (Ed.), *Studies of psychosocial risk* (pp. 45–61). Cambridge, UK: Cambridge University Press.

Malinosky-Rummell, R., & Hansen, D. J. (1993). Long-term consequences of childhood physical abuse. *Psychological Bulletin, 114,* 68–79.

Marshall, L. A., & Cooke, D. J. (1999). The childhood experiences of psychopaths: A retrospective study of familial and social factors. *Journal of Personality Disorders, 13,* 211–225.

Maxfield, M. G., & Widom, C. S. (1996). The cycle of violence revisited six years later. *Archives of Pediatrics and Adolescent Medicine, 150,* 390–395.

McCord, J. (1977). A comparative study of two generations of native Americans. In R. F. Meier (Ed.), *Theory in criminology* (pp. 83–92). Beverly Hills, CA: Sage.

McCord, J. (1979). Some child-rearing antecedents of criminal behavior in adult men. *Journal of Personality and Social Psychology, 37,* 1477–1486.

McCord, J. (1982). A longitudinal view of the relationship between paternal absence and crime. In J. Gunn & D. P. Farrington (Eds.), *Abnormal offenders, delinquency, and the criminal justice system* (pp. 113–128). Chichester, UK: Wiley.

McCord, J. (1983). A forty year perspective on effects of child abuse and neglect. *Child Abuse and Neglect, 7,* 265–270.

McCord, J. (1997). On discipline. *Psychological Inquiry, 8,* 215–217.

McCord, J. (2001). Psychosocial contributions to psychopathy and violence. In A. Raine & J. Sanmartin (Eds.), *Violence and psychopathy* (pp. 141–169). New York: Kluwer/Plenum Press.

McCord, W., & McCord, J. (1964). *The psychopath: An essay on the criminal mind.* Princeton, NJ: Van Nostrand.

Moffitt, T. E., Caspi, A., Rutter, M., & Silva, P. A. (2001). *Sex differences in antisocial behaviour.* Cambridge, UK: Cambridge University Press.

Morash, M., & Rucker, L. (1989). An exploratory study of the connection of mother's age at childbearing to her children's delinquency in four data sets. *Crime and Delinquency, 35,* 45–93.

Nagin, D. S., Pogarsky, G., & Farrington, D. P. (1997). Adolescent mothers and the criminal behavior of their children. *Law and Society Review, 31,* 137–162.

Nelson, S. E., & Dishion, T. J. (2004). From boys to men: Predicting adult adaptation from middle childhood sociometric status. *Development and Psychopathology, 16,* 441–459.

Newson, J., & Newson, E. (1989). *The extent of parental physical punishment in the UK.* London: Approach.

Olds, D. L., Eckenrode, J., Henderson, C. R., Kitzman, H., Powers, J., Cole, R., et al. (1997) Long-term effects of home visitation on maternal life course and child abuse and neglect: Fifteen-year follow-up of a randomized trial. *Journal of the American Medical Association, 278,* 637–643.

Olds, D. L., Henderson, C. R., Chamberlin, R., & Tatelbaum, R. (1986). Preventing child abuse and neglect: A randomized trial of nurse home visitation. *Pediatrics, 78,* 65–78.

Olds, D. L., Henderson, C. R., Cole, R., Eckenrode, J., Kitzman, H., Luckey, D., et al. (1998). Long-term effects of nurse home visitation on children's criminal and antisocial behavior: 15-year follow-up of a randomized controlled trial. *Journal of the American Medical Association, 280,* 1238–1244.

Patrick, C. J., Zempolich, K. A., & Levenston, G. K. (1997). Emotionality and violent behavior in psychopaths: A biosocial analysis. In A. Raine, P. A. Brennan, D. P. Farrington, & S. A. Mednick (Eds.), *Biosocial bases of violence* (pp. 145–161). New York: Plenum Press.

Patterson, G. R. (1982). *Coercive family process.* Eugene, OR: Castalia.

Patterson, G. R. (1995). Coercion as a basis for early age of onset for arrest. In J. McCord (Ed.), *Coercion and punishment in long-term perspectives* (pp. 81–105). Cambridge, UK: Cambridge University Press.

Patterson, G. R., Chamberlain, P., & Reid, J. B. (1982). A comparative evaluation of a parent training program. *Behavior Therapy, 13,* 638–650.

Patterson, G. R., Reid, J. B., & Dishion, T. J. (1992). *Antisocial boys.* Eugene, OR: Castalia.

Raine, A., Brennan, P. A., Farrington, D. P., & Mednick, S. A. (Eds.). (1997). *Biosocial bases of violence.* New York: Plenum Press.

Raine, A., Brennan, P. A., & Mednick, S. A. (1994). Birth complications combined with early maternal rejection at age 1 year predispose to violent crime at age 18 years. *Archives of General Psychiatry, 51,* 984–988.

Rasanen, P., Hakko, H., Isohanni, M., Hodgins, S., Jarvelin, M., & Tilhonen, J. (1999). Maternal smoking during pregnancy and risk of criminal behavior among adult male offspring in the Northern Finland 1966 birth cohort. *American Journal of Psychiatry, 156,* 857–862.

Reiss, A. J., & Farrington, D. P. (1991). Advancing knowledge about co-offending: Results from a prospective longitudinal survey of London males. *Journal of Criminal Law and Criminology, 82,* 360–395.

Robins, L. N. (1966). *Deviant children grown up.* Baltimore: Williams & Wilkins.

Robins, L. N. (1979). Sturdy childhood predictors of adult outcomes: Replications from longitudinal studies. In J. E. Barrett, R. M. Rose, & G. L. Klerman (Eds.), *Stress and mental disorder* (pp. 219–235). New York: Raven Press.

Robins, L. N. (1992). The role of prevention experiments in discovering causes of children's antisocial behavior. In J. McCord & R. E. Tremblay (Eds.), *Preventing antisocial behavior* (pp. 3–18). New York: Guilford Press.

Rothbaum, F., & Weisz, J. R. (1994). Parental caregiving and child externalizing behavior in nonclinical samples: A meta-analysis. *Psychological Bulletin, 116,* 55–74.

Rutter, M. (1981). The city and the child. *American Journal of Orthopsychiatry, 51,* 610–625.

Sampson, R. J., Raudenbush, S. W., & Earls, F. (1997). Neighborhoods and violent crime: A multilevel study of collective efficacy. *Science, 277,* 918–924.

Sanders, M., Markie-Dadds, C., Tully, L. A., & Bor, W. (2000). The Triple P-Positive parenting program: A comparison of enhanced, standard, and self-directed behavioral family intervention for parents of children with early onset conduct problems. *Journal of Consulting and Clinical Psychology, 68,* 624–640.

Scott, S., Spender, Q., Doolan, M., Jacobs, B., & Aspland, H. (2001). Multicentre controlled trial of parenting groups for child antisocial behaviour in clinical practice. *British Medical Journal, 323,* 194–196.

Shaw, C. R., & McKay, H. D. (1969). *Juvenile delinquency and urban areas* (rev. ed.). Chicago: University of Chicago Press.

Smith, C. A., Krohn, M. D., Lizotte, A. J., McCluskey, C. P., Stouthamer-Loeber, M., & Weiher, A. (2000). The effect of early delinquency and substance use on precocious transitions to adulthood among adolescent males. In G. L. Fox & M. L. Benson (Eds.), *Families, crime and criminal justice* (Vol. 2, pp. 233–253). Amsterdam: JAI Press.

Smith, C. A., & Stern, S. B. (1997). Delinquency and antisocial behavior: A review of family processes and intervention research. *Social Service Review, 71,* 382–420.

Smith, J. R., & Brooks-Gunn, J. (1997). Correlates and consequences of harsh discipline for young children. *Archives of Pediatrics and Adolescent Medicine, 151,* 777–786.

Stern, S. B., & Smith, C. A. (1995). Family processes and delinquency in an ecological context. *Social Service Review, 69,* 705–731.

Stone, W. L., Bendell, R. D., & Field, T. M. (1988). The impact of socioeconomic status on teenage mothers and children who received early intervention. *Journal of Applied Developmental Psychology, 9,* 391–408.

Strayhorn, J. M., & Weidman, C. S. (1991). Follow-up one year after parent–child interaction training: Effects on behavior of preschool children. *Journal of the American Academy of Child and Adolescent Psychiatry, 30,* 128–143.

Thornberry, T. P., Huizinga, D., & Loeber, R. (1995). The prevention of serious delinquency and violence: Implications from the program of research on the causes and correlates of delinquency. In J. C. Howell, B. Krisberg, J. D. Hawkins, & J. J. Wilson (Eds.), *Sourcebook on serious, violent and chronic juvenile offenders* (pp. 213–237). Thousand Oaks, CA: Sage.

Verona, E., Patrick, C. J., & Joiner, T. E. (2001). Psychopathy, antisocial personality, and suicide risk. *Journal of Abnormal Psychology, 110,* 462–470.

Wadsworth, M. E. J. (1976). Delinquency, pulse rates and early emotional deprivation. *British Journal of Criminology, 16,* 245–256.

Wasserman, G. A., & Miller, L. S. (1998). The prevention of serious and violent juvenile offending. In R. Loeber & D. P. Farrington (Eds.), *Serious and violent juvenile offenders: Risk factors and successful interventions* (pp. 197–247). Thousand Oaks, CA: Sage.

Webster-Stratton, C., & Hammond, M. (1997). Treating children with early-onset conduct problems: A comparison of child and parent training interventions. *Journal of Consulting and Clinical Psychology, 65,* 93–109.

Weiler, B. L., & Widom, C. S. (1996). Psychopathy and violent behavior in abused and neglected young adults. *Criminal Behavior and Mental Health, 6,* 253–271.

Wells, L. E., & Rankin, J. H. (1991). Families and delinquency: A meta-analysis of the impact of broken homes. *Social Problems, 38,* 71–93.

Werner, E. E., & Smith, R. S. (1982). *Vulnerable but invincible: A longitudinal study of resilient children and youth.* New York: McGraw-Hill.

West, D. J., & Farrington, D. P. (1973). *Who becomes delinquent?* London: Heinemann.

Widiger, T. (1998). Psychopathy and normal personality. In D. J. Cooke, A. E. Forth, & R. D. Hare (Eds.), *Psychopathy: Theory, research, and implications for society* (pp. 47–68). Dordrecht, The Netherlands: Kluwer.

Widom, C. S. (1989). The cycle of violence. *Science, 244,* 160–166.

Widom, C. S. (1994). Childhood victimization and adolescent problem behaviors. In R. D. Ketterlinus & M. E. Lamb (Eds.), *Adolescent problem behaviors* (pp. 127–164). Hillsdale, NJ: Erlbaum.

Widom, C. S., & Ames, M. A. (1994). Criminal consequences of childhood sexual victimization. *Child Abuse and Neglect, 18,* 303–318.

Wikström, P-O. H. (1985). *Everyday violence in contemporary Sweden.* Stockholm: National Council for Crime Prevention.

Wootton, J. M., Frick, P., Shelton, K. K., & Silverthorn, P. (1997). Ineffective parenting and childhood conduct problems: The moderating role of callous–unemotional traits. *Journal of Consulting and Clinical Psychology, 65,* 301–308.

13

Neurochemistry and Pharmacology of Psychopathy and Related Disorders

MICHAEL J. MINZENBERG
LARRY J. SIEVER

In reviewing the empirical knowledge base that exists for an aspect of psychopathy, an initial brief discussion of nomenclature and nosological issues is warranted. The term "psychopathy" is said to have originated in Germany in the late 19th century, initially covering the range of what we currently recognize as disorders of personality (Dolan, 1994). Later, in North America and England the term came to be used in a more restricted manner, more or less synonymously with antisocial behavior. With the widespread acceptance of the *Diagnostic and Statistical Manual of Mental Disorders* (DSM, currently in its 4th edition), antisocial personality disorder (APD) is the nosological entity applied most commonly to clinical cases characterized primarily by socially deviant behavior.

Currently, there are a few generally recognized problems with this construct. First, the current threshold for the APD diagnosis requires only 3 of 15 possible criteria exhibited in childhood, together with 3 of 7 in adulthood, and as a result the population of individuals with this diagnosis varies considerably in phenomenological profiles. This heterogeneity tends to limit the investigator's ability to identify brain–behavior relationships as they may pertain to the phenomenology of interest. Second, DSM-IV criteria

for APD consist almost exclusively of behavioral indicators, neglecting the affective–interpersonal features that appear to reflect much of the notion of a distinct personality type as described by Cleckley (1941/1976).

To address these issues, Hare and colleagues revived the construct of psychopathy, operationally defined by the Psychopathy Checklist, presently available in a revised version (PCL-R; Hare, 1991, 2003). This instrument includes assessment of the affective–interpersonal characteristics that reflect the emotional detachment thought to lie at the core of this personality type. Indeed, factor analyses of data generated with the PCL-R (cf. Hare, 1991, 2003) have identified two distinct underlying factors: one reflecting the affective–interpersonal features of psychopathy (Factor 1), and the other reflecting impulsive, antisocial deviance (Factor 2). (As described by Hare & Neumann, Chapter 4, and Cooke, Michie, & Hart, Chapter 5, this volume, alternative three- and four-factor models have recently been proposed—but here, we focus our discussion of PCL-R subcomponents mainly on the best-known two-factor model.)

In the review of the literature that follows, it is evident that the bulk of investigations of the neurobiology underlying this range of clinical phenomena are targeted at behavioral disturbance. Much of what is known of the relevant neurobiology is derived from studies of populations characterized by APD, impulsive aggression, criminality, type II alcoholism, and, in children, conduct disorders and oppositional defiant disorder (ODD), as well as behaviorally oriented constructs such as externalizing disorders, novelty seeking, and sensation seeking. This emphasis on behavior likely reflects both the recent historical predominance of the DSM construct of APD, as well as the tradition (largely surviving from the era of behaviorism) that observable, quantifiable behaviors hold privilege over internal subjective states or interpersonal phenomena, which have historically been much harder to define and operationalize in a rigorous manner.

The affective–interpersonal factor of psychopathy, as a result, has received relatively little attention as a topic of empirical investigation in studies of neurochemistry. Models that do exist of the neurobiology of social and emotion-related deficits in psychopathy have generally emphasized neurocognitive or psychophysiological disturbances, such as the consistent finding of deficits in autonomic responses and information processing of social and emotional stimuli (see Fowles & Dindo, Chapter 2; Blair, Chapter 15; and Rogers, Chapter 16, this volume). The relationship between this line of work and that of neurochemical dysfunction has generally not been addressed. This is in contrast to the considerable empirical evidence presently available implicating monoamine neurotransmitter dysfunction in behavioral syndromes of impulsivity and aggression (discussed in detail below). It may be that these two factors of psychopathy are expressions of independent (but frequently coexisting) neurobiological disturbances (Fowles & Dindo, Chapter 2, this volume; Patrick, 2001, in press).

With the foregoing caveats in mind, we present findings from a range of investigations indicating that individuals with these kinds of clinical problems have disturbances in a number of neurochemical systems found in the brain and periphery. These notably include the monoamine neurotransmitters and hormones such as testosterone, cortisol, and thyroid hormone; there are indicators of disturbances in glucose and lipid metabolism as well. The current state of knowledge has been derived from studies with diverse methodologies, including measurement of basal and drug-stimulated levels of these signaling molecules, and activity of elements of these neurochemical systems, such as synthetic enzymes, receptors and synaptic reuptake mechanisms, using biochemical assays and functional brain imaging. A promising approach to these research problems involves the identification of genetic variants (such as single nucleotide polymorphisms, or SNPs) of these elements that confer varying degrees of functional activity (Reif & Lesch, 2003).

We wish to emphasize, however, that the study of genetic aspects in no way diminishes the role of environmental factors in the etiology of these clinical problems. These are complex psychiatric disorders that have important antecedents in experiences such as childhood adversity (Raine, 2002). Indeed, some of the most exciting recent findings in the psychiatric literature address the complex interaction of genes and environment in the genesis of adult psychopathology such as antisocial behavior (Caspi et al., 2002).

SEROTONIN

While clinical depictions of psychopathy emphasize the instrumental nature of violent acts perpetrated against others, empirical studies suggest that psychopaths exhibit significant impulsivity in the expression of aggressive behavior as well, leading Hart and Dempster (1997) to conclude that they are "impulsively instrumental." In addition, the base rate of completed suicide may be 5% in APD (Frances, Fyer, & Clarkin, 1986). In a large sample of male prison inmates, a history of suicide attempts was related to PCL-R Factor 2 scores (Verona, Patrick, & Joiner, 2001).

Both self- and other-directed aggression has been strongly associated with dysfunction of the central serotonin system (see Gurvits, Koenigsberg, & Siever, 2000, for an earlier review). Early studies consistently demonstrated that aggressive, criminal and suicidal behavior was associated with decreased levels of overall activity in the serotonin system, indexed by lower levels of the major serotonin degradation product, 5-hydroxyindoleacetic acid (5-HIAA), found in the cerebrospinal fluid (CSF). Lower CSF

5-HIAA has been associated with suicidal behavior across psychiatric diagnoses (Asberg, Traskman, & Thoren, 1976), in patients with histories of violent suicidal or homicidal behavior (Lidberg, Tuck, Asberg, Scalia-Tomba, & Bertilsson, 1985; Siever et al., 1991).

Lower CSF 5-HIAA has also been found in each of the following samples of criminal or aggressive subjects: offenders who had committed violent, impulsive crimes versus those committing nonviolent premeditated crimes (Linnoila et al., 1983); alcoholic offenders with either APD or intermittent explosive disorder (Virkkunen et al., 1994); male arsonists (Virkkunen, Nuutila, Goodwin, & Linnoila, 1987); and aggressive patients without a history of suicide attempts (Stanley et al., 2000). CSF 5-HIAA was also lower in a mixed sample of violent offenders and arsonists (Virkkunen, De Jong, Bartko, Goodwin, & Linnoila, 1989), and recidivism to these crimes was associated with lower 5-HIAA in a larger sample extended from the 1989 study and followed for 4½ years on average (Virkkunen, Eggert, Rawlings, & Linnoila, 1996). Lower CSF 5-HIAA has also been associated with lifetime aggression history (Brown, Goodwin, Ballenger, Goyer, & Major, 1979; Limson et al., 1991). CSF 5-HIAA is also lower in newborns with a family history of APD (Constantino, Morris, & Murphy, 1997), and subjects with neonatal CSF 5-HIAA levels below the group median exhibited more aggressive behavior at 30 months of age than those above the median (Clarke, Murphy, & Constantino, 1999). Lower 5-HIAA levels were also observed in plasma of boys with disruptive behavior disorders (Kruesi et al., 1990) and in CSF of boys with ODD (van Goozen, Matthys, Cohen-Kettenis, Westenberg, & van Egeland, 1999), and were associated with the degree of aggression in both studies; lower CSF 5-HIAA levels also predicted severity of physical aggression at 2-year follow-up (Kruesi et al., 1992).

These studies suggest that disturbances in central serotonergic turnover appear early in life and are closely related to behaviors that often progress to adult antisocial behavior. Serotonergic dysregulation of dopaminergic activity may be partly responsible for the relationship with impulsive/aggressive behavior in adults with psychopathy, as the ratio of CSF HVA (homovanillic acid, a dopamine metabolite) to 5-HIAA is significantly higher in psychopaths (Soderstrom, Blennow, Manhem, & Forsman, 2001; Soderstrom, Blennow, Sjodin, & Forsman, 2003). In these two latter studies the HVA:5-HIAA ratio was similarly correlated with both PCL-R Factor 1 and Factor 2. In contrast, 5-HIAA levels alone were only modestly correlated with Factor 2 and not with Factor 1 in one study, and more strongly correlated with Factor 2 only in subgroups either without medication or without Axis I comorbidity in the other study. These findings suggest that serotonergic deficits are more fundamentally linked to the impulsive–antisocial (Factor 2) features of psychopathy, but that such deficits may exert effects in the affective–interpersonal domain of psychopathy (Factor 1) via interactions with dopamine.

The functional status of the central serotonin system can also be evaluated with the use of exogenous agents that activate this system, such as d-fenfluramine, which releases synaptic serotonin to activate postsynaptic serotonin receptors. These include serotonin receptors in the hypothalamus, which inhibit dopaminergic cells, removing tonic dopaminergic inhibition of prolactin-releasing cells. The functional status of central serotonin is then measured by levels of peripheral prolactin. Blunted prolactin response to fenfluramine has been observed in convicted murderers with APD (O'Keane et al., 1992) and detoxified heroin-dependent subjects with APD (Gerra et al., 2003). The degree of attenuation of this response is correlated with the level of impulsive aggression across personality disorder diagnoses (Coccaro et al., 1989, 1996; Coccaro, Kavoussi, Cooper, et al., 1997), and in a study of children with disruptive behavior disorders, the low-prolactin responder group had a higher incidence of first- and second-degree relatives with aggressive and antisocial characteristics (Halperin, Schulz, McKay, Sharma, & Newcorn, 2003).

The precise relationship of prolactin response in psychopathy is unclear: Dolan and colleagues (Dolan, Anderson, & Deakin, 2001; Dolan, Deakin, Roberts, & Anderson, 2002) did not find prolactin response to fenfluramine to be related to psychopathy as assessed by the Special Hospital Assessment of Personality and Socialization (SHAPS). In another study (Dolan & Anderson, 2003), this group used a three-factor solution to the PCL: Screening Version (Cooke et al., Chapter 5, this volume; Hart, Cox, & Hare, 1995) and found the prolactin response to fenfluramine to be inversely related to the impulsive–antisocial factor yet positively related to the arrogant–deceitful factor. The authors interpreted this second, counterintuitive finding as reflecting a possible adaptive component of psychopathy. This study highlights the need for careful analyses of facets of psychopathy, which may be associated with varying states of neurochemical function.

Unfortunately the serotonergic probes utilized in the aforementioned studies cited do not confer specificity for the site of disturbance within the serotonin system. Decreased activity in the central serotonergic system may be due to alterations at any point along the pathway of serotonin precursor uptake, synthesis, release, pre- and postsynaptic receptor activation, or reuptake and degradation. Preliminary studies measuring plasma tryptophan (TRYP) levels offer intriguing evidence that deficient serotonin precursor uptake or synthesis may be one feature of altered serotonergic activity. These studies have found higher TRYP or free: total TRYP levels in violent criminals (Eriksson & Lidberg, 1997; Tiihonen et al., 2001; Virkkunen & Narvanen, 1987), and in alcoholics with either APD (Swann, Johnson, Cloninger, & Chen, 1999) or a violent criminal history compared to those without that history (Buydens-Branchey, Branchey, Noumair, & Lieber, 1989). High plasma TRYP is associated with trait aggression in nonclinical populations (Moeller et al., 1996; Wingrove, Bond, Cleare, & Sherwood, 1999), and TRYP depletion increases aggressive responding by healthy males in a laboratory test of aggression (Bjork, Dougherty, Moeller, Cherek, & Swann, 1999; Moeller et al., 1996). These studies suggest that decreased serotonin precursor uptake, or activity of serotonergic synthetic enzymes (which could be reflected in elevated plasma TRYP levels), may play a role in the decreased serotonin turnover observed as reduced 5-HIAA in CSF.

Studies evaluating the activity of monoamine oxidase (MAO), the major degradative enzyme for brain serotonin (and also important for catechoamine metabolism), have also repeatedly found group differences in populations related to psychopathy, relative to control groups. These studies have examined MAO enzymatic activity in platelets, which contain one of the two MAO forms (MAO-B) contained in the brain (Lesch et al., 1993). Most of the studies have examined type II alcoholics, with several research groups finding significantly lower platelet MAO activity relative to both type I alcoholics and healthy controls (Devor, Cloninger, Hoffman, & Tabakoff, 1993; Hallman, von Knorring, & Oreland, 1996; Sherif, Hallman, & Oreland, 1992; Sullivan et al., 1990; von Knorring, Hallman, von Knorring, & Oreland, 1991).

However, other studies have found type II alcoholics to have MAO activity similar to type I alcoholics (Soyka et al., 2000; Yates, Wilcox, Knudson, Myers, & Kelly, 1990). Another study (Anthenelli, Smith, Craig, Tabakoff, & Schuckit, 1995) found the association of low MAO activity with alcoholism to be highly dependent on the criteria for identifying subtypes of alcoholism.

Other studies have examined subject samples with psychopathy-related symptoms in the absence of alcohol-use disorders. One study found the low-MAO group to exhibit a personality profile of high impulsiveness and irritability and low socialization (Schalling, Asberg, Edman, & Oreland, 1987). Lower MAO activity has been demonstrated in subject groups defined by Cleckley psychopathy criteria (Lidberg, Modin, Oreland, Tuck, & Gillner, 1985), adult offenders (Garpenstrand et al., 2002), and violent versus nonviolent offenders (Belfrage, Lidberg, & Oreland, 1992). In studies of criminal recidivism, lower MAO activity was observed among former juvenile "delinquents" with adult recidivism and high PCL scores (relative to nonrecidivists and noncriminal controls; Alm et al., 1996b), and in both early criminality (before age 15) and late criminality (after age 15) groups (Alm et al., 1994). In this second study, those in the early criminality group who had low MAO activity had a relative risk of 3.1 for later criminal behavior (Alm et al., 1994). High scores on the Psychopathy and Aggression factors of the Karolinska Scale of Personality (KSP) are also associated with low MAO activity among violent recidivists but not among non-violent recidivists or nonrecidivists (Stalenheim, 2004; Stalenheim, von Knorring, & Oreland, 1997). However, in the first of these studies the low-MAO group (at study entry) did not differ from a high-MAO group on PCL Factor 1 or 2 scores, and on follow-up it was reported that no association was seen overall between PCL scores and MAO activity.

Low MAO activity has also been consistently associated with the trait of sensation seeking, which is highly correlated with novelty seeking and associated with antisocial and criminal behavior, and psychopathy (reviewed in Zuckerman, 1993). Overall, there appears to be considerable evidence that low MAO activity is related to aggressiveness and criminality (including recidivism), and to antisocial behavior and affiliated personality traits, though the direct relationship to psychopathy per se remains poorly addressed. The precise role of low MAO activity is unclear, because lower rates of serotonin degradation in the brain would be expected to result in tonically *higher* levels of activity. It has been suggested that low MAO activity in platelets may reflect the density, size, or functional capacity of the central serotonin system (Oreland & Shaskan, 1983), but this remains an untested hypothesis. There is, however, some evidence that mice with an MAO-A gene promoter knockout display aberrant organization of projections from thalamus to somatosensory cortex (Vitalis et al., 1998) and accumulation of serotonin in atypical regions of the brain during development (Cases et al., 1998)—suggesting that the effects of altered serotonin degradative activity may be exerted during brain development, with behavioral sequelae manifest later in life.

A variety of methods have been used to target serotonin receptors and reuptake (i.e. transporter) sites. Platelet serotonin receptors (e.g., 5-HT$_{2A}$) and transporter sites are similar to those in the brain (Lesch et al., 1993) and are easily accessed, providing a model for central serotonergic function. The binding of serotonin to platelet membranes is higher in patients with suicidal behavior (Pandey et al., 1990) and self-reported aggressive behavior (Coccaro, Kavoussi,

Sheline, et al., 1997); if found in the brain as well, this deviation could reflect a receptor upregulation in response to blunted levels of synaptic serotonergic activity. In addition, platelet serotonin transporter numbers are inversely related to self-injurious behavior (Simeon et al., 1992) and lifetime aggression histories (Coccaro et al., 1996) in personality-disordered patients.

Receptor-binding studies in postmortem brain tissue provide a more direct assessment of central serotonergic receptor and transporter function. In suicide victims decreased serotonin transporter binding has been found (Arango, Underwood, & Mann, 1997), as well as a higher density of 5-HT$_{2A}$ receptors in prefrontal cortex (Arango et al., 1990). These differences could reflect an upregulation of these postsynaptic receptors in response to lower levels of synaptic serotonin. Suicide victims also have increased 5-HT$_{1A}$ binding in the midbrain, which, in contrast to 5-HT$_{2A}$ receptors (which are exclusively postsynaptic), may primarily lead to increased 5-HT$_{1A}$ autoreceptor-mediated inhibition of action potential generation in serotonergic cell bodies located in the raphe nuclei (Stockmeier et al., 1998).

Other studies have used agents having more specific serotonin receptor-binding activity, including direct serotonin agonists such as *m*-chlorophenylpiperazine (m-CPP, which has a complex profile of activity at numerous serotonin receptors), 5-HT$_{1A}$ partial agonists such as buspirone, and the more potent and selective 5-HT$_{1A}$ agonist ipsapirone. These studies have generally found reduced central serotonin function associated with aggressiveness and impulsivity, consistent with the literature cited earlier. Reduced prolactin response to m-CPP was observed in men with APD and substance abuse, compared to healthy controls (Moss, Yao, & Panzak, 1990), and prolactin response to m-CPP was inversely related to both self-reported violence and irritability (Coccaro et al., 1990) and to assaultiveness in a sample of subjects with personality disorder (Coccaro, Kavoussi, Trestman, et al., 1997). The oral temperature response to ipsapirone has been inversely related to aggressive behavior on a laboratory measure of aggression, the Point Subtraction Aggression Paradigm (Moeller et al., 1998). These studies indicate that impaired serotonin receptor-mediated activity is related to aggressive behavior. In the case of 5-HT$_{1A}$ active agents it remains unclear whether the crucial site of action is the postsynaptic serotonin 5-HT$_{1A}$ receptor on nonserotonergic cells (distributed widely throughout the brain), versus the cell–body 5-HT$_{1A}$ receptor on serotonin cells themselves, located primarily in the midbrain raphe nuclei.

Neuroimaging methods have recently come into use in order to specify more clearly the regional anatomy of neural activity. Positron emission tomography (PET) studies have found decreased resting glucose utilization (related local neural activity) in orbitofrontal cortex of murderers (Raine et al., 1994) and in adjacent areas of inferior and middle frontal cortex and temporal lobes of patients with personality disorder with aggressive behavior (Goyer et al., 1994). These brain regions integrate emotional and incentive-related information in behavioral control (Miller & Cummings, 1999) and appear to be related to clinical features of aggressiveness, impulsivity, and emotional disturbance.

PET imaging technology has also been used together with serotonergic agents to investigate impulsive and aggressive behavior. This represents a significant advance in the study of serotonin, which is distributed virtually throughout the entire brain of humans and other mammals (Cooper, Bloom, & Roth, 1996). Untreated depressed patients with personality disorder with a history of suicidal behavior exhibited an impaired response to fenfluramine in prefrontal cortex (Mann et al., 1996), and among a similar subject group the high-lethality suicide attempters exhibited a blunted response to fenfluramine in ventral, medial, and lateral regions of prefrontal cortex, compared to the low-lethality subgroup (Oquendo et al., 2003). Patients with impulsive aggression also showed blunted activation of orbitofrontal, ventral inferior, and cingulate cortices in response to fenfluramine (but normal activation in the inferior parietal cortex), compared to controls (Siever et al., 1999). Patients with impulsive aggression have altered metabolic responses to m-CPP in the orbitofrontal, anterior, and posterior cingulate cortices, suggesting that altered postsynaptic activity in these brain regions may mediate the blunted responses to fenfluramine (New et al., 2002).

Candidate Genes Related to Central Serotonin System

Genetic analysis of these central serotonergic system elements has been considered in relation to these disorders (Lesch & Merschdorf, 2000). These biochemical elements are commonly products of genes that exhibit polymorphisms, which are variations in the DNA sequences coding for the gene product; this variation may or may not confer differences in the functional activity of the gene product. The different copies of the gene are called "alleles." In order to associate a candidate gene of interest with the phenomenology or disorder of interest, covariation between the two is evaluated. Several promising candidate genes coding for elements of the serotonin system are described below (for a review of this issue with regard to type II alcoholism in particular, see Hill, Stoltenberg, Burmeister, & Closser, 1999).

Tryptophan Hydroxylase

Tryptophan hydroxylase (TPH) is the initial enzyme involved in the synthesis of neuronal serotonin. Two common alleles of a TPH polymorphism have been identified. The L allele is associated with reduced CSF 5-HIAA, a history of severe suicide attempts, and lower KSP socialization scale scores according to work by Nielsen and colleagues (1994, 1998). The U allele has also been associated with suicide attempts (Mann et al., 1997). However, some studies have not found an association of TPH genotype with suicide (Abbar et al., 2001; Geijer et al., 2000; Kunugi et al., 1999). The LL genotype has been associated with impulsive aggression in patients with personality disorder, in comparison to the UL and UU genotypes (New et al., 1998), although another study associated the U allele with measures of anger and aggression (Manuck et al., 1999). A polymorphism of the TPH gene promoter has also been associated with suicide attempts in a Finnish offender sample (Rotondo et al., 1999).

Serotonin Transporter

A polymorphism in the promoter region of the serotonin transporter gene (5-HTTP) has been identified, coding for transporter proteins with varying rates of functional activity. The "s" allele is less active than the "l" allele and is associated with measures of impulsivity and neuroticism (N), including the Angry Hostility facet of N (measured by a five-factor personality inventory), in a nonclinical sample (Greenberg et al., 2000; Lesch et al., 1996). Others have not replicated this finding (Ebstein et al., 1997; Gelernter, Kranzler, Coccaro, Siever, & New, 1998). Higher rates of the s,s genotype have been found in type II alcoholics compared to type I alcoholics and controls (Hallikainen et al., 1999), and in violent suicidal behavior (Bellivier et al., 2000; Bondy, Erfurth, DeJonge, Kruger, & Meyer, 2000), although other studies have found no association of the 5-HTTP polymorphism with suicidal behavior (Geijer et al., 2000; Mann et al., 2000; Russ, Lachman, Kasdan, Saito, & Bajmakovic-Kacila, 2000). The s allele has also been associated with lower harm avoidance and higher novelty seeking on the Tridimensional Personality Questionnaire among alcoholics diagnosed with "dissocial" personality disorder according to the criteria of the 10th edition of *International Classification of Diseases* (Sander et al., 1998). In addition, the s allele has been related to symptom counts for conduct disorder and aggressiveness among male adoptees (Cadoret et al., 2003).

These reports provide some evidence that variation in genetic regulation of serotonin transporter production is related to impulsive and aggressive behavior, although some inconsistencies remain to be resolved. In particular, the relationship of a low-transporter activity variant of serotonin transporter to mood and behavior disturbances appears paradoxical, because lower serotonin reuptake into neuron terminals would lead to elevated synaptic activity. However, serotonin transporter is associated with brain development in rodents and nonhuman primates, and altered patterns of serotonin reuptake early in life may have deleterious effects on serotonin function later in life, perhaps in a manner analogous to the developmental effects of the MAO-A gene promoter knock-

out described earlier (and discussed in Lesch & Merschdorf, 2000).

5-HT$_{1B}$ Receptor

Mice with a 5-HT$_{1B}$ receptor gene knockout display increased aggressive behavior (Saudou et al., 1994). A study of antisocial alcoholics (with comorbid APD or IED) from two different ethnic samples showed evidence for sib-pair linkage to a 5-HT$_{1B}$ receptor gene polymorphism (Lappalainen et al., 1998). However, differences in 5-HT$_{1B}$ receptor allele frequencies have not been associated with groups of alcoholics or alcoholic subtypes in other studies (Kranzler, Hernandez-Avila, & Gelernter, 2002; Sinha, Cloninger, & Parsian, 2003), and Soyka, Preuss, Koller, Zill, and Bondy (2004) found a *lower* frequency of this polymorphism in association with antisocial personality traits and conduct disorder history in a clinical alcoholic sample. This polymorphism is associated with differing susceptibility to suicidal behavior in patients with personality disorders (New et al., 2001), and nondepressed suicide victims show decreased 5-HT$_{1B}$ receptor binding in the frontal cortex (Arranz, Eriksson, Mellerup, Plenge, & Marcusson, 1994). However, another postmortem study found no difference in allele frequency of the 5-HT$_{1B}$ receptor gene polymorphism between suicide and nonsuicide victims, although there was some indication that the presence of this polymorphism was associated with reduced 5-HT$_{1B}$ receptor numbers (Huang, Grailhe, Arango, Hen, & Mann, 1999).

MAO-A

Transgenic mice with an MAO-A gene knockout are characterized by increased aggressive behavior, and the male mice exhibit increased attempts to copulate with nonreceptive females (Cases et al., 1995). In addition, a large Dutch kindred has been described which contains a prevalent point mutation in the MAO-A gene, leading to an absence of MAO-A activity (Brunner, Nelen, Breakefield, Ropers, & van Oost, 1993; Brunner, Nelen, van Zanvoort, et al., 1993). All affected males have mild mental retardation with decreased urinary 5-HIAA levels and exhibit impulsive–aggressive and hypersexual behavior; histories of arson and attempted suicide have been documented among affected individuals as well.

Affected males also have increased levels of catecholamine MAO substrates and decreased levels of catecholamine metabolites such as HVA and MHPG (3-methoxy-4-hydroxyphenylglycol), indicating altered catecholamine degradative activity as well. Because MAO-A is more strongly localized to the locus ceruleus than the raphe nuclei in primates, and to a lesser extent in midbrain dopaminergic neurons (Finberg, 1995), the behavioral effects of MAO-A deficiency may be partly or largely mediated by catecholamine excess (see following sections for discussion of the role of catecholamines in these disorders). However, pharmacological evidence suggests that the behavioral phenotype of the MAO-A knockout may be primarily due to effects on metabolism of serotonin rather than that of catecholamines. Another research group has found that mutation frequencies in the same exon of the human MAO-A gene, along with the most common associated haplotype, were observed more frequently in a sample of unrelated adults with alcoholism and APD compared to a control group (Parsian, 1999).

However, marked MAO-A deficiency may be very rare (Schuback et al., 1999). Low-transcription polymorphisms of the promoter for the MAO-A gene have also been identified (Sabol, Hu, & Hamer, 1998). One of these is more frequent in alcoholics with APD compared to alcoholics without APD or healthy controls (Samochowiec et al., 1999; Schmidt et al., 2000), and antisocial alcoholism symptom severity has been associated with homozygotes and hemizygotes for a low-activity MAO-A allele (Hill, Stoltenberg, Bullard, Li, Zucker, & Burmeister, 2002). However, other groups have failed to find an increased frequency of these polymorphisms in type II alcoholics (Lu, Lin, Lee, Ko, & Shih, 2003; Saito et al., 2002), APD without alcoholism (Lu et al., 2003), or adolescents with conduct disorder (Vanyukov, Moss, Yu, & Deka, 1995). In addition, in a community sample of men the low-transcription polymorphisms have been associated with *lower* scores on an aggression–impulsivity factor (derived from factor

analysis of the Barratt Impulsivity Scale, Buss–Durkee Hostility Inventory, and Life History of Aggression), along with greater prolactin response to fenfluramine (Manuck, Flory, Ferrell, Mann, & Muldoon, 2000). Also, the low-transcription polymorphisms were neither associated with high scores on these same impulsivity, irritability, and assaultiveness scales in a general alcoholic sample (Koller, Bondy, Preuss, Bottlender, & Soyka, 2003), nor associated with psychoticism or negative affect in a community sample in Australia (Jorm et al., 2000). In sum, although the functional significance of variations in MAO-A transcription in human populations remains unclear, the consistent finding of impaired MAO activity in the biochemical studies reviewed in the previous section, together with the effects of MAO deficiency on both monoamine levels and behavior in animal models, suggests a role for MAO in impulse control disorders.

In addition, a recent line of investigation suggests an intriguing link between monoaminergic disturbances and a neurocognitive deficit that may underlie the social and emotional dysfunction that is a hallmark of psychopathy. Harmer and colleagues have shown that recognition of facial expressions of fear can be specifically increased with tryptophan (Attenburrow et al., 2003) or selective serotonin reuptake inhibitor (SSRI) administration (Harmer, Bhagwagar, et al., 2003), decreased with tryptophan depletion (Harmer, Rogers, Tunbridge, Cowen, & Goodwin, 2003), and normalized in remitted depressed subjects with SSRIs (Bhagwagar, Cowen, Goodwin, & Harmer, 2004)—all in double-blind, placebo-controlled studies. These findings indicate a role for serotonergic activity in the recognition of fearful facial expressions, a neurocognitive function that is necessary for the development of moral behavior in children, and which is impaired in children and adults with psychopathic features (Blair, 2003).

In light of this work, the investigation of serotonergic deficits in other aspects of the phenomenology of psychopathy might be usefully extended to the emotion-related deficits characteristic of Factor 1, in order to test for a link between the pathophysiology of the two phenomenological factors that frequently co-occur in this illness. Nevertheless, at present, the main evidence for an association between serotonergic dysfunction and psychopathy lies with the impulsive, aggressive, antisocial features of the disorder (i.e., Factor 2). The role of neurochemical dysfunction in the affective–interpersonal factor remains to be directly investigated.

DOPAMINE

Dopamine systems in the brain subserve a variety of functions, including motor activity and higher cognitive functions such as working memory. Dopamine excess associated with the use of stimulants frequently leads to aggressive and impulsive behavior, and dopamine antagonists (neuroleptics) have a well-established role in treating hostility and aggressive behavior across a range of psychiatric disorders (Buckley, 1999). Nevertheless, the role of altered dopaminergic function in the clinical syndromes of impulsive aggression, APD, psychopathy, and others presently under consideration has received relatively little empirical attention. Early studies demonstrated lower levels of CSF HVA (indicating lower rates of dopamine turnover, analogous to 5-HIAA levels for serotonin turnover) in recidivist criminals compared to nonrecidivist criminals (Virkkunen et al., 1989), though this finding was not replicated by this group in a prospective follow-up study (Virkkunen et al., 1996). An inverse relationship of CSF HVA to lifetime aggression scores in alcoholics has also been reported (Limson et al., 1991).

However, more recent studies have observed *higher* levels of CSF HVA to be related to psychopathy scores in samples of violent offenders (Soderstrom et al., 2001, 2003). In the earlier study CSF HVA levels were strongly associated with both PCL-R Factor 1 and 2 scores, and the ratio of HVA:5-HIAA was also strongly associated with Factor 1 and 2 scores. The second study (with a different sample of violent offenders) found these indices to be much more strongly related to Factor 2 than Factor 1 scores, suggesting a clearer role for serotonin–dopamine interaction in the antisocial behavioral facet than the affective–interpersonal facet of psychopathy. Elevated blood HVA levels have also been observed in

youths (under 12 years old) with disruptive behavioral disorders who have substance-abusing fathers compared to those without this paternal history (Gabel, Stadler, Bjorn, & Schindledecker, 1995), providing preliminary evidence for dopamine dysfunction in the transgenerational transmission of substance use/behavioral disorders.

Dopamine receptor polymorphisms have been related to personality traits that are elevated in psychopathy, APD, and substance abuse, such as novelty seeking (Goldman, Skodol, McGrath, & Oldham, 1994; Svrakic, Whitehead, Przybeck, & Cloninger, 1993). A polymorphism of the dopamine D_4 receptor (DRD4) has been associated with novelty seeking (Ebstein et al., 1996). This finding is consistent with the behavioral phenotype of a DRD4 gene knockout mouse, which exhibits not only a decreased response to novel stimuli (Dulawa, Grandy, Low, Paulus, & Geyer, 1999) but supersensitivity to alcohol, cocaine, and methamphetamine as well (Rubinstein et al., 1997). The DRD4 polymorphism has also been positively related to extraversion and negatively related to conscientiousness (Benjamin et al., 1996). A number of groups have attempted to replicate these findings, with mixed results (see Reif & Lesch, 2003, for detailed summary). Some of this work has indicated interactions between the DRD4 and other monoaminergic polymorphisms (reviewed in Ebstein, Benjamin, & Belmaker, 2000); it has also been suggested (Reif & Lesch, 2003) that the results overall indicate that this DRD4 polymorphism is likely not a susceptibility gene for novelty seeking but, rather, in linkage disequilibrium with another gene variant, which may include a polymorphism in the DRD4 promoter region (Okuyama et al., 2000; Ronai et al., 2001).

Other dopamine receptor subtypes have been investigated in association with antisocial behavior. Two polymorphisms of the dopamine D_2 receptor (DRD2) have been identified. In one study of alcoholics, a group carrying one of these (the A1 allele) had a higher prevalence of comorbid APD than the group without this allele (Ponce et al., 2003). In another study, a group of alcoholics with APD had a stronger association with both DRD2 polymorphisms compared to alcoholics without APD or controls (Hill, Zezza,

Wipprecht, Locke, & Neiswanger, 1999), and the association of both polymorphisms has also been observed in alcoholism with conduct disorder (Lu, Lee, Ko, & Lin, 2001). However, other studies have not observed increased rates of these DRD2 polymorphisms in type II alcoholics (Bolos et al., 1990; Parsian et al., 1991; Parsian, Cloninger, & Zhang, 2000) or in PCL-R psychopathy among incarcerated substance abusers (Smith et al., 1993). Therefore, the status of DRD2 polymorphisms in these disorders remains undetermined.

Other studies have found a DRD3 polymorphism to be associated with impulsiveness in a group of violent offenders but not in a normal control group (Retz, Rosler, Supprian, Retz-Junginger, & Thome, 2003), and a DRD5 polymorphism to be associated with childhood symptom counts for ODD in men and women and adult APD symptom counts in women (mediated by ODD history; Vanyukov, Moss, Kaplan, Kirillova, & Tarter, 2000). Brain imaging studies have also been conducted to visualize the dopamine transporter (DAT) *in vivo* with single photon emission computed tomography (SPECT) using a ligand (β-CIT), which binds both the dopamine and serotonin transporter, together with pretreatment with citalopram to prevent β-CIT binding to serotonin transporter. Using this method, one study found violent alcoholics to have slightly higher striatal DAT binding than controls, who in turn had significantly higher DAT binding than a group of nonviolent alcoholics (Tiihonen et al., 1995). A follow-up study by these investigators found the same group differences, with a sample comprised primarily of violent type II alcoholic offenders (Tiihonen et al., 1997). These findings regarding DRD3, DRD5 and DAT must be regarded as preliminary, and await replication.

NOREPINEPHRINE

The norepinephrine (NE) system in the brain mediates states of vigilance, with effects on signal detection and widespread effects on cognition in general, as well as mediating behavioral activation, primarily in response to novel or threatening stimuli in the environment (Berridge & Waterhouse, 2003). It is also activated by exogenous amphetamine administration and appears to mediate many of the behavioral and subjective effects of this substance (Berridge & Waterhouse, 2003). Despite the well-established role of central NE in fight-or-flight responses, and the behavioral effects of NE activation by stimulants, the NE system has received little empirical attention in relation to aggressive or antisocial behavior.

Early studies of NE function in aggressive or criminal behavior found both higher plasma levels of phenylethylamine metabolites in violent prisoners compared to nonviolent prisoners and controls (Sandler, Ruthven, Goodwin, Field, & Matthews, 1978) and lower urinary levels of NE in arrested men awaiting trial who scored above the median on a scale derived from Cleckley criteria (Lidberg, Levander, Schalling, & Lidberg, 1978). The significance of these early findings is unclear, as phenylethylamine is a trace amine without a clear physiological role in the nervous system; blunted peripheral NE levels in response to a stressful event may be related to the well-described attenuation in stress reactivity observed clinically in psychopathy, but this relationship has not been addressed directly. Another early study found CSF levels of the major NE metabolite, MHPG, to be positively associated with lifetime aggression scores (Brown et al., 1979), though Virkkunen and colleagues (1987) reported lower CSF MHPG in a group of violent offenders and arsonists compared to healthy controls. Other studies found no relationship between CSF MHPG and aggressive behavior (Brown et al., 1982; Lidberg, Tuck, et al., 1985; Roy, Adinoff, & Linnoila, 1988).

More recent attention has been focused on a major degradative enzyme for NE, catechol-O-Methyl Transferase (COMT, which also catabolizes dopamine). Mice heterozygous for COMT deficiency display increased aggressive behavior (Gogos et al., 1998). Among schizophrenic patients, those with the low-activity (met/met) polymorphism of COMT are more aggressive compared to those with the high-activity COMT polymorphism (Lachman, Nolan, Mohr, Saito, & Volavka, 1998; Strous, Nolan, Lapidus, Libna, & Saito, 2003). Patients with schizophrenia with a history of homicide (Kotler et al., 1999) or violent suicide attempts (Nolan et al., 2000) have higher rates of the low-activity genotype versus nonviolent schizophrenics or nonpatient controls. This polymorphism was also more prevalent in a sample of aggressive inpatients with various Axis I and II diagnoses (Rujescu, Giegling, Gietl, Hartmann, & Moller, 2003).

TESTOSTERONE

Testosterone is a gonadal hormone with multiple physiological roles. It is primarily responsible for sexual maturation and sexual behavior in male mammals but has widespread effects on cognition, subjective experience, and behavior in both sexes. This includes aggressive behavior, particularly that exhibited by males. Circulating testosterone levels rise at puberty in boys, corresponding with a significant increase in aggressive behavior. A considerable literature exists relating peripheral testosterone levels (measured in serum or saliva) in nonclinical populations to aggressive behavior and hostility, particularly when behavior is assessed in the laboratory rather than with self-report measures (reviewed in Archer, 1991; Harris, 1999). A smaller set of studies has related testosterone to personality traits such as sensation seeking and extraversion (Daitzman & Zuckerman, 1980; Gerra et al., 1999).

Studies of forensic populations have found higher serum total and free testosterone levels among offenders with personality disorder compared to offenders with schizophrenia; within the personality disorder group the recidivists had higher total and free testosterone levels than did the non-recidivists (Rasanen et al., 1999). Adolescent male delinquents had higher plasma (Mattson, Schalling, Olweus, Low, & Svensson, 1980) and salivary free (Banks & Dabbs, 1996) testosterone levels than age-matched normal groups, and within the delinquent group in Mattson and colleagues (1980), those with an armed-robbery history had higher levels than did the less violent group. A study of clinic-referred children with disruptive behavior found salivary testosterone levels correlated with staff ratings of the children's aggressive behavior (Scerbo & Kolko, 1994), and among adolescents enrolled in a longitudinal study of children at

risk for psychopathology as the result of perinatal events or psychosocial adversity (Maras et al., 2003), higher plasma testosterone and 5α-dihydrotestosterone was found in a group of 14-year-old boys with elevated scores of externalizing behavior. In a study of young adult forensic psychiatric patients (uncharacterized diagnostically), the group with a violent criminal history had higher plasma testosterone levels than did the group with a nonviolent criminal history, though when grouped by history of fighting while in prison, the "fighters" testosterone levels were similar to that of the "nonfighters" (Kreuz & Rose, 1972).

Other studies of adult male prisoners found aggressive or violent groups to have higher testosterone levels in plasma (Ehrenkranz, Bliss, & Sheard, 1974), saliva (Dabbs, Carr, Frady, & Riad, 1995) and CSF (Virkkunen et al., 1994) than nonaggressive groups, offenders with higher salivary-free testosterone levels to have a greater history of violent crime than low-testosterone offenders (Dabbs, Frady, Carr, & Besch, 1987), and plasma testosterone levels to be correlated with antisocial symptom counts among a group of violent offenders (Aromaki, Lindman, & Eriksson, 1999). A study of psychopathy among violent criminals undergoing forensic examination found serum total testosterone and sex-hormone binding globulin to be associated with type II alcoholism and APD diagnoses, as well as with PCL-R Factor 2 scores; free testosterone was associated with high KSP psychopathy factor scores (Stalenheim, Eriksson, von Knorring, & Wide, 1998). A single study of female inmates found salivary testosterone levels to be associated with criminal behavior as well as aggressiveness in prison (Dabbs & Hargrove, 1997).

The role of testosterone in sexual crimes has also been addressed specifically in a few studies. Giotakos, Markianos, Vaidakis, and Christodoulou (2003) found a group of men convicted of rape to have higher testosterone than a normal control group, though testosterone levels were not associated with aggression scores. A study of a forensic psychiatric population with convictions for sexual crimes found the subgroup of rapists who used more violence during commission of the crime to have higher plasma testosterone levels than either less violent rapists, a group of nonviolent child molesters, or healthy controls (Rada, Laws, & Kellner, 1976). In another study involving a combined group of rapists and child molesters (50% with APD), salivary testosterone was associated with an index of antisocial behaviors (Aromaki, Lindman, & Eriksson, 2002), though the group on average had testosterone levels similar to a control group—possibly (in light of the Rada et al. results) due to heterogeneity in the target sample.

Testosterone has also been studied in the context of domestic violence. In a mixed group of male alcoholics, the subgroup with histories of violence and physical abuse had higher serum testosterone than the subgroup without that history (Bergman & Brismar, 1994). A study of domestic violence perpetrators showed the group with alcohol dependence (11/13 with comorbid Cluster B personality disorders) to have higher CSF testosterone than the group without alcohol dependence (5/10 with Cluster B personality disorders) (George et al., 2001). A study of men recruited from the community on the basis of risk factors for HIV (human immunodeficiency virus) infection found salivary testosterone levels to be associated with self-reported domestic violence using the Conflict Tactics Scale (CTS), including verbal and physical aggression (Soler, Vinayak, & Quadagno, 2000). Interestingly, another study of adult males from the community, using the CTS to assess domestic violence, found that whereas plasma testosterone was associated with high scores on the CTS physical assault and injury scales, plasma estradiol was associated with the emotional negotiation scale, suggesting that estradiol in men may serve to mitigate the adverse interpersonal effects of high testosterone (Eriksson, Pahlaen, Sarkola, & Seppa, 2003).

The mechanism by which testosterone may exert its effects on aggressive behavior is poorly understood at present. Animal models, in which rodents are first castrated and then administered various regimens of exogenous testosterone or other androgens, may involve a number of changes in other hormonal systems and may not be an appropriate model for psychiatric syndromes in which no clear gonadal pathology exists. If testosterone plays an etiological role of some kind in the development of aggressive or antisocial behavior, a critical period may need to be identified given the well-established effects of testosterone on the developing brain, which would not be well modeled by varying the hormone levels to which an adult animal is exposed. In addition, social factors appear even more important in their effects on testosterone levels than on many other neurochemical systems. For example, the preexistence or formation of dominance relationships is associated with varying testosterone levels (Mazur & Booth, 1998). In humans, the experience of success can cause testosterone levels to rise, with the reverse upon failure; this effect is apparent even in sports fans' responses to winning and losing (Mazur & Booth, 1998). Socioeconomic status, diet, alcohol intake, body fat content, and psychological stress can all have effects on testosterone levels. Testosterone also exhibits circadian and circannual rhythms and may vary with women's menstrual cycle. Testosterone effects may also be mediated by interactions with brain monoaminergic systems. These and other common methodological issues are reviewed in Harris (1999) and Archer (1991).

CORTISOL

Empirical studies addressing the hypothalamic–pituitary–adrenal (HPA) axis in psychopathy and related adult disorders such as APD have been scant. This is remarkable, given the strong emphasis in the psychopathy literature on disturbances in the subjective experience of anxiety, as well as stress and autonomic reactivity (Arnett, 1997). An early study of offenders at a maximum-security hospital in England found this group (which had twice the rate of fatalities resulting from their crimes, compared to the hospital's total population) to exhibit a blunted urinary cortisol response to a varied set of emotional and stressful stimuli compared to mentally ill or normal control groups (Woodman et al., 1978). Another study found a group of habitually violent offenders with APD to have lower 24-hour urinary-free cortisol levels compared to other violent offenders, APD subjects without violent behavior, and normal controls (Virkkunen, 1985). Lower salivary (free) cortisol levels have been found in other samples of violent versus nonviolent offenders (Brewer-Smyth,

Burgess, & Shults, 2004), and serum cortisol levels were lower in a subgroup of alcoholics with repeated physically abusive behavior, compared to alcoholics without that behavior (Bergman & Brismar, 1994). Lower cortisol nadirs have also been associated with self-reported antisocial behavior and aggressiveness (Fishbein, Dax, Lozovsky, & Jaffe, 1992). Not all studies have found lower cortisol associated with violent behavior, however (Buydens-Branchey & Branchey, 1992; van Heeringen, Audenaert, Van de Wiele, & Verstraete, 2000).

Overall, this literature suggests that violent and antisocial adults exhibit lower cortisol levels, though it remains unclear whether this represents primarily a blunted basal output or, possibly, also a blunted cortisol response to stress—such as that associated with incarceration, for example. Unfortunately, in the aforementioned studies, the effects of current or past stressors, and possible comorbid mood symptoms, posttraumatic stress disorder, traumatic brain injury, or other medical illness (all of which may affect cortisol levels) have not generally been evaluated (for a notable exception, see Brewer-Smyth et al., 2004).

Cortisol levels have also been evaluated in child and adolescent behavioral disorders related to psychopathy. Salivary cortisol levels have been inversely related to aggressive conduct disorder symptoms in preadolescent boys (McBurnett, Lahey, Rathouz, & Loeber, 2000; Vanyukov et al., 1993); to teachers' ratings of delinquent, aggressive, and externalizing behaviors in boys with ODD (van Goozen et al., 1998); and to APD symptom counts in the fathers of boys with conduct disorder who themselves have lower cortisol compared to controls (Vanyukov et al., 1993). Salivary cortisol levels are also lower in adolescent girls with conduct disorder compared to controls (Pajer, Gardner, Rubin, Perel, & Neal, 2001). In addition, higher adrenocorticotropin (ACTH) levels were found in a 10–13-year-old subgroup of a 10–18-year-old sample with conduct disorder, compared to an age-matched normal control group (Dmitrieva, Oades, Hauffa, & Eggers, 2001), offering some evidence consistent with a compensatory ACTH response to low circulating cortisol in this population. Low cortisol in preadolescent boys was a predictor of aggressive behavior 5 years later

in adolescence (Shoal, Giancola, & Kirillova, 2003); and an ODD subgroup characterized by low anxiousness and high externalizing behavior exhibited a paradoxical decrease in cortisol to a stressful scenario involving an unsolvable task and an interpersonal provocation (van Groozen et al., 1998). In addition, a study of a nonclinical population of young adults found the salivary cortisol response to a novel laboratory-controlled social stressor to be inversely related to self-reported social deviance and sexual risk-taking (Halpern, Campbell, Agnew, Thompson, & Udry, 2002). These findings suggest that disturbances in the HPA axis appear early, at least by the time of emergence of problematic behaviors in childhood, and may disrupt the socializing effects of affect experienced in an interpersonal setting, perhaps particularly with regard to anxiety and associated fear conditioning (see Arnett, 1997, for detailed discussion).

THYROID HORMONE, GLUCOSE, AND CHOLESTEROL

A small set of studies has examined neurochemical abnormalities in other systems. In a study of thyroid hormones in former juvenile delinquents ages 38–46, serum T3 levels were associated with criminality but not psychopathy-related personality traits; those who persisted with criminal behavior had higher T3 levels than those who did not (Alm et al., 1996a). A study of men undergoing forensic psychiatric examination found higher serum T3 levels in a subgroup with repeated violent criminality; the repeated nonviolent criminality subgroup showed normal T3 levels (Stalenheim, von Knorring, & Wide, 1998). The subgroup high on PCL-R Factor 2 had significantly higher T3 compared to those low on Factor 2, whereas the high Factor 1 subgroup did not differ from the low Factor 1 group in T3 levels. Serum free T4 (FT4) levels in these groups showed a generally similar pattern, though in the opposite direction. This suggests that the reciprocal changes in T3 and FT4 could reflect an increase in the conversion of FT4 to T3. In a prospective study by this same research group (Stalenheim, 2004), criminal recidivists had higher serum T3 and lower FT4 levels at follow-up than did nonrecidivists;

T3 levels were correlated with psychopathy- and aggression-related personality traits on the KSP, though not with PCL-R factor scores. Adult levels of thyroid hormones have also been associated with a history of childhood conduct disorder (Ramklint, Stalenheim, von Knorring, & von Knorring, 2000), and free T3 was also found to be higher in a preadolescent subgroup of conduct disorder patients compared to an age-matched group (Dmitrieva et al., 2001).

It should be noted that in the studies of adult populations, comorbid substance use (even in the absence of liver impairment) and differential rates of exposure to stressors are likely confounding effects. Of potential etiological interest is the relationship between stress and thyroid function (Mason, 1968). Thyroid hormone disturbances can be observed as much as 50 years after traumatic experiences that give rise to chronic post-traumatic stress disorder (Wang & Mason, 1999), and given the high rate of childhood adversity in APD and psychopathy, elevated T3 levels may index the severity or duration of childhood abuse, for example. This possibility remains unaddressed, as does the pathophysiological mechanism by which altered thyroid function may exert effects on behavior in these disorders.

Lower blood glucose nadirs during the glucose tolerance test are found among violent offenders with APD compared to those without APD (Virkkunen & Huttunen, 1982) and have been associated with measures of antisocial personality and aggressiveness among a group of substance abusers (Fishbein et al., 1992). This second study also found recovery from the glucose test to be slower for violent offenders compared to normal controls—an effect that has been shown for truancy as well as a paternal history of alcohol-related violence (Virkkunen, 1982). Enhanced insulin secretion was found among a group of offenders with intermittent explosive disorder (Virkkunen & Narvanen, 1987) and among a subgroup of young adult males with APD (Virkkunen, 1983a). However, physiological and nutritional factors that may affect insulin activity and glucose levels have not generally been evaluated in these studies, and it is unclear how altered peripheral glucose pharmacokinetics may affect central neuronal processes to lead to antisocial behaviors in the absence of clinically evident disturbances in glucose metabolism.

On the other hand, disturbances in cholesterol metabolism may be a more promising line of investigation. In the early 1990s, reports appeared suggesting a link between low serum cholesterol and an increased rate of "nonillness" deaths (primarily due to suicide, violence, or accident) in large studies of cardiovascular risk factors. Cohort studies with a combined N of 700,000 indicated a significantly increased rate of violent deaths in men with low cholesterol (Jacobs et al., 1992; Lindberg, Rastam, Gullberg, & Eklund, 1992; Neaton et al., 1992). In addition, an early meta-analysis of clinical trials of serum cholesterol-lowering drugs (Muldoon, Manuck, & Matthews, 1990) suggested a relationship between lowered cholesterol and violence as well, though a later meta-analysis from this research group did not support the earlier finding (Muldoon, Manuck, Mendelsohn, Kaplan, & Belle, 2001).

Several studies have examined serum cholesterol in psychiatric or offender populations. Serum cholesterol has been found to be lower among individuals with APD compared to those without APD in samples of both criminals (Virkkunen, 1979) and U.S. Army veterans (Freedman et al., 1995). In a sample of offenders with APD, those with low cholesterol had a more frequent history of early-onset conduct disorder, and a higher rate of early and non-illness-related death (Repo-Tiihonen, Halonen, Tiihonen, & Virkkunen, 2002). Lower cholesterol has also been observed in homicidal offenders who exhibit violence while intoxicated with alcohol (Virkkunen, 1983b), in adolescents with aggressive conduct disorder (Virkkunen & Penttinen, 1984), and in borderline personality disorder (New, Sevin, et al., 1998). Low cholesterol has also been associated with criminal violence in a large Swedish community cohort (Golomb, Stattin, & Mednick, 2000), and with more frequent aggression in male forensic patients (Hillbrand, Spitz, & Foster, 1995; Spitz, Hillbrand, & Foster, 1994). Some studies, however, have failed to demonstrate low cholesterol in APD (Stewart & Stewart, 1981) or in association with violence (Apter et al., 1999; Gray et al., 1993).

Low serum cholesterol has also been investigated in relation to suicide. Lower cholesterol has been associated with increasing degrees of suicidality (Sullivan, Joyce, Bulik, Mulder, & Oakley-Browne, 1994), parasuicide (Gallerani et al., 1995), suicide attempts (Golier, Marzuk, Leon, Weiner, & Tardiff, 1995; Modai, Valevski, Dror, & Weizman, 1994), and suicide completion (Lindberg et al., 1992). It has also been found to be lower in violent suicide attempters compared to nonviolent suicide attempters (Alvarez et al., 2000; Vevera, Zukov, Morcinek, & Papezova, 2003). The relationship of low serum cholesterol to both violence and suicide is similar to that of low central serotonergic function, and the mechanism of cholesterol effects on behavior may be mediated by decreased serotonergic activity. Monkeys fed a low-cholesterol diet have not only a lower plasma cholesterol level and increased aggressive behavior but lower CSF 5-HIAA as well (Kaplan et al., 1994). There is evidence that neuronal membrane cholesterol content can influence membrane fluidity with effects on serotonergic receptor availability (Heron, Shinitzky, Hershkowitz, & Samuel, 1980). In addition, rats with low brain concentrations of docosahexaenoic acid, a fatty acid that is an essential component of synaptic membranes and is processed in a manner similar to cholesterol, have increased 5-HT$_{2A}$ receptor numbers (DeLion et al., 1994)—which could be consistent with decreased synaptic serotonin levels. Plasma levels of this fatty acid have been inversely related to CSF 5-HIAA among a violent subgroup of alcoholics (Hibbeln et al., 1998). In addition, among a group of detoxified cocaine-dependent subjects, those with a history of aggression (all with comorbid APD) had both lower levels of high-density lipoprotein (HDL) cholesterol and blunted cortisol responses to m-CPP (Buydens-Branchey, Branchey, Hudson, & Fergeson, 2000).

Taken together with the extensive evidence for impaired serotonergic function in disorders of aggression and antisocial behavior (reviewed earlier), these findings, although correlational in nature, implicate central serotonergic function as the neuronal substrate mediating the behavioral effects of low serum cholesterol.

PSYCHOPHARMACOLOGICAL TREATMENT OF DISORDERS RELATED TO PSYCHOPATHY

As with the literature evaluating the pathophysiology underlying these disorders, very little empirical work has addressed the pharmacological treatment of psychopathy per se. Instead, efforts have been made to identify medications that effectively treat behavioral symptoms found in these disorders, such as aggression and impulsivity, and comorbid disorders such as substance abuse. Most of this literature has involved research subject samples that exhibit these behaviors as a part of psychiatric disorders unrelated to psychopathy, such as schizophrenia or neurological diseases. However, there are a number of studies involving personality disorder subjects or aggressive criminals.

In any event, a general rule in the pharmacotherapy of psychiatric conditions is that specific symptoms should be the target of treatment rather than clinical syndromes or diagnostic entities. This clinical rule is probably valid to the extent that individual symptoms (such as impulsive aggression) reflect a common underlying neurobiological basis, regardless of the syndrome or diagnosis in which they are found. This observation offers a partial remedy for the widespread sense of futility among clinicians regarding the treatment responsivity of APD and psychopathy (cf. Harris & Rice, Chapter 28, this volume). However, it should also be acknowledged that an essential element in any psychiatric treatment is the therapeutic alliance between clinician and patient, which is generally a challenge as a matter of course in these disorders. With these considerations in mind, we review the small existing empirical literature on the pharmacological treatment of the symptom dimensions and disorders addressed throughout this review, excluding studies of populations unrelated to psychopathy, as well as case reports and retrospective studies.

Lithium is probably the medication that received the earliest attention to its efficacy in treating aggression. In a double-blind, placebo controlled study of 66 nonpsychotic prisoners with chronic impulsive aggressive behavior, Sheard, Marini, Bridges, and Wagner (1976) found that lithium significantly reduced the commission of infractions involving violence in the prison setting. Lithium has also shown efficacy with nonbipolar impulsive aggressive adolescents (Lena, 1979), impulsive aggressive schoolboys who were unmanageable in a community setting (Siassi, 1982), and children hospitalized for aggressive behavior (Malone, Delaney, Luebbert, Cater, & Campbell, 2000).

SSRIs have also shown efficacy with impulsive aggression, as one might expect given the considerable evidence reviewed previously for central serotonergic deficits in this disorder. Decreased irritability and aggression as assessed by the Overt Aggression Scale (OAS) was associated with both sertraline (Kavoussi, Liu, & Coccaro, 1994) and fluoxetine (Coccaro & Kavoussi, 1997) treatment in open-label studies of patients with personality disorder. While early anecdotal reports suggested that fluoxetine may be associated with a paradoxical increase in aggressive behavior, a comprehensive meta-analysis of fluoxetine efficacy trials clearly demonstrated that overt hostility and antisocial behavior were four times more likely in placebo-treated individuals (Heiligenstein, Beasley, & Potvin, 1993).

A range of other psychotropic medications has been evaluated for antiaggressive effects in these populations. An 8-week, open-label trial of divalproex sodium found decreases in irritability and overt aggression after 4 weeks in 10 patients with personality disorder who had failed an SSRI trial (Kavoussi & Coccaro, 1998). A large, multisite double-blind placebo study of 12-week treatment with divalproex in 246 patients with impulsive aggression found that the subgroup of 96 subjects with Cluster B personality disorders exhibited a decrease in OAS aggression scores in the last 4 weeks of treatment compared to placebo (Hollander et al., 2003). Valproic acid was also found to decrease explosiveness and mood lability in a double-blind, placebo-controlled crossover study of 15 children with ODD or conduct disorder (Donovan et al., 2000). A placebo-controlled trial of phenytoin in prisoners also found efficacy for this drug in treating aggression (Barratt, Stanford, Felthous, & Kent, 1997). Although both typical and atypical antipsychotics have demonstrated utility in treating aggression in a range of disorders, particularly those characterized by psychosis

(Buckley, 1999), they have not been studied in relation to personality disorders. One study of risperidone, however, found improvement on multiple measures of aggression in a 10-week, randomized, double-blind placebo-controlled study of 20 boys with conduct disorder (Findling et al., 2000).

Substance use disorders are common in APD and are likely to exacerbate impulsivity and aggression and consequently impair prognosis, as they appear to when comorbid with psychiatric illness in general. As a consequence, the treatment of substance use is essential to optimizing the outcome of these disorders. A number of medications appear to show efficacy in reducing rates of substance use, craving, or sequelae of substance use such as criminality or HIV exposure (for reviews, see Kreek, LaForge, & Butelman, 2002; Schuckit, 1996). These notably include multiple opioidergic medications such as methadone, naltrexone, and buprenorphine, as well as other medications such as acamprosate. However, remarkably little work has addressed the clinical heterogeneity found in substance use disorders, and it is essentially unknown at present whether those comorbid for APD or psychopathy (such as type II alcoholics) exhibit treatment responses similar to those of substance abusers in general. Preliminary studies suggest that early-onset alcoholics (characteristic of type II) may experience reduced intake with a treatment combination of ondansetron and naltrexone (Ait-Daoud, Johnson, Prihoda, & Hargita, 2001), but that alcoholics with APD may improve on drinking measures in response to antidepressant treatment only when experiencing a current comorbid mood or anxiety disorder (Penick et al., 1996).

Finally, a somewhat controversial yet interesting area of pharmacological treatment involves the use of antiandrogens for the treatment of sexual offenders (reviewed in Briken, Hill, & Berner, 2003). Cyproterone acetate and medroxyprogesterone acetate have been used for decades in Europe to reduce recidivism rates in sexual offenders, yet are associated with a range of significant side effects that limit their use. More recently, long-acting agonists of luteinizing hormone-releasing hormone have been considered more tolerable alternatives. Several open-label trials, many in forensic settings and many with identified personality disorder subjects, suggest that medications such as leuprolide or triptorelin show efficacy in reducing the characteristic thoughts and behaviors associated with paraphilias and sexual offenses (Briken et al., 2003). These medications are generally reported as well-tolerated by the subjects, suggesting a possible role for these medications in the treatment of syndromes that are likely associated with a significant public health impact.

CONCLUSION

Psychopathy is a clinical construct that has experienced a recent resurgence of interest among researchers. However, the preponderance of empirical research on the neurochemical basis of this disorder remains targeted at disorders associated with the antisocial deviance (Factor 2) component of psychopathy, such as impulsive aggression, criminality, and other behavioral manifestations of antisociality, as well as affiliated personality dimensions. These studies reveal a consistent finding of impaired central serotonergic activity related to impulsivity and aggressive behavior, with multiple elements of the serotonergic system involved. Interesting though less consistent evidence suggests a role for other monoaminergic disturbances such as altered receptor and neurotransmitter activity in dopamine and norepinephrine systems. Other neurochemical systems appear to be altered in association with these behaviors, such as testosterone and lipids, which may interact with serotonergic activity. Many of these disturbances can be observed in childhood disorders that serve as antecedents of adult antisocial and psychopathic disorders, and in some cases even in infants of parents with these disorders. Nevertheless, significant childhood adversity is also a common antecedent and there is evidence that genetic and environmental factors may interact in the genesis of these adult disorders.

The neurobiological basis for the affective–interpersonal (Factor 1) component, in contrast, may be found independently at the level of impaired neurocognitive or information processing of social and emotional stimuli. However, the neurochemical aspects of the affective–interpersonal factor remain to be fully investigated, and there is some intriguing circumstantial evidence suggesting that the social neurocognitive disturbances seen in psychopathy may also be related to monoamine dysfunction. Few scientifically rigorous studies have yet addressed the pharmacological treatment of impulsive aggression or features of psychopathy, yet the principles of symptom-targeted pharmacotherapy, using the existing knowledge base derived from studies of other psychiatric disorders, may remain useful for the clinician.

REFERENCES

Abbar, M., Courtet, P., Bellivier, F., Leboyer, M., Boulenger, J. P., Castelhau, D., et al. (2001). Suicide attempts and the tryptophan hydroxylase gene. *Molecular Psychiatry*, 6, 268–273.

Ait-Daoud, N., Johnson, B. A., Prihoda, T. J., & Hargita, I. D. (2001). Combining ondansetron and naltrexone reduces craving among biologically predisposed alcoholics: Preliminary clinical evidence. *Psychopharmacology*, 154, 23–27.

Alm, P. O., Alm, M., Humble, K., Leppert, J., Sorensen, S., Lidberg, L., & Oreland, L. (1994). Criminality and platelet monoamine oxidase activity in former juvenile delinquents as adults. *Acta Psychiatrica Scandinavica*, 89(1), 41–45.

Alm, P. O., af Klinteberg B., Humble, K., Leppert, J., Sorensen, S., Tegelman, R., et al. (1996a). Criminality and psychopathy as related to thyroid activity in former juvenile delinquents. *Acta Psychiatrica Scandinavica*, 94(2), 112–117.

Alm, P. O., af Klinteberg, B., Humble, K., Leppert, J., Sorensen, S., Thorell, L. H., et al. (1996b). Psychopathy, platelet MAO activity and criminality among former juvenile delinquents. *Acta Psychiatrica Scandinavica*, 94(2), 105–111.

Alvarez, J. C., Cremniter, D., Gluck, N., Quintin, P., Leboyer, M., Berlin, I., et al. (2000). Low serum cholesterol in violent but not in non-violent suicide attempters. *Psychiatry Research*, 95, 103–108.

Anthenelli, R. M., Smith, T. L., Craig, C. E., Tabakoff, B., & Schuckit, M. A. (1995). Platelet monoamine oxidase activity levels in subgroups of alcoholics: Diagnostic, temporal, and clinical correlates. *Biological Psychiatry*, 38, 361–368.

Apter, A., Laufer, N., Bar-Sever, M., Har-Even, D., Ofek, H., & Weizman, A. (1999). Serum cholesterol, suicidal tendencies, impulsivity, aggression, and depression in adolescent psychiatric inpatients. *Biological Psychiatry*, 46(4), 532–41.

Arango, V., Ernsberger, P., Marzuk, P. M., Chen, J. S., Tierney, H., Stanley, M. et al. (1990). Autoradiographic demonstration of increased serotonin 5-HT2 and beta-adrenergic receptor binding sites in the brain of suicide victims. *Archives of General Psychiatry*, 47, 1038–1047.

Arango, V., Underwood, M. D., & Mann, J. J. (1997). Postmortem findings in suicide victims. Implications for in vivo imaging studies. *Annals of the New York Academy of Sciences, 836*, 269–287.

Archer, J. (1991). The influence of testosterone on human aggression. *British Journal of Clinical of Psychology, 82*, 1–28.

Arnett, P. A. (1997). Autonomic responsivity in psychopaths: A critical review and theoretical proposal. *Clinical Psychology Review, 17*(8), 903–936.

Aromaki, A. S., Lindman, R. E., & Eriksson, C. J. P. (1999). Testorsterone, aggressiveness, and antisocial personality. *Aggressive Behavior, 25*, 113–123.

Aromaki, A. S., Lindman, R. E., & Eriksson, C. J. P. (2002). Testosterone, sexuality and antisocial personality in rapists and child molesters: A pilot study. *Psychiatry Research, 110*, 239–247.

Arranz, B., Eriksson, A., Mellerup, E., Plenge, P., & Marcusson, J. (1994). Brain 5-HT1A, 5-HT 1D and 5-HT2 receptors in suicide victims. *Biological Psychiatry, 35*, 457–463.

Asberg, M., Traskman, L., & Thoren, P. (1976). 5-HIAA in the cerebrospinal fluid: A biochemical suicide predictor? *Archives of General Psychiatry, 33*, 1193–1197.

Attenburrow, M. J., Williams, C., Odontiadis, J., Reed, A., Powell, J., Cowen, P. J., & Harmer, C. J. (2003). Acute administration of nutritionally sourced tryptophan increases fear recognition. *Psychopharmacology, 169*, 104–107.

Banks, T., & Dabbs, J. M., Jr. (1996). Salivary testosterone and cortisol in a delinquent and violent urban subculture. *Journal of Social Psychology, 136*(1), 49–56.

Barratt, E. S., Stanford, M. S., Felthous, A. R., & Kent, T. A. (1997). The effects of phenytoin on impulsive and premeditated aggression: A controlled study. *Journal of Clinical Psychopharmacology, 17*, 341–349.

Belfrage, H., Lidberg, L., & Oreland, L. (1992). Platelet monoamine oxidase activity in mentally disordered violent offenders. *Acta Psychiatrica Scandinavica, 85*(3), 218–221.

Bellivier, F., Szoke, A., Henry, C., LaCoste, J., Bottos, C., Nosten-Bertrand, M., et al. (2000). Possible association between serotonin transporter gene polymorphism and violent suicidal behavior in mood disorders. *Biological Psychiatry, 48*, 319–322.

Benjamin, J., Li, L., Patterson, C., Greenberg, B. D., Murphy, D. L., & Hamer, D. H. (1996). Population and familial association between the D4 dopamine receptor gene and measures of Novelty seeking. *Nature Genetics, 12*, 81–84.

Bergman, B., & Brismar, B. (1994). Hormone levels and personality traits in abusive and suicidal male alcoholics. *Alcoholism: Clinical and Experimental Research, 18*(2), 311–316.

Berridge, C. W., & Waterhouse, B. D. (2003). The locus coeruleus-noradrenergic system: Modulation of behavioral state and state-dependent cognitive processes. *Brain Research Reviews, 42*, 33–84.

Bjork, J. M., Dougherty, D. M., Moeller, F. G., Cherek, D. R., & Swann, A. C. (1999). The effects of tryptophan depletion and leading on laboratory aggression in men: Time course and a food-restricted control. *Psychopharmacology, 142*, 24–30.

Blair, R. J. R. (2003). Facial expressions, their communicatory functions and neuro-cognitive substrates. *Philosophical Transactions of the Royal Society of London B, 358*, 561–572.

Bolos, A. M., Dean, M., Sucas-Derse, S., Ramsburg, M., Brown, G. L., & Goldman, D. (1990). Population and pedigree studies reveal a lack of association between the dopamine D2 receptor gene and alcoholism. *Journal of the American Medical Association, 264*(24), 3156.

Bondy, B., Erfurth, A., DeJonge, S., Kruger, M., & Meyer, H. (2000). Possible association of the short allele of the serotonin transporter promoter gene polymorphism (5-HTTLPR) with violent suicide. *Molecular Psychiatry, 5*, 193–195.

Brewer-Smyth, K., Burgess, A. W., & Shults, J. (2004). Physical and sexual abuse, salivary cortisol, and neurologic correlates of violent criminal behavior in female prison inmates. *Biological Psychiatry, 55*, 21–31.

Briken, P., Hill, A., & Berner, W. (2003). Pharmacotherapy of Paraphilas with long-acting agonists of luteinizing hormone-releasing hormone: A systematic review. *Journal of Clinical Psychiatry, 64*, 890–897.

Brown, G. L., Goodwin, F. K., Ballenger, J. C., Goyer, P. F., & Major, L. F. (1979). Aggression in humans correlates with cerebrospinal fluid amine metabolites. *Psychiatry Research, 1*(2), 131–139.

Brown, G. L., Ebert, M. H., Goyer, P. F., Jimerson, D. C., Klein, W. J., Bunney, W. E., & Goodwin, F. K. (1982). Aggression, suicide, and serotonin: Relationships to CSF amine metabolites. *American Journal of Psychiatry, 139*, 741–746.

Brunner, H. G., Nelen, M., Breakefield, X. O., Ropers, H. H., & van Oost, B. A. (1993). Abnormal behavior associated with a point mutation in the structural gene for monoamine oxidase A. *Science, 262*, 578–580.

Brunner, H. G., Nelen, M. R., van Zanvoort, P., Abeling, N. G., van Gennip, A. H., Wolters, E. C., et al. (1993). X-linked borderline mental retardation with prominent behavioral disturbance: Phenotype, genetic localization, and evidence for disturbed monoaminҫe metabolism. *American Journal of Human Genetics, 52*, 1032–1039.

Buckley, P. F. (1999). The role of typical and atypical antipsychotic medications in the management of agitation and aggression. *Journal of Clinical Psychiatry, 60*(Suppl. 10), 52–60.

Buydens-Branchey, L., & Branchey, M. H. (1992). Cortisol in alcoholics with a disordered aggression control. *Psychoneuroendocrinology, 17*(1), 45–54.

Buydens-Branchey, L., Branchey, M., Hudson, J., & Fergeson, P. (2000). Low HDL cholesterol, aggression and altered central serotonergic activity. *Psychiatry Research*, *93*, 93–102.

Buydens-Branchey, L., Branchey, M. H., Noumair, D., & Lieber, C. S. (1989). Age of alcoholism onset, II. Relationship to susceptibility to serotonin precursor availability. *Archives of General Psychiatry*, *46*, 231–236.

Cadoret, R. J., Langbehn, D., Caspers, K., Troughton, E. P., Yucuis, R., Sandhu, H. K., & Philibert, R. (2003). Associations of the serotonin transporter promoter polymorphism with aggressivity, attention deficit, and conduct disorder in an adoptee population. *Comprensive Psychiatry*, *44*(2), 88–101.

Cases, O., Seif, I., Grimsby, J., Gaspar, P., Chen, K., Pournin, S., et al. (1995). Aggressive behavior and altered amounts of brain serotonin and norepinephrine in mice lacking MAOA. *Science*, *268*, 1763–1766.

Cases, O., Lebrand, C., Giros, B., Vitalis, T., De Maeyer, E., Caron, M. G., et al. (1998). Plasma membrane transporters of serotonin, dopamine, and norepinephrine mediate serotonin accumulation in atypical locations in the developing brain of monoamine oxidase A knock-outs. *Journal of Neuroscience*, *18*(17), 6914–6927.

Caspi, A., McClay, J., Moffitt, T. E., Mill, J., Martin, J., Craig, I. W., et al. (2002). Role of genotype in the cycle of violence in maltreated children. *Science*, *297*, 851–854.

Clarke, R. A., Murphy, D. L., & Constantino, J. N. (1999). Serotonin and externalizing behavior in young children. *Psychiatry Research*, *86*(1), 29–40.

Cleckley, H. (1976). *The mask of sanity*. St. Louis, MO: Mosby. (Original work published 1941)

Coccaro, E. F., Gabriel, S., & Siever, L. J. (1990). Buspirone challenge: preliminary evidence for a role of 5-HT1A receptors in impulsive aggressive behavior in humans. *Psychopharmacology Bulletin*, *26*, 393–405.

Coccaro, E. F., & Kavoussi, R. J. (1997). Fluoxetine and impulsive aggressive behavior in personality disordered subjects. *Archives of General Psychiatry*, *54*(12), 1081–1088.

Coccaro, E. F., Berman, M. E., Kavoussi, R. J., & Hauger, R. L. (1996). Relationship of prolactin response to D-fenfluramine to behavioral and questionnaire assessments of aggression in personality disordered males. *Biological Psychiatry*, *40,157–164*.

Coccaro, E. F., Kavoussi, R. J., Cooper, T. B., & Hauger, R. L. (1997). Central serotonin activity and aggression: Inverse relationship with prolactin response to D-fenfluramine, but not with CSF 5-HIAA concentration in human subjects. *American Journal of Psychiatry*, *154*, 1430–1435.

Coccaro, E. F., Kavoussi, R. J., Sheline, Y. I., Berman, R. E., & Csernansky, J. G. (1997). Impulsive aggression in personality disorders: correlates with 125-I-LSD binding in the platelet. *Neuropsychopharmacology*, *16*, 211–216.

Coccaro, E. F., Kavoussi, R. J., Trestman, R. L., Gabriel, S. M., Cooper, T. B., & Siever, L. J. (1997). Serotonin function in human subjects: Intercorrelations among central 5-HT indices and aggressiveness. *Psychiatry Research*, *73*, 1–14.

Coccaro, E. F., Siever, L. J., Klar, H. M., Maurer, G., Cochrane, K., Cooper, T. B., et al. (1989). Serotonergic studies in patients with affective and personality disorders: correlates with suicidal and impulsive aggressive behavior. *Archives of General Psychiatry*, *46*, 587–599.

Constantino, J. N., Morris, J. A., & Murphy, D. L. (1997). CSF 5-HIAA and family history of antisocial personality disorder in newborns. *American Journal of Psychiatry*, *154*, 1771–1773.

Cooper, J. R., Bloom, F. E., & Roth, R. H. (Eds.). (1996). *The biochemical basis of neuropharmacology* (7th ed.). New York: Oxford University Press.

Dabbs, J. M., Jr., Carr, T. S., Frady, R. L., & Riad, J. (1995). Testosterone, crime, and misbehavior among 692 male prison inmates. *Personality and Individual Differences*, *18*(5), 627–633.

Dabbs, J. M., Jr., Frady, R. L., Carr, T. S., & Besch, N. F. (1987). Saliva testosterone and criminal violence in young adult prison inmates. *Psychosomatic Medicine*, *49*(2), 174–182.

Dabbs, J. M., Jr., & Hargrove, M. F. (1997). Age, testosterone, and behavior among female prison inmates. *Psychosomatic Medicine*, *59*(5), 477–480.

Daitzman, R., & Zuckerman, M. (1980). Disinhibitory sensation seeking, personality and gonadal hormones. *Personality and Individual Differences*, *1*, 103–110.

DeLion, S., Chalon, S., Herault, J., Guilloteau, D., Besnard, J., & Durand, G. (1994). Chronic dietary a-linolenic acid deficiency alters dopaminergic and serotonergic neurotransmission in rats. *Journal of Nutrition*, *124*, 2466–2467.

Devor, E. J., Cloninger, C. R., Hoffman, P. L., & Tabakoff, B. (1993). Association of monoamine oxidase (MAO) activity with alcoholism and alcoholic subtypes. *American Journal of Medical Genetics*, *48*, 209–213.

Dmitrieva, T. N., Oades, R. D., Hauffa, B. P., & Eggers, C. (2001). Dehaydroepiandrosterone sulphate and corticotrophin levels are high in young male patients with conduct disorder: Comparisons for growth factors, thyroid and gonadal hormones. *Neuropsychobiology*, *43*(3), 134–140.

Dolan, M. (1994). Psychopathy—A neurobiological perspective. *British Journal of Psychiatry*, *165*, 151–159.

Dolan, M. C., & Anderson, I. M. (2003). The relationship between serotonergic function and the Psychopathy Checklist: Screening Version. *Journal of Psychopharmacology*, *17*(2), 216–222.

Dolan, M., Anderson, I. M., & Deakin, F. W. (2001). Relationship between 5-HT function and impulsivity and aggression in male offenders with personality disorders. *British Journal of Psychiatry*, *178*, 352–359.

Dolan, M., Deakin, W. J., Roberts, N., & Anderson, I. (2002). Serotonergic and cognitive impairment in impulsive aggressive personality disordered offenders: Are there implications for treatment? *Psychological Medicine*, *32*(1), 105–117.

Donovan, S. J., Stewart, J. W., Nunes, E. V., Stewart, J. W., Quitkin, F. M., & Parides, M. (2000). Divalproex treatment for youth with explosive temper and mood ability: A double-blind, placebo-controlled crossover design. *American Journal of Psychiatry*, *157*, 818–820.

Dulawa, S. C., Grandy, D. K., Low, M. J., Paulus, M. P., & Geyer, M. A. (1999). Dopamine D4 receptor-knock-out mice exhibit reduced exploration of novel stimuli. *Journal of Neuroscience*, *19*, 9550–9556.

Ebstein, R. P., Benjamine, J., & Belmaker, R. H. (2000). Personality and polymorphisms of genes involved in aminergic neurotransmission. *European Journal of Pharmacology*, *410*, 205–214.

Ebstein, R. P., Gritsenko, I., Nemanov, L., Frisch, A., Osher, Y., & Belmaker, R. H. (1997). No association between the serotonin transporter gene regulation region polymorphism and the tridimensional personality questionnaire (TPQ) temperament of harm avoidance. *Molecular Psychiatry*, *2*, 224–226.

Ebstein, R. P., Novick, O., Umansky, R., Priel, B., Osher, Y., Blaine, D., et al. (1996). Dopamine D4 receptor (D4DR) exon III polymorphism associated with the human personality trait of Novelty Seeking. *Nature Genetics*, *12*, 78–80.

Ehrenkranz, J., Bliss, E., & Sheard, H. (1974). Plasma testosterone: correlation with aggressive behavior and social dominance in man. *Psychosomatic Medicine*, *36*(6), 469–475.

Eriksson, C. J. P., Pahlaen, B., Sarkola, T., & Seppa, K. (2003). Oestradiol and human male alcohol-related aggression. *Alcohol and Alcoholism*, *38*(6), 589–596.

Eriksson, T., & Lidberg, L. (1997). Increased plasma concentrations of the 5-HT precursor amino acid trytophan and other large neutral amino acids in violent criminals. *Psychological Medicine*, *27*, 477–481.

Finberg, J. P. M. (1995) Pharmacology of reversible and selective inhibitors of monoamine oxidase type A. *Acta Psychiatrica Scandinavica*, *91*(Suppl. 386), 8–13.

Findling, R. L., McNamara, N. K., Branicky, L. A., Schluchter, M. D., Lemon, E., & Blumer, J. L. (2000). A double-blind pilot study of risperidone in the treatment of conduct disorder. *Journal of the Academy of Child and Adolescent Psychiatry*, *39*(4), 509–516.

Fishbein, D. H., Dax, E., Lozovsky, D. B., & Jaffe, J. H. (1992). Neuroendocrine responses to a glucose challenge in substance users with high and low levels of aggression, impulsivity, and antisocial personality. *Neuropsychobiology*, *25*(2), 106–114.

Frances, A. J., Fyer, M. R., & Clarkin, J. (1986). Personality and suicide. In J. J. Mann & M. Stanley (Eds.), *Annals of the New York Academy of Science*, *487*, 281–293.

Freedman, D. S., Byers, T., Barrett, D. H., Stroup, N. E., Eaker, E., & Monroe-Blum, H. (1995). Plasma lipid levels and psychologic characteristics in men. *American Journal of Epidemiology*, *141*(6), 507–517.

Gabel, S., Stadler, J., Bjorn, J., & Shindledecker, R. (1995). Homovanillic acid and dopamine-beta-hydroxylase in male youth: Relationships with paternal substance abuse and antisocial behavior. *American Journal of Drug and Alcohol Abuse*, *21*(3), 363–378.

Gallerani, M., Manfredini, R., Caracciolo, S., Scapoli, C., Molinari, S., & Fersini, C. (1995). Serum cholesterol concentrations in parasuicide. *British Medical Journal*, *310*(6995), 1632–1636.

Garpenstrand, H., Longato-Stadler, E., af Klinteberg, B., Grigorenko, E., Damberg, M., Oreland, L., & Hallman, J. (2002). Low platelet monoamine oxidase activity in Swedish imprisoned criminal offenders. *European Neuropsychopharmacology*, *12*(2), 135–140.

Geijer, T., Frisch, A., Persson, M. L., Wasserman, D., Rockah, R., Michaelovsky, E., et al. (2000). Search for association between suicide attempt and serotonergic polymorphisms. *Psychiatric Genetics*, *10*, 19–26.

Gelernter, J., Kranzler, H., Coccaro, E. F., Siever, L. J., & New, A. S. (1998). Serotonin transporter protein gene polymorphism and personality measures in African American and European American subjects. *American Journal of Psychiatry*, *155*, 1332–1338.

George, D. T., Umhau, J. C., Phillips, M. J., Emmela, D., Ragan, P.W., Shoaf, S. E., & Rawlings, R. R. (2001). Serotonin, testosterone and alcohol in the etiology of domestic violence. *Psychiatry Research*, *104*, 27–37.

Gerra, G., Avanzini, P., Zaimovic, A., Sartori, R., Bocchi, S. R., Timpano, M., et al. (1999). Neurotransmitters, neuroendocrine correlates of sensation-seeking temperament in normal humans. *Neuropsychobiology*, *39*(4), 207–213.

Gerra, G., Zaimovic, A., Moi, G., Bussandri, M., Delsignore, R., Caccavari, R., & Brambilla, F. (2003). Neuroendocrine correlates of antisocial personality disorder in abstinent heroin-dependent subjects. *Addiction Biology*, *8*(1), 23–32.

Giotakos, O., Markianos, M., Vaidakis, N., & Christodoulou, G. N. (2003). Aggression, impulsivity, plasma sex hormones, and biogenic amine turnover in a forensic population of rapists. *Journal of Sex and Marital Therapy*, *29*(3), 215–225.

Gogos, J. A., Morgan, M., Luine, V., Santha, M., Ogawa, S., Pfaff, D., & Karayiorgou, M. (1998). Catechol-O-methyltransferase-deficient mice exhibit sexually dimorphic changes in catecholamine levels and behavior. *Proceedings of the National Academy of Sciences*, *95*, 9991–9996.

Goldman, R. G., Skodol, A. E., McGrath, P. J., & Oldham, J. M. (1994). Relationship between the Tridimensional Personality Questionnaire and DSM-III-R personality traits. *American Journal of Psychiatry*, 151, 274–276.

Golier, J. A., Marzuk, P. M., Leon, A. C., Weiner, C., & Tardiff, K. (1995). Low serum cholesterol level and attempted suicide. *American Journal of Psychiatry*, 152(3), 419–423.

Golomb, B. A., Stattin, H., & Mednick, S. (2000). Low cholesterol and violent crime. *Journal of Psychiatric Research*, 34, 301–309.

Goyer, P. F., Andreason, P. J., Semple, W. E., Clayton, A. H., King, A. C., Compton-Toth, B. A., et al. (1994). Positron-emission tomography and personality disorders. *Neuropsychopharamacology*, 10, 21–28.

Gray, R. F., Corrigan, F. M., Strathdee, A., Skinner, E. R., van Rhijin, A. G., & Horrobin, D. F. (1993). Cholesterol metabolism and violence: A study of individuals convicted of violent crimes. *Neuroreport*, 4, 754–6.

Greenberg, B. D., Li, Q., Lucas, F. R., Hu, S., Sirota, L. A., Benjamin, J., et al. (2000). Association between the serotonin transporter promoter polymorphism and personality traits in a primarily female population sample. *American Journal of Medical Genetics*, 96(2), 202–216.

Gurvits, I. G., Koenigsberg, H. W., & Siever, L. J. (2000). Neurotransmitter dysfunction in patients with borderline personality disorder. *Psychiatric Clinics of North America*, 23(1), 27–40.

Hallikainen, T., Saito, T., Lachman, H. M., Volavka, J., Pohjalainen, T., Ryynanen, O. P., et al. (1999). Association between low activity serotonin transporter promoter genotype and early onset alcoholism with habitual impulsive violent behavior. *Molecular Psychiatry*, 4(4), 385–388.

Hallman, J., von Knorring, L., & Oreland, L.(1996). Personality disorders according to DSM-III-R and thromboctye monoamine oxidase activity in Type 1 and Type 2 alcoholics. *Journal of Studies on Alcohol*, 57, 155–161.

Halperin, J. M., Schulz, K. P., McKay, K. E., Sharma, V., & Newcorn, J.H. (2003). Familial correlates of central serotonin function in children with disruptive behavior disorders. *Psychiatry Research*, 119(3), 205–216.

Halpern, C. T., Campbell, B., Agnew, C. R., Thompson, V., & Udry, J. R. (2002). Associations between stress reactivity and sexual and nonsexual risk taking in young adult human males. *Hormones Behavior*, 42, 387–398.

Hare, R. D. (1991). *The Hare Psychopathy Checklist—Revised*. Toronto, ON, Canada: Multi-Health Systems.

Hare, R. D. (2003). *The Psychopathy Checklist—Revised* (2nd ed.). Toronto, ON, Canada: Multi-Health Systems.

Harmer C. J., Bhagwagar, Z., Perrett, D. I., Vollm, B. A., Cowen P. J., & Goodwin G. M. (2003) Acute SSRI administration affects the processing of social cues in healthy volunteers. *Neuropsychopharmacology*, 28, 148–152.

Harmer C. J., Rogers, R. D., Tunbridge, E., Cowen P. J., & Goodwin G. M. (2003). Tryptophan depletion increases the recognition of fear in female volunteers. *Psychopharmacology*, 167, 411–417.

Harris, J. A. (1999). Review and methodological considerations in research on testosterone and aggression. *Aggressive Violent Behavior*, 4, 273–291.

Hart, S. D., Cox, D. N., & Hare, R. D. (1995). *Hare Psychopathy Checklist: Screening Version (PCL: SV)*. Toronto, ON, Canada: Multi-Health Systems.

Hart, S. D., & Dempster, R. J. (1997). Impulsivity and psychopathy. In C. D. Webster & M. A. Jackson (Eds.). *Impulsivity: Theory, assessment and treatment* (pp. 212–232). New York: Guilford Press.

Heiligenstein, J. H., Beasley, C. M., Jr., & Potvin, J. H. (1993). Fluoxetine not associated with increased aggression in controlled clinical trials. *International Clinical Psychopharmacology*, 8, 277–280.

Heron, D. S., Shinitzky, M., Hershkowitz, M., & Samuel, D. (1980). Lipid fluidity markedly modulates the binding of serotonin to mouse brain membranes. *Proceedings of the National Academy of Sciences*, 77, 7463–7467.

Hibbeln, J. R., Umhau, J. C., Linnoila, M., George, D. T., Ragan, P. W., Shoaf, S. E., et al. (1998). A replication study of violent and nonviolent subjects: Cerebrospinal fluid metabolites of serotonin and dopamine are predicted by plasma essential fatty acids. *Biological Psychiatry*, 44, 243–249.

Hill, E. M., Stoltenberg, S. F., Burmeister, M., & Closser, M. (1999). Potential associations among genetic markers in the serotonergic system and the antisocial alcoholism subtype. *Experimental Clinical Psychopharmacology*, 7(2), 103–121.

Hill, E. M., Stoltenberg, S. F., Bullard, K. H., Li, S., Zucker, R. A., & Burmeister, M. (2002). Antisocial alcoholism and serotonin—related polymorphisms: Association tests. *Psychiatric Genetics*, 12(3), 143–153.

Hill, S. Y., Zezza, N., Wipprecht, G., Locke, J., & Neiswanger, K. (1999). Personality traits and dopamine receptors (D2 and D4): Linkage studies in families of alcoholics. *American Journal of Medical Genetics*, 88, 634–641.

Hillbrand, M., Spitz, R. T., & Foster, H. G. (1995). Serum cholesterol and aggression in hospitalized male forensic patients. *Journal of Behavioral Medicine*, 18(1), 33–43.

Hollander, E., Tracy, K. A., Swann, A. C., Coccaro, E. F., McElroy, S. L., Wozniak, P., et al. (2003). Divalproex in the treatment of impulsive aggression: Efficacy in cluster B personality disorders. *Neuropsychopharmacology*, 28, 1186–1197.

Huang, Y., Grailhe, R., Arango, V., Hen, R., & Mann, J. J. (1999). Relationship of pathology to the human serotonin 1B genotype and receptor binding kinetics in postmortem brain tissue. *Neuropsychopharmacology*, *21*, 238–246.

Jacobs, D., Blackburn, H., Higgins, M., Reed, D., Iso, H., McMillan, G., et al. (1992). Report of the Conference on Low Blood Cholesterol: Mortality associations. *Circulation*, *86*, 1046–1060.

Jorm, A. F., Henderson, A. S., Jacomb, P. A., Christensen, H., Korten, A. E., Rodgers, B., et al. (2000). Association of a functional polymorphism of the monoamine oxidase A gene promoter with personality and psychiatric symptoms. *Psychiatric Genetics*, *10*, 87–90.

Kaplan, J. R., Shively, C. A., Fontenot, M. B., Morgan, T. M., Howell, S. M., Manuck, S. B., et al. (1994). Demonstration of an association among dietary cholesterol, central serotonergic activity, and social behavior in monkeys. *Psychosomatic Medicine*, *56*, 479–484.

Kavoussi, R. J., & Coccaro, E. F. (1994). An open trial of sertraline in personality disordered patients with impulsive aggression. *Journal of Clinical Psychiatry*, *55*(4), 137–141.

Kavoussi, R. J., & Coccaro, E. F. (1998). Divalproex sodium for impulsive aggressive behavior in patients with personality disorder. *Journal of Clinical Psychiatry*, *59*(12), 676–680.

Koller, G., Bondy, B., Preuss, U. S., Bottlender, M., & Soyka, M. (2003). No association between a polymorphism in the promoter region of the MAOA gene with antisocial personality traits in alcoholics. *Alcohol and Alcoholism*, *38*(1), 31–34.

Kotler, M., Barak, P., Cohen, H., Averbuch, I. E., Grinshpoon, A., Gritsenko, I., et al. (1999). Homicidal behavior in schizophrenia associated with a genetic polymorphism determining low catechol O-methyltransferase (COMT) activity. *American Journal of Medical Genetics*, *88*, 628–633.

Kranzler, H. R., Hernandez-Avila, C. A., & Gelernter, J. (2002). Polymorphism of the 5-HT1B receptor gene (HTR1B): Strong within-locus linkage disequilibrium without association to antisocial substance dependence. *Neuropsychopharmacology*, *26*(1), 115–122.

Kreek, M. J., LaForge K. S., & Butelman, E. (2002). Pharmacotherapy of addictions. *Nature Reviews Drug Discovery*, *1*(9), 710–726.

Kreuz, L. E., & Rose, R. M. (1972). Assessment of aggressive behavior and plasma testosterone in a young criminal population. *Psychosomatic Medicine*, *34*(4), 321–332.

Kruesi, M. J., Hibbs, E. D., Zahn, T. P., Keysor, C. S., Hamburger, S. D., Bartko, J. J., & Rapoport, J. L. (1992). A 2-year prospective follow-up study of children and adolescents with disruptive behavior disorders. Prediction by cerebrospinal fluid 5-hydroxyindoleacetic acid, homovanillic acid, and autonomic measures? *Archives of General Psychiatry*, *49*(6).

Kruesi, M. J., Rapoport, J. L., Hamburger, S., Hibbs, E., Potter, W. Z., Lenane, M., & Brown, G. L. (1990). Cerebrospinal fluid monoamine metabolites, aggression, and impulsivity in disruptive behavior disorders

of children and adolescents. *Archives of General Psychiatry*, *47*(5).

Kunugi, H., Ishida, S., Kato, T., Sakai, T., Tatsumi, M., Hirose, T., & Nanko, S. (1999). No evidence for an association of polymorphisms of the tryptophan hydroxylase gene with affective disorders of attempted suicide among Japanese patients. *American Journal of Psychiatry*, *156*, 774–776.

Lachman, H. M., Nolan, K. A., Mohr, P., Saito, T., & Volavka, J. (1998). Association between catechol-O-metyltransferase genotype and violence in schizophrenia and schizoaffective disorder. *American Journal of Psychiatry*, *155*, 835–837.

Lappalainen, J., Long, J. C., Eggert, M., Ozaki, N., Robin, R. W., Brown, G. L., et al. (1998). Linkage of antisocial alcoholism to the serotonin 5-HT1B receptor gene in 2 populations. *Archives of General Psychiatry*, *55*, 989–994.

Lena, B. (1979). The use of lithium in child and adolescent psychiatry. In T. B. Cooper, S. Gershon, N. S. Kline, & M. Sehon (Eds.), *Lithium: Controversies and unresolved issues* (pp. 30–33). Princeton, NJ: Excerpta Modiera.

Lesch, K. P., Wolozin, B. L., Murphy, D. L., & Reiderer, P. (1993). Primary structure of the human platelet serotonin uptake site: Identity with the brain serotonin transporter. *Journal of Neurochemistry*, *60*, 2319–2322.

Lesch, K., Bengel, D., Heils, A., Sabol, S. Z., Greenberg, B. D., Petri, S., et al. (1996). Association of anxiety-related traits with a polymorphism in the serotonin transporter gene regulatory region. *Science*, *274*, 1527–1531.

Lesch, K. P., & Merschdorf, U. (2000). Impulsivity, aggression, and serotonin: A molecular psychobiological perspective. *Behavioral Sciences and the Law*, *18*, 581–604.

Lidberg, L., Levander, S., Schalling, D., & Lidberg, Y. (1978). Urinary catecholamines, stress, and psychopathy: A study of arrested men awaiting trial. *Psychosomatic Medicine*, *40*(2), 116–125.

Lidberg, L., Modin, I., Oreland, L., Tuck, J. R., & Gillner, A. (1985). Platelet monoamine oxidase activity and psychopathy. *Psychiatric Research*, *16*, 339–343.

Lidberg, L., Tuck, J. R., Asberg, M., Scalia-Tomba, G. P., & Bertilsson, L. (1985). Homicide, suicide and CSF 5HIAA. *Acta Psychiatrica Scandinavica*, *71*, 230–236.

Limson, R., Goldman, D., Roy, A., Lamparski, D., Ravitz, B., Adinoff, B., & Linnoila, M. (1991). Personality and cerebrospinal fluid monoamine metabolites in alcoholics and controls. *Archives of General Psychiatry*, *48*, 437–441.

Lindberg, G., Rastam, L., Gullberg, B., & Eklund, G. A. (1992). Low serum cholesterol concentration and short term mortality from injuries in men and women. *British Medical Journal*, *305*, 277–279.

Lindberg, L., Asberg, M., Sunquist-Stensman, et al. (1984). 5-hydroxyindoleacetic acid levels in attempted suicides who have killed their children [letter]. *Lancet, 2*, 928.

Linnoila, M., Virkkunen, M., Schwannian, M., Nuutila, A., Rimon, R., & Goodwin, F. K. (1983). Low cerebrospinal fluid 5-fydroxyindoleacetic acid concentration differentiates impulsive from non-impulsive violent behavior. *Life Sciences, 33*, 2609–2614.

Lu, R. B., Lee, J. F., Ko, H. C., & Lin, W. W. (2001). Dopamine D2 receptor gene (DRD2) is associated with alcoholism with conduct disorder. *Alcoholism: Clinical and Experimental Research, 25*(2), 177–184.

Lu, R. B., Lin, W. W., Lee, J. F., Ko, H. C., & Shih, J. C. (2003). Neither antisocial personality disorder nor antisocial alcoholism is associated with the MAO-A gene in Han Chinese males. *Alcoholism: Clinical and Experimental Research, 27*(6), 889–893.

Malone, R. P., Delaney, M. A., Luebbert, J. F., Cater, J., & Campbell, M. A. (2000). A double-blind placebo-controlled study of lithium in hospitalized aggressive children and adolescents with conduct disorder. *Archives of General Psychiatry, 57*, 649–654.

Mann, J. J., Malone, K. M., Diehl, D. J., Perel, J., Cooper, T. B., & Minton, M. A. (1996). Demonstration in vivo of reduced serotonin responsivity in the brain of untreated depressed patients. *American Journal of Psychiatry, 153*, 174–182.

Mann, J. J., Malone, K. M., Nielson, D. A., Goldman, D., Erdos, J., & Gelernter, J. (1997). Possible association of a polymorphism of the tryptophan hydroxylase gene with suicidal behavior in depressed patients. *American Journal of Psychiatry, 154*, 1451–1453.

Mann, J. J., Huang, Y. Y., Underwood, M. D., Kassir, S. A., Oppenheim, S., Kelly, T. M., et al. (2000). A serotonin transporter gene promoter polymorphism (HTTLPR) and prefrontal cortical binding in major depression and suicide. *Archives of General Psychiatry, 57*, 729–738.

Manuck, S. B., Flory, J. D., Ferrell, R. E., Dent, K. M., Mann, J. J., & Muldoon, M. F. (1999) Aggression and anger-related traits associated with a polymorphism of the tryptophan hydroxylase gene. *Biological Psychiatry, 45*, 603–614.

Manuck, S. B., Flory, J. D., Ferrell, R. E., Mann, J. J., & Muldoon, M. F. (2000). A regulatory polymorphism of the monoamine oxidase-A gene may be associated with variability in aggression, impulsivity, and central nervous system serotonergic responsivity. *Psychiatry Research, 95*(1), 9–23.

Maras, A., Laucht, M., Gerdes, D., Wilhelm, C., Lewicka, S., Haack, D., et al. (2003). Association of testosterone and dihydrotestosterone with externalizing behavior in adolescent boys and girls. *Psychoneuroendocrinology, 28*, 932–940.

Mason, J. W. (1968). A review of psychoendocrine research on the pituitary–adrenal cortical system. *Psychosomatic Medicine, 30*, 576–606.

Mattson, A., Schalling, D., Olweus, D., Low, H., & Svensson, J. (1980). Plasma testosterone, aggressive behavior, and personality dimensions in young male delinquents. *Journal of the American Academy of Child Psychiatry, 19*, 476–490.

Mazur, A., & Booth, A. (1998). Testosterone and dominance in men. *Behavioral Brain Sciences, 21*(3), 353–363.

Mazur, A. (1995). Biosocial models of deviant behavior among male army veterans. *Biological Psychology, 41*, 271–293.

McBurnett, K., Lahey, B. B., Rathouz, P. J., & Loeber, R. (2000). Low salivery cortisol and persistent aggression in boys referred for disruptive behavior. *Archives of General Psychiatry, 57*, 38–43.

Miller, B. L., & Cummings, J. L. (1999). *The human frontal lobes: Functions and disorders*. New York: Guilford Press.

Modai, I., Valevski, A., Dror, S., & Weizman, A. (1994). Serum cholesterol levels and suicidal tendencies in psychiatric inpatients. *Journal of Clinical Psychiatry, 55*(6), 252–254.

Moeller, F. G., Dougherty, D. M., Swann, A. C., Colling, D., Davis, C. M., & Cherek, D. R. (1996). Tryptophan depletion and aggressive responding in healthy males. *Psychopharmacology, 126*, 97–103.

Moeller, F. G., Allen, T., Cherek, D. R., Dougherty, D. M., Lane, S., & Swann, A. C. (1998) Ipsapirone neuroendocrine challenge: Relationship to aggression as measured in the human laboratory. *Psychiatry Research, 81*, 31–38.

Moss, H. B., Yao, J. K., & Panzak, G. L. (1990). Serotonergic responsivity and behavioral dimensions in antisocial personality disorder with substance abuse. *Biological Psychiatry, 28*, 325–338.

Muldoon, M. F., Manuck, S. B., Mendelsohn, A. B., Kaplan, J. R., & Belle, S. H. (2001). Cholesterol reduction and non-illness mortality: Meta-analysis of randomized clinical trials. *British Medical Journal, 322*, 11–15.

Muldoon, M. F., Manuck, S. M., & Mathews, K. M. (1990). Lowering cholesterol concentrations and mortality: A quantitative review of primary prevention trials. *British Medical Journal, 301*, 309–314.

Neaton, J., Blackburn, H., Jacobs, D., Kuller, L., Lee, D., Sherwin, R., et al. (1992). Serum cholesterol level and mortality findings for men screened in the multiple risk factor intervention trial. *Archives of Internal Medicine, 152*, 1490–1500.

New, A. S., Gelernter, J., Goodman, M., Mitropoulou, V., Koenigsberg, H., Silverman, J., & Siever, L. J. (2001). Suicide, impulsive aggression, and HTR1B genotype. *Biological Psychiatry, 50*(1), 62–65.

New, A. S., Gelernter, J., Yovell, Y., Trestman, R. L., Nielsen, D. A., Silverman, J., et al. (1998). Tryptophan hydroxylase genotype is associated with impulsive–aggression measures: A preliminary study. *American Journal of Medical Genetics, 81*, 13–17.

New, A. S., Hazlett, E. A., Buchsbaum, M. S., Goodman, M., Reynolds, D., Mitropoulou, V., et al. (2002). Blunted prefrontal cortical 18fluorodeoxyglucose positron emission tomography response to meta-chlorophenylpiperazine in impulsive aggression. *Archives of General Psychiatry, 59*(7), 621–629.

New, A. S., Sevin, E. M., Mitropoulou, V., Reynolds, D., Novotny, S. L., Callahan, A., et al. (1998). Serum cholesterol and impulsivity in personality disorders. *Psychiatry Research, 85,* 145–150.

Nielsen, D. A., Goldman, D., Virkkunen, M., Tokola, R., Rawlings, R., & Linnoila, M. (1994). Suicidality and 5-hydroxyindoleacetic acid concentration associated with a tryptophan hydroxylase polymorphism. *Archives of General Psychiatry, 51,* 34–38.

Nielsen, D. A., Virkkunen, M., Lappalainin, J., Eggert, M., Brown, G. L., Long, J. C., et al. (1998). A tryptophan hydroxylase gene marker for suicidality and alcoholism. *Archives of General Psychiatry, 55,* 593–602.

Nolan, K. A., Volavka, J., Czobor, P., Czobor, P., Cseh, A., Lachman, H., et al. (2000). Suicidal behavior in patients with schizophrenia is related to COMT polymorphism. *Psychiatric Genetics, 10,* 117–124.

O'Keane, V., Moloney, E., O'Neill, H., O'Conner, A., Smith, C., & Dinan, T. G. (1992). Blunted prolactin responses to d-fenfluramine in sociopathy. Evidence for subsensitivity of central serotonergic function. *British Journal of Psychiatry, 160,* 643–6.

Okuyama, Y., Ishiguro, H., Nankai, M., Shibuya, H., Watanabe, A., & Arinami, T. (2000). Identification of a polymorphism in the promoter region of DRD4 associated with the human novelty seeking personality trait. *Molecular Psychiatry, 5,* 64–69.

Oquendo, M. A., Placidi, G. P., Malone, K. M., Campbell, C., Keilp, J., Brodsky, B., et al. (2003). Positron emission tomography of regional brain metabolic responses to a serotonergic challenge and lethality of suicide attempts in major depression. *Archives of General Psychiatry, 60*(1), 14–22.

Oreland, L., & Shaskan, E. G. (1983, August). Monoamine oxidase activity as a biological marker. *Trends in Pharmacological Sciences,* pp. 339–341.

Pajer, K., Gardner, W., Rubin, R. T., Perel, J., & Neal, S. (2001). Decreased cortisol levels in adolescent girls with conduct disorder. *Archives of General Psychiatry, 58,* 297–302.

Pandey, G. N., Pandey, S. C., Janicak, P. G., Marks, R. C., & Davis, J. M. (1990). Platelet serotonin-2 receptor binding sites in depression and suicide. *Biological Psychiatry, 28,* 215–222.

Parsian, A. (1999). Sequence analysis of exon 8 of MAO-A gene in alcoholics with antisocial personality and normal controls. *Genomics, 55*(3), 290–295.

Parsian, A., Cloninger, C. R., & Zhang, Z. H. (2000). Functional variant in the DRD2 receptor promoter region and subtypes of alcoholism. *American Journal of Medical Genetics (Neuropsychiatric Genetics), 86,* 407–411.

Parsian, A., Todd, R. D., Devor, E. J., O'Malley, K. L., Suarez, B. K., Reich, T., & Cloninger, C. R. (1991). Alcoholism and alleles of the human D2 dopamine receptor locus. Studies of association and linkage. *Archives of General Psychiatry, 48*(7), 655–663.

Patrick, C. J. (2001). Emotional processes in psychopathy. In A. Raine & J. Sanmartin (Eds.), *Violence and psychopathy* (pp. 57–77). New York: Kluwer.

Patrick, C. J. (in press). Getting to the heart of psychopathy. In H. Herve & J. C. Yuille (Eds.), *Psychopathy: Theory, research, and social implications.* Hillsdale, NJ: Erlbaum.

Patrick, C. J., Bradley, M. M., & Lang, P. J. (1993). Emotion in the criminal psychopath: Startle reflex modulation. *Journal of Abnormal Psychology, 102,* 82–92.

Penick, E. C., Powell, B. J., Campbell, J., Liskow, B. I., Nickel, E. J., Dale, T. M., et al. (1996). Pharmacological treatment for antisocial personality disorder alcoholics: A preliminary study. *Alcoholism, Clinical and Experimental Research, 20*(3), 477–484.

Ponce, G., Jimenez-Arriero, M. A., Rubio, G., Hoenicka, J., Ampuiero, I., Ramos, J. A., & Palomo, T. (2003). The A1 allele of the DRD2 gene (TaqI A polymorphisms) is associated with antisocial personality in a sample of alcohol-dependent patients. *European Psychiatry, 18,* 356–360.

Rada, R. T., Laws, D. R., & Kellner, R. (1976). Plasma testosterone levels in the rapist. *Psychosomatic Medicine, 38,* 257–268.

Rada, R. T., Laws, D. R., Kellner, R., Stivastava, L., & Peake, G. (1983). Plasma androgens in violent and nonviolent sex offenders. *Bulletin of the American Academy of Psychiatry and Law, 112,* 149–158.

Raine, A., Buchsbaum, M., Stanley, J., Lottenberg, S., Abel, L., 7 Stoddard, J. (1994). Selective reductions in prefrontal glucose metabolism in murderers. *Biological Psychiatry, 36,* 365–373.

Raine, A. (2002). Biosocial studies of antisocial and violent behavior in children and adults: A review. *Journal of Abnormal Child Psychology, 30,* 311–326.

Ramklint, M., Stalenheim, E., von Knorring, A-L., & von Knorring, L. (2000). Triiodothyronine(T3) related to conduct disorder in a forensic psychiatric population. *European Journal of Psychiatry, 14,* 33–41.

Rasanen, P., Hakko, H., Visuri, S., Paanila, J., Kapanen, P., Suomela, T., & Tiihonen, J. (1999). Serum testosterone levels, mental disorders and criminal behavior. *Acta Psychiatrica Scandinavica, 99*(5), 348–352.

Reif, A., & Lesch, K-P. (2003). Toward a molecular architecture of personality. *Behavior Brain Research, 139,* 1–20.

Repo-Tiihonen, E., Halonen, P., Tiihonen, J., & Virkkunen, M. (2002). Total serum cholesterol level, violent criminal offences, suicidal behavior, mortality and the appearance of conduct disorder in Finnish male criminal offenders with antisocial personality disorder. *European Archives of Psychiatry and Clinical Neuroscience, 252*(1), 8–11.

Retz, W., Rosler, M., Supprian, T., Retz-Junginger, P., & Thome, J. (2003). Dopamine D3 receptor gene-polymorphism and violent behavior: Relation to impulsiveness and ADHD-related psychopathology. *Journal of Neural Transmittors, 110,* 561–572.

Ronai, Z., Szekely, A., Nemoda, Z., Lakatos, K., Gervai, J., Staub, M., et al. (2001). Association between novelty seeking and the –521 C/T polymorphism in the promoter region of the DRD4 gene. *Molecular Psychiatry*, 6, 35–38.

Rotondo, A., Schuebel, K. E., Bergen, A. W., Aragon, R., Virkkunen, M., Linnoila, M., et al. (1999). Identification of four variants in the tryptophan hydroxylase promoter and association to behavior. *Molecular Psychiatry*, 4, 360–368.

Roy, A., Adinoff, B., & Linnoila, M. (1988). Acting out hostility in normal volunteers: Negative corrleation with levels of 5 HIAA in cerebrospinal fluid. *Psychiatry Research*, 24, 187–194.

Rubinstein, M., Phillips, T. J., Bunzow, J. R., Falzone, T. L., Dziewczapolski, G., Zhang, G., et al. (1997). Mice lacking dopamine D4 receptors are supersensitive to ethanol, cocaine, and methamphetamine. *Cell*, 90, 991–1001.

Rujescu, D., Giegling, I., Gietl, A., Hartmann, A. M., & Moller, H-J. (2003). A functional single nucleotide polymorphism (V158M) in the COMT gene is associated with aggressive personality traits. *Biological Psychiatry*, 54, 34–39.

Russ, M. J., Lachman, H. M., Kasdan, T., Saito, T., & Bajmakovic-Kacila, S. (2000). Analysis of catechol-o-methyltransferase and 5-hydroxytryptamine transporter polymorphisms in patients at risk for suicide. *Psychiatry Research*, 93, 73–78.

Sabol, S. Z., Hu, S., & Hamer, D. (1998). A functional polymorphism in the monoamine oxidase A gene promoter. *Human Genetics*, 103(3), 273–279.

Saito, T., Lachman, H.M., Diaz, L., Hallikainen, T., Kauhanen, J., Salonen, J. T., et al. (2002). Analysis of monoamine oxidase A (MAOA) promoter polymorphism in Finnish male alcoholics. *Psychiatry Research*, 109(2), 113–119.

Samochowiec, J., Lesch, K. P., Rottmann, M., Smolka, M., Syagailo, Y. V., Okladnova, O., et al. (1999). Association of a regulatory polymorphism in the promoter region of the monoamine oxidase A gene with antisocial alcoholism. *Psychiatry Research*, 86(1), 67–72.

Sander, T., Harms, H., Dufeu, P., Kuhn, S., Hoehe, M., Lesch, K., et al. (1998). Serotonin transporter gene variants in alcohol-dependent subjects with dissocial personality disorder. *Biological Psychiatry*, 43, 908–912.

Sandler, M., Ruthven, C. R., Goodwin, B. L., Field, H., & Matthews, R. (1978). Phenylethylamine overproduction in aggressive psychopaths. *Lancet*, 2(8103) 1269–1270.

Saudou, F., Amara, D. A., Dierich, A., LeMeur, M., Ramboz, S., Seog, L., et al. (1994). Enhanced aggressive behavior in mice lacking 5-HT1B receptor. *Science*, 265, 1875–1878.

Scerbo, A. S., & Kolko, D. J. (1995). Salivary testosterone and cortisol in disruptive children: Relationship to aggressive, hyperactive, and internalizing behav-

iors. *Journal of the American Academy of Child and Adolescent Psychiatry*, 34(5), 535–536.

Schalling, D., Asberg, M., Edman, G., & Oreland, L. (1987). Markers for vulnerability to psychopathology: Temperament traits associated with platelet MAO activity. *Acta Psychiatrica Scandinavica*, 76, 172–182.

Schuckit, M. A. (1996). Recent developments in the pharmacotherapy of alcohol dependence. *Journal of Consulting Clinical Psychology*, 64(4), 669–676.

Schmidt, L. G., Sander, T., Kuhn, S., Smolka, M., Rommelspacher, H., Samochowiec, J., & Lesch, K. P. (2000). Different allele distribution of a regulatory MAOA gene promoter polymorphism in antisocial and anxious–depressive alcoholics. *Journal of Neural Transmission*, 107(6), 681–689.

Schuback, D. E., Mulligan, E. L., Sims, K. B., Tivol, E. A., Greenberg, B. D., Chang, S. F., et al. (1999). Screen for MAOA mutations in target human groups. *American Journal of Medical Genetics*, 88(1), 25–28.

Sheard, M. H., Marini, J. L., Bridges, C. I., & Wagner, E. (1976). The effect of lithium on impulsive aggressive behavior in man. *American Journal of Psychiatry*, 133(12), 1409–1413.

Sherif, F., Hallman, J., & Oreland, L. (1992). Low platelet gamma-aminobutyrate aminotransferase and monoamine oxidase activities in chronic alcoholic patients. *Alcoholism, Clinical and Experimental Research*, 16(6), 1014–1020.

Shoal, G. D., Giancola, P. R., & Kirillova, G. P. (2003). Salivary cortisol, personality, and aggressive behavior in adolescent boys: A 5-year longitudinal study. *Journal of the American Academy of Child and Adolescent Psychiatry*, 42(9), 1101–1107.

Siassi, I. (1982). Lithium treatment of impulsive behavior in children. *Journal of Clinical Psychiatry*, 43, 482–484.

Siever, L. J., Kahn, R. S., Lawlor, B. A., Trestman, R. L., Lawrence, T. L., & Coccario, E. F. (1991). Critical issues in defining the role of serotonin in psychiatric disorders. *Pharmacology Review*, 43, 509–525.

Siever, L. J., Buchsbaum, M. S., New, A. S., Spiegel, Cohen, J., Wei, T., Hazlett, E. A., et al. (1999). d,l-fenfluramine response in impulsive personality disorder assessed with [18F] flurodeoxyglucose positron emission tomomgraphy. *Neuropsychopharmacology*, 20, 413–423.

Simeon, D., Stanley, B., Frances, A., Mann, J. J., Winchel, R., & Stanley, M. (1992). Self-mutilation in personality disorders: psychological and biological correlates. *American Journal of Psychiatry*, 149, 221–226.

Sinha, R., Cloninger, C. R., & Parsian, A. (2003). Linkage disequilibrium and haplotype analysis between serotonin receptor 1B gene variations and subtypes of alcoholism. *American Journal of Medical Genetics*, 121B(1), 83–88.

Smith, S. S., Newman, J. P., Evans, A., Pickens, R., Wydeven, J., Uhl, G. R., & Newlin, D. B. (1993).

Comorbid Psychopathy is not associated with increased D2 dopamine receptor TaqI A or B gene marker frequencies in incarcerated substance abusers. *Biological Psychiatry*, *33*, 845–848.

Soderstrom, H., Blennow, K., Manhem, A., & Forsman, A. (2001). CSF studies in violent offenders: 5-HIAA as a negative and HVA as a positive predictor of psychopathy. *Journal of Neural Transmission*, *108*, 869–878.

Soderstrom, H., Blennow, K., Sjodin, A-K., & Forsman, A. (2003). New evidence for an association between the CSF HVA: 5-HIAA ratio and psychopathic traits. *Journal of Neural Neurosurgery and Psychiatry*, *74*, 918–921.

Soler, H., Vinayak, P., & Quadagno, D. (2000). Bioxocial aspects of domestic violence. *Psychoneuroendocrinology*, *25*, 721–739.

Soyka, M., Bondy, B., Benda, E., Preuss, U., Hegerl, U., & Moller, H. (2000). Platelet monoamine oxidase activity in alcoholics with and without a family history of alcoholism. *European Addiction Research*, *6*(2), 57–63.

Soyka, M., Preuss, U. W., Koller, G., Zill, P., & Bondy, B. (2004). Association of 5-HT1B receptor gene and antisocial behavior in alcoholism. *Journal of Neural Transmittors*, *111*(1), 101–109.

Spitz, R. T., Hillbrand, M., Foster, & H. G., Jr. (1994). Serum cholesterol levels and frequency of aggression. *Psychology Report*, *74*(2), 622.

Stalenheim, E. G. (2004). Long-term validity of biological markers of psychopathy and criminal recidivism: Follow-up 6–8 years after forensic psychiatric investigation. *Psychiatry Research*, *121*, 281–291.

Stalenheim, E. G., Eriksson, E., von Knorring, L., & Wide, L. (1998). Testosterone as a biological marker in psychopathy and alcoholism. *Psychiatry Research*, *77*, 79–88.

Stalenheim, E. G., von Knorring, L. V., & Oreland, L. (1997). Platelet monoamine oxidase activity as a biological marker in Swedish forensic psychiatric population. *Psychiatry Research*, *69*, 79–87.

Stalenheim, E. G., von Knorring, L., & Wide, L. (1998). Serum levels of thyroid hormones as biological markers in a Swedish forensic psychiatric population. *Biological Psychology*, *43*, 755–761.

Stanley, B., Molcho, A., Stanley, M., Winchel, R., Gameroff, M. J., Parsons, B., & Mann, J. J. (2000). Association of aggressive behavior with altered serotonergic function in patients who are not suicidal. *American Journal of Psychiatry*, *157*(4), 609–14.

Stewart, M. A., & Stewart, S. G. (1981). Serum cholesterol in antisocial personality: A failure to replicate earlier findings. *Neuropsychobiology*, *7*, 9–11.

Stockmeier, C. A., Shapiro, L. A., Dilley, G. E., Kolli, T. N., Friedman, L., & Rajkowska, G. (1998). Increase in serotonin-1A autoreceptors in the midbrain of suicide victims with major depression–postmortem evidence for decreased serotonin activity. *Journal of Neuroscience*, *18*, 7394–7401.

Strous, R. D., Nolan, K. A., Lapidus, R., Libna, D., &

Saito, T. (2003). Aggressive behavior in schizophrenia is associated with the low enzyme activity COMP polymorphism: A replication study. *American Journal of Medical Genetics Part B (Neuropsychiatric Genetics)*, *120B*, 29–34.

Sullivan, J. L., Baenziger, J. C., Wagner, D. L., Rauscher, F. P., Nurnberger, J. I., Jr., & Holmes, J. S. (1990). Platelet MAO in subtypes of alcoholism. *Biological Psychiatry*, *27*(8), 911–22.

Sullivan, P. F., Joyce, P. R., Bulik, C. M., Mulder, R. T., & Oakley-Browne, M. (1994). Total cholesterol and suicidality in depression. *Biological Psychiatry*, *36*(7), 472–7.

Svrakic, D. M., Whitehead, C., Przybeck, T. R., & Cloninger, C. R. (1993). Differential diagnosis of personality disorders by the seven factor model of temperament and character. *Archives of General Psychiatry*, *50*, 991–999.

Swann, A. C., Johnson, B. A., Cloninger, C. R., & Chen, Y. R. (1999). Relationship of plasma tryptophan availability to course of illness and clinical features of alcoholism: preliminary study. *Psychopharmacology*, *143*, 380–384.

Tiihonen, J., Kuikka, J., Bergstrom, K., Hakola, P., Karhu, J., Ryynanen, O. P., & Fohr, J. (1995). Altered striatal dopamine re-uptake site densities in habitually violent and non-violent alcoholics. *Nature Medicine*, *1*(7), 654–657.

Tiihonen, J., Kuikka, J. T., Bergstrom, K. A., Karhu, J., Viinamaki, H., Lehtonen, J., et al. (1997). Single-photon emission tomography imaging of monoamine transporters in impulsive violent behavior. *European Journal of Nuclear Medicine*, *24*(10), 1253–1260.

Tiihonen, J., Virkkunen, M., Rasanen, P., Pennanen, S., Sainio, E. L., Callaway, J., et al. (2001). Free L-tryptophan plasma levels in antisocial violent offenders. *Psychopharmacology*, *157*, 395–400.

van Goozen, S. H., Matthys, W., Cohen-Kettenis, P. T., Westenberg, H., & van Egeland, H. (1999). Plasma monoamine metabolites and aggression: Two studies of normal and oppositional defiant disorder children. *European Neuropsychopharmacology*, *9*(1–2), 141–147.

van Goozen, S. H. M., Matthys, W., Cohen-Kettenis, R. P., Wied, C. G., Wiegand, V. M., & van Egeland, H. (1998). Salivary cortisol and cardiovascular activity during stress in oppositional-defiant disorder boys and normal controls. *Biological Psychiatry*, *43*, 531–539.

van Heeringen, K., Audenaert, K., Wiele, L. V., & Verstraete, A. (2000). Cortisol in violent suicidal behaviour: Association with personality and monoaminergic activity. *Journal of Affective Disorders*, *60*, 181–189.

Vanyukov, M. M., Moss, H. B., Kaplan, B. B., Kirillova, G. P., & Tarter, R. E. (2000). Antisociality, substance dependence, and the DRD5 gene: A preliminary study. *American Journal of Medical Genetics*, *96*(5), 654–658.

Vanyukov, M. M., Moss, H. B., Plail, J. A., Blackson, T.,

Mezzich, A. C., & Tarter, R. E. (1993). Antisocial symptoms in preadolescent boys and in their parents: Associations with cortisol. *Psychiatry Research, 46,* 9–17.

Vanyukov, M. M., Moss, H. B., Yu, L. M., & Deka, R. (1995). A dinucleotide repeat polymorphism at the gene for monoamine oxidase A and measures of aggressiveness. *Psychiatry Research, 59*(1–2), 35–41.

Verona, E., Patrick, C. J., & Joiner, T. E. (2001). Psychopathy, antisocial personality, and suicide risk. *Journal of Abnormal Psychology, 110*(3), 462–470.

Vevera, J., Zukov, I., Morcinek, T., & Papezova, H. (2003). Cholesterol concentrations in violent and non-violent women suicide attempters. *European Psychiatry, 18*(1), 23–27.

Virkkunen, M. (1979). Serum cholesterol in antisocial personality. *Neuropsychobiology, 5,* 27–30.

Virkkunen, M. (1982). Reactive hypoglycemic tendency among habitually violent offenders: A further study by means of the glucose tolerance test. *Neuropsychobiology, 8,* 35–40.

Virkkunen, M. (1983a). Insulin secretion during the glucose tolerance test in antisocial personality. *British Journal of Psychiatry, 142,* 598–604.

Virkkunen, M. (1983b). Serum cholesterol levels in homicidal offenders. A low cholesterol level is connected with a habitually violent tendency under the influence of alcohol. *Neuropsychobiology, 5,* 27–30.

Virkkunen, M. (1985). Urinary free cortisol secretion in habitually violent offenders. *Acta Psychiatrica Scandinavica, 72*(1), 40–44.

Virkkunen, M., De Jong, J., Bartko, J., Goodwin, F. K., & Linnoila, M. (1989). Relationship of psychobiological variables to recidivism in violent offenders and impulsive fire setters. A follow-up study. *Archives of General Psychiatry, 46*(7), 600–603.

Virkkunen, M., Eggert, M., Rawlings, R., & Linnoila, M. (1996). A prospective follow-up study of alcoholic violent offenders and fire setters. *Archives of General Psychiatry, 53*(6), 523–529.

Virkkunen, M., & Huttunen, M. O. (1982). Evidence for abnormal glucose tolerance test among violent offenders. *Neuropsychobiology, 8,* 30–34.

Virkkunen, M., & Narvanen, S. (1987). Plasma insulin, tryptophan and serotonin levels during the glucose tolerance test among habitually violent and impulsive offenders. *Neuropsychobiology, 17*(1–2), 19–23.

Virkkunen, M., Nuutila, A., Goodwin, F. K., & Linnoila, M. (1987). Cerebrospinal fluid monoamine metabolite levels in male arsonists. *Archives of General Psychiatry, 44,* 241–247.

Virkkunen, M., & Penttinen, H. (1984). Serum cholesterol in aggressive conduct disorder: A preliminary study. *Biological Psychiatry, 19,* 435–439.

Virkkunen, M., Rawlings, R., Tokola, R., Poland, R. E., Cuidotti, A., Nemweroff, C., et al. (1994). CSF biochemistries, glucose metabolism, and diurnal activity rhythms in alcoholic, violent offenders, fire setters, and healthy volunteers. *Archives of General Psychiatry, 51,* 20–27.

Vitalis, T., Cases, O., Callebert, J., Launay, J. M., Price, D. J., Seif, I., & Gaspar, P. (1998). Effects of monoamine oxidase A inhibition on barrel formation in the mouse somatosensory cortex: Determination of a sensitive developmental period. *Journal of Comparative Neurology, 393*(2), 169–184.

von Knorring, A-L., Hallman, J., von Knorring, L., & Oreland, L. (1991). Platelet monoamine oxidase activity in type 1 and type 2 alcoholism. *Alcohol and Alcoholism, 26,* 409–416.

Wang, S., & Mason, J. (1999). Elevations of serum T3 levels and their association with symptoms in World War II veterans with combat-related posttraumatic stress disorder: Replication of findings in Vietnam combat veterans. *Psychosomatic Medicine, 61,* 131–138.

Wingrove, J., Bond, A. J., Cleare, A. J., & Sherwood, R. (1999). Plasma trypophan and trait aggression. *Journal of Psychopharmacology, 13,* 235–237.

Woodman, D. D., Hinton, J. W., & O'Neill, M. T. (1978). Cortisol secretion and stress in maximum security hospital patients. *Journal of Psychosomatic Research, 22,* 133–136.

Yates, W. R., Wilcox, J., Knudson, R., Myers, C., & Kelly, M. W. (1990). The effect of gender and subtype on platelet MAO in alcoholism. *Journal of Studies in Alcohol, 51,* 463–467.

Zuckerman, M. (1993). P-Impulsive sensation seeking and its behavioral, psychophysiological and biochemical correlates. *Neuropsychobiology, 28,* 30–36.

14

The Neuroanatomical Bases of Psychopathy

A Review of Brain Imaging Findings

ADRIAN RAINE
YALING YANG

A decade ago, brain imaging research on antisocial behavior was in its infancy. Today, a burgeoning body of brain imaging evidence now attests to the fact that links exist between brain deficits and antisocial, violent behavior. Most of this research has assessed the functioning of the brain using PET (positron emission tomography, measuring glucose metabolism), SPECT (single photon emission computerized tomography, assessing blood flow), MRS (magnetic resonance spectroscopy, assessing neural density) or fMRI (functional magnetic resonance imaging, measuring blood flow). Some recent studies have employed MRI to assess brain structure (anatomic MRI [aMRI]). These supersede the older imaging studies using computed tomography (CT), which suffer from relatively poor spatial resolution. To date, the key brain areas that have been shown to be abnormal in antisocial individuals include the prefrontal cortex, temporal cortex, the amygdala–hippocampal complex, the corpus callosum, and the angular gyrus.

Despite this developing knowledge base, there has been surprisingly little brain imaging research on the specific construct of psychopathic behavior. Not surprisingly there-fore, within this small corpus of research there are very few imaging studies specifically on structural brain impairments in psychopaths. Consequently, the empirical basis for any discussion of the neuroanatomical basis of psychopathy based on imaging is very limited. As such, this chapter relies on the somewhat larger database of brain imaging research on antisocial and violent behavior. Although the emphasis is on structural brain impairments in psychopaths, fMRI research is also discussed as findings from such research may provide a context within which to evaluate the more limited research on psychopathic behavior and thus directions for future anatomical MRI research on psychopaths. Specific questions are posed even though complete answers cannot as yet be given. In particular, which brain regions are implicated in violent, antisocial, and psychopathic behavior? Do different brain deficits predispose to different features of psychopathy? What role does the environment play? Do brain deficits actually cause psychopathy? More theoretically, how do they cause psychopathy? What causes the brain deficits? And can they be treated or prevented?

WHAT BRAIN AREAS ARE IMPLICATED?

Psychopathy is a complex clinical construct that, according to one current definition (the Psychopathy Checklist—Revised [PCL-R]), is made up of 20 signs and symptoms (Hare, 1991). Given such complexity, it is highly likely that the neuroanatomical basis to psychopathy is not simple, and that abnormalities to multiple brain mechanisms contribute to the behavioral, cognitive, and emotional characteristics that make up the psychopath. This section briefly outlines what we have learned to date from structural (and functional) imaging studies covering the entire brain.

Prefrontal Cortex

The historical starting point for suspecting structural impairments to the prefrontal cortex as a predisposition to psychopathy is embodied in the case study of Phineas Gage, a foreman working for the Great Western Railways who, in 1848, had a tamping rod blown through his face and forehead. An MRI reconstruction of the resulting damage indicated that the trajectory of the rod selectively damaged the prefrontal cortex, in particular the ventromedial region including the orbitofrontal cortex (Damasio, Grabowski, Frank, Galaburda, & Damasio, 1994). The accident transformed Gage from a reliable, well-liked, respected, and organized individual into a man who was garrulous, sexually promiscuous, reckless, unreliable, and irresponsible—essentially a pseudo-psychopathic individual (Damasio, 1994). While only a single case study, this example nevertheless sets up the hypothesis that damage (or even functional impairment) within the prefrontal cortex may predispose an individual to psychopathic behavior. However, the key question to be asked concerns whether this proposition is supported by brain imaging studies of antisocial and psychopathic populations.

Indeed, there are reasons to believe that it may not be. For example, past neuropsychological research has suggested that findings on frontal dysfunction in psychopaths are inconsistent (e.g., Hare, 1984). This may be due to the fact that neuropsychological tests are indirect and relatively nonspecific indicates of frontal dysfunction, or alternatively because frontal dysfunction may be specific to the antisocial lifestyle but not the affective / interpersonal factor of psychopathy. Alternatively, a more recent meta-analysis of neuropsychological findings by Morgan and Lilienfeld (2000) supports both the notion of frontal dysfunction in antisocial behavior in general as well as psychopathy in particular. Given this debate in the field, findings from brain imaging research are of particular importance.

Antisocial/Violent Behavior: Functional Imaging

Reviews of brain imaging studies of violent and antisocial populations have been conducted by Raine (1993), Raine and Buchsbaum, (1996), Henry and Moffitt (1997), and Davidson, Putnam, and Larson (2000). These reviews all converge on the conclusion that the brain region most likely to be compromised in antisocial, violent populations is the prefrontal cortex.

Several examples of such studies are available from just the past few years. Goyer, Andreason, Semple, and Clayton (1994), using PET in an auditory activation condition, showed that an increased number of impulsive–aggressive acts was associated with reduced glucose in the frontal cortex of 17 patients with personality disorders. Volkow and colleagues (1995) using PET in a nonactivation, eyes open, resting state observed reduced glucose metabolism in both prefrontal and medial temporal regions in eight psychiatric patients (three with schizophrenia) with a history of violence. Kuruoglu, Arikan, Vural, and Karatas (1996) using SPECT in a resting state found that 15 alcoholics with antisocial personality disorder (APD) showed significantly reduced frontal regional cerebral blood flow (rCBF) compared to 4 alcoholics with other personality disorders and 10 nonalcoholic controls. Raine and colleagues (1994) using PET and a sustained attention challenge task observed reduced glucose metabolism in the prefrontal cortex of 22 murderers compared to 22 normal controls. In an extension of this study incorporating additional participants, Raine, Buchsbaum, and LaCasse (1997) found reduced prefrontal glucose metabolism in 41 murderers compared to 41 age- and sex-matched normal controls. Using SPECT,

Soderstrom, Tullberg, Wikkelsoe, Ekholm, and Forsman, (2000) found reduced blood flow in both the frontal and temporal lobes of 21 individuals convicted of impulsive violent offences. Using MRS, Critchley and colleagues (2000) found lower prefrontal concentrations of N-acetyl aspartate (NAA) and creatine phosphocreatine in 10 mildly retarded repetitively violent offenders compared to controls.

Psychopathy: Functional Imaging

In contrast to antisocial/criminal/violence studies, there are surprising few studies of frontal functioning in psychopaths. Those that have been conducted implicate abnormalities to negative affect stimuli, but not in the direction that might intuitively be expected based on the neuropsychological literature. Drug-abusing psychopaths compared to drug-abusing nonpsychopaths and controls show *increased* rCBF bilaterally in frontotemporal regions during the processing of negative affect words (Intrator, Hare, Stritzke, & Brichtswein, 1997). Similarly, during an aversive conditioning paradigm, psychopaths with APD show atypically *increased* activation in the dorsolateral prefrontal cortex. Similarly, in an affective memory task, psychopaths show overactivation of frontotemporal regions (Kiehl et al., 2001), although in this fMRI study they also showed decreased activation in subcortical regions during an affective memory task. Furthermore, psychopaths have shown *increased* activation to negative affect pictures in the right prefrontal cortex but decreased activation to positive affect pictures in the right medial prefrontal cortex along with increased left orbitofrontal activation (Muller et al., 2003). In a resting state using SPECT, no significant correlations were observed between frontal blood flow and total psychopathy scores in a group of violent offenders (Soderstrom et al., 2002). Taken together, all four studies using a negative affect emotional challenge indicate if anything *increased*, not decreased, frontal activation in psychopaths (Schneider et al., 2000). It is possible that psychopaths may paradoxically show enhanced activity because they have fear conditioning and emotion deficits; thus, to perform the behavioral activation task as well as controls, greater neurophysiological activation is required.

Structural Impairments in Psychopaths and APD

There appear to be only four studies that bear on the question of whether prefrontal structural impairments characterize antisocial and psychopathic personality. The first aMRI brain imaging study of antisocial behavior involved a sample of 21 community participants with diagnoses of APD who also had high scores on the PCL-R. This sample of antisocial psychopathic individuals showed an 11% reduction in the volume of gray matter in the prefrontal cortex compared with both normal controls and a substance dependence control group (Raine, Lencz, Bihrle, LaCasse, & Colletti, 2000). This deficit was relative in that no difference in whole brain volume was observed, and the deficit was specific to prefrontal gray matter as opposed to white.

In some support of these findings, Laakso and colleagues (2002) found reduced MRI left prefrontal gray volumes (dorsolateral, orbitofrontal, and medial) in alcoholics with antisocial personalities compared to controls. These authors argued for an abolition of these three area effects when duration of alcoholism was controlled, but because this covariate is very heavily correlated with group membership (i.e., all controls have a zero age of onset and all alcoholic antisocial subjects have some age of onset), this conclusion does not seem entirely warranted. Woermann and colleagues (2000) did find reduced left prefrontal gray volumes in aggressive epileptic patients. On the other hand, Dolan, Deakin, Roberts, and Anderson (2002) did not find reduced frontal volumes in patients with impulsive–aggressive patients with personality disorders. In contrast to antisocial personality, there appear to be no structural imaging studies of carefully defined psychopaths (but see section on correlations between psychopathy scores and prefrontal gray volume).

Temporal Cortex

Antisocial and Violent Behavior

Relatively poor cortical functioning in the temporal lobe is another finding emerging from the brain imaging literature with respect to antisocial behavior. Reduced glucose metabolism has been found in medial temporal regions of violent patients (Volkow et al.,

1995). The number of localized temporal lobe changes identified through electroencephalograph (EEG) and CT has also been positively associated with severity ratings for preadmission violence among offenders with mental disorders (Wong, Lumsden, Fenton, & Fenwick, 1994). In two other brain imaging studies, temporal lobe abnormalities were found to be more prevalent in aggressive versus nonaggressive psychiatric patients (Amen, Stubblefield, Carmichael, & Thisted, 1996; Wong, Lumsden, Fenton, & Fenwick, 1997). Aggressive dementia patients have also been found to show reduced blood flow in the left anterior temporal lobe as measured by SPECT (Hirono, Mega, Dinov, Mishkin, & Cummings, 2000).

It should be noted that many of the reported temporal lobe functional abnormalities in aggressive populations may reflect frontotemporal dysfunction, as evidenced by the fact that most of the aforementioned studies found coexisting frontal deficits. A second notable point is that different imaging technologies using different activation states may be sensitive to dysfunction in different brain regions. For example, Gatzke-Kopp, Raine, Buchsbaum, and LaCasse (2001) found resting EEG abnormalities in the temporal lobes of murderers, even though PET activation testing did not reveal evidence for temporal lobe dysfunction. In terms of structure, one aMRI study observed a 20% reduction in temporal lobe volume in impulsive–aggressive patients with personality disorders (Dolan et al., 2002).

Psychopathy

As discussed previously, Intrator and colleagues (1997) using SPECT found that psychopaths show *increased* bilateral blood flow in frontotemporal regions during the processing of emotional words. Two other studies suggest that this effect may, however, be specific to the frontal contribution to the effect. In a resting state using SPECT, no significant correlations were observed between left or right temporal lobe blood flow and total psychopathy scores in a group of violent offenders (Soderstrom et al., 2002). Activation was, however, *reduced* (not increased) in the right temporal gyrus in psychopaths in response to negative affect stimuli (Muller et al., 2003). Consequently, unlike broad-based antisocial personality, psychopathy in partic-

ular may not be associated with temporal lobe functioning.

Amygdala and Hippocampus

Functional impairments in the hippocampus and amygdala have been observed in violent offenders. For example, abnormal asymmetries of functioning were found in a PET study of murderers, with murderers showing lower left and increased right functioning in both the amygdala and hippocampus compared to controls (Raine et al., 1997). Soderstrom and colleagues (2000) in a SPECT study found bilaterally reduced hippocampal functioning in violent offenders. In a study of repetitively violent patients, Critchley and colleagues (2000) showed reduced NAA in the amygdala–hippocampal complex, which in turn indicates reduced neural density. Laakso and colleagues (2000) demonstrated reduced right hippocampal volume reductions in violent offenders with APD who were also early-onset alcoholics compared to controls. With respect to the amygdala, however, one structural imaging study has shown that aggressive and nonaggressive epileptic patients did not differ on amygdala volume or amygdala pathology as measured by MRI (Elst, Woermann, Lemieux, Thompson, & Trimble, 2000).

Psychopathy

Regarding function, during an aversive conditioning paradigm, psychopaths with APD show atypically *increased* activation in the amygdala (Schneider et al., 2000). In contrast, Kiehl and colleagues (2001) using fMRI found *reduced* activation in the amygdala–hippocampal complex in criminal psychopaths when processing affective stimuli. Relatedly, Muller and colleagues (2003) observed reduced activation in the left parahippocampal gyrus in psychopaths in response to negative affect stimuli. Alternatively, Soderstrom and colleagues (2000) failed to observe significant correlations between both amygdala and hippocampal frontal blood flow in relation to total psychopathy scores (Soderstrom et al., 2002).

With regard to structure, one aMRI study found reductions in the volume of the posterior hippocampus to be associated with increased psychopathy scores in antisocial alcoholics (Laakso et al., 2001). However, more complex structural abnormalities have been reported by Raine and colleagues (2004), which implicate abnormal asymmetry in the *anterior* hippocampus (see section on unsuccessful psychopaths for further details). One study has also reported reduced amygdala volume to be associated with increased psychopathy scores within a sample of violent offenders (Tiihonen, Hodgins, & Vaurio, 2000).

Corpus Callosum

Antisocial/Violent Behavior:
Functional Imaging

Although damage to the corpus callosum has long been hypothesized to represent a neurological predisposition to violence, only one imaging study to date appears to have assessed for such a relationship. Raine and colleagues (1997) using PET found that murderers exhibited decreased metabolic activity in the corpus callosum compared to normal controls.

Psychopathy: Structural Imaging

There appears to be only one study on the corpus callosum in psychopaths. Raine, Lencz, and colleagues (2003) assessed 15 male subjects with both high psychopathy scores and APD, and 25 matched controls from a larger sample of 83 community volunteers on aMRI measures of the corpus callosum (volume estimate of callosal white matter, thickness, length, area of genu and splenium), electrodermal and cardiovascular activity during a social stressor, and personality measures of affective and interpersonal deficits. Compared with controls, psychopathic antisocial individuals showed a 22.6% increase in estimated callosal white matter volume ($p = .0001$), a 6.9% increase in callosal length ($p = .002$), a 15.3% reduction in callosal thickness ($p = .043$), and increased functional interhemispheric connectivity ($p = .02$). Correlational analyses in the larger unselected sample of 83 subjects confirmed the association between psychopathic personality and callosal structural abnormalities. Larger callosal volumes were associated with affective and interpersonal deficits, low autonomic stress reactivity, and low spatial ability.

Angular Gyrus

Only two studies appear to have assessed functioning in the angular gyrus within the parietal lobe, although none have studied psychopaths in particular. Using PET, Raine and colleagues (1997) found reduced glucose metabolism in the left but not right angular gyrus in murderers. In a SPECT study, Soderstrom and colleagues (2000) also found that violent offenders showed reduced functioning in the angular gyrus, but in this case the deficit was lateralized to the right (not left) hemisphere (see also section on correlations between reduced left angular gyrus functioning and increased Factor 1 psychopathy scores).

ARE DIFFERENT BRAIN DEFICITS ASSOCIATED WITH DIFFERENT FORMS OF PSYCHOPATHY?

Impulsive versus Predatory Aggression

A number of researchers have suggested that there may be different brain bases to impulsive, affective violence versus predatory, planned violence (Davidson et al., 2000; Raine, Meloy, et al., 1998; Scarpa & Raine, 2000). Specifically, frontal abnormalities may be more pronounced in individuals engaging in impulsive rather than premeditated aggression. One study found prefrontal dysfunction to be specific to affective, impulsive murderers as opposed to predatory, instrumental murderers (Raine, Meloy, et al., 1998). Common to both sets of impulsive and planned murderers was *increased* subcortical activity (midbrain, amygdala, hippocampus, and thalamus) compared to controls. While predatory, controlled murderers may have sufficient prefrontal regulation to control the excess aggressive feelings generated subcortically, this inhibitory control may be lacking in the affective, impulsive murderers. Two other studies converge with this frontal finding. Frequency of impulsive aggression is associated with reduced glucose metabolism in the frontal cortex of patients with personality disorders (Goyer et al., 1994). Impulsive violent offenders also exhibit reduced frontotemporal cerebral blood flow (Soderstrom et al., 2000).

In contrast to impulsive affective violent offenders, psychopaths (who are more likely to commit predatory violence than non-psychopathic criminals) appear to show either normal or increased (not decreased) patterns of brain activation compared to nonpsychopathic offenders and controls. As outlined earlier, psychopaths show *increased* bilateral blood flow in frontotemporal regions during the processing of emotional words (Intrator et al., 1997), *increased* activation in both the dorsolateral prefrontal cortex and amygdala during an aversive conditioning paradigm (Schneider et al., 2000), and *overactivation* of frontotemporal regions (Kiehl et al., 2001) Similarly, predatory murderers who may more resemble psychopaths show relatively normal prefrontal activation (Raine, Meloy, et al., 1998), again suggesting relatively greater brain activation in predatory psychopaths. This issue needs to be assessed more carefully in subgroups of psychopaths (i.e. predatory/planned vs. impulsive psychopathic subgroups) in order to address this issue more precisely in the psychopathy domain.

Lying, Conning, and Manipulation

Several important fMRI studies have recently revealed informative clues on the brain mechanisms subserving lying in normal individuals. Spence and colleagues (2001) using a computer-based interrogation procedure found that lying was associated with both a longer response time and greater activation in bilateral ventrolateral prefrontal cortices. Lee and colleagues (2002) found normals who feign memory impairments when tested using a forced-choice format showed greater activation in a prefrontal–parietal–subcortical circuit. A third study on two different types of lying (well-rehearsed lies vs. spontaneous lies) found that both types elicited more bilateral activation in the anterior prefrontal cortex, bilateral parahippocampal gyrus, the right precuneus, and the left cerebellum (Ganis, Kosslyn, Stose, Thompson, & Yurgelun-Todd, 2003). Common to all of these studies is increased activation in the prefrontal cortex during lying.

While these fMRI studies have shown increased bilateral activation in the prefrontal cortex when normal subjects lie, there have been no imaging studies of deceitful, manipulative, conning individuals assessing whether they have *structural* abnormalities

to this same brain region. One recent study has attempted to address this issue. Prefrontal gray and white matter volumes were assessed using structural MRI in 12 liars, 16 antisocial controls, and 21 normal controls (Yang et al., in press). Subjects were defined as liars if (1) they fulfilled criteria for pathological lying on the PCL-R, or (2) they fulfilled criteria for conning/manipulative on the PCL-R, or (3) they met the deceitfulness criterion for DSM-IV APD (lifelong repeated lying, use of aliases, or conning others for personal profit or please), or (4) they admitted to malingering (i.e., telling lies to obtain sickness benefits). Liars showed a 22–26% increase in prefrontal white matter and a 36–42% reduction in prefrontal gray/white ratios compared to both antisocial controls and normal controls. Findings provide the first evidence of a structural brain deficit in liars and indicate that excessive prefrontal white matter relative to gray may act as a predisposition to these specific features of psychopathy.

Factors of Psychopathy and Prefrontal Gray Volume

Very few studies have assessed structural integrity of the prefrontal cortex and factors of psychopathy. Laakso and colleagues (2002) using aMRI found no significant correlations between Total, Factor 1, and Factor 2 scores on the PCL-R and either prefrontal gray or white matter. On the other hand, this null effect could be due to a restriction of range as the sample was restricted to violent offenders who had a diagnosis of APD and were also alcoholic.

In contrast to these null findings, Yang and colleagues (2005), using aMRI in a community sample with a wide range of psychopathy scores, found significant negative correlations between prefrontal gray volume and total PCL-R scores, Factor 1 scores, and Factor 2 scores, indicating reduced prefrontal gray volume in those with high psychopathy scores. In addition, similar correlations were observed between prefrontal gray volume and the three factors of psychopathy delineated by Cooke and Michie (2001) as Arrogant and Deceitful Interpersonal Style, Deficient Affective Experience, and Impulsive and Irresponsible Behavioral Style. The size of the correlations was similar across the psychopathy factors, indicating that reduced prefrontal gray was a common denominator to all features of psychopathy.

Factors of Psychopathy and Brain Functioning

One study deserves detailed attention because it correlated both the two-factor and the three-factor psychopathy structure to resting blood flow throughout the brain and observed effects for subfactors that were not observed for total psychopathy scores. In this SPECT study of 32 violent offenders (Soderstrom et al., 2002), significant correlations were observed between high scores on Hare's Factor 1 (affective/interpersonal) and reduced left basal prefrontal, left overall prefrontal, and bilateral temporal blood flow. This pattern of result was replicated for the Cooke Factor 1 scores (arrogant/deceptive) with the addition that high Cooke Factor 1 scores were associated with reduced blood flow in the right (but not left) basal prefrontal cortex, reduced left (but not right) angular gyrus, the right head of the caudate, and the left hippocampus. High scores on Cooke's Factor 2 scores (affective) were also associated with reduced left hippocampal and caudate functioning. No other effects were observed for Hare Factor 2 (antisocial lifestyle) or Cooke's Factors 2 (affective) and 3 (impulsive/unstable).

Successful versus Unsuccessful Psychopaths

Extremely few studies have assessed for differences between successful (i.e., nonconvicted) and unsuccessful (i.e., convicted) psychopaths on any type of measure. With respect to brain imaging research, Raine and colleagues (2004) assessed left and right hippocampal volumes using aMRI in 23 controls, 16 unsuccessful (caught) psychopaths, and 12 successful (uncaught) community psychopaths. Unsuccessful psychopaths showed an exaggerated structural hippocampal asymmetry (right > left) relative to both successful psychopaths and controls, findings which were localized to the anterior region. This effect could not be explained by environmental and diagnostic confounds. Atypical anterior hippocampal asymmetries in unsuccessful psychopaths may reflect an underlying neurodevelopmental abnormality that disrupts hippocampal–prefrontal circuitry, resulting in affect dysregulation, poor contextual fear conditioning, and insensitivity to cues predicting capture.

Using the same population, Yang, Raine, Lencz, LaCasse, and Colletti (2005) revealed a significant 18–23% reduction in prefrontal gray matter only in unsuccessful psychopaths compared to both successful psychopaths and controls. These findings may be best understood in the context of the somatic marker hypothesis of Damasio (1994), which argues that intact prefrontal functioning plays a central role in good decision making, autonomic anticipatory fear, and social regulation. Ishikawa, Raine, Lencz, Bihrle, and LaCasse (2001) had previously shown reduced autonomic stress reactivity and executive function deficits in this same group of unsuccessful psychopaths. Poor decision making, reduced autonomic reactivity to cues predictive of punishment, and reduced prefrontal gray may render unsuccessful psychopaths less sensitive to environmental cues signaling danger and capture and hence make them more prone to conviction. These findings place a caveat on the findings reported previously on correlations between high psychopathy scores and reduced prefrontal gray volume in that such relationships may be specific to unsuccessful (not successful) psychopaths.

THE ROLE OF THE ENVIRONMENT: A BIOSOCIAL PERSPECTIVE

One of the limitations of brain imaging studies on psychopaths and antisocial/violent offenders is that very few to date have addressed the role of psychosocial risk and protective factors for violence. Nevertheless, the few studies that have addressed this issue are beginning to develop knowledge on two related but different issues. The first concerns whether home background moderates the relationship between violence and brain functioning. The second concerns whether brain deficits combine with psychosocial deficits in predisposing to violence.

Regarding the first issue, two studies have demonstrated a moderating effect of home background, but in opposing directions. In one PET study, frontal deficits were found to be particularly pronounced in violent individuals who had not been exposed to significant social stressors. Murderers from nondeprived home backgrounds showed a 14.2% reduction in functioning of the right orbitofrontal cortex relative to murderers from deprived home backgrounds characterized by abuse, neglect, and marital violence (Raine, Stoddard, Bihrle, & Buchsbaum, 1998). It was argued that neurobiological deficits are more pronounced among violent individuals who lack the psychosocial deprivation that normally provides a "social push" toward violence. In contrast, a more recent fMRI study showed that violent offenders who had been severely abused as children were more likely to show poor temporal lobe functioning compared to violent offenders lacking abuse (Raine, Park, et al., 2001). In these two examples, it should be noted that the dependent (outcome) variable is brain functioning.

Turning to the second issue, when instead the outcome variable is psychopathy/violence, it appears that brain deficits can combine with family deficits in the prediction of antisocial behavior. An aMRI study of individuals with APD and high psychopathy scores (Raine et al., 2000) showed that the combination of reduced prefrontal gray volume, low autonomic responsivity, and a set of 10 psychosocial deficits (e.g., abuse, single-parent family, and parental criminality) correctly classified 88.5% of subjects into APD or control groups (compared to 73.0% for psychosocial predictors only and 76.9% for biological predictors only). A second structural imaging study on the corpus callosum in psychopaths showed that the combination of psychosocial risk factors with callosal measures accounted for 81.5% of the variance. However, in both studies, it should be noted that structural brain measures accounted for a significant increase in the variance in psychopathic/antisocial behavior *over and above* psychosocial risk factors.

While more brain imaging studies are needed to obtain greater clarification on the role of the social environment in relation to brain deficits and violence, neurological case studies hint at a possible role of a structured, benign home background in buffering against an antisocial outcome after prefrontal damage. Although Phineas Gage became irritable and irresponsible after his ac-

cident, there is no clear evidence (to the authors' knowledge) that he engaged in significant criminal or violent activities; part of the reason that this was not the outcome may be because he was eventually taken into care by his family. An intriguing case study from Spain of a man who had an iron spike pass through his head, selectively destroying the prefrontal cortex, showed that unlike other cases, this individual did not have an outcome over the next 60 years of antisocial or criminal behavior (Mataro et al., 2001). The subject in question had wealthy parents who owned a family business in which he could be employed for the rest of his life, and also a fiancé (a childhood sweetheart) who stood by him after the accident and married him, producing two healthy children and a family which, in the words of one of the children "protected" him throughout his life. It can be argued that this individual did not develop antisocial behavior and psychosocial dysfunction because his family environment buffered him against these negative outcomes. Without such psychosocial support, a very different outcome may have resulted. Similarly, patient MGS (Dimitrov, Phipps, Zahn, & Grafman, 2002) suffered from the frontal lesions in early adulthood but was rehabilitated and cared for in a structured, supportive environment and did not exhibit criminal, violent behavior. These three case studies raise intriguing questions that future brain imaging studies may help to address.

DO BRAIN DEFICITS *CAUSE* PSYCHOPATHIC BEHAVIOR?

While brain deficits are reliably found in antisocial and psychopathic individuals, brain imaging studies by themselves do not demonstrate that these deficits actually cause psychopathy. Nevertheless, findings from adult neurological patients, child neurological cases, head injury studies, and patients with degenerative brain diseases converge with brain imaging studies on the conclusion that damage to the brain can indeed directly contribute to the etiology of psychopathic and antisocial behavior.

Neurological research on individuals who were once normal but who then suffered brain lesions allows temporal cause–effect relationships to be teased out. Damasio and colleagues (Damasio, 1994; Damasio, Tranel, & Damasio, 1990) have convincingly demonstrated that damage to the ventral regions of the prefrontal cortex results in poor decision making, autonomic deficits, and sociopathic behavior. A quasi-experimental group study on head injuries in soldiers revealed that individuals with ventromedial lesions showed greater aggressive, violent, and/or antisocial behavior than individuals with nonfrontal lesions, or non-lesion controls (Grafman et al., 1996). Of these ventromedial patients, those with focal frontal medial lesions were generally aware of and able to self-report the increase in their aggressive behavior whereas those with focal orbitofrontal lesions were unaware of the behavioral change.

Another line of evidence supporting a causative role of brain dysfunction in predisposing to violent/psychopathic behavior comes from several studies of patients who suffered degenerating brain diseases and who thereafter became aggressive (Raine, 2002b). For example, patients diagnosed with frontotemporal dementia (FTD) are significantly more likely to engage in inappropriate aggressive, sexual, and antisocial behavior than are patients diagnosed with Alzheimer's disease (Miller, Darby, Benson, & Cummings, 1997). In addition, aggressive dementia patients (i.e., Alzheimer's disease and vascular dementia) show significant hypoperfusion (i.e., left activation) in the left and right dorsolateral frontal areas, left anterior temporal cortex, and right superior parietal areas compared to nonaggressive dementia patients (Hirono et al., 2000). Finally, a SPECT study of patients with right-sided (but not left-sided) frontotemporal dementia revealed evidence of socially undesirable behavior, including criminality, aggression, and sexually deviant behavior among these patients (Mychack, Kramer, Boone, & Miller, 2001). Nevertheless, further studies are required to extend this analysis to psychopathic behavior in particular.

While structural brain imaging studies of children with conduct disorder are lacking, there are studies of the behavioral sequelae that follow head injuries in children. Overwhelmingly, studies on head injuries occurring in childhood reveal that conduct disorder and externalizing behavior problems are common after head trauma (Raine, 2002a),

although some children develop internalizing rather than externalizing behavior problems while others remain relatively unaffected.

Studies of children with lesions to the prefrontal cortex early in life lend further support to the view that head (and therefore brain) trauma can directly lead to antisocial and aggressive behavior. Anderson, Damasio, Tranel, and Damasio (2001) reported on two individuals (one female, one male) who suffered selective lesions to the prefrontal cortex in the first 16 months of life (bilateral polar and ventromedial in the female, and right polar–medial–dorsal in the male). Both showed early antisocial behavior that progressed into delinquency in adolescence and criminal behavior in adulthood and included impulsive–aggressive and non-aggressive forms of antisocial behavior. Both had autonomic deficits, poor decision-making skills, and deficits on learning from feedback. Pennington and Bennetto (1993) reported on nine other cases of children suffering frontal brain lesions in the first 10 years of life. They noted that all nine suffered behavioral problems following the injuries; seven of the nine having conduct disorder, and the remaining two exhibiting impulsive, labile, or uncontrollable behavior. These cases when taken together strongly suggest that damage to the prefrontal cortex can directly lead to antisocial, aggressive, and criminal behavior. Again, further studies are required to assess the early neuroanatomical antecedents of psychopathic behavior in particular.

HOW DO BRAIN IMPAIRMENTS CAUSE PSYCHOPATHIC BEHAVIOR?

What are the mechanisms and processes by which structural brain impairments predispose an individual to psychopathy? This question is considered in the context of the multiple brain mechanisms implicated in psychopathic and antisocial from prior imaging studies.

Prefrontal Cortex

There are multiple pathways by which prefrontal impairments may predispose to psychopathic behavior. Patients with prefrontal damage fail to give anticipatory autonomic responses to choice options that are risky and make bad choices even when they are aware of the more advantageous response option (Bechara, Damasio, Tranel, & Damasio, 1997). This inability to reason and to make appropriate decisions in risky situations is likely to contribute to the impulsivity; rule breaking; poor behavioral control; lack of realistic, long-term goals; and irresponsible behavior that characterize psychopaths (Hare, 1991).

Second, prefrontal abnormalities may result in the poor fear conditioning which has been consistently found in psychopathic and antisocial groups (Hare & Quinn, 1971; Lykken, 1957; Raine, 1993; Patrick, 1994). The prefrontal cortex is part of a neural circuit that plays a central role in fear conditioning and stress responsivity (Frysztak & Neafsey, 2002; Hugdahl, 1998). Poor conditioning is theorized to be associated with poor conscience development (Eysenck, 1977; Raine, 1993), and individuals who are less autonomically responsive to aversive stimuli such as parental verbal and physical punishment during childhood would be less susceptible to socializing punishments and hence become predisposed to psychopathy.

Third, prefrontal dysfunction may result in abnormalities in arousal regulation which in turn predispose to psychopathy. The prefrontal cortex is involved in the regulation of arousal (Dahl, 1997). Low physiological arousal has been associated with stimulation-seeking behavior to compensate for such underarousal (Eysenck, 1977; Zuckerman, 1994), behavior which characterizes both psychopathic and antisocial populations (Gatzke, Raine, Loeber, Steinhauer, & Stouthamer-Loeber, 2002; Raine, 1993). Raine and colleagues (2000) reported that individuals with APD have reduced prefrontal gray volume (Raine et al., 2000) and also showed lower autonomic activity (both skin conductance and heart rate) during a social stressor task in which subjects had to prepare and give a speech about their worst faults—a task particularly well suited to eliciting secondary emotions such as shame, guilt, and embarrassment, which are thought to be mediated by the ventromedial prefrontal cortex (Damasio, 1994). Furthermore, individuals with the lowest prefrontal gray volumes had the lowest skin conductance arousal, indicating an intrinsic link between electrodermal arousal and prefrontal gray integrity in this group. This arousal and stress reactivity dysregulation produced by damage to the prefrontal cortex may contribute to emotion regulation problems that in turn contribute to aggressive and psychopathic behavior (Davidson et al., 2000; Scarpa & Raine, 2000).

Corpus Callosum

Deficits to the corpus callosum and the consequent abnormal interhemispheric transfer may result in the right hemisphere, which has been implicated in the generation of negative affect (Davidson & Fox, 1989), undergoing less regulation and control by left-hemisphere inhibitory processes. This impairment in affect regulation may in turn contribute to the expression of aggressive, unregulated behavior. As an example, rats that are stressed early in life are right-hemisphere dominant for mice killing (Garbanati et al., 1983). Severing the corpus callosum in these rats leads to an increase in muricide (Denenberg, Gall, Berrebi, & Yutzey, 1986), indicating that the left hemisphere acts to inhibit the right-hemisphere mediated killing via an intact corpus callosum. Both Sperry (1974) and Dimond (1979) commented on the inappropriate nature of emotional expression and the inability to grasp long-term implications of a situation in split-brain patients. Parallel influences may contribute to the inappropriate emotional expression of violent psychopaths and their lack of long-term planning. However, callosal dysfunction per se is unlikely to cause aggression and psychopathy; instead, it may contribute to psychopathy in those with concurrent limbic and cortical abnormalities.

A key feature of psychopathy is blunted affect, and low autonomic activity during emotional and social stressors is a well-replicated correlate of psychopathy (Hare, 1982; Patrick, Zempolich, & Levenston, 1997). In the study of Raine, Lencz, and colleagues (2003), callosal white matter volume was significantly related to the Deficient Affect factor of psychopathy, and to a lesser extent the Impulsive–Irresponsible factor, but not the Arrogant/Deceptive factor. Similarly, autonomic measures and personality measures reflecting blunted affect, lack of social closeness, and no close friends were related to callosal abnormalities. Individuals who suffer from neurodevelopmental failure of the corpus callosum, while not showing gross psychopathology, do show deficits in social insight and self-perception (Brown & Paul, 2000), deficits which also characterize psychopaths. As such, abnormal interhemispheric connectivity may partly account for the social, insight, autonomic, and emotion deficits observed in psychopaths.

Parietal Cortex

Reductions in glucose metabolism in the left angular gyrus in violent offenders (Raine et al., 1997) have been correlated with reduced verbal ability (Gur et al., 1994), while damage to the left angular gyrus has been linked to deficits in reading and arithmetic. Such cognitive dysfunction could predispose to educational and occupational failure, which in turn might predispose to crime and violence. Such learning deficits have been found to be common in violent offenders who also have low verbal IQs (Raine, 1993).

Neurodevelopmental Processes

Finally, consideration should be given to the developmental context within which brain deficits may give rise to psychopathy. No matter what brain deficits are observed in psychopaths, and irrespective of the ways in which impairments to specific brain regions can give rise to cognitive and behavioral alterations that predispose to psychopathy, one single process may underlie these multiple processes. Specifically, structural and functional brain impairments in psychopaths may be caused by abnormal neurodevelopment (Raine et al., 1995, 2004; Raine, Lencz, et al., 2003). For example, with respect to callosal structural abnormalities in psychopaths, research with moneys, cats, and hamsters has shown that approximately two-thirds of callosal axons are eliminated postnatally through adulthood, with most of this pruning being to excitatory rather than inhibitory fibers (Raine, Lencz, et al., 2003). Early arrest of this normal process of axonal pruning could therefore contribute to the increased callosal white matter volume and functional overconnectedness of the hemispheres observed in psychopaths (Raine, Lencz, et al., 2003).

In a similar fashion, the asymmetry in the structure of the anterior hippocampus in psychopaths may have a neurodevelopmental explanation (Raine et al., 2004). Atypical brain asymmetries are thought to in part reflect disrupted neurodevelopmental processes. Such disruption probably occurs early in life because brain asymmetries first emerge during fetal development and the overall degree of structural change attributable to environmental influences is limited by early morphogenesis. A neurodevelopmental perspective of psychopathy is consistent with the facts that it has its roots early in life, unfolds relatively consistently over childhood and adolescence, is impervious to conventional treatments, and is in part genetically determined (Raine et al., 2004).

Regarding frontal impairments, it has been hypothesized (Raine, 2002b) that the social and executive function demands of late adolescence place an overload on the late-developing prefrontal cortex, giving rise to a lack of inhibitory control over antisocial, aggressive behavior which reaches maximal expression at this age. This prefrontal overload is hypothesized to be particularly likely in individuals with developmental delays in prefrontal maturation or in hyperactive children with preexisting prefrontal deficits. Furthermore, persistence into adulthood of antisocial and psychopathic behavior is thought to be especially likely in those who have suffered head trauma that may prevent a maturational catchup of the prefrontal cortex in adulthood.

WHAT *CAUSES* THE BRAIN DEFICITS IN PSYCHOPATHS?

Environmental factors may play a role in shaping structural brain deficits in psychopaths. As outlined earlier, head injuries from physical child abuse, car and motorcycle accidents, fights, and sports are an important source of brain damage. Closed head injuries are particularly likely to create damage to the frontal and temporal poles, and thus it is not surprising that anterior (frontal and temporal) abnormalities are particularly implicated in psychopathic and antisocial behavior. Surprisingly, few studies have attempted to directly assess whether accidents and child abuse mediate brain dysfunction in offenders. One study of murderers revealed a trend

($p < .08$) for murderers with a history of head injury to have lower functioning of the corpus callosum than murderers without head injury (Raine et al., 1997) and it is known that long white nerve fibers are susceptible to sheering during closed head injury. On the other hand, other brain deficits found in these murderers, including reduced prefrontal glucose metabolism, were *not* linked to a history of head injury. Nevertheless, one fMRI study found that violent offenders with a history of child abuse had greater brain dysfunction than nonabused violent offenders (Raine, Park, et al., 2001), suggesting the potential importance of environmental factors in the etiology of functional brain impairments. There are important caveats to this conclusion. Murderers with a history of serious abuse early in childhood were *not* found to suffer from brain deficits relative to murderers without such abuse (Raine, Stoddard, et al., 1998). Importantly, the only *structural* brain imaging study of psychopathy that has examined the issue of environmental etiology has shown that structural abnormalities of the corpus callosum in this group are not attributable to head injury, child abuse, and other psychosocial risk factors (Raine, Lencz, et al., 2003). More studies that specifically focus on psychopaths are needed to further address this potentially important issue.

Drug and alcohol abuse could in theory also contribute to the brain deficits found in psychopaths. On the other hand, these factors may not be as salient as they at first appear. For example, individuals with APD and high psychopathy scores show significant prefrontal gray reductions not only compared to normal controls but also compared with a group with alcohol- and drug-dependent individuals not diagnosed with APD—indicating that substance abuse does not account for the structural brain deficits (Raine et al., 2000). Other studies have also shown structural and functional brain deficits in antisocial and violent offenders when alcohol and drug use is controlled for (e.g., Critchley et al., 2000; Hirono et al., 2000; Kuruoglu et al., 1996). While alcohol and drug use could be a cause of brain deficits in violent offenders, to date the evidence argues against this conclusion.

Early health factors could be another source of brain impairment. Birth complications have been associated with violence (Raine, 2002b), and lack of oxygen at birth leads to cell death, particularly in the hippocampus, a brain region linked to violence and psychopathy (Laakso et al., 2001; Raine et al., 2004). Protein is essential for brain development and protein deficiency has been recently linked to antisocial behavior problems (Liu, Raine, Venablis, & Mednick, 2004; Neugebauer, Hoek, & Susser, 1999). Rats fed a low-protein diet during pregnancy show impairments in corpus callosum functioning (Soto-Moyano et al., 1998) and reduction in DNA concentration in the forebrain (Bennis-Taleb, Remacle, Hoet, & Reusens, 1999), two brain areas found to be impaired in psychopaths. Fetal alcohol syndrome in which the fetus is exposed to alcohol *in utero* results in significant structural and functional brain deficits and could contribute to brain deficits in psychopaths. Smoking during pregnancy is linked to outcome for adult violence (Brennan, Mednick, & Hodgins, 2000) and can lead to brain impairments by reducing oxygen to the fetal brain (Raine, 2002b). Although these early health factors are likely to contribute to brain dysfunction in psychopaths, their role needs to be formally tested in future studies.

In all likelihood, brain deficits in psychopaths are likely to be caused by a combination of both early environmental health factors *and* genetic processes. Twin and adoption studies have demonstrated beyond doubt that there is heritability for criminal behavior (Raine, 2002a), and although there have been very few such studies on psychopathy, it is likely that psychopathic behavior has a significant heritable component (cf. Waldman & Rhee, Chapter 11, this volume). One recent MRI twin study has demonstrated that 90–95% of the variance in prefrontal volume is determined by genetic factors (Thompson et al., 2001). Consequently, genetic factors are likely to play some role in producing the type of structural prefrontal gray deficits previously found in those with psychopathic behavior and APD.

CAN BRAIN DEFICITS IN PSYCHOPATHS BE REMEDIATED OR PREVENTED?

The question whether the brain deficits seen in psychopaths can be reversed or prevented is of major societal importance. If brain deficits cause psychopathy, and if they can be remediated, it would be predicted that psychopathy could be significantly reduced in society. This issue can be viewed through past, present, and future lenses.

In the past, neurosurgery has been used on sociopaths, but such frontal lobectomies later fell into disrepute as being crude and unethical in many cases. Nevertheless, destructive brain surgery has been and still is used in severe, intractable cases of aggression, with some degree of success. For example, amygdalectomy has been used successfully in rare cases to "tame" individuals with intractable aggression (Lee et al., 1998). It has also been claimed that prefrontal lobotomy was successful in reducing aggression in 16 schizophrenic patients (da Costa, 1997), and there are similar reports of the success of amygdalo–hippocampectomy for the control of rage (Sachdev, Smith, Matheson, & Last, 1992). Clearly, however, such drastic psychosurgery intervention will rarely if ever be warranted for the treatment of psychopathy.

More recent studies have begun to show that brain structure and function are significantly shaped by environmental processes. For example, we have recently shown that an enrichment program involving nutritional, physical exercise, and educational components administered for 2 years between ages 3 and 5 is associated with better brain functioning 8 years later (i.e., at age 11). Specifically, recipients of this intervention showed greater EEG activation and increased skin conductance orienting responses to simple tone stimuli (Raine, Venables, et al., 2001). Nutrition is critical to brain development, and in animals physical exercise by itself has been shown to promote neurogenesis—the growth of new brain cells—within the hippocampus in animals (van Praag, Kempermann, & Gage, 1999). This environmental enrichment was also successful in reducing conduct disorder at age 17 and criminal behavior at age 23 (Raine, Mellingen, Liu, Venables, & Mednick, 2003).

It is also conceivable that children who show both frontal brain deficits and psychopathic-like personalities may benefit from attempts to cognitively remediate the executive function deficits that some believe contribute to psychopathy. In particular, researchers are beginning to explore the effectiveness of emotion regulation and executive function training in young children. Because brain function is more easily shaped and influenced early in life, such intervention programs may be much more successful in remediating cognitive deficits in young rather than old psychopaths. Any such attempts must by necessity be tempered by sensitivity to protecting the rights of children and avoiding negative effects of labeling.

In the future, the key question concerns whether *reparative* brain surgery could be used to remediate the structural and functional brain deficits observed in psychopathic offenders. Lesions to the hippocampus impair spatial learning in rats, but grafting of stem cells into these animals reverses these cognitive deficits (Grigoryan, Gray, Rashid, Chadwick, & Hodges, 2000). Similarly, transplants of stem cells from human brains into old rats results in migration of these cells to the hippocampus, improving cognitive ability in old rats within 4 weeks of transplantation (Qu, Brannen, Kim, & Sugaya, 2001). It is conceivable that in the long term, adult offenders with damage to the hippocampus and prefrontal cortex might receive treatment to literally "repair" these brain structures, opening up the possibility of reversal of cognitive and behavioral brain deficits implicated in the etiology of violence. Whether this future scientific possibility ever becomes acceptable, ethically or morally, to candidate offenders and to the public at large remains to be seen.

CONCLUSIONS AND SUMMARY

This chapter has attempted to delineate findings on the neuroanatomical basis of psychopathic behavior based on brain imaging research and to discuss broader conceptual issues stemming from these empirical findings. In essence, anatomical research on psychopathy is nearly nonexistent, and for this reason recourse has been made to fMRI research, as well as aMRI research on antisocial conditions broader than psychopathy.

Initial, preliminary structural imaging research on psychopathic groups has so far indicated (1) enlargement of the corpus callosum (Raine, Lencz, et al., 2003), (2) volume reduction in the posterior hippocampus (Laakso et al., 2001), (3) an exaggerated right > left asymmetry to the anterior hippocampus (Raine et al., 2004), and (4) reduced prefrontal gray volume (Yang, Raine, Lencz, LaCasse, & Colletti, 2005). Nevertheless, these latter two findings are specific to "unsuccessful" psychopaths and are not found in "successful" psychopaths. Research on subfeatures and dimensions of psychopathy has indicated (1) increased prefrontal white matter in deceitful/conning/manipulative individuals (Yang et al., in press), (2) reduced amygdala volume in violent offenders with high (nonspecific) psychopathy scores (Tiihonen et al., 2000), and (3) reduced prefrontal gray volume common to all factors of psychopathy (Yang et al., 2005) (although one study does not support the latter findings; Laakso et al., 2002). Supplementing these findings on psychopathy, structural imaging research on the broader construct of APD and violent behavior has revealed reduced prefrontal gray (Raine et al., 2000), reduced temporal lobe volume (Dolan et al., 2002), reduced posterior hippocampal volumes (Laakso et al., 2001), increased callosal volume (Raine, Lencz, et al., 2003), but a failure to find amygdala volume deficits (Elst et al., 2000). These initial anatomical findings at the very least provide an initial empirical basis for replication and extension on which future aMRI studies may build.

Because little prior aMRI research has been conducted, one way to provide directions for future anatomical research in psychopathy is to assess which brain regions reliably show *functional* impairment. Although by no means definitive, such evidence of impairment would be at least suggestive of anatomical abnormalities that could be further researched. Intriguingly, four studies have found *increased* functioning of the prefrontal cortex in psychopaths during activation conditions, even though *decreased* frontal functioning is now a reasonably well-replicated imaging correlate of general antisocial and aggressive behavior. Findings on frontotemporal and amygdala functioning are much more mixed. Although there is some limited evidence for reduced hippocampal and parahippocampal functioning,

firm conclusions on this structure are to date not warranted. Functional research on subfeatures of psychopathy have to date implicated higher Cooke Factor 1 scores (arrogant/deceptive) in association with lower functioning in the prefrontal cortex, the temporal cortex, the hippocampus and caudate, with null findings for total psychopathy scores and both the amygdala and hippocampus.

These structural and functional findings lead to two broad conclusions. First, the very basic and fundamental question of which brain regions may be anatomically impaired in psychopathy has been greatly underresearched and is in great need of even the simplest studies to further address this question. Second, the field is understandably even more removed from being able to answer the more complex questions of why brain impairment may cause psychopathy, what causes the impairments, and how they may be remediated.

Despite these limitations, initial suggestions can been made here which may guide future studies in this field. Clearly, any future imaging studies, whether anatomical or functional, would benefit from additional analyses into the features and subtypes of psychopathy which drive the overall finding for psychopathic behavior as such knowledge would help to further pinpoint potential etiological processes. Future studies that combine structural with functional imaging techniques would clearly help address the pivotal but unanswered question of how structural and functional impairments are related, and if not, why not? If future anatomical studies could incorporate basic environmental and early health processes hypothesized to be of etiological significance to psychopathy, it could enrich our understanding of possible interactions between brain and social influences in shaping psychopathic behavior, to date another greatly underresearched question (Patrick et al., 1997). The likelihood of undertaking future aMRI studies of psychopathy in a genetically informative design does not seem likely from a behavioral genetic standpoint, although molecular genetic approaches could conceivably research the future question of which specific genes predispose to which specific brain risk factors for psychopathy. Finally, developmental prospective aMRI research on the early brain antecedents of psychopathic behavior could yield extremely informative information on the etiological significance of structural brain abnormalities and a neurodevelopmental theory of psychopathy.

At the least, future research may explore, extend/modify, and explain empirically the strongest conclusion that can be drawn to date: abnormalities to the prefrontal cortex in both psychopathic and antisocial behavior. Such research could focus on the intriguing finding to date of reduced structure and function in antisocial/violent behavior yet increased prefrontal functioning in the context of reduced structure in psychopathy. Again, the caveat has to be emphasized that even here, research findings are sparse and this conclusion will inevitably need modification. In addition, there is some evidence for both reduced structure and function in the hippocampus. While findings for the amygdala are currently mixed, future research on this theoretically relevant structure, particularly with reference to prefrontal impairments, also seems warranted (Blair, 2003). Similarly, the corpus callosum is a clear candidate for further attention.

From a theoretical standpoint, anatomical prefrontal impairments in psychopathic and antisocial populations could help explain the disinhibited, impulsive behavior of psychopaths and underpin the classic low arousal/fearlessness/conditioning theories of psychopathic behavior. Callosal structural abnormalities give rise to a "faulty wiring" hypothesis of psychopathy and in part account for social, autonomic, and emotional impairments observed in psychopaths. Hippocampal impairments may predispose to affect dysregulation and poor contextual fear conditioning in psychopaths, in part by disruption to prefrontal–hippocampal circuits. In this context, while research on single brain structures provides a starting point for understanding the neuroanatomical basis of psychopathy, future research needs to better understand impairments to more specific neural *circuits* which give rise to biobehavioral abnormalities which result in specific psychopathic symptoms. As such, the neuroanatomy of psychopathy is a research field in its infancy but with a great deal of potential for providing an exponential leap in our understanding of the causes of psychopathy.

ACKNOWLEDGMENTS

This chapter was written with the support of Independent Scientist Award No. K02 MH01114-01 from the National Institute of Mental Health to Adrian Raine.

REFERENCES

Amen, D. G., Stubblefield, M., Carmichael, B., & Thisted, R. (1996). Brain SPECT findings and aggressiveness. *Annals of Clinical Psychiatry, 8,* 129–137.

Anderson, S. W., Damasio, H., Tranel, D., & Damasio, A. R. (2001). Long-term sequelae of prefrontal cortex damage acquired in early childhood. *Developmental Neuropsychology, 18,* 281–296.

Bechara, A., Damasio, H., Tranel, D., & Damasio, A. R. (1997). Deciding advantageously before knowing the advantageous strategy. *Science, 275,* 1293–1294.

Bennis-Taleb, N., Remacle C., Hoet, J. J., & Reusens, B. (1999). A low-protein isocaloric diet during gestation affects brain development and alters permanently cerebral cortex blood vessels in rat offspring. *Journal of Nutrition, 129,* 1613–1619.

Blair, R. J. R. (2003). Neurobiological basis of psychopathy. *British Journal of Psychiatry, 182,* 5–7.

Brennan, P. A., Mednick, S. A., & Hodgins, S. (2000). Major mental disorders and criminal violence in a Danish birth cohort. *Archives of General Psychiatry, 57,* 494–500.

Brown, W. S., & Paul, L. K. (2000). Cognitive and psychosocial deficits in agenesis of the corpus callosum with normal intelligence. *Cognitive Neuropsychiatry, 5,* 135–157.

Cooke, D. J., & Michie, C. (2001). Refining the construct of psychopathy: Towards a hierarchical model. *Psychological Assessment, 13,* 171–188.

Critchley, H. D., Simmons, A., Daly, E. M., Russell, A., van Amelsvoort, T., & Robertson, D. M. (2000). Prefrontal and medial temporal correlates of repetitive violence to self and others. *Biological Psychiatry, 47,* 928–934.

da Costa, D. A. (1997). The role of psychosurgery in the treatment of selected cases of refractory schizophrenia: A reappraisal. *Schizophrenia Research, 28,* 223–230.

Dahl, R. E. (1997). The regulation of sleep and arousal: Development and psychopathology. In M.E. Hertzig & E. A. Farber (Eds.), *Annual progress in child psychiatry and child development* (pp. 3–28). Philadelphia: Brunner/Mazel.

Damasio, A. (1994). *Descartes' error: Emotion, reason, and the human brain.* New York: G.P. Putnam's Sons.

Damasio, A. R., Tranel, D., & Damasio, H. (1990). Individuals with sociopathic behavior caused by frontal damage fail to respond autonomically to social stimuli. *Behavioural Brain Research, 41,* 81–94.

Damasio, H., Grabowski, T. J., Frank, R., Galaburda, A. M., & Damasio, A. (1994). Clues about the brain from the skull of a famous patient. *Science, 264,* 1102–1105.

Davidson, R. J., & Fox, N. A. (1989). Frontal brain asymmetry predicts infants' response to maternal separation. *Journal of Abnormal Psychology, 98,* 127–131.

Davidson, R. J., Putnam, K. M., & Larson, C. L. (2000). Dysfunction in the neural circuitry of emotion regulation—A possible prelude to violence. *Science, 289,* 591–594.

Denenberg, V. H., Gall, J. S., Berrebi, A., & Yutzey, D. A. (1986). Callosal mediation of cortical inhibition in the lateralized rat brain. *Brain Research, 397,* 327–332.

Dimitrov, M., Phipps, M., Zahn, T. P., & Grafman, J. (2002). A thoroughly modern Gage. *Neurocase, 5,* 345–354.

Dimond, S. J. (1979). Disconnection and psychopathology. In J.H. Gruzelier & P. Flor-Henry (Eds.), *Hemisphere asymmetries of function in psychopathology* (pp. 35–46). Amsterdam: Elsevier.

Dolan, M. C., Deakin, J. F. W., Roberts, N., & Anderson, I. M. (2002). Quantitative frontal and temporal structural MRI studies in personality-disordered offenders and control subjects. *Psychiatry Research Neuroimaging, 116,* 133–149.

Elst, L. T. V., Woermann, F. G., Lemieux, L., Thompson, P. J., & Trimble, M. R. (2000). Affective aggression in patients with temporal lobe epilepsy: A quantitative MRI study of the amygdala. *Brain, 123,* 234–243.

Eysenck H. J. (1977) Psychosis and psychoticism: A reply to Bishop. *Journal of Abnormal Psychology, 86,* 427–430.

Frysztak, R. J., & Neafsey, E. J. (2002). The effect of medial frontal cortex lesions on respiration, "freezing," and ultrasonic vocalizations during conditioned emotional responses in rats. *Cerebral Cortex, 1,* 418–425.

Ganis G., Kosslyn S. M., Stose S., Thompson W. L., & Yurgelun-Todd D. A. (2003). Neural correlates of different types of deception: An fMRI investigation. *Cerebral Cortex, 13,* 830–836.

Garbanati, J. A., Sherman, G. F., Rosen, G. D., Hofmann, M. J., Yutzey, D. A., & Denenberg, V. H. (1983). Handling in infancy, brain laterality and muricide in rats. *Behavioural Brain Research, 7,* 351–359.

Gatzke, L., Raine, A., Loeber, R., Steinhauer, S., & Stouthamer-Loeber, M. (2002). Serious delinquent behavior, sensation-seeking, and electrodermal arousal. *Journal of Abnormal Child Psychology, 30,* 477–486.

Gatzke-Kopp, L. M., Raine, A., Buchsbaum, M. S., & LaCasse, L. (2001). Temporal lobe deficits in murderers: EEG findings undetected by PET. *Journal of Neuropsychiatry and Clinical Neurosciences, 13,* 486–491.

Goyer, P. F., Andreason, P. J., Semple, W. E., & Clayton, A. H. (1994). Positron-emission tomography and personality disorders. *Neuropsychopharmacology, 10,* 21–28.

Grafman, J., Schwab, K., Warden, D., Pridgen, A., Brown, H. R., & Salazar, A. M. (1996). Frontal lobe injuries, violence, and aggression: A report of the Vietnam Head Injury Study. *Neurology, 46,* 1231–1238.

Grigoryan, G. A., Gray, J. A., Rashid, T., Chadwick, A., & Hodges, H. (2000). Conditionally immortal neuroepithelial stem cell grafts restore spatial learning in rats with lesions at the source of cholinergic forebrain projections. *Restorative Neurology and Neuroscience, 17,* 183–201.

Gur, R. C., Ragland, J. D., Resnick, S. M., Skolnick, B. E., Jaggi, J., & Muencz, L. (1994). Lateralized increases in cerebral blood flow during performance of verbal and spatial tasks: Relationship with performance level. *Brain and Cognition, 24,* 244–258.

Hare, R. D. (1982). Psychopathy and physiological activity during anticipation of an aversive stimulus in a distraction paradigm. *Psychophysiology 19,* 266–271.

Hare, R. D. (1984). Performance of psychopaths on cognitive tasks related to frontal lobe function. *Journal of Abnormal Psychology, 93,* 133–140.

Hare, R. D. (1991). *The Hare Psychopathy Checklist—Revised (PCL-R).* Toronto, ON, Canada: Multi-Health Systems.

Hare, R. D., & Quinn, M. J. (1971). Psychopathy and autonomic conditioning. *Journal of Abnormal Psychology, 77,* 223–235.

Henry, B., & Moffitt, T. E. (1997). Neuropsychological and neuroimaging studies of juvenile delinquency and adult criminal behavior. In D. M. Stoff, J. Breiling, & J. D. Maser (Eds.), *Handbook of antisocial behavior* (pp. 280–288). New York: Wiley.

Hirono, N., Mega, M. S., Dinov, I. D., Mishkin, F., & Cummings, J. L. (2000). Left fronto-temporal hypoperfusion in associated with aggression in patients with dementia. *Archives of Neurology, 57,* 861–866.

Hugdahl, K. (1998). Cortical control of human classical conditioning: Autonomic and positron emission tomography data. *Psychophysiology, 35,* 170–178.

Intrator, J., Hare, R., Stritzke, P., & Brichtswein, K. (1997). A brain imaging (single photon emission computerized tomography) study of semantic and affective processing in psychopaths. *Biological Psychiatry, 42,* 96–103.

Ishikawa, S. S., Raine, A., Lencz, T., Bihrle, S., & LaCasse, L. (2001). Autonomic stress reactivity and executive functions in successful and unsuccessful criminal psychopaths from the community. *Journal of Abnormal Psychology, 110,* 423–432.

Kiehl, K. A., Smith, A. M., Hare, R. D., Mendrek, A., Forster, B. B., & Brink, J. (2001). Limbic abnormalities in affective processing by criminal psychopaths as revealed by functional magnetic resonance imaging. *Biological Psychiatry, 50,* 677–684.

Kuruoglu, A. C., Arikan, Z., Vural, G., & Karatas, M. (1996). Single photon emission computerised tomography in chronic alcoholism: Antisocial personality disorder may be associated with decreased frontal perfusion. *British Journal of Psychiatry, 169,* 348–354.

Laakso, M. P., Gunning-Dixon, F., Vaurio, O., Repo-Tiihonen, E., Soininen, H., & Tiihonen, J. (2002). Prefrontal volumes in habitually violent subjects with antisocial personality disorder and type 2 alcoholism. *Psychiatry Research: Neuroimaging, 114,* 95–102.

Laakso, M. P., Vaurio, O., Koivisto, E., Savolainen, L., Eronen, M., & Aronen, H. J. (2001). Psychopathy and the posterior hippocampus. *Behavioural Brain Research, 118,* 187–193.

Laakso, M. P., Vaurio, O., Savolainen, L., Repo, E., Soininen, H., Aronen, H. J., & Tiihonen, J. (2000). A volumetric MRI study of the hippocampus in type 1 and 2 alcoholism. *Behavioural Brain Research, 109,* 177–186.

Lee, G. P., Bechara, A., Adolphs, R., Arena, J., Meador, K. J., & Loring, D. W. (1998). Clinical and physiological effects of stereotaxic bilateral amygdalotomy for intractable aggression. *Journal of Neuropsychiatry and Clinical Neurosciences, 10,* 413–420.

Lee, T. M. C., Liu, H. L., Tan, L. H., Chan, C. C. H., Mahankali, S., Feng, C. M., et al. (2002). Lie detection by functional magnetic resonance imaging. *Human Brain Mapping, 15,* 157–164.

Liu, J. H., Raine, A., Venables, P. H., & Mednick, S. A. (2004). Malnutrition at age 3 years predisposes to externalizing behavior problems at ages 8, 11 and 17 years. *American Journal of Psychiatry, 161,* 2005–2013.

Lykken, D. T. (1957). A study of anxiety in the sociopathic personality. *Journal of Abnormal Psychology, 55,* 6–10.

Mataro, M., Jurado, M. A., Garcia-Sanchez, C., Barraquer, L., Costa-Jussa, F. R., & Junque, C. (2001). Long-term effects of bilateral frontal brain lesion 60 years after injury with an iron bar. *Archives of Neurology, 58,* 1139–1142.

Miller, B. L., Darby, A., Benson, D. F., & Cummings, J. L. (1997). Aggressive, socially disruptive and antisocial behaviour associated with fronto-temporal dementia. *British Journal of Psychiatry, 170,* 150–155.

Morgan, A. B., & Lilienfeld, S. O. (2000). A metaanalytic review of the relation between antisocial behavior and neuropsychological measures of executive function. *Clinical Psychology Review, 20,* 113–156.

Muller J. L., Sommer, M., Wagner, V., Lange, K., Taschler, H., Roder, C. H., et al. (2003). Abnormalities in emotion processing within cortical and subcortical regions in criminal psychopaths: Evidence from a functional magnetic resonance imaging study using pictures with emotional content. *Biological Psychiatry, 54,* 152–162.

Mychack, P., Kramer, J. H., Boone, K. B., & Miller, B. L. (2001). The influence of right frontotemporal dysfunction on social behavior in frontotemporal dementia. *Neurology, 56,* S11–S15.

Neugebauer, R., Hoek, H. W., & Susser, E. (1999). Prenatal exposure to wartime famine and development of antisocial personality disorder in early adulthood. *Journal of the American Medical Association, 282,* 455–462.

Patrick, C. J. (1994). Emotion and psychopathy: Startling new insights. *Psychophysiology, 31,* 319–330.

Patrick C. J., Zempolich, K. A., & Levenston, G. K. (1997). Emotionality and violent behavior in psychopaths: A biosocial analysis. In A. Raine, P. Brennan, D. P. Mednick, & S. A. Mednick (Eds.), *Biosocial bases of violence* (pp. 145–161). New York: Plenum Press.

Pennington, B. F., & Bennetto, L. (1993). Main effects or transactions in the neuropsychology of conduct disorder? Commentary on "The neuropsychology of conduct disorder." *Development and Psychopathology, 5,* 153–164.

Qu, T., Brannen, C. L., Kim, H. M., & Sugaya, K. (2001). Human neural stem cells improve cognitive function of aged brain. *Neuroreport: For Rapid Communication of Neuroscience Research, 12,* 1127–1132.

Raine, A. (1993). *The psychopathology of crime: Criminal behavior as a clinical disorder.* San Diego, CA: Academic Press.

Raine, A. (2002a). Annotation: The role of prefrontal deficits, low autonomic arousal, and early health factors in the development of antisocial and aggressive behavior in children. *Journal of Child Psychology and Psychiatry, 43,* 417–434.

Raine, A. (2002b). The biological basis of crime. In J. Q. Wilson & J. Petersilia (Eds.), *Crime: Public policies for crime control* (pp. 43–74). San Francisco: ICS Press.

Raine, A., & Buchsbaum, M. S. (1996). Violence, brain imaging, and neuropsychology. In D. M. Stoff & R. B. Cairns (Eds.), *Aggression and violence: Genetic, neurobiological, and biosocial perspectives* (pp. 195–217). Mahwah, NJ: Erlbaum.

Raine, A., Buchsbaum, M., & LaCasse, L. (1997). Brain abnormalities in murderers indicated by positron emission tomography. *Biological Psychiatry, 42,* 495–508.

Raine, A., Buchsbaum, M. S., Stanley, J., Lottenberg, S., Abel, L., & Stoddard, J. (1994). Selective reductions in prefrontal glucose metabolism in murderers. *Biological Psychiatry, 36,* 365–373.

Raine, A., Ishikawa, S. S., Arce, E., Lencz, T., Knuth, K. H., Bihrle, S., et al. (2004). Hippocampal structural asymmetry in unsuccessful psychopaths. *Biological Psychiatry, 55,* 185–191.

Raine, A., Lencz, T., Bihrle, S., LaCasse, L., & Colletti, P. (2000). Reduced prefrontal gray matter volume and reduced autonomic activity in antisocial personality disorder. *Archives of General Psychiatry, 57,* 119–127.

Raine, A., Lencz, T., & Scerbo, A. (1995). Antisocial personality: Neuroimaging, neuropsychology, neurochemistry, and psychophysiology. In J. H. Ratey

(Ed.), *Neuropsychiatry of behavior disorders* (pp. 50–78). Oxford, UK: Blackwell.

Raine, A., Lencz, T., Taylor, K., Hellige, J. B., Bihrle, S., Lacasse, L., et al. (2003). Corpus callosum abnormalities in psychopathic antisocial individuals. *Archives of General Psychiatry, 60*, 1134–42.

Raine, A., Meloy, J. R., Bihrle, S., Stoddard, J., LaCasse, L., & Buchsbaum, M. S. (1998). Reduced prefrontal and increased subcortical brain functioning assessed using positron emission tomography in predatory and affective murderers. *Behavioral Sciences and the Law, 16*, 319–332.

Raine, A., Mellingen, K., Liu, J., Venables, P. H., & Mednick, S. A. (2003). Effects of environmental enrichment at 3–5 years on schizotypal personality and antisocial behavior at ages 17 and 23 years. *American Journal of Psychiatry, 160*, 1627–1635.

Raine, A., Park, S., Lencz, T., Bihrle, S., LaCasse, L., Widom, C. S., et al. (2001). Reduced right hemisphere activation in severely abused violent offenders during a working memory task: An fMRI study. *Aggressive Behavior, 27*, 111–129.

Raine, A., Stoddard, J., Bihrle, S., & Buchsbaum, M. (1998). Prefrontal glucose deficits in murderers lacking psychosocial deprivation. *Neuropsychiatry, Neuropsychology, and Behavioral Neurology, 11*, 1–7.

Raine, A., Venables, P. H., Dalais, C., Mellingen, K., Reynolds, C., & Mednick, S. A. (2001). Early educational and health enrichment at age 3–5 years is associated with increased autonomic and central nervous system arousal and orienting at age 11 years: Evidence from the Mauritius Child Health Project. *Psychophysiology, 38*, 254–266.

Sachdev, P., Smith, J. S., Matheson, J., & Last, P. (1992). Amygdalo-hippocampectomy for pathological aggression. *Australian and New Zealand Journal of Psychiatry, 26*, 671–676.

Scarpa, A., & Raine, A. (2000). Violence associated with anger and impulsivity. In J. Borod (Ed.), *The neuropsychology of emotion* (pp. 320–339). New York: Oxford University Press.

Schneider, F., Habel, U., Kessler, C., Posse, S., Grodd, W., & Muller-Gartner, H. W. (2000). Functional imaging of conditioned aversive emotional responses in antisocial personality disorder. *Neuropsychobiology, 42*, 192–201.

Soderstrom, H., Hultin, L., Tullberg, M., Wikkelso, C., Ekholm, S., & Forsman, A. (2002). Reduced frontotemporal perfusion in psychopathic personality. *Psychiatry Research Neuroimaging, 114*, 81–94.

Soderstrom, H., Tullberg, M., Wikkelsoe, C., Ekholm, S., & Forsman, A. (2000). Reduced regional cerebral blood flow in non-psychotic violent offenders. *Psychiatry Research: Neuroimaging, 98*, 29–41.

Soto-Moyano, R., Alarcon, S., Belmar, J., Kusch, C., Perez, H., Ruiz, S., et al. (1998). Prenatal protein restriction alters synaptic mechanisms of callosal connections in the rat visual cortex. *International Journal of Developmental Neuroscience, 16*, 75–84.

Spence, S. A., Farrow, T. F., Herford, A. E., Wilkinson, I. D., Zheng, Y., & Woodruff, P. W. (2001). Behavioural functional anatomical correlates of deception in humans. *Neuroreport, 12*, 2849–53

Sperry, R. W. (1974). Lateral specialization in the surgically separated hemispheres. In F. O. Schmitt & F. G. Worden (Eds.), *The neurosciences: Third study program* (pp. 5–19). Cambridge, MA: MIT Press.

Thompson, P. M., Cannon, T. D., Narr, K. L., van Erp, T., Poutanen, V. P., Huttunen, M., et al. (2001). Genetic influences on brain structure. *Nature Neuroscience, 4*, 1253–1258.

Tiihonen, J., Hodgins, S., & Vaurio, O. (2000). Amygdaloid volume loss in psychopathy. *Society for Neuroscience Abstracts*, 20017.

van Praag, H., Kempermann, G., & Gage, F. H. (1999). Running increases cell proliferation and neurogenesis in the adult mouse dentate gyrus. *Nature Neuroscience, 2*, 266–270.

Volkow, N. D., Tancredi, L. R., Grant, C., Gillespie, H., Valentine, A., Nullani, N., et al. (1995). Brain glucose metabolism in violent psychiatric patients: A preliminary study. *Psychiatry Research: Neuroimaging, 61*, 243–253.

Woermann, F. G., Van Elst, L. T., Koepp, M. J., Free, S. L., Thompson, P. J., Trimble, M. R., et al. (2000). Reduction of frontal neocortical grey matter associated with affective aggression in patients with temporal lobe epilepsy: An objective voxel by voxel analysis of automatically segmented MRI. *Journal of Neurology, Neurosurgery, and Psychiatry, 68*, 162–169.

Wong, M. T. H., Lumsden, J., Fenton, G. W., & Fenwick, P. B. C. (1994). Electroencephalography, computed tomography and violence ratings of male patients in a maximum-security mental hospital. *Acta Psychiatrica Scandinavica, 90*, 97–101.

Wong, M. T. H., Lumsden, J., Fenton, G. W., & Fenwick, P. B. C. (1997). Neuroimaging in a mentally abnormal offenders. *Issues in Criminological and Legal Psychology, 27*, 49–58.

Yang, Y. L., Raine, A., Lencz, T., Bihrle, S., Lacasse, L., & Colletti, P. (in press). Prefrontal structural abnormalities in liars. *British Journal of Psychiatry*.

Yang, Y., Raine, A., Lencz, T., Lacasse, L., & Colletti, P. (2005). Volume reduction in prefrontal gray matter in unsuccessful criminal psychopaths. *Biological Psychiatry, 57*, 1109–1116.

Zuckerman, M. (1994). *Behavioral expression and biosocial bases of sensation seeking*. New York: Cambridge University Press.

15

Subcortical Brain Systems in Psychopathy

The Amygdala and Associated Structures

R. J. R. BLAIR

The goal of this chapter is to consider the amygdala, its connections with related structures, and how amygdala pathology might be related to the development of psychopathy. The fundamental claim of this chapter is that psychopathy is indeed associated with early amygdala dysfunction (Blair, 2001, 2003b; Blair, Morris, Frith, Perrett, & Dolan, 1999; Patrick, 1994). This, of course, does not mean that other structures, such as the orbital frontal cortex, which are interconnected with the amygdala, are unaffected (Damasio, 1994; LaPierre, Braun, & Hodgins, 1995; Mitchell, Colledge, Leonard, & Blair, 2002; Raine, 2002). Indeed, we have argued that regions of orbital frontal cortex and ventrolateral prefrontal cortex may also be dysfunctional in this population, particularly in adults with the disorder (Blair, 2003a; Mitchell et al., 2002).

It is even possible that structures that are relatively independent of the amygdala may be affected. Individuals with psychopathy have been found to be more impaired in some forms semantic processing (Hare & Jutai, 1988; Kiehl, Hare, McDonald, & Brink, 1999). These effects have been related, through recent functional magnetic resonance imaging (fMRI) work, to reduced activity in right anterior temporal gyrus and surrounding cortex in individuals with psy-

chopathy (Kiehl et al., 2004). Of course, given the unclear relevance of these semantic difficulties in abstract word processing to the emergence of the disorder, it is possible that they reflect educational differences between the individuals with psychopathy and comparison individuals. It will certainly be interesting to determine whether these impairments are also seen in individuals who show the emotional difficulties but do not express the full behavioral syndrome because of material advantage.

In this chapter, I develop a model of psychopathy that has as its core the hypothesis of amygdala dysfunction in this population. I develop this model within the affective cognitive neuroscience literature. In addition, I attempt to make the components of this model as computationally tractable as possible to aid their formal modeling in the future.

THE AMYGDALA AND ITS CONNECTIONS WITH THE REST OF THE BRAIN

Burdach (1819–1822) is credited with first using the term "amygdala" to describe an almond-shaped mass of gray matter in the anterior portion of the human temporal lobe.

In later, seminal work, Johnston (1923) investigated the amygdala region in several mammalian and nonmammalian vertebrates as well as in human embryos and named its constituent nuclei on the basis of their relative positions within his "amygdaloid complex." These were the central, medial, cortical, basal, accessory basal, and lateral nuclei. Burdach's "amygdala" corresponds to the basolateral nuclei later identified by Johnston. Johnston claimed that the amygdala consisted of two parts: the central and medial nuclei constituting and the basal, lateral, and cortical nuclei (Johnston, 1923). This dichotomy between the basolateral and central nuclei is prevalent in the amygdala literature today.

The amygdala has long been implicated in emotional processing. For some time, the general view was that the basolateral nuclei received sensory input and allowed the formation of conditioned stimulus–unconditioned stimulus associations. These associations then allowed the basolateral amygdala (BLA) to control the activity of the central nucleus (CeN) which in turn allowed the control of hypothalamic and brainstem structures to orchestrate behavioral, autonomic, and neuroendocrine responses (LeDoux, 1998, 2000). While the activity of the amygdala can be characterized in this way in relation to some phenomena (Davis, 2000; LeDoux, 1998, 2000), it is clear that the BLA does more than control the CeN (Everitt, Cardinal, Parkinson, & Robbins, 2003). The BLA projects to ventral striatum and prefrontal cortex, allowing it a crucial role in goal-directed behavior. The CeN, in turn, receives direct sensory input as well as projections from other cortical areas such as the cingulate (LeDoux, Farb, & Ruggiero, 1990; McDonald, 1998) and appears able to learn behavioral expression independently of the BLA (Everitt et al., 2003); see Figure 15.1.

Three major connectional "systems" have been established that involve the amygdala with other regions of the brain (Price, 2003; see Figure 15.1).

1. A largely forebrain system providing sensory input to the amygdala. Structures include olfactory cortex, ascending taste/visceral pathways, posterior thalamus, and sensory association cortical areas.

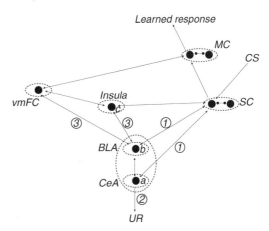

FIGURE 15.1. The integrated emotion systems (IES) model. Arrows indicate the transfer of information. Bidirectional arrows indicate that this transfer is reciprocal. (1) Corresponds to the transfer of information to both the basolateral (BLA) and central (CeN) nuclei of the amygdala from a subset of the systems providing sensory input to the amygdala. Sensory association cortex (SC) is depicted, but other structures would include olfactory cortex, ascending taste/visceral pathways, and posterior thalamus. (2) Corresponds to projections to the brainstem. (3) Corresponds to the transfer of information to forebrain systems including the depicted ventromedial frontal cortex (vmFC) and insula. MC, motor cortex, but also includes other regions necessary for the implementation of a motor response (e.g., basal ganglia); CS, conditioned stimulus; UR, unconditioned response. Hebbian learning at *a* allows a represented CS to become associated with a UR (i.e., the formation of a CS–UR association). Hebbian learning at *b* allows a represented CS to become associated with an affect representation (i.e., the formation of a CS–affect representation association). CS-valenced sensory properties of the UR associations are at *c*.

Many of these connections are reciprocal probably allowing the amygdala to modulate sensory processing. These connections are with both BLA and CeN.

2. A system of projections to the brainstem (extending from the hypothalamus, to the medulla, and even the spinal cord). These pathways are implicated in the modulation of visceral function in relation to emotional stimuli and mostly extend from the CeN.

3. A second forebrain system including ventromedial frontal, rostral insular, and rostral temporal cortex, the medial thala-

mus, and the ventromedial basal ganglia. These reciprocal connections allow the amygdala to influence goal-directed behavior and mostly extend from the BLA.

LEARNING FUNCTIONS OF THE AMYGDALA

It has been claimed that the amygdala is crucially involved in three types of conditioned stimulus association (Everitt et al., 2003). It is important to note that these associations can be either appetitive or aversive. The types of association are:

1. *Conditioned stimulus (CS)–unconditioned response (UR) associations.* Examples of behavior generated as a result of a CS–UR association are salivation to a tone that has been previous associated with food or a galvanic skin response to a colored shape that has previously been associated with the presentation of a loud noise. The CeN, but not the BLA, is necessary for the formation of CS–UR associations (Everitt et al., 2003; Killcross, Robbins, & Everitt, 1997).
2. *Conditioned stimulus (CS)–affect representation associations* (e.g., fear, or the expectation of reward). The concept is one of "an emotional 'tone' that is tagged to a stimulus" (Everitt et al., 2003, p. 234). Such a concept is widely used in theories of emotional learning (e.g., Dickinson & Dearing, 1979). The BLA, but not the CeN, is necessary for the formation of these associations (Everitt et al., 2003).
3. *Conditioned stimulus (CS)–valenced sensory properties of the unconditioned stimulus (US) associations.* The CS can be associated with specific sensory properties of the US (e.g., visual appearance, sound, and smell) and also "consummatory" qualities such as its taste. The BLA, but not the CeN, is necessary for the formation of these associations (Everitt et al., 2003). However, the suggestion from reinforcer devaluation studies is that these associations are not stored in the amygdala (Pickens et al., 2003). We believe, as is depicted in Figure 15.1, that they are stored within the insula.

For the purposes of the arguments to be developed here, we contrast the foregoing types of association with stimulus–response associations. In reference to this, it is important to note that the amygdala is not necessary for all forms of emotional learning. Earlier models of psychopathy suggested that the disorder was marked by reduced sensitivity to punishment, punishment-based learning, or fear (Fowles, 1988; Lykken, 1995; Patrick, 1994). Such models now require refinement. The empirical literature suggests that there is no single fear system but rather a series of at least partially separable neural systems that are engaged in specific forms of processing that can be subsumed under the umbrella term "fear" (Amaral, 2001; Blair & Cipolotti, 2000; Killcross et al., 1997; Prather et al., 2001). Specifically, punishment information can be used when learning about an object (i.e., when forming a CS–affect representation association). But it can also be used when learning about how to respond to an object (i.e., when forming a CS–response association, such as if you make response 1 to stimulus A you will be punished, but if you make response 2 you will not be punished). The amygdala is crucially involved in the formation of CS–affect representations, but it is not necessary for the formation of CS–(learned) response associations (Baxter & Murray, 2002). Thus, punishment-oriented theories need to distinguish learned threats from specific types of social threat (Amaral, 2001; Blair & Cipolotti, 2000) and recognize the different forms of association that can be established with a CS as a function of punishment information (Baxter & Murray, 2002; Killcross et al., 1997). The argument I make here is that it is only those forms of punishment-based learning that are dependent on the amygdala that are impaired in individuals with psychopathy.

In summary, the amygdala is necessary for the formation of stimulus–UC response associations and stimulus–reinforcement associations. These types of associations can be either appetitive or aversive. My position, developed in the sections that follow, is that individuals with psychopathy are impaired in the formation of both of these types of association, but the dysfunction is more substantial for aversive than appetitive associations.

BEHAVIORAL EXPRESSION AND THE AMYGDALA

The architecture depicted in Figure 15.1 is a simplification of the systems that allow the amygdala to express CS–UR associations. These mediate basic aversive/ appetitive conditioning, defined as the learning process through which a CS can come to elicit UR. This can either occur either (1) as a direct association of the CS through the CeN to a specific UR (e.g., salivation to the bell that has been paired with food); or (2) following the formation of a CS–affect representation association through BLA and then onto CeN (e.g., a rat experiencing a shock will demonstrate escape behaviors, but when presented with a tone that was previously paired with the shock, the rat will freeze; in this case, the rat has not learned a CS–UR association that would cause it to flee the tone but, rather, a CS–affect representation association that controls behavior through the CeN, resulting in freezing to the potential threat; Everitt et al., 2003).

With regard to my position that amygdala dysfunction is a central focus of the pathology associated with psychopathy (Blair, 2001; Blair et al., 1999), the initial evidence came from studies demonstrating impaired aversive conditioning in individuals with psychopathy (Flor, Birbaumer, Hermann, Ziegler, & Patrick, 2002; Hare, 1970; Lykken, 1957). Although we currently cannot be sure whether the failure of individuals with psychopathy to demonstrate a conditioned skin conductance response to, for example, a neutral face CS paired with a noxious odor (Flor et al., 2002) represents reduced ability to form CS–UR or CS–affect representation associations, either possibility is consistent with amygdala dysfunction. Relevant to this, recent neuroimaging work has indeed demonstrated reduced amygdala activity during aversive conditioning in individuals with psychopathy (Veit et al., 2002). It has also been reported that the ability of a child to perform aversive conditioning at age 15 can be used to predict their probability of displaying antisocial behavior in adulthood (Raine, Venables, & Williams, 1996). Similarly, there has been a recent demonstration that adolescent males with a persistently reduced response to a standardized stressor are overrepresented in the delinquent population

and that this pattern of results is a predictor of exceedingly high rates of criminal recidivism (Karnik, Delizonna, Miller, & Steiner, 2003).

There have been several investigations of the modulation of the startle reflex by visual appetitive and aversive picture primes in individuals with psychopathy (Levenston, Patrick, Bradley, & Lang, 2000; Pastor, Molto, Vila, & Lang, 2003; Patrick, Bradley, & Lang, 1993). Considerable data suggest that the amygdala is necessary for the modulation of the startle response by CSs (Angrilli et al., 1996; Davis, 2000). On the basis of Figure 15.1, the suggestion is that a visual prime, a CS, can increase the activity of brainstem neurons mediating the startle reflex through the CeN via the BLA as a result of a CS–affect representation (a CS–UR association would mean that the CS itself induced a startle response). This would suggest that if individuals with psychopathy present with amygdala dysfunction, they should show reduced modulation of the startle reflex by visual CS primes. Individuals with psychopathy do show strikingly reduced levels of augmentation of the startle reflex by visual threat primes (Levenston et al., 2000; Pastor et al., 2003; Patrick et al., 1993; for a review of these studies, see Fowles & Dindo, Chapter 2, this volume).

As depicted in Figure 15.1, one route to the activation of autonomic responding is through the amygdala. However, it is not the only route (Tranel & Damasio, 1994). The existence of these multiple routes may explain some of the inconsistent findings with respect to autonomic responses to CSs in individuals with psychopathy. Individuals with psychopathy show appropriate skin conductance responses (SCRs) to visual threats, even to the same visual threats that fail to prime their startle responses (Blair, Jones, Clark, & Smith, 1997; Levenston et al., 2000; Pastor et al., 2003; Patrick et al., 1993). In contrast, individuals with psychopathy show reduced SCRs to facial expressions of sadness (Blair, 1999; Blair et al., 1997), imagined threat scenes (Patrick, Cuthbert, & Lang, 1994), anticipated threat (Hare, 1965, 1982; Hare, Frazell, & Cox, 1978; Ogloff & Wong, 1990) and emotionally evocative sounds (e.g., a male attack sound or a baby's laugh; Verona, Patrick, Curtin, Bradley, & Lang, 2004). Relevant to this, it has been shown that SCRs to visual threats appear to be more disrupted by lesions of orbital frontal cortex rather than lesions of the amygdala (Tranel & Damasio, 1994). As yet, it is unknown whether amygdala lesions disrupt SCRs to facial expressions of sadness, imagined threat scenes, or emotionally evocative sounds. However, the model makes the clear prediction that they would. In line with the model, recent neuroimaging work has indicated that the amygdala plays a crucial role in generating SCRs to *anticipated* threat (Phelps et al., 2001).

It is important to note here that Verona and colleagues (2004) found reduced SCRs in individuals with psychopathy to both positive and negative emotional sounds, while all three studies examining the modulation of the startle reflex by visual primes (i.e., pictures) in individuals with psychopathy found reduced augmentation of the startle reflex by aversive primes but appropriate levels of suppression of the startle reflex by appetitive primes (Levenston et al., 2000; Pastor et al., 2003; Patrick et al., 1993). These data are apparently inconsistent: The SCR data to evocative sounds suggest dysfunctional reward-related processing, whereas the affect-modulated startle findings suggest intact reward processing. This apparent contradiction may prove of crucial significance. Early models of psychopathy made reference to unitary reward/ punishment systems suggesting dysfunction within the punishment systems and, occasionally, superior reward processing (Fowles, 1988; Lykken, 1995; Patrick, 1994). As noted previously, with respect to punishment processing, such models are currently being refined; indeed, the integrated emotion systems (IES) model (Blair, 2003a, 2004) can be considered such a refinement. According to this view, there is no single fear system but rather partially separable systems, only some of which are impaired in individuals with psychopathy (see also Patrick & Lang, 1999). Reward-related processing is somewhat less understood. However, concepts of reward-related processing are likely to be refined into separable systems as well. The contrast between the Verona and colleagues SCR findings and the affect-modulated startle findings may be highly informative in this regard (cf. Peschardt, Leonard, Morton, & Blair, 2004).

The systems depicted in Figure 15.2 are crucially involved in the individual's basic, gradated response to threat or stress. Low levels of threat from a distant potential predator initiate freezing. Higher levels of threat as the potential predator closes in lead to the animal attempting to escape its environment. At higher levels still, when the threat is very close and escape is impossible, the animal will display reactive aggression (Blanchard, Blanchard, & Takahashi, 1977). These systems which allow the expression of reactive aggression are shared with other mammalian species (Gregg & Siegel, 2001; Panksepp, 1998).

Individuals with psychopathy present with elevated levels of reactive aggression. They are not alone in this. A wide variety of other psychiatric and neurological conditions are associated with elevated levels of reactive aggression, including childhood bipolar disorder (Leibenluft, Blair, Charney, & Pine, 2003), borderline personality disorder (Edwards, Scott, Yarvis, Paizis, & Panizzon, 2003), posttraumatic stress disorder (Pavic et al., 2003), and acquired sociopathy (Anderson, Bechara, Damasio, Tranel, & Damasio, 1999; Blair & Cipolotti, 2000; Grafman, Schwab, Warden, Pridgen, & Brown, 1996). Reactive aggression is more likely if the responsiveness of the basic threat circuitry is elevated either due to sensitization of this circuitry by prior threat (e.g., physical/sexual abuse) or endogenous factors or due to reduced regulation of this circuitry by the frontal regions depicted in Figure 15.2 (for a review, see Blair & Charney, 2003). Individuals with psychopathy are unlikely to display heightened reactive aggression because of overactive brainstem threat circuitry. Indeed, in line with the hypothesis of amygdala dysfunction, this population is less responsive to environmental threat rather than more responsive. Certainly, they show no difference with comparison individuals in their basic startle response to an auditory probe (Patrick et al., 1993), an index of the responsiveness of the basic threat circuitry that bypasses the amygdala.

The suggestion here is that the elevated level of reactive aggression shown by individuals with psychopathy is due to dysfunction in frontal executive systems involved in the regulation of brainstem threat circuitry. Frustration has long been linked to the

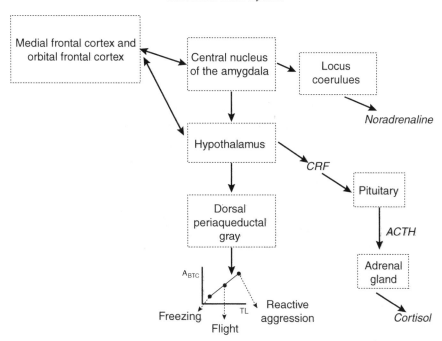

FIGURE 15.2. Neural and neurotransmitter systems involved in the basic response to threat. The figure relates threat level (TL) to activation of the basic threat circuitry (A_{BTC}) in a simple linear fashion. The points on the graph reflect levels of activation of the basic threat circuitry necessary for specific threat-related behaviors.

display of reactive aggression (Berkowitz, 1993). Frustration occurs following the initiation of a behavior to achieve an expected reward and the subsequent absence of this reward. Both medial and orbital frontal cortex (including ventrolateral prefrontal cortex; Brodmann's area 47) are involved in expectation violation computations and the error detection necessary to induce frustration (Blair, 2004; Rolls, 1997). Crucially, both are involved in changing behavioral responding when the initial attempt to reach a goal is unsuccessful and an alternative behavioral response needs to be initiated. Human neuropsychological studies (e.g., Rogers et al., 1999; Rolls, 1997; Rolls, Hornak, Wade, & McGrath, 1994) indicate that damage to medial and orbital frontal cortex impairs extinction (stopping a response to a stimulus that previously had been rewarded but which is now either not rewarded or punished) and response reversal (learning to make an alternative response to a stimulus array to gain reward after the previously learned response to the stimulus array is either not rewarded or punished).

Thus, damage to medial and orbital frontal cortex gives rise to an individual predisposed to frustration and, in consequence, reactive aggression. Individuals with psychopathy present with both impairments in extinction, as evidenced by performance on Newman's card playing task (Newman, Patterson, & Kosson, 1987), and in response reversal (Mitchell et al., 2002; Peschardt, Leonard, et al., 2004). On the basis of these data, we postulate that individuals with psychopathy (particularly adults with the disorder) present with orbital frontal cortex dysfunction, and this leads to heightened reactive aggression in this population (Blair, 2004).

Figure 15.2 also depicts two important neurochemical systems that respond to stress/ threat (Charney, 2003; Francis & Meaney, 1999):

1. *The hypothalamic–pituitary–adrenal (HPA) axis.* Stress stimulates release of corticotropin-releasing factor (CRF) from the paraventricular nucleus (PVN) of the hypothalamus. CRF is released by the PVN neurons into the portal blood supply of

the anterior pituitary, where it provokes the synthesis and release of adreno-cor-ticotropin hormone (ACTH) from the pi-tuitary. This results in increased secretion of cortisol from the adrenal gland. High levels of cortisol, through negative feed-back, decrease both CRF and norepin-ephrine (NE) synthesis at the level of the PVN, and thereby constrain the PVN.

2. *The noradrenergic system.* There is a sec-ond population of CRF neurons in the central nucleus of the amygdala. These neurons project to the locus coeruleus, re-sulting in increased noradrenaline release from the terminal fields of this ascending noradrenergic system.

If the sensitivity of the amygdala to threat is suppressed in individuals with psychopa-thy, we would predict reduced cortisol and noradrenaline levels in these individuals. To my knowledge these predictions remain un-tested. However, reduced cortisol levels have been reported in life-course persistent of-fenders (a subset of whom are likely to be in-dividuals with psychopathy; Moffitt, 1993) and are predictive of future aggression levels (Shoal, Giancola, & Kirillova, 2003). Sim-ilarly, reduced noradrenaline levels have frequently been associated with elevated levels of antisocial behavior (Raine, 1993; Rogeness, Cepeda, Macedo, Fischer, & Harris, 1990; Rogeness, Javors, Mass, & Macedo, 1990). In this regard it is interesting to note that NE function appears to be *in-creased* in a variety of anxiety disorders (Charney, Heninger, & Breier, 1984). These patients show the opposite affective impair-ment to individuals with psychopathy: a heightened responsiveness to aversive cues.

THE ROLE OF THE AMYGDALA IN STIMULUS SELECTION ("ATTENTION")

In Figure 15.3 the suggested role of the amygdala in biasing stimulus selection (i.e., in "attention") is depicted. Recent formula-tions suggest that attention is the result of the competition for neural representation which occurs when multiple stimuli are pres-ent (Desimone & Duncan, 1995; Duncan, 1998). Which stimuli win this competition and are "attended to" is determined by both

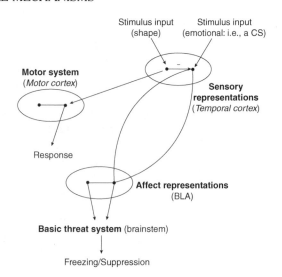

FIGURE 15.3. A subset of components of the integrated emotion systems (IES) model involved in the emotional modulation of attention.

bottom-up sensory processes such as emo-tional salience, and top-down influences such as directed attention (Desimone & Duncan, 1995). Past research has implicated the amygdala in processes involving en-hanced attention for emotional information relative to neutral information, even when the emotional information is peripheral to ongoing behavior (Anderson & Phelps, 2001; Vuilleumier, Armony, Driver, & Dolan, 2001). We hypothesize that the insula may also play a role in this respect. In rela-tion to the model depicted in Figure 15.3, the suggestion is that a CS will activate CS–affect representation associations. As the connections of these representations with the representation of the CS are reciprocal, the activation of the CS in turn will be aug-mented. All other things being equal, repre-sentations of the CS will therefore be more salient (strongly activated) than the repre-sentations of any competing environmental stimuli.

The foregoing model suggests that if in-dividuals with psychopathy present with amygdala dysfunction, they will receive markedly reduced augmentation of the rep-resentation of the CS from the reciprocal connections with the amygdala and insula. This means that if the CS is the target stimu-lus, performance will be impaired in individ-uals with psychopathy relative to comparison individuals (i.e., a weaker representation should be less able to control behavior); on the other hand, if the CS is a distracter to ongoing behavior, performance will be superior in individuals with psychopathy relative to comparison individuals (i.e., a weaker representation will be less of a competitor for the stimulus that should be controlling behavior). Both of these predictions have been supported by research findings (Day & Wong, 1996; Lorenz & Newman, 2002; Mitchell, Richell, Leonard, & Blair, in press; Williamson, Harpur, & Hare, 1991).

Emotional words (e.g., murder) can be considered CSs, and they should, and do, activate the amygdala and insula (Hamann & Mao, 2002); Nakic, Mitchell, Vythilingham, & Blair, 2005). Consistent with prediction, this activation in turn augments the representation of such words in temporal cortex (Nakic et al., 2005). Augmentation of the representation of affective word "stimuli" should make lexical decisions easier for these words; that is, it should be easier to state that an emotional word is a word than it is to identify a neutral word as a word. Experimental data indeed indicate that healthy participants are faster to state that an emotional word is a word than a neutral word (Graves, Landis, & Goodglass, 1981; Strauss, 1983). Moreover, they show larger cortical event-related potentials (ERPs) over central and parietal cortical sites to emotional words than neutral words (Begleiter, Gross, & Kissin, 1967). In contrast, but again in line with the hypothesis developed here, psychopathic individuals fail to show reaction time or ERP differences between neutral and emotional words (Day & Wong, 1996; Lorenz & Newman, 2002; Williamson et al., 1991).

In the emotional interrupt task (Mitchell et al., in press), participants are instructed to make one response if a square is presented and another response if a triangle is presented on a computer screen. The participant is presented with a positive, negative, or neutral visual image for 200 milliseconds before the target stimulus (presented for 150 milliseconds) and for 400 milliseconds after the target stimulus. Healthy participants are slower to respond to the square/triangle if it is temporally bracketed by an emotional stimulus rather than a neutral stimulus. In terms of the model, the representation of the emotional CS is boosted by reciprocal feedback from the valence representations and stimulus-affect representation associations. It therefore becomes a more effective competitor for attention with the square/triangle target stimulus. Individuals with psychopathy, in contrast, perform similarly whether the square/ triangle is temporally bracketed by an emotional stimulus or a neutral stimulus (Mitchell et al., in press).

THE ROLE OF THE AMYGDALA IN INSTRUMENTAL LEARNING

Instrumental learning requires the individual either to learn to perform an action to a stimulus if this action results in reward or to withhold performing an action to a stimulus if this action results in punishment; the latter form of learning is referred to as passive avoidance learning. The amygdala (particularly the BLA) is necessary for some (e.g., passive avoidance learning; Ambrogi Lorenzini, Bucherelli, Giachetti, Mugnai, & Tassoni, 1991), but not all forms of instrumental learning (e.g., object discrimination learning and conditional learning; Baxter & Murray, 2002; Burns, Everitt, & Robbins, 1999; Malkova, Gaffan, & Murray, 1997; Petrides, 1982, 1985). Importantly, the amygdala mediates these specific forms of instrumental learning in interaction with other brain regions; notably, in this case, regions involved in coding motor responses (i.e., basal ganglia and motor cortex) and specific forms of decision making (medial orbital frontal cortex/rostral anterior cingulate).

In the IES model depicted in Figure 15.1, two modules of nonlinear, identical computational units were depicted that have not received much attention until now. The first of these corresponds to units coding motor responses (implemented by regions that include basal ganglia and premotor cortex). The second corresponds to units coding expectation of reward (implemented by medial orbital frontal cortex/rostral anterior cingulate). These units allow rapid decision making on the basis of expected reinforcement information provided by the amygdala.

In regard to the second module, implemented by medial orbital frontal cortex, here a claim is being made about a commonality of function of the medial orbital frontal cortex with other regions of the frontal cortex.

There have been several recent suggestions that the left dorsolateral prefrontal cortex is involved in the selection of a verbal response option when more than one is in competition (Frith, 2000; Robinson, Blair, & Cipolotti, 1998). These have been elegantly modeled computationally (Usher & Cohen, 1999). Very briefly, the Usher and Cohen (1999) model assumes the existence of modality-specific posterior units that are limited by temporal decay while anterior units use active reverberations which can sustain themselves and which are limited by displacement from competing new information. The anterior units, by being self-excitatory but mutually inhibitory allow rapid selection between competing, multiple active posterior response options (Usher & Cohen, 1999). The suggestion here is that the "decision" units in orbital frontal cortex may serve a similar function over units in premotor cortex that mediate motor responses. The "decision" units would receive information in order to solve response competition on the basis of not only the activation of units coding the motor response but also expectations of reinforcement as a result of previously formed CS–affect representations and CS-valenced sensory representations (i.e., from the amygdala and insula). The more active a unit from expectation information, the more likely it will "win" the representational competition and the response associated with this unit will be initiated.

In line with the hypothesis of amygdala dysfunction in psychopathy, individuals with psychopathy only present with impairment for those instrumental learning tasks that rely on the amygdala. For example, individuals with psychopathy show impairment on passive avoidance learning tasks (Blair et al., 2004; Newman & Kosson, 1986; Newman & Schmitt, 1998) but not on object discrimination or conditional learning tasks (Blair, Colledge, & Mitchell, 2001; Mitchell et al., 2002).

In their recent review, Baxter and Murray (2002) provided a theoretical basis for the distinction between instrumental learning tasks that require the amygdala (e.g., passive avoidance learning) and those that do not (object discrimination and conditional learning). They argued that the amygdala is necessary for instrumental learning tasks requiring the formation of stimulus–rein-forcement associations (i.e., the CS–affect representations and CS-valenced sensory representations discussed previously), but not for tasks that require, or at least can easily be solved by, the formation of stimulus–response associations (i.e., the formation of an association between a stimulus and a motor response). For example, in passive avoidance learning, the participant is presented with differing stimuli. Some stimuli, if responded to, engender reward. Other stimuli, if responded to, engender punishment. The participant's task is to learn to respond to the good stimuli and avoid responding to the bad stimuli. Computationally, the participant must code the valence associated with a particular stimulus (i.e., the participant must learn which stimuli to approach and which to avoid). In terms of the model depicted in Figure 15.1, passive avoidance learning can be solved on the basis of stored CS–affect representations. If the individual has formed a CS–positive affect association, the individual will approach (respond to) this stimulus. If the individual has formed a CS–negative affect association, the individual will avoid (fail to respond to) this stimulus.

In contrast, Baxter and Murray (2002) argued that object discrimination and conditional learning are solved through stimulus–response associations. Object discrimination involves learning to respond to one of two objects (one rewarded and one not rewarded) repeatedly presented in a pairwise fashion over a series of trials. In other words, participants must learn that when Stimulus A and Stimulus B are present they should respond to A. Conditional learning involves learning to perform a particular motor response in the presence of a particular stimulus; in this case, participants must learn that when Stimulus A is present they should enact Response 1, and when Stimulus B is present they should enact Response 2 (e.g., press left button if green light is on, but right button if red light is on).

In object discrimination and conditional learning tasks, unlike passive avoidance learning tasks, the participant cannot learn that some of the stimuli are "good" or "bad" and thus should be approached or avoided. In object learning tasks, the compound stimulus (A plus B) can either be "good" or "bad"—what determines its valence is not the quality of the stimulus (this is always repeated) but the quality of the response made to the stimulus. This is even clearer with respect to conditional learning tasks. Again the value of the stimulus is determined by the individual's action to the stimulus; the same stimulus can give rise to reward or punishment depending on the individual's actions. Such tasks cannot be solved by stimulus–affect representation associations.

The foregoing argument is important for two main reasons. First, the earlier generation of emotion learning-based accounts of psychopathy, the fear dysfunction positions (Fowles, 1988; Lykken, 1995; Patrick, 1994), were challenged by Newman and colleagues on the basis of results with variants of the passive avoidance paradigm (e.g., (Newman, 1998). As stated previously, in the standard passive avoidance paradigm, participants must learn to respond to some stimuli (to gain reward) while not responding to others (to avoid punishment). In "punishment-only" passive avoidance learning, participants must learn to respond to some stimuli (if they do not, they are punished) and not to respond to others (if they do, they are punished). While individuals with psychopathy present with impairment on standard passive avoidance learning tasks (Blair et al., 2004; Newman & Kosson, 1986; Newman & Schmitt, 1998), they show no impairment on punishment-only passive avoidance learning tasks (Newman, 1998).

These data are problematic for the fear dysfunction positions because these positions should predict difficulties whenever punishment information needs to be processed (Newman, 1998). If these positions were correct, individuals with psychopathy should learn poorly in both the standard passive avoidance paradigm and the punishment-only paradigm. However, the model developed above provides a plausible explanation for this dissociation: punishment-only task variants cannot be solved through the formation of CS–affect representation associations. In these variants of the passive avoidance task, there are no "good" or "bad" stimuli; both S+ and S– stimuli can give rise to reward or punishment. Instead of forming a stimulus–reinforcement association, the participant must form a stimulus–response association: If S+, do R1 (respond); if S–, do R2 (respond differently). In short, the punishment-only versions of the task are very similar to conditional learning tasks and, given their dependence on stimulus–response associations, should be, and are, solvable by individuals with psychopathy.

Second, the foregoing argument is important because it allows new predictions. On the basis of this model, some recent, novel multiple stimulus/reward instrumental learning paradigms have been developed; e.g., the Snake, Tokens, and Differential Reward and Punishment Learning tasks (Fine et al., 2004; Peschardt, Leonard, et al., 2004). We hypothesize that these tasks require the integrity of the valence units (amygdala), sensory-valence representations (insula), and "decision" units that represent expected levels of reinforcement (medial frontal cortex). In these tasks, the participant is presented with a series of stimuli, any of which can be paired with any other stimulus. For example, in the Snake task, and the very similar Tokens task, the participant is presented with pairs of stimuli but, unlike object discrimination, it is not the same pair presented trial after trial. Rather, pairs are derived from a set of four test stimuli. Two of the four stimuli, when chosen, give rise to a reward; the other two, when chosen, give rise to a punishment. Each of the four stimuli can be paired with any of the others, including itself (i.e., there may be two blue tokens on the screen and the participant has to choose one of these two). This task presumably could be solved through the formation of stimulus–response associations. However, given that there are 10 different stimulus combinations, this is not a very efficient solution. A more efficient solution is to learn that there are two rewarding stimuli and two punishing stimuli (i.e., to solve the task by the formation of stimulus–reinforcement associations). In line with our hypotheses, we reported a case of a patient with a congenital amygdala lesion who presented with impairment on a version of the Tokens task (Fine et al., 2004). In contrast, two patients with acquired lesions involving the orbital frontal cortex showed intact acquisition during the instrumental learning phase but were severely impaired on the reversal phase of the task. Individuals with psychopathy also present with pronounced impairment on this task (Fine et al., 2004).

In the Differential Reward and Punishment Learning task (Peschardt, Leonard, et al., 2004), the participant also has to choose between two objects presented on a computer screen. However, in this task there are 10 different objects to choose among (versus only four in the Tokens task). Each of these 10 objects is randomly assigned a value at the beginning of the testing session (–1,600, –800, –400, –200, –100, 100, 200, 400, 800, or 1,600). The two objects presented to the participant on any one trial can either comprise one rewarding and one punishing object, two objects with different levels of punishment, or two objects with different levels of rewards. The participant has to choose the object that will gain the most points or lose the least points. This task allows an assessment of an individual's sensitivity to variations in reward/punishment levels. For example, choosing between the object that gives 1,600 points and the object giving 100 points is generally easier than choosing between the object that gives 1,600 points and the object giving 800 points. Individuals with psychopathy show pronounced difficulty with this task (Peschardt, Leonard, et al., 2004). Strikingly, and very unlike comparison individuals, their impairment is far more pronounced when choosing between objects that give rise to different levels of punishment as opposed to choosing between objects that give rise to different levels of reward.

THE AMYGDALA AND THE DEVELOPMENT OF PSYCHOPATHY

In this chapter, I have developed the hypothesis that there is amygdala dysfunction in individuals with psychopathy. However, a further important question is why amygdala dysfunction should give rise to the development of this disorder. Such an account is the focus of this final section.

As noted earlier, individuals with psychopathy present with elevated levels of reactive aggression (Cornell et al., 1996; Williamson et al., 1987). However, as also noted earlier, elevated levels of reactive aggression are found in a wide variety of mood disorders. We relate this to either dysfunctional over-responsiveness in the basic threat circuitry or dysfunctional frontal regulatory systems (Blair & Charney, 2003)—with the latter,

particularly dysfunction of the ventral lateral prefrontal cortex (BA 47), postulated to underlie enhanced reactive aggression in psychopathy. What is remarkable about psychopathy, a feature noted in no other psychiatric condition (other than, of course, conduct disorder/antisocial personality disorder), is that individuals with the disorder present with elevated levels of instrumental aggression also (Cornell et al., 1996; Porter & Woodworth, Chapter 24, this volume; Williamson et al., 1987). Instrumental aggression, also referred to as proactive aggression, is purposeful and goal directed: The aggression is used instrumentally to achieve a specific desired goal (Berkowitz, 1993). The goal is not usually the pain of the victim but, rather, the victim's possessions, or increased status within a group hierarchy.

Importantly, instrumental aggression is a motor response made to achieve a particular goal. However, in contrast with other forms of goal-directed behavior (e.g., placing a card in an ATM machine to extract money), it causes distress and in some cases harm to others. The willingness of some individuals to employ aggressive, antisocial behavior to achieve goals can be understood as a failure of moral socialization. Moral socialization is the term given to the process by which caregivers, and others, reinforce behaviors they wish to encourage and punish behaviors they wish to discourage. The ease with which a child can be socialized has been related to the temperamental variable of fearfulness (Fowles & Dindo, Chapter 2, this volume; Kochanska, 1993, 1997). Fearful children have been found to show higher levels of moral development or conscience using a variety of measures (Asendorpf & Nunner-Winkler, 1992; Kochanska, 1997; Kochanska, De Vet, Goldman, Murray, & Putnam, 1994; Rothbart, Ahadi, & Hershey, 1994). The punishment that normally promotes moral socialization in relation to instrumental antisocial behavior is the victim's resulting pain and distress; empathy induction, focusing the transgressor's attention on the victim, particularly fosters moral socialization (Eisenberg, 2002; Hoffman, 1994).

The claim here is that the amygdala dysfunction present in individuals with psychopathy specifically interferes with their ability to process the sadness and fear of victims, and to engage in victim empathy, and disrupts core emotional learning processes that are crucial for moral socialization. The temperamental variable of fearfulness, related to the ease with which the child can be socialized (Fowles & Dindo, Chapter 2, this volume; Kochanska, 1993, 1997), can be understood as an index of the integrity of the amygdala (Blair, 2003a). While fear conditioning is not necessarily important in socialization (Brody & Shaffer, 1982; Hoffman, 1994), it is argued that the amygdala's response to the fear and sadness of victims, during empathy induction, is crucial for socialization (Blair, 1995). For normal moral socialization to occur, the developing child needs to associate harmful transgressions with the punishment of the distress of the victim. However, individuals with psychopathy are less able to form these associations and so are at greater risk to choose antisocial behavioral options. Indeed, whereas positive parenting techniques are associated with reduced antisocial behavior levels in healthy children, they have no impact on the level of antisocial behavior expressed by children who present with the emotional dysfunction associated with psychopathy (Wootton, Frick, Shelton, & Silverthorn, 1997).

CONCLUSIONS

In this chapter, I have reviewed a body of data that strongly suggests that individuals with psychopathy present with amygdala dysfunction. The argument is that this amygdala dysfunction reduces (1) the individual's responsiveness to the sadness and fear of potential victims and (2) the individual's ability to learn the stimulus–reinforcement associations that are crucial for moral socialization. Because of this, children with amygdala dysfunction do not learn to avoid using antisocial behaviors to achieve their goals. Of course, this does not mean that such children will *necessarily* learn to rely on antisocial behaviors to reach their goals; if other behaviors prove effective, they will tend to use these instead. The argument is simply that children with psychopathic tendencies are more likely to learn to use antisocial behavior to achieve their goals.

The stress on the amygdala does not imply that there are not other dysfunctional regions of the brain in psychopathy. Currently,

there are clear indications of pathology in orbital frontal and ventrolateral regions of prefrontal cortex in this population, especially in adults (LaPierre et al., 1995; Mitchell et al., 2002). There are also suggestions of anomalies in right anterior temporal gyrus and surrounding cortex in individuals with psychopathy (Kiehl et al., 2004). However, it is currently unclear whether these additional pathologies reflect the fundamental disorder or whether they are secondary consequences of the disorder. The orbital frontal/ventrolateral prefrontal cortex dysfunction may be at least partially a result of drug use in this population (Mitchell et al., 2002). The reduced activation of right anterior temporal gyrus and surrounding cortex in relation to abstract words in individuals with psychopathy could easily be a result of their reduced educational exposure.

One issue that needs to be considered carefully in the future is the extent to which individuals with psychopathy are impaired in the processing of both aversive and appetitive information—in particular, whether are they equivalently impaired in forming stimulus–reward and stimulus–punishment associations (cf. Peschardt et al., 2004). Early suggestions that individuals with psychopathy are overly responsive to reward information (Fowles, 1988) have not been supported. Although there have been studies indicating that reward processing is less impaired (Peschardt et al., 2003, 2004) or unimpaired (Blair et al., 2004; Levenston et al., 2000; Pastor et al., 2003; Patrick et al., 1993) in individuals with psychopathy, there have been no reports that reward processing is superior in psychopathic individuals. Indeed, some reports have indicated that the impairment in reward processing is comparable to that in punishment processing (Mitchell et al., in press; Verona et al., 2004; Williamson et al., 1991). If this proved true, a potential explanation would be that the amygdala is involved in the formation of both stimulus–reward and stimulus–punishment associations (Baxter & Murray, 2002; Everitt et al., 2003). However, other findings indicating that reward processing in psychopathy is less impaired than punishment processing, for comparable tasks, suggest that the amygdala dysfunction is selective. Such a suggestion is more consistent with a neurochemical model (cf. Peschardt, Leonard, et al., 2004) than a neurological model positing a general dysfunction in the amygdala. That is, the functioning of neurotransmitter(s) involved in specific aspects of amygdala functioning, in particular coding of punishment information, may be dysfunctional in psychopathy (Blair, 2003; Peschardt, Leonard, et al., 2004; Peschardt, Morton, & Blair, 2003). Pertinent to this, there is evidence that polymorphisms of particular genes can alter the functioning of specific neurotransmitter systems (Lichter et al., 1993; Shih, Chen, & Ridd, 1999; Vandenbergh et al., 1992).

Currently, it remains unclear which neurotransmitter systems might be dysfunctional in individuals with psychopathy (cf. Minzenberg & Siever, Chapter 13, this volume). However, one possibility is that the noradrenergic response to stress or threat stimuli, described earlier, is disturbed in individuals with psychopathy (Blair, 2003; Peschardt, Leonard et al., 2004). Interestingly, there have been recent suggestions that noradrenaline is involved in mediating the impact of aversive cues in human choice (Rogers, Lancaster, Wakeley, & Bhagwager, 2004). Moreover, recent pharmacological data imply that noradrenergic manipulations selectively affect the processing of sad facial expressions (Harmer, Perrett, Cowen, & Goodwin, 2001; Sustrik, Coupland, & Blair, 2004). Thus, it can be hypothesized that the genetic anomalies considered to be present in individuals with psychopathy disrupt the functioning of the noradrenergic system such that the impact of aversive stimuli is muted.

Finally, it is worth noting that considerable advances are being made with respect to the pathophysiology underlying psychopathy. Understanding the neural and neurochemical systems involved in the emergence of the disorder will be invaluable for the development of future treatment strategies. Currently, most emotional disorders are considered to be at least manageable through treatment. It is high time that this perspective also be taken toward the emotional disorder of psychopathy.

REFERENCES

Amaral, D. G. (2001). *The amygdaloid complex and the neurobiology of social behaviour.* Paper presented at the meeting of the Society for Research in Child Development, Minneapolis.

Ambrogi Lorenzini, C. G., Bucherelli, C., Giachetti, A., Mugnai, L., & Tassoni, G. (1991). Effects of nucleus basolateralis amygdalae neurotoxic lesions on aversive conditioning in the rat. *Physiology and Behavior, 49*, 765–770.

Anderson, A. K., & Phelps, E. A. (2001). Lesions of the human amygdala impair enhanced perception of emotionally salient events. *Nature, 411*, 305–309.

Anderson, S. W., Bechara, A., Damasio, H., Tranel, D., & Damasio, A. R. (1999). Impairment of social and moral behaviour related to early damage in human prefrontal cortex. *Nature Neuroscience, 2*, 1032–1037.

Angrilli, A., Mauri, A., Palomba, D., Flor, H., Birhaumer, N., Sartori, G., et al. (1996). Startle reflex and emotion modulation impairment after a right amygdala lesion. *Brain, 119*, 1991–2000.

Asendorpf, J. B., & Nunner-Winkler, G. (1992). Children's moral motive strength and temperamental inhibition reduce their immoral behaviour in real moral conflicts. *Child Development, 63*, 1223–1235.

Baxter, M. G., & Murray, E. A. (2002). The amygdala and reward. *Nature Reviews Neuroscience, 3*, 563–573.

Begleiter, H., Gross, M. M., & Kissin, B. (1967). Evoked cortical responses to affective visual stimuli. *Psychophysiology, 3*, 336–344.

Berkowitz, L. (1993). *Aggression: Its causes, consequences, and control.* Philadelphia: Temple University Press.

Blair, R. J. R. (1995). A cognitive developmental approach to morality: Investigating the psychopath. *Cognition, 57*, 1–29.

Blair, R. J. R. (1999). Responsiveness to distress cues in the child with psychopathic tendencies. *Personality and Individual Differences, 27*, 135–145.

Blair, R. J. R. (2001). Neuro-cognitive models of aggression, the antisocial personality disorders and psychopathy. *Journal of Neurology, Neurosurgery and Psychiatry, 71*, 727–731.

Blair, R. J. (2003a). Neurobiological basis of psychopathy. *British Journal of Psychiatry, 182*, 5–7.

Blair, R. J. R. (2003b). A neurocognitive model of the psychopathic individual. In M. A. Ron & T. W. Robbins (Eds.), *Disorders of brain and mind 2* (pp. 400–420). Cambridge, UK: Cambridge University Press.

Blair, R. J. R. (2004). The roles of orbital frontal cortex in the modulation of antisocial behavior. *Brain and Cognition, 55*, 198–208.

Blair, R. J. R., & Charney, D. S. (2003). Emotion regulation: An affective neuroscience approach. In M. P. Mattson (Ed.), *Neurobiology of aggression: Understanding and preventing violence* (pp. 21–32). Totowa, NJ: Humana Press.

Blair, R. J. R., & Cipolotti, L. (2000). Impaired social response reversal: A case of "acquired sociopathy." *Brain, 123*, 1122–1141.

Blair, R. J., Colledge, E., & Mitchell, D. G. (2001). Somatic markers and response reversal: Is there orbitofrontal cortex dysfunction in boys with psychopathic tendencies? *Journal of Abnormal Child Psychology, 29,* 499–511.

Blair, R. J. R., Jones, L., Clark, F., & Smith, M. (1997). The psychopathic individual: A lack of responsiveness to distress cues? *Psychophysiology, 34,* 192–198.

Blair, R. J. R., Mitchell, D. G. V., Leonard, A., Budhani, S., Peschardt, K. S., & Newman, C. (2004). Passive avoidance learning in psychopathic individuals: Modulation by reward but not by punishment. *Personality and Individual Differences, 37,* 1179–1192.

Blair, R. J. R., Morris, J. S., Frith, C. D., Perrett, D. I., & Dolan, R. (1999). Dissociable neural responses to facial expressions of sadness and anger. *Brain, 122,* 883–893.

Blanchard, R. J., Blanchard, D. C., & Takahashi, L. K. (1977). Attack and defensive behaviour in the albino rat. *Animal Behavior, 25,* 197–224.

Brody, G. H., & Shaffer, D. R. (1982). Contributions of parents and peers to children's moral socialisation. *Developmental Review, 2,* 31–75.

Burdach, K. F. (1819–1822). *Vom baue und Leben des Gehirns.* Leipzig, Germany.

Burns, L. H., Everitt, B. J., & Robbins, T. W. (1999). Effects of excitotoxic lesions of the basolateral amygdala on conditional discrimination learning with primary and conditioned reinforcement. *Behavioural Brain Research, 100,* 123–133.

Charney, D. S. (2003). Neuroanatomical circuits modulating fear and anxiety behaviors. *Acta Psychiatrica Scandinavica, 417*(Suppl.), 38–50.

Charney, D. S., Heninger, G. R., & Breier, A. (1984). Noradrenergic function in panic anxiety. Effects of yohimbine in healthy subjects and patients with agoraphobia and panic disorder. *Archives of General Psychiatry, 41,* 751–763.

Cornell, D. G., Warren, J., Hawk, G., Stafford, E., Oram, G., & Pine, D. (1996). Psychopathy in instrumental and reactive violent offenders. *Journal of Consulting and Clinical Psychology, 64,* 783–790.

Damasio, A. R. (1994). *Descartes' error: Emotion, rationality and the human brain.* New York: Putnam .

Davis, M. (2000). The role of the amygdala in conditioned and unconditioned fear and anxiety. In J. P. Aggleton (Ed.), *The amygdala: A functional analysis* (pp. 289–310). Oxford, UK: Oxford University Press.

Day, R., & Wong, S. (1996). Anomalous perceptual asymmetries for negative emotional stimuli in the psychopath. *Journal of Abnormal Psychology, 105,* 648–652.

Desimone, R., & Duncan, J. (1995). Neural mechanisms of selective visual attention. *Annual Review of Neuroscience, 18,* 193–222.

Dickinson, A., & Dearing, M. F. (1979). Appetitive-aversive interactions and inhibitory processes. In A. Dickinson & R. A. Boakes (Eds.), *Mechanisms of learning and motivation* (pp. 203–231). Hillsdale, NJ: Erlbaum.

Duncan, J. (1998). Converging levels of analysis in the cognitive neuroscience of visual attention. *Philosophical Transactions of the Royal Society of London, Series B, Biological Sciences, 353,* 1307–1317.

Edwards, D. W., Scott, C. L., Yarvis, R. M., Paizis, C. L., & Panizzon, M. S. (2003). Impulsiveness, impulsive aggression, personality disorder, and spousal violence. *Violence and Victims, 18,* 3–14.

Eisenberg, N. (2002). Empathy-related emotional responses, altruism, and their socialization. In R. J. Davidson & A. Harrington (Eds.), *Visions of compassion: Western scientists and Tibetan Buddhists examine human nature* (pp. 131–164). Oxford: Oxford University Press.

Everitt, B. J., Cardinal, R. N., Parkinson, J. A., & Robbins, T. W. (2003). Appetitive behavior: Impact of amygdala-dependent mechanisms of emotional learning. *Annals of the New York Academy of Sciences, 985,* 233–250.

Fine, C., Richell, R. A., Mitchell, D. G. V., Newman, C., Lumsden, J., & Blair, R. J. R. (2004). *Instrumental learning and response reversal: The involvement of the amygdala and orbital frontal cortex and implications for psychopathy.* Manuscript submitted for publication.

Flor, H., Birbaumer, N., Hermann, C., Ziegler, S., & Patrick, C. J. (2002). Aversive Pavlovian conditioning in psychopaths: Peripheral and central correlates. *Psychophysiology, 39,* 505–518.

Fowles, D. C. (1988). Psychophysiology and psychopathy: A motivational approach. *Psychophysiology, 25,* 373–391.

Francis, D. D., & Meaney, M. J. (1999). Maternal care and the development of stress responses. *Current Opinions in Neurobiology, 9,* 128–134.

Frith, C. (2000). The role of dorsolateral prefrontal cortex in the selection of action, as revealed by functional imaging. In S. Monsell & J. Driver (Eds.), *Control of cognitive processes: Attention and performance* (Vol. 18, pp. 549–567). Cambridge, MA: MIT Press.

Grafman, J., Schwab, K., Warden, D., Pridgen, B. S., & Brown, H. R. (1996). Frontal lobe injuries, violence, and aggression: A report of the Vietnam head injury study. *Neurology, 46,* 1231–1238.

Graves, R., Landis, T., & Goodglass, H. (1981). Laterality and sex differences for visual recognition of emotional and non-emotional words. *Neuropsychologia, 19,* 95–102.

Gregg, T. R., & Siegel, A. (2001). Brain structures and neurotransmitters regulating aggression in cats: Implications for human aggression. *Progress in Neuropsychopharmacology and Biological Psychiatry, 25,* 91–140.

Hamann, S., & Mao, H. (2002). Positive and negative emotional verbal stimuli elicit activity in the left amygdala. *Neuroreport, 13,* 15–19.

Hare, R. D. (1965). Temporal gradient of fear arousal in psychopaths. *Journal of Abnormal Psychology, 70,* 442–445.

Hare, R. D. (1970). *Psychopathy: Theory and research.* New York: Wiley.

Hare, R. D. (1982). Psychopathy and physiological activity during anticipation of an aversive stimulus in a distraction paradigm. *Psychophysiology, 19,* 266–271.

Hare, R. D., Frazelle, J., & Cox D. N. (1978). Psychopathy and physiological responses to threat of an aversive stimulus. *Psychophysiology, 15,* 165–172.

Hare, R. D., & Jutai, J. W. (1988). Psychopathy and cerebral asymmetry in semantic processing. *Personality and Individual Differences, 9,* 329–337.

Harmer, C. J., Perrett, D. I., Cowen, P. J., & Goodwin, G. M. (2001). Administration of the beta-adrenoceptor blocker propranolol impairs the processing of facial expressions of sadness. *Psychopharmacology (Berlin), 154,* 383–389.

Hoffman, M. L. (1994). Discipline and internalisation. *Developmental Psychology, 30,* 26–28.

Johnston, J. B. (1923). Further contributions to the study of the evolution of the forebrain. *Journal of Comparative Neurology, 35,* 337–481.

Karnik, N., Delizonna, L., Miller, S., & Steiner, H. (2003). Psychological characteristics of adolescent males with low heart rates. *Scientific Proceedings of the Annual Meeting of the American Academy of Child and Adolescent Psychiatry, 19,* 172.

Kiehl, K. A., Hare, R. D., McDonald, J. J., & Brink, J. (1999). Semantic and affective processing in psychopaths: An event-related potential (ERP) study. *Psychophysiology, 36,* 765–774.

Kiehl, K. A., Smith, A. M., Mendrek, A., Forster, B. B., Hare, R. D., & Liddle, P. F. (2004). Temporal lobe abnormalities in semantic processing by criminal psychopaths as revealed by functional magnetic resonance imaging. *Psychiatry Research, 130,* 27–42.

Killcross, S., Robbins, T. W., & Everitt, B. J. (1997). Different types of fear-conditioned behaviour mediated by separate nuclei within amygdala. *Nature, 388,* 377–380.

Kochanska, G. (1993). Toward a synthesis of parental socialization and child temperament in early development of conscience. *Child Development, 64,* 325–347.

Kochanska, G. (1997). Multiple pathways to conscience for children with different temperaments: From toddlerhood to age 5. *Developmental Psychology, 33,* 228–240.

Kochanska, G., De Vet, K., Goldman, M., Murray, K., & Putman, P. (1994). Maternal reports of conscience development and temperament in young children. *Child Development, 65,* 852–868.

LaPierre, D., Braun, C. M. J., & Hodgins, S. (1995). Ventral frontal deficits in psychopathy: Neuropsychological test findings. *Neuropsychologia, 33,* 139–151.

LeDoux, J. (1998). *The emotional brain.* New York: Weidenfeld & Nicolson.

LeDoux, J. E. (2000). Emotion circuits in the brain. *Annual Review of Neuroscience, 23,* 155–184.

LeDoux, J. E., Farb, C., & Ruggiero, D. A. (1990). Topographical organisation of neurons in the acoustic thalamus that project to the amygdala. *Journal of Neuroscience, 10,* 1043–1054.

Leibenluft, E., Blair, R. J., Charney, D. S., & Pine, D. S. (2003). Irritability in pediatric mania and other childhood psychopathology. *Annals of the New York Academy of Sciences, 1008,* 201–218.

Levenston, G. K., Patrick, C. J., Bradley, M. M., & Lang, P. J. (2000). The psychopath as observer: Emotion and attention in picture processing. *Journal of Abnormal Psychology, 109,* 373–386.

Lichter, J. B., Barr, C. L., Kennedy, J. L., Van Tol, H. H., Kidd, K. K., & Livak, K. J. (1993). A hypervariable segment in the human dopamine receptor D4 (DRD4) gene. *Human Molecular Genetics, 2,* 767–773.

Lorenz, A. R., & Newman, J. P. (2002). Deficient response modulation and emotion processing in low-anxious caucasian psychopathic offenders: Results from a lexical decision task. *Emotion, 2,* 91–104.

Lykken, D. T. (1957). A study of anxiety in the sociopathic personality. *Journal of Abnormal and Social Psychology, 55,* 6–10.

Lykken, D. T. (1995). *The antisocial personalities.* Hillsdale, NJ: Erlbaum.

Malkova, L., Gaffan, D., & Murray, E. A. (1997). Excitotoxic lesions of the amygdala fail to produce impairment in visual learning of auditory secondary reinforcement but interfere with reinforcer devaluation effects in rhesus monkeys. *Journal of Neuroscience, 17,* 6011–6020.

McDonald, A. J. (1998). Cortical pathways to the mammalian amygdala. *Progress in Neurobiology, 55,* 257–332.

Mitchell, D. G. V., Colledge, E., Leonard, A., & Blair, R. J. R. (2002). Risky decisions and response reversal: Is there evidence of orbitofrontal cortex dysfunction in psychopathic individuals? *Neuropsychologia, 40,* 2013–2022.

Mitchell, D. G. V., Richell, R. A., Leonard, A., & Blair, R. J. R. (in press). Emotion at the expense of cognition: Psychopathic individuals outperform controls on an operant response task. *Journal of Abnormal Psychology.*

Moffitt, T. E. (1993). Adolescence-limited and life-course-persistent antisocial behavior: A developmental taxonomy. *Psychological Review, 100,* 674–701.

Nakic, M., Mitchell, D. G. V., Vythilingham, M., & Blair, R. J. R. (2005). *Neural correlates of lexical decision: The impact of emotion and frequency.* Manuscript in preparation.

Newman, J. P. (1998). Psychopathic behaviour: An information processing perspective. In D. J. Cooke, A. E. Forth, & R. D. Hare (Eds.), *Psychopathy: Theory, research and implications for society* (pp. 81–105). Dordrecht, The Netherlands: Kluwer.

Newman, J. P., & Kosson, D. S. (1986). Passive avoidance learning in psychopathic and nonpsychopathic offenders. *Journal of Abnormal Psychology, 95*, 252–256.

Newman, J. P., Patterson, C. M., & Kosson, D. S. (1987). Response perseveration in psychopaths. *Journal of Abnormal Psychology, 96*, 145–148.

Newman, J. P., & Schmitt, W. A. (1998). Passive avoidance in psychopathic offenders: A replication and extension. *Journal of Abnormal Psychology, 107*, 527–532.

Ogloff, J. R., & Wong, S. (1990). Electrodermal and cardiovascular evidence of a coping response in psychopaths. *Criminal Justice and Behaviour, 17*, 231–245.

Panksepp, J. (1998). *Affective neuroscience: The foundations of human and animal emotions*. New York: Oxford University Press.

Pastor, M. C., Molto, J., Vila, J., & Lang, P. J. (2003). Startle reflex modulation, affective ratings and autonomic reactivity in incarcerated Spanish psychopaths. *Psychophysiology, 40*, 934–938.

Patrick, C. J. (1994). Emotion and psychopathy: Startling new insights. *Psychophysiology, 31*, 319–330.

Patrick, C. J., Bradley, M. M., & Lang, P. J. (1993). Emotion in the criminal psychopath: Startle reflex modulation. *Journal of Abnormal Psychology, 102*, 82–92.

Patrick, C. J., Cuthbert, B. N., & Lang, P. J. (1994). Emotion in the criminal psychopath: Fear image processing. *Journal of Abnormal Psychology, 103*, 523–534.

Patrick, C. J., & Lang, A. R. (1999). Psychopathic traits and intoxicated states: Affective concomitants and conceptual links. In M. Dawson, A. Schell, & A. Böhmelt (Eds.), *Startle modification: Implications for neuroscience, cognitive science, and clinical science* (pp. 209–230). Cambridge, UK: Cambridge University Press.

Pavic, L., Gregurek, R., Petrovic, R., Petrovic, D., Varda, R., Vukusic, H., et al. (2003). Alterations in brain activation in posttraumatic stress disorder patients with severe hyperarousal symptoms and impulsive aggressiveness. *European Archives of Psychiatry and Clinical Neuroscience, 253*, 80–83.

Peschardt, K. S., Leonard, A., Morton, J., & Blair, R. J. R. (2004). *Differential stimulus–reward and stimulus–punishment learning in individuals with psychopathy*. Manuscript under revision.

Peschardt, K. S., Morton, J., & Blair, R. J. R. (2003). *They know the words but don't feel the music: Reduced affective priming in psychopathic individuals*. Manuscript under revision.

Peschardt, K. S., Newman, C., Mitchell, D. G. V., Richell, R. A., Leonard, A., Morton, J., et al. (2004). *Differentiating among prefrontal substrates in psychopathy: Neuropsychological test findings*. Manuscript under revision.

Petrides, M. (1982). Motor conditional associative-learning after selective prefrontal lesions in the monkey. *Behavior Brain Research, 5*, 407–413.

Petrides, M. (1985). Deficits on conditional associative-learning tasks after frontal- and temporal-lobe lesions in man. *Neuropsychologia, 23*, 601–614.

Phelps, E. A., O'Connor, K. J., Gatenby, J. C., Gore, J. C., Grillon, C., & Davis, M. (2001). Activation of the left amygdala to a cognitive representation of fear. *Nature Neuroscience, 4*, 437–441.

Pickens, C. L., Saddoris, M. P., Setlow, B., Gallagher, M., Holland, P. C., & Schoenbaum, G. (2003). Different roles for orbitofrontal cortex and basolateral amygdala in a reinforcer devaluation task. *Journal of Neuroscience, 23*, 11078–11094.

Prather, M. D., Lavenex, P., Mauldin-Jourdain, M. L., Mason, W. A., Capitanio, J. P., Mendoza, S. P., et al. (2001). Increased social fear and decreased fear of objects in monkeys with neonatal amygdala lesions. *Neuroscience, 106*, 653–658.

Price, J. L. (2003). Comparative aspects of amygdala connectivity. *Annual Review of the New York Academy of Sciences, 985*, 50–58.

Raine, A. (1993). *The psychopathology of crime: Criminal behavior as a clinical disorder*. San Diego, CA: Academic Press.

Raine, A. (2002). Annotation: the role of prefrontal deficits, low autonomic arousal, and early health factors in the development of antisocial and aggressive behavior in children. *Journal of Child Psychology and Psychiatry, 43*, 417–434.

Raine, A., Venables, P. H., & Williams M. (1996). Better autonomic conditioning and faster electrodermal half-recovery time at age 15 years as possible protective factors against crime at age 29 years. *Developmental Psychology, 32*, 624–630.

Robinson, G., Blair, J., & Cipolotti, L. (1998). Dynamic aphasia: An inability to select between competing verbal responses? *Brain, 121*, 77–89.

Rogeness, G. A., Cepeda, C., Macedo, C. A., Fischer, C., & Harris, W. R. (1990). Differences in heart rate and blood pressure in children with conduct disorder, major depression, and separation anxiety. *Psychiatry Research, 33*, 199–206.

Rogeness, G. A., Javors, M. A., Mass, J. W., & Macedo, C. A. (1990). Catecholamines and diagnoses in children. *Journal of the American Academy of Child and Adolescent Psychiatry , 29*, 234–241.

Rogers, R. D., Everitt, B. J., Baldacchino, A., Blackshaw, A. J., Swainson, R., Wynne, K., et al. (1999). Dissociable deficits in the decision-making cognition of chronic amphetamine abusers, opiate abusers, patients with focal damage to prefrontal cortex, and tryptophan-depleted normal volunteers: Evidence for monoaminergic mechanisms. *Neuropsychopharmacology, 20*, 322–339.

Rogers, R. D., Lancaster, M., Wakeley, J., & Bhagwager Z. (2004). The effects of beta-adrenoceptor blockade on components of human decision-making. *Psychopharmacology, 172*, 157–164.

Rolls, E. T. (1997). The orbitofrontal cortex. *Philosophical Transactions of the Royal Society of London, Series B, Biological Sciences, 351*, 1433–1443.

Rolls, E. T., Hornak, J., Wade, D., & McGrath J. (1994). Emotion-related learning in patients with social and emotional changes associated with frontal lobe damage. *Journal of Neurology, Neurosurgery, and Psychiatry, 57,* 1518–1524.

Rothbart, M., Ahadi, S., & Hershey, K. L. (1994). Temperament and social behaviour in children. *Merrill-Palmer Quarterly, 40,* 21–39.

Shih, J. C., Chen, K., & Ridd, M. J. (1999). Monoamine oxidase: From genes to behavior. *Annual Review of Neuroscience, 22,* 197–217.

Shoal, G. D., Giancola, P. R., & Kirillova, G. P. (2003). Salivary cortisol, personality, and aggressive behavior in adolescent boys: A 5–year longitudinal study. *Journal of the American Academy of Child and Adolescent Psychiatry, 42,* 1101–1107.

Strauss, E. (1983). Perception of emotional words. *Neuropsychologia, 21,* 99–103.

Sustrik, R., Coupland, N., & Blair, R. J. R. (2004). *Noradrenergic drugs and emotion recognition.* Manuscript in preparation.

Tranel, D., & Damasio, H. (1994). Neuroanatomical correlates of electrodermal skin conductance responses. *Psychophysiology, 31,* 427–438.

Usher, M., & Cohen, J. D. (1999). *Short term memory and selection processes in a frontal-lobe model. Connectionist models in cognitive neuroscience.* London: Springer-Verlag.

Vandenbergh, D. J., Persico, A. M., Hawkins, A. L., Griffin, C. A., Li, X., Jabs, E. W., et al. (1992). Human dopamine transporter gene (DAT1) maps to chromosome 5p15.3 and displays a VNTR. *Genomics, 14,* 1104–1106.

Veit, R., Flor, H., Erb, M., Hermann, C., Lotze, M., Grodd, W., et al. (2002). Brain circuits involved in emotional learning in antisocial behavior and social phobia in humans. *Neuroscience Letters, 328,* 233–236.

Verona, E., Patrick, C. J., Curtin, J. J., Bradley, M. M., & Lang, P. J. (2004). Psychopathy and physiological response to emotionally evocative sounds. *Journal of Abnormal Psychology, 113,* 99–108.

Vuilleumier, P., Armony, J. L., Driver, J., & Dolan, R. J. (2001). Effects of attention and emotion on face processing in the human brain: An event-related fMRI study. *Neuron, 30,* 829–841.

Williamson, S., Hare, R. D., & Wong, S. (1987). Violence: Criminal psychopaths and their victims. *Canadian Journal of Behavioral Science, 19,* 454–462.

Williamson, S., Harpur, T. J., & Hare, R. D. (1991). Abnormal processing of affective words by psychopaths. *Psychophysiology, 28,* 260–273.

Wootton, J. M., Frick, P. J., Shelton, K. K., & Silverthorn, P. (1997). Ineffective parenting and childhood conduct problems: The moderating role of callous-unemotional traits. *Journal of Consulting and Clinical Psychology, 65,* 292–300.

16

The Functional Architecture
of the Frontal Lobes

Implications for Research with Psychopathic Offenders

ROBERT D. ROGERS

Modern conceptions of psychopathy have emphasized a complex of personality traits involving callousness, egocentricity, and poverty of emotion, combined with behavioral traits such as impulsiveness, poor behavioral controls, and irresponsibility (Cleckley, 1955; Hare, 1991). The development of reliable techniques for assessing these features—organized around factor structures reflecting interpersonal/affective facets and propensity toward a socially deviant lifestyle (Cooke & Michie, 2001; Hare, 1991, 2003; Harpur, Hare, & Hakstian, 1989)—opens up possibilities for investigating more precisely the neurobiological substrates of the disorder. The frontal lobes play a pivotal role in cognitive control and emotional regulation. Therefore, researchers have naturally proposed that psychopathy is associated with both structural (Raine & Yang, Chapter 14, this volume) and functional (Kiehl, Smith, Hare, & Liddle, 2000) abnormalities within anterior neural systems. However, evidence that psychopathy, as opposed to antisocial behavior defined more generally, is specifically associated with frontal lobe impairment remains sparse. This chapter reviews evidence relevant to this claim and prospects for further progress in this important area of investigation.

First, I describe pertinent anatomical features of the frontal lobes, focusing on connectivity with other cortical and subcortical systems, relevant neurochemistry, and maturational factors. Second, I describe currently prominent models of how anterior cortical systems mediate cognitive control, what is currently known about the functional architecture of these systems, and recent proposals that the representation of affective states and the *regulation* of these states are mediated by distinct but interacting corticolimbic pathways. Third, I consider the strengths and weaknesses of neuropsychological test instruments as a means of assessing frontal lobe dysfunction in psychiatric disorder before considering in detail the extant evidence for specific deficits in psychopathic as compared to nonpsychopathic offenders. These sections consider the evidence for neuropsychological deficits associated with distinct frontal sectors, as well as evidence that psychopathy is associated with response control deficits. I argue that recent studies, exploiting contemporary neuropsychology, provide encouraging evidence for altered functioning in corticolimbic circuitry mediating emotional signaling and regulation. Finally, I comment on prospects for further progress. Comparison with developments in the schizophrenia literature suggests that progress depends on identification of neurobiological mechanisms that can be linked to cognitive and emotional deficits associated with psychopathy ("endophenotypes") with plausible biological roles in the etiology of the disorder.

ANATOMY OF THE FRONTAL LOBES

Traditionally, the frontal lobes are divided into three sectors: a primary motor sector, a premotor sector, and a prefrontal sector—the prefrontal cortex (PFC) being widely proposed as being at the top of a hierarchy of control and mediating the most uniquely human of cognitive and emotional functions (Fuster, 1989). The cortical surface of the frontal lobes, accounting for roughly 30% of the cerebrum, consists of a number of subregions that differ in terms of their cytoarchitectonic properties and interconnections. These subregions have marked homologies (as well as moderate differences) between humans and monkeys (Brodmann, 1925; see Petrides & Pandya, 1999); however, their functional significance in health and in psychiatric disorder, such as psychopathy, remains an area of highly active, and often controversial, research.

Several features of frontal lobe anatomy are relevant to understanding its function. First, sectors of the frontocortical surface have distinctive patterns of connections with other frontal sectors, with subcortical/limbic nuclei, and with posterior cortical systems. These patterns of interconnectivity provide significant clues as to the cognitive and emotional functions subserved by PFC regions (Barbas, 2000). Caudal lateral areas of the PFC receive projections from visual, auditory, and somatosensory association cortices; from intraparietal and posterior cingulate; and from the thalamic structures including the mediodorsal nucleus (Petrides & Pandya, 1999). Cortical afferents tend to overlap, so that this part of the PFC can process converging information from multimodal sensory systems. In turn, caudal lateral prefrontal areas project to premotor and supplementary motor cortex involved in the control of head, body, and limb movements; the PFC does not project to primary motor cortex. There are direct connections from

lateral PFC to rostral cingulate cortex and to the frontal eye fields, suggesting a role for this region of PFC in the control of gaze and overt attention (Passingham, 1993). Lateral PFC also projects to the major neurochemical nuclei within the brainstem reticular formation, consistent with a role in oculomotor control, motor planning, arousal, and attention.

By contrast, the caudal orbitofrontal cortex is richly innervated by cortical areas that support relatively late stages of unimodal visual, auditory, and somatosensory processing (Barbas, 2000; Carmichael & Price, 1996). Other afferents convey olfactory and gustatory inputs (Ongur & Price, 2000). Notably, caudal orbitofrontal cortex receives information from medial temporal cortical structures including the hippocampal–amygdala complex. In turn, efferent connections from the medial orbitofrontal cortex project to the ventral striatum and the medial caudate nucleus as well as hypothalamic visceromotor centers (Ongur & Price, 2000). These connections form part of a larger distributed network of neural stations—including the insula cortex, amygdala, anterior cingulate cortex (ACC), and periaquaductal gray—that is closely implicated in the control of autonomic and visceral function (Ongur & Price, 2000).

Second, the PFC is richly innervated by the ascending arousal systems of the reticular formation, and there is now abundant evidence from experiments with both animal and human subjects that the cognitive and emotional functions of dorsolateral and orbital sectors of the PFC are highly sensitive to changes in the neuromodulatory activity of the monoamine and catecholamine systems (Robbins, 1996). For example, the ability to maintain information within short-term or "working" memory depends on dopaminergic modulation within dorsolateral PFC (mediated by D_1 receptor activity; Sawaguchi & Goldman-Rakic, 1991), whereas the ability to maintain memory performance under stress or distraction depends on noradrenergic action (mediated by α_1- and α_2-adrenoceptors; Arnsten, 2000). By contrast, relearning stimulus–reward associations—a function largely dependent on the orbitofrontal cortex (Rolls, 1999)—is impaired by reductions in central serotonergic activity (Rogers, Blackshaw, et al., 1999).

Clinical evidence suggests that particular personality traits present in impulsive personality disorders (and likely to be shared with psychopathy) are associated with dysfunction within these systems (Coccaro et al., 1989; Soderstrom, Blennow, Sjodin, & Forsman, 2003). Such dysfunction may be associated with cognitive impairments, reflecting altered neuromodulation of PFC, but detectable by neuropsychological assessment.

Anatomical studies suggest that the processing of the PFC recruits identifiable circuits or "cortico–striatal–thalamic" loops that have dissociable functions in cognitive control and affective regulation (Alexander, Delong, & Strick, 1986). Discrete areas of the frontocortical surface send excitatory (glutamate) fibers to the neostriatum (caudate, putamen), which in turn sends inhibitory (GABAergic) fibers to the globus pallidus/substantia nigra. These nuclei project onto discrete thalamic targets. Finally, glutamate pathways from these thalamic nuclei project back to the original cortical area to form partially closed loops. Because the striatal targets of these circuits receive input from cortical association areas, these circuits provide a mechanism for integrating information from various cortical sources and other cortico–striatal–thalamic loops, which can be relayed back to the original cortical regions and/or output mechanisms. Several "cortico–striatal–thalamo–cortical" loops have been identified; including two linking dorsolateral and orbitofrontal areas to discrete striatothalamic pathways, and a third that originates in the ACC. The functioning of these loops is influenced at several neural stations by neuromodulatory systems, including the mesocortical and mesostriatal dopamine systems, serotonergic systems, and the cholinergic system originating in the nucleus basalis of Meynert (Haber, Kunishio, Mizobuchi, & Lynd-Balta, 1995).

The precise functional significance of the loops and the degree to which they either integrate or segregate information remains controversial (Robbins & Rogers, 2001). However, it is clear that cortico–striatal–thalamic loops are involved in the cognitive control mediated by PFC. Studies have shown comparable impairments in the performance of behavioral tasks when lesions are made at different sites within the same loop (Goldman & Rosvold, 1972). Moreover, patients with early-in-the-course Parkinson's disease demonstrate deficits comparable to patients with focal lesions of the frontal lobes, suggesting that reduced catecholamine activity disrupts fronto–striatal–thalamic functioning involved in cognitive control (Owen et al., 1992).

Finally, the time course of cortical maturation within specific regions of the frontal lobes continues well into adolescence. Recent data, acquired using magnetic resonance imaging obtained every 2 years between the ages of 4 and 21 years to map the dynamic sequence of cortical gray matter development, suggest that higher-order association cortices (including the PFC) mature only after lower-order sensory cortices have developed, and that maturation of PFC continues well into late adolescence (Gogtay et al., 2004). Therefore, disrupted maturation of PFC may occur within a relatively extended interval to undermine specific cognitive and emotional processes required for the effective organization and control of behavior—thereby increasing the risk of psychiatric disorder and serious delinquency (Bauer & Hesselbrock, 2004).

FRONTAL LOBES AND MODELS OF COGNITIVE CONTROL

Lesions of the frontal lobes have been shown to be associated with problems in the control of behavior at least since the early 19th century. In 1922, Bianchi noted that large frontal lesions in monkeys induced an inability to combine different actions appropriately in a complex activity. Other subsequent studies found that frontal lobe damage was associated with changes in fear and anxiety (Anderson & Hanvik, 1950; Moniz, 1937), as well as reductions in drive and energy and increased irritability (Miller, 1959). However, the failure to demonstrate consistent changes in IQ following frontal lobe damage (e.g., Mettler, 1949) engendered the view that the frontal lobes support few intellectual functions (Hebb, 1945). This view was successfully challenged by the work of Milner (1964) and Luria (1969), who investigated task-specific changes in cognitive function following frontal lobe damage and reported a tendency toward perseveration and a failure to use external cues to adjust behavior, as well as deficient verbal fluency.

Since Milner (1964) and Luria (1969), the dominant view has been that the frontal lobes are the site of a broad "executive" system that mediates flexible control of cognitive and motor resources for the attainment of distal goals (see Shallice, 1982, 1988, for a full statement of this position). Fuster (1989) suggested that the frontal lobes have a "superordinate function . . . to form temporal structures of behaviour with a unifying purpose or goal." Norman and Shallice (1986) advanced a model that exemplifies the metaphor. In this model, the lowest level of control consists of routines or schemas that govern discrete patterns of thought or action that can be triggered by appropriate environmental stimuli; these schemas can then "run off" with little or no input from higher levels of control. Schemas can be organized into hierarchies through learning, so that more complicated action sequences can be acquired and triggered by activation of a "source" schema that then recruits component schemas into motor output.

According to Norman and Shallice (1986), two kinds of control are available to this system. First, there is a "contention scheduling" mechanism by which mutual inhibition between schemas at each level of the hierarchy ensures that only the schema with the strongest activation—determined by the presence of stimulus triggers, and the recency and frequency with which the schema has been activated—can win out at that level of control. Second, there is a supervisory attentional system (SAS) that "has access to a representation of the environment and of the organism's intentions and cognitive capacities" and is able to activate or inhibit activity within source schemas to bias contention scheduling so that the appropriate schema gains control of the system. Critically, the SAS is active in situations involving novelty, novel actions in a familiar context (e.g., overcoming temptation); troubleshooting, danger or technical difficulty, and decision making and planning. This list has been taken as a prototypical specification of the so-called executive control functions. In its original conception, the SAS was thought to be a unitary, limited capacity resource and was incorporated into other models of control including Baddeley's central executive (Baddeley, 1986); a similar construct was

also apparent in the distinction between controlled and automatic processing (Shiffrin & Schneider, 1977). However, recent developments have sought to fractionate the SAS and establish distinct underlying neural substrates for its components (Shallice & Burgess, 1996; see below).

The metaphor that cognitive control is achieved by biasing input that acts to increase or decrease activity in specialized modules has survived in more recent theoretical accounts of the role of the PFC in cognitive control. Miller and Cohen (2001) recently proposed that the PFC mediates representations of both goals and the action sequences needed to achieve them. These representations provide biasing signals to other brain structures so that the relative patterns of activity along neural pathways establish appropriate mappings between sensory inputs, internal states (of all kinds), and output mechanisms. In this context, Miller and Cohen identified features of the architecture and cellular properties of PFC that make it suitable for this purpose.

First, as noted earlier, the PFC has interconnections with virtually all sensory, cortical, and subcortical motor systems, as well as limbic systems controlling affective, reinforcement, and autonomic information. Second, PFC cells exhibit a high degree of plasticity that promotes flexible links between input and output to facilitate the expression of motivationally appropriate behaviour. For example, Assad, Rainer, and Miller (1998) reported that the majority of cells within the PFC were able to acquire patterns of activity that reflected the rule governing a conditional response ("if object A, saccade left") rather than just the presentation of the cue or execution of the response (see also Thorpe, Rolls, & Maddison, 1983). Third, the efferent connections of the PFC are able to provide feedback to influence activity in other brain systems. Fourth, PFC activity reflects the representation of goals that can be maintained over intervals when task-relevant stimuli are absent (Goldman & Rakic, 1987). Finally, PFC supports information processing relevant to anticipated events and the priming of output mechanisms. There is abundant evidence that PFC neurons code the expected size and valence of anticipated reinforcers and mediate choice between actions associated with these reinforcers (Tremblay & Schultz, 1999).

Cognitive neuroscience research now uses a wide variety of techniques for generating convergent evidence concerning the contribution of these features of frontal lobe function to the control of cognition and affect. Accordingly, research indicates that the PFC plays a prominent role in an extraordinarily broad range of cognitive activity, including (but not limited to) short-term spatial and object-based memory (Goldman-Rakic, 1987); encoding and retrieval processes in episodic and prospective memory (Burgess, Scott, & Frith, 2003); control of attentional set (Dias, Robbins, & Roberts, 1996); the initiation of voluntary action (Passingham, 1993); the representation of intention (Lau, Rogers, Haggard, & Passingham, 2004); decision making under uncertainty (Bechara, Tranel, Damasio, & Damasio, 1996; Rogers, Everitt, et al., 1999); pain processing and conditioning of anticipatory anxiety (Ploghaus et al., 1999); the representation of affective responses to primary and secondary reinforcers (Rolls, 1999); the perception of others' mental states and aspects of social cognition (Frith & Frith, 2003); response inhibitory processes (Aron, Robbins, & Poldrack, 2004); and even the cortical representation of Spearman's g (Duncan et al., 2000).

Despite these advances, localization of function within the PFC has proven highly controversial so that there remain very few demonstrations of double dissociations of distinct cognitive processes within the PFC or the frontal lobes more broadly (Dias et al., 1996). Indeed, there has been some suggestion that only general task difficulty consistently recruits dorsolateral PFC circuits (Duncan & Owen, 2000). Alternative proposals (see Owen, 1997, for review; Petrides, 1996) include the suggestion that the PFC mediates the same set of cognitive operations (e.g., working memory) over distinct types of information represented in PFC fields (e.g., spatial information in dorsolateral PFC and object information in ventrolateral PFC), and the suggestion that different sectors of PFC mediate different *processes* on the same kinds of information (e.g., monitoring of information in dorsolateral PFC and retrieval from longer-term storage in ventrolateral PFC).

The foregoing discussion highlights a multiplicity of mechanisms by which the frontal lobes contribute to the cognitive control. However, it is also possible to evaluate what is known about the function of circuitries involving different portions of the PFC with a view to postulating distinct but interacting functional systems. Importantly, Phillips, Drevets, Rauch, and Lane (2003) have proposed that a ventral anterior system—encompassing orbitofrontal PFC, insula, ventral striatum, rostrocingulate cortex, and amygdala—plays a predominant role in the identification and appraisal of emotional stimuli and the mediation of resultant affective states, while a dorsal system—encompassing dorsal PFC regions, the hippocampus, and dorsal ACC—plays a role in *regulating* such affective experiences and modulating behavior. The role of the PFC (involving these dorsal and ventral subdivisions) in emotion regulation is considered in the next section.

LOCALIZATION OF FRONTAL LOBE FUNCTION AND THE REGULATION OF AFFECT

Evidence for the involvement of the anterior cortical system in the perception and appraisal of emotional stimuli includes findings that the ventral PFC represents the affective value of both primary and secondary reinforcers in relation to motivational states (Rolls, 1999), mediates learning revised stimulus–reward associations (Thorpe et al., 1983), and interacts with the amygdala to inhibit sympathetic autonomic arousal and defensive reactions elicited by amygdala stimulation (e.g., Timms, 1977) and the presentation of fear-conditioned stimuli (Sullivan & Grattan, 1999). Evidence for the involvement of the insula cortex includes findings that lesions in this cortical area impair identification of facial and vocal expressions of disgust (Calder, Lawrence, & Young, 2001), whereas stimulation of this area induces perception of unpleasant tastes (Penfield & Faulk, 1955). Lesions of the rostrocingulate cortex abolish autonomic responses to conditioned stimuli and vocalized responses to painful stimuli, and can result in reduced aggression and emotional blunting (MacLean & Newman, 1988). As noted previously, the orbitofrontal and rostrocingulate cortices interact, by cortico–striatal–thalamic loops, with the ventral striatum in reward prediction and incentive-motivation (see Schultz, Tremblay, & Hollerman, 2000, for a review).

Support for the proposal that dorsal PFC, ACC, and the hippocampus support the *regulation* of affective states includes demonstrations that the hippocampal system is involved in both activation and inhibition of behavior in response to aversive environmental stimuli (Gray, 1982), and in the inhibition of stress responses via inhibitory connections with other stress-related centers (Lopez, Akil, & Watson, 1999). Evidence for the involvement of dorsal PFC includes findings that this cortical region is involved in overriding attentional bias toward stimulus dimensions associated with reinforcement (e.g., Rogers, Andrews, Grasby, Brooks, & Robbins, 2000). Involvement of the dorsal medial PFC and dorsal ACC in the regulation of affective states is indicated by their involvement in error processing as indicated by the "error-related negativity" (ERN; Kiehl, Liddle, & Hopfinger, 2000), the representation of arousal and uncertainty (Critchley, Elliott, Mathias, & Dolan, 2000), attention to subjective emotional experiences (Gusnard, Akbudak, Shulman, & Raichle, 2001), and self-reflective thought (Johnson et al., 2002). Similarly, activation of the dorsal medial PFC is specifically associated with lowered blood flow during exposure to anxiety-inducing stimuli (Simpson, Drevets, Snyder, Gusnard, & Raichle, 2001) and induction of sad mood (Mayberg et al., 1999). (See Phillips et al., 2003, for a statement of these proposals and review of the supportive evidence.)

NEUROPSYCHOLOGICAL ASSESSMENT AND FRONTAL LOBE DYSFUNCTION

In the light of the foregoing discussion, it is unsurprising that research into the neural substrates of psychopathy should focus on the role of the frontal lobes. Specifically, the wider role of the PFC in organizing cognitive and motor resources to achieve behavioral flexibility suggests that PFC dysfunction may mediate facets of psychopathy associated with an antisocial lifestyle (Factor 2; Hare, 1991). However, equally, the role of the PFC in representing emotional information and regulating emotional response may also be important for understanding the interpersonal–affective features of the disorder (Factor 1; Hare, 1991). Systematic investigation

of these hypotheses, exploiting our increasing understanding of the anatomical and functional characteristics of the frontal lobes, has barely begun. Rather, much clinical research in this area has relied on traditional neuropsychological instruments such as the Wisconsin Card Sorting Task (WCST; Grant & Berg, 1948) or the Stroop Color–Word Interference task (Stroop, 1935) to assess executive control functions. Royall and colleagues (2002) provide a comprehensive review of the methodological assumptions behind this work and highlight important issues that need to be borne in mind when considering the use of frontal lobe tests in psychiatric populations. As pointed out previously, PFC sectors contribute to distributed networks involving subcortical and posterior systems that mediate control over particular cognitive and motor resources involved in a given task. Consequently, impairment may reflect compromised control function mediated by that portion of PFC circuitry (rather than an overarching, unitary executive system) or dysfunction in task-specific component resources themselves.

Attempts to compile definitive lists of executive functions and identify tasks that load on stable factor structures reflecting underlying dimensions of control have identified factors such as rule discovery, working memory, attentional control, and response inhibition (Grozinksy & Diamond, 1992). However, traditional clinical neuropsychological tasks do not tap these factors selectively (Royall et al., 2002). Therefore, the *psychological* meaning of impairments on such tasks in terms of specific underlying control mechanisms often remains unclear.

In addition, the specificity and sensitivity of neuropsychological tests with respect to underlying neural dysfunction in frontal lobe systems is uncertain. The WCST is widely cited as the quintessential measure of executive control. Subjects/patients are asked to match response cards to one of four stimulus cards on the basis of a rule that must be inferred from experimenter feedback. The stimulus cards differ by values on three stimulus dimensions (color, number, and shape). After 10 correct sorts, the experimenter changes the rule and the subject must learn the new sorting principle (Milner, 1964). Several studies have shown that patients with focal damage to the frontal lobes do not identify (achieve) as many sorting rules (categories) as do patients with posterior lesions, and their behavior is characterized by a tendency to continue to sort by the previously correct sorting rule (Milner, 1964). However, the specificity and sensitivity of the WCST for frontal dysfunction remain doubtful. One careful neuropsychological investigation found no differences in performance between 49 frontal lobe patients and 42 control-lesion patients, while optimal cutoff scores correctly classified only 62% of patients as having frontal lobe damage (Anderson, Damasio, Jones, & Tranel, 1991; see also van den Broek, Bradshaw, & Szabadi, 1993).

Similarly, Reitan and Wolfson (1995) found that neither the Category Test (a concept formation task related to the WCST) nor Part B of the Trail Making-Test (TMT)—tasks that require repeated switches of attentional and response sets (Lezak, 1995)—discriminated adequately between patients with frontal and nonfrontal damage. Finally, analyses of the usefulness of the Stroop task (Stroop, 1935) for establishing frontal lobe damage revealed evidence of impairments associated with posterior cortical dysfunction (Pujol et al., 2001), suggesting that at least some aspects of efficient Stroop performance—such as selective attention and response inhibition—recruit cortical systems outside the frontal lobes (Andres, 2003; but see Stuss, Floden, Alexander, Levine, & Katz, 2001). These, and other findings, indicate that impaired performance on neuropsychological tests is a relatively inaccurate and *indirect* guide to the presence of frontal lobe dysfunction. For this reason, there has been recognition of the need to supplement data from such tasks with convergent information reflecting more directly the functioning of underlying neural substrates, such as that provided by brain-imaging and electrophysiological techniques.

NEUROPSYCHOLOGICAL EVIDENCE FOR FRONTAL LOBE DYSFUNCTION IN ANTISOCIAL GROUPS

The proposal that psychopathy is associated with impairments in frontal lobe functioning originated with neurological observations of altered mood, affect, and behavior after neurological damage to this region (see Kandel

& Freed, 1989, for a review). More recently, it has been suggested that it is damage to the orbitofrontal cortex specifically that is associated with behavioral and affective changes that might relate to antisocial personality and psychopathy (e.g., Meyers, Berman, Schiebel, & Hayman, 1992). This view was most clearly expressed by the proposal that orbitofrontal lesions induce "pseudopsychopathy" (characterized by thoughtlessness, impulsivity, and a disregard for social norms) whereas lesions of the dorsolateral cortex induce a "pseudodepression" (apathy, lowered mood, and psychomotor slowing; Blumer & Benson, 1975).

However, while lesions of the orbitofrontal cortex—particularly when sustained early in life (Anderson, Bechara, Damasio, Tranel, & Damasio, 1999)—can profoundly compromise social function, the comparison with psychopathy is frequently overstated. Reviews of the neurological data have highlighted enormous variation in the localization of damage within affected individuals, suggesting that the relationship between frontal lobe damage and changes in mood and affect remains highly uncertain (Nauta, 1971). Moreover, attempts to establish such links have tended to ignore premorbid personality in affected individuals and to dwell on a subset of features associated with psychopathy, such as poor behavioural controls and impulsivity (Elliot, 1978; Hare, 1984; but see Eslinger, 1997). These latter features are as likely to involve dysfunction in wider circuitry such as medial temporal cortices (Raine, Buchsbaum, & LaCasse, 1997).

Even so, repeated observations that frontal lobe damage can be associated with impairments in the control of behavior in both clinical settings (e.g., Meyers et al., 1992) and experimental settings (e.g., Hornak, Rolls, Wade, & McGrath, 1994) have sustained neuropsychological research into the presence and possible importance of frontal lobe deficits in various delinquent and antisocial populations. Early studies demonstrated significantly impaired performance on the Halstead–Reitan Neuropsychological Battery in adult offender and delinquent groups in comparison with either healthy nonoffender controls or individuals with depressive disorder (Yeudall & Fromm-Auch, 1979; Yeudall, Fromm-Auch, & Davis, 1982). Anticipating contemporary perspectives (Blair, 2003), these results were interpreted as suggesting an association between antisocial behavior and frontotemporal dysfunction. Subsequent studies involving similar comparisons of prison and hospitalized offenders identified as suffering from DSM-IV antisocial personality disorder (APD) with nonoffender controls have tended to confirm these findings (e.g., Dinn & Harris, 2000; Dolan & Park, 2002). In an influential meta-analytic review of 39 studies of executive control function in diverse antisocial samples, Morgan and Lilienfeld (2000) reported effects of medium to large size on putative frontal lobe tasks including the WCST, Stroop task, Part B of the TMT, verbal fluency, Category Test of the Halstead–Reitan Neuropsychological Battery, and the Porteus Maze task. The variability of impairment across studies was interpreted as reflecting varying methods of defining antisocial groups (i.e., delinquency, conduct disorder, or APD according to DSM-III or DSM-III-R criteria) as well as uncontrolled differences in substance abuse and associated illness (e.g., attention-deficit/hyperactivity disorder [ADHD]).

Overall, the pattern of effects reported by Morgan and Lilienfeld (2000) supports the view that marked impairments in neuropsychological test performance are evident in comparisons between various antisocial sample and healthy nonoffending control samples. Consequently, in assessing differences between psychopathic offenders and nonpsychopathic offenders (see below), it should be borne in mind that such differences may be attributable to, or superimposed on, a basal level of performance deficits associated with APD per se. Such deficits are likely to reflect widely reported reductions in general intelligence or IQ (Wilson & Herrnstein, 1985), in more specific left-hemisphere mediated verbal functions (as evidenced by discrepant performance and verbal IQs; West & Farrington, 1973), as well as impairments in executive functions such as planning, response sequencing, and inhibition (Skoff & Libon, 1987). Such impairments are probably not attributable to sampling bias, poor clinical assessment, or comorbid psychiatric disorder. For instance, Moffitt and Silva (1988) found impairments in verbal, visuospatial, *visuomotor, and* cognitive flexibility measures in delinquents (identified by self-report and informant data)

with *and without* comorbid ADHD (identified by interview and informants) in comparison to healthy controls. In the following sections, I critically review the existing evidence for frontal lobe deficits in relation to psychopathy more narrowly defined.

NEUROPSYCHOLOGICAL EVIDENCE FOR FRONTAL DYSFUNCTION IN PSYCHOPATHIC OFFENDERS

Although serious controversy concerning frontal lobe deficits in psychopathic offenders developed only in the early 1980s through the early 1990s, findings of studies prior to this time provided at least suggestive evidence (Lidberg, Levander, Schalling, & Lidberg, 1978). Typifying early studies, Schalling and Rosen (1968) found that criminals rated high in psychopathy according to the criteria provided by Cleckley (1955) were less diligent in their performance of the Porteus Maze task, which requires subjects to trace a pathway through a maze presented on a sheet of paper, and less accurate as indicated by the task's Q-score (Lezak, 1995) compared to criminals with low psychopathy ratings. However, while between-group differences in age and alcohol abuse do not appear to have influenced these particular results, interpretation of these data, and that from other similar studies, is complicated by variation in diagnostic procedures and task sensitivity.

The first systematic investigation of frontal lobe function in psychopathic offenders was provided by Gorenstein (1982). The rationale for this study derived from analysis of the behavioral changes observed following septal–hippocampal lesions in experimental animals, and the proposal that disruption of a wider circuitry incorporating the PFC may account for disinhibition in psychopathy and other forms of psychopathology (Gorenstein & Newman, 1980; Patterson & Newman, 1983). Forty-three patients, recruited from substance abuse programs, and 18 college student controls participated. Patients were categorized as psychopathic (n = 23) and nonpsychopathic (n = 20) on the basis of two diagnostic indicators: a diagnosis of DSM-III APD (American Psychiatric Association, 1980) according to a self-report version of the Research Diagnostic Criteria (Spitzer, Endicott & Robins, 1975) and a score of 27 or less on the Socialization (*So*) Scale of the California Psychological Inventory (CPI; Gough, 1960). The test battery consisted of the WCST, Stroop Color–Word task, Sequential Matching Memory Task (SMMT; Lezak, 1995), Necker cube task (Teuber, 1964), and a control anagram task.

The SMMT requires subjects to monitor a series of visually presented numbers and, on each trial, repeat the sign (plus or minus) of the number presented three places earlier in the series. It involves the maintenance of information within working memory and, in modern forms, has consistently been shown to depend on lateral PFC function (Owen, 1997). There is less consistent evidence that focal damage to the frontal lobes affects the stability of perceptual experience while viewing the Necker cube (a visual illusion involving alterations in depth/figure perception); however, both Teuber (1964) and Cohen (1959) reported significant deficits after bilateral damage. Planned comparisons showed that psychopathic offenders did not differ in their performance of the Stroop Color–Word task or the anagram task compared to the controls and nonpsychopathic offenders. However, psychopathic offenders made more errors on the WCST and the SMMT and more spontaneous reversals on the Necker cube compared to both the nonpsychopathic offender group and the college controls. Gorenstein (1982) interpreted these results as support for the proposal that psychopathic offenders show impairments in frontal function.

Gorenstein's interpretation of his data was forcefully challenged by Hare (1984), who raised concerns about the reliability of the diagnostic procedures used and the consistency with which they were applied. Given that both DSM-III-R APD and the *So* scale of the CPI are both selectively associated with an antisocial lifestyle (Factor 2 of the PCL-R; Hare, 1991), the psychopathic offenders in Gorenstein (1982) were differentiated from the control group mainly on the antisocial deviance component of psychopathy and not on the affective–interpersonal component. Consequently, Hare noted that patients in Gorenstein's study would have shown only low-to-moderate ratings of psychopathy on the recently developed Psychopathy Checklist (PCL; Hare, 1980). Other concerns included a lack of matching on demographic and educational variables and the possibility that the deficits in the psychopathic compared to nonpsychopathic patients might have been attributable to comorbid substance abuse (cf. Rogers, Everitt, et al., 1999). In his own study, Hare compared the performance of high (*n* = 14), medium (*n* = 16), and low (*n* = 16) psychopathic offender groups identified by application of the PCL; the groups were balanced for age, education, cognitive ability, and scores on the *So* scale. Analysis showed that high, medium, and low psychopathic offenders showed no significant differences in performance on the three principal tasks: the WCST, Necker cube, and SMMT. Citing these findings, together with unpublished data indicating normal performance of psychopaths on the Stroop task, Hare successfully cast doubt on Gorenstein's findings as a basis for inferring frontal lobe deficits in psychopathy.

Subsequent studies of frontal lobe function in psychopathic offenders focused on the importance of diagnostic procedures and have tended to sustain researchers' skepticism (e.g., Blair & Frith, 2000). Hoffman, Hall, and Bartsch (1987) attempted a direct replication of Gorenstein (1982) by administering a battery of neuropsychological tests consisting of the SMMT (and a related memory test involving interference between items), the Necker cube, the WCST, and the Mazes subtest of the Weschler Intelligence Scale for Children (WISC) to 81 substance abusers assessed for psychopathy using exactly the same procedure as described in Gorenstein. Surprisingly, given that this diagnostic classification procedure would tend to define subgroups of offenders with high versus low levels of antisociality (as opposed to groups differing in the interpersonal–affective features of psychopathy), there were no significant differences between the groups on frontal lobe measures.

Similarly, Sutker and Allain (1987; see also Sutker, Moan, & Allain, 1983) administered the WCST, the Porteus Maze, and a card-based visual–verbal test sensitive to frontal lobe damage (Stuss & Benson, 1984) to 19 psychopaths and 15 age- and IQ-matched nonpsychopathic offenders. The psychopaths were diagnosed according to the following composite criteria: a score above the

70th percentile on the Psychopathic Deviate (Pd) scale, or on both the Pd and Hypomania scales, of the Minnesota Multiphasic Personality Inventory (MMPI; Hathaway & McKinley, 1943); a score of 32 or *above* on the "MMPI Pd minus CPI *So*" index of psychopathy (on which higher scores reflect greater deviance; Heilbrun, 1982); and a diagnosis of DSM-III APD. Again, there was no indication that psychopathic offenders performed worse on the frontal lobe tasks than did nonpsychopathic offenders. It should be noted that all three diagnostic measures used in this study (MMPI Pd/Hypomania scales, Pd minus *So* index; DSM-III APD) are primarily indicators of antisociality, as opposed to the core interpersonal–affective features of psychopathy (Hare, 1991, 2003; Lilienfeld & Fowler, Chapter 6, this volume). Consequently, the relevance of these findings to an understanding of frontal lobe function in psychopathy is uncertain.

Finally, Devonshire, Howard, and Sellars (1988) examined performance of the WCST in mentally disordered offenders held in a British maximum-security hospital. Comparison of those stipulated as suffering from a "psychopathic disorder" according to the Mental Health Act (1983; UK) with those stipulated as "mentally ill," and comparison of offenders scoring high as compared to low on the PCL, failed to show significant differences in performance on the WCST. In fact, those offenders diagnosed as "primary" psychopaths achieved significantly *more* sorting categories than those diagnosed as "secondary" psychopaths using Blackburn's (1974)criteria.

Integrating the findings of Gorenstein (1982), Hare (1984), and Devonshire and colleagues (1988), together with the meta-analysis provided by Morgan and Lilienfeld (2000), suggests that the antisocial deviance features of psychopathy (Factor 2; Hare, 1991) are associated with relatively poor frontal lobe function, whereas the affective–interpersonal features (Factor 1; Hare, 1991) are associated with normal or perhaps even better frontal function. Assessment procedures that result in groups differing primarily on Factor 2 (e.g., Gorenstein, 1982) are likely to yield differences on frontal lobe tasks, whereas assessment procedures that result in groups differing primarily on Factor 1 or on both factors together (Devonshire et

al., 1988; Hare, 1984) are likely to yield null or opposing findings. From this perspective, the failure of Hoffman and colleagues (1987) and Sutker and Allain (1987) to replicate the findings of Gorenstein is somewhat inexplicable given that the assessment methods used in these studies would have favored the formation of groups differing markedly on the antisocial deviance component of psychopathy.

In any case, the foregoing findings provide little evidence that psychopathy as indexed by overall scores on the PCL is associated with deficits in frontal lobe function. Further support for this conclusion comes from a study by Smith, Arnett, and Newman (1992), who administered a comprehensive battery of frontal lobe tasks to a larger sample of 69 inmate offenders assessed with the PCL (Hare, 1980). Psychopathic offenders were identified as those exhibiting high levels of both the affective–interpersonal and antisocial deviance features. The neuropsychological battery included the TMT, the fluency measure from the Controlled Word Association Test (CWAT; Benton & Hamsher, 1976), the Stroop task, and a shortened Category Test. Although there were a number of performance differences between high and low anxious offenders, only performance on the TMT differed between the psychopathic (n = 32) and nonpsychopathic offenders (n = 37).

More definitively, Hart, Forth, and Hare (1990) administered comprehensive neuropsychological test batteries to two independent samples of inmates (N = 90; N = 167) assessed for high, medium, and low levels of psychopathy using the Psychopathy Checklist—Revised (PCL-R; Hare, 1991). One test battery consisted of the TMT (see above), together with memory tests including the Visual Retention Test (Benton, 1974), Auditory–Verbal Learning Test (AVLT; Lezak, 1995; Rey, 1964), and Visual Organization Test (Hooper, 1958). The second test battery consisted of the TMT, verbal fluency from the CWAT, and the vocabulary and block design subtests of the Wechsler Adult Intelligence Scale—Revised (WAIS-R; Weschler, 1998). Substance abuse history and self-report depression and anxiety were carefully matched across subject groups. Test performance indicated equivalent and low rates of impairment in comparison with published norms, and no indication that offenders with high PCL-R scores were impaired on either the TMT or the fluency measure of the CWAT relative to offenders with medium or low PCL-R scores.

While the foregoing studies provide little evidence that psychopathic offenders exhibit widespread frontal lobe impairments, none of these studies examined relations separately for the two factors of the PCL, and none of these studies distinguished adequately among the different cognitive and emotional functions mediated by the frontal lobes or between the differences in the anterior corticolimbic systems that subserve these functions. As noted in earlier sections, the frontal lobes do not support a unitary supervisory or control system recruited in equal measure by neuropsychological tests thought to be sensitive to frontal lobe damage or dysfunction. Moreover, the traditional neuropsychological tests used in the aforementioned studies of psychopathy and frontal lobe function are predominantly cognitive in character, reflecting processes of selective attention (Stroop), manipulation of information within short-term memory (SMMT), response planning (Maze learning), cognitive control (WCTS and TMT), and strategic search within longer-term storage (CWAT). In view of contemporary conceptions of psychopathy that emphasize the importance of emotional deficits (Blair, Chapter 15, this volume; Fowles & Dindo, Chapter 2, this volume; Patrick, 1994; Williamson, Harpur, & Hare, 1991), an alternative strategy entails investigating cognitive and emotional functions that recruit corticolimbic circuitries encompassing PFC pathways implicated in processing of emotional signals and the regulation of affect.

NEUROPSYCHOLOGICAL EVIDENCE FOR ORBITOFRONTAL DYSFUNCTION IN PSYCHOPATHIC OFFENDERS

Only three published studies have examined neuropsychological test performance associated with orbitofrontal cortex function in psychopathy. In a well-controlled study, LaPierre, Braun, and Hodgins (1995) compared the performance of 30 psychopathic and 30 nonpsychopathic drug-free offenders on a battery of neuropsychological tests explicitly constructed to tap functions subserved by the orbitofrontal cortex. The two groups of offenders were matched in terms of age, years of education, socioeconomic status, and measures of previous alcohol consumption and daily cigarette use. Measures of orbitofrontal cortex function included a go/no-go task (in which participants viewed a series of visually presented squares and crosses, and were required to make fast motor responses selectively to crosses having previously been trained to respond to the squares), the error score on the Porteus Maze, and an index of anosmia provided by the Modular Smell Identification Test (Doty, Shaman, & Dann, 1984). The single measure of dorsolateral PFC function was the number of perseverative errors on the WCST. The authors also administered an odor detection task to control for basic sensory deficits and mental rotation and block design tasks previously shown to be sensitive to right and left posterior cortical function, respectively.

In comparison with the nonpsychopaths, the psychopathic offenders exhibited significant increases in the number of errors of commission, but not omission, on the go/no-go task and qualitative (rule-breaks), but not quantitative, errors on the Porteus Maze. They were reliably less accurate at discriminating between odors and showed a *nonsignificant trend* toward a greater number of perseverative responses on the WCST; however, psychopaths showed no significant impairments on either the mental rotation task or the block design measure.

Taken as a whole, the aforementioned pattern of deficits provides encouraging support for the proposal that psychopathy is associated with cognitive deficits mediated by orbitofrontal cortex dysfunction. In the case of the go/no-go task, studies with experimental animals and neurological patients indicate that lesions of the ventrolateral PFC impair performance of such tasks (Drewe, 1975; Iversen & Mishkin, 1970), with some suggestion that the inhibition of current responding is lateralized to the right inferior frontal gyrus (Aron et al., 2004). Similarly, odor processing is known to recruit neural systems within the orbitofrontal cortex (Rolls, 1999), and lesions in this area are associated with deficits in odor identification tasks (Jones-Gotman & Zatorre, 1988). Therefore, problems on tasks of this kind in psychopathy are at least suggestive of dysfunction in orbitofrontal cortex. On the other hand, as noted previously, the lack of specificity of neuropsychological tasks for cortical subsystems inevitably limits the interpretation of these and other data sets. First, interpreting rule breaks on the Porteus Maze as reflecting dysfunction within orbitofrontal cortex is controversial. There is evidence that indifference to rules is associated with orbitofrontal damage or disconnection syndromes (Crown, 1952), and with altered metabolism in this specific region of PFC in patients with a variety of frontal lobe pathologies (see Sarazin et al., 2003); however, rule-breaking behavior is also commonly observed after damage to dorsolateral and dorsomedial frontal areas (Roberts & Wallis, 2000).

Second, although the tendency toward a reduced number of categories achieved and increased perseverative errors on the WCST in psychopathic offenders might be interpreted as evidence of dorsolateral PFC deficits, theoretical and empirical work has shown that performance of the WCST depends on multiple cognitive and affective processes subserved by distinct cortical and neurochemical systems (Robbins, 1996). Shifting sorting rules in the WSCT requires the use of trial-by-trial feedback to redirect the focus of attention away from a previously relevant but now irrelevant stimulus dimension (such as shape) toward a newly relevant dimension (such as number), *as well as* relearning new associations between specific stimulus exemplars and reinforcement values (reward or punishment). Research with visual discrimination–learning paradigms such as intra-/extradimensional set shifting (Dias et al., 1996) in which these processes are separated suggests that shifting an attentional bias depends on dorsolateral PFC, whereas relearning stimulus–reward associations recruits orbitofrontal cortex. Therefore, using the WCST to identify dysfunction in PFC subsystems is highly problematic.

Roussy and Toupin (2000) sought to replicate the findings of LaPierre and colleagues (1995) in 25 psychopathic and 29 nonpsychopathic juvenile offenders assessed with the PCL-R (Hare, 1991). Two tasks were added to the battery: the CWAT as a test of dorsolateral PFC function and a "stop-signal" paradigm in which participants performed a choice reaction time task involving letters and digits but were required to stop responding on the presentation of an auditory "Stop" signal (see Logan, 1994). The dependent measures in the stop-signal task were the mean reaction time for responding to targets and the number of errors of commission. Paralleling the findings of LaPierre and colleagues, the psychopathic offenders made significantly more errors of commission on the go/no-go task (errors of omission and mean reaction time were not significantly different) and more errors of commission on the stop-signal task (mean reaction times were unaffected), and they showed a nonsignificant trend toward increased qualitative errors on the Porteus Maze compared to nonpsychopathic offenders. However, in contrast to LaPierre and colleagues, the psychopathic offenders were not impaired in the discrimination of odors, nor did they show any significant change in the number of categories obtained, the number of perseverative responses on the WCST, or the number of items generated in the fluency measure on the CWAT. Notwithstanding the lack of matching for psychometric measures of cognitive ability, the results of this study tend to confirm the view that psychopathic offenders do exhibit impairments in the control of prepotent responses (as in go/no-go tasks) or the inhibition of already initiated actions (as in the stop-signal task), possibly reflecting dysfunction in ventrolateral PFC mechanisms. However, the data cast at least some doubt on whether such impairments also include odor discrimination difficulties.

Mitchell, Colledge, Leonard, and Blair (2002) provided further evidence that psychopathy is associated with cognitive and emotional processes associated with the orbitofrontal cortex. These authors compared decision making and visual discrimination learning in psychopathic and nonpsychopathic offender groups. All offenders were assessed with the PCL-R (Hare, 1991) and the groups were matched for age and cognitive ability as measured by the Raven's Progressive Matrices. Much empirical work now suggests that making decisions between actions associated with uncertain rewards and punishments invokes the functioning of neural circuitry incorporating orbitofrontal cortex (Bechara et al., 1996; Rogers, Owen, Middleton, Pickard, & Robbins, 1999c), the striatum (Rogers et al., 2004), the amygdala (Bechara, Damasio, Damasio, & Lee, 1999), and other cortical centers implicated in the representation of emotion. In view of the hypothesis that psychopathy involves dysfunction of circuitry interconnecting these systems (Blair, 2003), the possibility that psychopaths show impairments in risky decision making has impressive face validity. Following Bechara and colleagues (1996), offenders in the Mitchell and colleagues study drew cards from four decks to earn facsimile money. Two decks were "bad" in that they offered large gains but larger losses, while two decks were "good" in that they offered small gains but smaller losses; the two "bad" and two "good" decks differed from each other in terms of the rate at which the losses were delivered across the 100 trials of the task.

Mitchell and colleagues (2002) also examined performance on a visual discrimination learning task, the intra-/extradimensional shift learning task. As noted earlier, performance of the WCST can be decomposed into at least two separate cognitive processes: shifting attention from the now-irrelevant stimulus dimensions toward the newly relevant dimension, and relearning which specific stimulus-exemplars within a dimension are associated with reward or punishment. There is now extensive evidence to suggest that affective learning in the form of acquiring and reacquiring new stimulus–reward associations—reversal learning—is mediated by the orbitofrontal cortex (Dias et al., 1996; Thorpe et al., 1983), with some indication that deficits in reversal learning are in turn associated with the degree of social impairment consequent to frontal lobe lesions (Hornak et al., 1994). Mitchell and colleagues hypothesized that psychopathic offenders would exhibit deficits in risky decision making for uncertain rewards or penalties, and in the acquisition of reversal discriminations but not in extradimensional shift discriminations.

The results largely supported these predictions. In the decision-making task, the nonpsychopathic offenders (in common with healthy nonforensic samples) began by choosing cards from the bad decks (because of their frequent large rewards) but gradu-

ally altered their choices in favor of the good decks. By contrast, the psychopathic offenders continued to choose cards from the bad decks throughout the course of the task. In the case of the visual discrimination–learning task, the psychopathic offenders showed consistently higher rates of errors compared to the nonpsychopathic offenders during all stages of the task; however, they made significantly more errors only during the learning of reversal discriminations.

Mitchell and colleagues' (2002) finding that psychopathic offenders were impaired in the performance of Bechara's card gambling task contrasts with the negative results of an earlier study by Schmitt, Brinkley, and Newman (1999), in which data on the same task were collected from a sample of 157 Caucasian and African American inmates assessed for psychopathy using the PCL-R (Hare, 1991). Inmates diagnosed with high, medium, and low levels of psychopathy were equally proficient in completing the task, with no evidence that psychopathic offenders retained their preference for the bad decks compared to nonpsychopathic offenders. However, low anxious offenders as assessed by the self-report Welsh Anxiety Scale (Welsh, 1956) continued to choose from the bad decks more frequently than high anxious offenders. Possible reasons for the discrepancy between findings of this study and those of Mitchell and colleagues include differences in experimenter instructions and differences in the reinforcers (large but fictitious monetary rewards in Mitchell et al., 2002; small amounts of real money in Schmitt et al., 1999).

Overall, the findings of LaPierre and colleagues (1995), Roussy and Toupin (2000), and Mitchell and colleagues (2002) provide encouraging support for the hypothesis that psychopathy involves dysfunction in the cognitive and emotional processes subserved by the neural circuitry of the orbitofrontal cortex. Each of these studies used the PCL-R as the method for assessing psychopathy. Also, in the case of the LaPierre and colleagues and Mitchell and colleagues studies, groups were matched on certain crucial age and psychometric variables. In each case, deficits in psychopathic offenders were demonstrated on more than one outcome measure linked in some way to orbitofrontal function.

As noted earlier, the orbitofrontal cortex plays an important role in representing emotional information and in a variety of motivational and reinforcement processes (Phillips et al., 2003). It is positioned within a distributed network that plays a critical role in affect. Its afferent projections allow it to integrate information from other parts of the PFC and from subcortical structures such as the amygdala that are critical for processing emotional signals (Barbas, 2000). Its efferent projections allow it to influence both autonomic reactivity and action selection systems. Therefore, further research on the links between the cognitive and emotional facets of psychopathy, with an emphasis on the orbitofrontal cortex, is warranted.

RESPONSE MODULATION AND ERROR PROCESSING DEFICITS IN PSYCHOPATHIC OFFENDERS

Both LaPierre and colleagues (1995) and Roussy and Toupin (2000) reported that psychopaths exhibited increases in the number of errors of commission on a successive discrimination go/no-go task, as well as impairments in the ability to interrupt an already initiated action in a stop-signal task. The most theoretically developed account of response control deficits in psychopathy has been that proposed by Joseph Newman (Newman, 1998; Newman & Lorenz, 2002). In its most recent formulation, the theory states that self-regulation involves "temporary suspension of a dominant response set and a brief concurrent shift of attention from the organization and implementation of goal-directed responding to its evaluation" (Patterson & Newman, 1993, p. 717). The mechanism that supports this shift of attention is mobilized automatically without active control and facilitates processing of contextual information as part of reappraising the current response set. Failure to activate this shift of attention means that psychopaths are not able to interrupt maladaptive behavior and regulate ongoing behavior. Crucially, the theory proposes that the core deficit is attentional and involves a failure to balance appetitive motivational states with the regulatory impact of extraneous stimuli.

Several reviews of response modulation theory are available (e.g., Lykken, 1995; see also Blackburn, Chapter 3, and Hiatt & Newman, Chapter 17, this volume), and thus details of studies conducted within this framework are not described here. Probably the most replicated finding arising out of this research is that psychopathic offenders show difficulties in attending to feedback information or using that information to modulate current cognitive or motor activity. Specifically, psychopaths continue to play the Newman card playing task, which entails learning to inhibit a previously rewarded response when contingencies change, despite increasing levels of punishing feedback (Newman & Kosson, 1986)—and, under some conditions, they actually emit faster responses after punished trials than after rewarded ones (Newman, 1998). Surprisingly little research has been conducted into the neural substrates of continued instrumental responding in the face of increasing punishment or into the neural bases of response modulation deficits in psychopathic offenders. However, these substrates are likely to include elements of the network identified by Phillips and colleagues (2003) as mediating regulation of affective states—namely, dorsal medial PFC regions, hippocampus, and dorsal ACC.

Supportive evidence for this proposal has been provided by brain event-related potential (ERP) studies showing that incorrect responses on a variety of sensory-motor tasks, involving multimodal sensory and motor outputs, are associated with a response-locked negative potential (the so-called ERN), which peaks between 50 and 150 milliseconds after an erroneous response has been made (Falkenstein, Hohnshein, Hoorman, & Blanke, 1991). Source localization research suggests that the ERN originates from generators within an area encompassing the anterior cingulate and medial frontal gyrus and an area within the lateral frontal cortex (Dehaene, Posner, & Tucker, 1994). This interpretation was supported by a recent event-rated functional magnetic resonance imaging study of performance of go/no-go task performance in healthy volunteers which demonstrated increased neural activity as measured by the blood-oxygenation-level-dependent response within ACC and left lateral PFC when participants erroneously responded to distractors (see Kiehl, Liddle, & Hopfinger, 2000).

At the time of this writing, differences in ERN response have not yet been investigated in psychopathic individuals assessed with the PCL-R (Hare, 1991). However, Dikman and Allen (2000) examined the ERN in 18 high- and 16 low-socialized participants as defined by scores on the *So* scale. In one study condition, participants were punished for every error of commission or omission; in the other condition, they were rewarded for every correct response. Low-socialized participants showed smaller ERNs than high-socialized participants in the former condition (punished responding) but not in the latter condition (rewarded responding), suggesting that error processing within medial PFC is altered in individuals with antisocial features of psychopathy.

Other data suggest that psychopathic individuals may show altered attention to targets and distracters in a visual go/no-go task. Kiehl, Liddle, and Hopfinger (2000) examined performance in 12 medicated and stable schizophrenic patients, 13 psychopathic offenders, and 16 nonpsychopathic offenders. Psychopathy was assessed using the PCL-R (Hare, 1991). These groups were balanced for age and years of education. The schizophrenic offenders, but not the psychopathic offenders, made more errors of commission than did the nonpsychopathic offenders. The nonpsychopathic offenders showed greater early brain response negativity (N275) in frontal locations after distracters compared to targets, but this difference was attenuated in the schizophrenic patients and largely absent in the psychopathic offenders. In addition, while later brain positivity (P375) was larger following targets than distracters in the nonpsychopathic offenders, this effect was reduced in the schizophrenic patients and reversed in the psychopaths.

In summary, data from available ERP studies suggest that low socialization and psychopathy are associated with altered processing of errors of commission within medial PFC and anterior cingulate structures, perhaps reflecting altered functioning within an extended circuitry associated with the regulation of affect and behavior (Phillips et al., 2003).

SUMMARY AND FUTURE DIRECTIONS

Proposals that the PFC supports a limited-capacity, unitary executive system have been superseded by increasing recognition that the anatomy of the PFC and the functional properties of its cytoarchitectural fields support sets of control operations over diverse types of information via processes involving interconnected subcortical and cortical systems (Miller & Cohen, 2001).

The foregoing review suggests that our understanding of the role and importance of PFC dysfunction in psychopathy is at an extremely formative stage. Early neuropsychological studies provide only inconsistent support for possible frontal lobe deficits in psychopathy and are complicated by variations in assessment methods, the use of behavioral tasks with uncertain sensitivity and specificity for frontal lobe damage, and relatively small sample sizes (Hare, 1984). In the main, the totality of research to date provides very little evidential support for the proposal that psychopathy is associated with generalized PFC impairments—in contrast with delinquent offenders or individuals with APD (Morgan & Lilienfeld, 2000).

However, recent studies suggest that psychopathy as defined by the PCL-R (Hare, 1991) is associated with impairments that may reflect dysfunction in PFC pathways specifically implicated in emotional processing and regulation. These deficits include problems in response control (as indexed by go/no-go discrimination tasks; LaPierre et al., 1995; Roussy & Toupin, 2000), difficulties with selecting actions associated with uncertain rewards and penalties (as indexed by risky decision making; Mitchell et al., 2002), and error monitoring (as indexed by choice reaction time tasks and ERN, and the Newman card playing task; see, respectively, Dikman & Allen, 2000; Newman, Patterson, & Kosson, 1987). These deficits suggest that psychopathy involves dysfunction in both a ventral system—encompassing orbitofrontal PFC, insula, ventral striatum, rostrocingulate cortex, and amygdala—that identifies emotional signals *and* a dorsal system—encompassing dorsal PFC, hippocampus, and ACC—that mediates *regulation* of affective states.

Future research will need to demonstrate that neuropsychological impairments involving the PFC have some specificity for the disorder and its associated affective–interpersonal and antisocial deviance factors rather then just the severity of an underlying APD diagnosis or constellation of diagnoses within DSM-IV clusters. At the current time, very little research has attempted to relate neuropsychological impairment to the distinct factors of the PCL-R (for an example of how this might be done, see Verona, Patrick, Curtin, Bradley, & Lang, 2004). Given the association between frontal lobe dysfunction and APD, one might hypothesize that PFC deficits relate principally to the antisocial deviance compoment of psychopathy (reflecting dysfunction in systems of emotional regulation). However, the foregoing discussion has highlighted the role of the medial and orbitofrontal cortex, in tandem with anterior temporal lobe structures, in the representation of emotional and social information (Rolls, 1999). Therefore, it remains entirely possible that the emotional shallowness and interpersonal style characteristic of the Cleckley psychopath are mediated by dysfunction in dorsomedial and ventral PFC sectors.

Finally, future research will need to integrate demonstrations of neuropsychological impairment with emerging evidence of structural and functional changes within frontotemporal circuitry (see Raine & Yang, Chapter 14, this volume; Soderstrom et al., 2002) and link these changes with the etiology of the disorder and its time course. In this context, comparison with recent developments in the schizophrenia area may be pertinent. Schizophrenia has consistently been demonstrated to involve PFC impairments (Weinberger, Berman, & Illowsky, 1988). Because unaffected but genetically at risk individuals show related deficits (Weinberger et al., 2001) and alterations to neural responses within dorsolateral PFC associated with cognitive activity (Callicott et al., 2003), PFC dysfunction may represent an endophenotype for the disorder (Weinberger et al., 2001). Recent research has isolated susceptibility genes (e.g., neuregulin, dysbindin, and COMT) that appear to be linked to PFC dysfunction, and other intermediate phenotypes involving the hippocampus function, and appear to involve biological processes that might be plausibly implicated in the development of clinically significant illness—namely, the regulation of synaptic plasticity. Such advances are facilitating research strategies that explore how multiple susceptibility genes influence schizophrenia risk via converging influences on the development of neural circuitries implicated in the disorder (Harrison & Weinberger, 2004).

In the case of psychopathy, research has not yet identified stable endophenotypes (which may or may not involve PFC dysfunction). However, as the genetic bases of the disorder's constituent traits become clearer (cf. Waldman & Rhee, Chapter 11, this volume), future research strategies may be able to identify genotypical variation associated with information-processing deficits characteristic of psychopathy, operating via influence on frontotemporal neural substrates. Such developments would provide opportunities for an improved understanding of development and early intervention.

REFERENCES

Alexander, G. E., Delong, M. R., & Strick, P. (1986). Parallel organization of functionally segregated circuits linking basal ganglia and cortex. *Annual Review of Neuroscience, 9,* 357–381.

American Psychiatric Association. (1980). Diagnostic and statistical manual of mental disorders (3rd ed.). Washington, DC: Author.

Anderson, A. L., & Hanvik, L. J. (1950). The psychmetric localization of brain lesions: the differential of frontal and parietal lesions on MMPI profiles. *Journal of Clinical Psychology, 6,* 177–180.

Anderson, S. W., Bechara, A., Damasio, H., Tranel, D., & Damasio, A. R. (1999). Impairment of social and moral behavior related to early damage in human prefrontal cortex. *Nature Neuroscience, 2*(11), 1032–1037.

Anderson, S. W., Damasio, H., Jones, R. D., & Tranel, D. (1991). Wisconsin Card Sorting Test performance as a measure of frontal lobe damage. *Journal of Clinical and Experimental Neuropsychology, 13*(6), 909–922.

Andres, P. (2003). Frontal cortex as the central executive of working memory: time to revise our view. *Cortex, 39*(4-5), 871–895.

Arnsten, A. F. T. (2000). Catecholamine modulation of prefrontal cortical cognitive function. *Trends in Cognitive Sciences, 2*(11), 436–447.

Aron, A. R., Robbins, T. W., & Poldrack, R. A. (2004). Inhibition and the right inferior frontal cortex. *Trends in Cognitive Neurscience, 8*(4), 170–177.

Assad, W.F., Rainer, G., & Miller, E. K. (1998). Neural activity in the primate prefrontal cortex during associative learning. *Neuron, 21,* 1399–1407.

Baddeley, A. D. (1986). *Working memory*. Oxford, UK: Clarendon Press.

Barbas, H. (2000). Connections underlying the synthesis of cognition, memory and emotion in primate prefrontal cortices. *Brain Research Bulletin, 52*(5), 319–300.

Bauer, L. O., & Hesselbrock, V.M. (2004). Brain maturation and subtypes of conduct disorder: interactive effects on p300 amplitude and topography in male adolescents. *Journal of the American Academy of Child and Adolescent Psychiatry, 42*(1), 106–115.

Bechara, A., Damasio, H., Damasio, A. R., & Lee, G. P. (1999). Different contributions of the human amygdala and ventromedial prefrontal cortex to decision-making. *Journal of Neuroscience, 19*(13), 5473–5481.

Bechara, A., Tranel, D., Damasio, H., & Damasio, A. R. (1996). Failure to respond autonomically to anticipated future outcomes following damage to prefrontal cortex. *Cerebral Cortex, 6*, 215–225.

Benton, A. L. (1974). The revised visual retention test (4th ed.). New York: Psychological Corporation.

Benton, A. L., & Hamsher, K. (1976). *Multilingual Aphasia Examination*. Iowa City: University of Iowa.

Bianchi, L. (1922). *The mechanisms of the brain, and the function of the frontal lobes*. Edinburgh: Livingstone.

Blackburn, R. (1975). An empirical classification of psychopathic personality. *British Journal of Psychiatry, 127*, 456–460.

Blair, R. J. (2003). Neurobiological basis of psychopathy. *British Journal of Psychiatry, 182*, 5–7.

Blair, R. J. R., & Frith, U. (2000). Neurocognitive explanations of the antisocial personality disorders. *Criminal Behaviour and Mental Health, 10*, S66–S81.

Blumer, D., & Benson, D. F. (1975). Personality changes with frontal and temporal lobe lesions. In D. F. Benson & D. Blumer (Eds.), *Psychiatric aspects of neurological disease*. New York: Grune & Stratton.

Brodmann, K. (1925). *Vergleichende localisationslehre der grosshirnrinde* (2nd ed.). Leipzig, Germany: Barth.

Burgess, P. W., Scott, S. K., & Frith, C. D. (2003). The role of the rostral frontal cortex (area 10) in prospective memory: A lateral versus medial dissociation. *Neuropsychologia, 41*(8), 906–918.

Calder, A. J., Lawrence, A. D., & Young, A. W. (2001). Neuropsychology of fear and loathing. *Nature Neuroscience Review, 2*, 352–363.

Callicott, J. H., Mattay, V. S., Verchinski, B. A., Marenco, S., Egan, M. F., & Weinberger, D. R. (2003). Abnormal fMRI response of the dorsolateral prefrontal cortex in cognitively intact siblings of patients with schizophrenia. *American Journal of Psychiatry, 160*(4), 709–719.

Carmichael, S. T., & Price, J. L. (1996). Connectional networks within the orbital and medial prefrontal cortex of macaque monkeys. *Journal of Comparative Neurology, 371*(2), 179–207.

Cleckley, H. (1955). *The mask of sanity*. St Louis, MO: Mosby.

Coccaro, E. F., Siever, L. J., Klar, H. M., Maurer, G., Cochrane, K., Cooper, T. B., et al. (1989). Serotonergic studies in affective and personality disorders: Correlates with suicidal and impulsive aggressive behavior. *Archives of General Psychiatry, 46*, 587–599.

Cohen, L. (1959). Perception of reversible figures after brain injury. *Archives of Neurology and Psychiatry, 81*, 37–46.

Cooke, D. J., & Michie, C. (2001). Refining the construct of psychopathy: Towards a hierarchical model. *Psychological Assessment, 13*(2), 171–188.

Critchley, H. D., Elliott, R., Mathias, C. J., & Dolan, R. J. (2000). Neural activity relating to generation and representation of galvanic skin conductance responses: A functional magnetic resonance imaging study. *Journal of Neuroscience, 20*, 3033–3040.

Crown, S. (1952). An experimental study of psychological changes following frontal lobotomy. *Journal of General Psychology, 47*, 3–41.

Dehaene, S., Posner, M. I., & Tucker, D. M. (1994). Localization of a neural system for error detection and compensation. *Psychological Science, 5*(5), 303–305.

Devonshire, P. A., Howard, R. C., & Sellars, C. (1988). Frontal lobe functions and personality in mentally abnormal offenders. *Personality and Individual Differences, 9*(2), 339–344.

Dias, R., Robbins, T. W., & Roberts, A. C. (1996). Dissociation in prefrontal cortex of affective and attentional shifts. *Nature, 380*, 69–72.

Dikman, Z. V., & Allen, J. J. (2000). Error monitoring during reward and avoidance learning in high- and low-socialized individuals. *Psychophysiology, 37*(1), 43–54.

Dinn, W. M., & Harris, C. L. (2000). Neurocognitive function in antisocial personality disorder. *Psychiatry Research, 97*, 173–190.

Dolan, M., & Park, I. (2002). The neuropsychology of antisocial personality disorder. *Psychological Medicine, 32*, 417–427.

Doty, R. L., Shaman, P., & Dann, M. (1984). Development of the UPSIT: a standardized microencapsulated test of olfactory function. *Physiology and Behavior, 32*, 481–502.

Drewe, E. A. (1975). Go–no go learning after front lobe lesions in humans. *Cortex, 11*(1), 8–16.

Duncan, J., & Owen, A. M. (2000). Common regions of the human frontal lobe recruited by diverse cognitive demands. *Trends in Neuroscience, 23*(10), 475–483.

Duncan, J., Seitz, R. J., Kolodny, J., Bor, D., Herzog, H., Ahmed, A., et al. (2000). A neural basis for general intelligence. *Science, 289*, 457–60.

Elliott, F. A. (1978). Neurological aspects of antisocial behavior. In W. H. Reid (Ed.), *The psychopath* (pp. 146–189). New York: Brunner/Mazel.

Eslinger, P. J. (1997). Neurological and neuropsychological bases of empathy. *European Neurology, 39*, 193–199.

Falkenstein, M., Hohnsbein, J., Hoormann, J., & Blanke, L. (1991). Effects of crossmodal divided attention on late ERP components. II. Error processing in choice reaction tasks. *Electroencephalography and Clinical Neurophysiology, 78*(6), 447–55.

Frith, U., & Frith, C. (2003). Development and neurophysiology of mentalizing. *Philosophical transactions of the Royal Society of London, Series B, Biological sciences, 358*(1431), 459–73.

Fuster, J. M. (1989). *The prefrontal cortex: Anatomy, physiology, and neuropsychology of the frontal lobe.* New York: Raven Press.

Gogtay, N., Giedd, J. N., Lusk, L., Hayashi, K. M., Greenstein, D., Vaituzis, A. C., et al. (2004). Dynamic mapping of human cortical development during childhood through early adulthood. *Proceedings of the National Academy of Sciences USA, 101*(21), 8174–8179.

Goldman, P. S., & Rosvold, H. E. (1972). The effects of selective caudate lesions in infant and juvenile thersus monkeys. *Brain Research, 43*, 53–66.

Goldman-Rakic, P. S. (1987). Circuitry of primate prefrontal cortex and regulation of behavior by representational memory. In F. Plum (Ed.), *Handbook of physiology: The nervous system* (pp. 373–417). Bethesda, MD: American Physiology Society.

Gorenstein, E. E. (1982). Frontal lobe functions in psychopaths. *Journal of Abnormal Psychology, 91*(5), 368–379.

Gorenstein, E. E., & Newman, J.P. (1980). Disinhibitory psychopathology: A new perspective and model for research. *Psychological Review, 87*, 301–315.

Grant, D. A., & Berg, E. A. (1948). A behavioral analysis of degree of reinforcement and ease of shifting to new responses in a Weigl-type card-sorting. *Journal of Experimental Psychology, 38*, 404–411.

Gray, J. A. (1982). *The neuropsychology of anxiety: An enquiry in to the functions of the septo-hippocampal system.* Oxford, UK: Oxford University Press.

Grozinsky, G. M., & Diamond, R. (1992). Frontal lobe functioning in boys with attention-deficit hyperactivity disorder. *Developmental Neuropsychology, 8*, 427–445.

Gusnard, D. A., Akbudak, E., Shulman, G. L., & Raichle, M. E. (2001): Medial prefrontal cortex and self-referential mental activity: Relation to a default mode of brain function. *Proceedings of the National Academy of Science, USA, 98*, 4259–4264.

Haber, S. N., Kunishio, K., Mizobuchi, M., & Lynd-Balta, E. (1995). The orbital and medial prefrontal circuit through the primate basal ganglia. *Journal of Neuroscience, 15*(7), 4851–4867.

Hare, R. D. (1991). *The Psychopathy Checklist—Revised.* Toronto, ON, Canada: Multi-Health Systems.

Hare, R. D. (2003). *Manual for the revised Psychopathy Checklist* (2nd ed.). Toronto, ON, Canada: Multi-Health Systems.

Hare, R. D. (1984). Peformance of psychopaths on cognitive tasks related to frontal lobe function. *Journal of Abnormal Psychology, 93*(2), 133–140.

Hare, R. D. (1980). A research scale For the assessment of psychopathy in criminal populations. *Personality and Individual Differences, 1*, 111–119.

Harpur, T. J., Hare, R. D., & Hakstian, A. R. (1989). Two-factor conceptualization of psychopathy: Construct validity and assessment implications. *Psychological Assessment, 1*, 6–17.

Harrison, P. J., & Weinberger, D. R. (2004). Schizophrenia genes, gene expression, and neuropathology: On the matter of their convergence. *Molecular Psychiatry, 10*(1), 1–29.

Hart, S. D., Forth, A. E., & Hare, R. D. (1990). Performance of criminal psychopaths on selected neuropsychological tests. *Journal of Abnormal Psychology, 99*(4), 374–379.

Hathaway, S. R., & McKinley, J. C. (1943). *Minnesota Multiphasic Personality Inventory.* Minneapolis: University of Minnesota Press.

Hebb, D. O. (1945). Man's frontal-lobes. *Archives of Neurological Psychiatry, 54*, 10–13.

Heilbrun, A. B. (1982). Cognitive models of criminal violence based upon intelligence and psychopathy levels. *Journal of Consulting and Clinical Psychology, 50*, 546-557.

Hoffman, J. J., Hall, R. W., & Bartsch, T. W. (1987). On the relative importance of "psychopathic" personality and alcoholism on neuropsychological measures of frontal lobe dysfunction. *Journal of Abnormal Psychology, 96*(2), 158–160.

Hooper, H. E. (1958). *The Hooper Visual Organisation Test.* Los Angeles: Western Psychological Services.

Hornak, J., Rolls, E. T., Wade, D., & McGrath, J. (1994). Emotion-related learning in patients with social and emotional changes associated with frontal lobe damage. *Journal of Neurology Neurosurgery and Psychiatry, 57*(12), 1518–1524.

Iversen, S. D., & Mishkin, M. (1970). Perseverative interference in monkey following selective lesions of the prefrontal convexity. *Experimental Brain Research, 11*, 376–386.

Johnson, S. C., Baxter, L. C., Wilder, L. S., Pipe, J. G., Heiserman, J. E., & Prigatano, G. P. (2002). Neural correlates of self-reflection. *Brain, 125*(8), 1808–1814.

Jones-Gotman, M., & Zatorre, R. J. (1988). Olfactory identification deficits in patients with focal cerebral excision. *Neuropsychologia, 26*, 387–400.

Kandel, E., & Freed, D. (1989). Frontal-lobe dysfunction and antisocial behavior: A review. *Journal of Clinical Psychology, 45*(3), 404–413.

Kiehl, K. A., Liddle, P. F., & Hopfinger, J. B. (2000). Error processing and the rostral anterior cingulate: An event-related fMRI study. *Psychophysiology, 37*, 216–223.

Kiehl, K. A., Smith, A. M., Hare, R. D., & Liddle, P. F. (2000). An event-related (ERP) potential investigation of response inhibition in schizophrenia and psychopathy. *Biological Psychiatry, 48*(3), 210–221.

LaPierre, D., Braun, C., & Hodgins, S. (1995). Ventral frontal deficits in psychopathy: neuropsychological findings. *Neuropsychologia, 33*(2), 139–151.

Lau, H. C., Rogers, R. D., Haggard P., & Passingham, R.E. (2004). Attention to intention. *Science 303,* 1208–1210.

Lezak, M.D. (1995). Neuropsychological assessment (3rd ed.). New York: Oxford University Press.

Lidberg, L., Levander, S. E., Schalling, D., & Lidberg, Y. (1978). Necker cube reversals, arousal and psychopathy. *British Journal of Clinical and Social Psychology, 17,* 355–361.

Logan, G. D. (1994). On the ability to inhibit thought and action: a users' guide to the Stop Signal paradigm. In D. Dagenbach & T. H. Carr (Eds.), *Inhibitory processes in attention, memory and language,* (pp. 189–239). New York: Academic Press.

Lopez, F., Akil, H., & Watson, S. J. (1999). Neural circuits mediating stress. *Biological Psychiatry, 46,* 1461–1471.

Luria, A. R. (1969). The frontal lobe syndromes. In P. J. Vinken & G. W. Bruyn (Eds.), *Handbook of clinical neurology* (Vol. 2, pp. 725–757). Amsterdam: North-Holland.

Lykken, D. T. (1995). *The antisocial personalities.* Hillsdale, NJ: Erlbaum.

MacLean, P. D., & Newman, J. D. (1988). Role of midline frontolimbic cortex in production of the isolation call of squirrel monkeys. *Brain Research, 450,* 111–123.

Mayberg, H. S., Liotti, M., Brannan, S. K., McGinnis, S., Mahurin, R. K., Jerabek, P.A., et al. (1999). Reciprocal limbic-cortical function and negative mood: Converging PET findings in depression and normal sadness. *American Journal of Psychiatry, 156*(5), 675–682.

Mettler, F. A. (1949). *Selective partial ablation of the frontal cortex. A correlative study of its effects on human psychotic subjects.* New York: Hoeber.

Meyers, C., Berman, S. A., Schiebel, R. S., & Hayman, A. (1992). Acquired antisocial personality disorder associated with unilateral orbital frontal lobe damage. *Journal of Psychiatry Neuroscience, 17,* 121–125.

Miller, E. K., & Cohen, J. D. (2001). An integrative theory of prefrontal function. *Annual Review of Neuroscience, 24,* 167–202.

Miller, N. E. (1959). Liberalization of basis S-R concepts: Extensions to conflict behavior, motivation and social learning. In S. Koch (Ed.), *Psychology: A study of science.* New York: McGraw-Hill.

Milner, B. (1964). Some effects of frontal lobotomy in man. In J. M. Warren & K. Akert (Eds.), *The frontal granular cortex and behavior.* New York: McGraw-Hill.

Mitchell, D. G. V., Colledge, E., Leonard, A., & Blair, R. J. R. (2002). Risky decisions and response reversal: Is there evidence of orbitofrontal cortex dysfunction in psychopathic individuals? *Neuropsychologia, 40*(12), 2013–2022.

Moffitt, T. E., & Silva, P. A. (1988). Self-reported delinquency, neuropsychological deficit, and history of attention deficit disorder. *Journal of Abnormal Child Psychology, 16,* 553–569.

Moniz, E. (1937). Prefrontal leucotomy in the treatment of mental disorders. *American Journal of Psychiatry, 93,* 1379–1385.

Morgan, A. B., & Lilienfeld, S. O. (2000). A meta-analytic review of the relation between antisocial behaviour and neuropsychological measures of executive function. *Clinical Psychology Review, 20,* 113–136.

Nauta, W. J. M. (1971). The problem of the frontal lobe: a reinterpretation. *Journal of Psychiatric Research, 8,* 167–187.

Newman, J. P. (1998). Psychopathic behavior: An information processing perspective. In D. J. Cooke, A. E. Forth, & R. D. Hare (Eds.), *Psychopathy: Theory, research, and implications for society* (pp. 81–104). Dordrecht, The Netherlands: Kluwer.

Newman, J. P., & Kosson, D. S. (1986). Passive avoidance learning in psychopathic and nonpsychopathic offenders. *Journal of Abnormal Psychology, 95,* 257–263.

Newman, J. P., & Lorenz, A. R. (2002). Response modulation and emotion processing: Implications for psychopathy and other dysregulatory psychopathology. In R. J. Davidson, K. Scherer, & H. H. Goldsmith (Eds.), *Handbook of affective sciences* (pp. 1043–1067). New York: Oxford University Press.

Newman, J. P., Patterson, C. M., & Kosson, D. S. (1987). Response perseveration in psychopaths. *Journal of Abnormal Psychology, 96,* 145–148.

Norman, D. A., & Shallice, T. (1986). Attention to action: willed and autonomic control of behaviour. In G. E. Schwartz & D. Shapiro (Eds.), *Consciousness and self-regulation* (Vol. 4). New York: Plenum Press.

Ongur, D., & Price, J. L. (2000). The organization of networks within the orbital and medial prefrontal cortex of rats, monkeys and humans. *Cerebral Cortex, 10,* 206–219.

Owen, A. M. (1997). The functional organization of working memory processes within human lateral frontal cortex: The contribution of functional neuroimaging. *European Journal of Neuroscience, 9*(7), 1329–1339.

Owen, A. M., James, M., Leigh, P. N., Summers, B. A., Marsden, C. D., Quinn, N. P., et al. (1992). Frontostriatal cognitive deficits at different stages of Parkinson's disease. *Brain, 115*(6), 1727–1751.

Passingham, R. E. (1993). *The frontal lobes and voluntary action.* Oxford, UK: Oxford University Press.

Patrick, C. J. (1994). Emotion and psychopathy: Startling new insights. *Psychophysiology, 31,* 319–330.

Patterson, C.M., & Newman, J.P. (1993). Reflectivity and learning from aversive events: Toward a psychological mechanism for the syndromes of disinhibition. *Psychological Review, 100,* 716–736.

Penfield, W., & Faulk, M. E. (1955). The insula: Further observations of its function. *Brain, 78,* 445–470.

Petrides, M. (1996). Specialized systems for the processing of mnemonic information within the primate frontal cortex. *Philosophical Transactions of the Royal Society of London, Series B, Biological Sciences, 351*, 1455–1461.

Petrides, M., & Pandya, D. N. (1999). Dorsolateral prefrontal cortex: Comparative cytoarchitectonic analysis in the human and the macaque brain and corticocortical connection patterns. *European Journal of Neuroscience, 11*, 1011–1036.

Phillips, M. L., Drevets, W. C., Rauch, S. L., & Lane, R. (2003). Neurobiology of emotion perception I: the basis of normal emotion perception. *Biological Psychiatry, 54*(5), 515–528.

Ploghaus, A., Tracey, I., Gati, J. S., Clare, S., Menon, R. S., Matthews, P. M., & Rawlins, J. N. (1999). Dissociating pain from its anticipation in the human brain. *Science, 284*, 1979–1981.

Pujol, J., Vendrell, P., Deus, J., Junque, C., Bello, J., Marti-Vilalta, J. L., & Capdevila, A. (2001). The effect of medial frontal and posterior parietal demyelinating lesions on Stroop interference. *Neuroimage, 13*(1), 68–75.

Raine, A., Buchsbaum, M., & LaCasse, L. (1997). Brain abnormalities in murderers indicated by positron emission tomography. *Biological Psychiatry, 42*, 495–508.

Reitan, R. M., & Wolfson, D. (1995). Category Test and Trail Making Test as measures of frontal lobe functions. *Clinical-Neuropsychologist, 9*(1), 50–56.

Rey, A. (1964). *L'examen clinique en psychologie [The clinical test in psychology]*. Paris: Presses Universitaires de France.

Robbins, T. W. (1996). Dissociating executive functions of the prefrontal cortex. *Philosophical Transactions of the Royal Society of London, Series B, Biological Sciences, 351*, 1463–1454.

Robbins, T.W., & Rogers, R.D. (2001). Functioning of fronto-striatal anatomical loops in mechanisms of attentional control. In S. Monsell & J. Driver (Eds.), *Control of cognitive processes: Attention and performance* (Vol. 18). Cambridge, MA: MIT Press.

Rogers, R. D., Andrews, T. C., Grasby, P. M., Brooks, D., & Robbins, T. W. (2000). Contrasting cortical and sub-cortical PET activations produced by reversal learning and attentional-set shifting in humans. *Journal of Cognitive Neuroscience, 12*(1), 1–21.

Rogers, R. D., Blackshaw, A.J., Middleton, H. C., Matthews, K., Deakin, J. F. W., Sahakian, B. J., & Robbins, T. W. (1999). Tryptophan depletion impairs stimulus–reward learning while methylphenidate disrupts attentional control in healthy young adults: Implications for the monoaminergic basis of impulsive behaviour. *Psychopharmacology, 146*, 482–491.

Rogers, R. D., Everitt, B. J., Baldacchino, A., Blackmore, A. J., Swainson, R., London, M., et al. (1999). Dissociating deficits in the decision-making cognition of chronic amphetamine abusers, opiate abusers, patients with focal damage to prefrontal cortex, and tryptophan-depleted normal volunteers: Evidence for monoaminergic mechanisms. *Neuropsychopharmacology, 20*(4), 322–329.

Rogers, R. D., Owen, A. M., Middleton, H. C., Pickard, J., & Robbins, T. W. (1999). Decision-making in humans activates multiple sites within orbital prefrontal cortex: A PET study. *Journal of Neuroscience, 20*(19), 9029–9038.

Rogers, R. D., Ramnani, N., Mackay, C., Wilson, J., Jezzard, P. J., Carter, C. S., & Smith, S. M. (2004). Distinct portions of anterior cingulate cortex and medial prefrontal cortex are activated during separable phases of decision-making. *Biological Psychiatry 55*(6), 594–602.

Rolls, E. T. (1999). *The brain and emotion*. Oxford, UK: Oxford University Press.

Roussy, S., & Toupin, J. (2000). Behavioral inhibition deficits in juvenile psychopaths. *Aggressive Behavior, 26*, 413–424.

Royall, D. R., Lauterbach, E. C., Cummings, J. L., Reeve, A., Rummans, T. A., Kaufer, D. I., LaFrance, et al. (2002). Executive control function: A review of its promise and challenges for clinical research. A report from the Committee on Research of the American Neuropsychiatric Association. *Journal of Neuropsychiatry and Clinical Neuroscience, 14*(4), 377–405.

Sarazin, M., Michon, A., Pillon, B., Samson, Y., Canuto, A., Gold, G., et al. (2003). Metabolic correlates of behavioral and affective disturbances in frontal lobe pathologies. *Journal of Neurology, 250*(7), 827–833.

Sawaguchi, T., & Goldman-Rakic, P. S. (1991). D1 dopamine receptors in prefrontal cortex. *Science, 251*, 947–950.

Schalling, D., & Rosen, A. S. (1968). Porteus Maze differences between psychopathic and non-psychopathic criminals. *British Journal of Social and Clinical Psychology, 7*(3), 224–228.

Schmitt, W. A., Brinkley, C. A., & Newman, J. P. (1999). Testing Damasio's somatic marker hypothesis with psychopathic individuals: Risk takers or risk averse? *Journal of Abnormal Psychology, 108*(3), 538–543.

Schultz, W., Tremblay, L., & Hollerman, J. R. (2000). Reward processing in primate orbitofrontal cortex and basal ganglia. *Cerebral Cortex, 10*, 272–283.

Shallice, T. (1982). Specific impairments in planning. *Philosophical Transactions of the Royal Society of London, Series B, Biological Sciences, 298*, 199–209.

Shallice, T. (1988). *From neuropsychology to mental structure*. Cambridge, MA: Cambridge University Press.

Shallice, T., & Burgess, P. (1996). The domain of supervisory processes and temporal organization of behaviour. *Philosophical Transactions of the Royal Society of London, Series B, Biological Sciences, 351*, 1405–1412.

Shiffrin, R. M., & Schneider, W. (1977). Controlled and automatic information processing: II. Perceptual learning, autonomic attending, and a general theory. *Psychological Review, 84*, 127–190.

Simpson, J. R., Drevets, W. C., Snyder, A. Z., Gusnard D. A., & Raichle, M. E. (2001) Emotion-induced changes in human medial prefrontal cortex II. During anticipatory anxiety. *Proceeding of the National Academy of Sciences USA, 98,* 688–693.

Skoff, B. F., & Libon, J. (1987). Impaired executive functions in a sample of male juvenile delinquents. *Journal of Clinical and Experimental Neuropsychology, 9,* 60.

Smith, S. S., Arnett, P.A., & Newman, J. P. (1992). Neuropsychological differentiation of psychopathic and nonpsychopathic criminal offenders. *Personality and Individual Differences, 13,* 1233–1243.

Soderstrom, H., Blennow, K., Sjodin, A-K., & Forsman, A. (2003). New evidence for an association between the CSF HVA: 5-HIAA ratio and psychopathic traits. *Journal of Neural Neurosurgery and Psychiatry, 74,* 918–921.

Soderstrom, H., Hultin, L., Tullberg, M., Wikkelso, C., Ekholm, S., & Forsman, A. (2002). Reduced frontotemporal perfusion in psychopathic personality. *Psychiatry Research Neuroimaging, 114,* 81–94.

Spitzer, R. L., Endicott J., & Robins, E. (1975). *Research diagnostic criteria.* New York: Biometrics Research, New York State Psychiatric Institute.

Stroop, J. R. (1935). Studies of interference in serial verbal reactions. *Journal of Experimental Psychology, 18,* 643–662.

Stuss, D. T., & Benson, D. F. (1984). Neuropsychological studies of the frontal lobes. *Psychological Bulletin, 95,* 3–28.

Stuss, D. T., Floden, D., Alexander, M. P., Levine, B., & Katz, D. (2001). Stroop performance in focal lesion patients: dissociation of processes and frontal lobe lesion location. *Neuropsychologia, 39*(8), 771–786.

Sullivan, R. M., & Gratton, A. (1999). Lateralised effects of medial prefrontal cortex lesions on neuroendocrine and autonomic stress in rats. *Journal of Neuroscience, 19,* 2834–2840.

Sutker, P. B., & Allain, A. N. (1987). Cognitive abstraction, shifting, and control: Clinical sample comparisons of psychopaths and non-psychopaths. *Journal of Abnormal Psychology, 96*(1), 73–75.

Sutker, P. B., Moan, C. E., & Allain, A. N. (1983). Assessment of cognitive control in psychopathic and normal prisoners. *Journal of Behavioral Assessment, 5,* 275–287.

Teuber, H. L. (1964). The riddle of frontal lobe function in man. In J. M. Warren & K. Akert (Eds.), *The frontal granular cortex and behavior.* New York: McGraw-Hill.

Thorpe, S. J., Rolls, E. T., & Maddison, S. (1983). The orbitofrontal cortex: Neuronal activity in the behaving monkey. *Experimental Brain Research, 49,* 93–115.

Timms, R. J. (1977). Cortical inhibition and facilitation of the defence reaction. *Journal of London, 266,* 98P–99P.

Tremblay, L., & Schultz, W. (1999). Relative reward preference in primate orbitofrontal cortex. *Nature, 398,* 704–708.

van den Broek, M. D., Bradshaw, C. M., & Szabadi, E. (1993). Utility of the Modified Wisconsin Card Sorting Test in neuropsychological assessment. *British Journal of Clinical Psychology, 32*(3), 333–343.

Verona, E., Patrick, C. J., Curtin, J. J., Bradley, M. M., & Lang, P. J. (2004). Psychopathy and physiological response to emotionally evocative sounds. *Journal of Abnormal Psychology, 113*(1), 99–108.

Wechsler, D. (1981). *Wechsler Adult Intelligence Scale—Revised.* New York: Psychological Corporation.

Weinberger, D. R., Berman, K. F., & Illowsky, B. P. (1988). Physiological dysfunction of dorsolateral prefrontal cortex in schizophrenia. III. A new cohort and evidence for a monoaminergic mechanism. *Archives of General Psychiatry, 45*(7), 609–615.

Weinberger, D. R., Egan, M. F., Bertolino, A., Calicott, J. H., Mattay, V. S., & Lipska, B. K. (2001). Prefrontal neurons and the genetics of schizophrenia. *Biological Psychiatry, 50*(11), 825–844.

Welsh, G. (1956). Factor dimensions A and R. In G. S. Welsh & W. G. Dahlstrom (Eds.), *Basic readings on the MMPI in psychology and medicine* (pp. 264–281). Minneapolis: University of Minnesota Press.

West, D. J., & Farrington, D. P. (1973). *Who becomes delinquent? Second report of the Cambridge study in delinquent development.* Oxford, UK: Crane, Russak.

Williamson, S., Harpur, T. J., & Hare, R. D. (1991). Abnormal processing of affective words by psychopaths. *Journal of Abnormal Psychology, 28*(5), 260–273.

Wilson, J. Q., & Herrnstein, R. J. (1985). *Crime and human nature.* New York: Simon & Schuster.

Yeudall, L. T., & Fromm-Auch, D. (1979). Neuro-psychological impairment in various psychopathological populations. In J. Gruzilier & P. Flor-Henry (Eds.), *Hemisphere asymmetrics of function and psychopathology* (pp. 5–13). New York: Elsevier/North Holland.

Yeudall, L. T., Fromm-Auch, D., & Davis, P. (1982). Neuropsychological impairment of persistent delinquency. *Journal of Nervous and Mental Disease, 170*(5), 257–265.

17

Understanding Psychopathy

The Cognitive Side

KRISTINA D. HIATT
JOSEPH P. NEWMAN

Psychopathy is a complex disorder of un-known etiology. Clinically, psychopathic individuals are striking for their shallow affect, lack of meaningful relationships, irresponsibility, impulsivity, and lack of insight into their disorder. Empirical studies of psychopathy have revealed emotion-processing deficits, such as poor fear conditioning (e.g., Flor, Birbaumer, Hermann, Ziegler, & Patrick, 2002; Hare & Quinn, 1971; Lykken, 1957) and reduced startle potentiation (e.g., Levenston, Patrick, Bradley, & Lang, 2000; Patrick, Bradley, & Lang, 1993; Patrick, Cuthbert, & Lang, 1994; Sutton, Vitale, & Newman, 2002), as well as deficits in broader cognitive processing, such as dual-task attention (e.g., Jutai, Hare, & Connolly, 1987; Kosson, 1996) and behavioral inhibition (e.g., Newman & Kosson, 1986; Newman, Patterson, Howland, & Nichols, 1990). Although both popular and empirical characterizations of psychopathy have tended to emphasize the emotion-processing deficits, the information-processing deficits associated with psychopathy provide critical insight into the disorder. A primary challenge for researchers attempting to understand the psychopathic syndrome is to elaborate the relationship between psychopaths' cognitive and emotional deficits such that the disorder can be viewed within one theoretical framework. Toward this end, this chapter (1) provides a review of the major cognitive deficits that have been associated with psychopathy, and (2) suggests possible avenues for integrating these cognitive deficits with psychopaths' emotion-processing deficits, with the aim of promoting the development of a unified understanding of psychopathy.

STUDY SELECTION

The following review is restricted to studies that identify psychopathic participants by means of the Psychopathy Checklist (PCL; Hare, 1980) or Psychopathy Checklist—Revised (PCL-R; Hare, 1991). This restriction of studies is based on our strong belief that etiological understanding of psychopathy depends on the identification of a well-defined, relatively homogenous population. Because of the phenotypical overlap but presumed etiological differences among psychopathy and other externalizing-spectrum disorders (e.g., antisocial personality disorder), we feel that it is critical to use diagnostic methods that can reliably differentiate psychopathic and nonpsychopathic individuals. The PCL-R and its predecessor were derived from

Cleckley's (1982) classic description of the disorder, and the PCL-R is generally considered to be the premier instrument for assessing psychopathy among incarcerated populations. By restricting our review to studies employing this reliable and valid measure of psychopathy, we hope to provide a clear picture of the deficits that have been specifically associated with psychopathy. However, we acknowledge the contributions of research using alternative methods of psychopathy assessment, such as research involving community or adolescent populations, and we look forward to further validation of the psychopathy construct in these samples and the eventual integration of this work with the literature on traditional, PCL/PCL-R psychopathy.

For similar reasons, we also restrict the following literature review to studies involving male participants. Although empirical studies of PCL-R psychopathy among female populations are increasing, the generality of the construct across gender has yet to be firmly established (see Verona & Vitale, Chapter 21, this volume). Furthermore, there appear to be important performance differences between male and female PCL-R psychopaths (Vitale & Newman, 2001; Vitale, Smith, Brinkley, & Newman, 2002). Although we encourage further investigation of the similarities and differences among male and female psychopathic individuals, current knowledge is insufficient to allow straightforward integration of findings across male and female samples. Therefore, studies using female samples are excluded from this review.

LITERATURE REVIEW

Psychopathy has not traditionally been associated with cognitive dysfunction, at least with regard to intelligence, memory, and executive ability (e.g., Cleckley, 1982). Indeed, psychopaths are notorious for the contrast between their good explicit knowledge and their profound failures when put to the test of daily life. However, it is possible that the assumption of intact cognitive ability is based on an overly simplified model of cognitive and executive functions. It is widely recognized that cognitive control and adaptive self-regulation depend on much more

than adequate intelligence or the ability to perform well on traditional measures of executive ability. For example, what determines how top-down cognitive or executive resources will be directed, and which stimuli will become the focus of, and benefit from, the available cognitive resources? Clearly, the appropriate allocation of cognitive resources is as important to successful cognitive control and self-regulation as traditional executive functions such as goal maintenance. Thus, despite their good overall intelligence and cognitive ability, psychopaths may be impaired in more subtle aspects of cognition. Indeed, the existing literature on cognitive functioning among psychopaths reveals subtle but important abnormalities in several broad domains. These domains include attention, language processing, behavioral inhibition, and neuropsychological functioning.

ATTENTION

Interest in psychopaths' attentional functioning arose in part from their demonstrated insensitivity to incidental punishment cues (e.g., Lykken, 1957). In response to psychopaths' poor passive avoidance learning and aversive conditioning, Hare (1986) proposed that psychopaths, when not forced to attend to warning cues, "may be able to focus attention on things of immediate interest, effectively ignoring warning cues and other stimuli not of immediate interest to them" (p. 12). Consistent with this proposal, many studies indicate that psychopaths fail to accommodate secondary or unattended information.

Jutai and Hare (1983) found that psychopaths showed reduced physiological responsivity to irrelevant auditory stimuli when their attention was focused elsewhere, although they showed normal responsivity during passive listening. Autonomic and electrocortical activity was recorded while inmates with high and low ratings of psychopathy were presented with a series of binaural tone pips, either by themselves (passive attention) or while video games were being played (selective attention). During selective attention the subjects were told that the tone pips were irrelevant to the primary task. The N100 component of the auditory evoked potential was used as an index of attention paid to the tone pips, while performance on the video games was considered to be a reflection of attentiveness to the primary task. Psychopaths displayed normal N100 responses to the tone pips presented alone. However, psychopaths gave small N100 responses to the tone pips during each trial, including the first one, when they were engaged in playing the video game. In contrast, nonpsychopaths gave large N100 responses to tone pips during the first trial and small responses during later trials. Jutai and Hare interpreted this result in terms of limited-capacity models of attention and suggested that psychopaths allocate a relatively large proportion of their attentional resources to events of immediate interest, effectively ignoring other stimuli.

Similarly, Newman and colleagues (Hiatt, Schmitt, & Newman, 2004; Newman, Schmitt, & Voss, 1997; Smith, Arnett, & Newman, 1992) have demonstrated that psychopaths show reduced interference from irrelevant distractors on certain Stroop-like paradigms. Newman, Schmitt, and Voss (1997) presented psychopaths and nonpsychopaths with a picture–word interference task. At the start of each trial, the relevant (to-be-attended) dimension was indicated by the letter P or W. A compound picture–word stimulus (line drawing with superimposed word) was then presented, followed by a test stimulus (a picture on P trials, a word on W trials). Participants were to judge whether the relevant dimension of the compound stimulus was semantically related to the test stimulus. Nonpsychopaths showed significant reaction time interference for trials in which the irrelevant, but not the relevant, dimension of the compound stimulus was related to the test stimulus (i.e., correct response "unrelated"), particularly when the irrelevant stimulus was a word. Psychopaths failed to show this interference effect, indicating decreased sensitivity to unattended contextual information.

However, Smith and colleagues (1992) found normal Stroop interference among psychopaths on the standard color–word Stroop. To further examine psychopaths' selective attention, Hiatt and colleagues (2004) presented psychopathic and nonpsychopathic inmates with three different Stroop-like tasks: the standard color–word Stroop, a picture–word Stroop, and the "box" Stroop,

in which color–words appeared inside a colored rectangular frame, thereby spatially separating the color and color–word components. Hiatt and colleagues found that psychopaths showed normal Stroop interference on the standard, spatially coincident color–word Stroop but reduced interference on the spatially separated picture–word and box Stroop tasks.

The Stroop interference displayed by healthy participants indicates that incongruent but task-irrelevant information interferes with primary task performance, despite participants' attempts to ignore this information. Psychopaths show normal Stroop interference when the target and distractor overlap spatially (e.g, the word *BLUE* written in green ink) but show dramatically reduced interference when the target and distractor are spatially separated (e.g., the word *BLUE* in white ink, surrounded by a green rectangle). In the spatially separated condition, the primary task information (e.g., the color of the rectangle) can be attended separately from the secondary task information (e.g., the word *BLUE*). Nevertheless, the interference demonstrated by healthy controls indicates that focused attention is modulated by the secondary information that occurs outside the deliberate attentional focus. Psychopaths, however, fail to show this attentional modulation, consistent with poor accommodation of secondary or contextual information that occurs outside their primary attentional focus.

Similarly, Christianson and colleagues (1996) found that psychopaths failed to show the typical emotion-modulated narrowing of attention when they were unexpectedly presented with a slide depicting an aversive scene. Controls showed poorer recall for peripheral details on the aversive relative to neutral slides, whereas psychopaths showed good recall of both central and peripheral details, regardless of emotional content. Thus, despite reporting a typical emotional reaction to the scene and showing good recall for the details of the slide, psychopaths' attentional processing did not appear to be affected by the emotional nature of the slide. This finding indicates that psychopaths' performance on the primary task of attending to slides was unaffected by the unexpected emotional information and is consistent with deficient modulation of attention by secondary or contextual information.

Also consistent with poor processing of information that occurs outside the attentional focus, psychopaths show abnormal event-related potential (ERP) responses to auditory "oddball" targets when they are engaged in a distractor task. Jutai and colleagues (1987) recorded ERPs to phonemic stimuli while psychopaths and nonpsychopaths performed a speech discrimination "oddball" paradigm in which participants were required to respond whenever the target (oddball) phoneme occurred. ERPs were recorded while participants performed the oddball task alone (single-task condition) and simultaneously performed a distractor video-game task (dual-task condition). There were no group differences in performance or on measures of central arousal (N100) during the single- or dual-task conditions. However, psychopaths' P300 responses to the target under dual-task conditions were notable for an overlapping positive slow wave, primarily at vertex and left-hemisphere sites. Jutai and colleagues interpreted this positive slow wave as evidence of unusual speech processing in psychopaths under conditions of distraction. They proposed that psychopaths' large slow wave may reflect increased processing effort and suggested that psychopaths may have had some difficulty keeping track of the sequential probabilities of the speech stimuli (e.g., that two targets never occurred in a row) when engaged in the video game.

In addition to poor processing of secondary or incidental information, there is some evidence that psychopaths allocate excessive attention to their primary task. Forth and Hare (1989) recorded electrocortical responses among psychopathic and nonpsychopathic inmates during the interval between a warning tone and an imperative tone. Participants were instructed to press a response button as quickly as possible on hearing the imperative tone and were also informed that the pitch of the warning tone on each trial indicated whether they would win money for a fast response, lose money for a slow response, or neither win nor lose money on that trial. Forth and Hare found no group differences in N100 or P300 responses but did find that the early (600–1,500 milliseconds) contingent negative variation (CNV) response was larger among psychopaths than controls. Forth and Hare interpreted the early CNV as a reflection of attention to the warning stimulus and task demands and suggested that psychopaths may be more proficient than nonpsychopaths at focusing attention on events that interest them.

There is also evidence that incidental processing of contextual information may be relatively uncoupled from primary attention among psychopaths relative to controls. Bernstein, Newman, and Wallace (2000) asked participants to memorize a series of eight words that were presented one at a time, with two words appearing in each corner of the video display. This explicit word recall task produced the expected left-hemisphere advantage among both psychopaths and controls, with better recall for words that were presented on the right versus the left side of the monitor. Following the word recall task, participants were unexpectedly asked to recall the spatial position in which each word had appeared. This incidental recall of locations followed the pattern of word recall among controls, with better accuracy for the spatial locations of words that had appeared on the right side of the monitor. This finding suggests that controls' processing of the incidental spatial information was to some extent coupled with their primary focus of attention. Among psychopaths, however, recall accuracy was equally distributed across both visual fields. According to Bernstein and colleagues, secondary attention appears to be more closely tied to primary attention among controls than among psychopathic individuals. One consequence of this group difference is that controls may be more likely to process multiple dimensions of a stimulus (or event) that is the focus of primary attention.

The preceding findings provide consistent evidence that psychopathy is associated with rigid task-focused attention that is poorly modulated by secondary or incidental information. However, the picture becomes somewhat more complex when psychopaths are presented with demanding dual-task paradigms. Kosson and Newman (1986) presented participants with a visual search task, in which participants counted the number of targets that appeared across each set of 8 test frames, and a go/no-go task, in which they were to respond as quickly as possible to low-pitched but not high-pitched tones. In one condition, participants were told to focus on the visual search task, while in the other condition they were told to divide attention equally between the two tasks. Psychopaths made more visual-search errors than nonpsychopaths under the divided attention condition, and they tended to make fewer visual-search errors than nonpsychopaths in the focused condition. Across conditions, psychopaths responded slower than nonpsychopaths to the target tones.

Psychopaths' increase in visual-search errors under divided attention conditions does not immediately appear to be consistent with poor accommodation of secondary information when attention is allocated elsewhere, which suggests that psychopaths may have a more general difficulty in distributing attention across multiple complex response contingencies. However, it is possible that nonpsychopaths make use of relatively automatic attentional processing (as opposed to top-down effortful attention) to manage multiple response contingencies, and that psychopaths' difficulty accommodating secondary or peripheral information requires them to compensate by using a more effortful, top-down approach to the task. A more effortful, top-down approach to this complex dual-task paradigm may account for psychopaths' slower responses to the target tones and tendency to commit visual-search errors under divided attention conditions. This proposal is consistent with Kosson and Newman's (1986) suggestion that psychopaths may incur relatively large-capacity costs in attempting to shift their attentional resources between processing tasks.

In a second dual-task study, Kosson (1996) presented participants with two simultaneous classification tasks. Participants were asked to classify symbol strings as all numbers, all letters, or a mixture (50%), but only if the string appeared in a horizontal rather than vertical frame. They were also asked to classify a four-tone sequence as increasing in pitch, maintaining constant pitch, or a mixture, but only if the tones were relatively low pitched. The relative priority of each task was manipulated by target frequency rather than by explicit instructions; visual targets were more likely than auditory targets. In the dual-task condition, some tri-

als had two targets (i.e., both a visual and an auditory target) and some trials had one target. Kosson found no group differences in responses to either primary- or secondary-task targets under dual-task conditions, nor were there any group differences when either the visual or the auditory task was presented alone. However, psychopaths overresponded to secondary-task distractors, especially when they followed a primary-task target. Kosson interpreted psychopaths' responses to distractors as consistent with a failure to "process peripheral stimulus features in attention-demanding situations" (p. 398). Psychopaths also displayed a trend toward a performance deficit in primary task accuracy when the primary-task target followed a secondary-task target and they were responding with their right hand to the primary task, which Kosson interpreted as consistent with a deficit in "shifting attention under conditions involving left hemisphere processing resources" (p. 398).

These findings by Kosson and colleagues (Kosson, 1996; Kosson & Newman, 1986) are consistent with poor use of secondary information but also suggest a possible hemispheric asymmetry such that attentional processing is disrupted by phasic left-hemisphere activation. Kosson (1998) examined psychopaths' performance on a divided visual field task with two lateralized stimuli per trial and provided further evidence for the importance of left-hemisphere activation. Participants were to classify symbol strings as all numbers, all letters, or a mixture, but only if the string appeared in green rather than yellow type. Attention to the two stimuli was manipulated by target frequency; in one condition (relatively focused attention) targets were more frequent in one visual field, while in the other condition (equally divided attention) targets were equally likely to occur in either visual field. When the majority of the targets were presented in the right visual field (RVF), psychopaths misclassified more left-visual-field (LVF) targets and marginally more RVF targets than nonpsychopaths. Psychopaths also overresponded to distractors on both tasks under focusing conditions. There were no group differences in performance under single-task conditions (i.e., when only one stimulus was presented per trial). Kosson proposed that "reduced breadth of attention under focusing conditions and cognitive deficits given left hemisphere activation appear viable explanations of psychopaths' performance deficits" (p. 373).

Howland, Kosson, Patterson, and Newman (1993) also found evidence that psychopaths' attentional abnormalities may be exacerbated by left-hemisphere activation. Howland et al. examined the attentional performance of psychopaths and nonpsychopaths on an exogenously cued Posner task. They found that psychopaths made more errors than nonpsychopaths following invalid RVF cues. Given that RVF cues are initially processed by the left hemisphere, and vice versa, this finding indicates that psychopaths had difficulty shifting attention from left-hemisphere (RVF) cues to right-hemisphere (LVF) targets and provides further evidence that left-hemisphere activation may contribute to psychopaths' attentional abnormalities. Howland and colleagues also found that psychopaths made more errors than controls on neutral trials for which the imperative stimulus appeared in the RVF.

Kiehl, Hare, Liddle, and McDonald (1999) found that psychopaths' P300 differentiation between targets and nontargets was reduced relative to nonpsychopaths on a visual oddball task, although psychopaths' behavioral performance was comparable to that of controls. Participants were instructed to respond as quickly as possible to the infrequent target stimulus by pressing a response key with their right hand. Psychopaths showed normal ERPs to nontarget stimuli, but, unlike controls, they failed to show reliable P300 amplitude differences between the target and nontarget conditions. P300 responses were generally greater in the right than the left hemisphere, but psychopaths' P300 responses were less lateralized to the right hemisphere than those of controls. In contrast, psychopaths showed larger left-hemisphere N550 responses than controls to target stimuli. Thus, psychopaths showed reduced P300 differentiation between targets and nontargets, showed less P300 lateralization to the right hemisphere, and showed a greater left-hemisphere N550 response to target stimuli. Consistent with psychopaths' proposed difficulty modulating task-focused attention, Kiehl, Hare, Liddle, and colleagues (1999) interpreted psychopaths'

poor P300 differentiation as consistent with deficient sustained attention or unusual allocation of attentional resources to task demands and suggested that psychopaths' attention, once focused, may be difficult to remobilize. This study provides physiological evidence that is consistent with both poor distribution of attention and unusual lateralization of processing across the cerebral hemispheres.

Thus, both behavioral and physiological investigations of psychopaths' attentional functioning are largely consistent with rigid task-focused attention that is poorly modulated by secondary or contextual information. In addition, these studies suggest that psychopaths' attentional insensitivity to secondary or contextual information may be exacerbated by left-hemisphere activation. The possible contribution of left-hemisphere activation suggests a potential refinement of psychopaths' difficulty accommodating unattended contextual information. We return to this possibility in the discussion section.

LANGUAGE

Psychopaths' notorious abilities to manipulate, and the apparent disconnect between their statements and their intentions, has led to substantial interest in the ways in which psychopaths use and understand language. As paraphrased by Hare (1986), "Cleckley long held that the speech of psychopaths appears to be a mechanically correct artifact that masks a semantic disorder in which the formal, semantic, and affective components of language are dissociated from one another" (p. 21). Hare suggested that this disorder may involve "unusual or abnormal interactions among the cortical, subcortical, and limbic mechanisms responsible for the integration of verbal, emotional, and social behavior" (p. 22). Empirical studies of psychopaths' language processing have revealed abnormalities that fall into two major categories: (1) the use of associative or contextual aspects of language such as connotation, affect, abstract meanings, and metaphor; and (2) unusual functional cerebral asymmetries for processing verbal stimuli.

Hare, Williamson, and Harpur (1988) reported that psychopaths, when asked to choose the two words in a triad that were most similar in meaning, tended to group words on the basis of denotation and literal meaning (e.g., antonyms). In contrast, nonpsychopathic controls tended to group words on the basis of their connotations (e.g., metaphorical relationships and emotional polarity). Based on these data, Hare and colleagues suggested that psychopaths may be less sensitive than controls to the connotative meanings of language. Similarly, Herve, Hayes, and Hare (2003) reported that incarcerated PCL-R psychopaths made significantly more sorting errors than nonpsychopaths on an emotional metaphor Q-sort task, despite having good literal understanding of the metaphors. They concluded that these results support the hypothesis that "incarcerated psychopaths do not understand or make effective use of the emotional content of language" (p. 1497).

Williamson, Harpur, and Hare (1991) demonstrated that psychopaths fail to show the normal reaction time facilitation for emotional words on a lexical-decision task, indicating poor accommodation of unexpected affective information. Psychopaths also showed poor ERP differentiation between neutral and emotional words. In addition, the positive slow wave component of the ERP was relatively small and brief among psychopaths relative to controls, and was preceded for both neutral and emotional words by a large centrofrontal negative wave (N500). Williamson et al. suggested that psychopaths' slow lexical-decision reaction times, short-lived late positive ERP, and abnormal N500 reflect difficulty integrating word meanings within broader linguistic or conceptual structures.

Lorenz and Newman (2002) replicated Williamson and colleagues' (1991) finding of reduced emotion facilitation among psychopaths on a lexical-decision task. However, Lorenz and Newman found that psychopaths' lack of emotion facilitation was specific to right-handed responses. When performing the lexical-decision task with their left hand, psychopaths' emotion facilitation was equivalent to that of controls. As right-handed responses are controlled by the left hemisphere, this result is reminiscent of Kosson's (1996, 1998) findings that the failure of psychopaths to accommodate contextual or secondary information is exacerbated by left-hemisphere activation.

Kiehl, Hare, McDonald, and Brink (1999) examined psychopaths' ERP responses to semantic and affective verbal information, using lexical-decision and word discrimination tasks with either concrete (e.g., "chair") and abstract (e.g., "justice") or positive and negative words. Kiehl and colleagues found that psychopaths made more errors identifying abstract than concrete words. On all tasks, psychopaths failed to show the normal ERP differentiation between types of word stimuli. In addition, the ERPs of psychopaths included a large centrofrontal negative-going wave (N350) that was absent or very small among nonpsychopaths.

Psychopaths also show relative deficits in the global coherence of their language. Brinkley, Newman, Harpur, and Johnson (1999) found that psychopaths' narratives included fewer cohesive ties per clause than those of nonpsychopaths. Brinkley, Bernstein, and Newman (1999) asked participants to generate stories including specific plot units (i.e., story elements or themes), and found that psychopaths closed fewer plot units than nonpsychopaths. Gillstrom and Hare (1988) examined psychopaths' use of hand gestures during speech. They recorded hand gestures that served to illustrate what was being said (iconic gestures) and small, repetitive, apparently unintentional gestures (beats) during videotaped interview segments in which participants discussed their family life and criminal offenses. Participants with high PCL scores used significantly more beats than those with low or moderate PCL scores, and the latter two groups did not differ from one another.

Although psychopaths' language abilities are grossly intact, the preceding studies indicate that psychopaths have difficulty using the more subtle or contextual aspects of language. In many instances, this difficulty involves the use of emotional connotation in language, although psychopaths also have difficulty with abstract concepts and global cohesion. While the neural bases of these connotative and contextual components of language are not fully understood, it is reasonable to presume that they depend on broad and relatively automatic activation of semantic networks. In this sense, they may be considered "secondary" aspects of language that automatically influence processing in normal controls. Consistent with their difficulty using secondary information in other domains, psychopaths may have difficulty making use of these broad linguistic associations without deliberately attending to them. Importantly, psychopaths are able to accurately evaluate and use emotion and connotation in language when explicitly required to do so (e.g., Levenston et al., 2000; Patrick et al., 1993; Williamson et al., 1991).

In addition to their poor use of secondary or contextual aspects of language, psychopaths also show abnormal cerebral asymmetries on certain language processing tasks. Although psychopaths show a normal left-hemisphere advantage for the identification (Hare, 1979), detection (Hiatt, Lorenz, & Newman, 2002), and recall (Bernstein et al., 2000) of common words, other studies have revealed abnormal language lateralization among psychopathic individuals. Hare and McPherson (1984) found a reduced right-ear advantage among psychopaths on a dichotic listening task in which participants were asked, at the end of each set of three word pairs, to report all the words they could recall hearing. Hare and Jutai (1988) examined psychopaths' cerebral asymmetries for the categorization of words into specific (four-footed animal, vehicle, bird, or weapon) or abstract (living or nonliving) categories. Words were briefly presented in either the LVF or RVF, and participants indicated whether or not the word was a member of the specified category by pressing the appropriate response button. On the simple categorization task, both psychopaths and nonpsychopaths showed the expected RVF advantage. On the abstract categorization task, nonpsychopaths continued to show a RVF advantage while psychopaths showed a large LVF advantage. Thus, psychopaths displayed a normal RVF/left-hemisphere advantage for the classification of words into concrete, but not abstract, categories. Together, these studies suggest that the processing of complex language-based tasks is less lateralized to the left hemisphere among psychopaths than controls, although psychopaths show normal left-hemisphere lateralization for simple linguistic tasks.

Although the number of studies is limited, the available evidence suggests that psychopaths' use of language tends to be unelaborated and lacking in associative depth.

In addition to this poor use of secondary aspects of language, psychopaths show a reduced left-hemisphere advantage for the classification of abstract words and for the delayed recall of dichotically presented word pairs but a normal left-hemisphere advantage for simple word identification, recognition, and recall, as well as for the classification of concrete words. These laterality findings suggest that psychopaths have reduced lateralization of processing for language tasks that require the use of broad associations (e.g., categorizing abstract words) or entail heavy processing demands (e.g., recall of dichotically presented word pairs). Note that unusual asymmetry effects (i.e., poor distribution of attention under left-hemisphere activating conditions; unusual ERP lateralization) were also observed in physiological and behavioral studies of psychopaths' attentional processing, suggesting that abnormal functional cerebral asymmetries may be a consistent feature of psychopathy.

BEHAVIORAL INHIBITION

Poor behavioral inhibition is one of the hallmark features of psychopathy and has been the focus of numerous investigations. Many of these investigations have used passive avoidance paradigms, which require participants to inhibit responses in order to avoid punishment. The earliest study of passive avoidance in psychopaths was conducted by Lykken (1957). Lykken used a "mental maze" in which participants were required to navigate choice points in a maze by pressing one of four response levers. There was one correct lever at each decision point. The passive avoidance component of the task involved a latent shock contingency: At each decision point, one of the three incorrect response levers was paired with an electric shock. Passive avoidance was measured by the increased avoidance of shocked responses across trials. Lykken found that psychopaths committed more passive avoidance errors than nonpsychopathic controls.

Attempts to replicate Lykken's (1957) finding have produced mixed results and have revealed that psychopaths' passive avoidance deficits are context dependent. Schmauk (1970) used a modified version of

Lykken's task, and examined passive avoidance under conditions involving verbal punishment ("wrong"), tangible punishment (loss of 25 cents), or physical punishment (electric shocks). In the conditions involving verbal and physical punishment, low-anxious psychopaths displayed smaller skin conductance responses, poorer passive avoidance learning, and less awareness of the punishment contingencies than did nonincarcerated controls. However, the groups did not differ on any of these measures when the punishment contingency involved loss of money.

Later studies by other researchers have found passive avoidance deficits even with loss of money (Newman & Kosson, 1986; Newman, Patterson, & Kosson, 1987; Siegel, 1978). Newman and colleagues (1990) argued that, unlike Schmauk (1970), each of the studies demonstrating poor passive avoidance under conditions of monetary loss also involved a competing reward contingency. They argued that a competing reward contingency is an important component of psychopaths' poor passive avoidance.

Several studies have explicitly investigated the effect of reward contingencies on psychopaths' passive avoidance performance. Newman and Kosson (1986) presented participants with two versions of a passive avoidance task. In one version (reward + punishment), participants received both reward and punishment feedback. If their response was incorrect, they heard a tone and lost 10 cents. If their response was correct, they heard a different tone and earned 10 cents. In the other version (punishment only), participants received only punishment feedback; they lost money if they responded to a punished stimulus or failed to respond to a rewarded stimulus. No feedback was given after correct responses. Psychopaths made more passive avoidance (commission) errors than controls in the version involving competing reward and punishment contingencies but performed comparably to controls in the punishment-only condition. Newman and Kosson concluded that psychopaths show poor passive avoidance only in the presence of competing reward contingencies.

Similarly, Newman and colleagues (1990) found poor passive avoidance among psychopaths relative to controls when participants were engaged in a task that emphasized obtaining rewards, but psychopaths performed comparably to controls when punishment and reward contingencies were salient from the start of the task and given equal emphasis. Furthermore, using subject-terminated response feedback, they found that in the task emphasizing rewards, psychopaths paused less than controls following negative feedback, and the extent to which participants paused following negative feedback was correlated with passive avoidance learning. Newman and colleagues concluded that it is not the presence of reward per se but, rather, the need to interrupt a dominant reward-seeking set in order to process and learn from punishment feedback that disrupts psychopaths' passive avoidance learning.

Arnett, Smith, and Newman (1997) provided further evidence that psychopaths show normal avoidance of explicit punishment contingencies. They employed a simple stop-signal task, in which participants were required to respond to targets as quickly as possible but refrain from responding if an inhibitory cue was also present. Psychopaths showed normal behavioral inhibition on this task. Similarly, Newman, Wallace, Schmitt, and Arnett (1997) found normal response inhibition among psychopaths when participants were instructed to search a letter string and respond to targets unless the letter "Q" also appeared in the letter string. These studies demonstrate that psychopaths show good behavioral inhibition when the inhibitory cues or punishment contingencies are made explicit. Kiehl, Smith, Hare, and Liddle (2000) also found good behavioral inhibition among psychopaths on an explicit go/no-go task. However, they found that psychopaths' ERP responses to the go and no-go stimuli were abnormal, with less differentiation between the go and no-go stimuli at the N275 and reversed differentiation (no-go greater than go) at the P375 component. This finding suggests that psychopaths' processing of straightforward inhibition tasks may differ from that of nonpsychopaths, despite their good performance.

As mentioned previously, Newman and colleagues (1990) found that psychopaths paused less than controls following negative feedback, and they proposed that the need to interrupt a dominant reward-seeking set is a critical feature of psychopaths' passive avoidance deficits. Providing support for this proposal, Newman and colleagues (1987) demonstrated that forced pauses can remedy psychopaths' poor behavioral inhibition in the presence of prepotent reward contingencies. They presented psychopaths and controls with three different versions of a card-playing task. In each task, the probability of reward declined steadily across trials while the probability of punishment increased steadily. To perform successfully (i.e., maximize winnings), participants needed to stop playing cards approximately halfway through the 100-trial task. The three task versions differed in the feedback given to participants. In the first version, participants received feedback after each response but no cumulative feedback. In the second version, cumulative results were displayed on the screen after each response. In the third version, cumulative results were displayed and participants were forced to pause for 5 seconds before the start of the next trial. Newman and colleagues found normal response inhibition among psychopaths only in the third condition, when they were forced to pause for 5 seconds following feedback.

A study by Mitchell, Colledge, Leonard, and Blair (2002) suggests that psychopathic individuals also perform more poorly than controls on Bechara, Damasio, Damasio, and Lee's (1999) four-pack gambling task (Mitchell, Colledge, Leonard, & Blair, 2002). This task allows participants to play cards from any of four decks. Two decks are "risky," with occasional large rewards but an overall net loss, and two desks are "safe," with smaller rewards and an overall net gain. Mitchell and colleagues found that controls learned to avoid the "risky" decks over time, whereas psychopaths did not. Thus, psychopaths failed to modify their reward-seeking behavior in accord with punishment feedback.

However, an earlier study by Schmitt, Brinkley, and Newman (1999) found no evidence of group differences on the four-pack gambling task, although their procedure differed from that of Mitchell and colleagues (2002) in that they did not explicitly instruct participants that some decks were better than others and they used a small amount of real money rather than play money to represent losses and gains. A recent study by Lösel and Schmucker (2004) used the same methods as Mitchell and colleagues and again found no evidence of group differences. Lösel and Schmucker suggested that the performance of psychopathic individuals is moderated by attentional skills, with "less attentive" psychopaths making poorer decisions than those with strong attention skills. The factors driving psychopaths' performance on the four-pack gambling task and the reliability of psychopaths' disinhibition on this task remain to be resolved.

Mitchell and colleagues (2002) reported a second experiment that provides additional evidence of disinhibition among psychopaths. This second study employed an instrumental learning task that required participants to use feedback ("correct" or "incorrect") to learn which of two stimuli they should select on each trial. The stimuli and the correct choices were periodically altered, requiring participants to adjust their response strategies. Psychopaths did not differ from controls in their ability to learn which stimulus should be responded to when new pairs of stimuli were presented. However, psychopaths made more errors than controls when the stimulus pairs remained the same but the reward contingencies were reversed. These findings suggest that psychopaths are adept at learning reward contingencies for novel stimuli but may have difficulty withholding responses to previously rewarded stimuli.

The foregoing studies reveal consistent behavioral disinhibition among psychopaths, but these deficits appear to be quite sensitive to task conditions. In general, psychopaths' behavioral disinhibition is most evident when there is a predominant reward contingency for responding and when participants are not required to pause for feedback between responses. Thus, psychopaths appear to have difficulty inhibiting previously punished responses when they are actively engaged in reward-seeking approach behavior. As argued by Newman, Schmitt, and Voss (1997), psychopaths appear to have no difficulty avoiding punishment when (1) avoidance learning is their only goal (i.e., there is no approach contingency; Newman & Kosson, 1986); (2) the avoidance contingency is made salient from the outset of the task (Newman et al., 1990); or (3) positive and negative feedback are provided during an extended intertrial interval, thereby reducing the need for efficient processing of negative/ avoidance feedback (Arnett, Howland, & Smith, 1993; Newman et al., 1987).

It should be noted that these findings are most robust in comparisons involving low-anxious psychopaths and controls; high-anxious controls are frequently as disinhibited or more disinhibited than high-anxious psychopaths. The reason for this specificity has yet to be fully explained. One possibility is suggested by Gray's (1982; see also Fowles, 1980) model of behavioral inhibition system (BIS) functioning, which corresponds to the anxiety dimension assessed by the Welsh Anxiety Scale (Welsh, 1956). According to this model, higher levels of anxiety are associated with increasing arousal and inhibition in response to cues for punishment. Trait anxiety may therefore be a particularly important moderator of psychopaths' performance on tests of behavioral inhibition, which directly assess responses to punishment cues. Regardless, psychopaths' behavioral disinhibition has also been observed irrespective of anxiety (e.g., Mitchell et al., 2002; Newman & Kosson, 1986; Newman et al., 1987).

As with psychopaths' attentional and language-processing abnormalities, psychopaths' behavioral inhibition deficits reveal evidence of difficulty using information that occurs outside the primary focus of attention. Thus, poor accommodation of secondary or incidental information appears to be a consistent feature of psychopaths' cognitive functioning. Although psychopaths' hemispheric processing asymmetries have not been investigated within the domain of behavioral inhibition, it is worth noting that reward-seeking behaviors may differentially activate the left hemisphere (e.g., Davidson 1995; Miller & Tomarken, 2001; Sobotka, Davidson, & Senulis, 1992). The exacerbation of psychopaths' disinhibition in the presence of a reward-seeking response set may therefore be consistent with Kosson's (1996, 1998) findings of attentional dysfunction under left-hemisphere activating conditions.

NEUROPSYCHOLOGICAL FUNCTIONING

A number of researchers have examined the performance of psychopathic individuals on standardized neuropsychological tests. Consistent with Cleckley's clinical insight, these tests generally fail to reveal clinically significant deficits among psychopathic populations. However, psychopaths do display circumscribed abnormalities relative to nonpsychopathic controls on a minority of neuropsychological tests.

Hare (1984), following Gorenstein's (1982) report of poor frontal functioning among inpatients with psychopathic features, administered the Wisconsin Card Sorting Test (WCST), Necker cube, and a sequential matching memory task to incarcerated PCL psychopaths and controls. Hare found no evidence of group differences on any of these measures, and concluded that "the performance of both the inmates in general and the psychopaths in particular was very similar to that of normal or non-criminal individuals and not at all like that of frontal lobe patients" (p. 138).

Hart, Forth, and Hare (1990) administered neuropsychological batteries to two large samples of incarcerated PCL-R psychopaths and nonpsychopaths. One battery consisted of the Trail-Making Test, Visual Retention Test, Auditory–Verbal Learning Test, and Visual Organization Test. A second battery included the Trail-Making Test, Controlled Word Association Test, Vocabulary and Block Design subtests of the Wechsler Adult Intelligence Scale—Revised (WAIS-R), and the Wide Range Achievement Test, Second Edition, Reading. Hart and colleagues found no group differences on any of the tests, and concluded that the results "offer no support for traditional brain-damage interpretations of psychopathy" (p. 377).

However, Smith, Arnett, and Newman (1992) found evidence for circumscribed neuropsychological deficits among low-anxious psychopaths. They administered tests of executive (Controlled Word Association Test, Trail-Making Test, Category Test, Stroop), memory (Digit Span, Paired Associate Learning), motor (Finger Tapping), and visuospatial (Block Design) functions to a large sample of incarcerated PCL psychopaths and controls. They found no group differences in performance among high-anxious psychopaths and controls, but low-anxious psychopaths performed more poorly than controls on Block Design and Trails-B. These findings stand in contrast to those of Hart and colleagues (1990) and suggest that anxiety may moderate the expression of neuropsychological deficits among psychopaths. Interestingly, and as noted by Smith and colleagues, the specificity of low-anxious psychopaths' deficits to the Block Design and Trails-B subtests suggests that they may be "less adept at cognitively demanding activities mediated primarily by the right hemisphere—at least while actively engaged in motor responding" (p. 9).

LaPierre, Braun, and Hodgins (1995) administered tests associated with orbitofrontal/ventromedial functions (a go/no-go discrimination task, the Porteus Maze task, and the Modular Smell Identification Test), frontodorsolateral function (WCST perseverative errors), and right posterior cortex (mental rotation) to PCL-R psychopaths and incarcerated nonpsychopaths. They found that psychopaths made more olfactory identification errors, more commission errors on the go/no-go task, and more qualitative errors on the Porteus Maze. Psychopaths and controls did not differ on any other measures. The authors concluded that these findings are "concordant with the hypothesis of a specific ventral frontal dysfunction in psychopathy" (p. 146).

Pham, Vanderstukken, Philippot, and Vanderlinden (2003) administered a letter cancellation task, the Porteus Maze task, the Tower of London Test (TOL), the Stroop, the Trail-Making Test, and a modified WCST to PCL-R psychopaths and controls. Psychopaths committed more qualitative errors on the Porteus Maze (e.g., crossed walls), made more errors on the letter cancellation test and had more variability in the number of items read per line, and made excessive "moves" and took more time on misleading TOL problems. The authors interpreted these findings as consistent with a selective attention deficit and poor control of attention when exposed to distracters.

The foregoing studies reveal that psychopaths perform normally on the majority of neuropsychological tasks. However, two studies have reported greater qualitative errors (e.g., crossing walls) among psychopaths relative to controls on the Porteus Maze task, and poor performance relative to controls has also been reported for the Modular Smell Identification Test, Trail-Making Test—Part B, and the Block Design subtest of the WAIS-R. The Modular Smell Identification Test has been linked to orbitofrontal cortex (OFC) and might suggest OFC impairment among psychopaths. The remaining tests on which psychopaths have shown deficits relative to controls all involve visuospatial processing and suggest that psychopaths may have difficulty performing complex visuospatial processing, at least while engaged in active motor responding.

These neuropsychological findings are not obviously congruent with the attentional deficits or abnormal cerebral asymmetries observed in studies of psychopaths' functioning in the domains of attention, language, and behavioral inhibition. However, further consideration reveals possible connections. As argued by Newman and Wallace (1993), psychopaths' specific difficulty with tasks that involve perceptual–motor integration may relate to their attentional difficulties, as these tasks require frequent shifts of attention between planning motor behavior and analyzing stimulus materials. Further, visuospatial tasks are likely to rely heavily on right-hemisphere processing and again suggest a possible influence of cerebral asymmetries upon psychopaths' performance.

DISCUSSION

The extensive literature on cognitive and language processing among psychopathic individuals reveals a broad array of deficits. Although emotion deficits are often emphasized in etiological models of the disorder, it is clear that psychopathy is also associated with reliable and specific cognitive abnormalities.

One intriguing aspect of psychopaths' cognitive deficits is their circumscribed, context-specific nature. Psychopaths' attentional functioning is characterized by good performance on explicit tasks presented in isolation but poor distribution of attention on complex dual-task paradigms and poor modulation of attention by unexpected or secondary information. Psychopaths' language processing is characterized by poor spontaneous use of cohesion, elaborative associations, and connotation. Psychopaths' performance on tests of behavioral inhibition reveals poor inhibition of punishable responses only in the presence of a dominant reward-seeking response set and in the absence of instructions to pause and process performance feedback. Finally, psychopaths show normal performance on a broad array of neuropsychological tasks but have difficulty with olfactory identification and with complex visuospatial tasks that require concurrent motor responses. Together, these deficits indicate that psychopaths generally perform well on primary, explicit tasks that are the focus of effortful attention but have difficulty using information that occurs outside their focus of attention.

Because of the expected impact of psychopaths' cognitive functioning on their functioning in other domains, it is useful to examine the literature on psychopaths' cognitive and language function with an eye toward identifying principles that may play a broad role in psychopaths' processing style. In this regard, the preceding review has revealed two consistent themes that may lend insight into mechanisms underlying psychopathy. These themes involve poor accommodation of secondary or peripheral information when attention is focused elsewhere and unusual distribution of processing across the cerebral hemispheres. Next, we expand on these themes and consider their implications for understanding the syndrome of psychopathy.

Accommodation of Secondary Cues

As discussed throughout the preceding review, and consistent with multiple prior reviews (e.g., Newman, 1998) and theoretical statements (e.g., Newman & Wallace, 1993), many of the cognitive deficits exhibited by psychopaths are consistent with poor accommodation of secondary or unattended information. One influential perspective on this deficit has been provided by the response modulation hypothesis of Newman and colleagues (Newman, 1998; Newman & Wallace, 1993). Here, we briefly review the

evidence for poor accommodation of secondary information and then consider the potential relevance of this deficit to psychopaths' functioning in other, noncognitive, domains.

Before proceeding, it is useful to clarify the concept of secondary or unattended information. To this end, we find it helpful to invoke the concepts of top-down and bottom-up processing. Top-down, or voluntary, goal-directed processing is assumed to be capacity limited and to correspond to a dominant set, primary task, or effortful attention. Bottom-up, or stimulus-driven, processing is presumed to be involved in the processing of aspects of the internal or external environment that are not explicitly relevant to the ongoing task. Bottom-up processing proceeds without effortful attention and would include spreading activation among related neural networks. It is presumed that normal processing involves the continual reciprocal influence of top-down and bottom-up processes. Adaptive behavior is presumed to depend on an appropriate balance between top-down and bottom-up processes, such that top-down, deliberate processing is neither too vulnerable nor too insulated from the influence of unexpected bottom-up information (see Corbetta & Shulman, 2002, for further discussion). Using this framework, psychopaths' proposed difficulty accommodating secondary information can be understood as difficulty accommodating bottom-up, stimulus-driven information, especially when the bottom-up information is inconsistent with or unrelated to the current top-down, effortful focus of attention (see MacCoon, Wallace, & Newman, 2004, for further discussion).

Consistent with poor accommodation of unattended or bottom-up information, psychopaths' performance on attentional paradigms is associated with reduced physiological responsivity to irrelevant or secondary information (Jutai & Hare, 1983; Jutai et al., 1987), increased physiological reactivity to attended information (Forth & Hare, 1989), decreased interference from incongruent but irrelevant information that is spatially separated from the attentional focus (Hiatt et al., 2004; Newman, Schmitt, & Voss, 1997), and poor modulation of attention by unexpected emotional content (Christianson et al., 1996).

Psychopaths' language processing is also potentially consistent with poor accommodation of secondary, bottom-up information. Whereas control participants spontaneously use metaphor, affect, and elaborative associations when engaged in a linguistic task, psychopaths often fail to incorporate these secondary or contextual aspects of language, despite having good explicit awareness and understanding on direct examination (Hare et al., 1988; Lorenz & Newman, 2002; Williamson et al., 1991). Psychopaths also appear to have difficulty using abstract concepts (e.g., Kiehl, Hare, McDonald, & Brink, 1999), and their speech has less global cohesiveness than that of nonpsychopaths (Brinkley, Bernstein, & Newman, 1999; Brinkley, Newman, et al., 1999). Although the neural bases of these connotative and contextual components of language are not fully understood, it is reasonable to presume that they depend on broad activation of semantic networks, and that this activation typically proceeds in an automatic, bottom-up fashion.

On tests of behavioral inhibition, psychopaths routinely display deficits (i.e., commission errors) when the avoidance of punishable responses is secondary to an approach- or reward-based response contingency (e.g., Lykken, 1957; Newman et al., 1990; Newman & Kosson, 1986). Thus, psychopaths appear to have difficulty accommodating secondary or contextual cues that indicate the need to suspend responding and self-evaluate behavior when already engaged in a primary, goal-directed task.

The foregoing findings are quite consistent with regard to psychopaths' difficulty accommodating incidental information that occurs outside their focus of attention. Together, they suggest that poor accommodation of secondary or contextual information may be an important factor underlying psychopaths' processing deficits.

Given its prominence in the cognitive literature, this deficit might also be expected to moderate psychopaths' performance in other domains, such as emotion processing. Indeed, the foregoing review of cognitive deficits reveals several instances in which psychopaths have difficulty using affective information that is incidental to an ongoing task (e.g., Christianson et al., 1996; Hare et al., 1988; Lorenz & Newman, 2002; Wil-

liamson et al., 1991). Several of these same studies report evidence of good explicit use of emotional information. This "emotion paradox" is a common feature of psychopaths' emotion processing deficits (see Newman & Lorenz, 2003) and is consistent with good "top-down" but poor "bottom-up" use of affective information. In addition, imaging studies have identified abnormalities in the relative balance of top-down (e.g., frontal) and bottom-up (e.g., limbic) processing among psychopathic individuals (Kiehl et al., 2001; Muller et al., 2003) on emotion-processing tasks.

Psychopaths' difficulty accommodating bottom-up information can also be assumed to contribute to general difficulties with behavioral regulation. As mentioned earlier, the ability to maintain an appropriate balance between top-down and bottom-up processes is essential to adaptive executive control. If psychopaths are relatively insensitive to contextual information that occurs outside their top-down focus of attention, they can be expected to have difficulty interrupting or modifying ongoing behavior in response to cues that this behavior is no longer adaptive or appropriate (see MacCoon et al., 2004, for further discussion).

Hemispheric Processing

Another theme that emerges from the literature on psychopaths' cognitive deficits is the presence of unusual hemispheric processing. The existing studies reveal at least three components of this abnormality: (1) unusual cerebral processing asymmetries, (2) exacerbation of deficits under left-hemisphere activating conditions, and (3) context-specific failures to use information that is typically processed by the right hemisphere.

Cerebral Processing Asymmetries

As with psychopaths' attentional deficits, psychopaths' unusual processing asymmetries appear to occur only under particular conditions. Direct investigations of psychopaths' cerebral processing asymmetries have primarily used language-based tasks, and these studies indicate that psychopaths show abnormal asymmetries for word categorization, word detection, and oddball phoneme detection, but only when the task is relatively complex (e.g., assigning words to abstract categories; detecting but also remembering dichotically presented words, and identifying rare targets when engaged in a concurrent distractor task). Together, these studies suggest that psychopaths' abnormal functional asymmetries may be specific to tasks that involve the integration of multiple task components. Hiatt and colleagues (2002) noted that task complexity has been shown to promote interhemispheric processing (Banich & Belger, 1990; Weissman & Banich, 2000), and they proposed that psychopaths' abnormal processing asymmetries may be related to the efficiency with which they can coordinate interhemispheric processing (see also Hare, 1998; Mills, 1995, as cited in Hare, 1998).

Left-Hemisphere Activation

Across several studies, Kosson and colleagues have demonstrated that psychopaths' attentional processing is disrupted under conditions that preferentially activate the left hemisphere (e.g., right-handed responses and RVF targets). Similarly, Howland and colleagues (1993) found that psychopaths had difficulty detecting LVF/right-hemisphere targets following misleading RVF/left-hemisphere cues. Interestingly, reward-seeking response sets may also preferentially engage the left hemisphere (Davidson, 1995; Miller & Tomarken, 2001, Sobotka et al., 1992), suggesting that the context-specificity of psychopaths' disinhibition and poor passive avoidance may be due in part to left hemisphere activation.

Poor Accommodation of Right-Hemisphere Processing

Psychopaths' performance on neuropsychological tests reveals deficits on several tasks that involve concurrent visuospatial processing and motor responses (e.g., TMT-B, Block Design, and Porteus Maze task). As visuospatial processing is believed to rely preferentially on the right hemisphere (Hellige, 1993), these deficits raise the possibility of right-hemisphere dysfunction. Interestingly, many of psychopaths' deficits in other domains are at least superficially consistent with right-hemisphere dysfunction. For example, the aspects of language overlooked

by psychopaths, such as metaphor, context, and connotations, are also dysfunctional among patients with right-hemisphere lesions (see Beeman, 1998; Fiore & Schooler, 1998). However, direct tests of psychopaths' right-hemisphere processing reveal no evidence of dysfunction (e.g., Day & Wong, 1996; Hiatt et al., 2002; LaPierre et al., 1995). It appears that psychopaths are most likely to show evidence of right-hemisphere dysfunction on tasks that involve concurrent goal-directed motor responses (e.g., Smith et al., 1992) or language processing (e.g., Hare et al., 1988). Goal-directed behaviors and language processing appear to rely preferentially on left-hemisphere processing, suggesting that psychopaths' deficits on right-hemisphere tasks, like their poor accommodation of secondary cues, may depend in part on the degree of concurrent left-hemisphere involvement.

It is not entirely clear how psychopaths' unusual cerebral processing asymmetries, sensitivity to left-hemisphere activation, and poor accommodation of right-hemisphere processing are related to each other. However, each of these abnormalities suggests a disruption in the coordination of processing across the cerebral hemispheres. One possibility is that psychopaths have difficulty efficiently integrating information across the cerebral hemispheres when the left hemisphere is strongly activated. A deficit of this sort could be expected to lead to an abnormal distribution of processing (i.e., unusual cerebral asymmetries) on tasks that normally elicit interhemispheric coordination (see Banich & Belger, 1990; Hiatt et al., 2002) as well as poor utilization of right-hemisphere processes under left-hemisphere activating conditions. As noted previously, psychopaths' deficits in language and visuospatial processing are potentially consistent with a context-specific failure to use right-hemisphere processing. Interestingly, the right hemisphere has also been implicated in emotion processing (Borod, Cicero, & Obler, 1998; Jansari, Tranel, & Adolphs, 2000; Lang, Bradley, & Cuthbert, 1990), behavioral inhibition (Davidson, 1995; Kawashima et al., 1996; Schiff & Bassel, 1996; Swartzburg, 1983) and attention to unexpected secondary cues (e.g., Corbetta & Shulman, 2002), suggesting that psychopaths' context-specific deficits in these domains may also be consistent with poor utilization of right-hemisphere processing under left-hemisphere activating conditions (see also Hiatt & Newman, 2005).

The connections between psychopaths' cerebral processing abnormalities and their difficulty accommodating unattended secondary cues are especially intriguing and suggest that these two major components of psychopaths' cognitive deficits may arise from a common mechanism. Corbetta and Shulman (2002) argue that the "detection of behaviorally relevant stimuli, particularly when they are salient or unexpected" (p. 201) is largely lateralized to the right hemisphere, and they propose that this right-hemisphere based attentional system acts as a "circuit breaker" for top-down, goal-directed attentional systems. Thus, the right hemisphere may be particularly involved in the processing of secondary or unattended information. Psychopaths' context-specific failures to accommodate secondary or bottom-up information may therefore be closely related to psychopaths' difficulty using right-hemisphere processes under left-hemisphere activating conditions.

Regardless of the underlying mechanism, cerebral processing abnormalities appear to be a consistent feature of psychopaths' cognitive processing. Given the relative right-hemisphere lateralization of emotion processing, including startle responsivity (see, e.g., Bradley, Cuthbert, & Lang, 1991, 1996; Funayama, Grillon, Davis, & Phelps, 2001), cerebral processing abnormalities provide a potentially important link between psychopaths' cognitive and affective deficits.

SUMMARY

The literature on psychopaths' cognitive functioning is extensive and reveals a variety of consistent and compelling deficits. We have reviewed the existing findings with an eye toward identifying common themes that run throughout psychopaths' performance on cognitive tasks. Two major themes that emerge are difficulty accommodating secondary or bottom-up information and abnormal hemispheric processing. As noted previously, it is possible that these two broad deficits arise from a common mechanism. Regardless, each of these deficits appears to

have a strong influence upon psychopaths' cognitive processing, and each can also be expected to affect psychopaths' functioning in other domains, such as emotion processing. To the extent that these broad deficits apply to psychopaths' deficits in other, non-cognitive domains, they have the potential to lend coherence to the existing literature and promote greater understanding of the fundamental causes of the disorder.

It is intriguing that psychopaths' cognitive deficits do not fit established models of cognitive dysfunction, such as executive deficits or difficulty with sustained attention. Psychopaths appear to have adequate cognitive resources and capacity but difficulty maintaining an adaptive balance between top-down and bottom-up processing. The influence of bottom-up, automatic activation appears to be restricted among psychopaths when it is inconsistent with or occurs outside their top-down focus of attention. Currently, relatively little is known about how top-down and bottom-up networks interact. Nevertheless, psychopaths' cognitive functioning suggests that the mechanisms governing this interaction may play a central role in the psychopathic syndrome. Psychopaths' deficits also indicate that context-specific failures in the appropriate, adaptive allocation of available resources can contribute to profound failures of self-regulation, despite the absence of traditional cognitive or executive deficits.

REFERENCES

Arnett, P. A., Howland, E. W., & Smith, S. S. (1993). Autonomic responsivity during passive avoidance in incarcerated psychopaths. *Personality and Individual Differences, 14*(1), 173–184.

Arnett, P. A., Smith, S. S., & Newman, J. P. (1997). Approach and avoidance motivation in psychopathic criminal offenders during passive avoidance. *Journal of Personality and Social Psychology, 72,* 1413–1428.

Banich, M. T., & Belger, A. (1990). Interhemispheric interaction: How do the hemispheres divide and conquer a task? *Cortex, 26,* 77–94.

Beeman, M. (1998). Course semantic coding and discourse comprehension. In M. Beeman & C. Chiarello (Eds.), *Right hemisphere language comprehension: Perspectives from cognitive neuroscience* (pp. 255–284). Mahwah, NJ: Erlbaum.

Bernstein, A., Newman, J. P., & Wallace, J. F. (2000). Left-hemisphere activation and deficient response modulation in psychopaths. *Psychological Science, 11*(5), 414–418.

Borod, J. C., Cicero, B. A., & Obler, L. K. (1998). Right hemisphere emotional perception: Evidence across multiple channels. *Neuropsychology, 12*(3), 446–458.

Bradley, M., Cuthbert, B. N., & Lang, P. J. (1991). Startle and emotion: Lateral acoustic probes and the bilateral blink. *Psychophysiology, 28*, 285–295.

Bradley, M., Cuthbert, B. N., & Lang, P. J. (1996). Lateralized startle probes in the study of emotion. *Psychophysiology, 33*, 156–161.

Brinkley, C. A., Bernstein, A., & Newman, J. P. (1999). Coherence in the narratives of psychopathic and nonpsychopathic criminal offenders. *Personality and Individual Differences, 27*, 519–530.

Brinkley, C. A., Newman, J. P., Harpur, T. J., & Johnson, M. M. (1999). Cohesion in texts produced by psychopathic and nonpsychopathic criminal inmates. *Personality and Individual Differences, 26*, 873–885.

Christianson, S. A., Forth, A. E., Hare, R. D., Strachan, C., Lidberg, L., & Thorell, L. H. (1996). Remembering details of emotional events: A comparison between psychopathic and nonpsychopathic offenders. *Personality and Individual Differences, 20*, 437–443.

Cleckley, H. (1982). *The mask of sanity.* St. Louis, MO: Mosby.

Corbetta, M., & Shulman, G. L. (2002). Control of goal-directed and stimulus-driven attention in the brain. *Nature Reviews Neuroscience, 3*, 201–215.

Davidson, R. J. (1995). Cerebral asymmetry, emotion, and affective style. In R. J. Davidson & K. Hugdahl (Eds.), *Brain asymmetry* (pp. 361–383). Cambridge, MA: MIT Press.

Day, R., & Wong, S. (1996). Anomalous perceptual asymmetries for negative emotional stimuli in the psychopath. *Journal of Abnormal Psychology, 105*(4), 648–652.

Fiore, S. M., & Schooler, J. W. (1998). Right hemisphere contributions to creative problem solving: Converging evidence for divergent thinking. In M. Beeman & C. Chiarello (Eds.), *Right hemisphere language comprehension: Perspectives from cognitive neuroscience* (pp. 349–371). Mahwah, NJ: Erlbaum.

Flor, H., Birbaumer, N., Hermann, C., Ziegler, S., & Patrick, C. J. (2002). Aversive Pavlovian conditioning in psychopaths: Peripheral and central correlates. *Psychophysiology, 39*, 505–518.

Forth, A. E., & Hare, R. D. (1989). The contingent negative variation in psychopaths. *Psychophysiology, 26*, 676–682.

Fowles, D. C. (1980). The three arousal model: Implications of Gray's two factor learning theory for heart rate, electrodermal activity, and psychopathy. *Psychophysiology, 17*, 87–104.

Funayama, E. S., Grillon, C., Davis, M., & Phelps, E. A. (2001). A double dissociation in the affective modulation of startle in humans: Effects of unilateral temporal lobectomy. *Journal of Cognitive Neuroscience, 13*, 721–729.

Gillstrom, B. J., & Hare, R. D. (1988). Language related hand gestures in psychopaths. *Journal of Personality Disorders, 2*, 21–27.

Gorenstein, E. E. (1982). Frontal lobe functions in psychopaths. *Journal of Abnormal Psychology, 91*, 368–379.

Gray, J. A. (1982). Precis of the neuropsychology of anxiety: An enquiry into the functions of the septo-hippocampal system. *Behavioral and Brain Sciences, 5*, 469–534.

Hare, R. D. (1979). Psychopathy and laterality of cerebral function. *Journal of Abnormal Psychology, 88*, 608–610.

Hare, R. D. (1980). A research scale for the assessment of psychopathy in criminal populations. *Personality and Individual Differences, 1*, 111–119.

Hare, R. D. (1984). Performance of psychopaths on cognitive tasks related to frontal lobe function. *Journal of Abnormal Psychology, 93*, 133–140.

Hare, R. D. (1986). Twenty years of experience with the Cleckley psychopath. In W. H. Reid, D. Dorr, J. I. Walker, & J. W. Bonner, III (Eds.), *Unmasking the psychopath: Antisocial personality and related syndromes* (pp. 3–27). New York: Norton.

Hare, R. D. (1991). *The Hare Psychopathy Checklist—Revised.* Toronto, ON, Canada: Multi-Health Systems.

Hare, R. D. (1998). Psychopathy, affect, and behavior. In D. J. Cooke, R. D. Hare, & A. Forth (Eds.), *Psychopathy: Theory, research and implications for society* (pp. 105–137). Dordrecht, The Netherlands: Kluwer.

Hare, R. D., & Jutai, J. W. (1988). Psychopathy and cerebral asymmetry in semantic processing. *Personality and Individual Differences, 9*, 329–337.

Hare, R. D., & McPherson, L. M. (1984). Psychopathy and perceptual asymmetry during verbal dichotic listening. *Journal of Abnormal Psychology, 93*, 141–149.

Hare, R. D., & Quinn, M. J. (1971). Psychopathy and autonomic conditioning. *Journal of Abnormal Psychology, 77*, 223–235.

Hare, R. D., Williamson, S. E., & Harpur, T. J. (1988). Psychopathy and language. In T. E. Moffitt & S. A. Mednick (Eds.), *Biological contributions to crime causation* (pp. 68–92). Dordrecht, The Netherlands: Kluwer.

Hart, S. D., Forth, A. E., & Hare, R. D. (1990). Performance of criminal psychopaths on selected neuropsychological tests. *Journal of Abnormal Psychology, 99*, 374–379.

Hellige, J. B. (1993). *Hemispheric asymmetry: What's right and what's left.* Cambridge, MA: Harvard University Press.

Herve, H. F., Hayes, P. J., & Hare, R. D. (2003). Psychopathy and sensitivity to the emotional polarity of metaphorical statements. *Personality and Individual Differences, 35*, 1497–1507.

Hiatt, K. D., Lorenz, A. R., & Newman, J. P. (2002). Assessment of emotion and language processing in psychopathic offenders: Results from a dichotic listening task. *Personality and Individual Differences, 32,* 1255–1268.

Hiatt, K. D., & Newman, J. P. (2005). *Interhemispheric integration: A proximal mechanism for psychopathy.* Manuscript in preparation.

Hiatt, K. D., Schmitt, W. A., & Newman, J. P. (2004). Stroop tasks reveal abnormal selective attention among psychopathic offenders. *Neuropsychology, 18*(1), 50–59.

Howland, E. W., Kosson, D. S., Patterson, C. M., & Newman, J. P. (1993). Altering a dominant response: Performance of psychopaths and low socialization college students on a cued reaction time task. *Journal of Abnormal Psychology, 102,* 379–387.

Jansari, A., Tranel, D., & Adolphs, R. (2000). A valence-specific lateral bias for discriminating emotional facial expressions in free field. *Cognition and Emotion, 14*(3), 341–353.

Jutai, J. W., & Hare, R. D. (1983). Psychopathy and selective attention during performance of a complex perceptual motor task. *Psychophysiology, 20,* 146–151.

Jutai, J. W., Hare, R. D., & Connolly, J. F. (1987). Psychopathy and event related brain potentials (ERPs) associated with attention to speech stimuli. *Personality and Individual Differences, 8,* 175–184.

Kawashima, R., Satoh, K., Itoh, H., Ono, S., Furumoto, S., Gotoh, R., et al. (1996). Functional anatomy of GO/NO GO discrimination and response selection: A PET study in man. *Brain Research, 728,* 79–89.

Kiehl, K. A., Hare, R. D., Liddle, P. F., & McDonald, J. J. (1999). Reduced P300 responses in criminal psychopaths during a visual oddball task. *Biological Psychiatry, 45,* 1498–1507.

Kiehl, K. A., Hare, R. D., McDonald, J. J., & Brink, J. (1999). Semantic and affective processing in psychopaths: An event related potential (ERP) study. *Psychophysiology, 36,* 765–774.

Kiehl, K. A., Smith, A. M., Hare, R. D., & Liddle, P. F. (2000). An event-related potential investigation of response inhibition in schizophrenia and psychopathy. *Biological Psychiatry, 48,* 210–221.

Kiehl, K. A., Smith, A. M., Hare, R. D., Mendrek, A., Forster, B. B., Brink, J., et al. (2001). Limbic abnormalities in affective processing by criminal psychopaths as revealed by functional magnetic resonance imaging. *Biological Psychiatry, 50,* 677–684.

Kosson, D. S. (1996). Psychopathy and dual task performance under focusing conditions. *Journal of Abnormal Psychology, 105,* 391–400.

Kosson, D. S. (1998). Divided visual attention in psychopathic and nonpsychopathic offenders. *Personality and Individual Differences, 24,* 373–391.

Kosson, D. S., & Newman, J. P. (1986). Psychopathy and the allocation of attentional capacity in a divided-attention situation. *Journal of Abnormal Psychology, 95,* 257–263.

Lang, P. J., Bradley, M. M., & Cuthbert, B. N. (1990).

Emotion, attention, and the startle reflex. *Psychological Review, 97*(3), 377–395.

LaPierre, D., Braun, C. M. J., & Hodgins, S. (1995). Ventral frontal deficits in psychopathy: Neuropsychological test findings. *Neuropsychologia, 33,* 139–151.

Levenston, G. K., Patrick, C. J., Bradley, M. M., & Lang, P. J. (2000). The psychopath as observer: Emotion and attention in picture processing. *Journal of Abnormal Psychology, 109,* 373–385.

Lorenz, A. R., & Newman, J. P. (2002). Deficient response modulation and emotion processing in low anxious Caucasian psychopathic offenders: Results from a lexical decision task. *Emotion, 2,* 91–104.

Lösel, F., & Schmucker, M. (2004). Psychopathy, risk taking, and attention: A differentiated test of the somatic marker hypothesis. *Journal of Abnormal Psychology, 113*(4), 522–529.

Lykken, D. T. (1957). A study of anxiety in the sociopathic personality. *Journal of Abnormal and Social Psychology, 55,* 6–10.

MacCoon, D. G., Wallace, J. F., & Newman, J. P. (2004). Self-regulation: Context-appropriate balanced attention. In R. F. Baumeister & K. D. Vohs (Eds.), *Handbook of self-regulation: Research, theory, and applications* (pp. 422–444). New York: Guilford Press.

Miller, A., & Tomarken, A. J. (2001). Task dependent changes in frontal brain asymmetry: Effects of incentive cues, outcome expectancies, and motor responses. *Psychophysiology, 38,* 500–511.

Mitchell, D. G. V., Colledge, E., Leonard, A., & Blair, R. J. R. (2002). Risky decisions and response reversal: Is there evidence of orbito-frontal cortex dysfunction in psychopathic individuals? *Neuropsychologia, 40,* 2013–2022.

Muller, J. L., Sommer, M., Wagner, V., Lange, K., Taschler, H., Roder, C. H., et al. (2003). Abnormalities in emotion processing within cortical and subcortical regions in criminal psychopaths: Evidence from a functional magnetic resonance imaging study using pictures with emotional content. *Biological Psychiatry, 54,* 152–162.

Newman, J. P. (1998). Psychopathic behavior: An information processing perspective. In D. J. Cooke, R. D. Hare, & A. Forth (Eds.), *Psychopathy: Theory, research and implications for society* (pp. 81–104). Dordrecht, The Netherlands: Kluwer.

Newman, J. P., & Kosson, D. S. (1986). Passive avoidance learning in psychopathic and nonpsychopathic offenders. *Journal of Abnormal Psychology, 95,* 252–256.

Newman, J. P., & Lorenz, A. R. (2003). Response modulation and emotion processing: Implications for psychopathy and other dysregulatory psychopathology. In R. J. Davidson, K. Scherer, & H. H. Goldsmith (Ed.), *Handbook of affective sciences* (pp. 1043–1067). New York: Oxford University Press.

Newman, J. P., Patterson, C. M., Howland, E. W., & Nichols, S. L. (1990). Passive avoidance in psychopaths: The effects of reward. *Personality and Individual Differences, 11*, 1101–1114.

Newman, J. P., Patterson, C. M., & Kosson, D. S. (1987). Response perseveration in psychopaths. *Journal of Abnormal Psychology, 96*, 145–148.

Newman, J. P., Schmitt, W. A., & Voss, W. D. (1997). The impact of motivationally neutral cues on psychopathic individuals: Assessing the generality of the response modulation hypothesis. *Journal of Abnormal Psychology, 106*, 563–575.

Newman, J. P., & Wallace, J. F. (1993). Psychopathy and cognition. In P. C. Kendall & K. S. Dobson (Eds.), *Psychopathology and cognition* (pp. 293–349). New York: Academic Press.

Newman, J. P., Wallace, J. F., Schmitt, W. A., & Arnett, P. A. (1997). Behavioral inhibition system functioning in anxious, impulsive and psychopathic individuals. *Personality and Individual Differences, 23*, 583–592.

Patrick, C. J., Bradley, M. M., & Lang, P. J. (1993). Emotion in the criminal psychopath: Startle reflex modulation. *Journal of Abnormal Psychology, 102*, 89–92.

Patrick, C. J., Cuthbert, B. N., & Lang, P. J. (1994). Emotion in the criminal psychopath: Fear image processing. *Journal of Abnormal Psychology, 103*, 523–534.

Pham, T. H., Vanderstukken, O., Philippot, P., & Vanderlinden, M. (2003). Selective attention and executive functions deficits among criminal psychopaths. *Aggressive Behavior, 29*, 393–405.

Schiff, B. B., & Bassel, C. (1996). Effects of asymmetrical hemispheric activation on approach and withdrawal responses. *Neuropsychology, 10*, 557–564.

Schmauk, F. J. (1970). Punishment, arousal, and avoidance learning in sociopaths. *Journal of Abnormal Psychology, 76*, 325–335.

Schmitt, W. A., Brinkley, C. A., & Newman, J. P. (1999). Testing Damasio's somatic marker hypothesis with psychopathic individuals: Risk takers or risk averse? *Journal of Abnormal Psychology, 108*(3), 538–543.

Siegel, R. A. (1978). Probability of punishment and suppression of behavior in psychopathic and nonpsychopathic offenders. *Journal of Abnormal Psychology, 87*, 514–522.

Smith, S. S., Arnett, P. A., & Newman, J. P. (1992). Neuropsychological differentiation of psychopathic and nonpsychopathic criminal offenders. *Personality and Individual Differences, 13*, 1233–1243.

Sobotka, S. S., Davidson, R. J., & Senulis, J. A. (1992). Anterior brain electrical asymmetries in response to reward and punishment. *Electroencephalography and Clinical Neurophysiology, 83*, 236–247.

Sutton, S. K., Vitale, J. E., & Newman, J. P. (2002). Emotion among women with psychopathy during picture perception. *Journal of Abnormal Psychology, 111*, 610–619.

Swartzburg, M. (1983). Hemispheric laterality and EEG correlates of depression. *Research Communications in Psychology, Psychiatry and Behavior, 8*, 187–205.

Vitale, J. E., & Newman, J. P. (2001). Response perseveration in psychopathic women. *Journal of Abnormal Psychology, 110*, 644–647.

Vitale, J. E., Smith, S. S., Brinkley, C. A., & Newman, J. P. (2002). The reliability and validity of the Psychopathy Checklist—Revised in a sample of female offenders. *Criminal Justice and Behavior, 29*, 202–231.

Weissman, D. H., & Banich, M. T. (2000). The cerebral hemispheres cooperate to perform complex but not simple tasks. *Neuropsychology, 14*, 41–59.

Welsh, G. (1956). Factor dimensions A and R. In G. S. Welsh & W. G. Dahlstrom (Ed.), *Basic readings on the MMPI in psychology and medicine* (pp. 264–281). Minneapolis: University of Minnesota Press.

Williamson, S., Harpur, T. J., & Hare, R. D. (1991). Abnormal processing of affective words by psychopaths. *Psychophysiology, 28*, 260–273.

18

Psychopathy and Developmental Pathways to Antisocial Behavior in Youth

PAUL J. FRICK
MONICA A. MARSEE

The constellation of affective (e.g., poverty of emotions, lack of empathy, and guilt), interpersonal (e.g., callous use of others for one's own gain), self-referential (e.g., inflated sense of ones own importance), and behavioral (e.g., impulsivity and irresponsibility) traits associated with the construct of psychopathy have proven to be quite important for designating a distinct group of antisocial adults. Research has consistently shown that incarcerated adults who also show psychopathic traits show a more severe and violent pattern of antisocial behavior, both within the institution and after release (Gendreau, Goggin, & Smith, 2002; Hemphill, Hare, & Wong, 1998; Walters, 2003). In addition, incarcerated adults with and without psychopathic features show a number of distinct cognitive (Newman & Lorenz, 2003), affective (Hare, 1998; Patrick, 2001), and neurological (Kiehl et al., 2001) correlates that could implicate different causal processes involved in the development of antisocial behavior for the two groups of individuals.

To date, most published research on psychopathic traits has been conducted in adult samples and, even more specifically, in incarcerated adult samples. This is unfortunate for a number of reasons. First, incarcerated adults with psychopathic traits often have a long history of antisocial behavior beginning in childhood (Hare, McPherson, & Forth, 1988; Marshall & Cooke, 1999). Therefore, by the time the individual is incarcerated as an adult, the lifelong pattern of antisocial behavior has already been quite costly to society (Loeber & Farrington, 2000). In addition, if early manifestations of psychopathic traits can be identified, it is quite possible that interventions may be more effective in changing these traits earlier in development when personality tends to be more changeable (Roberts & DelVecchio, 2000). Second, studying these traits earlier in development may provide an important method for disentangling the causal processes related specifically to this constellation of personality traits, as compared to those processes related to antisocial behavior more generally. That is, it is difficult to determine in incarcerated adult samples what might be causally related to psychopathic traits and what might be a cause or a consequence of a lifelong pattern of antisocial behavior and the concomitant problems in adjustment (e.g., low educational achievement, extended periods of incarceration, and substance abuse) that often accompanies such behavior. Third, the study of psychopathic traits earlier in development allows for the study of protective factors that may enhance the adjustment of individuals who are at risk for developing these traits (e.g., Frick, Kimonis, Dandreaux, & Farrell, 2003). Such findings could be critical for causal theory by uncovering the mechanisms through which the expression of these traits may be moderated in individuals at risk for psychopathy. More important, understanding potential protective factors for persons at risk for psychopathy could provide critical information for designing more effective preventive interventions.

Perhaps the most important benefit of extending the construct of psychopathy to youth, however, is that this research could help in developing better causal models for severe antisocial and aggressive behavior in youth. As with adult antisocial behavior, research has clearly indicated that antisocial youth are a very heterogeneous group (Frick & Ellis, 1999). For example, the most persistent 5–6% of youthful offenders account for about 50% of reported crimes (Farrington, Ohlin, & Wilson, 1986; Moffitt, 1993). Recent causal theories of antisocial behavior have also recognized that there may be many different causal processes that can lead to the development of childhood conduct problems (Dodge & Petit, 2003; Frick & Morris, 2004; Raine, 2002). For example, the affective (Frick & Morris, 2004), cognitive (Dodge & Petit, 2003), and psychophysiological (Raine, 2002) correlates of antisocial and aggressive behavior may differ substantially across subgroups of antisocial youth. Based on this research, there have been a number of approaches to subtyping antisocial youth (Frick & Ellis, 1999). Unfortunately, no approach has garnered widespread acceptance over an extended period. Given the utility that the construct of psychopathy has shown for designating an important subgroup of antisocial adults (Hare, 1998), it is quite possible that extending the construct earlier in development could similarly enhance attempts to define meaningful subtypes of antisocial youth.

Based on these considerations, the purpose of this chapter is to review research that has attempted to define meaningful subgroups of antisocial and aggressive youth, focusing on approaches that appear to be particularly important for extending the construct of psychopathy to youth. In reviewing these approaches, we attempt to highlight their similarities and points of divergence with the construct of psychopathy and their potential relevance for developmental models of psychopathy. In the final section, we discuss some conceptual, methodological, ethical, and developmental issues that are important to consider in extending the construct of psychopathy to youth.

SUBTYPES BASED ON AGGRESSIVE BEHAVIOR

Aggressive behavior, defined as behavior that is intended to hurt or harm others (Berkowitz, 1993), is an important dimension of childhood conduct problems in most classification systems (American Psychiatric Association, 2000). Specifically, many approaches to subtyping children with conduct problems make a distinction between children with aggressive and nonaggressive forms of conduct problems (American Psychiatric Association, 1980; Loeber, Keenan, & Zhang, 1987; Quay, 1987). The importance of this distinction is supported by research showing that aggressive behavior in children is often quite stable across the lifespan (Huesmann, Eron, Lefkowitz, & Walder, 1984) and is very difficult to treat (Kazdin, 1995; Quay, 1987). This distinction could also be important for understanding developmental precursors to psychopathy because research in adult samples has shown that adults with psychopathy show a particularly violent and aggressive pattern of antisocial behavior (Gendreau et al., 2002; Hemphill et al., 1998; Walters, 2003; Porter & Woodworth, Chapter 24, this volume).

Research on aggressive behavior in youth has indicated that there are several distinct patterns of aggressive behavior that may be displayed by children. The distinctions among aggressive behaviors have typically focused on differences in the form (i.e., overt and relational aggression) and the function (i.e., reactive and proactive aggression) of aggressive behavior (see Dodge & Petit, 2003; Little, Jones, Henrich, & Hawley, 2003; Poulin & Boivin, 2000, for reviews). Overt and relational forms of aggression can be descriptively distinguished by (1) their method of harm and (2) the goals they serve. Overt aggression harms others by damaging their physical well-being and consists of physically and verbally aggressive behaviors such as hitting, pushing, kicking, and threatening (Coie & Dodge, 1998). In contrast, relational aggression harms others through damage to their social relationships, their friendships, or their feelings of inclusion and acceptance in the peer group (Crick et al., 1999). Relational aggression consists of behaviors such as gossiping about others, excluding target children from a group, spreading rumors, or telling others not to be friends with a target child (Crick & Grotpeter, 1995).

A major focus of research on relational and overt aggression has been the study of gender differences in aggressive behaviors. Research has consistently shown that boys are significantly more overtly aggressive than girls, whereas girls may be more relationally aggressive (Crick, Casas, & Mosher, 1997; Crick & Grotpeter, 1995). Regardless of gender, however, both relational and overt aggression have been shown to predict social, psychological, and school-related adjustment problems in children and adolescents (Crick, 1996; Crick et al., 1997; Prinstein, Boergers, & Vernberg, 2001). Unfortunately, the relationship between relational aggressive behavior and characteristics associated with psychopathy has not been directly studied in either adults or youth. This limitation in research is likely due to the limited research that has been conducted on psychopathic traits in women (e.g., Lorenz & Newman, 2002; Verona & Vitale, Chapter 21, this volume). As a result, the relevance of the distinction between relational and overt aggression to developmental models of psychopathy is difficult to evaluate.

On the other hand, the second distinction among types of aggressive behaviors could have quite important implications for developmental models of psychopathy. This distinction separates aggressive behavior into reactive and proactive dimensions (Dodge & Petit, 2003; Poulin & Boivin, 2000). Reactive aggression, also referred to as hostile or impulsive aggression, is generally defined as aggression that occurs as an angry response to provocation or threat (Dodge & Petit, 2003; Poulin & Bouvin, 2000). Aggressive acts of this type often occur in the context of high emotional arousal, such as in an argument and fight, and they are typically not planned. In contrast, proactive aggression, also referred to as instrumental aggression or

premeditated aggression, is generally defined as aggression that is unprovoked and typically involves planning and forethought. Most important, however, this form of aggression is used for some sort of instrumental gain, such as to obtain goods or services, to obtain dominance over others, or to enhance one's social status (Dodge & Petit, 2003).

Factor analyses have consistently identified separate dimensions of aggressive behavior related to these two functional categories in samples of children and adolescents (Brown, Atkins, Osborne, & Milnamow, 1996; Dodge & Coie, 1987; Poulin & Bouvin, 2000; Salmivalli & Nieminen, 2002). However, these studies have also shown that the dimensions of reactive and proactive aggression are highly correlated, with estimates ranging from .40 to .90 and typically being about .70 (e.g., Brown et al., 1996). These substantial correlations suggest that a large number of aggressive children show both types of aggression. Research has indicated that there is some asymmetry in the high degree of association between the two types of aggression. Specifically, there appears to be a significant number of children who only show reactive forms of aggression, whereas most children who show high levels of proactive aggression also show high rates of reactive aggression (Brown et al., 1996; Dodge & Coie, 1987; Pitts, 1997). Therefore, there appears to be a group of highly aggressive children who show both types of aggressive behavior and another group of children who are less aggressive overall and who show only reactive types of aggression (Frick, Cornell, Barry, Bodin, & Dane, 2003).

Research on these different patterns of aggressive behavior is somewhat difficult to interpret because studies have not consistently controlled for the overlap between the two types of aggression. However, there is growing evidence for a number of distinct characteristics between children in these aggressive subgroups. First, children in the two aggressive groups have different risk for problems later in adolescence and adulthood. Specifically, children who show proactive aggression are at higher risk for delinquency and alcohol abuse in adolescence, as well as criminality in adulthood (Pulkkinen, 1996; Vitaro, Brendgen, & Tremblay, 2002; Vitaro, Gendreau, Tremblay, & Oligny, 1998).

Second, the social adjustment of children

in these two aggressive subgroups appears to be different. Reactively aggressive children show greater school adjustment problems, higher rates of peer rejection, and more peer victimization than do proactively aggressive children (Dodge, Lochman, Harnish, Bates, & Pettit, 1997; Poulin & Boivin, 2000; Schwartz et al., 1998; Waschbusch, Willoughby, & Pelham, 1998). These social problems may be related to deficits in social cognition that have been related to reactive aggression, such as a tendency to attribute hostile intent to ambiguous provocations by peers and difficulty developing nonaggressive solutions to problems in social encounters (Crick & Dodge, 1996; Dodge, Price, Bachorowski, & Newman, 1990; Hubbard, Dodge, Cillessen, Coie, & Schwartz, 2001). In contrast, children who show proactive aggression are less rejected and victimized, have more friends, and are often perceived as leaders in social groups (Dodge & Coie, 1987; Poulin & Boivin, 2000; Price & Dodge, 1989; Schwartz et al., 1998). However, proactively aggressive children overestimate the possible positive consequences of their aggressive behavior (e.g., the likelihood that it will produce tangible rewards and reduce adverse treatment from others) and are less likely to believe that they will be punished because of their behavior (Dodge et al., 1997; Price & Dodge, 1989; Schwartz et al., 1998).

Third, the two patterns of aggressive behavior have been related to distinct emotional correlates. Reactively aggressive children show high rates of angry reactivity, low frustration tolerance, and a propensity to react with high levels of negative emotion to aversive stimuli (Hubbard et al., 2002; Little et al., 2003; Shields & Cicchetti, 1998; Vitaro et al., 2002). Consistent with these problems in emotional regulation, reactively aggressive children exhibit high rates of depression and anxiety, and they score higher on measures impulsivity (Day, Bream, & Pal, 1992; Dodge et al., 1997; Vitaro et al., 1998, 2002). In contrast, children who are high on proactive aggression do not show these problems in emotional regulation (Crick & Dodge, 1996; Dodge & Coie, 1987; Dodge et al., 1997; Vitaro et al., 2002). In fact, they often show reduced levels of emotional reactivity (Hubbard et al., 2002; Pitts, 1997). For example, Pitts (1997) reported on a group of

103 boys (grades 3–6) who were placed into three groups: nonaggressive ($N = 38$), reactive aggressive ($N = 19$), and reactive–proactive aggressive ($N = 38$). Both groups of aggressive children exhibited lower rates of resting heart rate than did the nonaggressive group. However, in response to a simulated provocation from peers, the heart rate of the reactive group increased significantly compared to control children, whereas the heart rate of the proactive–reactive group remained low.

In summary, research comparing children with different patterns of aggressive behavior has uncovered a number of important differences between children who show purely reactive aggression and those who show both proactive and reactive aggression. These include many differences in their social, cognitive, and affective characteristics. Most important, it appears that the group high on both reactive and proactive aggression shows a number of characteristics that are similar to adults with psychopathy, such as the severe and pervasive nature of their aggression, their risk for adult criminality, their insensitivity to potential punishment for their aggressive behavior, and deficits in their emotional reactivity. This link between the pervasive pattern of aggression in children and characteristics associated with psychopathy is consistent with research on incarcerated adults that has shown that severe patterns of violence that include instrumental and premeditated aggression are associated with psychopathic traits (Cornell et al., 1996; Patrick, Zempolich, & Levenston, 1997; Woodworth & Porter, 2002).

A few studies have provided an even more direct link between proactive and instrumental forms of aggression and psychopathic traits in youth. For example, violent sex offenders, who tend to show more instrumental and premeditated violence, showed higher rates of psychopathic traits compared to other violent offenders and nonviolent juvenile offenders (Caputo, Frick, & Brodsky, 1999). Similarly, in a sample of juvenile offenders incarcerated in adult prison, offenders who showed more severe, repeated, instrumental, and sadistic violence against their victims scored higher on a self-report measure of psychopathic traits (Kruh, Frick, & Clements, 2005). In a sample of 169 adjudicated adolescents, psychopathic traits were associated with a tendency to emphasize the positive aspects (e.g., obtaining rewards and gaining dominance) of aggression and de-emphasize the negative aspects (e.g., getting punished) of these acts (Pardini, Lochman, & Frick, 2003). As noted previously, this particular social cognitive style has been linked specifically to instrumental aggression. Finally, in a nonreferred community sample of children, youth with conduct problems and psychopathic traits exhibited more aggression overall, and more proactive aggression specifically, than other children with conduct problems (Frick, Cornell, Bodin, et al., 2003). Taken together, this research provides growing support for the contention that children who show a combination of proactive and reactive patterns of aggression show a number of characteristics consistent with the construct of psychopathy.

CHILDHOOD- AND ADOLESCENT-ONSET CONDUCT PROBLEMS

Another approach to designating subgroups of children with severe conduct problems that has been the subject of substantial research (see Moffitt, 2003, for a review) and that has been incorporated into the most recent versions of the *Diagnostic and Statistical Manual of Mental Disorders* (DSM-IV-TR; American Psychiatric Association, 2000) to classify children with conduct disorder distinguishes between children who begin showing severe conduct problems in childhood versus those whose onset of severe antisocial behavior coincides with the onset of puberty. Children in the childhood-onset group often begin showing mild oppositional and defiant behaviors early in childhood (i.e., preschool or early elementary school). Their behavioral problems tend to increase in rate and severity throughout childhood and into adolescence (Lahey & Loeber, 1994). In contrast, the adolescent-onset group does not show significant behavioral problems in childhood, but this group begins exhibiting significant antisocial and delinquent behavior during adolescence (Hinshaw, Lahey, & Hart, 1993; Moffitt, 1993). In addition to different patterns of onset, there are important differences in the severity of behavior and outcome for the two groups of antisocial youth. Specifically, chil-

dren in the childhood-onset group are more likely to show aggressive behaviors in childhood and adolescence and they are more likely to continue to show antisocial and criminal behavior through adolescence and into adulthood (Frick & Loney, 1999; Moffitt & Capsi, 2001).

More relevant to causal theory, however, is the finding that the two groups differ on a number of the risk factors related to antisocial behavior. Specifically, most of the dispositional (e.g., neuropsychological abnormalities and low intelligence) and contextual (e.g., family dysfunction and poverty) correlates that have been associated with severe antisocial behavior seem primarily associated with the childhood-onset subtype (Moffitt, 1993; Moffitt & Caspi, 2001). In contrast, youth in the adolescent-onset subtype do not consistently show these same risk factors. This group primarily differs from children without conduct problems in showing more affiliation with delinquent peers and in scoring higher on measures of rebelliousness and authority conflict (Moffitt & Caspi, 2001; Moffitt, Caspi, Dickson, Silva, & Stanton, 1996).

The different characteristics of children in the two groups of antisocial youth have led to theoretical models that propose very different causal mechanisms operating across the two groups. For example, Moffitt (1993, 2003) has proposed that children in the childhood-onset group develop their problem behavior through a transactional process involving a difficult and vulnerable child (e.g., impulsive, with verbal deficits and a difficult temperament) who experiences an inadequate rearing environment (e.g., poor parental supervision and poor-quality schools). This dysfunctional transactional process disrupts the child's socialization leading to poor social relations with persons both inside (e.g., parents and siblings) and outside the family (e.g., peers and teachers). These disruptions lead to enduring vulnerabilities that can negatively affect the child's psychosocial adjustment across multiple developmental stages (see also Hinshaw et al., 1993; Patterson, Reid, & Dishion, 1992).

In contrast, Moffitt (1993, 2003) has proposed a very different causal model to explain the development of conduct problems for children in the adolescent-onset pathway. Because children in this subgroup are more likely to have their problems limited to adolescence, and because they show fewer dispositional and contextual risk factors, this group is conceptualized as showing an exaggeration of the normative process of adolescent rebellion. That is, most adolescents show some level of rebelliousness to parents and other authority figures. This behavior is part of a process by which the adolescent begins to develop his or her autonomous sense of self and his or her unique identity. According to Moffitt (1993), children in the adolescent-onset group engage in antisocial and delinquent behaviors as a misguided attempt to obtain a subjective sense of maturity and adult status in a way that is maladaptive (e.g., breaking societal norms) but encouraged by an antisocial peer group. Given that their behavior is viewed as an exaggeration of a process specific to adolescence, and not due to enduring vulnerabilities, their antisocial behavior is less likely to persist beyond adolescence. However, they may still have impairments that persist into adulthood due to the consequences of their adolescent antisocial behavior (e.g., a criminal record, dropping out of school, and substance abuse; Moffitt & Caspi, 2001).

It is important to note that the clear differences between the childhood-onset and adolescent-onset groups have not been found in all samples (Lahey et al., 2000) and the applicability of this model to girls requires further testing (Silverthorn & Frick, 1999). However, given the consistency of findings across samples (Moffitt, 2003), any model of the development of severe antisocial behavior, including those attempting to extend the construct of psychopathy to youth, must consider the childhood- and adolescent-onset distinction. Furthermore, the childhood-onset group shows a number of characteristics that would be consistent with the construct of psychopathy, such as showing a severe, chronic, and aggressive pattern of antisocial behavior that is likely to persist into adulthood. Two studies have directly tested the association between age of onset of conduct problems and features associated with the construct of psychopathy. First, in their study of a representative birth cohort of New Zealand children, Moffitt and colleagues (1996) reported that boys who showed a preadolescent onset to their conduct problems and showed a continuous level of con-

duct problem behavior across development (i.e., life-course persistent) were more likely to show a personality style characterized by a suspicious and cynical stance toward others and cold and callous behavior toward others than boys whose conduct problems started in adolescence. Second, in an adjudicated sample, Silverthorn, Frick, and Reynolds (2001) reported that boys who showed serious conduct problems prior to adolescence (prior to age 10) showed higher rates of impulsivity, narcissism, and callous and unemotional traits than boys whose antisocial behavior emerged after age 11.

Taken together, this research suggests that the childhood-onset group shows a number of characteristics that are consistent with the construct of psychopathy. However, this group also shows a number of features that are not consistent with psychopathy, such as verbal intelligence deficits (Moffitt, 1993), high levels of family dysfunction (Frick, 1998), and high levels of anxiety (Walker et al., 1991) Furthermore, not all children with early-onset delinquency show a chronic pattern of antisocial deviance that extends into adulthood (Frick & Loney, 1999). For example, only 43% of a sample of boys with an early onset to their conduct problems self-reported severe violent behavior as an adult, and only 55% had a conviction in adult court by the age of 26 years (Moffit, Caspi, Harrington, & Milne, 2002). Therefore, the childhood-onset category may be too broad of a category to represent a developmental precursor to psychopathy.

COMORBIDITY BETWEEN CONDUCT DISORDER AND ATTENTION-DEFICIT/HYPERACTIVITY DISORDER

Past research on conduct problems in children has consistently shown that these problems co-occur with a large number of other disorders and problems in adjustment (Frick, 1998). Furthermore, the presence of certain comorbid conditions has been a common criterion for designating important subgroups of youth with conduct problems (Loeber & Keenan, 1994). One of the most common overlapping disorders in children with conduct problems is attention-deficit/hyperactivity disorder (ADHD), for which rates of diagnosis range from 36% in community samples (Waschbush, 2002) to as high as 90% in some clinic-referred samples of children with conduct problems (Abikoff & Klein, 1992). This overlap between conduct problems and ADHD seems to be particularly strong for children in the childhood-onset group (Moffitt, 2003).

There have been a number of reviews of the extensive body of research investigating the overlap between conduct problems and ADHD (Hinshaw, 1987; Lilienfeld & Waldman, 1990; Newcorn & Halperin, 2000; Waschbusch, 2002). These reviews have documented a number of consistent differences between children with conduct problems and ADHD compared to those with conduct problems alone. First, research has consistently shown that youth with both conduct problems and ADHD show a more severe and aggressive pattern of antisocial behavior than youth with conduct problems alone (Waschbusch, 2002). Second, children with ADHD and conduct problems have poorer outcomes than children with conduct problems alone, such as showing higher rates of police contact, delinquency, theft, and overall offending in adolescence (Loeber, Brinthaupt, & Green, 1990), as well as higher rates of arrests and convictions in adulthood (Babinski, Hartsough, & Lambert, 1999; Magnusson, 1987). Third, youth with co-occurring ADHD and conduct problems also exhibit a number of distinct neuropsychological deficits. For example, antisocial youth with ADHD are more impaired on tasks measuring verbal and auditory memory (Moffitt & Silva, 1988), show greater deficits in verbal intelligence (Moffitt, 1990), show greater deficits in executive functioning (Moffitt & Henry, 1989), and have more problems inhibiting a dominant response (Halperin, O'Brien, & Newcorn, 1990).

This evidence clearly suggests that the combination of ADHD and conduct problems designates an important subgroup of antisocial and aggressive youth. However, there is considerable disagreement as to the best way to conceptualize this co-occurrence in causal theories. For example, it has been proposed that the symptoms of ADHD (or, more specifically, the impulsivity or hyperactivity symptoms) may be the primary causal factor leading to the development of serious conduct problems for many children with childhood-onset conduct problems (Burns &

Walsh, 2002). Alternatively, it has been suggested that the comorbidity of ADHD and conduct problems represents an additive combination of two separate domains that, when combined, leads to a particularly severe and impairing pattern of behavior (Waschbusch, 2002). Finally, it has been proposed that the combination of ADHD and conduct problems designates a distinct disorder that is qualitatively different from either disorder alone (Lynam, 1996).

This latter view is potentially important for developmental models of psychopathy because Lynam (1996) has proposed that the combination of symptoms of ADHD and conduct problems may represent a disorder in children similar to psychopathy in adults. Lynam suggests that the combination of these behavioral problems arises from a "psychopathic deficit" that consists of difficulty incorporating feedback from the environment and using this information to modulate responses when pursuing rewards. This deficit purportedly leads to hyperactive, inattentive, and impulsive behaviors in early childhood, which then develops into oppositional and defiant behaviors as the child acquires verbal and motor skills. In adolescence and adulthood, the psychopathic deficit can result in the manipulative and callous behaviors that are characteristic of adults who show psychopathic traits. In a test of this model, Lynam (1998) found that children with both ADHD symptoms and conduct problems differed from other children with conduct problems by showing greater deficits on laboratory tasks assessing response modulation, delay of gratification, and executive functioning. These characteristics of children with co-occurring conduct problems and ADHD are similar to those found for adults with psychopathic traits (Brinkley, Newman, Widiger, & Lynam, 2004).

Lynam's model could explain why children with childhood-onset conduct problems are more likely to show the cold and callous features associated with psychopathy. As noted previously, children with both ADHD and conduct problems are more common among this subgroup of antisocial youth. Importantly, Lynam's (1996) model provides even greater specificity by suggesting that within the childhood-onset group, those with co-occurring ADHD are most likely to develop these traits. Furthermore, this theory makes use of a great deal of existing research by embedding its model of developmental precursors to psychopathy within the existing diagnostic definitions of disruptive behavior disorders for youth (Burns, 2000). However, the focus on ADHD and conduct problems places primary emphasis on an impulsive–antisocial dimension of behavior, which has not proven to be specific to adults with psychopathy. That is, impulsive–antisocial tendencies appear to be elevated in most adults with significant criminal histories and/or a diagnosis of antisocial personality disorder (Hare, 1985).

What has been critical to adult definitions of psychopathy is the presence of a specific affective (e.g., lack of guilt or empathy) and interpersonal (e.g., using others for own gain and manipulating others) style that may accompany this impulsive and antisocial lifestyle (Hare, 2003). It is possible that, as suggested by Lynam (1996), the affective and interpersonal features emerge later in development and are secondary to the problems in inhibitory control. However, there is evidence that the affective components of conscience and inhibitory control represent separable dimensions very early in development (Kochanska, 1995, 1997; Kochanska, Gross, Lin, & Nichols, 2002). Therefore, it is also possible that a specific focus on the affective and interpersonal features of the construct of psychopathy may provide even greater specificity for developmental models of psychopathy.

In support of this contention, Barry, Frick, DeShazo, McCoy, Ellis, and Loney (2000) divided clinic-referred children (ages 6–13) with both ADHD symptoms and a conduct problem diagnosis into those elevated and not elevated on a measure of callous and unemotional (CU) traits. Only those children who also showed CU traits showed higher levels of thrill-seeking behaviors and deficits in response modulation compared to a control group with ADHD alone or a group without behavior problems. Similarly, in a sample of nonreferred, elementary-age schoolchildren, those with conduct problems and CU traits showed greater levels of aggression and self-reported delinquency (Frick, Cornell, Barry, et al., 2003). The group with CU traits also showed higher rates of ADHD symptoms. However, the higher rates of aggression and delinquency could not be accounted for by the ADHD symptoms. In fact, those children high on CU traits and conduct problems but without significant ADHD symptoms showed the highest level of aggressive and delinquent behaviors.

UNDERSOCIALIZED AND SOCIALIZED SUBGROUPS OF ANTISOCIAL YOUTH

These findings suggest that a specific focus on the affective and interpersonal dimensions of psychopathy could be critical for developmental models of psychopathy. One of the earliest attempts to explicitly extend the construct of psychopathy to youth divided juvenile offenders into categories labeled "psychopathic" and "socialized" (Quay, 1964). The psychopathic group was characterized by such traits as a lack of concern for others, untrustworthiness, a lack of bonding with others, and destructive and assaultive behaviors. This group was contrasted with a socialized delinquent group that was less aggressive and less interpersonally alienated and often committed nonaggressive delinquent acts (e.g., truancy, stealing, and drug use) with antisocial peers. In an attempt to avoid the pejorative connotations associated with the label "psychopathy," the name of the former subgroup was later changed to "undersocialized aggressive" (Quay, 1986)

A number of subsequent studies tested the validity and clinical utility of this subtyping approach. The results of this research were quite promising in terms of designating a group of antisocial youth who may be showing a developmental precursor to psychopathy. Specifically, undersocialized aggressive youth showed more adjustment problems in juvenile facilities, were less successful in institutional work-release programs, and were more likely to violate probation and be rearrested than socialized aggressive youth (Quay, 1987). Furthermore, undersocialized aggressive youth were characterized by low autonomic arousal, diminished serotonergic functioning, response perseveration on laboratory tasks, and stimulation-seeking behaviors (Lahey, Hart, Pliszka, Applegate, & McBurnett, 1993; Quay, 1987, 1993; Raine, 2002). These results are all similar to findings for adults with psychopathy (Brinkley et al., 2004).

Because of these promising findings, DSM-III (American Psychiatric Association, 1980) included in its diagnosis of conduct disorder a distinction between "socialized" or "undersocialized" subtypes. The following quote from DSM-III illustrates its link to adult conceptualizations of psychopathy:

> The *Undersocialized* types [of CD] are characterized by a failure to establish a normal degree of affection, empathy, or bond with others. Peer relationships are generally lacking, although the youngster may have superficial relationships with other youngsters. Characteristically, the child does not extend himself or herself for others unless there is an obvious immediate advantage. Egocentrism is shown by readiness to manipulate others for favors without any effort to reciprocate. There is generally a lack of concern for the feelings, wishes, and well-being of others, as shown by callous behavior. Appropriate feelings of remorse are generally absent. Such a child may readily inform on his or her companions and try to place blame on them. (American Psychiatric Association, 1980, p. 45)

Unfortunately, the change in name from psychopathy to undersocialized aggressive resulted in considerable confusion as to the core features of this subtype and as to the best way to operationalize these features (Hinshaw et al., 1993; Lahey, Loeber, Quay, Frick, & Grimm, 1992). Some definitions focused on the child's ability to form and maintain social relationships, whereas others focused primarily on the context (alone or as a group) in which the antisocial acts were typically committed (see Frick & Ellis, 1999, for examples). Very few definitions focused directly on the interpersonal and affective characteristics that were central to the clinical descriptions of psychopathic individuals on which this method of subtyping was purportedly based.

As a result of this definitional confusion, the next revision of DSM (DSM-III-R; American Psychiatric Association, 1987) revised its criteria for subtyping conduct disorder (Lahey et al., 1992). Specifically, the criteria for the undersocialized subtype were changed to focus solely on whether the antisocial acts were committed alone and whether the pattern included aggressive

symptoms. It was renamed the solitary–aggressive subtype. The criteria for the second subtype focused solely on whether the antisocial acts were committed with other antisocial peers, and this subtype was assumed to be primarily nonaggressive in nature. It was renamed the group subtype. The rationale for defining subtypes in this way was twofold. First, children of the undersocialized type tended to be highly aggressive, whereas most children identified as falling within the socialized type tended to show nonaggressive symptoms. Second, it was assumed that reliability would be enhanced because there was less ambiguity in measuring physical aggression and in determining who was typically present when a child engaged in antisocial behavior than in measuring more subjective personality traits related to a child's empathic concern for others and feelings of guilt (Hinshaw et al., 1993; Lahey et al., 1992). This rationale, while eliminating some of the confusion inherent in assessing the earlier DSM-III criteria, moved this subtyping approach away from a focus on the interpersonal and affective dimensions that are considered hallmarks of adult psychopathy (see Hare, Hart, & Harpur, 1991, for a similar trend in definitions used to define psychopathy in adults).

CU TRAITS AND DEVELOPMENTAL PATHWAYS TO CONDUCT PROBLEMS

Explicitly Extending the Construct of Psychopathy to Youth

Another attempt to explicitly extend the construct of psychopathy to youth has focused on using the CU dimension of psychopathy to designate a distinct subgroup of antisocial and aggressive youth. This interpersonal–affective dimension, which involves a lack of guilt, lack of empathy, and a basic poverty of emotional reaction, is just one of several dimensions that have emerged as being related to psychopathy in adult samples (Cooke & Michie, 2001; Hare, 2003). Similarly, factor analyses of psychopathic features in youth have typically resulted in two (Frick, O'Brien, McBurnett, & Wootton, 1994) or three dimensions (Frick, Bodin, & Barry, 2000). For example, Frick and colleagues (2000) conducted a factor analysis of teacher and parent ratings of psychopathic traits in a community sample of 1,136 elementary school–age and 160 clinic-referred children. In both samples, a separate CU dimension emerged. In the community sample, there was clear evidence for two other dimensions, one involving narcissistic traits (e.g., thinks he or she is more important than others; brags excessively) and the other involving impulsive behaviors (e.g., acts without thinking, does not plan ahead). Although this same three-factor solution could fit in the clinic-referred sample, there was less evidence for a divergence between the narcissism and impulsivity dimensions in this sample (see also Frick et al., 1994).

Although all three dimensions emerged in these samples of youth, in clinic-referred samples of children (e.g., Christian, Frick, Hill, Tyler, & Frazer, 1997) and adjudicated samples of adolescents (e.g., Caputo et al., 1999), the narcissism and impulsivity dimensions do not appear to differentiate within severely antisocial youth. For example, a cluster analysis of psychopathic traits and conduct problems in a clinic-referred sample of children ages 6–13 revealed two distinct conduct problem clusters (Christian et al., 1997). These clusters did not differ on their level of impulsivity and narcissism, but they did differ on their level of CU traits, with the group high on CU traits showing more severe patterns of antisocial behavior. Similarly, in a sample of adjudicated adolescents, narcissistic and impulsive traits did not differentiate among nonviolent offenders, violent offenders, and violent sex offenders (Caputo et al., 1999). In contrast, the violent sex offenders did show significantly higher levels of CU traits. Across both studies, children who were high on CU traits also tended to be high on the impulsive and narcissistic dimensions. However, there were children with childhood-onset conduct problems and serious adolescent offenders who showed high levels of impulsive and narcissistic traits but without CU traits (see Frick et al., 2000, for similar findings in a community sample).

Before reviewing research on the importance of this group of antisocial youth high on CU traits, and its relevance to extending the construct of psychopathy, it is important to consider the stability of these traits in youth (Seagrave & Grisso, 2002). That is, it is important to test whether these traits designate a stable pattern behavior that would

warrant them being considered "personality traits." Frick, Kimonis, Dandreaux, and colleagues (2003) examined the stability of parent ratings of CU traits over a 4-year study period in a sample of 98 children who were in grades 3, 4, 6, and 7 at the time of initial assessment. The intraclass correlation coefficients across 2 (.76), 3 (.86), and 4 years (.71) were quite high, indicating a substantial degree of stability in parent ratings of these traits. These estimates are substantially higher than those that have been reported for parent ratings of other forms of childhood psychopathology. For example, in two studies of the stability of parent ratings of children's adjustment in community samples over 3 years (McConaughy, Stanger, & Achenbach, 1992) or 4 years (Verhulst, Koot, & Berden, 1990), the mean stability estimates across different types of child adjustment were .46 (range of .30–.58) and .41 (range of .11 to .67), respectively.

The Importance of CU Traits for Defining Subgroups of Antisocial Youth

The utility of CU traits for designating a distinct group of antisocial youth has been supported by a number of studies. Specifically, in juvenile forensic facilities (Caputo et al., 1999; Silverthorn et al., 2001), in outpatient mental health clinics (Christian et al., 1997; Frick et al., 1994), and in school-based samples (Frick, Cornell, Barry, et al., 2003; Frick, Stickle, Dandreaux, Farrell, & Kimonis, in press), antisocial youth with CU traits seem to show an especially severe, aggressive, and stable pattern of conduct problems. For example, clinic-referred youth who met criteria for a conduct problem diagnosis showed a more severe and varied pattern of conduct problems and were more likely to have contact with the police prior to adolescence if they were also high on CU traits (Christian et al., 1997). Similar results were found in a sample of nonreferred community children in which children who showed both conduct problems and CU traits exhibited more aggression overall and were more likely to show proactive and instrumental patterns of aggression than children with conduct problems but not CU traits (Frick, Cornell, Barry, et al., 2003).

As reviewed previously, one of the key findings supporting the importance of psychopathy in adult samples is its ability to predict later antisocial behavior (Gendreau et al., 2002; Hemphill et al., 1998; Walters, 2003). Unfortunately, research extending the construct of psychopathy to youth has largely been cross-sectional in nature (Edens, Skeem, Cruise, & Cauffman, 2001). There are several notable exceptions in which the predictive utility of psychopathic traits has been tested in samples of institutionalized adolescents. These studies have documented that psychopathic features predict subsequent delinquency, aggression, number of violent offenses, and a shorter length of time to violent reoffending in antisocial youth (Brandt, Kennedy, Patrick, & Curtin, 1997; Forth, Hart, & Hare, 1990; Toupin, Mercier, Dery, Cote, & Hodgins, 1995). In one of the only studies to test the predictive utility of CU traits in a nonreferred sample of children, Frick and colleagues (in press) reported that children with conduct problems who also showed CU traits exhibited the highest rates of conduct problems, self-reported delinquency, and police contacts across a 4-year study period. In fact, this group with CU traits accounted for at least half of all of the police contacts reported in the sample across the last three waves of data collection. In contrast, children with conduct problems who were low on CU traits did not report higher rates of self-reported delinquency than nonconduct problem children. In fact, the second highest rate of self-reported delinquency in the sample was found for the group of children who were high on CU traits but without conduct problems at the start of the study. This latter finding suggests that CU traits may designate a group of children at risk for delinquency, even in the absence of significant conduct problems.

Besides showing a more severe, aggressive, and stable pattern of conduct problems, there is also evidence to suggest that the subgroup of antisocial youth with CU traits may have different causal processes underlying their behavior problems compared to other antisocial youth. One of the strongest pieces of evidence for potential differences in causal processes across the two groups comes from a study of 6,330 7-year-old twins (3,165 twin pairs; Viding, Blair, Moffitt, & Plomin, in press). In this study, children scoring in the top 10% of the sample on a measure of conduct problems were further divided into those with ($N = 359$) and without ($N = 333$) significant levels of CU traits. Estimates of the genetic and environmental effects on variations in conduct problems were very different for the two groups. Specifically, the heritability estimate for the group high on both conduct problems and CU traits (.81) was over twice that for the group low on CU traits (.30). This finding is consistent with research from adult samples showing significant heritability for measures of psychopathic traits (Blonigen, Carlson, Krueger, & Patrick, 2003).

While this finding suggests that genetic factors may play a larger role in the development of conduct problems for children with CU traits, it does not provide clues as to the mechanism by which heredity may exert its effects. There is, however, a growing body of research to suggest that children with conduct problems and CU traits exhibit a temperamental style that is distinct from other conduct problem youth. Specifically, in both mental health (Frick, Lilienfeld, Ellis, Loney, & Silverthorn, 1999) and school-based (Frick, Cornell, Bodin, et al., 2003) samples, children with conduct problems who also show CU traits exhibit a preference for novel, exciting, and dangerous activities. In addition, children with CU traits and conduct problems have been shown to be less reactive to threatening and emotionally distressing stimuli than other antisocial youth (Blair, 1999; Frick, Cornell, Bodin, et al., 2003; Kimonis, Frick, Fazekas, & Loney, in press; Loney, Frick, Clements, Ellis, & Kerlin, 2003). For example, in a sample of adolescents referred to a diversion program for delinquent behavior, youth high on CU traits showed reduced emotional reactivity on a lexical decision task that assessed facilitation in the speed of a child's recognition of words with negative emotional content compared to emotionally neutral words (Loney et al., 2003). In contrast, adjudicated youth who were high on impulsivity but not CU traits actually showed evidence for heightened emotional reactivity on the lexical-decision task. Similarly, in a sample of nonreferred children between ages 6 and 13, those with conduct problems and CU traits showed reduced reactivity to pictures involving distressing content (e.g., a child in pain and a hurt animal) using a dot-probe paradigm, whereas children high on a measure of conduct problems but low on CU traits showed a heightened level of reactivity to these stimuli (Kimonis et al., in press).

These findings for a deficit in emotional processing for children with both conduct problems and CU traits is very similar to findings with antisocial adults who are high on psychopathic traits (Levenston, Patrick, Bradley, & Lang, 2000; Williamson, Harpur, & Hare, 1991). Another finding that is consistent with adult research on psychopathy (e.g., Newman, Patterson, & Kosson, 1997) is that children with CU traits and conduct problems show response perseveration on computer tasks in which a reward-oriented response set is primed (Barry et al., 2000; Fisher & Blair, 1998; Frick, Cornell, Bodin, et al., 2003; O'Brien & Frick, 1996). That is, on tasks in which responding leads to a high rate of rewards initially but then leads to a high rate of punishment (e.g., loss of points) later in the task, children with conduct problems and CU traits continue to respond despite the increasing rate of punishment. Importantly, this reward-oriented response set not only appears in computerized laboratory tests but also in social situations. In sample of adjudicated adolescents, CU traits were related to a tendency to emphasize the positive aspects (e.g., obtaining rewards and gaining dominance) of solving peer conflicts with aggression and to deemphasize the negative aspects (e.g., getting punished; Pardini et al., 2003).

Developmental Models to Explain CU Traits

The preference for novel and dangerous activities, the lack of emotional responsiveness to negative emotional material, and the lack of sensitivity to cues to punishment are all consistent with a temperamental style that has been variously labeled as "low fearfulness" (Rothbart & Bates, 1998), "low behavioral inhibition" (Kagan & Snidman, 1991), "low harm avoidance" (Cloninger, 1987), or "high daring" (Lahey & Waldman, 2003). Importantly, several studies of normally developing children have linked this temperamental style to lower scores on measures of conscience development in both concurrent (Asendorpf & Nunner-Winkler, 1992; Kochanska et al., 2002) and prospective studies (Rothbart, Ahadi, & Hershey,

1994). These findings have led to a number of theories as to how this temperamental disposition may be involved in conscience development (see Frick & Morris, 2004, for a more extended review).

For example, some theories suggest that moral socialization and the internalization of parental and societal norms are partly dependent on the negative arousal evoked by potential punishment for misbehavior (e.g., Fowles & Kochanska, 2000; Kagan, 1998; Kochanska, 1993). Guilt and anxiety associated with actual or anticipated wrongdoing can be impaired if the child has a temperament in which the negative arousal to cues of punishment is attenuated, resulting in a diminished experience of anxiety (Kagan, 1998; Kochanska, 1993). Blair and colleagues (Blair, 1995; Blair, Colledge, Murray, & Mitchel, 2001; Blair, Jones, Clark, & Smith, 1997) have proposed a similar model of moral socialization that also emphasizes the importance of negative emotional arousal. However, this model focuses more specifically on the development of empathetic concern in response to the distress in others. According to this model, early negative emotional reactivity to the distress of others becomes conditioned to behaviors on the part of the child that prompted the distress in others (Blair, 1995). Through a process of conditioning, the child learns to inhibit such behaviors as a means of avoiding this negative arousal. This process of avoidance learning can be impaired by a temperamental deficit in negative emotional arousal.

The primacy of negative emotional arousal in the development of conscience has been questioned by a number of theorists (Grusec & Goodnow, 1994; Hoffman, 1994). The primary criticism is that it ignores the importance of parental socialization strategies that do not rely on punishment to evoke negative emotions. These criticisms have led to theories that consider a more complex role of emotional arousal and fearful inhibitions in conscience development. One example is the model proposed by Kochanska and colleagues (Kochanska, 1993, 1995, 1997; Kochanska et al., 2002). This model focuses on emotional arousal as key to conscience development. However, it proposes that the optimal level of arousal for moral socialization is achieved through an interaction between the child's temperament and the type of parenting he or she receives. To illustrate this assumption, Kochanska and colleagues reported that relatively fearful toddlers showed enhanced scores on measures of conscience development later in childhood if they experienced gentle, consistent, and nonpower assertive parenting (Kochanska, 1995, 1997). In contrast, relatively fearless children did not respond with improved scores on measures of conscience development when they experienced gentle discipline in the home. Presumably, such discipline did not lead to an optimal state of arousal for conscience development.

Although all these theories differ somewhat in the developmental mechanisms involved, they each propose a developmental process through which low levels of fearful inhibitions can impair moral socialization in general, and the development of conscience specifically. These theories are consistent with many of the characteristics of antisocial youth with CU traits. Specifically, children with conduct problems and CU traits appear to be less responsive to typical parental socialization practices than other children with conduct problems (Oxford, Cavell, & Hughes, 2003; Wootton, Frick, Shelton, & Silverthorn, 1997), they are less distressed by the negative effects of their behavior on others (Blair et al., 1997; Frick et al., 1999; Pardini et al., 2003), they are more impaired in their moral reasoning and empathic concern toward others (Blair, 1999; Fisher & Blair, 1998; Pardini et al., 2003), and they are less able to recognize expressions of sadness in the faces and vocalizations of other children (Blair et al., 2001; Stevens, Charman, & Blair, 2001). Furthermore, the emphasis of such theories on impairments in the affective components of conscience is consistent with many theories of psychopathic behavior in adults (Hare, 1993).

Potential Benefits of Using CU Traits over Other Methods

Research on the use of CU traits to designate a distinct group of youth with conduct problems has great promise for extending the construct of psychopathy earlier in development. It offers a number of advantages over other methods of subtyping antisocial youth for this purpose. First, it explicitly focuses on the affective and interpersonal features that have been critical to defining the construct of psychopathy in adult samples and, more important, for differentiating persons with psychopathy from other antisocial individuals (Cleckley, 1976; Hare, 1998). As noted previously, CU traits, but not other dimensions of psychopathy, seem to designate a distinct subgroup of children within severely antisocial youth as well. Second, characteristics of children with CU traits can be integrated with theories of the normal development of conscience (Frick & Morris, 2004). Such an integration between normal and abnormal development could benefit causal theory by highlighting when and how the normal process of conscience development can go awry. Third, the use of CU traits could help to integrate and explain some of the findings from research using other methods to designate distinct subgroups of antisocial youth. Specifically, CU traits seem to designate a subgroup of children within the childhood-onset group (e.g., Christian et al., 1997; Viding et al., in press) and within the group of children who exhibit both ADHD symptoms and serious conduct problems (e.g., Barry et al., 2000; Frick, Cornell, Barry, et al., 2003) who show characteristics consistent with psychopathy. Furthermore, CU traits are associated with severe aggression involving both proactive and reactive forms of aggression (e.g., Frick, Cornell, Barry, et al., 2003). Finally, the explicit delineation of the core features of CU traits (e.g., Frick et al., 2000) and the explicit link to the adult literature on psychopathy could avoid some of the definitional confusion associated with the undersocialized aggressive method for subtyping antisocial youth that has been used in past research.

One additional and very important advantage of the use of CU traits to designate a distinct group of antisocial youth is that it also designates a group of children without these traits who show some of the features that are often associated with psychopathy (i.e., narcissism and impulsivity) but who show other characteristics that do not fit with traditional conceptualizations of psychopathy (Frick & Morris, 2004). For example, children with conduct problems who are not elevated on CU traits are less aggressive than children high on CU traits, and, when they do act aggressively, it is more likely to be reactive in nature (Frick, Cornell, Barry, et al., 2003) and in response to real or perceived provocation by others (Frick, Cornell, Bodin, et al., 2003). Also, antisocial children without CU traits have conduct problems that are more strongly associated with dysfunctional parenting practices (Oxford et al., 2003; Wooton et al., 1997) and with deficits in verbal intelligence (Loney, Frick, Ellis, & McCoy, 1998). Finally, antisocial youth *without* CU traits appear to show problems regulating their emotions. They exhibit high levels of self-reported emotional distress (Frick et al., 1999; Frick, Cornell, Bodin, et al., 2003), they are more reactive to the distress of others in social situations (Pardini et al., 2003), and they are highly reactive to negative emotional stimuli (Kimonis et al., 2004; Loney et al., 2003).

Overall, these findings suggest that different mechanisms are operating in the development of conduct problems for children with and without high levels of CU traits. A significant proportion of children with conduct problems who lack CU traits seem to have difficulty regulating their emotions (Frick & Morris, 2004). This difficulty in emotion regulation can lead to a number of problems in adjustment. It can result in the child's committing impulsive and unplanned aggressive acts for which he or she may be remorseful afterward, but still has difficulty controlling in the future (Pardini et al., 2003). Difficulty in emotion regulation can also render a child particularly susceptible to becoming angry in response to perceived provocations from peers, leading to aggressive acts within the context of high emotional arousal, such as in arguments and fights with parents, teachers, and peers (Hubbard et al., 2002; Kruh et al., 2005; Loney et al., 2003; Shields & Cicchetti, 1998). Given these problems of behavioral and emotional dysregulation, such children may require a very different approach to treatment compared to other children with conduct problems (Frick, 1998, 2001). More important to the current discussion, however, is that the fact that many of the characteristics of this group of youth (e.g., lower verbal intelligence, dysfunctional family backgrounds, and high levels of emotional reactivity) appear to be consistent with adults who show criminal and antisocial behavior but who lack the concomitant affective–interpersonal features of psychopathy (Hare et al., 1991).

IMPORTANT CONSIDERATIONS IN EXTENDING THE CONSTRUCT OF PSYCHOPATHY TO YOUTH

This research on the use of CU traits to designate a distinct group of antisocial youth may be important for developmental models of psychopathy and for advancing our understanding of the multiple causal pathways through which children may develop severe antisocial and aggressive behaviors. However, an explicit extension of the construct of psychopathy involves a number of important conceptual, methodological, ethical, and developmental considerations that have been the subject of published critiques of this line of research.

First, there has been an emerging consensus about the basic features of psychopathy in adult samples that include the interpersonal, affective, self-referential, and behavioral traits described previously. However, there is still great debate as to how many psychological dimensions best summarize these traits, with factor analyses of these traits in adults finding from two (Harpur, Hare, & Hakstian, 1989) to eight (Lilienfeld & Andrews, 1996) factors underlying these traits (see Hare & Neumann, Chapter 4, and Cooke, Michie, & Hart, Chapter 5, this volume). More importantly, there is great disagreement about which of these dimensions are core to the definition of psychopathy (Cooke & Michie, 2001) and even whether any of these dimensions is either necessary or sufficient for defining the construct psychopathy (Brinkley et al., 2004; Skeem, Poythress, Edens, Lilienfeld, & Cale, 2003). Further, there is disagreement as to whether some characteristics associated with psychopathy, like fearlessness (Lilienfeld & Andrews, 1996) and antisocial behavior (Hare, 2003), should be considered part of the defining features of the construct or whether they should be considered as a temperamental risk factor for psychopathy or one possible outcome for individuals with psychopathy, respectively (Cooke & Miche, 2001; Frick, Bodin, & Barry, 2000; Frick, Cornell, Bodin, et al., 2003). These basic, yet unresolved, conceptual issues make it very difficult to extend the construct of psychopathy to youth. It necessitates some operational definition of the construct of psychopathy that is being extended to youth. Such operational definitions are likely to meet with significant disagreement as to whether what is specified to be "core" to psychopathy is sufficiently covered or covered in a way that is developmentally appropriate (Johnstone & Cooke, 2004).

Second, the most common methods for assessing psychopathic traits have been based on techniques developed for use in adult samples and, even more specifically, for use in incarcerated adult samples. For example, the most common measure used to assess adults, the Psychopathy Checklist—Revised (Hare, 2003), employs data from a semistructured interview and from institutional files to assign a rating of psychopathy. However, when studying youth in nonincarcerated samples, the availability of extensive historical data may be limited. Furthermore, the reliability and validity of child (i.e., preadolescent) self-report for assessing most forms of psychopathology has been questioned, especially when assessing antisocial attitudes and behaviors (Kamphaus & Frick, 2002). Unfortunately, some critiques of the extension of the psychopathy construct to youth have focused on differences in the methods of assessment between adults and children, without considering that such differences in procedures may be needed because of the different age groups and settings studied (Johnstone & Cooke, 2004).

Third, concern has been expressed over the fact that some level of psychopathic traits (e.g., irresponsibility, egocentrism, lack of planning, and forethought) may be normative in youth and that extending the construct of psychopathy to this age group runs the risk of labeling as disordered some youth who show a transient and normative pattern of behavior (Seagreave & Grisso, 2002; Skeem & Cauffman, 2003). This is a critical issue in all areas of child psychopathology in which there are often normative variants of the indicators or "symptoms" of the disorder and the level of these symptoms in normal samples may vary over the course of development due to changing demands across developmental stages (Cicchetti & Richters, 1997). This feature of psychopathology makes it critical to have some method of determining when the level of symptoms is non-normative and/or predicts significant impairment within a specific developmental stage (Kamphaus & Frick, 2002).

Unfortunately, some critiques have suggested that because of the normative varia-

tion in indicators of psychopathy, measures of this construct in youth should only include indicators that are not found in normal development (Seagrave & Grisso, 2002) or that are uncorrelated with normative measures of personality that change across development (Skeem & Cauffman, 2003). Other critiques have suggested that the construct of psychopathy needs to be as stable in youth as it is in adulthood for it to be a useful extension of the construct (Hart, Watt, & Vincent, 2002; Seagrave & Grisso, 2002). These assumptions are antithetical to a developmental perspective on psychopathology that explicitly acknowledges the often artificial boundaries between normal developmental and pathological processes (Cicchetti & Richters, 1997). Such artificial boundaries make it unlikely that one could develop a list of indicators for any form of psychopathology that would not have normative variants that may change in rate across development (Frick, 2002). Furthermore, such arguments do not recognize that personality processes may be intrinsically less stable in youth than in adulthood (Roberts & DelVecchio, 2000). As mentioned previously, one of the reasons for extending the construct of psychopathy to youth is to identify developmental precursors to the construct, so that interventions may be instituted at a point at which the traits are hopefully more changeable (Frick, 2001).

A final important issue that has been raised concerning research extending the construct of psychopathy to youth is that the term "psychopath" is a highly pejorative label that implies a biologically based and untreatable condition (Steinberg, 2002; see Edens & Petrila, Chapter 29, this volume). As a result, there is a distinct risk that the term will be used in many settings to make important and potentially harmful decisions concerning youth, such as their risk for future offending, their likelihood to be unresponsive to treatment, or their need for more restrictive placements. The validity of existing measures of psychopathic traits in youth for making such decisions has not been established and, thus, there is great potential for misuse of such measures in many applied settings (Edens et al., 2001). This is a critically important issue given the early stage of research extending the construct of psychopathy to youth, in that many of the important uses of the construct in adult samples (e.g., assessing recidivism risk) have not been as extensively studied in younger age groups (Frick, 2002). Our hope is that this important caveat will encourage cautious and skeptical use of the construct in applied settings but will not discourage additional research extending the construct to youth. It is only through such research that we can eventually determine the appropriate uses for the construct in applied settings with youth.

SUMMARY AND IMPLICATIONS

These concerns with regard to extending the construct of psychopathy to youth suggest that such research needs to proceed very cautiously. If one assumes that psychopathy by definition is a biologically based personality disposition that is highly stable and relatively difficult to change, then it is unlikely that such a construct will be found in children. Such a definition would be antithetical to developmental perspectives on personality development that recognize the interplay between biological predispositions and environmental influences for all forms of personality, and which recognize that personality in youth tends to be much more changeable than that found in adults. Furthermore, if methods for assessing these traits are extended to youth without considering changes mandated by the child's developmental level and context, or if measures are assumed to possess the same validity in adults and youth for making important decisions without directly testing such assumptions, such research could have quite harmful effects on youth. Finally, it is critically important to note that no prospective study to date has followed any of the subgroups of antisocial youth reviewed in this chapter into adulthood to determine what percentage will show significant levels of psychopathic traits and/or be diagnosed as "psychopathic" using traditional definitions (Frick, Kimonis, et al., 2003). It is open to question whether any of the subgroups described in this review should be considered a "developmental precursor" to psychopathy until such predictive utility has been established.

Despite these very important cautions, there is also great potential gain to be realized by investigating whether certain aspects of the construct of psychopathy can be used to differentiate subgroups of antisocial youth. As noted in this chapter, there is a long history of research attempting to define subgroups of antisocial and delinquent youth that differ in terms of the type, severity, and chronicity of their antisocial behavior, and that differ in the causal processes presumed to underlie their antisocial and aggressive behavior. Unfortunately, no subtyping approach for antisocial youth has garnered widespread acceptance over an extended period. However, the usefulness of the construct of psychopathy for designating a distinct subgroup of antisocial adults has withstood several decades of research scrutiny. Furthermore, the rich theoretical models that have been proposed and tested for explaining psychopathic behaviors in adults (e.g., Hare, 1998; Lykken, 1995; Newman, 1998; Patrick, 2001) could be quite helpful for guiding theoretical models of antisocial and aggressive behavior in youth.

Not only could research on psychopathy in adults prove to be useful for advancing causal models of antisocial behavior in youth, but the study of psychopathic traits in youth could greatly advance causal theories of psychopathy. For example, the two most prominent theories of psychopathy based on research with adults place emphasis on either (1) a cognitive deficit involving the ability of the person with psychopathy to use contextual cues that are peripheral to a dominant response set to modulate his or her behavior (Brinkley et al., 2004; Newman, 1998) or (2) a deficit in the experience of certain critical emotions that guide prosocial behavior and inhibit deviance (Hare, 1993; Lykken, 1995; Patrick, 2001). Both theories can explain a number of the characteristics of adults with psychopathy. Testing predictions consistent with these theories in youth and integrating these findings with research on the normal development of prosocial behavior could be critical for advancing these causal models. It could provide evidence for which of these (or other) deficits may be present earlier in development and which may develop later. Furthermore, research in childhood could uncover factors, both environmental (e.g., parenting variables) and dispositional (e.g., verbal intelligence), that might protect children with these deficits from showing the full pattern of affective, interpersonal, self-referential, and behavioral traits associated with psychopathy in adults.

This last point provides perhaps the most important reason for extending the construct of psychopathy to youth, despite the many potential pitfalls involved. If the construct can be integrated into developmentally informed causal theories of antisocial behavior and the processes that enhance and reduce the risk for later problems across different groups of antisocial youth can be identified, it is quite possible that more effective interventions for these youth can be developed (Frick, 2001; see also Seto & Quinsey, Chapter 30, this volume). Clearly, this provides great incentive for additional research extending the construct of psychopathy to youth.

REFERENCES

Abikoff, H., & Klein, R. G. (1992). Attention-deficit hyperactivity and conduct disorder: Co-morbidity and implications for treatment. *Journal of Consulting and Clinical Psychology*, 60, 881–892.

American Psychiatric Association. (1980). *The diagnostic and statistical manual of mental disorders* (3rd ed.). Washington, DC: Author.

American Psychiatric Association. (1987). *The diagnostic and statistical manual of mental disorders* (3rd ed. rev). Washington, DC: Author.

American Psychiatric Association. (2000). *The diagnostic and statistical manual of mental disorders* (4th ed., text rev.). Washington, DC: Author.

Asendorpf, J. B., & Nunner-Winkler, G. (1992). Children's moral motive strength and temperamental inhibition reduce their egoistic behavior in real moral conflicts. *Child Development*, 63, 1223–1235.

Babinski, L. M., Hartsough, C. S., & Lambert, N. M. (1999). Childhood conduct problems, hyperactivity-impulsivity, and inattention as predictors of adult criminal activity. *Journal of Child Psychology and Psychiatry*, 40, 347–355.

Barry, C. T., Frick, P. J., DeShazo, T. M., McCoy, M. G., Ellis, M., & Loney, B. R. (2000). The importance of callous-unemotional traits for extending the concept of psychopathy to children. *Journal of Abnormal Psychology*, 109, 335–340.

Berkowitz, L. (1993). *Aggression: Its causes, consequences, and control*. New York: Academic Press.

Blair, R. J. R. (1995). A cognitive developmental approach to morality: Investigating the psychopath. *Cognition*, 57, 1–29.

Blair, R. J. R. (1999). Responsiveness to distress cues in the child with psychopathic tendencies. *Personality and Individual Differences*, 27, 135–145.

Blair, R. J. R., Colledge, E., Murray, L., & Mitchell, D.

G. V. (2001). A selective impairment in the processing of sad and fearful expressions in children with psychopathic tendencies. *Journal of Abnormal Child Psychology*, 29, 491–498.

Blair, R. J. R., Jones, L., Clark, F., & Smith, M. (1997). The psychopathic individual: A lack of responsiveness to distress cues? *Psychophysiology*, 34, 192–198.

Blonigen, D. M., Carlson, R. F., Krueger, R. F., & Patrick, C. J. (2003). A twin study of self-reported psychopathic personality traits. *Personality and Individual Differences*, 35, 179–197.

Brandt, J. R., Kennedy, W. A., Patrick, C. J., & Curtin, J. J. (1997). Assessment of psychopathy in a population of incarcerated adolescent offenders. *Psychological Assessment*, 9, 429–435.

Brinkley, C. A., Newman, J. P., Widiger, T. A., & Lynam, D. R. (2004). Two approaches to parsing the heterogeneity of psychopathy. *Clinical Psychology: Research and Practices*, 11, 69–94.

Brown, K, Atkins, M. S., Osborne, M. L., & Milnamow, M. (1996). A revised teacher rating scale for reactive and proactive aggression. *Journal of Abnormal Child Psychology*, 24, 473–480.

Burns, G. L. (2000). Problem of item overlap between the Psychopathy Screening Device and attention deficit hyperactivity disorder, oppositional defiant disorder, and conduct disorder rating scales. *Psychological Assessment*, 12, 447–450

Burns, G. L., & Walsh, J. A. (2002). The influence of ADHD-hyperactivity/impulsivity symptoms on the development of oppositional defiant disorder symptoms in a 2-year longitudinal study. *Journal of Abnormal Child Psychology*, 30, 245–256

Caputo, A. A., Frick, P. J., & Brodsky, S. L. (1999). Family violence and juvenile sex offending: Potential mediating roles of psychopathic traits and negative attitudes toward women. *Criminal Justice and Behavior*, 26, 338–356.

Christian, R., Frick, P. J., Hill, N., Tyler, L. A., & Frazer, D. (1997). Psychopathy and conduct problems in children: II. Subtyping children with conduct problems based on their interpersonal and affective style. *Journal of the American Academy of Child and Adolescent Psychiatry*, 36, 233–241.

Ciccheti, D., & Richters, J. E. (1997). Examining the conceptual and scientific underpinnings of research in developmental psychopathology. *Development and Psychopathology*, 9, 189–192.

Cleckley, H. (1976). *The mask of sanity* (5th ed.). St. Louis, MO: Mosby.

Cloninger, C. R. (1987). A systematic method for clinical description and classification of personality variants. *Archives of General Psychiatry*, 44, 573–588.

Coie, J. D., & Dodge, K. A. (1998). Aggression and antisocial behavior. In W. Damon & N. Eisenberg (Eds.), *Handbook of child psychology: Social, emotional, and personality development* (pp. 779–862). Toronto, ON, Canada: Wiley.

Cooke, D. J., & Michie, C. (2001). Refining the construct of psychopathy: Towards a hierarchical model. *Psychological Assessment, 13,* 171–188.

Cornell, D. G., Warren, J., Hawk, G., Stafford, E., Oram, G., & Pine, D. (1996). Psychopathy in instrumental and reactive violent offenders. *Journal of Consulting and Clinical Psychology, 64,* 783–790.

Crick, N. R. (1996). The role of overt aggression, relational aggression, and prosocial behavior in the prediction of children's future social adjustment. *Child Development, 67,* 2317–2327.

Crick, N. R., Casas, J. F., & Mosher, M. (1997). Relational and overt aggression in preschool. *Developmental Psychology, 33,* 579–588.

Crick, N. R., & Dodge, K. A. (1996). Social information-processing mechanisms in reactive and proactive aggression. *Child Development, 67,* 993–1002.

Crick, N. R., & Grotpeter, J. K. (1995). Relational aggression, gender, and social–psychological adjustment. *Child Development, 66,* 710–722.

Crick, N. R., Werner, N. E., Casas, J. F., O'Brien, K. M., Nelson, D. A., Grotpeter, J. K., & Markon, K. (1999). Childhood aggression and gender: A new look at an old problem. In D. Bernstein (Ed.), *The 45th Nebraska Symposium on Motivation: Gender and motivation* (pp. 75–141). Lincoln: Nebraska University Press.

Day, D. M., Bream, L. A., & Pal, A. (1992). Proactive and reactive aggression: An analysis of subtypes based on teacher perceptions. *Journal of Clinical Psychology, 2,* 210–217.

Dodge, K. A., & Coie, J. D. (1987). Social-information-processing factors in reactive and proactive aggression in children's peer groups. *Journal of Personality and Social Psychology, 53,* 1146–1158.

Dodge, K. A., Lochman, J. E., Harnish, J. D., Bates, J. E., & Pettit, G. S. (1997). Reactive and proactive aggression in school children and psychiatrically impaired chronically assaultive youth. *Journal of Abnormal Psychology, 106,* 37–51.

Dodge, K. A., & Pettit, G. S. (2003). A biopsychosocial model of the development of chronic conduct problems in adolescence. *Developmental Psychology, 39,* 349–371.

Dodge, K. A., Price, J. M., Bachorowski, J., & Newman, J. P. (1990). Hostile attributional biases in severely aggressive adolescents. *Journal of Abnormal Psychology, 99,* 385–392.

Edens, J., Skeem, J., Cruise, K., & Cauffman, E. (2001). The assessment of juvenile psychopathy and its association with violence: A critical review. *Behavioral Sciences and the Law, 19,* 53–80.

Farrington, D. P., Ohlin, L., & Wilson, J. Q. (1986). *Understanding and controlling crime.* New York: Springer-Verlag.

Fisher, L., & Blair, R. J. R. (1998). Cognitive impairment and its relationship to psychopathic tendencies in children with emotional and behavioral difficulties. *Journal of Abnormal Child Psychology, 26,* 511–519.

Forth, A. E., Hart, S. D., & Hare, R. D. (1990). Assessment of psychopathy in male young offenders. *Psychological Assessment, 2,* 342–344.

Fowles, D. C., & Kochanska, G. (2000). Temperament as a moderator of pathways to conscience in children: The contribution of electrodermal activity. *Psychophysiology, 37,* 788–795

Frick, P. J. (1998). *Conduct disorders and severe antisocial behavior.* New York: Plenum Press.

Frick, P. J. (2001). Effective interventions for children and adolescents with conduct disorder. *Canadian Journal of Psychiatry, 46,* 26–37.

Frick, P. J. (2002). Juvenile psychopathy from a developmental perspective: Implications for construct development and use in forensic assessments. *Law and Human Behavior, 26,* 247–253.

Frick, P. J., Bodin, S. D., & Barry, C. T. (2000). Psychopathic traits and conduct problems in community and clinic-referred samples of children: Further development of the Psychopathy Screening Device. *Psychological Assessment, 12,* 382–393.

Frick, P. J., Cornell, A. H., Barry, C. T., Bodin, S. D., & Dane, H. A. (2003). Callous–unemotional traits and conduct problems in the prediction of conduct problem severity, aggression, and self-report of delinquency. *Journal of Abnormal Child Psychology, 31,* 457–470..

Frick, P. J., Cornell, A. H., Bodin, S. D., Dane, H. A., Barry, C. T., & Loney, B. R. (2003). Callous–unemotional traits and developmental pathways to severe conduct problems. *Developmental Psychology, 39,* 246–260.

Frick, P. J., & Ellis, M. L. (1999). Callous–unemotional traits and subtypes of conduct disorder. *Clinical Child and Family Psychology Review, 2,* 149–168.

Frick, P. J., Kimonis, E. R., Dandreaux, D. M., & Farrell, J. M. (2003). The four-year stability of psychopathic traits in non-referred youth. *Behavioral Sciences and the Law, 21,* 713–736.

Frick, P. J., Lilienfeld, S. O., Ellis, M. L., Loney, B. R., & Silverthorn, P. (1999). The association between anxiety and psychopathy dimensions in children. *Journal of Abnormal Child Psychology, 27,* 381–390.

Frick, P. J., & Loney, B. R. (1999). Outcomes of children and adolescents with conduct disorder and oppositional defiant disorder. In H. C. Quay & A. Hogan (Eds.), *Handbook of disruptive behavior disorders* (pp. 507–524). New York: Plenum Press.

Frick, P. J., & Morris, A. S. (2004). Temperament and developmental pathways to conduct problems. *Journal of Clinical Child and Adolescent Psychology, 33,* 54–68.

Frick, P. J., O'Brien, B. S., Wootton, J. M., & McBurnett, K. (1994). Psychopathy and conduct problems in children. *Journal of Abnormal Psychology, 103,* 700–707.

Frick, P. J., Stickle, T. R., Dandreaux, D. M., Farrell, J. M., & Kimonis, E. R. (in press). Callous–unemotional traits in predicting the severity and stability of conduct problems and delinquency. *Journal of Abnormal Child Psychology.*

Gendreau, P., Goggin, C., & Smith, P. (2002). Is the PCL-R really the "unparalleled" measure of offender risk? A lesson in knowledge accumulation. *Criminal Justice and Behavior, 29,* 397–426.

Grusec, J. E., & Goodnow, J. J. (1994). Impact of parental discipline methods on the child's internalization of values: A reconceptualization of current points of view. *Developmental Psychology, 30,* 4–19.

Halperin, J. M., O'Brien, J. D., & Newcorn, J. H. (1990). Validation of hyperactive, aggressive, and mixed hyperactive/aggressive childhood disorders: A research note. *Journal of Child Psychology and Psychiatry, 81,* 455–459.

Hare, R. D. (1985). A comparison of procedures for the assessment of psychopathy. *Journal of Consulting and Clinical Psychology, 53,* 716.

Hare, R. D. (1993). *Without a conscience: The disturbing world of the psychopaths among us.* New York: Pocket.

Hare, R. D. (1998). Psychopathy, affect, and behavior. In D. J. Cooke, A. E. Forth, & R. D. Hare (Eds.), *Psychopathy: Theory, research, and implications for society* (pp. 105–138). Dordrecht, The Netherlands: Kluwer.

Hare, R. D. (2003). *Hare Psychopathy Checklist—Revised (PCL-R): Second edition, technical manual.* Toronto, ON, Canada: Multi-Health Systems.

Hare, R. D., Hart, S. D., & Harpur, T. J. (1991). Psychopathy and the DSM-IV criteria for antisocial personality disorder. *Journal of Abnormal Psychology, 100,* 391–398.

Hare, R. D., McPherson, L. E., & Forth, A. E. (1988). Male psychopaths and their criminal careers. *Journal of Consulting and Clinical Psychology, 56,* 710–714.

Harpur, T. J., Hare, R. D., & Hakstian, A. R. (1989). Two-factor conceptualization of psychopathy: Construct validity and assessment implications. *Psychological Assessment, 1,* 6–17.

Hart, S. D., Watt, K. A., & Vincent, G. M. (2002). Commentary on Seagrave and Grisso: Impressions of the state of the art. *Law and Human Behavior, 26,* 241–246.

Hemphill, J. F., Hare, R. D., & Wong, S. (1998). Psychopathy and recidivism: A review. *Legal and Criminological Psychology, 3,* 139–170.

Hinshaw, S. P. (1987). On the distinction between attentional deficits/hyperactivity and conduct problems/aggression in child psychopathology. *Psychological Bulletin, 101,* 443–463.

Hinshaw, S. P., Lahey, B. B., & Hart, E. L. (1993). Issues of taxonomy and co-morbidity in the development of conduct disorder. *Development and Psychopathology, 5,* 31–50.

Hoffman, M. L. (1994). Discipline and internalization. *Developmental Psychology, 30,* 26–28.

Hubbard, J. A., Dodge, K. A., Cillessen, A. H. N., Coie, J. D., & Schwartz, D. (2001). The dyadic nature of social information processing in boys' reactive and proactive aggression. *Journal of Personality and Social Psychology, 80,* 268–280.

Hubbard, J. A., Smithmyer, C. M., Ramsden, S. R., Parker, E. H., Flanagan, K. D., Dearing, K. F., et al. (2002). Observational, physiological, and self-report measures of children's anger: Relations to reactive versus proactive aggression. *Child Development, 73,* 1101–1118.

Huesmann, L. R., Eron, L. D., Lefkowitz, M. M., & Walder, L. O. (1984). Stability of aggression over time and generations. *Developmental Psychology, 20,* 1120–1134.

Johnstone, L., & Cooke, D. J. (2004). Psychopathic-like traits in childhood: Conceptual and measurement concerns. *Behavioral Sciences and the Law, 22,* 103–125.

Kagan, J. (1998). Biology and the child. In N. Eisenberg (Ed.) & W. Damon (Series Ed.), *Handbook of child psychology: Vol. 3. Social, emotional, and personality development* (pp. 177–235). New York: Wiley.

Kagan, J., & Snidman, N. (1991). Temperamental factors in human development. *American Psychologist, 46,* 856–862.

Kamphaus, R. W., & Frick, P. J. (2002). *Clinical assessment of child and adolescent personality and behavior* (2nd ed.). Boston: Allyn & Bacon.

Kazdin, A. E. (1995). *Conduct disorder in childhood and adolescence* (2nd ed.). Thousand Oaks, CA: Sage.

Kiehl, K. A., Smith, A. M., Hare, R. D., Mendrek, A., Forster, B. B., Brink, J., & Liddle, P. F. (2001). Limbic abnormalities in affective processing by criminal psychopaths as revealed by functional magnetic resonance imaging. *Biological Psychiatry, 50,* 677–684.

Kimonis, E. R., Frick, P. J., Fazekas, H., & Loney, B. R. (in press). Psychopathy, aggression, and the processing of emotional stimuli in non-referred children. *Behavioral Sciences and the Law.*

Kochanska, G. (1993). Toward a synthesis of parental socialization and child temperament in early development of conscience. *Child Development, 64,* 325–347.

Kochanska, G. (1995). Children's temperament, mothers' discipline, and security of attachment: Multiple pathways to emerging internalization. *Child Development, 66,* 597–615.

Kochanska, G. (1997). Multiple pathways to conscience for children with different temperaments: From toddlerhood to age 5. *Developmental Psychology, 33,* 228–240.

Kochanska, G., Gross, J. N., Lin, M. H., & Nichols, K. E. (2002). Guilt in young children: Development, determinants, and relations with a broader system of standards. *Child Development, 73,* 461–482.

Kruh, I. P., Frick, P. J., & Clements, C. B. (2005). Historical and personality correlates to the violence patterns of juveniles tried as adults. *Criminal Justice and Behavior, 32,* 69–96.

Lahey, B. B., Hart, E. L., Pliszka, S., Applegate, B., & McBurnett, K. (1993). Neurophysiological correlates of conduct disorder: A rationale and a review of research. *Journal of Clinical Child Psychology*, 22, 141–153.

Lahey, B. B., & Loeber, R. (1994). Framework for a developmental model of oppositional defiant disorder and conduct disorder. In D. K. Routh (Ed.), *Disruptive behavior disorders in childhood* (pp. 139–180). New York: Plenum Press.

Lahey, B. B., Loeber, R., Quay, H. C., Frick, P. J., & Grimm, J. (1992). Oppositional defiant disorder and conduct disorders: Issues to be resolved for DSM-IV. *Journal of the American Academy of Child and Adolescent Psychiatry*, 31, 539–546.

Lahey, B. B., Schwab-Stone, M., Goodman, S. H., Waldman, I. D., Canino, G., Rathouz, P. J., et al. (2000). Age and gender differences in oppositional behavior and conduct problems: A cross-sectional household study of middle childhood and adolescence. *Journal of Abnormal Psychology*, 109, 488–503.

Lahey, B. B., & Waldman, I. D. (2003). A developmental propensity model of the origins of conduct problems during childhood and adolescence. In B. B. Lahey, T. E. Moffitt, & A. Caspi (Eds.), *Causes of conduct disorder and juvenile delinquency* (pp. 76–117). New York: Guilford Press.

Levenston, G. K., Patrick, C. J., Bradley, M. M., & Lang, P. J. (2000). The psychopath as observer: Emotion and attention in picture processing. *Journal of Abnormal Psychology*, 109, 373–385.

Lilienfeld, S. O., & Andrews, B. P. (1996). Development and preliminary validation of a self-report measure of psychopathic personality. *Journal of Personality Assessment*, 66, 488–524.

Lilienfeld, S. O., & Waldman, I. D. (1990). The relation between childhood attention-deficit disorder and adult antisocial behavior reexamined: The problem of heterogeneity. *Clinical Psychology Review*, 10, 699–725.

Little, T. D., Jones, S. M., Henrich, C. C., & Hawley, P. H. (2003). Disentangling the "whys" from the "whats" of aggressive behavior. *International Journal of Behavioral Development*, 27, 122–133.

Loeber, R., Brinthaupt, V. P., & Green, S. M. (1990). Attention deficits, impulsivity, and hyperactivity with or without conduct problems: Relationships to delinquency and unique contextual factors. In R. J. McMahon & R. D. Peters (Eds.), *Behavior disorders of adolescence: Research, intervention, and policy in clinical and school settings* (pp. 39–61). New York: Plenum Press.

Loeber, R., & Farrington, D. P. (2000). Young children who commit crime: Epidemiology, developmental origins, risk factors, early interventions, and policy implications. *Development and Psychopathology*, 12, 737–762.

Loeber, R., & Keenan, K. (1994). Interaction between conduct disorder and its comorbid conditions: Effects of age and gender. *Clinical Psychology Review*, 14, 497–523.

Loeber, R., Keenan, K., & Zhang, Q. (1997). Boys'

experimentation and persistence in developmental pathways toward serious delinquency. *Journal of Child and Family Studies*, 6, 321–357.

Loney, B. R., Frick, P. J., Clements, C. B., Ellis, M. L., & Kerlin, K. (2003). Callous–unemotional traits, impulsivity, and emotional processing in antisocial adolescents. *Journal of Clinical Child and Adolescent Psychology*, 32, 66–80.

Loney, B. R., Frick, P. J., Ellis, M., & McCoy, M. G. (1998). Intelligence, psychopathy, and antisocial behavior. *Journal of Psychopathology and Behavioral Assessment*, 20, 231–247.

Lorenz, A. R., & Newman, J. P. (2002). Utilization of emotion cues in male and female offenders with antisocial personality disorder: Results from a lexical decision task, *Journal of Abnormal Psychology*, 111, 513–516.

Lykken, D. T. (1995). *The antisocial personalities.* Hillsdale, NJ: Erlbaum.

Lynam, D. R. (1996). The early identification of chronic offenders: Who is the fledgling psychopath? *Psychological Bulletin*, 120, 209–234.

Lynam, D. R. (1998). Early identification of the fledgling psychopath: Locating the psychopathic child in the current nomenclature. *Journal of Abnormal Psychology*, 107, 566–575.

Magnusson, D. (1987). Adult delinquency in the light of conduct and physiology at an early age: A longitudinal study. In D. Magnusson & A. Ohman (Eds.), *Psychopathology: An interactional perspective* (pp. 221–253). New York: Academic Press.

Marshall, L., & Cooke, D. J. (1999). The childhood experiences of psychopaths: A retrospective study of familial and societal factors. *Journal of Personality Disorders*, 13(3), 211–225.

McConaughy, S., Stanger, C., & Achenbach, T. M. (1992). Three-year course of behavioral/emotional problems in a national sample of 4- to 16-year olds: I. Agreement among informants. *Journal of the American Academy of Child and Adolescent Psychiatry*, 31, 932–94

Moffitt, T. E. (1990). Juvenile delinquency and attention-deficit disorder: Developmental trajectories from age 3 to 15. *Child Development*, 61, 893–910.

Moffitt, T. E. (1993). Adolescence-limited and life-course persistent antisocial behavior: A developmental taxonomy. *Psychological Review*, 100, 674–701.

Moffitt, T. E. (2003). Life-course persistent and adolescence-limited antisocial behavior: A 10-year research review and research agenda. In B. B. Lahey, T. E. Moffitt, & A. Caspi (Eds.), *Causes of conduct disorder and juvenile delinquency* (pp. 49–75). New York: Guilford Press.

Moffitt, T. E., & Caspi, A. (2001). Childhood predictors differentiate life-course persistent and adolescence-limited antisocial pathways in males and females. *Development and Psychopathology*, 13, 355–376.

Moffitt, T. E., Caspi, A., Dickson, N., Silva, P., & Stanton, W. (1996). Childhood-onset versus adolescent-onset antisocial conduct problems in males: Natural history from ages 3 to 18 years. *Development and Psychopathology, 8,* 399–424.

Moffitt, T. E., Caspi, A., Harrington, H., & Milne, B. J. (2002). Males on the lifes-course persistent and adolescence-limited pathways: Follow-up at age 26 years. *Development and Psychopathology, 14,* 179–207.

Moffitt, T. E., & Henry, B. (1989). Neuropsychological assessment of executive functions in self-reported delinquents. *Development and Psychopathology, 1,* 105–118.

Moffitt, T. E., & Silva, P. A. (1988). Self-reported delinquency, neuropsychological deficit, and history of attention deficit disorder. *Journal of Abnormal Child Psychology, 16,* 553–569.

Newcorn, J. H., & Halperin, J. M. (2000). Attention-deficit disorders with oppositionality and aggression. In T. E. Brown (Ed.), *Attention-deficit disorders and comorbidities in children, adolescents, and adults* (pp. 171–207). Washington, DC: American Psychiatric Press.

Newman, J. P. (1998). Psychopathic behavior: An information processing perspective. In D. J. Cooke, A. E. Forth, & R. D. Hare (Eds.), *Psychopathy: Theory, research, and implications for society* (pp. 81–104). Dordrecht, The Netherlands: Kluwer.

Newman, J. P., & Lorenz, A. R. (2003). Response modulation and emotion processing: Implications for psychopathy and other dysregulatory psychopathology. In R. J. Davidson, K. Scherer, & H. H. Goldsmith (Eds.), *Handbook of affective sciences* (pp. 1043–1067). London: Oxford University Press.

Newman, J. P., Patterson, C. M., & Kosson, D. S. (1987). Response perseveration in psychopaths. *Journal of Abnormal Psychology, 96,* 145–148.

O'Brien, B. S., & Frick, P. J. (1996). Reward dominance: Associations with anxiety, conduct problems, and psychopathy in children. *Journal of Abnormal Child Psychology, 24,* 223–240.

Oxford, M., Cavell, T. A., & Hughes, J. N. (2003). Callous–unemotional traits moderate the relation between ineffective parenting and child externalizing problems: A partial replication and extension. *Journal of Clinical Child and Adolescent Psychology, 32,* 577–585.

Pardini, D. A., Lochman, J. E., & Frick, P. J. (2003). Callous/Unemotional traits and social cognitive processes in adjudicated youth. *Journal of the American Academic of Child and Adolescent Psychiatry, 42,* 364–371.

Patrick, C. J. (2001). Emotional processes in psychopathy. In A. Raine & J. Sanmartin (Eds.), *Violence and psychopathy* (pp. 57–77). New York: Kluwer.

Patrick, C. J., Zempolich, K. A., & Levenston, G. K. (1997). Emotionality and violent behavior in psychopaths: A biosocial analysis. In A. Raine, D. Farrington, P. Brennan, & S. A. Mednick (Eds.), *The biosocial bases of violence* (pp. 145–161). New York: Plenum Press.

Patterson, G. R., Reid, J. B., & Dishion, T. J. (1992). *Antisocial boys.* Eugene, OR: Castilia.

Pelham, W. E., Milich, R., Cummings, M. E., Murphy, D. A. Schaughency, E. A., & Greiner, A. R. (1991). Effects of background anger, provocation, and methylphenidate on emotional arousal and aggressive-responding in attention-deficit hyperactivity disordered boys with and without concurrent aggressiveness. *Journal of Abnormal Child Psychology, 19,* 407–426.

Pitts, T. B. (1997). Reduced heart rate levels in aggressive children. In A. Raine, P. A. Brennan, D. P. Farrington, & S. A. Mednick (Eds.), *Biosocial bases of violence* (pp. 317–320). New York: Plenum Press.

Poulin, F., & Boivin, M. (2000). Reactive and proactive aggression: Evidence of a two-factor model. *Psychological Assessment, 12,* 115–122.

Price, J. M., & Dodge, K. A. (1989). Reactive and proactive aggression in childhood: Relations to peer status and social context dimensions. *Journal of Abnormal Child Psychology, 17,* 455–471.

Prinstein, M. J., Boergers, J., & Vernberg, E. M. (2001). Overt and relational aggression in adolescents: Social–psychological adjustment of aggressors and victims. *Journal of Clinical Child Psychology, 30,* 479–491.

Pulkkinen, L. (1996). Proactive and reactive aggression in early adolescence as precursors to anti- and prosocial behavior in young adults. *Aggressive Behavior, 22,* 241–257.

Quay, H. C. (1964). Dimensions of personality in delinquent boys as inferred from the factor analysis of case history data. *Child Development, 35,* 479–484.

Quay, H. C. (1986). Classification. In H. C. Quay & J. S. Werry (Eds.), *Psychopathological disorders of childhood* (3rd ed., pp. 1–42). New York: Wiley.

Quay, H. C. (1987). Patterns of delinquent behavior. In H. C. Quay (Ed.), *Handbook of juvenile delinquency* (pp. 118–138). New York: Wiley.

Quay, H. C. (1993). The psychobiology of undersocialized aggressive conduct disorder. *Development and Psychopathology, 5,* 165–180.

Raine, A. (2002). Biosocial studies of antisocial and violent behavior in children and adults: A review. *Journal of Abnormal Child Psychology, 30,* 311–326.

Roberts, B. W., & DelVecchio, W. F. (2000). The rank-order consistency of personality traits from childhood to old age: A quantitative review of longitudinal studies. *Psychological Bulletin, 126,* 3–25.

Rothbart, M. K., Ahadi, S. A., & Hershey, K. (1994). Temperament and social behavior in childhood. *Merrill-Palmer Quarterly, 40,* 21–39.

Rothbart, M. K., & Bates, J. E. (1998). Temperament. In W. Damon (Ed.), *Handbook of child psychology: Vol. 3. Social, emotional, and personality development* (pp. 105–176). New York: Wiley.

Salmivalli, C., & Nieminen, E. (2002). Proactive and reactive aggression among school bullies, victims, and bully-victims. *Aggressive Behavior, 28,* 30–44.

Schwartz, D., Dodge, K. A., Coie, J. D., Hubbard, J. A.,

Cillessen, A. H. N., Lemerise, E. A., & Bateman, H. (1998). Social-cognitive and behavioral correlates of aggression and victimization in boys' play groups. *Journal of Abnormal Child Psychology, 26,* 431–440.

Seagrave, D., & Grisso, T. (2002). Adolescent development and the measurement of juvenile of psychopathy. *Law and Human Behavior, 26,* 219–239.

Shields, A., & Cicchetti, D. (1998). Reactive aggression among maltreated children: The contributions of attention and emotion dysregulation. *Journal of Clinical Child Psychology, 27,* 381–395.

Silverthorn, P., & Frick, P. J. (1999). Developmental pathways to antisocial behavior: The delayed-onset pathway in girls. *Development and Psychopathology, 11,* 101–126.

Silverthorn, P., Frick, P. J., & Reynolds, R. (2001). Timing of onset and correlates of severe conduct problems in adjudicated girls and boys. *Journal of Psychopathology and Behavioral Assessment, 23,* 171–181.

Skeem, J. L., & Cauffman, E. (2003). Views of the downward extension: Comparing the youth version of the Psychopathy Checklist with the Youth Psychopathic Traits Inventory. *Behavioral Sciences and the Law, 21,* 689–846.

Skeem, J., Poythress, N., Edens, J., Lilienfeld, S., & Cale, E. (2003). Psychopathic personality or personalities? Exploring potential variants of psychopathy and their implications for risk assessment. *Aggression and Violent Behavior, 8,* 513–546.

Steinberg, L. (2002). The juvenile psychopath: Fads, fictions, and facts. In *National Institute of Justice Perspectives on Crime and Justice* (Vol. V). Washington, DC: National Institute of Justice.

Stevens, D., Charman, T., & Blair, R. J. R. (2001). Recognition of emotion in facial expressions and vocal tones in children with psychopathic tendencies. *Journal of Genetic Psychology, 16,* 201–211.

Toupin, J., Mercier, H., Dery, M., Cote, G., & Hodgins, S. (1995). Validity of the PCL-R for adolescents. *Issues in Criminological and Legal Psychology, 24,* 143–145.

Verhulst, F. C., Koot, H. M., & Berden, G. F. (1990). Four-year follow-up of an epidemiological sample. *Journal of the American Academy of Child and Adolescent Psychiatry, 29,* 440–448.

Viding, E., Blair, R. J. R., Moffitt, T. E., & Plomin, R. (in press). Psychopathic syndrome indexes strong genetic risk for antisocial behaviour in 7-year-olds. *Journal of Child Psychology and Psychiatry.*

Vitaro, F., Brendgen, M., & Tremblay, R. E. (2002). Reactively and proactively aggressive children: Antecedent and subsequent characteristics. *Journal of Child Psychology and Psychiatry and Allied Disciplines, 43,* 495–506.

Vitaro, F., Gendreau, P. L., Tremblay, R. E., & Oligny, P. (1998). Reactive and proactive aggression differentially predict later conduct problems. *Journal of Child Psychology and Psychiatry, 39,* 377–385,

Walker, J. L., Lahey, B. B., Russo, M. F., Frick, P. J., Christ, M. A. G., McBurnett, K., et al. (1991). Anxiety, inhibition, and conduct disorder in children: I. Relations to social impairment. *Journal of the American Academy of Child and Adolescent Psychiatry, 30,* 187–191.

Walters, G. D. (2003). Predicting criminal justice outcomes with the Psychopathy Checklist and Lifestyle Criminality Screening Form: A meta-analytic comparison. *Behavioral Sciences and the Law, 21,* 89–102.

Waschbusch, D. A. (2002). A meta-analytic examination of comorbid hyperactive–impulsive–attention problems and conduct problems. *Psychological Bulletin, 128,* 118–150.

Waschbusch, D. A., Willoughby, M. T., & Pelham, W. E. (1998). Criterion validity and the utility of reactive and proactive aggression: Comparisons to attention deficit hyperactivity disorder, oppositional defiant disorder, conduct disorder, and other measures of functioning. *Journal of Clinical Child Psychology, 27,* 369–405.

Williamson, S. E., Harpur, T. J., & Hare, R. D. (1991). Abnormal processing of affective words by psychopaths. *Psychophysiology, 28,* 260–273.

Woodworth, M., & Porter, S. (2002). In cold blood: Characteristics of criminal homicides as a function of psychopathy. *Journal of Abnormal Psychology, 111,* 436–445.

Wootton, J. M., Frick, P. J., Shelton, K. K., & Silverthorn, P. (1997). Ineffective parenting and childhood conduct problems: The moderating role of callous–unemotional traits. *Journal of Consulting and Clinical Psychology, 65,* 301–308.

19

Toward an Integrated Perspective on the Etiology of Psychopathy

ANGUS W. MACDONALD, III
WILLIAM G. IACONO

A PRESCRIPTION FOR PSYCHOPATHY RESEARCH

Systematic advances in psychopathology research designed to uncover the etiology of mental disorders have historically involved progress on multiple fronts. Research on the causes of psychopathy can be evaluated in part by how progress in this area parallels that of psychopathology research generally in terms of description, epidemiology, development, cognition, and neurobiology. The chapters in this section do a nice job of summarizing, integrating, and criticizing the existing literature, and these reviews serve as the basis for many of the observations we make here.

The message that emerges most clearly from these reviews is that much work remains to be done before we can claim to understand the "Cleckley psychopath" per se, or distinguish it from antisociality more generally in terms of its etiology. Although each of the preceding chapters covers a different method for understanding psychopathy, there is little convergence between the substantive hypotheses; each method lead to divergent conclusions about the nature of psychopathy. Although not uncommon in other psychopathology research, this has to be rec-

ognized as an uncomfortable state of affairs. This chapter takes a more abstract approach to the problem by emphasizing methodological snags and currents to facilitate progress. In doing so, we echo and emphasize many of the concerns sprinkled throughout these fine reviews.

DESCRIPTION

Psychopathy overlaps with, but is not the same as, antisociality, yet much of the etiologically relevant research deals broadly with antisocial behavior or specifically with selected antisocial traits and behaviors (e.g., aggression and violence). Although the significance of this body of work is considerable, given the toll antisocial individuals exact on society, it is nonetheless the case that even after a half century of systematic research on psychopathy, exactly how it may be etiologically distinct or overlapping with antisociality more generally remains unclear. A wealth of research supports the construct validity of psychopathy, but as the reviews in this and other sections of this volume indicate (e.g., Hare & Neumann, Chapter 4; Cooke, Michie, & Hart, Chapter 5; Lilienfeld & Fowler, Chapter 6; and Hall &

Benning, Chapter 23, this volume), uncertainty persists regarding the scope of the psychopathy construct and what its essential features are.

Most of the research that targets the study of psychopathy focuses on psychopathic offenders within prison settings. While this represents some of the finest research in the tradition of experimental psychopathology, the generally accepted Psychopathy Checklist—Revised (PCL-R) criteria used to identify incarcerated psychopaths are not broadly applicable outside prison settings (cf. Hall & Benning, Chapter 23, this volume). The typical definition of psychopathy that is operationalized by the PCL-R uses a cutoff score that requires the presence of both antisocial behavior and personality traits such as impulsivity and lack of remorse. Alternatives to the PCL-R typically stress the importance of antisocial deviance and effectively reduce psychopathy to a construct that is nested within criminality or antisocial personality disorder (APD). For instance, criminal behavior or delinquency may be considered a proxy for psychopathy. This approach, however, likely yields a diluted pool because only a fraction of criminals can be considered psychopaths.

Another option is to rely on the DSM definition of APD or its adolescent precursor, conduct disorder, to identify individuals who may be psychopaths. While this approach no doubt captures many psychopaths, most individuals satisfying criteria for these DSM disorders would not be considered psychopaths. In addition, relying on the DSM criteria is problematic in that persons with late-onset antisociality are omitted. These are individuals whom DiLalla and Gottesman (1989) call "late bloomers," that is, those who satisfy the adult criteria for the diagnosis of APD without evidence of conduct disorder (e.g., Elkins, Iacono, Doyle, & McGue, 1994; Tweed, George, Blazer, Swartz, & MacMillan, 1997). These individuals, who have avoided obvious acting out as adolescents, may be among the more cunning and successful psychopaths, but they would not be included in any study using APD to identify cases. As noted by Frick and Marsee (Chapter 18, this volume), there is also the question of how to identify psychopathy in

youth samples. Although important strides are being made in this area (e.g., Barry et al., 2000; Frick, Bodin, & Barry, 2000; Kosson et al., 2002; Murrie & Cornell, 2002), it is not clear at this point to what degree child and adolescent assessments of psychopathy are comparable to the adult PCL-R assessment, or to what degree these assessments are appropriate in community-based samples or in preadolescent children (see Salekin, Chapter 20, this volume, for a detailed discussion of these issues).

Although there is no question that identifying criminal psychopaths has enormous utility, it seems likely that there is also great value in the identification of noncriminal psychopaths—individuals who, without conscience, manipulate and con those around them but manage to elude detection when conventional DSM or PCL criteria are applied (see Lykken, 1995, for examples, which include Oskar Schindler, savior of hundreds of Jews in World War II; see also Hall & Benning, Chapter 23, this volume). Indeed, Cooke, Michie, Hart, and Clark (2004) have argued on the basis of their structural analyses of the PCL-R that psychopathy is fundamentally a constellation of personality features (comprising an arrogant and deceitful interpersonal style, deficient affective experience, and impulsive and irresponsible behavior) that in turn gives rise to antisociality. From this perspective, antisocial behavior is a consequence of psychopathy rather than a defining feature.

An advantage of DSM-III was that it established an unambiguous set of criteria for each mental disorder that all investigators could use as a starting point for identifying individuals with a given disorder. Despite the many limitations of DSM-III and its successors, it is difficult to argue with the conclusion that it has advanced our understanding of the etiology of many of the major disorders. Robert Hare and his colleagues have made great strides toward the development of standardized criteria for the diagnosis of psychopathy (the PCL and its offshoots like the PCL: Screening Version). However, there remains a need for a broadly applicable set of diagnostic criteria modeled after the disorder criterion sets found in DSM, that all researchers—both inside and outside forensic settings—could use as the diagnostic benchmark against which to compare and evaluate findings.

EPIDEMIOLOGY

An unfortunate consequence of not having an inclusive definition of psychopathy that is generally applicable outside prisons is that little epidemiological research on this phenomenon has been carried out. Conduct disorder and APD are relatively common in the population at large, but it is not clear what percentage of antisocial individuals are psychopaths, or to what degree psychopaths might be identifiable in individuals without these diagnoses. Left unanswered are important questions about psychopathy's prevalence outside prison settings, its gender and age distribution, and how it varies across ethnic and sociocultural groups. Antisocial behavior shows distinct patterns of variation across demographic subgroups in the population, and it would be interesting to know if psychopathy varies similarly in its distribution. Much also remains to be learned about patterns of comorbidity between psychopathy and other mental disorders (cf. Widiger, Chapter 8, this volume). Such basic information is often the cornerstone of etiologic theory building and is obviously important to understanding the significance of a disorder as well as designing appropriate research protocols.

DEVELOPMENTAL PSYCHOPATHOLOGY

An important approach to unraveling the etiology of psychopathy is to focus on individuals at high risk for the development of the disorder in large-scale population studies that are likely to include substantial numbers of those at risk. This includes both those who ultimately manifest psychopathology and those who, although at risk, do not. In this approach, emphasis is placed on understanding familial (genetic and environmental) risk factors and the underlying mechanisms and processes leading to disorder development. This approach is best realized through genetically informed lifespan longitudinal research that examines both continu-

ities and discontinuities in the trajectory of disorder development.

Familiality

The meta-analyses of twin studies in Chapter 11 (Waldman & Rhee, this volume) clearly point to the heritable nature of antisocial behavior, and the likely contribution of shared environmental factors. Less clear is the heritability of psychopathy. Although there are twin studies based on questionnaire measures of psychopathic characteristics, there are no studies of which we are aware that examine twin concordance for PCL-defined psychopathy. The twin studies of psychopathy examined by Waldman and Rhee rely on traditional self-report measures of psychopathy, such as the Minnesota Multiphasic Personality Inventory (MMPI) Pd scale, which predominantly assess antisocial tendencies (Lilienfeld & Fowler, Chapter 6, this volume), and consequently these studies may be addressing primarily the heritability of antisocial deviance. Surprisingly little is known about the familiality of psychopathy or APD. We are aware of no studies that deal with the risk to offspring of having a psychopathic parent, and there are only two studies that examine offspring risk as a function of parental APD (Foley et al, 2001; Kendler, Davis, & Kessler, 1997), neither of which deals with psychopathy. Family studies would also assist our understanding of the comorbidity of psychopathy, in terms of the extent to which it breeds true or is associated with other forms of psychopathology besides antisocial disorders. As Rutter, Caspi, and Moffitt (2003) have noted, understanding comorbidity has the potential to provide important clues to disorder etiology.

Endophenotypes

Waldman and Rhee (Chapter 11, this volume) noted the value of having endophenotypes to guide etiological theory building, and here we elaborate this theme. Studies designed to identify genes associated with the major psychopathologies such as schizophrenia or alcoholism were originally carried out with the reasonable belief that single genes could be identified that would have a major effect on the expression of these disorders.

The failure to find such genes has redirected the search toward genes with much smaller effect. These genes account for just a few percent of heritable variance. As such, they may come to explain individual facets of psychopathy, including specific behavioral tendencies (e.g., violence), traits (e.g., agression, fearlessness), or features correlated with psychopathy that may reflect underlying mechanisms (e.g., frontal lobe deficits).

These phenotype-related characteristics are sometimes referred to as alternative or intermediate phenotypes, terms that are often used interchangeably without precise definition and in ways that include the notion of the endophenotype. Many of the chapters in this section, by focusing on findings related to antisocial subtypes, personality features, and criminal behaviors, have pointed to the value of viewing psychopathy as a collection of facets and traits, each of which may be profitably studied in its own right. At present, it is not clear exactly how or to what degree each of these antisocial phenotype-related characteristics is related to psychopathy per se. Nevertheless, the chapters in this section point to their construct validity and the value of investigating further their association with psychopathy. As these reviews note, some of these characteristics have themselves been shown to be heritable, so they are worthy of study in their own right as well as in relation to psychopathy.

Lifespan Course

One cannot help but notice among the reviews in this section that most of what we know about the course of psychopathy has focused on what becomes of incarcerated psychopaths, most typically adult-adjudicated offenders. Although quite important, it is difficult to uncover how psychopaths came to be if the only opportunity to study them is after the fact. Fortunately, many longitudinal studies of antisocial youth are now underway, and some of these studies have incorporated psychopathy-related measures (e.g., Farrington, Chapter 12, this volume). In addition, there are several population-based longitudinal studies of twin children underway, some of which include over 1,000 twin pairs (e.g., Iacono & McGue, 2002). Such studies are especially informative as they provide the opportunity

to understand how the contribution of genetic and environmental factors is altered over the course of development. All large-scale longitudinal studies of children would be enriched if they included formal attempts to assess psychopathy or psychopathy-related traits.

The lack of information regarding familial risk makes it difficult to implement wisely familial high-risk designs with potential to identify etiologically relevant precursors to psychopathy. In one variant of these designs, unaffected children in high-risk families (defined by having one or more affected parents) are studied longitudinally and compared to children in low-risk families, but the yield from such studies focused on psychopathy would be uncertain without better understanding of the risk to offspring of psychopathic parents.

An alternative high-risk approach involves the study of unaffected first-degree biological relatives of affected individuals. Included here would be studies of twins discordant for psychopathy. This design follows from a diathesis-stress model. To take one common example, it is assumed that unaffected members of identical twin pairs, as well as some of their unaffected relatives, share genetic risk with the index twin (the diathesis) but have not succumbed to disorder (experienced the stress) despite their genetic risk. Their shared genes are nevertheless expected to exert detectable effects, and the study of these unaffected relatives thus provides the opportunity to identify variables related to the phenotype that are likely to be etiologically relevant.

When applied to psychopathy, this design would have a number of advantages. First, it would make it possible to identify variables (including endophenotypes) that are clearly associated with risk for disorder development rather than correlates that are possible consequences of having the disorder. Second, it would provide leads as to why some individuals at risk for psychopathy do not develop the disorder, as individuals with the risk indicator would presumably have life experiences and possible compensatory qualities that would separate them from their psychopathic relative. Another obvious advantage of this design is it has the potential to identify noncriminal psychopaths, including possibly those with the interpersonal–

affective personality characteristics in the absence of antisocial behavior, as a target for study.

Combining these two high-risk approaches has the value of increasing the yield of interesting cases. For instance, a high-risk longitudinal study could be designed to include groups defined by both the affected status of parents and the expression of a psychopathy related trait, such as evidence of fearlessness, in offspring.

The need for informative longitudinal studies highlights some of the problems inherent to the study of psychopathy. Any prospective research on the development of psychopathy would be well informed by epidemiological research on the distribution of psychopathy by age group. Absent information regarding the age of onset of psychopathy, it is difficult to understand the degree to which prospectively studied variables tap causally relevant contributions to the development of psychopathy or factors that emerge as consequences of psychopathy. Epidemiological studies of delinquency and adult criminality indicate that the rates of these antisocial behaviors vary substantially with age, and longitudinal studies suggest heterogeneity in the continuity of antisociality over the lifespan that varies as a function of the age of onset (Moffitt, 1993). As Waldman and Rhee found and others have noted (Slutske, 2001), behavior genetic research points to possible differences in the heritability of antisocial behavior that vary as a function of age. These findings point to the need for well-designed cross-sectional research, using age-appropriate criteria for the identification of psychopaths, which could be used both to estimate the prevalence of psychopathy over the lifespan and to identify the age range of risk for the onset of psychopathy.

Farrington's remarkable prospective study of risk factors that predict the development of psychopathy 40 years later is both an exemplar of the type of study that is desperately needed and a point of reference for some of the key problems inherent to psychopathy research. The criteria used to assess psychopathy in this study are based on the PCL:SV applied in middle adulthood. First, overall scores on this instrument, which are the basis for Farrington's primary analyses, do not distinguish the anti-social deviancy component of psychopathy from the personality component. That the antisocial deviancy component figures importantly in the psychopathy designation can be inferred from the fact that 96% of the most psychopathic men have been convicted of a criminal offense. Moreover, most of the risk factors listed in Farrington's Table 2 are well-known risk factors for the development of criminal behavior generally, so the specificity of these risk factors to psychopathy per se as opposed to severe antisociality remains unresolved. Second, in this community-based inner-city sample, 40% of whom had been convicted by age 48, only 8 of 304 followed-up men achieved the recommended PCL derived cutoff for psychopathy. This small fraction highlights either the rarity of psychopathy in this high-risk sample or, more likely, the restrictiveness of the PCL criteria when applied to community research participants. Third, these criteria can only reasonably be applied to adults, leaving unanswered at what age the participants developed psychopathy, or even if it was possible that they had already developed it at the time the risk factors were first measured at ages 8–11years. These various issues highlight the problems associated with the definition of psychopathy that all investigators face.

Risk Factors

What factors increase the risk that someone will become a psychopath? While much is known about risk factors associated with antisociality, the difficulty answering this question as it applies to psychopathy illustrates why it is important that psychopathy research address unanswered questions posed by the research agenda we have outlined above. Knowledge of the epidemiology of psychopathy, including its genetic epidemiology, would provide a foundation for the identification of risk factors. Endophenotypes and other alternative phenotypes related to psychopathy are types of risk factors, each with potential to shed light on the genetic and neurobiological etiology of psychopathy and psychopathy-related characteristics. Longitudinal research beginning in childhood can be used to identify etiologically relevant risk (and protective) factors, especially if genetically informative designs are used to identify risk factors differentially influenced by genes and environment. Risk factors are unlikely to be the same at all ages (e.g., Burt, Krueger, McGue, & Iacono, 2001, 2003), further pointing to the need for well-designed prospective studies with comprehensive assessments spanning childhood, adolescence, and early adulthood.

PSYCHOLOGICAL AND NEUROBIOLOGICAL INDICATORS

However genes and environment interact to influence the development of psychopathy, the result is reflected in core deficits in cognitive, affective, and affiliated neural processes that are likely to be both causes and consequences of psychopathy. The preceding chapters make clear that substantial headway has been made in the past decade toward understanding psychological and neurobiological aspects of psychopathy. However, this has not resulted in a coherent picture or a standard etiological model that can begin to be refined. Before a coherent picture can be expected to emerge, it is important to unpack some of the problems that arise when attempting to answer questions about the etiology of individual differences in brain structure and function.

Cognitive and Affective Markers

Abnormalities in cognition and emotion are a critical level of analysis for bridging biological processes (such as genetic expression or brain functions) and the behavioral manifestations of a disorder. At the same time, identifying the cognitive and affective abnormalities that underlie psychiatric disorders is especially challenging because of the complex nature of these processes and the quasi-experimental nature of psychopathology.

In the absence of true experimental designs, psychopathology research in general, and psychopathy research specifically, is reliant on correlational findings. By correlational, we also mean to include group difference findings in which group membership is measured rather than manipulated (i.e., "ex post facto" designs). In etiological research, such correlational designs rest on the assumption that the variables most highly correlated with one another are likely to be the most closely linked in a causal chain of events.

However, it is well recognized that this is a vulnerable assumption and a number of controls are required to permit inferences about etiology to be made on the basis of correlational findings.

First, as psychopathologists are well aware, correlational designs are subject to third-variable confounds. That is, we wish to conclude that if condition X is correlated with Y, X is somehow causally related to Y. However, factor Z may cause both X and Y, leading to a spurious, or misleading, correlation. As an example, demographic characteristics such as age may affect scores on both X and Y, leading to an illusory correlation between X and Y. Fortunately, psychopathologists in general are aware of and conscientious about controlling for such "nuisance" variables (but see also Meehl, 1970).

A more persistent concern is the *psychometric confound* (Chapman & Chapman, 1973; Knight, 1984), which still frequently infects quasi-experimental designs because it is difficult to address. The psychometric confound is the result of two interacting components. The first component is a *generalized deficit*, which is simply an impairment over a number of cognitive domains. This may be the downstream result of a single deficit required for performance on every task, or it may be due to multiple, heterogeneous impairments that may be motivational, interpersonal, or intellectual. Unsurprisingly, a number of studies suggest that psychopaths show deficits across a variety of domains including attentional and executive functioning tasks (see Morgan & Lilienfeld, 2000). Under the shadow of a generalized deficit, an observed difference on any single task is not readily interpretable; the effect may be due entirely to the generalized deficit. Therefore, it is important to show that one task is relatively more impaired than another. Consistent with this requirement, Hiatt and Newman (Chapter 17, this volume) discuss several studies in which psychopaths perform worse on Task A than on Task B relative to controls. Unfortunately, this form of argument raises the second component of the psychometric confound, which is differential task sensitivity.

Sensitivity, or discriminating power (Chapman & Chapman, 1978), is a property of a test that reflects how accurately the test measures individual differences in a sample, and it is therefore related to the probability of observing a group difference when a difference does in fact exist. In classic psychometrics, tasks with greater reliability and observed variance are generally more sensitive to group differences (Chapman & Chapman, 1978; Lord, 1952). The problem introduced by differential task sensitivity occurs whenever we hope to make etiological inferences on the basis of correlations or group differences. For example, if Task A and Task B are related to different cognitive processes, and those cognitive processes are related to different brain networks, we are tempted to use a relatively larger effect on Task A to justify studying brain network A rather than brain network B. This is a temptation we should resist, because the conclusion is vulnerable to the following critique. What if the cognitive processes and brain network associated with Task B are more closely linked to the causes of psychopathy, but Task A is simply a more sensitive measure of the generalized deficit? In this way, a generalized deficit and differential task sensitivity can collude to mislead even conscientious investigators. In other words, this psychometric confound represents a potential "nuisance" factor because differences in test sensitivity can result in a mental disorder appearing to have a higher correlation with a spurious but sensitively measured cognitive process, and a lower correlation with a causal but insensitively measured process. Thus, in the presence of a generalized deficit, sensitivity is a nuisance variable of a different stripe than a "third variable." It inheres in a test, not a sample.

This interpretive conundrum arising from behavioral measures unmatched for sensitivity is more generally appreciated in the schizophrenia, aging, and cognitive neuropsychology literatures, but because it is a thorny problem it is frequently ignored even there (cf. MacDonald & Carter, 2002). This psychometric confound cannot be addressed in the same way as a third-variable confound—for example, by measuring the extent of the generalized deficit and then controlling for it—for two different statistical reasons. The first is the recurrent problem associated with covariance procedures (Miller & Chapman, 2001). The second is that the measurement of the deficit itself requires measurement of and control over that measure's task sensitivity, which only serves

to nest the problem. Other common solutions from the clinical neuropsychology literature, such as statistically or demographically norming scores, are largely inadequate because these procedures serve to disguise the differences in sensitivity between the tasks without correcting them.

In contrast, the pattern of results that most convincingly overcomes the psychometric confound is that of a double dissociation (Strauss, 2001). This occurs when the experimental (or pathological) group scores higher than controls on one task, and the control group scores higher than the experimental group on a different task.[1] The inclusion of controls for the psychometric confound allows one to determine whether a particular tasks taps a differential, or specific, deficit rather than a generalized impairment. Unfortunately, demonstrations of specific deficits are rare in the psychopathology literature, and the psychopathy area is no exception. However, as Hiatt and Newman point out, one potential domain for demonstrating specific deficit through the use of a double dissociation is that of selective attention. Here, psychopaths show *less* interference from irrelevant distracters. Reduced interference is opposite to what one would expect from a generally impaired group, so these data provide a promising start. What is needed is evidence that psychopaths perform worse than the comparison group on a similar task that does not involve selective attention, or where better selective attention leads to inferior performance. Why is it important to demonstrate the other side of a double dissociation before drawing strong conclusions? Because it is plausible that some samples of nonpsychopathic prisoners will be more impaired than psychopaths across many cognitive tests, thereby detracting from the interpretability of the selective attention findings.

It is worth noting that resolving the psychometric confound and demonstrating a specific deficit is a necessary but not a sufficient condition for determining whether a cognitive process is relevant to the etiology of a disorder. The relationship between that process and the causes of the disorder must still be established. One way in which cross-sectional cognitive and affective data can be etiologically suggestive is to show within-group relationships. Demonstrating that among psychopathic participants more extreme scores are associated with more extreme symptom expression is useful. Additional information can be gleaned by demonstrating that one cognitive process is associated with one symptom cluster, whereas a different cognitive process is associated with another. Such within-group comparisons can provide vital validation for the cognitive basis of the dimensions of psychopathy discussed by Hare and Neumann (Chapter 4, this volume) and Cooke and colleagues (Chapter 5, this volume). This approach gains further etiological traction when combined with developmental, endophenotypic, and other strategies outlined earlier.

Functional Neuroanatomy

The bugbears of a quasi-experimental, correlational science so pervasive in behavioral studies of psychopathology also confront functional neuroimaging studies. For reasons described above, functional neuroimaging is likely to be most fruitful when applied to tasks that show specific deficits in performance. However, even when studies focus on a cognitive or affective process that is causally related to the manifestation of psychopathy symptoms, there remain a number of ways that spurious brain activations can arise in neuroimaging studies. One prominent and well-recognized problem is the causal confound, or performance confound. The performance confound occurs when differences in performance and differences in brain activity are present in the same sample (Ebmeier, Lawrie, Blackwood, Johnstone, & Goodwin, 1995; Gur & Gur, 1995). Intuitively, this is the point of a neuroimaging study—to discern abnormalities in brain activity that underlie the abnormalities in behavior. However, there is an interpretive ambiguity here. It might also follow that the group differences in brain activity are due to differences in how the groups perform the task. That is, psychopaths perform differently because they adopt a different strategy, they have different levels of motivation to perform the task, and so on—which leads in turn to different task demands and different brain activity. As a result, abnormal activation can be the result of cognitive differences rather than the other way around.

There are a number of clever approaches to this confound that have been developed by conscientious neuroimaging researchers. One approach is to focus on a task that is so easy that group differences in performance are not observed because all participants perform close to perfectly. However, we regard this as a form of capitulation: The approach precludes observing a specific deficit, obtaining interesting correlations between behavior and brain activation, and it may reduce group differences in brain activity in important regions of the brain (i.e., because these regions only become active with more challenging tasks). A second way to deal with this confound is to preselect participants for the different groups that are matched on performance on the task paradigm. While this allows one to study more challenging paradigms, it can also lead to some unexpected results. For example, psychopaths who perform at near-normal levels may perform that way because they are more readily able to activate their brains than poor-performing psychopaths (for other concerns about this design, see Kremen et al., 1996; Meehl, 1970). Other approaches include titrating task difficulty in order to match performance across groups and including only brain activity during correct trials in the analysis. Both of these techniques have their adherents and opponents.

The recent growth of interest among neuroimaging researchers in decision-making paradigms raises new questions about the performance confound. In many decision-making paradigms there are no right or wrong responses. Of course, this does not imply that groups can therefore differ only in interesting ways. For example, a performance confound could conceivably arise from participants in one group failing to understand their decisions as well as those in the other group. Under such circumstances, the impact of performance on brain activation could still be meaningfully evaluated through the inclusion of validity trials in which all participants are likely to make the same response if they are engaged in and understand the task. Such validity would not constitute a separate condition, but like validity questions in personality research, they would serve to indicate whether the participant was engaged in the task.

One conclusion is increasingly clear: Differences in brain activity derived from tasks involving no overt responses are difficult to attribute conclusively to cognitive or affective processing differences. The interpretive problem is the same as that associated with resting blood-flow studies: Biological differences are evident, but one cannot infer whether the differences are spurious or etiologically relevant because they cannot be related to a specifiable cognitive process. The use of tasks that require overt behavioral responses, particularly those that show specific deficits, increases interpretive leverage dramatically.

There are other difficulties in functional neuroimaging studies, such as group differences in movement and brain anatomy, which will be mentioned only briefly here. A fundamental challenge for expensive methodologies such as functional neuroimaging is to prove their worth in the marketplace of ideas. Although the prospect of localizing brain function to a specified neuroanatomical network has immediate appeal, the accumulated knowledge derived from neuroimaging experiments in psychopathology to date has probably not yet justified their expense. Neuroimaging in psychopathy is in its infancy, and deserves its time in the limelight. However, it may prove counterproductive to proceed with building a neuroimaging literature in this area without first addressing the basic methodological challenges identified in other forms of psychopathological research.

In this light, it is interesting to consider the competing hypotheses offered by Blair (Chapter 15) and Rogers (Chapter 16). The former posits that psychopathy is a bottom-up impairment, whereas the latter presents evidence for a top-down impairment. While one should not expect this debate to be settled soon, this is a useful example of where efforts toward a direct comparison of competing hypotheses using conscientious methods might benefit the field most.

Neurophysiology and Neuroanatomy

Consistent with the multiplicity of cognitive, affective, and functional neuroanatomical hypotheses regarding the etiology of psychopathy, Raine and Yang (Chapter 14) highlight abnormalities in diverse brain structures associated with different aspects of psychopathy—in particular, abnormalities in prefrontal and temporal lobe gray matter and in the white matter fibers of the corpus callosum that connect the two hemispheres. In addition to providing a good example of how dimensional indices of psychopathy can be used to bootstrap tenable hypotheses, this review highlights a growing realization among neuroimagers who study other forms of psychopathology—namely, that psychiatric or mental illnesses are unlikely to be localized in a way that parallels neurological illnesses. Instead, etiological researchers are faced with the daunting task of assembling plausible, transactional models of brain development. Such models will need to contend with the basic neuroscientific fact of brain plasticity, in terms of both migrations of function and putative changes in the size of brain structures associated with relative use or disuse (e.g., Maguire et al., 2000). From this perspective, the challenges of teasing apart upstream causes that lead to downstream changes in brain use and disuse appear to be daunting indeed. This enterprise would be greatly aided by the identification of specific genes that transmit a propensity for psychopathy and by elucidation of their primary modes of action in the brain.

CONCLUSION

As the various chapters in this section illustrate, a great deal is known about antisocial personality disorder, criminality, and the psychopathic offender as defined by the PCL-R. Much less is known about psychopathy, especially outside prison populations. This research area has benefited tremendously from the development and widespread use of the PCL-R, but to bring psychopathy into the mainstream of psychopathology research, a more broadly applicable set of diagnostic criteria is needed that can serve as a basis for larger-scale epidemiological, longitudinal, and high-risk studies. Crucial to the success of such an enterprise would be criteria that focus on the affective and interpersonal features of psychopathy. It is this focus that is often missing from much of the research examining antisociality generally, and it is these features that are most critical to the conceptualization of psychopathy.

The preceding review offers a prescription for etiological research in psychopathy. Rather than attempting to abstract a standard causal model of psychopathy from the current state of knowledge, we have identified five priorities that we hope to see emphasized in the next generation of research in this area:

1. Continuing efforts to explicitly define and broaden the concept of psychopathy to better guide research, which in turn should facilitate understanding of etiological mechanisms.
2. Epidemiological research that clarifies the degree to which psychopathy is likely to be an important problem outside of prison settings.
3. Basic high-risk and longitudinal studies that enable the identification of relevant risk factors prior to the development of psychopathy and that are not simply risk factors for delinquent and criminal behavior generally;
4. Continued development of cognitive and affective tasks that allow one to demonstrate and interpret specific deficits and that allow the comparison of competing, substantive hypotheses; and
5. Efforts aimed at relating biological markers of psychopathy not only to group differences but also to the degree of abnormality of cognitive functioning, symptomatology, and the expression of psychopathy-related traits.

NOTE

1. In addition to double dissociations, patterns wherein the experimental group scores higher on the first task than the second, whereas the control group scores higher on the second than the first generally rules out a psychometric confound. Other methods for addressing psychometric confounds include controlling for difficulty, reliability, and observed variance (Chapman & Chapman, 1978) and estimating latent trait scores (Coleman et al., 2002).

ACKNOWLEDGMENTS

This work was supported in part by the National Institutes of Health (Grant Nos. DA13240, DA05147, AA09367, and MH65137).

REFERENCES

Barry, C. T., Frick, P. J., DeShazo, T. M., McCoy, M. G., Ellis, M., & Loney, B. R (2000). The importance of callous–unemotional traits for extending the concept of psychopathy to children. *Journal of Abnormal Psychology, 109,* 335–340.

Burt, S. A., Krueger, R., McGue, M., & Iacono, W. (2001). Sources of covariation among ADHD, CD, and ODD: The importance of shared environment. *Journal of Abnormal Psychology, 110,* 516–525.

Burt, S. A., Krueger, R., McGue, M., & Iacono, W. (2003). Parent–child conflict and the comorbidity among childhood externalizing disorders. *Archives of General Psychiatry, 60,* 505–513.

Chapman, L. J., & Chapman, J. P. (1973). Problems in the measurement of cognitive deficit. *Psychological Bulletin, 79,* 380–385.

Chapman, L. J., & Chapman, J. P. (1978). The measurement of differential deficit. *Journal of Psychiatric Research, 14,* 303–311.

Coleman, M. J., Cook, S., Matthysse, S., Barnard, J., Lo, Y., Levy, D. L. et al. (2002). Spatial and object working memory impairments in schizophrenia patients: A bayesian item-response theory analysis. *Journal of Abnormal Psychology, 111*(3), 425–435.

Cooke, D. J., Michie, C., Hart, S. D., & Clark, D. A. (2004). Reconstructing psychopathy: Clarifying the significance of antisocial and socially deviant behavior in the diagnosis of psychopathic personality disorder. *Journal of Personality Disorders, 18,* 337–357.

DiLalla, L. F., & Gottesman, I. I. (1989). Heterogeneity of causes for delinquency and criminality. Lifespan perspectives. *Development and Psychopathology, 1,* 339–349.

Ebmeier, K. P., Lawrie, S. M., Blackwood, D. H. R., Johnstone, E. C., & Goodwin, G. M. (1995). Hypofrontality revisited: A high resolution single photon emission computer tomography study in schizophrenia. *Journal of Neurology, Neurosurgery and Psychiatry, 58,* 452–456.

Elkins, I. J., Iacono, W. G., Doyle, A. E., & McGue, M. (1997). Characteristics associated with the persistence of antisocial behavior: Results from recent longitudinal research. *Aggression and Violent Behavior, 2,* 101–124.

Foley, D. L., Pickles, A., Simonoff, E., Maes, H. H., Silberg, J. L., Hewitt, J. K., & Eaves, L. J. (2001). Parental concordance and comorbidity for psychiatric disorder and associate risks for current psychiatric symptoms and disorders in a community sample of juvenile twins. *Journal of Child Psychology and Psychiatry, 42,* 381–394.

Frick, P. J., Bodin, S. D., & Barry, C. T. (2000). Psychopathic traits and conduct problems in community and clinic-referred samples of children: Further development of the Psychopathy Screening Device. *Psychological Assessment, 12,* 382–393.

Gur, R. C., & Gur, R. E. (1995). Hypofrontality in schizophrenia: RIP. *Lancet, 345,* 1338–1340.

Iacono, W. G., & McGue, M. (2002). Minnesota Twin Family Study. *Twin Research, 5,* 482–487.

Kendler, K. S., Davis, C. G., & Kessler, R. C. (1997). The familial aggregation of common psychiatric and substance use disorders in the National Comorbidity Study: A family history study. *British Journal of Psychiatry, 170,* 541–548.

Knight, R. (1984). Converging models of cognitive deficits in schizophrenia. In W. Spaulding & J. Coles (Eds.), *Nebraska Symposium on Motivation: Theories of schizophrenia and psychosis* (Vol. 31, pp. 93–156). Lincoln: University of Nebraska Press.

Kosson, D. S., Cyterski, T. D., Steuerwald, B. L., Neumann, C. S., & Walker-Matthews, S. (2002). The reliability and validity of the psychopathy checklist: Youth version (PCL:YV) in nonincarcerated adolescent males. *Psychological Assessment, 14,* 97–109.

Kremen, W. S., Seidman, L. J., Faraone, S. V., Pepple, J. R., Lyons, M. J., & Tsuang, M. T. (1996). The "3Rs" and neuropsychological function in schizophrenia: An empirical test of the matching fallacy. *Neuropsychology, 10,* 22–31.

Lord, F. M. (1952). The relation of the reliability of multiple-choice tests to the distribution of item difficulties. *Psychometrika, 17*(2), 181–194.

Lykken, D. T. (1995). *The antisocial personalities.* Hillsdale, NJ: Erlbaum.

Maguire, E. A., Gadian, D. G., Johnsrude, I. S., Good, C. D., Ashburner, J., Frackowiak, R. S. J., & Frith, C. F. (2000). Navigation-related structural change in the hippocampi of taxi drivers. *Proceedings of the National Academy of Sciences, USA, 97,* 4398–4403.

MacDonald, A. W., III, & Carter, C. S. (2002). Cognitive experimental approaches to investigating impaired cognition in schizophrenia: A paradigm shift. *Journal of Clinical and Experimental Neuropsychology, 24,* 873–882.

Meehl, P. E. (1970). Nuisance variables and the ex post facto design. In M. Radner & S. Winokur (Eds.), *Minnesota studies in the philosophy of science* (pp. 373–402). Minneapolis: University of Minnesota Press.

Miller, G., & Chapman, J. (2001). Misunderstanding analysis of covariance. *Journal of Abnormal Psychology, 110*(1), 40–48.

Moffitt, T. E. (1993). Adolescence-limited and life course persistent antisocial behavior: A developmental taxonomy. *Psychological Review, 100,* 674–701.

Morgan, A. B., & Lilienfeld, S. O. (2000). A meta-analytic review of the relation between antisocial behavior and neuropsychological measures of executive function. *Clinical Psychology Review, 20*(1), 113–136.

Murrie, D. C., & Cornell, D. G. (2002). Psychopathy screening of incarcerated juveniles: A comparison of measures. *Psychological Assessment, 14,* 390–396.

Rutter, M., Caspi, A., & Moffitt, T. E. (2003). Using sex differences in psychopathology to study causal mechanisms: Unifying issues and research strategies. *Journal of Child Psychology and Psychiatry, 44,* 1092–1115.

Slutske, W. S. (2001). The genetics of antisocial behavior. *Current Psychiatry Reports, 3,* 158–162.

Strauss, M. E. (2001). Demonstrating specific cognitive deficits: A psychometric perspective. *Journal of Abnormal Psychology, 110*(1), 6–14.

Tweed, J. L., George, L. K., Blazer, D., Swartz, M., & MacMillan, J. (1994). Adult onset of severe and pervasive antisocial behavior: A distinct syndrome? *Journal of Personality Disorders, 8,* 192–202.

IV

PSYCHOPATHY IN SPECIFIC SUBPOPULATIONS

20

Psychopathy in Children and Adolescents

Key Issues in Conceptualization and Assessment

RANDALL T. SALEKIN

Interest and debate regarding the study of psychopathy in children and adolescents was sparked by the work of Frick (e.g., Frick, O'Brien, Wootton, & McBurnett, 1994) and Lynam (1996) in the mid-1990s and has grown in the last decade, with numerous journal articles and several special issues of leading journals being devoted to the topic (see Petrila & Skeem, 2003; Salekin & Frick, 2005; Skeem & Petrila, 2004; Wiener, 2002). While considerable construct validity has been established, concerns remain regarding the downward extension of psychopathy to children and adolescents. Concerns in this area center on the (1) applicability of the construct, (2) possible transient nature of psychopathy-like symptoms in adolescent samples (3) comorbidity that can occur in child and adolescent samples, (4) lack of temporal stability data, and, relatedly, (5) negative connotations that the term has for treatment success and overall long-term outcome (see Salekin, 2002; Skeem, Monahan, & Mulvey, 2002). In addition, researchers and clinicians have been concerned, legitimately so, about the potential misuse of the term with child and adolescent samples in primarily forensic settings (Hart, Watt, & Vincent, 2002; Murrie, Cornell, & McCoy, 2005; Seagrave & Grisso, 2002; Skeem & Cauffman, 2003; Skeem &

Petrila, 2004). Others (Cleckley, 1941; Frick, 1998, 2002; Frick & Ellis, 1999; Karpman, 1949; Lykken, 1995; Lynam, 1996, 1998, 2002; McCord & McCord, 1964; Salekin, Neumann, Leistico, DiCicco, & Duros, 2004) have argued, although acknowledging the concerns outlined previously, that there are clear benefits to studying psychopathy such as garnering further knowledge about the etiology of psychopathy and the development of prevention and intervention programs. Moreover, researchers contend that psychopathy may parse some of the heterogeneity of the disruptive behavior disorder categories of DSM-IV (American Psychiatric Association, 1994, 2000), and particularly conduct disorder (CD).

Clearly, much remains to be addressed with regard to the potential usefulness of the psychopathy construct as applied to children and adolescents. The purpose of this chapter is fourfold. First, differences between psychopathy and the disruptive behavior disorders of DSM-IV are delineated. This section places an emphasis on understanding the similarities and differences between DSM-IV disruptive disorders and psychopathy at the descriptive and conceptual level. In addition, this section attempts to address, briefly, whether psychopathy can be accommodated within DSM-IV disruptive behavior disorders. Second, developmental research on the extent to which psychopathy can be identified from an early age is reviewed. This section of the chapter asks whether psychopathy does emerge in childhood and adolescence and examines available developmental literature on the topic. Third, to further examine the appropriateness of applying the concept to youth, the structural properties and validity of alternative measures of child/adolescent psychopathy are covered. Fourth, directions for future research are outlined with an emphasis on developmental psychopathology and alternate pathways to conduct problems, and the need for further research on the ontogeny of conduct problems. In this latter section of the chapter, I also address issues such as the need to further delineate differences between psychopathy and the disruptive behavior disorders.

DIFFERENTIATING PSYCHOPATHY FROM DSM-IV DISRUPTIVE BEHAVIOR DISORDERS

The dividing line between oppositional defiant disorder (ODD), CD, and psychopathy has been a subject of some debate and controversy (Burke, Loeber, & Lahey, 2003; Burns, 2000; Frick, 2000; Frick et al., 1991; Lahey & Loeber, 1994; Loeber, 1991; Loeber, Lahey, & Thomas, 1991; Russo, Loeber, Lahey, & Keenan, 1994). However, the majority of research examining the definitional boundaries of psychopathy and the disruptive disorders of DSM has led scientists to the conclusion that certain aspects of psychopathy represent symptom constellations beyond what is offered with the current inclusion criteria sets etched in DSM-IV (Burns, 2000; Frick, 2000). In contrast with DSM's focus on overt behavioral symptoms for antisocial personality disorder (APD) and its childhood variants, early factor-analytic work on the psychopathy construct revealed that the syndrome may include distinctive interpersonal/affective and behavioral/antisocial components (Harpur, Hare, & Hakstian, 1989), and that such symptom parcels have been shown to vary in degree in youth with conduct problems (Frick, 1998). Researchers have also suggested that there exist important conceptual differences between psychopathy and the disruptive behavior disor-

ders of DSM-IV. For example, Kazdin (1997) has suggested that the crux of the difference between conduct problems and psychopathy has a great deal to do with interpersonal, affective, and perhaps motivational considerations. These important conceptual differences have to some extent also been reflected in research suggesting that psychopathy differs from youth with CD and others with conduct problems on important factors such as type of aggressive behavior exhibited (e.g., reactive and proactive aggression), social skills (Cleckley, 1976; Quay, 1964, 1986, 1987), and intellectual (Loney, Frick, Ellis, & McCoy, 1998; Salekin, Neumann, Leistico, & Zalot, 2004) and emotional functioning (Salekin & Frick, 2005).

Empirical research has also shown that at the adult level, the relation between psychopathy and APD is asymmetric (Forth & Burke, 1998; Forth & Mailloux, 2000). Specifically, approximately 90% of adult psychopathic offenders meet APD criteria, but only 25% of those diagnosed with APD are psychopathic (Hare, 1991, 2003). A similar asymmetric relation has emerged when comparing CD and psychopathy as measured by the Psychopathy Checklist: Youth Version (PCL:YV; Forth, Kosson, & Hare, 2003). Forth and Burke (1998) reported that nearly all adolescent offenders (97–100%) qualify for a diagnosis of CD whereas less than 30% of the young offenders with CD met diagnostic criteria for psychopathy on the PCL:YV.

Researchers have suggested that CD diagnoses, based on successive versions of DSM, have lacked predictive validity for identifying serious and chronic conduct problem youth (Frick, 2002; Loeber, Green, Keenan, & Lahey, 1995; Lynam, 1998; Moffitt, 1993; Salekin, Rogers, & Machin, 2001). One explanation for this lack of predictive validity is the lack of discriminability in the DSM inclusion criteria. Specifically, symptoms of CD are often common in childhood (Werry & Quay, 1971), and some level of delinquency in adolescence is normative (see Elliott et al., 1983; Feldman et al., 1983; Moffitt, 1993, 2003; Moffitt, Lynam, & Silva, 1994). Relying on behaviors commonly found in nonantisocial youth may diminish the predictive validity of CD. Although Moffitt's (1993) taxonomy has helped a great deal to parse some of the heterogeneity in CD, there continues to be some concern that psychopathy, as a classification scheme, is not easily accommodated within DSM-IV disruptive disorders. As such, the need to further establish a well-validated CD diagnosis, or CD subtype, that captures affective, interpersonal, and motivational factors continues to be recognized (Frick, 1998, 2002; Hinshaw, Lahey, & Hart, 1993; Kazdin, 1997; Lahey, Loeber, Quay, Frick, & Grimm, 1992; Loeber & Dishion, 1983; Lynam, 1998, 2002). Some have argued that Cleckley's model of psychopathy might be one diagnostic approach that would allow for greater specificity for designating a special class of conduct problem youth (see Table 20.1).

Despite the important need to parse the heterogeneity of youth with conduct problems, the ability to assess psychopathy in children and adolescents has been subject of considerable debate. A major question in personality research has been whether character disorders exist in child and adolescent samples and whether these personality styles can be assessed with modern psychometric technology. This question seems to take on a heightened sensitivity when we ask if particular personality styles, in this case psychopathy, can be identified and assessed in youthful populations (Salekin & Frick, 2005). This query has been debated recently from theoretical and empirical perspectives by leading researchers and scholars in the areas of developmental, clinical child and adolescent, and forensic psychology (Frick, 2002; Hart, Watt, & Vincent, 2002; Lynam, 2002; Seagrave & Grisso, 2002; Skeem & Petrila, 2004; Vincent & Hart, 2002). To further advance understanding in this area, researchers need to empirically address the important

TABLE 20.1. Criteria for Oppositional Defiant Disorder, Conduct Disorder, and Psychopathy

ODD	CD	Cleckley psychopath
1. Often loses temper	1. Often bullies, threatens, and intimidates	1. Superficial charm and good "intelligence"
2. Often argues with adults	2. Often initiates physical fights	2. Absence of delusions and irrational thinking
3. Often actively defies or refuses to comply with adults' requests or rules	3. Has used a weapon that can cause serious physical harm to others	3. Absence of "nervousness"
4. Often deliberately annoys people	4. Has been physically cruel to other people	4. Unreliability
5. Often blames others for his or her mistakes	5. Has been physically cruel to animals	5. Untruthfulness and insincerity
6. Is often touchy or easily annoyed	6. Has stolen while confronting a victim	6. Lack of remorse or shame
7. Is often angry or resentful	7. Has forced someone into sexual activity	7. Inadequately motivated antisocial behavior
8. Is often spiteful or vindictive	8. Has deliberately engaged in fire setting with the intention of causing serious damage	8. Poor judgment/failure to learn from experience
	9. Has deliberately destroyed others' property	9. Pathological egocentricity/incapacity for love
	10. Has broken into someone else's house, building, or car	10. General poverty in major affective reactions
	11. Often lies to obtain goods or favors or to avoid obligations	11. Specific loss of insight
	12. Has stolen items of nontrivial value without confronting a victim	12. Unresponsive in interpersonal relations
	13. Often stays out at night despite parental prohibitions	13. Fantastic and uninviting behavior
	14. Has run away from home overnight at least twice while living in parental or parental surrogate home	14. Suicide rarely carried out
	15. Is often truant from school	15. Sex life impersonal, trivial, poorly integrated
		16. Failure to follow any life plan

questions and concerns that have been raised about downward extensions of psychopathy to youthful populations. Because one of the major questions in this area is whether psychopathy is capable of starting at an early age, in the next section, I review developmental literature on the underlying trait elements of psychopathy that suggest the syndrome may emerge at an early age. Later in the chapter, I provide descriptions of alternative strategies that have been developed for assessing psychopathy in childhood and adolescence.

PSYCHOPATHY IN CHILDREN AND ADOLESCENTS

One major concern mentioned earlier regarding psychopathy has to do with the developmental appropriateness of diagnosing the syndrome in children and adolescents. Developmental research has been cited to support the contention that the disorder is inapplicable for youth (e.g., Seagrave & Grisso, 2002; Vincent & Hart, 2002). Despite some important considerations such as the work of Elkind (1967), which suggests that some forms of egocentricity may be typical at the adolescent stage of development, considerable evidence for distinct emotional, interpersonal, and possibly biological characteristics in psychopaths also suggests that the roots of this disorder may begin in early developmental periods. Moreover, researchers have made the cogent observation that the traits of a personality disorder presumably do not have a sudden onset at the moment the individual turns 18 years of age (see Forth et al., 2003; Frick & Hare, 2001; Salekin et al., 2004; Vincent & Hart, 2002). DSM reflects this notion of early development of personality and personality disorder. Specifically, across versions, DSM explicitly recognizes that personality disorders have their onset in childhood and/or adolescence and can be recognized from adolescence onward. Yet the study of psychopathy in youthful populations to date has largely progressed by attempting to extend research strategies and findings from the adult psychopathy literature downward to children and adolescents. As such, it is important to ask whether psychopathy actually does emerge at an early age according to existing data and how early deficits in interpersonal,

affective, and behavioral functioning can be accurately detected. That is, are the underlying trait elements of the disorder well enough in place for pathology to be manifested at an early age? And, if these traits are manifested at an early age, how can we best measure them? In the following section, I briefly review several relevant pieces of research from developmental science.

Development of Psychopathy from an Early Age: Hints from Empirical Research

To use computer terminology, there has been some concern that we are not going to notice interpersonal, affective, or perhaps even behavioral deficits of psychopathy until these systems come fully on line. Some researchers suggest that characteristics such as empathy and conscience development may not be sufficiently developed until one is older, perhaps even in adulthood (Hart et al., 2002; Seagrave & Grisso, 2002). However, the developmental research cited in these papers may tell only part of the story and there exists considerable developmental research to suggest that psychopathy may emerge at an early age. Specifically, we know from theoretical and empirical work that basic emotions are present from the earliest days of life (Izard, 1977; Izard & Harris, 1995; Plutchik, 1980). Thus, the capability to assess emotion and perhaps even psychopathy-related symptoms such as shallow affect, sensation seeking, and emotional responsiveness may be possible incrementally from an early age (see also Johnstone & Cooke, 2004).

Related to this, some evidence suggests that conscience development and the internalization of societal values starts as early as the toddler years (Kochanska, 1991, 1993). Theories of conscience development also acknowledge concerns regarding predispositions to psychopathy associated with individual differences in the internalization of conscience. Several researchers have underscored the importance of early social referencing, during which mothers and young children negotiate affective meanings of acts of conduct. Barret and Campos (1987) proposed that social referencing endows events with social significance, including emotional tagging of acts that parents consider undesirable or forbidden. Emde, Biringen, Clyman, and Oppenheim (1991) further pointed out that early social referencing is essential in establishing initial prohibitions against deviant acts. This research indicated that parental practices can either promote or undermine early elements of internalization of conscience, such as awareness of standards, the development of the self, early social emotions, and emerging self-regulation. Developmental science has shown that by 18 months of age the cognitive prerequisites for emotions such as perspective taking and differentiation between self and other are well in place, and indices of empathic responding have been recorded even in this early developmental period, with youth showing compassion and concern for others as well as moral sensitivity to the wishes and needs of others (Dunn, 1987; Eisenberg & Mussen, 1989; Haan, Aerts, & Cooper, 1987; Johnstone & Cooke, 2004; Radke-Yarrow & Zahn-Waxler, 1984; Zahn-Waxler & Radke-Yarrow, 1990; Zahn-Waxler, Radke-Yarrow, Wagner, & Chapman, 1992).

Developmental science has also delineated relations between arrogant and deceitful characteristics of youth, and preliminary research suggests that pathological levels of these symptoms do not appear to be a normal part of child or adolescent development. For example, Stouthamer-Loeber (1986) reviewed empirical studies on childhood lying, and although they reported that some experimentation with deceit is common at the age of 4 years (75% of parents and teachers reported an incidence of lying), prevalence rates for chronic lying were much lower (14.4% according to teacher reports, and 19.4% according to parent reports). Stouthamer-Loeber noted on the basis of the limited longitudinal studies available that the number of frequent liars stayed the same or increased slightly over time, and frequent or persistent lying is an important precursor for delinquency (Mitchell & Rosa, 1981). Barry, Frick, and Killian (2003) found significant differences between youth scoring high versus low on the interpersonal features of psychopathy and on a narcissism scale developed for children—indicating that children are capable of appraising their self-worth, that an exaggerated and/or distorted self-view may be observable from an early age, and that such distorted views may extend beyond developmental egocentricity experienced in adolescence (Johnstone & Cooke,

2004). These findings are concordant with those of Harter (1990), who showed that by the age of 8 years, children had developed a view of their general self-worth.

Further supportive evidence comes from research on temperament. In recent years, researchers have proposed that temperament may act to moderate the child's perception and acceptance of parental messages. In particular, the temperamental dimensions of fearfulness, anxiety, and inhibitory control have been implicated in the regulation of moral conduct and moral emotions (Kochanska, 1993). In this regard, some researchers have taken the extreme position that upbringing and parental practices have very little to do with the development of psychopathy, but rather the development of the disorder is set in motion from birth because of the genetic or biological makeup of the youth (Frick & Jackson, 1993; Wootton, Frick, Shelton, & Silverthorn, 1997). These views are now in some retreat as further research on parenting practices emerges in this area (e.g., Kochanska, 1993). However, these perspectives are important because temperament may, in part, set the stage for a psychopathic condition to develop. Furthermore, a recent large-scale twin study has indicated that there is evidence for substantial genetic risk for psychopathy in children (Viding, Blair, Moffitt, & Plomin, 2004; see also Waldman & Rhee, Chapter 11, this volume). Although it is clear that we need to build further bridges between research on parental practices, child temperament, genetics, early emotions, self-regulation, and psychophysiology, significant steps toward understanding some of the most fundamental issues regarding the etiology of psychopathy might well derive from the study of relevant trait dispositions in the very early years of life.

Concerns have also been raised regarding whether psychopathy can be measured in childhood and/or adolescence even if it does have its onset during childhood. Many have argued that the features that comprise the clinical concept of psychopathy can be considered as elements of normal development (see Hart et al., 2002; Seagrave & Grisso, 2002). For instance, as mentioned, some researchers have made the claim that "egocentricity" may be a normal part of adolescent development (e.g., Elkind, 1967; Seagrave & Grisso, 2002). In addition, researchers have also claimed that "impulsivity" and "irresponsible behavior" might also be part of normal adolescent development. Because of the "normalness" of these symptoms, one might expect that the prevalence of psychopathy would be artificially inflated during adolescence (Vincent, 2002). However, the research thus far does not support this supposition. Rather, the prevalence rates of adolescent psychopathy in incarcerated juvenile samples appear to be similar to, or slightly below, those of incarcerated adult samples (Cruise, 2000; Forth et al., 2003; Hare, 2003; Salekin et al., 2004; Salekin, Leistico, Trobst, Schrum, & Lochman, 2005). Therefore, in comparison to CD symptoms, which do evidence some degree of normalcy in adolescence (Moffitt, 2003), symptoms more specific to the syndrome of psychopathy appear to be much less common.

Research has also attempted to examine the appropriateness of the psychopathy construct to youth using methods of item response theory (IRT; for a summary of this methodology, see Hare & Neumann, Chapter 4; Cooke, Michie, & Hart, Chapter 5, this volume). This methodology can be used to address the appropriateness of items designed to measure the underlying trait, and to examine and determine whether age-related bias exists in such items. Using IRT, Vincent (2002) examined PCL:YV scores from a sample of young offenders ($N = 269$) and compared the properties of items in this sample to corresponding items of the PCL-R in adult offenders ($N = 444$). The analyses indicated that psychopathy items appeared to measure the same underlying trait, in the same manner, across age groups. Using confirmatory factor analysis, this research also indicated that psychopathy appeared to be a coherent construct in youth but that behavioral items might artificially inflate psychopathy classifications (see Schrum & Salekin, in press, for similar results with adolescent girls).

Finally, the applicability of psychopathy to younger populations might be evaluated via taxometric research. Although preliminary, it is important to note that recent taxometric research has produced evidence for both a broad conduct problem taxon consistent with CD in DSM-IV, and a much lower base rate taxon consistent with prevalence expectations for psychopathy (Skilling, Quinsey, & Craig, 2001; Vasey, Kotov, Frick, &

Loney, 2005). However, much more research is needed to determine whether psychopathy is best conceptualized as dimensional or taxonic.

Taken together, the findings of research on early conscience development, interpersonal style, prevalence rates, IRT, genetic predispositions, and taxometric analyses suggest that the disorder may manifest itself early in the developmental process. It is important to note that this evidence does not imply that the disorder is immutable or irreversible but, rather, that adult psychopathy likely has its roots in childhood and early adolescence. Also, these studies do not negate legitimate developmental concerns about the onset and maintenance of psychopathy that warrant further study (see Hart et al., 2002; Seagrave & Grisso, 2002; Vincent & Hart, 2002). Although the foregoing empirical studies reviewed provide us with some hints regarding the development of the disorder from an early age, the reliability and validity of the concept as indexed by childhood and adolescent measures must be demonstrated if we are to assume that psychopathy-like symptoms exist in these youthful populations (cf. Frick, 1998; Vincent & Hart, 2002).

The following sections build on earlier empirical work examining the reliability and validity of measures of the psychopathy construct in children and adolescents (Forth & Burke, 1998; Frick, 1998, 2002; Hart et al., 2002; Vincent & Hart, 2002). In light of the concerns raised by proponents of the APD diagnosis regarding the reliability of affective–interpersonal versus behavioral features of the psychopathy construct (Cloninger, 1978; Robins, 1966), it is important to examine the structure and validity of these measures, including the psychometric properties of the interpersonal and affective features of the syndrome. By doing so, concerns as to whether the hallmarks of psychopathy apply to this younger age group can be more systematically and comprehensively evaluated. In addition, more generally, issues related to measurement fidelity can be examined.

MEASUREMENT OF PSYCHOPATHY IN YOUTH

In an effort to measure psychopathy in youthful populations, a number of child and adolescent psychopathy tools have been developed. Three instruments are direct descendants of the Psychopathy Checklist—Revised (Hare, 1991). These are the PCL:YV (Forth et al., 2003), the Antisocial Process Screening Device (APSD; Frick & Hare, 2001), and the Child Psychopathy Scale (CPS; Lynam, 1997). At least one other recent child psychopathy measure also exists, namely the Youth Psychopathy Inventory (YPI; Andershed, Kerr, Stattin, & Levander, 2002). Because of the newness of this measure, and limits on the scope of this chapter, only the PCL derivatives are reviewed. Nonetheless, psychopathy researchers may want to incorporate the YPI in future child and adolescent psychopathy research. A brief descriptive summary, as well as reliability and validity data, are provided here for the PCL:YV, the CPS, and the APSD.

PCL:YV

Over a decade ago, Forth, Hart, and Hare (1990) examined the construct of psychopathy in a group of adolescent offenders using the PCL-R. This study used a modified PCL-R scale that was viewed as more appropriate for adolescent offenders. Because adolescents have limited work histories and few, if any, marital relationships, two items were dropped from the PCL-R: item 9 (parasitic lifestyle) and item 17 (any short-term marital relationships). In addition, because adolescents have less opportunity to come into contact with the law than adult offenders, the scoring criteria for two other items were modified: item 18 (juvenile delinquency) and item 20 (criminal versatility).

Several studies examining adolescent offenders were conducted with this modified version of the PCL-R (e.g., Sullivan & Gretton, 1996). On the basis of initial data gathered using this version of the inventory, and in order to further address the restricted time duration of adolescent offense behavior, three other modifications were made. First, a scoring system that relied more heavily on involvement with peers, family, and schools was developed. Second, two items (items 9 and 17, assessing parasitic lifestyle and impersonal relationships, respectively) were reincorporated but modified. Third, and perhaps most important, the scoring system was further modified to accommodate enduring

characteristics of youth across settings. This draft version, the PCL:YV (Forth, Kosson, & Hare, 1996/2003), was made available to researchers for use in a variety of empirical studies. Subsequently, the PCL:YV (Forth et al., 2003) was published with several other modifications. For example, "superficial charm" was changed to "impression management." According to the authors, this change was made because the item was confusing to some assessors and because its chief emphasis was to identify those who were attempting to influence the assessor's impression. Other items were also altered to be more developmentally appropriate for adolescent assessment (see Forth et al., 2003). The PCL:YV in its current form remains a 20-item inventory, with each of its items rated on a 3-point scale (0 = no; 1 = maybe; 2 = yes). It is intended for use with adolescents ages 13–18 years.

Two studies examined the factor structure of the PCL-R (modified for adolescents) and the PCL:YV with adolescent samples (Brandt, Kennedy, Patrick, & Curtin, 1997; Forth, 1995). Both studies reported similar two-factor models, replicating to some extent what had been found previously with adult offenders (Hare, 1991; Harpur et al., 1989). Factor 1 reflected the interpersonal and affective characteristics and Factor 2 reflected behavioral features and social deviance. More recently, three- and four-factor models have been proposed (cf. Cooke et al., Chapter 5, this volume; Hare & Neumann, Chapter 4, this volume). These models parse the two original factors as follows: Facet 1 of the four-factor model reflects an interpersonal–deceitful style, Facet 2 reflects deficiencies in affect, Facet 3 taps tendencies toward impulsive behavior and sensation seeking, and Facet 4 comprises indicators of antisocial behavior. Adequate fit results have been attained for both three- and four-factor solutions (see Forth et al., 2003).

Initial reports of the reliability and validity of the PCL:YV show that it has relatively high reliability. Specifically, using the standardization sample, Forth and colleagues (2003) found that the alpha coefficients for the four facets of psychopathy were acceptably high (facet 1 = .75, facet 2 = .71, facet 3 = .70, and facet 4 = .78). Interrater reliability for the PCL:YV has also appeared adequate in other independent investigations (Brandt et al., 1997; Gretton, 1998; McBride, 1998; Salekin et al., 2004). Initial validity data also appear to be promising (see Forth et al., 2003).

APSD

Frick and Hare (2001) developed the Psychopathy Screening Device (PSD) in the early 1990s in order to screen for psychopathy in childhood. The PSD, now named the APSD (Frick & Hare, 2001), was also an adaptation of the PCL-R. Items from the PCL-R were designed to be more developmentally sensitive to the concept of psychopathy in childhood. For example, the authors used items such as "concerned about schoolwork" to address responsibility rather than the corresponding item of "irresponsibility" on the PCL-R. Thus, to capture the dimensions of psychopathy in children, each of the 20 items included in the PCL-R was made into an analogous item thought to be more applicable to children.

The APSD is a 20-item rating scale that was originally designed to be completed by parents and teachers. The age range for the APSD is 6–13 years and the scale is rated on a 3-point system (0 = not at all true; 1 = sometimes true, and 2 = definitely true). The decision to design the APSD to incorporate both parent and teacher ratings was based on the concerns regarding the validity of children's self-report for assessing their emotional and behavioral functioning (Kamphaus & Frick, 1996). Moreover, research at the time suggested that parents and teachers are the optimal informants for assessing child aggression and conduct problems (Loeber, Green, Lahey, & Stouthamer-Loeber, 1991).

Recently, a self-report version of the APSD was developed. This measure has the same rating format as the child rating measure and is intended for youth ages 13–18 years. Loney, Frick, Clements, Ellis, and Kerlin (2003) contend that there are some compelling reasons for having a self-report version of psychopathy for adolescents. First, Loney et al. cite evidence indicating that the reliability of child report for assessing most types of psychopathology increases in adolescence, whereas the validity of parent and teacher report decreases (Kamphaus & Frick, 1996). Second, in cases in which youth

have spent significant time in out-of-home placements, parents may be unavailable or insufficiently knowledgeable about youth behavior to complete valid ratings. Finally, there is growing evidence that self-report measures can play a unique and valuable role in the assessment of psychopathy and antisocial deviance (cf. Lilienfeld & Fowler, Chapter 6, this volume). In this regard, the self-report version of the APSD has been successfully used to differentiate subgroups of juvenile offenders in adolescent samples (e.g., Caputo, Frick, & Brodsky, 1999; Kruh, Frick, & Clements, 2005; Loney et al., 2003; Silverthorn, Frick, & Reynolds, 2002), and other self-report measures have been found useful for assessing psychopathic traits in adolescents and young adult samples (Lilienfeld & Andrews, 1996; Lynam, Whiteside, & Jones, 1999; Poythress, Edens, & Lilienfeld, 1998; Salekin, Ziegler, Larrea, Anthony, & Bennett, 2003).

In an initial test of the APSD, Frick and colleagues (1994) obtained parent and teacher ratings on 92 clinic-referred children (age range = 6–13 years). The study sample consisted of consecutive referrals to two university-based outpatient clinics, and the participants were predominantly male (84%) and white (82%). A principal components analysis of the APSD items revealed two dimensions, one tapping poor impulse control, irresponsibility, narcissism, and antisocial behavior (Impulsive/Conduct Problems [I/CP] Factor), and the other reflecting a callous and unemotional (CU) interpersonal style. More recently, Frick, Bodin, and Barry (2000) conducted a factor analysis of the APSD using parent and teacher report of 1,136 elementary school–age children (M = 10.7 years). This study yielded alternative two- and three-factor solutions. In the three-factor solution, a similar CU factor emerged; this factor consisted of six items, four of which overlapped with items marking the CU factor in Frick and colleagues. The I/CP component was divided into two distinct factors, one reflecting impulsivity (five items) and the other reflecting interpersonal aspects of psychopathy (seven items), which the authors labeled narcissism.

Reliability estimates for the APSD have been modest to high, ranging from .82 to .92. Across four waves of assessment (each 1 year apart) involving different raters, alphas for the APSD were somewhat lower, ranging from .50 to .92 (Frick, Kimonis, Dandreaux, & Farell, 2003). Interrater reliability for the APSD between children and parents has not been particularly strong, ranging from .26 to .40 (e.g., Frick, Lilienfeld, Ellis, Loney, & Silverthorn, 1999; Loney et al., 1998). However, divergence in results for children and parents tends to be the norm for ratings of psychopathology. Also, direct comparisons between interrater reliabilities for the PCL and the APSD are complicated by the fact that the two forms of assessment are conducted in a very different manner. Nonetheless, to better understand the psychopathy construct in children and adolescents, future research should attempt to further address the question of why these differences are occurring. On balance, promising evidence of construct, concurrent, and predictive validity has been demonstrated for the APSD (see Frick & Hare, 2001).

CPS

Lynam (1997) modeled the 13-item Childhood Psychopathy Scale (CPS) after the PCL-R as a method for assessing psychopathy in children and adolescents (age range 6–17; personal communication, September 13, 2004). The CPS was originally based on archival data from a large-scale study of 430 boys ages 12–13 years. Specifically, data on behavior and personality that were completed by mothers were used to measure psychopathy. The items for the CPS (41 items) were drawn from the Child Behavior Checklist (CBCL; Achenbach, 1991) and the Common Language Q-Sort (CCQ; Caspi et al., 1992). Using these two measures, Lynam was able to operationalize 13 of the 20 PCL-R items.

Recently, a revision of the CPS was undertaken in order to (1) simplify complex items, (2) increase the reliability and validity of several constructs that were not optimally operationalized in the original version (i.e., shallow affect and glibness), (3) reduce overlap with explicit antisocial behavior (dropping an item assessing criminal versatility), and (4) increase representation of other personality traits thought to be important (i.e., items assessing boredom susceptibility; see Lynam et al., 2005). The revised CPS contains 55 items and continues to assess 13 of the PCL

items (i.e., glibness, untruthfulness, boredom susceptibility, manipulation, lack of guilt, poverty of affect, callousness, parasitic lifestyle, behavioral dyscontrol, lack of planning, impulsiveness, unreliability, and failure to accept responsibility). This most recent version of the CPS has both a caregiver and a self-report version, each consisting of identical items. The CPS items are rated on dichotomous scale (0 = no; 1 = yes).

Factor analysis of the original CPS resulted in a two-factor structure similar to that found using the PCL-R with adult offenders. However, because the two factors of the CPS were so highly correlated ($r = .95$), typically only total scores have been reported. Although factor-analytic studies have not yet clearly demarcated the dimensions of the CPS, some researchers have used rationally derived factor scores for the CPS patterned after the three-factor model of the PCL-R advanced by Cooke and Michie (2001; see also Cooke et al., Chapter 5, this volume). One study has indicated that these rationally derived CPS factor scores show meaningful relations with trait constructs from the Big Five and the interpersonal circumplex models of personality (Salekin, Leistico, et al., 2005).

Initial reports of the internal structure and reliability of the CPS based on caregivers' ratings are promising, with corresponding alphas of .87, .86, and .90 for Factor 1, Factor 2, and the Total score, respectively. However, interrater reliability figures for caregiver versus child ratings of the CPS are not yet available. Validation work for the CPS was primarily based on the original version of the measure. According to self-, teacher, and mother reports of delinquency collected at ages 10 and 13, boys who scored high on the CPS were found to be more impulsive on a multimethod, multiscore battery of impulsiveness. Psychopathic boys were also prone to disruptive behavior disorders but comparatively immune to internalizing disorders. Finally, scores on the CPS predicted serious delinquency above and beyond other known predictors (previous delinquency, socioeconomic status, IQ, and impulsivity) and alternate parsings of the item pool used to create the CPS. Thus, with regard to reliability and validity, the CPS has been shown, at least initially, to be a reliable and valid measure of psychopathy (Lynam, 1997; Lynam et al.,

2005; see also Salekin, Leistico, et al., 2005; Spain, Douglas, Poythress, & Epstein, 2004).

KEY ISSUES IN CONCEPTUALIZING AND ASSESSING PSYCHOPATHY IN YOUTH

Given that psychopathy may be an important construct that contributes to our understanding of youth with conduct problems, several other chief issues should be addressed in greater detail in order to facilitate further understanding and research in this area. Issues that have been of concern include the structural stability of psychopathy symptoms in youth, comorbidity, and the temporal stability of the syndrome. Also of concern are factors that might help differentiate youth with psychopathy from those exhibiting other conduct problems. Because these issues are all crucial to understanding in this area, the following section provides a review of evidence regarding the homogeneity, factor structure, and temporal stability of psychopathy in children and adolescents. The literature on comorbidity of child and adolescent psychopathy is also reviewed to determine whether psychopathy offers a refinement over current DSM disruptive disorders. In addition, I review evidence that psychopathy may be linked to intelligence as suggested by Cleckley (1941). Although there are certainly other variables that could differentiate psychopathic youth from those with conduct problems, intelligence is one salient factor that should, according to theory, clearly distinguish these groups.

Homogeneity of Psychopathy Symptoms

Vincent and Hart (2002) reviewed research on the structural stability of psychopathy and concluded that there was reasonable internal consistency for the studies that existed at the time. Subsequent research has continued to show that there is generally good internal consistency and item homogeneity for these child and adolescent psychopathy measures. Moreover, the reliability of scores on the distinctive interpersonal and affective factors underlying these psychopathy measures also tends to be high in terms of both internal consistency of items and interrater reliability of aggregate scores. Taken together, these data suggest that the assessment of the interpersonal and affective components of psychopathy appears to be more reliable than previously thought (Cloninger, 1978; Robins, 1966), and that these features of psychopathy can be reliably assessed even in youthful populations. However, it is important to note that with untrained raters, these reliability estimates may drop considerably.

Child and Adolescent Psychopathy and Factor Structures

The structure of psychopathic symptoms in young people shows some similarities and dissimilarities to that in adults, as can be seen from the foregoing review. Early reports supported a two-factor structure for the PCL:YV in adolescents (Brandt et al., 1997; Forth, 1995) and for the APSD (Frick et al., 1994) and CPS (Lynam, 1997) in children. But, as noted by Vincent and Hart (2002), the factor structures observed in studies examining the APSD differed in important ways from those reported in adults (i.e., some items loaded on different factors, and in Frick et al.'s, 1994, early factor-analytic study the I/CP factor accounted for the majority of the variance). Recently, Frick, Bodin, and Barry (2000) reported a three-factor solution for the APSD in community children, although once again its correspondence with the three-factor structure reported in adults was limited (cf. Vincent & Hart, 2002). Even more recently, Hare (2003) proposed a four-factor model for the PCL-R that comprises interpersonal, affective, lifestyle, and antisocial facets. This model, which reaffirms the antisocial component of the disorder, is supported by some recent research findings (see Forth et al., 2003; Hare & Neumann, Chapter 4, this volume; Salekin, Brannen, Zalot, Leistico, & Neumann, in press; Salekin, Rogers, & Machin, 2001).

Clearly, much more research is needed to resolve this important issue. Nevertheless, there appears to be little disagreement that the interpersonal and affective characteristics central to psychopathy in adults are measureable in children and adolescents. However, the extent to which irresponsible and antisocial characteristics belong to the construct may be somewhat dependent on the sample under investigation, as well as theoretical and tautological concerns.

Temporal Stability of Psychopathy in Children and Adolescents

A significant shortcoming of research on psychopathy in youth has been the absence of longitudinal studies examining the stability of psychopathic traits across time and prior to adulthood (Farrington, 1991, 2005; Frick, Kimonis, et al., 2003; Loeber, 1991; Rutter, 2005). Evidence for the chronicity of psychopathy has been derived almost exclusively from analyses of retrospective data from adults with APD. In her seminal study, Robins (1966, 1978) traced the onset of psychopathic symptoms back to the age of 6–10 years after a fortunate discovery of comprehensive case file information at a child guidance clinic in St. Louis. Review of case file information from individuals who had been assessed at this clinic revealed that many of these youth were considered to have sociopathic, delinquent, and conduct problem symptoms at the time of initial assessment. Robins set out to identify and interview this same sample of individuals as adults, 20 years after their assessment at the clinic. Robins (1966) reported that many (slightly over 50%) of these adults continued to have primarily antisocial lifestyles over two decades later in time.

A few other studies have also addressed the stability issue but did so in a less than direct way. Harpur and Hare (1994) compared the prevalence rates of psychopathy classifications and the mean level of psychopathy traits in six different age subgroups of adult offenders (overall age range of sample = 16 to 70 years). These authors found that overall rates of psychopathy declined with age, especially after the age of 45. This decline was strong for the impulsive and antisocial features of psychopathy (Factor 2), whereas the average level of interpersonal and affective traits (Factor 1) remained relatively constant across age groups. These findings suggest that the hallmark symptoms of psychopathy tend to be stable over time. It is important to note that this was a cross-sectional study in which variations in psychopathy levels were examined across different-age cohorts, and thus the study was not a direct test of temporal stability.

Two other studies have addressed the temporal stability of psychopathy directly, but test–retest intervals were relatively short. Schroeder, Schroeder, and Hare (1983) reported a stability coefficient of .89 for psychopathic traits over a 10-month period. Rutherford, Cacciola, Alterman, McKay, and Cook (1999) reported 2-year stability estimates of .60 for men and .65 for women within a sample of 200 male and 25 female patients receiving methadone treatment for drug abuse. However, a potential limitation of this study is that the lower (or higher) stability estimates in this substance-dependent sample could reflect changes (or stability) in drug-related symptomatology over time, rather than changes (or lack of changes) in features of psychopathy.

Frick, Kimonis, and colleagues (2003) recently conducted one of the most rigorous prospective studies yet of the temporal stability of psychopathy from childhood through late adolescence. Psychopathic traits were assessed using the APSD over a 4-year period in a sample of nonreferred children who were in the third, fourth, sixth, and seventh grades at the time of initial assessment. Assessments included parent- and self-report versions of the APSD. For parent ratings of overall psychopathic traits, stability estimates using intraclass correlation coefficients (ICCs) ranged from .80 to .88 across 2–4 years, with a stability estimate of .93 across all four assessments. These coefficients suggest that considerable variance in parent ratings is consistent across time. Stabilities for individual subscales of the APSD (narcissism, callous unemotional, and impulsivity) were also quite high based on parent report, ranging from .71 to .92.

The cross-informant stability estimates in this study were lower but still indicated that a considerable amount of variance was consistent across time. For instance, the ICC stability estimates for parent report at time 1 predicting later self-report of psychopathy by the child or adolescent ranged from .65 for the interpersonal (narcissism) scale of the APSD to .79 each for the total score and impulsivity scale of the APSD (p's < .001). The 4-year coefficients were lower but continued to account for significant variance; these ranged from .38 ($p < .05$) for the interpersonal (narcissism) scale, to .51 ($p <. 001$) for the total score. While these data support, to some extent, the stability of psychopathic traits in youth, they also clearly indicate that there is some variability in the level of these traits across time. In particular, the findings of Frick et al. suggest that the pattern of change tends to be one in which some youth high on psychopathic traits improve and show less severe levels of these traits over time. Equally important was the fact that it was less common for youth who scored initially low on these traits in childhood to develop significant levels of psychopathic traits later in childhood and adolescence.

Interestingly, the two most consistent predictors of stability across the different methods of estimation were factors related to the child's psychosocial context, including socioeconomic status and quality of parenting. This is consistent with research, reviewed earlier in this chapter, indicating the importance of parenting in the development of empathy, guilt, and conscience (Hoffman, 1991; Kochanska, 1994; Lykken, 1998). The only other variable that contributed to predicting the stability of psychopathic traits was the child's level of conduct problems. Frick, Kimonis, and colleagues (2003) concluded that "It is possible that chronically engaging in antisocial, aggressive, and criminal behavior over time further desensitizes individuals to the consequences of their behavior on themselves and others, making their callous personality traits more stable across time" (p. 731).

In summary, there is not a great deal of research on the temporal stability of child and adolescent psychopathy, and to date, no studies have examined the test–retest reliability of the CPS or the PCL:YV in children or adolescents, respectively (Forth et al., 2003; Vincent & Hart, 2002). However, even at the adult level where psychopathy has been researched extensively, few test–retest reliability studies have been conducted. Thus, it could be argued that there is currently greater evidence for stability at the child and adolescent levels than at the adult level (see Frick et al., 2003). More research is needed on the temporal stability of psychopathy across the lifespan, both to determine stability estimates and to understand de-

velopmental relations between psychopathy and other disorders (Caron & Rutter, 1991). Such investigations would help to address questions such as the following: Does one type of psychopathology tend to precede another in developmental time, thereby increasing the likelihood of the latter occurring? Do psychopathy and other disorders that are highly comorbid at early points in life emerge as more differentiated in development? Do psychopathy and other disorders such as CD tend to "wax and wane in concert over time" (Lahey, Loeber, Burke, Rathouz, & McBurnett, 2002, p. 556)? This latter question is partially addressed in the following section.

Psychopathy and Comorbidity: Unpacking the Overlap

A concern regarding the applicability of the psychopathy construct to children and adolescents has been that its overlap with other symptoms of psychopathology is so high that elevated psychopathy scores might simply mean that youth are exhibiting general dysfunction rather than a psychopathic condition. Available research indicates that comorbidity of mental disorder is normative in child and adolescent samples (Achenbach, 1995; Biederman, Newcorn, & Sprich, 1991; Caron & Rutter, 1991; Frick, 2002; Lahey et al., 2002). This is particularly true for youth who are diagnosed with externalizing disorders such as ODD or CD, and for samples drawn from clinical and child forensic settings (Lahey et al., 2002; Seagrave & Grisso, 2002). For example, disorders frequently co-occurring with CD include various forms of depression, anxiety, substance use/abuse, and attention problems (Hinshaw & Zupan, 1997). Some researchers have argued that because of the high comorbidity evident for CD and ODD, psychopathy may also show high overlap with other forms of pathology when diagnosed early in life (Hart et al., 2002; Seagrave & Grisso, 2002; Vincent & Hart, 2002).

However, to date, only two published investigations (Brandt et al., 1997; Myers, Burket, & Harris, 1995) and two conference presentations (Bauer & Kosson, 2000; Epstein, Douglas, Poythress, Spain, & Falkenbach, 2002) have examined the comorbidity of psychopathy in young individuals with conditions aside from other disruptive behavior disorders (CD, ODD, attention-deficit/hyperactivity disorder [ADHD]) or theoretically linked traits (e.g., anxiety). Brandt and colleagues (1997) investigated the reliability, validity, and factor structure of a modified version of the PCL-R with incarcerated male adolescent offenders. Two items of the PCL-R that were inapplicable to youth (parasitic lifestyle, many short-term marital relationships) were omitted, and the scoring of two other items (juvenile delinquency, criminal versatility) was modified (cf. Forth et al., 1990). Scores on the Minnesota Multiphasic Personality Inventory (MMPI) and the CBCL were also available in this adolescent sample. Significant correlations of modest magnitude were found between total scores on the PCL-R and scales 4 ($r = .17$) and 9 ($r = .23$) of the MMPI. Modest correlations were also found between the PCL-R and the aggressive and externalizing disorder subscales of the CBCL, r's = .31 and .23, respectively. Somewhat unexpectedly, the diffuse pathology scale of the CBCL, defined by overall elevations on its constituent scales, also correlated significantly with PCL-R total scores ($r = .24$). Comparable correlations were found for the immature ($r = .20$), self destructive ($r = .20$), and unpopular ($r = .18$) subscales of the CBCL.

Myers and colleagues (1995) examined relations among psychopathy as measured by the PCL-R, Axis I and II psychopathology, and delinquent behaviors in 30 psychiatrically hospitalized male and female adolescents. This study used the Diagnostic Interview for Children and Adolescents (DICA-R) and the Structured Interview for DSM-III-R Personality Disorders (SIDP-R). These authors found significant relations among psychopathy, CD, delinquent behaviors, substance abuse, and narcissistic personality disorder. However, this high comorbidity may be in part reflective of the setting (i.e., psychiatric hospital). The authors noted that many participants in this sample had multiple personality problems and, aside from age requirements, would have met criteria for many of the personality disorders on the SIDP-R (i.e., approximately one-third of the sample had met criteria for four or more personality disorders).

Epstein and colleagues (2002) investigated associations between two measures of psychopathy (PCL:YV, APSD) and various other mental disorders in a sample of 60 male adolescent offenders remanded for treatment. Overall, scores on the PCL:YV were associated positively with both alcohol dependence ($r = .29$) and substance dependence ($r = .51$), but not with anxiety ($r = .07$) or depression ($r = .04$). However, overall APSD scores showed significant positive relations with anxiety ($r = .28$) and ADHD ($r = .23$). In another recent study that focused on female offenders, Bauer and Kosson (2000) examined 80 adolescent girls detained at the Illinois Youth Center and reported that psychopathy as indexed by the PCL:YV was significantly and positively associated with number of psychiatric diagnoses, even after removing CD from the analyses. The rates of comorbidity that psychopathy (PCL:YV > 30) showed with other diagnoses in this sample were generally very high: alcohol dependence (61%), drug dependence (72%), ADHD (71%), dysthymia (22%), depression (52%), and posttraumatic stress disorder (19%).

Recently, Salekin and colleagues (2004) examined the construct of psychopathy as applied to 130 adolescent offenders utilizing three psychopathy measures (APSD; PCL:YV; modified version of the Self-Report Psychopathy Scale [Hare, 1991]) and a broad range of DSM-IV Axis I diagnoses and psychosocial problems (indexed by the Adolescent Psychopathology Scale; Reynolds, 1998). This study attempted to expand the knowledge base on the discriminant validity of psychopathy by comparing the extent of its comorbidity with other forms of child and adolescent psychopathology to that shown by ODD and CD. The data from this study indicated that psychopathy exhibited less comorbidity with internalizing problems (i.e., involving symptoms of anxiety or depression), as well as other forms of psychopathology, than did ODD or CD. This suggests that the psychopathy construct could offer a refinement over existing DSM-IV disruptive behavior disorders in terms of differentiation from other conditions (see also Lahey et al., 2002). However, it is important to note that comorbidity was not absent for the diagnosis of psychopathy; it merely evidenced lower rates of comorbidity with other conditions than the DSM-IV disruptive behavior disorders. Furthermore, anxiety and depression were evident at higher rates among psychopathic youth than would be expected based on theory (Cleckley, 1976; Kosson, Cyterski, Steuerwald, Neumann, & Walker-Matthews, 2002).

Psychopathy and Intelligence

Cleckley hypothesized that psychopaths had good intelligence; this is potentially an important demarcation between psychopathy and other subtypes of conduct problem youth. Specifically, Cleckley noted that psychopathic individuals showed indications of "good sense and sound reasoning," had "high abilities," and were individuals "whose outer perceptual reality is accurately recognized." In sum, Cleckley often described the psychopath as a person having "excellent rational powers" and being "in full possession of his rational faculties" (Cleckley, 1976, p. 240). Other researchers (e.g., Bullard, 1941; Hankoff, 1961; Lindner, 1943; MacDonald, 1966) have echoed Cleckley's sentiments by describing psychopaths as being above average or superior intelligence, appearing poised, competent, and having good rational powers. These descriptions mirror the sentiments of Pinel (1801/ 1962), whose descriptive term for psychopathy, *manie sans delire* ("madness without confusion"), connoted clarity of thought despite abnormalities in passion and affect.

At the adult level, there is some support for a positive association between intelligence and psychopathy. For example, Harris, Rice, and Lumiere (2001) used structural equation modeling techniques to examine associations among psychopathy, violence, and historic factors (neurodevelopmental insults, parenting) in a sample of 868 violent offenders assessed at a maximum-security psychiatric hospital. Neurodevelopmental insults and psychopathy were not directly related, but both were independently related to criminal violence. In addition, antisocial parenting was related to both neurodevelopmental insults and psychopathy but had no direct relationship to criminal violence. The authors concluded that there are two separate developmental pathways to violence originating early in life, one involving neurodevelopmental damage and the other involving psychopathy. A further finding in this study was that IQ and violence were positively corre-

lated within the high psychopathy group ($r = .19$). Although weak, this association implies greater violence among psychopaths with higher intelligence.

Recent studies using child and adolescent samples (Loney et al., 1998; Salekin, Kubak, Abboud, & Tomczak, 2005; Salekin et al., 2004) have yielded preliminary evidence that psychopathy is positively related to several different types of intelligence in youthful populations. Loney and colleagues (1998) examined whether deficits in intelligence (particularly in the verbal realm) occur only in certain subgroups of children with severe conduct problems. The sample consisted of 117 clinic-referred children between the ages of 6 and 13. Assessment measures included ODD and CD according to DSM-III-R criteria, CU traits as indexed by the APSD, and intelligence as measured by the Wechsler Intelligence Scales for Children, third edition (Wechsler, 1991). Loney and colleagues found that children with ODD or CD diagnoses who did not show CU traits scored poorly on subtests measuring verbal ability in comparison to a clinic control group. On the other hand, children who exhibited CU traits along with either ODD or CD did not show verbal deficits.

Salekin and colleagues (2004) examined the relation between psychopathy and intelligence in 122 children and adolescents residing at a southeastern detention center. The PCL:YV and two intelligence tests, one a standard measure (i.e., the Kaufman Brief Intelligence Test [K-BIT]; Kaufman & Kaufman, 1990) and the other a test of triarchic intelligence (Sternberg's Triarchic Abilities Test [STAT]; Sternberg, 1993), were administered to tap alternative operationalizations of the intelligence construct. Structural equation modeling indicated that dimensions of psychopathy and intelligence modeled as latent variables were related in unique and important ways. In particular, psychopathy traits reflecting a superficial and deceitful interpersonal style were positively related to intellectual skills in the verbal realm (KBIT) and to a nontraditional intellectual measure reflecting creativity, practicality, and analytic thinking (STAT; Sternberg, 1993). The results also suggested that psychopathy traits reflecting disturbances in affective processing were inversely associated with verbal intellectual abilities.

Thus, Cleckley's hypothesis was partially supported by the data in relation to particular facets of psychopathy and when examining intelligence from the perspective of traditional and contemporary intellectual models.

Taken together, the results just reviewed highlight the importance of recognizing distinct subgroups of children with severe conduct problems when evaluating effects of intellectual deficits in children. Moreover, the current findings have several research implications. First, understanding the relation between the hallmark symptoms of psychopathy and intelligence may facilitate our understanding of the potential etiology of the disorder. Second, intelligence may have important implications in terms of the severity of the psychopathic condition and affiliated tendencies toward criminality and violence. Individuals who lack normal emotional capacities (e.g., for remorse and empathy) but possess critical intellectual abilities such as premeditation, planning, foresight, creativity, manipulation, and the ability to create a positive impression on others, may commit crimes with greater precision and a decreased likelihood of detection. Finally, in contrast with earlier research findings suggesting impairments on traditional measures of intelligence among delinquent youth, more recent findings (e.g., Loney et al., 1998; Salekin et al., 2004) suggest that the hallmark symptoms of psychopathy may not be associated with cognitive deficits but, rather, with higher verbal and creative, practical, and analytic abilities. These results highlight the importance of considering distinct facets of the psychopathy construct (i.e., affective–interpersonal vs. antisocial deviance features) in relation to variables such as intelligence.

EVIDENCE FOR THE VALIDITY OF PSYCHOPATHY AS ASSESSED IN CHILDREN AND ADOLESCENTS

There are at least two other important considerations regarding the applicability of the psychopathy concept to children and adolescents. Specifically, there are concerns that psychopathy is associated with deficits in neurocognitive processing, and this issue certainly deserves attention with youthful populations. In addition, psychopathy has been noted to be a particularly effective predictor of antisocial behavior in adulthood (cf. Douglas, Vincent, & Edens, Chapter 27, this volume). Evidence that psychopathy is also predictive of negative outcomes with children and adolescents is important if the construct is to be downwardly extended. In the next section, research on the neurocognitive processing and antisocial behavior of children and adolescents scoring high on psychopathy scales is reviewed and compared to existing data on these two topics with adult samples.

Performance on Laboratory Measures of Neurocognitive Processing

An extensive body of research exists to suggest impairments in emotional reactivity (see Fowles & Dindo, Chapter 2, and Blair, Chapter 15, this volume) and response inhibition/modulation (cf. Hiatt & Newman, Chapter 17, this volume) in adult psychopathic individuals. Parallel investigations of affective and inhibitory deficits in younger participants are beginning to emerge, with some studies yielding results similar to those obtained in adults, and others showing dissimilarities.

Using a representative sample of 308 16-year-olds from the Child Development Project (Dodge, Bates, & Pettit, 1990), Vitale and colleagues (2005) tested and corroborated the hypotheses that participants with low anxiety and high APSD scores would display (1) poorer passive avoidance learning, and (2) less interference on a spatially separated, picture–word Stroop task than controls. Both of the aforementioned tasks require participants to make decisions in complex contexts. Paralleling results with adult prisoners, Vitale and colleagues found the expected group differences in picture–word Stroop interference with both male and female adolescent participants and predicted differences in passive avoidance for the males only.

In another study, Loney and colleagues (2003) examined the emotional reactivity of adolescents referred for antisocial behavior problems using the lexical-decision paradigm (Williamson, Harpur, & Hare, 1991), in which recognition times for emotional (positive and negative) and nonemotional words are compared under instructions to identify whether a visual character string is a word or a nonword. Consistent with findings for adult psychopathic participants, Loney and colleagues found that CU traits as indexed by the APSD were associated with slower reaction times for negative words. In contrast, the authors found that problems of impulse control were associated with faster recognition time for negative emotional words. The authors posited that different patterns of emotional reactivity may characterize distinct subgroups of youth with antisocial behavior problems.

Findings from other laboratory studies of children and adolescents have also shown parallels with studies of adult psychopathy. For instance, Frick and his colleagues found that among conduct problem children, only those with CU traits showed a reward dominant response style indicative of a failure to evaluate all pertinent information before making a decision (Barry et al., 2000; O'Brien & Frick, 1996). Conduct problem children with CU traits also show a preference for thrill- and adventure-seeking activities (Frick et al., 1994). Christian, Frick, Hill, Tyler, and Frazer (1997) reported that youth scoring high on the CU scale of the APSD were unable to inhibit a dominant response set, as has been frequently demonstrated in adult males with psychopathy (Hiatt & Newman, Chapter 17, this volume). Blair and colleagues, also using the APSD in children, have reported deficits related to both impulsivity and emotionality facets of psychopathy (Blair, 1999; Blair, Colledge, Murray, & Mitchell, 2001; Colledge & Blair, 2001; Stevens, Charman, & Blair, 2001). In addition, various investigators have reported deficits in empathy and moral reasoning among adolescents high in psychopathy as indexed by the PCL:YV (Chandler & Moran, 1990; Trevethan & Walker, 1989), and among children high in psychopathy as indexed by the APSD (Blair, Monson, & Frederickson, 2001).

In terms of neuropsychological test performance, research with adult psychopathic offenders has yielded reliable deficits on tasks designed to index orbitofrontal/vendromedial functioning (e.g., go/no-go, Porteus Maze, olfactory discrimination task), with no accompanying deficits on tests of dorsolateral prefrontal function (LaPierre, Braum, & Hodgins, 1995; Mitchell, Colledge, Leon-

ard, & Blair, 2002). Consistent with this, a recent study of adolescent offenders (Roussy & Toupin, 2000) reported a significant difference between high (> 30) and low (< 20) PCL:YV scorers on two of four orbitofrontal/ventromedial tasks: a go/no-go task, and a stopping task (i.e., high PCL:YV scorers committed more commission errors on both the go/no-go task and the stopping task than did the low PCL:YV group). In addition, the group difference on the qualitative score index of the Porteus Maze task approached significance ($p = .06$), with the high PCL:YV group committing more rule-breaking errors than the low PCL:YV group. No group differences were evident on an olfactory discrimination task, nor on any measures of frontal/dorsolateral function (i.e., Wisconsin Card Sorting test, Porteus Maze test/quantitative score, Controlled Oral Word Association Test). However, within a sample of 80 incarcerated female adolescents, Bauer (1999) found no psychopathy-related differences on any measures of executive or orbitofrontal functioning or on measures of verbal abilities.

The question of whether adolescents with psychopathic traits display difficulties in cognitive and emotional processing warrants further systematic investigation. Applications of neuroimaging technology may help to address this question. However, it is not clear whether such deficits would necessarily be apparent from an early age. An alternative possibility is that such deficits might accrue over time as children or adolescents encounter problems in their lives such as incarceration, drug and alcohol use, impaired relations, and the like. In any case, the foregoing results provide some evidence for differences in the processing and use of semantic and affective among children and adolescents diagnosed as psychopathic and signal the need for further research in this key area.

Associations with Criterion Variables Reflecting Antisocial Deviance and Aggression

An important aspect of the psychopathy construct is its relation to violent and nonviolent criminal behavior (Salekin, Rogers, & Sewell, 1996). In a recent meta-analytic study (Salekin, Leistico, Rogers, & DeCoster, 2005), we found that psychopathy had a similar magnitude of relation with violent crime among adolescents ($d = .54$) as in adults ($d = .57$), but a slightly lower relation with nonviolent recidivism ($d = .40$) than in adults ($d = .55$). On average, adolescent reoffenders scored about one-half of a standard deviation higher on the PCL than did nonreoffenders. A similar magnitude of effect was found for institutional infractions ($d = .60$), again paralleling findings with adults ($d = .58$).

There are now a considerable number of studies that have examined relations between psychopathy and antisocial behavior in children (e.g., Edens, Skeem, Cruise, & Cauffman, 2001; Frick, Cornell, Barry, Bodin, & Dane, 2003; Lynam, 1997), with the majority having focused on formal delinquency in adolescents (e.g., Brandt et al., 1997; Caputo et al., 1999; Cruise, 2000; Forth et al., 1990; Gretton, 1998; O'Neill, 2001; Ridenour, Marchant, & Dean, 2001). Consistent with the adult literature, adolescents with high scores on the PCL:YV engage in more antisocial behavior than do others, both in institutions (Bauer, 1999; Brandt et al., 1997; Cruise, 2000; Forth et al., 1990; Hicks, Rogers, & Cashel, 2000; Rogers, Johansen, Chang, & Salekin, 1997; Stafford & Cornell, 2003) and in the community (Brandt et al., 1997; Corrado, Vincent, Hart, & Cohen, 2004; Forth et al., 1990; Toupin, Mercier, Dery, Cote, & Hodgins, 1996; Vitacco, Neumann, Robertson, & Durant, 2002). Adolescents with high PCL:YV scores also commit more serious antisocial behavior—specifically more violence (Brandt et al., 1997; Forth et al., 1990; Gretton, 1998; Gretton, Hare, & Catchpole, 2001; Ridenour et al., 2001; Stafford & Cornell, 2003).

In addition, the predictive validity of the PCL:YV with respect to serious antisocial behavior is evident over periods as long as 1–10 years (e.g., Corrado et al., 2004; Forth et al., 1990; Gretton et al., 2003; Toupin et al., 1996). The results are generally robust, with moderate to large effect sizes obtained for a range of institutional infractions. The data from these studies indicate a similar magnitude of effect for PCL Factors 1 and 2 in predicting violent offending and institutional infractions among adolescent offenders. However, for general recidivism, Factor 2 was more predictive. These results suggest that the psychopathy construct has similar predictive power for adolescents and adults, with the exception that Factor 1 appears to be more predictive of dangerousness for adolescents. Although the bulk of research on the association between psychopathy and antisocial behavior has been conducted with the PCL and PCL:YV, the APSD appears to produce similar results (see Frick, Stickle, Dandreaux, Farell, & Kimonis, 2005).

RECOMMENDATIONS FOR SCIENCE AND PRACTICE

To this point in the chapter, evidence regarding application of the psychopathy construct to children and adolescents has been reviewed. In terms of supportive evidence, available data suggest that interpersonal, affective, and even behavioral deficits linked to psychopathy might very well be identified early in life. In addition, reliability and validity data indicate that psychopathy measures developed for use with children and adolescents do, in fact, measure a syndrome that is coherent and similar to psychopathy in adults, and that youth diagnosed as psychopathic may have some neurological abnormalities similar to adults. Research findings also suggest that psychopathy, in view of its lesser comorbidity with other syndromes, may provide a "purer" object of study than the disruptive behavior disorders of DSM-IV. Moreover, higher psychopathy levels in childhood and adolescence predict subsequent antisocial behavior, with both the interpersonal and affective components of the syndrome contributing to prediction.

Despite these compelling similarities in findings for psychopathy in adult and youth populations, some discrepancies were noted, particularly in the areas of comorbidity and neurological anomalies. Psychopathy at the child and adolescent levels tends to be positively correlated with depression and anxiety, and not all neurological impairments found with adult samples have been noted with adolescent samples. In addition, stability estimates for psychopathy across the early years appear to be modest. Some have even questioned whether it is possible to say with certainty that it is in fact psychopathy we are assessing when using youth psychopathy measures (Hart et al., 2002; Vincent & Hart, 2002). This is likely to be an issue of continuing importance as research on the psychopathy construct in children and adolescents progresses. The process of construct validation is invariably an ongoing one. With these aforementioned limitations in mind, there are several specific areas that researchers examining child and adolescent psychopathy may want to focus on to move the study of child and adolescent psychopathy forward. In the brief sections that follow, I delineate what I see to be the main priorities for future research in this area.

Clarifying Differences between Psychopathy and the Disruptive Behavior Disorders

Hare (2003) and others have argued that the diagnosis of APD in DSM-IV-TR, while offering high reliability, focuses excessively on the salient antisocial behaviors of the psychopath embodied in PCL-R Factor 2, while underemphasizing the callous, manipulative, and arrogant features of the disorder embodied in Factor 1. McBurnett and Pfiffner (1998) have argued that an analogous situation exists with the DSM criteria for CD. All CD behavioral criteria represent major violations of the basic rights of others or of age appropriate societal norms. Even when ADHD and ODD symptoms are included, the DSM disruptive behavior items predominantly tap the antisocial deviance (Factor 2) component of psychopathy, with minimal representation of the affective–interpersonal features (Factor 1). As a consequence, according to McBurnett and Pfiffner (1998), young people who meet diagnostic criteria for CD will have an elevated risk for being diagnosed with APD and receiving high ratings on PCL-R Factor 2 in adulthood, but these individuals will be heterogeneous with respect to their positions on Factor 1 (i.e., many will be diagnosable as APD in adulthood, but most will not be psychopaths). Thus, although psychopathy is a construct of potential importance for differentiating among subgroups of conduct problem youth, the work of these authors suggests that it can not easily be accommodated within existing DSM-IV categories.

Also important, and perhaps related to some of the mixed neurocognitive findings noted in this review, are concerns currently being raised about the PCL itself, and the variants of the PCL that have been developed for use with young participants. For example, it has been noted that the first three of Cleckley's (1976) diagnostic criteria for psychopathy (good intelligence, absence of nervousness, and absence of delusions/clarity of thought) are not explicitly included in the PCL (Brinkley, Newman, Widiger, & Lynam, 2004; Rogers, 2001; Salekin, 2002; Skeem, Mulvey, & Grisso, 2003). Moreover, the current version of the PCL:YV has replaced another key Cleckley criterion ("superficial charm") with an alternative indicator ("impression management"). Changes of this sort may result in drift from the construct originally articulated by Cleckley (1941, 1976) and may cause changes in the nomological net we expect to surround psychopathy.

Brinkley and colleagues (2004) have argued that although the PCL instruments provide an excellent starting point for assessment of psychopathy, they may also provide for a heterogenous group of individuals with differing etiologies because they include distinctive subsets of items and they exclude certain criteria that Cleckley used to delineate the disorder. In assessing psychopathy in childhood and adolescence, it may be useful to include evaluation of features such as "superficial charm," "absence of delusions" (clarity of thought), and "absence of nervousness" in order to more sharply differentiate children/adolescents with psychopathy from those who have other disorders (e.g., CD and ODD). This would provide for a more expected nomological net around the concept of psychopathy in childhood and adolescence, assuming the syndrome thus defined does indeed emerge in younger individuals.

Moffitt's Taxonomy: Are Two Groups Enough?

Although Moffitt's (1993) model of delinquent subtypes has added substantially to our understanding of youth with conduct disorder, it is unclear how the phenomenon of psychopathy can be accommodated within this dual-subtype scheme. Although there has been some suggestion that the life-course persistent offender category is likely to capture the youthful psychopathic individual, there are several lines of evidence that suggest that such individuals do not fit neatly into this offender subgroup. For instance, life-course persistent adolescents have been found to have a host of neurological deficits including low intelligence. This runs counter to classic conceptualizations of psychopathy and is inconsistent with recent data suggest ing positive associations between psychopathy and various aspects of intelligence (Harris et al., 2001; Loney, Frick, Ellis, & McCoy, 1998; Salekin et al., 2004). Moreover, Vincent Vitacco, Grisso, and Corrado (2003), based on a cluster analysis of distinctive facets of the psychopathy construct (affective, interpersonal, and behavioral), identified four different juvenile offender subtypes. The cluster group highest on all three facets of psychopathy was the most chronic and severe. Impulsive features alone were strongly associated with severe antisocial behaviors, retrospectively, but not prospectively. Findings from this study suggest that there may be more than two juvenile offender subtypes. Further research is needed to substantiate this, and to further elucidate the position of psychopathic individuals within the taxonomy of delinquent subtypes.

Ontogeny of Conduct Problems, Antisocial Behavior, and Psychopathy

Much more research on the ontogeny of conduct problems, and on the distinctive phenomenon of psychopathy in young people, is needed. There are numerous compelling theories that are in the early stages of development and require further research (cf. Frick & Marsee, Chapter 18, this volume; Lahey & Waldman, 2003; Silverthorn & Frick, 1999). However, causal models have not adequately accounted for the interpersonal aspects of psychopathy thus far, and much more research is needed in this specific area if we are to better understand the nature of the syndrome. What distinguishes psychopathy from other personality disorders is its specific symptom pattern of deficits in affect accompanied by strong rational and intellectual capacities—a clinical picture that led Cleckley to his conclusion that these individuals had a "mask of sanity."

In addition, developmental psychopathology models are likely to be key in understanding the ontogeny of psychopathy (Cicchetti & Richters, 1993; Richters & Cicchetti, 1993). Specifically, for many indi-

viduals, high stability or continuity of antisocial behavior over time is evident (Hinshaw et al., 1993), but the specific expression of antisocial tendencies is more likely than not to change over the individual's lifespan. Moreover, factors such as level of comorbidity may change as one moves through childhood to adolescence and adulthood. Thus, it is possible for individuals to look somewhat different at varying developmental stages of the disorder. One fundamental error in the application of psychopathy to children and adolescents is to assume that studying different age groups cross-sectionally will result in highly similar findings across groups. Similarly, an unreasonable assumption in the past has been that the disorder in childhood should look the same as it does in adulthood, when it is fully developed. It is probably more accurate to suppose that a disorder, whether it be psychopathy or something else, will look "generally the same" in childhood as in adulthood, rather than the same or virtually identical. This is not a conceptual stretch if one accepts the notion that disorders follow a developmental course. As one example of this, Lahey and colleagues (2002) found anxiety to be comorbid with CD, but the degree of comorbidity declined substantially across waves of this longitudinal study. Thus, the disorder appeared somewhat similar in childhood to how it appeared in later developmental stages, but there were some notable developmental changes across time (e.g., less anxiety). Similar findings suggesting developmental shifts in the association between *psychopathy* and anxiety are beginning to emerge in the child literature.

With respect to causal inferences, a final word of caution is warranted regarding the danger of assuming biological primacy or biological determinism on the basis of a statistical association between some biological factor and overt antisocial behavior. As Rutter (1997) cogently pointed out, biological changes can be associated with events that are relatively benign. For example, winners in closely matched chess or tennis games show a rise in testosterone whereas losers show a drop. Similarly, in animals, changes in social status lead to changes in hormone levels. According to Rutter, phenomena such as these indicate "a complex two-way interplay between soma and psyche, and it cannot be assumed that the biological feature is primary." In a related vein, Johnstone and Cooke (2004) noted that although there is clear evidence that youth with certain temperaments are more likely to engage in antisocial behavior, it might be the impact of particular experiences coupled with extreme temperament that accounts the brain dysfunction characteristic of psychopathy. The basic point is that the route between brain and environment is not one way, and evidence of cortical plasticity across the lifespan is increasingly being recognized. This is an essential point to bear in mind in constructing causal models of psychopathy.

In closing, the issue of psychopathy in children and adolescents is a controversial one, and many questions remain to be resolved. On the basis of the findings reviewed, it can be concluded that psychopathy appears to be definitionally and conceptually distinct from DSM-IV disruptive disorders. In addition, available findings indicate that there is not an easy alliance between psychopathy and current DSM-IV categories, even when taking into consideration the life-course persistent subtype of CD. The weight of evidence also suggests that psychopathy likely has its roots in childhood. However, despite some supportive findings, it is important to note that not all the neurocognitive findings previously obtained with adults have been found for child and adolescent psychopathy, and this may in part be due to the heterogeneous class of psychopaths assessed by the PCL:YV and its derivatives. Alternatively, some of the differences in results might be attributable to developmental changes in the condition across time. Whatever the case, these findings signal the need for much more research on this topic—as continued study of child and adolescent psychopathy has great potential to provide us with deeper levels of knowledge regarding the ontogeny of psychopathy, and to advance our understanding of the best methods for prevention and intervention.

REFERENCES

Achenbach, T. M. (1991). *Manual for the Child Behavior Checklist and 1991 profile*. Burlington: University of Vermont Press.

Achenbach, T. M. (1995). Diagnosis, assessment, and comorbidity in psychological treatment research. *Journal of Abnormal Psychology, 23*, 45–65.

American Psychiatric Association. (1994). *Diagnostic and statistical manual of mental disorders* (4th ed.). Washington, DC: Author.

American Psychiatric Association. (2000). *Diagnostic and statistical manual of mental disorders* (4th ed., text rev.). Washington, DC: Author.

Andershed, H., Kerr, M., Stattin, H., & Levander, S. (2002). Psychopathic traits in non-referred youths: A new assessment tool. In E. Blauuw & L. Sheridan (Eds.), *Psychopaths: Current international perspectives* (pp. 131–158). The Hague, The Netherlands: Elsevier.

Barrett, K. C., & Campos, J. J. (1987). Perspectives on emotional development: II. A functionalist approach to emotions. In J. D. Osofsky (Ed.), *Handbook of infant development* (pp. 555–578). New York: Wiley.

Barry, C. T., Frick, P. J., DeShazo, T. M., McCoy, M. G., Ellis, M., & Loney, B. R. (2000). The importance of callous–unemotional traits for extending the concept of psychopathy to children. *Journal of Abnormal Psychology, 109*, 335–340.

Barry, C. T., Frick, P. J., & Killian, A. L. (2003). The relation of narcissism and self-esteem to conduct problems in children: A preliminary investigation. *Journal of Clinical Child and Adolescent Psychology, 32*, 139–152.

Bauer, D. (1999). *Psychopathy in incarcerated adolescent females: Prevalence rates and individual differences in cognition, personality and behavior.* Unpublished doctoral dissertation, Finch University of Health Sciences/Chicago Medical School, North Chicago, IL.

Bauer, D., & Kosson, D. S. (2000, March). *Psychopathy in incarcerated females: Prevalence rates and individual differences in personality and behavior.* Paper presented at the conference of the American Psychology–Law Society, New Orleans.

Biederman, J., Newcorn, J., & Sprich, S. (1991). Comorbidity of attention deficit hyperactivity disorder with conduct, depressive, anxiety, and other disorders. *American Journal of Psychiatry, 148*, 564–577.

Blair, R. J. R. (1999). Responsiveness to distress cues in the child with psychopathic tendencies. *Personality and Individual Differences, 27*, 135–145.

Blair, R. J. R. (2001). Neuro-cognitive models of aggression, the antisocial personality disorders and psychopathy. *Journal of Neurology, Neurosurgery, and Psychiatry, 71*, 727–731.

Blair, R. J. R., Colledge, E. Murray, L., & Mitchell, D. G. V. (2001). A selective impairment in the processing of sad and fearful expressions in children with psychopathic tendencies. *Journal of Abnormal Child Psychology, 29*, 491–498.

Blair, R. J. R., Monson, J., & Fredrickson, N. (2001). Moral reasoning and conduct problems in children with emotional and behavioral difficulties. *Personality and Individual Differences, 31*, 799–811.

Brandt, J. R., Kennedy, W. A., Patrick, C. J., & Curtin, J. J. (1997). Assessment of psychopathy in a population of incarcerated adolescent offenders. *Psychological Assessment, 9,* 429–435.

Brinkley, C. A., Newman, J. P., Widiger, T. A., & Lynam, D. R. (2004). Two approaches to parsing the heterogeneity of psychopathy. *Clinical Psychology: Science and Practice, 11,* 69–94.

Bullard, D. M. (1941). Psychopathic personality in selective service psychiatry. *Psychiatry, 4,* 231–239.

Burke, J. D., Loeber, R., & Lahey, B. B. (2003). Course and outcomes. In C. A. Essau (Ed.), *Conduct and oppositional defiant disorders: Epidemiology, risk factors, and treatment,* (pp. 61–94). Mahwah, NJ: Erlbaum.

Burns, G. L. (2000). Problem of item overlap between the Psychopathy Screening Device and attention deficit hyperactivity disorder, oppositional defiant disorder, and conduct disorder rating scales. *Psychological Assessment, 12,* 447–450.

Caldwell, M., Skeem, J. L., Salekin, R. T., & Van Rybroek, G. (in press). Treatment response of adolescent offenders with psychopathy features: A two year follow-up. *Criminal Justice and Behavior.*

Caputo, A. A., Frick, P. J., & Brodsky, S. L. (1999). Family violence and juvenile sex offending: Potential mediating roles of psychopathic traits and negative attitudes toward women. *Criminal Justice and Behavior, 26,* 338–356.

Caron, C., & Rutter, M. (1991). Comorbidity in child psychopathology: Concepts, issues, and research strategies. *Journal of Child Psychology and Psychiatry, 32,* 1063–1080.

Caspi, A., & Bem, D. (1990). Personality continuity and change across the life course. In L. Pervin (Ed.), *Handbook of personality: Theory and research* (pp. 549–575). New York: Guilford Press.

Caspi, A., Block, J., Block, J. H., Lynam, D., Moffitt, T. E., & Stouthamer-Loeber, M. (1992). A "common language" version of the California Child Q-Set (CCQ) for personality assessment. *Psychological Assessment, 4,* 512–523.

Cicchetti, D., & Richters, J. E. (1993). Developmental considerations in the investigation of conduct disorder. *Development and Psychopathology, 5,* 331–344.

Chandler, M., & Moran, T. (1990). Psychopathy and moral development: A comparative study of delinquent and nondelinquent youth. *Development and Psychopathology, 2,* 227–246.

Christian, R., Frick, P. J., Hill, N., Tyler, A. L., & Frazer, D. (1997). Psychopathy and conduct problems in children: II. Implications for subtyping children with conduct problems. *Journal of the American Academy of Child and Adolescent Psychiatry, 36,* 233–241.

Cleckley, H. (1941). *The mask of sanity.* St. Louis, MO: Mosby.

Cleckley, H. (1976). *The mask of sanity* (5th ed.). St. Louis, MO: Mosby.

Cloninger, C. R. (1978). The antisocial personality. *Hospital Practice, 13,* 97–106.

Colledge, E., & Blair, R. J. R. (2001). The relationship between the inattention and impulsivity components of attention deficit and hyperactivity disorder and psychopathic tendencies. *Personality and Individual Differences, 30,* 1175–1187.

Cooke, D. J., & Michie, C. (2001). Refining the construct of psychopathy: Towards a hierarchical model. *Psychological Assessment, 13,* 171–188.

Corrado, R. R., Vincent, G. M., Hart, S. D., & Cohen, I. M. (2004). Predictive validity of the Psychopathy Checklist: Youth Version for general and violent recidivism. *Behavioral Sciences and the Law, 22,* 5–22.

Cruise, K. R. (2000). *Measurement of adolescent psychopathy: Construct and predictive validity in two samples of juvenile offenders.* Unpublished doctoral dissertation, University of North Texas.

Dodge, K. A., Bates, J. E., & Pettit, G. S. (1990). Mechanisms in the cycle of violence. *Science, 250,* 1678–1683.

Dunn, J. (1987). The beginnings of moral understanding: Development in the second year. In J. Kagan & S. Lamb (Eds.), *The emergence of morality in young children* (pp. 91–112). Chicago: University of Chicago Press.

Edens, J. F., Skeem, J. L., Cruise, K. R., & Cauffman, E. (2001). Assessment of "juvenile psychopathy" and its association with violence: A critical review. *Behavioral Sciences and the Law, 19,* 53–80.

Eisenberg, N., & Mussen, P. A. (1989). *The roots of prosocial behavior in children.* New York: Cambridge University Press.

Elkind, D. (1967). Egocentrism in adolescence. *Child Development, 38,* 1025–1034.

Emde, R. N., Biringen, Z., Clyman, R. B., & Oppenheim, D. (1991). The moral self of infancy: Affective core and procedural knowledge. *Developmental Review, 11,* 251–270.

Epstein, M., Douglas, D., Poythress, N., Spain, S., & Falkenbach, D. (2002, March). *A discriminant study of juvenile psychopathy and mental disorders.* Paper presented at the conference of the American Psychology–Law Society, Austin, TX.

Farrington, D. P. (1991). Antisocial personality from childhood to adulthood. *Psychologist, 4,* 389–394.

Farrington, D. P. (2005). The importance of child and adolescent psychopathy. *Journal of Abnormal Child Psychology, 33,* 489–498.

Forth, A. E. (1995). Psychopathy in adolescent offenders: Assessment, family background, and violence. *Issues in Criminological and Legal Psychology, 24,* 42–44.

Forth, A. E., & Burke, H. C. (1998). Psychopathy in adolescence: Assessment, violence, and developmental precursors. In D. J. Cooke, A. E. Forth, & R. D. Hare (Eds.), *Psychopathy: Theory, research and implications for society* (pp. 205–229). Boston: Kluwer.

Forth, A. E., Hare, R. D., & Hart, S. D. (1990). Assessment of psychopathy in male young offenders. *Psychological Assessment, 2,* 342–344.

Forth, A. E., Kosson, D. S., & Hare, R. D. (1996/2003). *The Psychopathy Checklist: Youth Version.* Toronto, ON, Canada: Multi-Health Systems.

Forth, A. E., & Mailloux, D. L. (2000). Psychopathy in youth: What do we know? In C. Gacono (Ed.), *The clinical and forensic assessment of psychopathy: A practitioner's guide* (pp. 25–54). Mahwah, NJ: Erlbaum.

Frick, P. J. (1998). Callous–unemotional traits and conduct problems: Applying the two-factor model of psychopathy to children. In D. J. Cooke, A. E. Forth, & R. D. Hare (Eds.), *Psychopathy: Theory, research and implications for society* (pp. 161–187). Boston: Kluwer.

Frick, P. J. (2000). The problems of internal validation without a theoretical context: The different conceptual underpinnings of psychopathy and the disruptive behavior disorder criteria. *Psychological Assessment, 12,* 451–456.

Frick, P. J. (2002). Juvenile psychopathy from a developmental perspective: Implications for construct development and use in forensic assessments. *Law and Human Behavior, 26,* 247–253.

Frick, P. J., Bodin, D., & Barry, C. (2000). Psychopathic traits and conduct problems in community and clinic-referred samples of children: Further development of the Psychopathy Screening Device. *Psychological Assessment, 12,* 382–393.

Frick, P. J., Bodin, D. S., & Barry, C. T. (2000). Applying the concept of psychopathy to children: Implications for the assessment of antisocial youth. In C. Gacono (Ed.), *The clinical and forensic assessment of psychopathy: A practitioner's guide* (pp. 3–24). Mahwah, NJ: Erlbaum.

Frick, P. J., Cornell, A., Barry, C. T., Bodin, S. D., & Dane, H. (2003). Callous–unemptional traits and conduct problems in the prediction of conduct problem severity, aggression, and self-report of delinquency. *Journal of Abnormal Child Psychology, 31,* 457–470.

Frick, P. J., & Ellis, M. L. (1999). Callous–unemotional traits and subtypes of conduct disorder. *Clinical Child and Family Psychology Review, 2,* 149–168.

Frick, P. J., & Hare, R. D. (2001). *Antisocial Process Screening Device.* Toronto, ON, Canada: Multi-Health Systems.

Frick, P. J., Kimonis, E. R., Dandreaux, D. M., & Farell, J. M. (2003). The 4 years stability of psychopathic traits in non-referred youth. *Behavioral Sciences and the Law, 21,* 1–24.

Frick, P. J., Lahey, B. B., Loeber, R., Stouthamer-Loeber, M., Green, S., Hart, E. L., & Christ, A. G. (1991). Oppositional defiant disorder and conduct disorder in boys: Patterns of behavioral covariation. *Journal of Clinical Child Psychology, 20,* 202–208.

Frick, P. J., Lilienfeld, S. O., Ellis, M., Loney, B., & Silverthorn, P. (1999). The association between anxiety and psychopathy dimensions in children. *Journal of Abnormal Child Psychology, 27,* 383–392.

Frick, P. J., & Jackson, Y. K. (1993). Family functioning and childhood antisocial behavior: Yet another reinterpretation. *Journal of Clinical Child Psychology, 22,* 410–419.

Frick, P. J., O'Brien, B. S., Wootton, J. M., & McBurnett, K. (1994). Psychopathy and conduct problems in children. *Journal of Abnormal Psychology, 103,* 700–707.

Frick, P. J., & Sheffield Morris, A. (2004). Temperament and developmental pathways to conduct problems. *Journal of Clinical Child and Adolescent Psychology, 33,* 54–68

Frick, P. J., Stickle, T. R., Dandreaux, D. M., Farell, J. M., & Kimonis, E. R. (2005). Callous–unemotional traits in predicting the severity and stability of conduct problems and delinquency. *Journal of Abnormal Child Psychology, 33,* 471–488.

Gretton, H. M. (1998). *Psychopathy and recidivism in adolescence: A ten year retrospective follow-up.* Unpublished doctoral dissertation, University of British Columbia, Vancouver.

Gretton, H. M., Hare, R. D., & Catchpole, R. E. H. (2004). Psychopathy and offending from adolescence to adulthood: A ten-year follow up. *Journal of Consulting and Clinical Psychology, 72,* 636–645.

Haan, N., Aerts, E., & Cooper, B. A. (1987). *On moral grounds.* New York: New York University Press.

Hankoff, L. D. (1961). The psychopath in the clinical interview. *Journal of Offender Therapy, 5,* 4–6.

Hare, R. D. (1991). *Manual for the Revised Psychopathy Checklist.* Toronto, ON, Canada: Multi-Health Systems.

Hare, R. D. (2003). *Manual for the Revised Psychopathy Checklist* (2nd ed.). Toronto, ON, Canada: Multi-Health Systems.

Harpur, T. J., & Hare, R. D. (1994). Assessment of psychopathy as a function of age. *Journal of Abnormal Psychology, 103,* 604–609.

Harpur, T. J., Hare, R. D., & Hakstian, A. R. (1989). Two-factor conceptualization of psychopathy: Construct validity and assessment implications. *Psychological Assessment, 1,* 6–17.

Harris, G. T., Rice, M. E., & Lalumiere, M. (2001). The roles of psychopathy, neurodevelopmental insults, and antisocial parenting. *Criminal Justice and Behavior, 28,* 402–426.

Hart, S. D., Watt, K. A., & Vincent, G. M. (2002). Commentary on Seagrave and Grisso: Impressions of the state of the art. *Law and Human Behavior, 26,* 241–245.

Harter, S. (1990). Causes, correlates and functional role of global self worth: A life span perspective. In R. J. Sternberg & J. Kolligan (Eds.), *Competence considered* (pp. 67–97). New Haven, CT: Yale University Press.

Hicks, B. M., Rogers, R., & Cashel, M. (2000). Predictions of violent and total infractions among institutionalized male juvenile offenders. *Journal of the American Academy of Psychiatry and Law, 28,* 183–190.

Hinshaw, S. P., Lahey, B. B., & Hart, E. L. (1993). Issues of taxonomy and co-morbidity in the development of conduct disorder. *Development and Psychopathology, 5,* 31–50.

Hinshaw, S. P., & Zupan, B. A. (1997). Assessment of antisocial behavior in children and adolescents. In E. J. Mash & R. A. Barkley (Eds.), *Child psychopathology* (pp. 36–50). New York: Guilford Press.

Hoffman, M. L. (1991). Empathy, social cognition and moral action. In W. M. Kurtines, & J. L. Gewirtz (Eds.), *Handbook of moral behavior and developmental theory* (pp. 275–301). Mahwah, NJ: Erlbaum.

Izard, C. E. (1977). *Human emotions*. New York: Plenum Press.

Izard, C. E., & Harris, P. (1995). Emotional development and developmental psychopathology. In D. Cicchetti & D. J. Cohen (Eds.), *Developmental psychopathology, Vol. 2: Risk, disorder, and adaptation* (pp. 467–503). New York: Wiley.

Johnstone, L., & Cooke, D. J. (2004). Psychopathic-like traits in childhood: Conceptual and measurement concerns. *Behavioral Sciences and the Law, 22,* 103–125.

Kamphaus, R. W., & Frick, P. J. (1996). *The clinical assessment of children's emotion, behavior, and personality*. Boston: Allyn & Bacon.

Karpman, B. (1949). The psychopathic delinquent child. *American Journal of Orthopsychiatry, 20,* 223–265.

Kaufman, A. S., & Kaufman, N. L. (1990). *Kaufman Brief Intelligence Test (K-BIT)*. Circle Pines, MN: American Guidance Service.

Kazdin, A. E. (1997). Conduct disorders across the lifespan. In S. S. Luthar, J. A. Burack, D. Cicchetti, & J. R. Weisz (Eds.), *Developmental psychopathy, perspectives on adjustment, risk, and disorder* (pp. 248–272). New York: Cambridge University Press.

Kochanska, G. (1991). Socialization and temperament in the development of guilt and conscience. *Child Development, 62,* 1379–1392.

Kochanska, G. (1993). Toward a synthesis of parental socialization and child temperament in early development of conscience. *Child Development, 64,* 325–347.

Kochanska, G. (1994). Beyond cognition: Expanding the search for the early roots of internalization and conscience. *Developmental Psychology, 30,* 20–22.

Kosson, D. S., Cyterski, T. D., Steuerwald, B. L., Neumann, C. S., & Walker-Matthews, S. (2002). The reliability and validity of the Psychopathy Checklist: Youth Version in nonincarcerated males. *Psychological Assessment, 14,* 97–109.

Kruh, I. P., Frick, P. J., & Clements, C. B. (2005). Historical and personality correlates to the violence patterns of juveniles tried as adults. *Criminal Justice and Behavior, 32,* 69–96.

Lahey, B. B., & Loeber, R. (1994). Framework for a developmental model of oppositional defiant disorder and conduct disorder. In D. K. Routh (Ed.), *Disruptive behavioral disorders in childhood* (pp. 139–180). New York: Plenum Press.

Lahey, B. B., Loeber, R., Burke, J., Rathouz, P. J., & McBurnett, K. (2002). Waxing and waning in concert: Comorbidity of conduct disorder with other disruptive and emotional problems over 7 years among clinic-referred boys. *Journal of Abnormal Psychology, 111,* 556–567.

Lahey, B. B., Loeber, R., Quay, H. C., Frick, P. J., & Grimm, J. (1992). Oppositional defiant and conduct disorders: Issues to be resolved for the DSM-IV. *Journal of the American Academy of Child and Adolescent Psychiatry, 31,* 539–546.

Lahey, B. B., & Waldman, I. D. (2003). A developmental propensity model of the origins of conduct problems during childhood and adolescence. In B. B. Lahey, T. E. Moffitt, & A. Caspi (Eds.), *Causes of conduct disorder and juvenile delinquency* (pp. 76–117). New York: Guilford Press.

LaPierre, D., Braum, C. M., & Hodgins, S. (1995). Ventral frontal deficits in psychopathy: Neuropsychological test findings. *Neuropsychologia, 33,* 139–151.

Lindner, R. M. (1943). Experimental studies in constitutional psychopathic inferiority. *Journal of Criminal Psychopathology, 4,* 484–500.

Lilienfeld, S. O., & Andrews, B. P. (1996). Development and preliminary validation of a self-report measure of psychopathic personality traits in noncriminal populations. *Journal of Personality Assessment, 66,* 488–524.

Loeber, R. (1991). Antisocial behavior: More enduring than changeable? *Journal of the American Academy of Child and Adolescent Psychiatry, 30,* 393–397.

Loeber, R., & Dishion, T. (1983). Early predictors of male delinquency: A review. *Psychological Bulletin, 94,* 68–99.

Loeber, R., Green, S. M., Keenan, K., & Lahey, B. B. (1995). Which boys will fare worse? Early predictors of the onset of conduct disorder in a six-year longitudinal study. *Journal of the American Academy of Child and Adolescent Psychiatry, 34,* 499–509.

Loeber, R., Green, S. M., Lahey, B. B., & Stouthamer-Loeber, M. (1991). Differences and similarities between children, mothers, and teachers as informants on disruptive child behavior. *Journal of Abnormal Child Psychology, 19,* 75–95.

Loeber, R., Lahey, B. B., & Thomas, C. (1991). Diagnostic conundrum of oppositional defiant disorder and conduct disorder. *Journal of Abnormal Psychology, 100,* 379–390.

Loney, B. R., Frick, P. J., Clements, C. B., Ellis, M. L., & Kerlin, K. (2003). Callous–unemotional traits, impulsivity, and emotional processing in antisocial adolescents. *Journal of Clinical Child and Adolescent Psychology, 32*(1), 66–80.

Loney, B. R., Frick, P. J., Ellis, M. L., & McCoy, M. G. (1998). Intelligence, psychopathy, and antisocial behavior. *Journal of Psychopathology and Behavioral Assessment, 20,* 231–247.

Lykken, D. T. (1995). *The antisocial personalities*. Hillsdale, NJ: Erlbaum.

Lynam, D. R. (1996). Early identification of chronic offenders: Who is the fledgling psychopath? *Psychological Bulletin, 120,* 209–234.

Lynam, D. R. (1997). Pursuing the psychopath: Capturing the psychopath in a nomological net. *Journal of Abnormal Psychology, 106,* 425–438.

Lynam, D. R. (1998). Early identification of the fledgling psychopath: Locating the psychopathic child in the current nomenclature. *Journal of Abnormal Psychology, 107,* 566–575.

Lynam, D. R. (2002). Fledgling psychopathy: A view from personality theory. *Law and Human Behavior, 26,* 255–259.

Lynam, D. R., Caspi, A., Moffitt, T. E., Raine, A., Loeber, R., & Stouthamer-Loeber, M. (2005). Adolescent psychopathy and the Big Five: Results from two samples. *Journal of Abnormal Child Psychology, 33,* 431–444.

Lynam, D. R., Whiteside, S., & Jones, S. (1999). Self-reported psychopathy: A validation study. *Journal of Personality Assessment, 73,* 110–132.

MacDonald, J. M. (1966). The prompt diagnosis of the psychopathic personality. *Journal of Psychiatry, 122*(Suppl.), 45–50.

McBride, M. (1998). *Individual and familial risk factors for adolescent psychopathy.* Unpublished doctoral dissertation, University of British Columbia, Vancouver.

McBurnett, K., & Pfiffner, L. (1998). Comorbidities and biological correlates of conduct disorder. In D. J. Cooke, A. E. Forth, & R. D. Hare (Eds.), *Psychopathy: Theory, research, and implications for society* (pp. 189–203). London: Kluwer.

McCord, W., & McCord, J. (1964). *The psychopath: An essay on the criminal mind.* New York: Van Nostrand Reinhold.

Mitchell, D. G. V., Colledge, E., Leonard, A., & Blair, R. J. R. (2002). Risky decisions and response reversal: Is there evidence of orbito-frontal cortex dysfunction in psychopathic individuals? *Neuropsychologia, 40,* 2013–2022.

Mitchell, S., & Rosa, P. (1981). Boyhood behavior problems as precursor of criminality: A fifteen year follow-up study. *Journal of Child Psychology and Psychiatry, 22,* 19–23.

Moffitt, T. E. (1993). Adolescence-limited and life-course-persistent antisocial behavior: A developmental taxonomy. *Psychological Review, 100,* 674–701.

Moffitt, T. E. (2003). Life course persistent and adolescent limited antisocial behavior: A ten year research review and a research agenda. In B. B. Lahey, T. E. Moffitt, & A. Caspi (Eds.), *Causes of conduct disorder and juvenile delinquency* (pp. 49–75). New York: Guilford Press.

Moffitt, T. E., Lynam, D. R., & Silva, P. A. (1994). Neuropsychological tests predict persistent male delinquency. *Criminology, 32,* 101–124.

Murrie, D. C., Cornell, D. G., & McCoy, W. K. (2005). Psychopathy, conduct disorder, and stigma: Does diagnostic labeling influence juvenile probation officer recommendation? *Law and Human Behavior, 29,* 323–342.

Myers, W. C., Burket, R. C., & Harris, H. E. (1995). Adolescent psychopathy in relation to delinquent behaviors, conduct disorder, and personality disorders. *Journal of Forensic Sciences, 40,* 436–440.

Newman, J. P. (1998). Psychopathic behavior: An information processing perspective. In D. J. Cooke, A. E. Forth, & R. D. Hare (Eds.), *Psychopathy: Theory, research and implications for society* (pp. 81–104). Boston: Kluwer.

O'Brien, B. S., & Frick, P. J. (1996). Reward dominance: Associations with anxiety, conduct problems, and psychopathy in children. *Journal of Abnormal Child Psychology, 24,* 223–240.

O'Neill, M. L. (2001). *Adolescents with psychopathic characteristics in a substance abusing cohort: Predictors, correlates, and treatment process and outcome.* Unpublished doctoral dissertation, MCP Hahnemann University, Philadelphia.

Patrick, C. J. (1994). Emotion and psychopathy: Startling new insights. *Psychophysiology, 31,* 319–330.

Petrila, J., & Skeem, J. L. (2003). An introduction to the special issues on juvenile psychopathy and some reflections on the current debate: Juvenile psychopathy: The debate. *Behavioral Sciences and the Law, 21,* 689–694.

Pinel, P. (1962). *A treatise on insanity* (D. D. Davis, Trans.). New York: Hafner. (Original work published 1801)

Plutchik, R. (1980). *Emotion: A psychoevolutionary synthesis.* New York: Harper & Row.

Poythress, N. G., Edens, J. F., & Lilienfeld, S. O. (1998). Criterion-related validity of the Psychopathic Personality Inventory in a prison sample. *Psychological Assessment, 10,* 426–430.

Quay, H. C. (1964). Dimensions of personality in delinquent boys as inferred from the factor analysis of case history data. *Child Development, 35,* 479–484.

Quay, H. C. (1986). Classification. In H. C. Quay & J. S. Werry (Eds.), *Psychopathological disorders of childhood* (3rd ed., pp. 1–42). New York: Wiley.

Quay, H. C. (1987). Patterns of delinquent behavior. In H. C. Quay (Ed.), *Handbook of juvenile delinquency* (pp. 118–138). New York: Wiley.

Radke-Yarrow, M., & Zahn-Waxler, C. (1984). Roots, motives and patterns in children's prosocial behaviour. In E. Staub, J. Bar-Tal, J. Karylowski, & J. Reykowski (Eds.), *Development and maintenance of prosocial behavior: International perspectives on positive behavior* (pp. 81–99). New York: Plenum Press.

Reynolds, W. M. (1998). *Adolescent Psychopathology Scale: Administration and interpretation manual.* Odessa, FL: Psychological Assessment Resources.

Richters, J. E., & Cicchetti, D. (1993). Mark Twain meets the DSM-III-R: Conduct disorder, development, and the concept of harmful dysfunction. *Development and Psychopathology, 5,* 5–29.

Ridenour, T. A., Marchant, G. J., & Dean, R. S. (2001). Is the Psychopathy Checklist—Revised clinically useful for adolescents? *Journal of Psychoeducational Assessment, 19,* 227–238.

Robins, L. N. (1966). *Deviant children grown up: A sociological and psychiatric study of sociopathic personality*. Baltimore: Williams & Wilkins.

Robins, L. N. (1978). Sturdy childhood predictors of adult antisocial behavior: Replications from longitudinal studies. *Psychological Medicine, 8*, 611–622.

Rogers, R. (2001). *Handbook of diagnostic and structured interviewing*. New York: Guilford Press.

Rogers, R. Johansen, J., Chang, J. J., & Salekin, R. T. (1997). Predictors of adolescent psychopathy: Oppositional and conduct-disordered symptoms. *Journal of the American Academy of Psychiatry and Law, 25*, 261–271.

Roussy, S., & Toupin, J. (2000). Behavioral inhibition deficits in juvenile psychopaths. *Aggressive Behavior, 26*, 413–424.

Russo, M. F., Loeber, R., Lahey, B. B., & Keenan, K. (1994). Oppositional defiant and conduct disorders: Validation of the DSM-III-R and alternative diagnostic option. *Journal of Clinical Child Psychology, 23*, 56–68.

Rutherford, M. J., Cacciola, J. S., Alterman, A. I., McKay, J. R., & Cook, T. G. (1999). Two-year test–retest reliability of the Psychopathy Checklist—Revised in methadone patients. *Assessment, 6*, 285–291.

Rutter, M. (1997). Nature–nurture integration: The example of antisocial behavior. *American Psychologist, 52*, 390–398.

Rutter, M. (2005). What is the meaning and utility of the psychopathy concept? *Journal of Abnormal Child Psychology, 33*, 499–503.

Salekin, R. T. (2002). Psychopathy and therapeutic pessimism: Clinical lore or clinical reality? *Clinical Psychology Review, 22*, 79–112.

Salekin, R. T., Brannen, D. N., Zalot, A. A., Leistico, A. R., & Neumann, C. S. (in press). Factor structure of psychopathy in youth: Testing the applicability of the new four factor model. *Criminal Justice and Behavior*.

Salekin, R. T., & Frick, P. J. (2005). Psychopathy in children and adolescents: The need for a developmental psychopathology perspective. *Journal of Abnormal Child Psychology, 33*, 403–409.

Salekin, R. T., Kabak, F., Abboud, B., & Tomczak, V. (2005, June). *Psychopathy and emotional processing in adolescents: Cleckley's formulation*. Paper presented at the annual meeting of the International Society for Research on Child and Adolescent Psychopathology, New York.

Salekin, R. T., Leistico, A. R., Rogers, R., & DeCoster, (2004, August). *Psychopathy, dangerousness, and risk management: An updated meta-analysis of the Psychopathy Checklist—Revised augmented with the Youth and Screening Versions*. Paper presented at the annual meeting of the American Psychological Association, Honolulu, HI.

Salekin, R. T., Leistico, A. R., Trobst, K. K., Schrum, C. L., & Lochman, J. E. (2005). Adolescent psychopathy and personality theory—the interpersonal circumplex: Expanding evidence of a nomological net. *Journal of Abnormal Child Psychology, 33*, 445–460.

Salekin, R. T., Neumann, C. S., Leistico, A. R., DiCicco, T., & Duros, R. L. (2004). Construct validity of psychopathy in a young offender sample: Taking a closer look at psychopathy's potential importance over disruptive behavior disorders. *Journal of Abnormal Psychology, 113*, 416–427.

Salekin, R. T., Neumann, C. S., Leistico, A. R., & Zalot, A. A. (2004). Psychopathy in youth and intelligence: An investigation of Cleckley's hypothesis. *Journal of Clinical Child and Adolescent Psychology, 33*, 731–742.

Salekin, R. T., Rogers, R., & Machin, D. (2001). Psychopathy in youth: Pursuing diagnostic clarity. *Journal of Youth and Adolescence, 30*, 173–195.

Salekin, R. T., Rogers, R., & Sewell, K. W. (1996). A review and meta-analysis of the Psychopathy Checklist and Psychopathy Checklist—Revised. *Clinical Psychology: Science and Practice, 3*, 203–215.

Salekin, R. T., Ziegler, T. A., Larrea, M. A., Anthony, V. L., & Bennett, A. D. (2003). Predicting psychopathy with two Millon Adolescent psychopathy scales. The importance of egocentric and callous traits. *Journal of Personality Assessment, 80*, 154–163.

Schroeder, M. L., Schroeder, K. G., & Hare, R. D. (1983). Generalizability of a checklist for the assessment of psychopathy. *Journal of Consulting and Clinical Psychology, 51*, 511–516.

Schrum, C. L., & Salekin, R. T. (in press). Psychopathy in adolescent female offenders: An item response theory analysis of the Psychopathy Checklist: Youth Version. *Behavioral Sciences and the Law*.

Seagrave, D., & Grisso, T. (2002). Adolescent development and the measurement of juvenile psychopathy. *Law and Human Behavior, 26*, 219–239.

Silverthorn, P., & Frick, P. J. (1999). Developmental pathways to antisocial behavior: The delayed onset pathway in girls. *Development and Psychopathology, 11*, 101–126.

Silverthorn, P., Frick, P. J., & Reynolds, R. (2002). Timing of onset and correlates of severe conduct problems in adjudicated girls and boys. *Journal of Psychopathology and Behavioral Assessment, 23*, 171–181.

Skeem, J. L., & Cauffman, E. (2003). Views of the downward extension: Comparing the youth version of the Psychopathy Checklist with the Youth Psychopathic Traits Inventory. *Behavioral Sciences and the Law, 21*, 737–770.

Skeem, J. L., Monahan, J., & Mulvey, E. P. (2002). Psychopathy, treatment involvement, and subsequent violence among civil psychiatric patients. *Law and Human Behavior, 26*, 577–603.

Skeem, J. L., Mulvey, E. P., & Grisso, T. (2003). Applicability of the traditional and revised models of psychopathy to the Psychopathy Checklist: Screening Version. *Psychological Assessment, 15*, 41–54.

Skeem, J. L., & Petrila, J. (2004). Introduction to the special issue on juvenile psychopathy, volume 2: Juvenile psychopathy: Informing the debate. *Behavioral Sciences and the Law*, 22, 1–4.

Skilling, T. A., Quinsey, V. L., & Craig, W. M. (2001). Evidence of a taxon underlying serious antisocial behavior in boys. *Criminal Justice and Behavior*, 28, 450–470.

Spain, S. E., Douglas, K. S., Poythress, N. G., & Epstein, M. A. (2004). The relationship between psychopathic features, violence, and treatment outcome: The comparison of three youth measures of psychopathic features. *Behavioral Sciences and the Law*, 22, 49–67.

Stafford, E., & Cornell, D. G. (2003). Psychopathy scores predict adolescent inpatient aggression. *Assessment*, 10, 102–112.

Sternberg, R. J. (1993). *Sternberg Triarchic Abilities Test, High School Level*. Unpublished psychological test, Yale University, New Haven, CT.

Stevens, D., Charman, T., & Blair, R. J. R. (2001). Recognition of emotion in facial expressions and vocal tones in children with psychopathic tendencies. *Journal of Genetic Psychology*, 162, 201–211.

Stouthamer-Loeber, M. (1986). Lying as a problem behavior in children: A review. *Clinical Psychology Review*, 6, 267–289.

Sullivan, L. E., & Gretton, H. (1996, March). *Concurrent validity of the MMPI-A and the PCL-R in an adolescent forensic population*. Poster presented at the meeting of the American Psychology–Law Society, Hilton Head, SC.

Trevethan, S. D., & Walker, L. J. (1989). Hypothetical versus real-life moral reasoning among psychopathic and delinquent youth. *Development and Psychopathology*, 1, 91–103.

Toupin, J., Mercier, H., Dery, M., Cote, G., & Hodgins, S. (1996). Validity of the PCL-R for adolescents. In D. J. Cooke, A. E. Forth, J. P. Newman, & R. D. Hare (Eds.), *Issues in criminological and legal psychology: No. 24, International perspectives on psychopathy* (pp. 143–145). Leicester, UK: British Psychological Society.

Vasey, M. W., Kotov, R., Frick, P. J., & Loney, B. R. (2005). The latent structure of psychopathy in youth: A taxometric investigation. *Journal of Abnormal Child Psychology*, 33, 411–430.

Viding, E., Blair, R. J. R., Moffitt, T. E., & Plomin, R. (2004). Evidence for substantial genetic risk for psychopathy in 7-year-olds. *Journal of Child Psychology and Psychiatry*, 45, 1–6.

Vincent, G. M. (2002). *Investigating the legitimacy of adolescent psychopathy assessments: Contributions of item response theory*. Unpublished doctoral dissertation, Simon Fraser University, Burnaby, British Columbia.

Vincent, G. M., & Hart, S. D. (2002). Psychopathy in childhood and adolescence: Implications for the assessment and management of multi problem youths. In R. R. Corrado, R. Coesch, S. D. Hart, & J. K. Gierowski (Eds.), *Multi-problem violent youth: A foundation for comparative research on needs, interventions, and outcomes* (NATO Science Series A: Life Sciences) (pp. 150–163). Amsterdam: IOS Press.

Vincent, G. M., Vitacco, M. J., Grisso, T., & Corrado, R. R. (2003). Subtypes of adolescent offenders: Affective traits and antisocial behavior patterns. *Behavioral Sciences and the Law*, 21, 695–712.

Vitacco, M. J., Neumann, C. S., Robertson, A. A., & Durant, S. L. (2002). Contribution of impulsivity and callousness in the assessment of adjudicated male adolescents: A prospective study. *Journal of Personality Assessment*, 78, 87–103.

Vitale, J. E., Newman, J. P., Bates, J. E., Goodnight, J., Dodge, K. A., & Pettit, G. S. (2005). Deficient behavioral inhibition and anomalous selective attention in a community sample of adolescents with psychopathic traits and low-anxiety traits. *Journal of Abnormal Child Psychology*, 33, 461–470.

Wechsler, D. (1991). *Wechsler Intelligence Scale for Children—Revised*. San Antonio, TX: Psychological Corporation.

Werry, J. S., & Quay, H. C. (1971). The prevalence of behavior symptoms in younger elementary school children. *American Journal of Orthopsychiatry*, 41, 136–143.

Wiener, R. L. (2002). Adversarial forum: Issues concerning the assessment of juvenile psychopathy. *Law and Human Behavior*, 26, 217–218.

Williamson, S. Harpur, T. J., & Hare, R. D. (1991). Abnormal processing of affective words by psychopaths. *Psychophysiology*, 28, 260–273.

Wootton, J. M., Frick, P. J., Shelton, K. K., & Silverthorn, P. (1997). Ineffective parenting and childhood conduct problems: The moderating role of callous–unemotional traits. *Journal of Consulting and Clinical Psychology*, 65, 301–308.

Zahn-Waxler, C., & Radke-Yarrow, M. (1990). The origins of empathic concern. *Motivation and Emotion*, 14, 107–130.

Zahn-Waxler, C., Radke-Yarrow, M., Wagner, E., & Chapman, M. (1992). Development of concern for others. *Developmental Psychology*, 28, 126–136.

21

Psychopathy in Women

Assessment, Manifestations, and Etiology

EDELYN VERONA
JENNIFER VITALE

Until recently, the study of psychopathy in women was all but ignored by psychopathologists and forensic psychologists. Since the development of Hare's Psychopathy Checklist (PCL; Hare, 1980) and its revision (PCL-R; Hare, 1991, 2003), only a few researchers have taken on the pioneering work of attempting to validate measures of psychopathy, and the construct itself, in women. The current chapter involves a comprehensive review of the admittedly sparse literature, encompassing most facets of research that have been conducted to understand psychopathy and related syndromes in women. More specifically, we review and evaluate the growing literature on the (1) validity of the construct of psychopathy and measures of the construct as it is currently conceptualized, (2) diagnostic syndromes associated with female antisocial behavior and psychopathy, and (3) distinct developmental and etiological factors contributing to psychopathic tendencies in women. In the process of reviewing this literature, we highlight similarities with and important departures from the male psychopathy literature. This chapter should serve to introduce researchers interested in this topic to important conceptual issues and fruitful directions to pursue in future research on female psychopathy.

GENDER DIFFERENCES IN EXTERNALIZING TRAITS AND SYNDROMES

Psychiatric epidemiological data confirm a heightened tendency for women to experience internalizing symptomatology (depression, anxiety) in relation to men, whereas men are more likely than women to present with externalizing psychopathology, including substance abuse/dependence, antisocial personality, and aggression (Kessler et al., 1994; Robins & Regier, 1991). Some have suggested that social sanctions against reporting feelings and attitudes that have been traditionally associated with the opposite sex, as well as sex biases in diagnoses by clinicians, may explain these differences (Ford & Widiger, 1989). Others, however, have suggested that gender differences in baserates for certain diagnoses are due to meaningful underlying cognitive (e.g., rumination) and biological (e.g., sex hormones) differences between the genders (Hankin &

Abramson, 2001; Nolen-Hoeksema, 1990; Widiger & Spitzer, 1991).

Research has also indicated that men and women may differ in evolutionarily influenced action tendencies involving activation and withdrawal. For example, women tend to report more intense negative emotions, particularly fear, and exhibit greater facial reactivity when exposed to aversive stimuli relative to men (Bradley, Codispoti, Sabatinelli, & Lang, 2001; Tobin, Graziano, Vanman, & Tassinary, 2000). Men are less likely than women to report anxiety in response to threatening situations (Carver & White, 1994), and they report more positive emotions and exhibit greater physiological arousal in response to pleasant images (Bradley et al., 2001). Men also report more frequent experiences of anger, a negatively valenced but activating emotion (cf. Harmon-Jones & Allen, 1998), than women or girls (Fabes & Eisenberg, 1992). Consistent with this hypothesis, developmental researchers have reported that boys tend to exhibit higher activity levels and more impulsivity during infancy, whereas girls show more stress reactivity and behavioral inhibition (Garstein & Rothbart, 2003; Sooyeon, Brody, & Murray, 2003).

Other developmental psychologists have speculated that emerging differences in aggression can arise from parental socialization practices that encourage internalizing and prosocial expressions of affect (e.g., empathy) in girls versus boys (see Keenan & Shaw, 1997). In addition, there is evidence that girls show earlier development of cognitive adaptive skills, including in language and social–emotional skills, than boys (Keenan & Shaw, 1997). These cognitive skills relate to the development of more efficient behavioral inhibition strategies in girls relative to boys.

This brief summary of findings on gender differences in externalizing behaviors and potential underlying causes highlights some reasons why prevalence rates for antisocial personality and psychopathy may be higher in men than women (Salekin, Rogers, & Sewell, 1997). More important, though, this literature may also be relevant to understanding (1) differential manifestations of the same underlying vulnerability for antisocial and psychopathic behaviors in men and women, and (2) unique etiological factors leading to the development of psychopathic traits in women versus men. These issues are addressed across different sections of this chapter.

EARLY WORK ON PSYCHOPATHIC FEMALES

Although men may be more likely to present with psychopathy than women, Cleckley (1976) included female clientele among the prototype cases in his monograph, indicating that the full syndrome of psychopathy does occur in both genders. The female clients he described, notably "Roberta" and "Anna," often exhibited many of the characteristics he had observed in his male clients (i.e., stealing, truancy, and pathological lying). At the same time, Cleckley also said:

> One of [Roberta's] most appealing qualities is, perhaps, her friendly impulse to help others. . . . She often went to sit with an ill neighbor, watched the baby of her mother's friend, and rather patiently helped her younger sister with her studies. In none of these things was she consistent. She often promised her services and, with no explanation, failed to appear. . . . She would stop to pet a puppy, take crumbs out to the birds, and comfort a stray cat. Yet, when her own dog was killed by an automobile, she showed only the most fleeting and superficial signs of concern. (p. 19)

This description of Roberta's shallow expressions of nurturance highlights potential differences in how judgments of psychopathy are made in women versus men, as well as distinctions between female and male expressions of psychopathic traits. First, the primary traits of psychopathy are antithetical to female socialization more so than male socialization, and for this reason, the kinds of traits exhibited by Roberta may seem more striking to observers who expect women to be nurturant, selfless, and emotional. Second, the contexts in which these psychopathic women displayed these traits—within the home and in their relationships—differed from the more public arenas (i.e., pubs, gambling houses, business, and military) in which Cleckley's psychopathic men wreaked havoc. In essence, Cleckley's female clientele exhibited similar personality traits to male psychopaths, but these traits were manifested more typically as violations of female role expectations.

Since Cleckley, few researchers have investigated female forms of antisocial behavior, and, until recently, most of this research focused on general criminality and violence rather than on the specific syndrome of psychopathy (e.g., Hoffman-Bustamante, 1973). However, there were some notable exceptions. For example, Widom (1978) was interested, among other things, in testing whether certain female prisoners would fit the profile of the psychopath as described by Cleckley (1976). Based on a cluster analysis of personality measures, she identified four offender subtypes in her sample of incarcerated women: (1) a psychopathic or undercontrolled type, exhibiting hostility and aggression, extensive criminal histories, and relatively low scores on anxiety; (2) a secondary or neurotic psychopath type, exhibiting high impulsivity and high levels of anxiety, depression and other maladjustment; (3) an overcontrolled type (Megargee, 1966), with hyponormal scores on hostility and anxiety, higher psychological defensiveness and fewer previous convictions; and (4) a "normal" criminal type, scoring in the midrange on most personality scales, with a peak in hostility. These offender groups, which have been identified to some extent in other female samples (Butler & Adams, 1966; Verona & Carbonell, 2000), resembled subtypes previously found in male delinquent samples (Megargee, 1966). From these data, Widom concluded that similar subtypes, including a psychopathic group, were present in female as well as male offenders. However, a notable difference is that undercontrolled and psychopathic types appear to be less prevalent in female than male offender samples, whereas overcontrolled offenders with less extensive criminal histories are more prevalent in female samples (Verona & Carbonell, 2000; Widom, 1978).

However, a limitation of the Widom (1978) study is that the indices of psychopathy used in this study reflected primarily the antisocial deviance aspects of the disorder as opposed to the affective–interpersonal features that have been emphasized in contemporary research. In the following section, we review studies that have attempted to assess psychopathy in women using recently validated measures of the construct.

VALIDITY AND MEASUREMENT OF FEMALE PSYCHOPATHY

In their recent reviews of the area, Cale and Lilienfeld (2002b) and Vitale and Newman (2001b) note that, despite the relatively lower baserates of psychopathy within many female samples, the reliability and factor structures of psychopathy measures appear to generalize across gender. However, these reviews highlight unanswered questions regarding differential symptom expression of psychopathy across gender, differential item functioning of psychopathy inventories across gender, and the criterion-related validity of psychopathy measures, particularly in regard to forensic criteria and laboratory variables.

Evidence for the utility of the PCL-R with female offenders was first reported in the PCL-R manual (Hare, 1991); this evidence was drawn primarily from unpublished sources (i.e., Neary, 1990; Strachan, Williamson, & Hare, 1990). Neary (1990) administered the PCL-R to 120 female inmates of a federal prison in Missouri, and found the interrater reliability for overall PCL-R scores ($r = .94$) to be comparable to that for male samples reported by Hare (1991). However, indices of scale homogeneity (internal consistency) were somewhat lower in this female offender sample (coefficient alpha = .77, vs. .87 for men; mean interitem correlation = .14, vs. .26 for men). Strachan and colleagues (1990), using a sample of 40 female prison inmates in British Columbia, reported comparable interrater reliability for PCL-R total scores in this sample ($r = .95$), but internal consistency figures were somewhat lower than those observed in men (coefficient alpha = .79; mean interitem correlation = .19). Hare (1991) has suggested that the lower internal consistency of the PCL-R in these female samples stemmed from problems with certain items, particularly items 18 (Juvenile Delinquency) and 19 (Revocation of Conditional Release), which showed weak correlations with PCL-R total scores.

In the next sections, we review more recent data pertaining to the prevalence of psychopathy across gender, the factor structure of psychopathy instruments across gender, and differential item functioning of the PCL-R across gender. Although much of this work has utilized the PCL-R, investigations using alternative measures of psychopathy, including the Screening Version of the PCL (PCL:SV), the Self-Report Psychopathy Scale (SRP-II; Hare, 1991), and the Psychopathy Personality Inventory (PPI; Lilienfeld & Andrews, 1996), will also be considered.

Prevalence Rates

The prevalence of aggressive behavior disorders such as antisocial personality disorder (APD) and conduct disorder (CD) is consistently lower in female samples than in male samples (e.g., Hartung & Widiger, 1998; Rutherford, Alterman, Cacciola, & Snider, 1995). In regard to the prevalence of psychopathy, however, results are similar but somewhat less consistent. For example, using a diagnostic cutoff of 30 on the PCL-R, several Canadian studies of incarcerated women have reported baserates well within the range for men (32–31%; Louth, Hare, & Linden, 1998; Strachan, 1993; Tien, Lamb, Bond, Gillstrom, & Paris, 1993). However, there are a number of studies of female offenders in which substantially lower baserates of psychopathy have been reported. Warren and colleagues (2003) reported a baserate of 17% in their sample of American prison inmates, and Salekin and colleagues (1997) reported a baserate of 15% in a sample from an American jail. Neary (1990) and Loucks (1995) each reported an 11% baserate, and Vitale, Smith, Brinkley, and Newman (2002) reported a 9% baserate in an American prison sample.

In an unpublished dissertation, O'Connor (2001) reported a baserate of 15.5% using the standard score of 30 as a cutoff. However, he also examined the effectiveness of different PCL-R diagnostic cutoff scores using receiver operating characteristic (ROC) curves (i.e., plot of true-positive rate [sensitivity] as a function of the false-alarm rate [one minus specificity]) and Cleckley's original ratings as criteria for group membership. The cutoff score on the PCL-R that produced the most comparable diagnostic efficiency between Hare's (1991) normative male offender sample and O'Connor's sample of female prisoners ($N = 226$) was 27 (sensitivity = .74, specificity = .90), which produced a baserate for psychopathy of 24%.

However, it should be noted that, even if diagnostic cut scores are not used, differ-

ences in the mean scores for males and females on a variety of psychopathy measures have been observed. For example, within a noninstitutionalized sample of abused or neglected young adults, Weiler and Widom (1996) found that males had higher mean PCL-R scores than females. Likewise, using the PCL:SV, Forth, Brown, Hart, and Hare (1996) reported that the mean score for undergraduate males was significantly higher than that of undergraduate females. In addition, a comparison of a male sample and a female sample composed of noninstitutionalized methadone patients revealed significantly lower mean PCL-R scores for the females (Rutherford, Cacciola, Alterman, & McKay, 1996) than for the males (Alterman, Cacciola, & Rutherford, 1993). Thus, when gender differences on psychopathy measures have been found in studies of nonincarcerated samples, mean scores appear generally to be higher for males than for females. However, there have also been null findings in regard to gender differences in PCL-R scores (Cooney, Kadden, & Litt, 1990; Stafford & Cornell, 2003).

In addition to the rater-based PCL, PCL-R, and PCL:SV, a handful of studies have examined psychopathy across gender using self-report measures of psychopathy. Results from these investigations also find evidence for generally higher psychopathy scores for males than females. For example, studies using the SRP-II (Hare, 1991) to assess psychopathy have found that males score significantly higher than females (Lilienfeld & Hess, 2001; Wilson, Frick, & Clements, 1999; Zagon & Jackson, 1994). Similarly, Lilienfeld and Andrews (1996) and Lilienfeld and Hess (2001) observed significantly higher scores for males, relative to females, on the self-report based PPI. However, in their study of the PPI in an undergraduate sample, Hamburger and colleagues (1996) found no significant gender differences in PPI scores.

In summary, studies that have examined whether psychopathy, like APD and CD, is less prevalent in females than males have yielded less consistent findings. Studies using rater-based measures of psychopathy, such as the PCL, PCL-R, and PCL:SV, have reported baserates for females that clearly overlap with the range observed in male samples. However, in the majority of these studies, baserates for females fall at the lower end of the range observed in male samples. Similarly, studies using self-report based measures of psychopathy suggest that males tend to score higher on these measures than females, although this pattern is qualified by the handful of studies finding no significant gender differences.

Factor Structure

To demonstrate the generality of psychopathy measures across gender, it is necessary also to consider the comparability of instrument structure and item functioning. To the extent that an instrument functions differently across groups, it becomes increasingly difficult to draw conclusions regarding the validity of the construct being assessed (Sue, 1999). However, the generalizability of the PCL-R and PCL:SV factor structure across gender will be influenced, in part, by the factor model being chosen to be tested.

There are a small number of studies testing the generality of the factor structure of psychopathy across gender; however, a number of these are limited by small sample size or an exclusive focus on only one of the three alternative factor models—that is, the original two-factor model (Hare, 1991; Harpur, Hare, & Hakstian, 1989), the three-factor model (Cooke & Michie, 2001), or Hare's (2003) new four-facet model (see also Hare & Neumann, Chapter 4, this volume). As a result, it is difficult to determine if failures to replicate the factor structure of the PCL-R and PCL:SV across gender stem from procedural limitation, the particular factor model chosen to be tested, or true gender differences in the structure of the instrument across gender.

In one of the first of studies of the generalizability of the two-factor model across gender, Salekin and colleagues (1997) conducted exploratory factor analysis of the PCL-R using a sample of 103 females. Results showed that although a two-factor structure similar to that originally proposed by Harpur and colleagues (1989) emerged, the individual PCL-R items did not load on these factors in the same way for women as they had for men. Specifically, the items "poor behavioral controls," "impulsivity," and "lack of realistic long-term goals" crossloaded on Factors 1 and 2, and the items "failure to accept responsibility," "many-short term marital relationships," and "revocation of conditional release" failed to load on either factor (Salekin et al., 1997). Salekin and colleagues' (1997) findings are qualified by the possibility that their sample size was insufficient for an exploratory factor analysis of an instrument of the PCL-R's length and structure (Cale & Lilienfeld, 2002b; Vitale & Newman, 2001b). Nonetheless, O'Connor (2001) also found similar deficiencies in fit for the two-factor model when he conducted confirmatory factor analysis on PCL-R items using a sample of 226 female prisoners drawn from a federal prison in Florida.

As noted, the inconsistency in factor structure across gender could reflect limitations of the original two-factor model. For example, Warren and colleagues (2003) conducted a detailed examination of the goodness of fit of the original two-factor model, the Cooke and Michie (2001) three-factor model, and Hare's (2003) four-facet model in their sample of 138 female inmates. Results of confirmatory factor analyses indicated that although the best fit to the data was achieved using the three-factor model, both the three-factor and four-factor models represented better fits to the data than the original two-factor model (Warren et al., 2003). Thus, Salekin and colleagues' (1997) failure to demonstrate the generality of the two-factor model across gender might have been due to limitations of the model itself, rather than to significant differences in the structure of the instrument across gender.

A test of the Cooke and Michie (2001) three-factor solution using the PCL:SV in a 42% female sample provided support for the generality of the factor structure of this psychopathy measure across gender. Skeem, Mulvey, and Grisso (2003) compared the original two-factor model with the Cooke and Michie three-factor model in a sample of 870 psychiatric inpatients. In addition to concluding that the three-factor model represented a better description of the PCL:SV than the original two-factor model, the authors noted that the fit of the three-factor model to the data was not reduced when factor loadings for items and the covariances among the three factors were constrained to be equal across gender (Skeem et al., 2003). However, potential limitations of the three-factor model (cf. Hare, 2003) should be considered in evaluating these findings.

Bolt, Hare, Vitale, and Newman (2004) investigated the functioning of the PCL-R in female samples using item response theory (IRT) analyses of differential item functioning (DIF). A detailed review of the application of IRT analyses to the PCL-R can be found elsewhere (see Hare & Neumann, Chapter 4, this volume). Briefly, IRT analyses examine the relationship between levels of the latent trait presumed to underlie a test instrument and the scores obtained on the individual items. When differences in this relationship occur across samples, the item is said to exhibit DIF. If a large proportion of the items display substantial amounts of DIF, the validity of the instrument may be called into question across the groups being compared.

Analyses of the PCL-R item scores of females versus males have demonstrated the presence of DIF for a number of items (Bolt, Hare, Vitale, & Newman, 2004). The largest differences in item functioning were found for the following items: conning/manipulative, early behavior problems, juvenile delinquency, and criminal versatility. Thus, when the PCL-R is used with female samples, there may be some differences in item functioning, particularly for items tapping antisocial or criminal behavior.

However, DIF is independent of directionality, and thus differences in item functioning can reflect both higher (positive DIF) and lower (negative DIF) scores for a comparison group relative to a reference group. If the number of individual items demonstrating positive DIF and the number of individual items demonstrating negative DIF is roughly equivalent, then the total effect of DIF on the Full-Scale scores will be minimal (Bolt et al., 2004). It was found in this study in that although there appear to be significant differences in the functioning of some of the PCL-R items as a function of gender, the overall impact of these differences on PCL-R scores may be mitigated in part by the canceling out of positive and negative DIF.

Although the effects of DIF observed by Bolt and colleagues (2004) on total PCL-R scores for females are likely to be negligible, it is useful to consider alternative indicators of differential test functioning. In a comparison of the test characteristic curves of the

PCL-R for male and female samples, Bolt and colleagues found that the curve for females differs significantly from that of a male offender reference group. However, the authors note that this group difference, although significant, translates to only small differences across each level of the latent psychopathy trait. For example, at the level of the latent trait roughly equivalent to the diagnostic cutoff of 30, the group difference is less than 2 score points (Bolt et al., 2004).

In sum, the results of the IRT analyses suggest that there is some difference in the item and test functioning of the PCL-R between males and females. However, given that these differences are relatively small and the effects of these differences on total PCL-R score are likely to be minimal, the authors argue that these results support PCL-R scalar equivalence across gender.

Correlates

Although many investigations have focused primarily on the structure and function of psychopathy measures, a number have also examined the generality of psychopathy correlates across gender. Such studies allow for comparisons of the psychopathy construct as it is assessed in women versus men.

Personality Correlates

Theoretical and empirical approaches to male psychopathy have historically placed great emphasis on the associations between psychopathy and the personality factors of constraint and socialization (e.g., Belmore & Quinsey, 1994; Benning, Patrick, Hicks, Blonigen, & Krueger, 2003; Hare, 1978). Research with incarcerated females has provided evidence that these important relations generalize across gender. In their sample of incarcerated female offenders, Vitale and colleagues (2002) found significant negative correlations between the PCL-R and scores on both the Socialization scale of the California Psychological Inventory (Gough, 1969) and the Constraint scale of the Multidimensional Personality Questionnaire (MPQ; Tellegen, 1982). Strachan (1993) also demonstrated a significant association between PCL-R scores and lower scores on the Socialization scale in a female offender sample. O'Connor (2001) reported that PCL-R total scores showed expected associations with trait scales on the MPQ, such as high aggressiveness, low social closeness, and low adherence to social norms (Traditionalism). Using partial correlations, he also found that Hare's (1991) original Factor 1 (F1) was associated with low anxiousness, but, unexpectedly, not with high dominance. Hare's original Factor 2 (F2) was associated with both higher negative emotionality and with lower constraint. These associations parallel, for the most part, those found among male prisoners (Patrick, 1994; Verona, Patrick, & Joiner, 2001).

Other studies have shown that psychopathy in female samples is associated with personality measures selected to reflect the glib, grandiose, callous, and unempathic characteristics emphasized in clinical descriptions of psychopathic individuals. For example, high PCL-R scores are associated with poor perspective taking (Rutherford et al., 1996; Strachan, 1993) and a lack of empathic concern (Rutherford et al., 1996) in women. Furthermore, Zagon and Jackson (1994) reported significant positive relations between SRP-II scores and measures of narcissism, social desirability, and lying and significant negative relations between SRP-II scores and anxiety in both male and female undergraduates. However, a negative relation between empathy and SRP-II scores was significant only for females. Forth and colleagues (1996) also reported that the PCL-R:SV was significantly positively correlated with self-ratings of arrogance and calculation and dominance and significantly negatively correlated with ratings of love and affection in both men and women, although PCL-R:SV scores were significantly negatively correlated with scores on the unassuming and ingenuous scales only in women.

On the basis of Cleckley's (1976) hypothesis that psychopathy entails an underlying deficit in emotion, Louth and colleagues (1998) examined the relation between psychopathy and alexithymia in a sample of female offenders. They found that the emotion deficits characteristic of F1 psychopathy were not related to alexithymia, as measured by the Alexithymia Scale (TAS; Taylor, Ryan, & Bagby, 1985); however, the antisocial and unstable behaviors comprising F2 were related to alexithymia. In contrast, in studies with male offenders, differences in physiological reactivity to emotional stimuli have more consistently been associated with PCL-R F1 (e.g., Patrick, Bradley, & Lang, 1993; Verona, Patrick, Curtin, Bradley, & Lang, 2004). These findings suggest that, despite some similarities, the emotion deficits characteristic of psychopathy and alexithymia are not synonymous. More broadly, associations between emotion and distinct facets of psychopathy may vary with the particular measure of emotion under investigation.

Taken together, these findings suggest that self-reported abnormalities in the expression and experience of emotion and empathy and deficits in self-control and socialization characterize both male and female psychopaths.

Behavioral Correlates

Studies with male samples have consistently revealed significant relations between PCL-R and the Youth Version (PCL:YV) scores and a variety of behavioral criterion measures, including poor treatment response, criminal behavior, poor institutional adjustment, alcoholism and recidivism (Catchpole & Gretton, 2003; Dolan & Doyle, 2000; Hare, 1999; Hemphill, Templeman, Hare, & Wong, 1998; Ogloff, Wong, & Greenwood, 1990; Walters, 2003). However, examinations of these variables in female samples have yielded less consistent results.

In a sample of female offenders, Salekin and colleagues (1997) reported a nonsignificant relation between PCL-R scores and the treatment rejection scale of the Personality Assessment Inventory (Morey, 1991). This finding runs counter to suggestions that psychopathic individuals may not benefit from treatment, and it raises the possibility of gender differences in treatment response. However, a distinction must be made between self-reported treatment motivation and actual treatment compliance. In their sample of 404 female substance abusers, Richards, Casey, and Lucente (2003) found that high PCL-R-assessed psychopathy predicted poor treatment response, including noncompliance, poor attendance, violent rule violations, and avoidance of urinalysis testing.

Research on the association between psychopathy and future violence in women has been similarly equivocal. On the one hand, higher PCL-R scores have been reliably associated with higher levels of prior violent and nonviolent criminal behavior in females, and with greater numbers of prior convictions for violent and nonviolent offenses (Strachan, 1993; Vitale et al., 2002), prior arrests (Rutherford et al., 1996; Weiler & Widom, 1996), and self-reported violence (Weiler & Widom, 1996). By contrast, in one of the few studies of psychopathy and recidivism in a female sample, Salekin, Rogers, Ustad, and Sewell (1998) concluded that when inmates were classified as psychopathic or nonpsychopathic on the basis of a cut score of 30 on the PCL-R, the classification accuracy of the PCL-R was "moderate to poor," with 90% of the women who recidivated being classified as nonpsychopathic, and 9% of the nonrecidivators classified as psychopathic. Furthermore, in prior male samples, both F1 and F2 were found to be significantly associated with recidivism. However, in Salekin and colleagues' female sample, only F1 showed a significant association with recidivism. Consistent with these weaker associations with future violence, Salekin and colleagues (1997) reported no significant associations between PCL-R scores and correctional officer ratings of female offenders' subsequent violent behavior, verbal aggression, and noncompliance in the prison institution.

The inconsistent findings across gender regarding the relation between psychopathy and criminal and violent behavior may reflect broader inconsistencies in the development of antisocial and aggressive behavior across gender. Conceptualizations and assessments of psychopathy often include a focus on violent and aggressive behavior and place particular emphasis on the presence of such behaviors in early childhood and adolescence. As discussed below, gender differences in the development of aggression across childhood and adolescence (e.g. Silverthorn & Frick, 1999) and in the types of aggression exhibited by girls and boys (Crick & Grotpeter, 1995) may contribute to differences in the baserates of psychopathy across gender as well as the construct's apparently less powerful prediction of violence in female than in male samples. The literature on differential manifestations of psychopathy and differences in its development is discussed in the next few sections.

CLINICAL PRESENTATION OF PSYCHOPATHY IN WOMEN

Diagnostic Comorbidity

Most studies have confirmed that incarcerated women experience higher rates of Axis I psychopathology compared to matched community women (Jordan, Schlenger, Fairbank, & Cadell, 1996; Teplin, Abram, & McClelland, 1996) and incarcerated men (Teplin, Abram, McClelland, Dulcan, & Mericle, 2002). However, in studies that have examined rates of various personality disorders in female offender samples, incarcerated women show *lower* rates of APD than male prisoners, and may be more likely than men in prison to be diagnosed with borderline personality disorder (BPD). For example, Hurley and Dunne (1991) reported approximately equal prevalence of APD and BPD (17–20%) among a sample of female Australian prisoners. Jordan and colleagues (1996) found that BPD was the most prevalent Axis II disorder (2-year prevalence of 28%) among North Carolina female felons, and the lifetime prevalence rate for APD was nearly 12% in this prison sample, which is similar to the rate of APD reported by Teplin and colleagues (1996) among female jail inmates.

Unfortunately, only a few studies have been conducted to examine the relationship between psychopathy per se, as opposed to criminality and incarceration more broadly, with other forms of psychopathology in women. In a recent study, Vitale and colleagues (2002) examined correlates of psychopathy in a large sample of female inmates and failed to find significant relationships between total scores on the PCL-R and scores on the Beck Depression Inventory, the Beck Anxiety Inventory, and the Symptom Checklist-90-R global functioning index. Piotrowski, Tusel, Sees, Banys, and Hall (1995) reported that high PCL-R scores were associated with an APD diagnosis, according to the Computerized Diagnostic Interview Schedule—Revised, among male but not female methadone patients. On the other hand, other researchers have found slightly different results when the factors of the PCL-R (F1 and F2) are examined separately. Warren and colleagues (2003) reported that F2 of the PCL-R was significantly correlated with all Cluster B personality disorders

(APD, BPD, histrionic and narcissistic personality) and paranoid personality disorder in their sample of female prisoners. The interpersonal–affective factor (F1), on the other hand, was negatively related to avoidant personality disorder, consistent with the idea that primary psychopathy involves tendencies toward social potency and extraversion in women as well as men (Patrick, 1995). Other research has shown positive relationships between PCL-R F2 and suicide risk in both men and women, whereas F1 is unrelated in men and negatively related to suicide attempts in women (Verona et al., 2001; Verona, Hicks, & Patrick, in press). In addition, consistent with prior findings in men (see Taylor & Lang, Chapter 25, this volume), O'Connor (2001) reported that whereas F2 was robustly and positively associated with both alcohol and drug abuse, F1 was not significantly related to drug abuse and was only weakly associated with alcohol abuse in female prisoners. These studies indicate that, for the most part, the types of disorders that show comorbidity with psychopathy are similar for men and women.

More recent work, however, has demonstrated differential relationships between psychopathy and comorbid psychopathology in men and women. Blonigen, Hicks, Kruger, Patrick, and Iacono (2005) examined etiological associations between facets of psychopathy and broad spectra of psychopathology (internalizing, externalizing) in a large sample of adolescent twins from the community. They reported that traits related to F1 showed a positive genetic correlation with externalizing syndromes in male but not female participants, whereas F2-related traits showed a positive genetic correlation with internalizing syndromes in females but not males. This study provides preliminary evidence that genetic liabilities associated with different elements of the psychopathy construct may confer risk for different forms of psychopathology in women versus men.

In summary, women with criminal histories (i.e., who are incarcerated) tend to experience a larger range of Axis I symptoms and disorders than do their male counterparts, are diagnosed most often with BPD, and show rates of APD (10–20%) that for the most part are lower than that reported in male prisoners (40–60%; see Hare, 1991; Widiger et al., 1996). On the other hand,

patterns of comorbidity associated with psychopathy, per se, in women appear similar in many ways to those for men. The DSM disorders that co-occur most often with psychopathy in women are APD and other Cluster B personality disorders including BPD and histrionic personality, and this association is particularly marked for PCL-R F2. In contrast, the affective–interpersonal factor (F1) of the PCL-R typically shows a negative association with internalizing psychopathology and suicidal behavior in women. In addition, the findings of a recent behavior genetic study (Blonigen et al., 2005) provide some evidence that underlying dispositions toward psychopathy may be expressed differently in women than in men, with stronger links between F2 and Axis I mood–anxiety symptoms in women than men. The next section reviews other available data that speak to differential manifestations of psychopathy in women and men.

Differential Manifestations of Psychopathy in Women versus Men

A vivid illustration of how psychopathy may be manifested differently in women comes from the Hollywood portrayal of an obsessively violent woman in the 1987 movie *Fatal Attraction*. Glenn Close's character in that movie exhibits psychopathic-like traits, including lack of empathy, manipulation, impulsivity, and violence; however, unlike most men who exhibit such traits, this female character manifested these traits in an effort to prevent abandonment by a romantic partner (and thus most clinicians would have diagnosed her as having BPD). In an empirical demonstration, Robbins, Monahan, and Silver (2003) found that although female and male psychiatric patients showed comparable rates of violence at postinstitutionalization, there were gender differences in the situational correlates of the violent behavior. Relative to men, the women tended to be violent in the home and toward family members, inflicted significantly less serious injury, and were less often arrested following their violent behavior. Consistent with these data, Goldstein, Powers, McCusker, and Mundt (1996) reported that women diagnosed with APD were more likely than APD men to be irresponsible as parents, to engage in prostitution, and to have been physically violent against sex partners and children. These data emphasize differences in the context in which the same underlying propensity (violence and antisocial traits) is manifested in men and women: The interpersonal context and the family become the major focus of women's mental health problems.

In this regard, some psychopathy researchers have advanced the view that certain disorders that are diagnosed more commonly in women, including BPD, histrionic personality disorder (HPD), and somatization disorder (SD), may represent female expressions of psychopathy (Lilienfeld, 1992). Early on, Cloninger and Guze (1970a, 1970b) reported that sociopathy in male family members was common among women diagnosed with hysteria, and that 40% of diagnosed sociopathic women received an additional diagnosis of hysteria. Subsequently, Cloninger and Guze (1973) reported that the male relatives of convicted women were more often diagnosed with sociopathy than the female relatives (31% vs. 11%, respectively), and hysteria was often diagnosed among the female relatives. Based on the familial clustering of sociopathy and hysteria, Cloninger, Reich, and Guze (1975) successfully tested a model that suggested that female hysteria, male sociopathy, and female sociopathy are increasingly severe expressions of the same vulnerability. In addition, adoption studies by Cadoret (1978) and colleagues (Cadoret, Cunningham, Loftus, & Edwards, 1978) confirmed the genetic association between hysteria and sociopathy. It should be noted that in these studies, "sociopathy" was defined mostly in terms of the behavioral features of the syndrome, including engaging in criminal and aggressive behaviors.

Recently, Lilienfeld, Van Valkenburg, Larntz, and Akiskal (1986) reported significant within-person associations between APD, SD, and HPD, and a high prevalence of APD in the families of patients with SD. In a more recent study that used the PPI to index psychopathy, Hamburger, Lilienfeld, and Hogben (1996) reported that college men showed a significantly stronger association between PPI psychopathy and APD, whereas psychopathy was more strongly related to HPD among college women. This study is notable because there is evidence that the PPI taps the affective–interpersonal component of psychopathy as well as the antisocial deviance component (Benning et al., 2003). Lilienfeld and Hess (2001) also reported that gender moderated the relationship between secondary psychopathy (akin to PCL-R F2) and somatization among university students, with women showing a stronger relationship than men. On the other hand, other work has failed to replicate these findings (Cale & Lilienfeld, 2002a; Wilson et al., 1999). In addition, Salekin and colleagues (1997) found that SD was actually negatively associated with psychopathy, assessed via the PCL-R, in a sample of female jail inmates. They also reported substantial discriminant validity for psychopathy and BPD and moderate discriminant validity for psychopathy and HPD.

To summarize, the data indicate that there is substantial familial and intraindividual overlap between APD, SD, and other Cluster B personality disorders, such as BPD and HPD, in women, potentially indicating gender differences in manifestations of vulnerability for general antisocial behavior. On the other hand, gender differences have not consistently been found when using measures designed to index psychopathy rather than antisocial deviance, and where positive findings have been obtained in studies of this kind, effect sizes have been quite small (Lilienfeld & Hess, 2001). In addition, most recent work has used self-report measures of psychopathy with college student and nonclinical participants who, for the most part, have low levels of psychopathology. Researchers can help clarify mixed findings by examining relationships between the separate facets of psychopathy (antisocial, impulsive, affective, and interpersonal) and various other diagnostic conditions in women (Lilienfeld & Hess, 2001). For example, Wilson and colleagues (1999) and Lilienfeld and Hess (2001) reported that measures of primary psychopathy (i.e., F1) were negatively related to SD, whereas measures of secondary psychopathy (i.e., F2) were positively related to SD. Thus, BPD, SD, or HPD may represent gender-specific manifestations of underlying risk for externalizing or disinhibitory problems (however, see Wilson et al., 1999, for negative findings). On the other hand, the emotional–interpersonal features relevant to primary psychopathy may have similar manifestations in men and women. The idea of gender differences in manifestation of general externalizing psychopathology is supported by the literature on differences in the development of antisocial and aggressive traits in girls and boys, which is discussed next.

GENDER DIFFERENCES IN THE DEVELOPMENT OF PSYCHOPATHY

Examinations of antisocial behavior in males have reliably identified two developmental pathways. Specifically, antisocial adolescent boys with a history of early-onset conduct problems differ from antisocial adolescent boys with no childhood history of conduct problems in that the former exhibit higher levels of callous–unemotional personality traits, greater diversity of criminal behaviors, poorer impulse control (Moffitt, 2003; see also Frick & Marsee, Chapter 18, this volume). Early-onset cases are also more likely to be labeled psychopaths in adulthood (Lahey & Loeber, 1994; Lynam, 1996). In their attempts to generalize these findings to females, Silverthorn and colleagues (Silverthorn & Frick, 1999; Silverthorn, Frick, & Reynolds, 2001) have found that, in contrast to males, childhood-onset conduct problems are rare among females. However, there is a subgroup of females whose *adolescent*-onset conduct problems resemble those exhibited by the early-onset males in that they show similar deficits in impulse control, heightened levels of callous and unemotional personality traits, and diversity in the types of antisocial behaviors in which they engage. Furthermore, like boys with early-onset CD, girls exhibiting the "delayed-onset" pattern are more likely be classified as psychopathic. On the basis of these findings, a delayed-onset pathway for conduct problems in girls has been proposed (Silverthorn & Frick, 1999; Silverthorn et al., 2001).

This conceptualization is bolstered by research examining the relations between CD, APD, and the interpersonal/emotional and behavioral factors of psychopathy in adult males and females. In a sample of adult male and female substance abusers, Rutherford, Alterman, Cacciola, and McKay (1998) found no difference between men and women in the correlation between total PCL-R scores and an APD diagnosis. However,

among men, childhood symptoms of APD were significantly related to F1 scores, whereas this was not the case for women. Thus, in this sample, childhood criminal involvement, rule breaking, and aggression seemed more predictive of primary psychopathy among men than among women.

However, these differences may be due partly to the types of antisocial behaviors chosen for study. Many aggression researchers have argued that males and females differ more in the quality of their aggressive behavior (i.e., specific forms engaged in) than in the quantity of their aggressive behavior. For example, Bjorkqvist and colleagues (Bjorkqvist, Osterman, & Kaukianen, 1992; Lagerspetz, Bjorkqvist, & Peltonen, 1988) have found that although men and boys are generally more likely to engage in overt forms of aggression (e.g., kicking, hitting, and punching) than women and girls, females are more likely than males to utilize covert forms of aggression involving the manipulation of their social network (e.g., gossip, refusal of friendship, and ostracism). The term "relational aggression" has been used to refer to these behaviors, which aim to cause harm by disenfranchising the victim from the social group (Crick & Grotpeter, 1995), and although relational aggression can be detected in both males and females, it is more common among females (Bjorkqvist et al., 1992; Lagerspetz et al., 1988).

There is evidence that relational aggression in women represents an alternative manifestation of antisocial traits. Grotpeter and Crick (1996) reported that relationally aggressive children seem to engage in highly intimate friendships that involve high levels of jealousy and exclusivity, and that these children also exhibit high levels of relational aggression *within* these friendships. In contrast, overtly aggressive children tend to aggress against children outside their friendship group. Werner and Crick (1999) found that relational aggression in college women predicted high levels of peer rejection, antisocial behavior, stimulus seeking, egocentricity, a number of BPD-related symptoms, and bulimic symptomatology. In men, relational aggression predicted peer rejection and egocentricity only.

In summary, preliminary evidence suggests that the antisocial behaviors associated with adult psychopathy and APD may differ between men and women both in their time course and in their specific manifestation (Rutherford et al., 1998), with important implications for the assessment of psychopathy across gender. Specifically, whereas early-onset antisocial behavior is associated with psychopathy in males (Frick & Marsee, Chapter 18, this volume; Salekin, Chapter 20, this volume), these behaviors may not emerge until adolescence in females. Furthermore, when these antisocial and aggressive behaviors do emerge, they may manifest differently across gender (e.g., Crick & Grotpeter, 1995). Such findings provide further impetus for evaluating psychopathy in women using other behavioral indicators.

PUTATIVE ETIOLOGICAL FACTORS

In the next few sections, we review existing research that has examined etiological processes that may contribute to the emergence of psychopathy in women.

Hormones and Neurotransmitters

Hormonal and neurochemical differences between men and women may be one important factor contributing to the differential prevalence of antisocial personality and psychopathy across the genders. Olweus, Mattson, Schalling, and Low (1988), for example, reported significant correlations between levels of testosterone and provoked aggression in men. In regard to the effects of androgens on women's behaviors, Benton (1992) reviewed the literature on characteristics associated with adrenogenital syndrome (AGS; also known as congenital adrenal hyperplasia), a condition which results from a recessive gene that induces the adrenal gland to produce abnormally high levels of androgens rather than cortisone. AGS girls tend to be "tomboys" and display many male characteristics, such as increased rough-and-tumble play activity (Meyer-Bahlburg & Ehrhardt, 1982); however, they do not display a tendency toward higher levels of aggression during adulthood compared to non-AGS girls (Benton, 1992). Similarly, a follow-up study of girls who had been exposed prenatally to diethylstilbestrol, a synthetic progestogen, revealed no differences in childhood play behavior or aggressiveness,

based on retrospective self-report, between these girls and nonexposed ("well") women (Lish, Meyer-Bahlburg, Erhardt, Travis, & Veridiano, 1992). Thus, abnormally high levels of androgens in girls appear to be associated with more male-typical behaviors during childhood, but socialization and developmental processes may override these effects in the long term.

Based on this previous work and on work by Ellis (1989), Baumgardner (1993) reported that higher PCL scores in female inmates were related to measures of sexual orientation and masculine gender identity, with predominance of left-handedness, and with right-hemisphere mediated skills—all of which are purportedly influenced by androgen effects on brain development. He interpreted these findings as indicating a role of androgen-influenced neurocognitive processes in the development of psychopathy in women, although other predicted associations were nonsignificant or contrary to predictions. Unfortunately, his research did not involve the actual measurement of hormones in these women, which would provide more direct evidence of a relation between hormone levels and PCL-R scores in women. In other work, however, van Honk and colleagues (1999, 2004) reported that women with high levels of testosterone or those given a single administration of testosterone exhibited enhanced vigilance to angry faces, as well as psychopathic-like deficits in decision making in the Bechara gambling task (i.e., relative insensitivity to punishment cues and higher reward dependence). These studies, however, did not involve the direct measurement of psychopathy in women.

With regard to neurochemistry, human studies have demonstrated reliable relationships between dysregulated serotonin (5-HT) neurotransmitter functioning and aggression, alcoholism, and criminality (see reviews by Roy, Virkkunen, & Linnoila, 1990; Minzenberg & Siever, Chapter 13, this volume). Most of this research has been conducted in men and has demonstrated that individuals exhibiting externalizing forms of psychopathology exhibit lower levels of blood platelet and central nervous system 5-HT. However, preliminary evidence suggests gender differences in the relationship between serotonin dysregulation and impulsivity (Soloff, Kelly, Strotmeyer, Malone, &

Mann, 2003), negative affect/neuroticism (Du, Bakish, & Hrdina, 2000), and anger/aggression (Manuck et al., 1999). For example, nonexperimental studies have shown that 5-HT functioning is more robustly related to aggression and impulsivity in men than in women (Manuck et al., 1999), and a recent laboratory study (Verona, Joiner, Johnson, & Bender, in press) found that the 5-HT transporter gene was related to increases in stress-induced aggression in men but not women. In a related vein, recent data indicate that the transporter gene for monoamine oxidase A (MAOA), an enzyme that metabolizes neurotransmitters including 5-HT and that has been tied to aggressive antisocial behavior in men (e.g., Samochowiec et al., 1999), is linked to mood disorders in women but not men (Hauser et al., 2002).

These gender differences could arise in part from the fact that female sex hormones, particularly estrogen, increase the density of certain 5-HT receptor sites and serotonin transporters in the brain (Fink, Sumner, Rosie, Wilson, & McQueen, 1999), which in turn may lead to greater efficiency in 5-HT neurotransmission in women as compared to men. One implication of this perspective is that the effects of sex hormones on serotonergic pathways may partly account for gender differences in antisociality and aggression. A second implication is that genotypic risk conferred by serotonin-related alleles may manifest itself more in terms of externalizing psychopathology (aggression and antisocial behavior) in men, and as internalizing psychopathology (depression and anxiety) in women.

In summary, although neurobiological contributions to aggression and antisocial behavior are well established in men, less research has been conducted on the neurobiological bases of externalizing behaviors in women. The few existing studies reviewed here provide limited support for the claim that male hormones are linked to aggression and other forms of antisocial behavior in women, and the weight of evidence indicates that there are gender differences in the role of 5-HT in aggressive and antisocial behavior. Although some research exists on associations between hormone/neurotransmitter levels and established measures of psychopathy in men (see Minzenberg & Siever, Chapter 13, this volume), no such studies have been conducted

with women, and there are no data comparing men and women in terms of such associations. Research of this kind represents an important priority for the future.

Genetic and Environmental Etiological Influences

As described by Waldman and Rhee (Chapter 11, this volume), the review of twin studies examining the heritability of general antisocial, criminal, and aggressive behaviors have failed to reveal clear gender differences. However, findings suggesting no gender differences in the heritability of antisocial and aggressive behaviors run contrary to the polygenic multiple threshold model, which suggests that sociopaths are on the extreme of a normal distribution whose genetic component is (1) polygenic and (2) to a large degree sex-limited (Cloninger et al., 1975; Cloninger, Christiansen, Reich, & Gottesman, 1978). Thus, women who do express psychopathic features must have greater dose or genetic load than males who express the trait.

In support of this, the Stockholm adoption study (Bohman, Cloninger, Sigvardsson, & von Knorring, 1982) indicated that the biological parents of adopted women with criminal histories were more likely to have repeated convictions than parents of adopted men. In addition, Baker, Mack, Moffitt, and Mednick (1989) found that offspring of female sociopaths were at greater risk for developing the syndrome than offspring of male sociopaths. On the other hand, family studies that have examined environmental and genetic liability for antisocial behavior show that familial influences to the development of antisocial personality are largely the same in men and women (Cloninger et al., 1978). Thus, adoption and family studies produce mixed findings in terms of differences in the magnitude of liability for sociopathy between men and women. Rhee and Waldman (2002) cautioned that the fact that females may need more liability (either genetic or environmental) to express antisocial behavior does not mean that genetic influences are of greater magnitude in females than males.

Only one twin study has been conducted that reports on gender differences in the heritability of psychopathy, using a measure of the construct that taps into the antisocial deviance and interpersonal–affective features. Based on results from a prior study (Benning et al., 2003), Blonigen and colleagues (2005) used scale scores on the MPQ (Tellegen, 1982) to estimate participants' scores on Lilienfeld's PPI, composed of two factors, Fearless Dominance (akin to PCL-R F1) and Impulsive Antisociality (akin to PCL-R F2). Twin data analyses revealed no sex differences in the magnitude of estimates of genetic and environmental influences on total psychopathy or the two factors. However, unpublished preliminary data from the Florida State Twin Registry (Taylor, 2004) indicate that psychopathy, as measured by the Minnesota Temperament Inventory (MTI), appears to be more influenced by shared environmental than additive genetic factors in young women. However, these data are questionable, given a very small sample of twins, and due to the fact that the MTI may not be the best proxy for self-reported psychopathy.

In summary, there are too few studies, using suboptimal measures of psychopathy, to make firm conclusions on gender differences in etiological influences on psychopathy or its different facets. Next, we describe evidence for the influence of environmental adversity in the development of psychopathy in women and men.

Adverse Background and Childhood Abuse

Research suggests that antisocial deviance and incarceration in women, as compared to men, may be more strongly associated with experiences of severe social and familial dysfunction (Mulder, Wells, Joyce, & Bushnell, 1994), even though women have lower rates of unlawful behavior (see also Cloninger & Guze, 1970b). Evidence also points to higher rates of abuse, particularly sexual abuse, among incarcerated women versus men (26% vs. 5%, respectively; McClellan, Farabee, & Crouch, 1997).

Researchers have, thus, compared the influence of childhood adversity and family background on the development of externalizing problems in men and women. McClellan and colleagues (1997) reported that early victimization was associated with a greater risk of adult substance abuse/de-

pendence among female than male inmates. Capaldi and Clark (1998) found that childhood family experiences were more predictive of female than male perpetration of intimate partner violence, and Magdol, Moffitt, Caspi, and Silva (1998) suggested that early family relations were more important in predicting partner violence for women than for men perpetrators. In a prospective study, White and Widom (2003) found that, controlling for demographic and familial variables, childhood abuse and neglect significantly predicted APD diagnosis in men but not other types of externalizing behavior such as early aggression, alcohol problems, and hostility. However, in women, abuse and neglect significantly predicted all forms of externalizing behavior except early aggression. These results may be partly attributable to the fact that when girls are victimized, they suffer more severe levels of abuse and are more likely to be sexually abused than boys (McClellan et al., 1997). Nonetheless, abuse experiences in women seem to predict higher levels of externalizing maladjustment than they do in men.

With regard to the prediction of psychopathy as measured by the PCL-R, Weiler and Widom (1996) reported that although victims of childhood abuse and/or neglect had significantly higher PCL-R scores than did nonabused controls, no gender differences in these relationships were found. Verona, Hicks, and Patrick (in press) found that, among a sample of female federal prisoners, a history of childhood physical and sexual abuse was associated with PCL-R F2 scores, but not to PCL-R F1 scores when F2 was partialed out. No men were included in this sample, so the authors could not compare the magnitude of the association between abuse and psychopathy in men versus women.

In summary, the fact that sexual abuse may be more predictive of psychopathological outcomes than physical abuse (Bryant & Range, 1995), and that girls are more likely to suffer from sexual abuse (and more severe forms of sexual abuse) than boys (McClelland et al., 1997), may suggest that sexual abuse may play an important role in the development of antisocial deviance and other forms of psychopathology in women relative to men. This hypothesis is mostly corroborated by existing evidence from studies on the effects of abuse on general antisociality and externalizing outcomes (Capaldi & Clark, 1998; White & Widom, 2003), although most have not been prospective studies. Unfortunately, minimal data are available for evaluating gender differences in the relationship between abuse and psychopathy as defined by established inventories such as the PCL-R and the PPI.

Laboratory Findings: Affective, Attentional, and Behavioral Deficits

Laboratory research with male participants (prisoners in particular) has revealed consistent deficits in specific emotional, attentional, and regulatory processes among psychopaths. The following section reviews findings from parallel studies with women.

Affective Processing Deficits

In view of Cleckley's (1976) observation that psychopaths lack the normal range and depth of emotion, numerous studies have been conducted to assess deficits in affective responding among psychopathic compared with nonpsychopathic individuals (see Fowles & Dindo, Chapter 2, and Blair, Chapter 15, this volume). Although most of these studies have involved male participants, some recent studies have been conducted with women.

Sutton, Vitale, and Newman (2002) examined acoustic startle reactions during viewing of emotional and neutral pictures in female prisoners. Consistent with previous findings for men (Levenston, Patrick, Bradley, & Lang, 2000; Patrick et al., 1993), women with high scores on the PCL-R, particularly those scoring low in trait anxiety, showed lesser startle potentiation (defined as augmentation of the startle reflex during unpleasant vs. neutral picture viewing) than women with low scores on the PCL-R; and reduced startle potentiation was associated with high scores on F1 but not F2. Nonetheless, psychopathic women did not show significant *inhibition* of the startle response to unpleasant relative to neutral pictures, as has been observed in male psychopaths (Patrick et al., 1993). Similarly, Patrick, Verona, and Sullivan (2000) reported that female inmates scoring high on the PCL-R showed decreased startle potentiation in comparison to non-

psychopaths, but again, the pattern among psychopaths was one of lesser potentiation for unpleasant versus neutral pictures rather than inhibition of startle for unpleasant pictures. However, within the psychopath group, those with the highest global ratings of psychopathy according to Cleckley's (1976) original criteria (i.e., those who matched the Cleckley prototype of the psychopath most closely) showed startle inhibition for both pleasant and unpleasant pictures, paralleling results reported for men in Patrick and colleagues (1993).

A further study by Lorenz and Newman (2002) that examined emotional facilitation in a lexical-decision task is worthy of mention here, although it focused on APD diagnosis in prisoners rather than PCL-R psychopathy. Unlike psychopathic men in prior research, who showed negligible facilitation for emotional versus neutral words (Williamson, Harpur, & Hare, 1991), incarcerated men with APD in this study did not differ from non-APD incarcerated men in their reaction times to emotional versus neutral words on this task. Importantly, incarcerated women with APD demonstrated *more* facilitation to the emotional words (both positive and negative) than non-APD incarcerated women. In addition, greater emotion facilitation among APD women was associated with higher levels of violent crimes committed, whereas the reverse was true for non-APD women (i.e., increased emotion facilitation was related to fewer violent crimes). These results indicate that the diagnosis of APD (which is strongly and selectively related to PCL-R F2; Hare, 1991, 2003) is not associated with emotional reactivity deficits; if anything, it may be associated with heightened negative affectivity reactivity, which in turn may dispose toward increased behavioral reactivity in the form of violence (Sher & Trull, 1994; Verona et al., 2001).

In summary, studies of psychopathy and emotional reactivity in women have yielded findings that parallel those reported in men: Reduced negative emotional reactivity and low levels of anxiety are associated with PCL-R F1 (Patrick, 1994), whereas PCL-R F2 is linked to increased negative emotionality and aggression (Verona et al., 2001). In addition, although psychopathy group differences in defensive startle responses were observed in women, the effects were not as robust as what has been reported in men (i.e., no startle inhibition to unpleasant pictures was observed in psychopathic women). Instead, findings from Patrick and colleagues (2000) suggest that this more deviant startle modulation pattern characterizes a distinct subset of psychopathic women, and that among female offenders the PCL-R may be less discriminating of this subset than the original Cleckley diagnostic criteria.

Attentional and Behavioral Abnormalities

A substantial body of research with male offenders has revealed attentional abnormalities in high-psychopathy individuals (cf. Hiatt & Newman, Chapter 17, this volume). Only a few studies have examined these attentional and behavioral responses in girls or women with psychopathy and related syndromes; however, results have been relatively consistent across them.

Segarra, Molto, and Torrubia (2000) found that extraverted women did not differ from introverted women in their reaction times during a passive avoidance task involving reward and punishment cues, a finding inconsistent with previous work on men (Patterson & Newman, 1993). Segarra and colleagues (2000) speculated that these results relate to gender differences in the functioning and degree of activation of the behavioral inhibition and behavioral activation systems. MacCoon and Newman (2004) also failed to find differences between high- and low-impulsive female inmates on a passive avoidance task, although anxious inmates did show greater passive avoidance errors than low anxious inmates. These authors suggested that anxiety, rather than impulsivity, predicts poor passive avoidance in Caucasian female prisoners. Similarly, Dougherty, Bjork, Huckable, Moeller, and Swann (1999) failed to find significant differences between BPD and non-BPD diagnosed women in their responses to laboratory tasks involving delay of gratification. However, Hochhausen, Lorenz, and Newman (2002) reported that BPD female offenders committed more passive avoidance errors on a go/no-go task than did non-BPD female offenders.

With regard to PCL-R assessed psychopathy, Vitale and Newman (2001a) examined the performance of 112 incarcerated women on a card-playing task previously used to demonstrate disinhibition in psychopathic men. They found, contrary to prediction but consistent with findings among impulsive females reported earlier, that psychopathic women did not exhibit perseverative responding on this task. In a follow-up study, Vitale and colleagues (2004) examined both selective attention and behavioral inhibition (or passive avoidance deficits) in a community sample of adolescents assessed for psychopathic traits using Frick's Antisocial Processes Screening Device (APSD; Frick & Hare, 2001). Girls as well as boys with psychopathic traits showed attentional abnormalities (lack of interference from irrelevant peripheral cues) in a picture–word Stroop task. On the other hand, only psychopathic boys showed behavioral disinhibition (increased passive avoidance errors) on a go/no-go task.

Thus, from the few studies conducted, it appears that although female psychopathy is also associated with attentional deficits, there is less evidence for response perseveration or behavioral disinhibition among women with psychopathic or related traits. Given that girls and women in these studies were targeted due to disinhibited and impulsive behaviors (i.e., the psychopath group), the assessment strategies and experimental tasks commonly used to measure response perseveration in psychopaths may not adequately tap into the underlying mechanisms associated with real-life psychopathic behaviors in females. Further studies, and perhaps newer technologies, are needed to resolve these differential findings involving response modulation and impulsivity in women as compared to men.

CONCLUSIONS AND FUTURE DIRECTIONS

There are some important conclusions to be made based on the review of the literature on female psychopathy. The first point is that the available evidence indicates slightly lower rates of psychopathy in women, in both self-report and interview-based assessments. The second major consideration is that although sex biases by diagnosticians may in part account for gender differences in baserates, data from diverse domains of study (including developmental, laboratory, and psychiatric research) suggest that these baserate differences also reflect distinct behavioral manifestations of antisociality in women versus men. For example, studies comparing male and female offenders have revealed salient differences in the expression of psychopathy among women, including less evidence of early behavior problems (Rutherford et al., 1998; Silverthorn & Frick, 1999); less evidence of overtly violent/aggressive symptoms (Crick & Grotpeter, 1995); higher rates of BPD, HPD, or somatization (Cloninger & Guze, 1970a, 1970b; Lilienfeld, 1992); and more evidence of sexual misbehavior such as prostitution (Robins, 1966).

We can also conclude, based on available assessment, comorbidity, and laboratory data on women, that the interpersonal–affective traits of the PCL-R are validly captured by current conceptualizations and measurements of psychopathy. For example, limited laboratory data suggest that abnormalities in emotional responding (associated with F1) theorized to contribute to psychopathy syndromes in males also underlie psychopathy in females. On the other hand, the processes underlying behavioral symptoms (e.g., impulsiveness and disinhibition) of psychopathy, as measured in the laboratory, appear to differ in men and women. In addition, some of the behavioral features (including early behavior problems and disinhibition) of psychopathy may be less pronounced in women than men, and emotional reactivity and mood–anxiety may be more strongly associated with antisocial (F2) traits in women than men. It is likely that although men and women have similar underlying deficits (emotional and attentional), these are manifested differently across the genders, or the measures currently available to assess disinhibition in the laboratory are inadequate in tapping into real-life psychopathic behaviors in women.

Does this mean that adjustments should be made to assessment instruments to better reflect gender differences in the manifestation of psychopathy? Studies conducted on the PCL-R suggest that the instrument shows adequate reliability and validity, and psychopathy is related to similar personality indices in men and women. On the other hand, the PCL-R does not do as well in predicting vio-

lence and is not associated with childhood conduct problems and aggression in women. There is indeed skepticism as to whether the PCL-R items adequately tap the characteristics that best discriminate psychopathic from nonpsychopathic women (Salekin et al., 1997; Vitale & Newman, 2001a); from this perspective, assessment strategies among women may need to be modified. One approach may be to include other indicators of psychopathy that tap uniquely female expressions of antisocial–externalizing tendencies (F2), such as prostitution, intimate partner violence, abuse and neglect of children, comorbid psychopathology (e.g., histrionic personality and somatization), and relational forms of aggression such as friendship betrayal and "backbiting."

It is not atypical for a comprehensive review to call for "future research" in a particular area, and this chapter is no exception. However, this research should not take place in a theoretical vacuum. To date, far more emphasis has been placed on generalizing findings from the male psychopathy literature to female psychopathy, but less conceptually motivated work, such as testing theoretically derived predictions concerning gender differences in the syndrome, has been conducted. Psychopathy research with male samples has yielded findings of greatest impact when it has been conducted and interpreted in relation to specific theories (e.g., tests of the low-fear hypothesis, specific hypotheses involving amygdala dysfunction, tests of the response modulation hypothesis). Discrepancies in patterns of findings between males and females may have different meanings for theorists from one theoretical perspective versus another.

Relatedly, we should begin applying the corpus of research on socialization influences, sex roles, and biological–developmental differences between genders to developing uniquely female theories of psychopathic and antisocial behavior. These theories can then be tested with innovative paradigms involving more female-relevant contexts (e.g., the interpersonal domain) and using alternative indicators of psychopathy that are specifically relevant to women (e.g., relational aggression). Simply put, a call for "more research" is insufficient; what is needed is more theory development, testing, and refinement that accommodate what is known about gender differences in developmental processes, temperament, biology, and socialization.

REFERENCES

Alterman, A. I., Cacciola, J. S., & Rutherford, M. J. (1993). Reliability of the Revised Psychopathy Checklist in substance abuse populations. *Psychological Assessment, 5*, 442–448.

Baker, L. A., Mack, W., Moffitt, T., & Mednick, S. (1989). Sex differences in property crime in a Danish adoption cohort. *Behavior Genetics, 16*, 127–142.

Baumgardner, T. L. (1993). *Neurobehavioral correlates of psychopathy in female inmates: Support for the contribution of prenatal androgens.* Unpublished doctoral dissertation, California School of Professional Psychology, Fresno.

Belmore, M. F., & Quinsey, V. L. (1994). Correlation of psychopathy in a noninstitutional sample. *Journal of Interpersonal Violence, 9*, 339–349.

Benning, S. D., Patrick, C. J., Hicks, B. M., Blonigen, D. M., & Krueger, R. F. (2003). Factor structure of the Psychopathic Personality Inventory: Validity and implications for clinical assessment. *Psychological Assessment, 15*, 340–350.

Benton, D. (1992). Hormones and human aggression. In K. Bjorkqvist & P. Niemela (Eds.), *Of mice and women: Aspects of female aggression* (pp. 37–46). San Diego, CA: Academic Press.

Bjorkqvist, K., Osterman, K., & Kaukiainen, A. (1992). The development of direct and indirect aggressive strategies in males and females. In K. Bjorkqvist & P. Niemela (Eds.), *Of mice and women: Aspects of female aggression* (pp. 51–64). San Diego, CA: Academic Press.

Blonigen, D. M., Hicks, B. M., Krueger, R. F., Patrick, C. J., & Iacono, W. G. (2005). Psychopathic personality traits: Heritability and genetic overlap with internalizing and externalizing psychopathology. *Psychological Medicine, 35*, 1–12.

Bohman, M., Cloninger, C. R., Sigvardsson, S., & von Knorring, A.-L. (1982). Predisposition to petty criminality in Swedish adoptees: I. Genetic and environment heterogeneity. *Archives of General Psychiatry, 39*, 1233–1241.

Bolt, D., Hare, R. D., Vitale, J. E., & Newman, J. P. (2004). A multigroup item response theory analysis of the Psychopathy Checklist—Revised. *Psychological Assessment, 16*(2), 155–168.

Bradley, M. M., Codispoti, M., Sabatinelli, D., & Lang, P. J. (2001). Emotion and motivation II: Sex differences in picture processing. *Emotion, 1*, 300–319.

Bryant, S. L., & Range, L. M. (1995). Suicidality in college women who were sexually and physically abused and physically punished by parents. *Violence and Victims, 10*, 195–201.

Cadoret, R. J. (1978). Psychopathology in adopted-away offspring of biologic parents with antisocial behavior. *Archives of General Psychiatry, 35*, 176–184.

Cadoret, R. J., Cunninghman, L., Loftus, R., & Edwards, J. (1976). Studies of adoptees from psychiatrically disturbed biological parents: III. Medical symptoms and illnesses in childhood and adolescence. *American Journal of Psychiatry, 133*, 1316–1318.

Cale, E. M., & Lilienfeld, S. O. (2002a). Histrionic personality disorder and antisocial personality disorder: Sex-differentiated manifestations of psychopathy? *Journal of Personality Disorders, 16*, 52–72.

Cale, E. M., & Lilienfeld, S. O. (2002b). Sex differences in psychopathy and antisocial personality: A review and integration. *Clinical Psychology Review, 22*, 1179–1207.

Capaldi, D. M., & Clark, S. (1998). Prospective family predictors of aggression toward female partners for at-risk young men. *Developmental Psychology, 34*, 1175–1188.

Carver, C. S., & White, T. L. (1994). Behavioral inhibition, behavioral activation, and affective responses to impending reward and punishment: The BIS/BAS Scales. *Journal of Personality and Social Psychology, 67*, 319–333.

Catchpole, R. E. H., & Gretton, H. M. (2003). The predictive validity of risk assessment with violent young offenders: A 1-year examination of criminal outcome. *Criminal Justice and Behavior, 30*, 688–708.

Cleckley, H. (1976). *The mask of sanity* (5th ed.). St. Louis, MO: Mosby.

Cloninger, C. R., Christiansen, K. O., Reich, T., & Gottesman, I. I. (1978). Implications of sex differences in the prevalences of antisocial personality, alcoholism, and criminality for familial transmission. *Archives of General Psychiatry, 35*, 941–951.

Cloninger, C. R., & Guze, S. B. (1970a). Female criminals: Their personal, familial, and social backgrounds. *Archives of General Psychiatry, 23*, 554–558.

Cloninger, C. R., & Guze, S. B. (1970b). Psychiatric illness and female criminality: The role of sociopathy and hysteria in the antisocial woman. *American Journal of Psychiatry, 127*, 303–311.

Cloninger, C. R., & Guze, S. B. (1973). Psychiatric illness in the families of female criminals: A study of 288 first-degree relatives. *British Journal of Psychiatry, 122*, 697–703.

Cloninger, C. R., Reich, T., & Guze, S. B. (1975). The multifactorial model of disease transmission: II. Sex differences in the familia transmission of sociopathy (antisocial personality). *British Journal of Psychiatry, 127*, 11–22.

Cooke, D. J., & Michie, C. (2001). Refining the construct of psychopathy: Towards a hierarchical model. *Psychological Assessment, 13*, 171–188.

Cooney, N. L., Kadden, R. M., & Litt, M. D. (1990). A comparison of methods for assessing sociopathy in male and female alcoholics. *Journal of Studies on Alcohol, 51,* 42–48.

Crick, N. R., & Grotpeter, J. K. (1995). Relational aggression, gender, and social-psychological adjustment. *Child Development, 66,* 710–722.

Dolan, M., & Doyle, M. (2000). Violence risk prediction: Clinical and actuarial measures and the role of the Psychopathy Checklist. *British Journal of Psychiatry, 177,* 303–311.

Dougherty, D. M., Bjork, J. M., Huckabee, H. C. G., Moeller, F. G., & Swann, A. C. (1999). Laboratory measures of aggression and impulsivity in women with borderline personality disorder. *Psychiatry Research, 85,* 315–326.

Du, L., Bakish, D., & Hrdina, P. D. (2000). Gender differences in association between serotonin transporter gene polymorphism and personality traits. *Psychiatric Genetics, 10,* 159–164.

Ellis, L. (1989). Sex hormones, r/K selection, and victimful criminality. *Mankind Quarterly, 29,* 329–340.

Fabes, R. A., & Eisenberg, N. (1992). Young children's coping with interpersonal anger. *Child Development, 63,* 116–128.

Fink, G., Sumner, B., Rosie, R., Wilson, H., & McQueen, J. (1999). Androgen action on central serotonin neurotransmission: Relevance for mood, mental state, and memory. *Behavioural Brain Research, 105,* 53–68.

Ford, M. R., & Widiger, T. A. (1989). Sex bias in the diagnosis of histrionic and antisocial personality disorders. *Journal of Consulting and Clinical Psychology, 57,* 301–305.

Forth, A. E., Brown, S. L., Hart, S. D., & Hare, R. D. (1996). The assessment of psychopathy in male and female noncriminals: Reliability and validity. *Personality and Individual Differences, 20,* 531–543.

Frick, P. J., & Hare, R. D. (2001). *The Antisocial Process Screening Device.* Toronto, ON, Canada: Multi-Health Systems.

Garstein, M. A., & Rothbart, M. K. (2003). Studying infant temperament via the Revised Infant Behavior Questionnaire. *Infant Behavior and Development, 26,* 64–86.

Goldstein, R. B., Powers, S. I., McCusker, J., & Mundt, K. A. (1996). Gender differences in the manifestations of antisocial personality disorder among residential drug abuse treatment clients. *Drug and Alcohol Dependence, 41,* 35–45.

Gough, H. G. (1969). *Manual for the California Psychological Inventory.* Palo Alto, CA: Consulting Psychologists Press.

Grotpeter, J. K., & Crick, N. R. (1996). Relational aggression, overt aggression, and friendship. *Child Development, 67,* 2328–2338.

Hamburger, M. E., Lilienfeld, S. O., & Hogben, M. (1996). Psychopathy, gender, and gender roles: Implications for antisocial and histrionic personality disorders. *Journal of Personality Disorders, 10,* 41–55.

Hankin, B. L., & Abramson, L. Y. (2001). Measuring cognitive vulnerability to depression in adolescence: Reliability, validity and gender differences. *Journal of Clinical Child and Adolescent Psychology, 31,* 491–504.

Hare, R. D. (1978). Electrodermal and cardiovascular correlates of psychopathy. In R. D. Hare & D. Schalling (Eds.), *Psychopathic behavior: Approaches to research* (pp. 107–143). Chichester, UK: Wiley.

Hare, R. D. (1980). A research scale for the assessment of psychopathy in criminal populations. *Personality and Individual Differences, 1,* 111–119.

Hare, R. D. (1991). *The Hare Psychopathy Checklist—Revised.* Toronto, ON, Canada: Multi-Heath Systems.

Hare, R. D. (1999). Psychopathy as a risk factor for violence. *Psychiatric Quarterly, 70,* 191–197.

Hare, R. D. (2003). *Manual for the Hare Psychopathy Checklist—Revised* (2nd ed.). Toronto, ON, Canada: Multi-Health Systems.

Harmon-Jones, E., & Allen, J. J. D. (1998). Anger and frontal brain activity: EEG asymmetry consistent with approach motivation despite negative affective valence. *Journal of Personality and Social Psychology, 74,* 1310–1316.

Harpur, T. J., Hare, R. D., & Hakstian, A. R. (1989). Two-factor conceptualization of psychopathy: Construct validity and assessment implications. *Psychological Assessment, 1,* 6–17.

Hartung, C. M., & Widiger, T. A. (1998). Gender differences in the diagnosis of mental disorders: Conclusions and controversies of the DSM-IV. *Psychological Bulletin, 213,* 260–278.

Hauser, J., Leszczynska, A., Samochowiec, J., Ostapowicz, A., Czerski, P., Jaracz, J., et al. (2002). The association study of a functional polymorphism of the monoamine oxidase A gene promoter in patients with affective disorders. *Archives of Psychiatry and Psychotherapy, 4,* 9–15.

Hemphill, J., Templeman, R., Wong, S., & Hare, R. D. (1998). Psychopathy and crime: Recidivism and criminal careers. In D. J. Cooke, A. E. Forth, & R. D. Hare (Eds.), *Psychopathy: Theory, research and implications for society* (pp. 375–398). Boston: Kluwer.

Hochhausen, N. M., Lorenz, A. R., & Newman, J. P. (2002). Specifying the impulsivity of female inmates with borderline personality disorder. *Journal of Abnormal Psychology, 111,* 495–501.

Hoffman-Bustamante, D. (1973). The nature of female criminality. *Issues in Criminology, 8,* 117–136.

Hurley, W., & Dunne, M. (1991). Psychological distress and psychiatric morbidity in women prisoners. *Australian and New Zealand Journal of Psychiatry, 25,* 461–470.

Jordan, B. K., Schlenger, W. E., Fairbank, J. A., & Caddell, J. M. (1996). Prevalence of psychiatric disorders among incarcerated women: II. Convicted felons entering prison. *Archives of General Psychiatry, 53,* 513–519.

Keenan, K., & Shaw, D. (1997). Developmental and social influences on young girls' early problem behavior. *Psychological Bulletin, 121,* 95–113.

Kessler, R. C., McGonagle, K. A., Zhao, S., Nelson, C. R., Highes, M., Eshleman, S., et al. (1994). Lifetime and 12-month prevalence of DSM-III-R psychiatric disorders in the United States: Results from the National Comorbidity Survey. *Archives of General Psychiatry, 51,* 8–19.

Lagerspetz, K. M. J., Bjorkqvist, K., & Peltonen, T. (1988). Is indirect aggression typical of females? Gender differences in aggressiveness in 11- to 12-year-old children. *Aggressive Behavior, 14,* 403–414.

Lahey, B. B., & Loeber, R. (1994). Framework for a developmental model of oppositional defiant disorder and conduct disorder. In D. K. Routh (Ed.), *Disruptive behavior disorders in childhood* (pp. 139–180). New York: Plenum Press.

Levenston, G. K., Patrick, C. J., Bradley, M. M., & Lang, P. J. (2000). The psychopath as observer: Emotion and attention in picture processing. *Journal of Abnormal Psychology, 109,* 373–389.

Lilienfeld, S. O. (1992). The association between antisocial personality and somatization disorders: A review and integration of theoretical models. *Clinical Psychology Review, 12,* 641–662.

Lilienfeld, S. O., & Andrews, B. P. (1996). Development and preliminary validation of a self-report measure of psychopathic personality traits in noncriminal populations. *Journal of Personality Assessment, 66,* 488–524.

Lilienfeld, S. O., & Hess, T. H. (2001). Psychopathic personality traits and somatization: Sex differences in the mediating role of negative emotionality. *Journal of Psychopathology and Behavioral Assessment, 23,* 11–24.

Lilienfeld, S. O., Van Valkenburg, C., Larntz, K., & Akiskal, H. S. (1986). The relationship of histrionic personality disorder to antisocial personality and somatization disorders. *American Journal of Psychiatry, 143,* 718–722.

Lish, J. D., Meyer-Bahlburg, H. F., Ehrhardt, A. A., Travis, B. G., & Veridiano, N. P. (1992). Prenatal exposure to diethylstilbestrol (DES): Childhood play behavior and adult gender-role behavior in women. *Archives of Sexual Behavior, 21,* 423–442.

Lorenz, A. R., & Newman, J. P. (2002). Utilization of emotion cues in male and female offenders with antisocial personality disorder: Results from a lexical decision task. *Journal of Abnormal Psychology, 111,* 513–516.

Loucks, A. D. (1995). *Criminal behavior, violent behavior, and prison maladjustment in federal female offenders.* Unpublished doctoral dissertation, Queen's University, Kingston, ON.

Louth, S. M., Hare, R. D., & Linden, W. (1998). Psychopathy and alexithymia in female offenders. *Canadian Journal of Behavioural Science, 30,* 91–98.

Lynam, D. R. (1996). The early identification of chronic offenders: Who is the fledgling psychopath? *Psychological Bulletin, 120,* 209–234.

MacCoon, D. G., & Newman, J. P. (2004). *Dysregulation in female prisoners: Anxiety and impulsivity.* Manuscript submitted for publication.

Magdol, L., Moffitt, T. E., Caspi, A., & Silva, P. A. (1998). Developmental antecedents of partner abuse: A prospective-longitudinal study. *Journal of Abnormal Psychology, 107,* 375–389.

Manuck, S. B., Flory, J. D., Ferell, R. E., Dent, K. M., Mann, J. J., & Muldoon, M. F. (1999). Aggression and anger-related traits associated with a polymorphism of the trytophan hydroxylase gene. *Biological Psychiatry, 45,* 603–614.

McClellan, D., Farabee, D., & Crouch, B. (1997). Early victimization, drug use and criminality. *Criminal Justice and Behavior, 24,* 455–477.

Megargee, E. I. (1966). Undercontrolled and overcontrolled personality types in extreme antisocial aggression. *Psychological Monographs, 80*(Whole No. 611), 1–29.

Meyer-Bahlburg, H. F., & Ehrhardt, A. A. (1982). Prenatal sex hormones and human aggression: A review, and new data on progestogen effects. *Aggressive Behavior, 8,* 39–62.

Moffitt, T. E. (2003). Life-course persistent and adolescence-limited antisocial behavior: A 10-year research review and research agenda. In B. B. Lahey, T. E. Moffitt, & A. Caspi (Eds.), *Causes of conduct disorder and juvenile delinquency* (pp. 49–75). New York: Guilford Press.

Morey, L. C. (1991). *An interpretive guide to the Personality Assessment Inventory (PAI).* Odessa, FL: Assessment Resources.

Mulder, R. T., Wells, J. E., Joyce, P. R., & Bushnell, J. A. (1994). Antisocial women. *Journal of Personality Disorders, 8,* 279–287.

Neary, A. (1990). *DSM-III and psychopathy checklist assessment of antisocial personality disorder in black and white female felons.* Unpublished doctoral dissertation, University of Missouri, St. Louis.

Nolen-Hoeksema, S. (1990). *Sex differences in depression.* Stanford, CA: Stanford University Press.

O'Connor, D. A. (2001). *The female psychopath: Validity and factor structure of the revised Psychopathy Checklist (PCL-R) in women inmates.* Unpublished doctoral dissertation, Florida State University, Tallahassee.

Ogloff, J. R., Wong, S., & Greenwood, A. (1990). Treating criminal psychopaths in a therapeutic community program. *Behavioral Sciences and the Law, 8,* 181–190.

Olweus, D., Mattsson, A., Schalling, D., & Low, H. (1988). Circulating testosterone levels and aggression in adolescent males. *Psychosomatic Medicine, 50,* 261–272.

Patrick, C. J. (1994). Emotion and psychopathy: Startling new insights. *Psychophysiology, 31,* 319–330.

Patrick, C. J. (1995, Fall). Emotion and temperament in psychopathy. *Clinical Science,* pp. 5–8.

Patrick, C. J., Bradley, M. M., & Lang, P. J. (1993). Emotion in the criminal psychopath: Startle reflex modulation. *Journal of Abnormal Psychology, 102,* 82–92.

Patrick, C. J., Verona, E., & Sullivan, E. A. (2000, October). *Emotion and psychopathy in female offenders.* Poster presented at the 40th annual meeting of the Society for Psychophysiological Research, San Diego, CA.

Patterson, C. M., & Newman, J. P. (1993). Reflectivity and learning from aversive events: Toward a psychological mechanism for the syndromes of disinhibition. *Psychological Review, 100,* 716–736.

Piotrowski, N. A., Tusel, D. J., Sees, K. L., Banys, P., & Hall, S. M. (1995). Psychopathy and antisocial personality in men and women with primary opioid dependence. *Issues in Criminological and Legal Psychology, 24,* 123–126.

Rhee, S. H., & Waldman, I. D. (2002). Genetic and environmental influences on antisocial behavior: A meta-analysis of twin and adoption studies. *Psychological Bulletin, 128,* 490–529.

Richards, H. J., Casey, J. O., & Lucente, S. W. (2003). Psychopathy and treatment response in incarcerated female substance abusers. *Criminal Justice and Behavior, 30,* 251–276.

Robbins, P. C., Monahan, J., & Silver, E. (2003). Mental disorders, violence, and gender. *Law and Human Behavior, 27,* 561–571.

Robins, L. N. (1966). *Deviant children grown up.* Baltimore: Williams & Wilkins.

Robins, L. N., & Regier, D. A. (1991). *Psychiatric disorders in America: The Epidemiological Catchment Area study.* New York: Free Press.

Roy, A., Virkkunen, M., & Linnoila, M. (1990). Serotonin in suicide, violence, and alcoholism. In E. F. Coccaro & D. L. Murphy (Eds.), *Serotonin in major psychiatric disorders* (pp. 185–208). Washington, DC: American Psychiatric Association.

Rutherford, M. J., Alterman, A. I., Cacciola, J. S., & McKay, J. R. (1998). Gender differences in the relationship of antisocial personality criteria to Psychopathy Checklist—Revised scores. *Journal of Personality Disorders, 12,* 69–76.

Rutherford, M. J., Alterman, A. I., Cacciola, J. S., & Snider, E. C. (1995). Gender differences in diagnosing antisocial personality disorder in methadone patients. *American Journal of Psychiatry, 152,* 1309–1316.

Rutherford, M. J., Cacciola, J. S., Alterman, A. I., & McKay, J. R. (1996). Reliability and validity of the Revised Psychopathy Checklist in women methadone patients. *Assessment, 3,* 145–156.

Samochowiec, J., Lesch, K. P., Rottman, M., Smoka, M., Syagailo, Y. V., Okladnova, O., et al. (1999). Association of a regulatory polymorphism in the promoter region of the monoamine oxidase A gene with antisocial alcoholism. *Psychiatry Research, 86,* 67–72.

Salekin, R. T., Rogers, R., & Sewell, K. W. (1997). Construct validity of psychopathy in a female offender sample: A multitrait–multimethod evaluation. *Journal of Abnormal Psychology, 106,* 576–585.

Salekin, R. T., Rogers, R., Ustad, K. L., & Sewell, K. W. (1998). Psychopathy and recidivism among female inmates. *Law and Human Behavior, 22,* 109–128.

Segarra, P., Molto, J., & Torrubia, R. (2000). Passive avoidance learning in extraverted females. *Personality and Individual Differences, 29,* 239–254.

Sher, K. J., & Trull, T. J. (1994). Personality and disinhibitory psychopathology: Alcoholism and antisocial personality disorder. *Journal of Abnormal Psychology, 103,* 92–102.

Silverthorn, P., & Frick, P. J. (1999). Developmental pathways to antisocial behavior: The delayed onset pathway in girls. *Development and Psychopathology, 11,* 101–126.

Silverthorn, P., Frick, P. J., & Reynolds, R. (2001). Timing of onset and correlates of severe problems in adjudicated girls and boys. *Journal of Psychopathology and Behavioral Assessment, 23,* 171–181.

Skeem, J. L., Mulvey, E. P., & Grisso, T. (2003). Applicability of traditional and revised models of psychopathy to the Psychopathy Checklist: Screening Version. *Psychological Assessment, 15,* 41–55.

Soloff, P. H., Kelly, T. M., Strotmeyer, S. J., Malone, K. M., & Mann, J. J. (2003). Impulsivity, gender and response to fenfluramine challenge in borderline personality disorder. *Psychiatry Research, 119,* 11–24.

Sooyeon, K., Brody, G. H., & Murray, V. M. (2003). Factor structure of the early adolescent temperament questionnaire and measurement invariance across genders. *Journal of Early Adolescence, 23,* 268–294.

Stafford, E., & Cornell, D. G. (2003). Psychopathy scores predict adolescent inpatient aggression. *Assessment, 10,* 102–112.

Strachan, C. E. (1993). *The assessment of psychopathy in female offenders.* Unpublished doctoral dissertation, University of British Columbia, Vancouver.

Strachan, K., Williamson, S., & Hare R. D. (1990). *Psychopathy and female offenders.* Unpublished data, Department of Psychology, University of British Columbia, Vancouver.

Sue, S. (1999). Science, ethnicity, and bias: Where have we gone wrong? *American Psychologist, 54,* 1070–1077.

Sutton, S. K., Vitale, J. E., & Newman, J. P. (2002). Emotion among females with psychopathy during picture presentation. *Journal of Abnormal Psychology, 111,* 610–619.

Taylor, G. J., Ryan, D., & Bagby, R. M. (1985). Toward the development of a new self-report alexithymia scale. *Psychotherapy and Psychosomatics, 44,* 191–199.

Taylor, J. (2004). *Florida State Twin Registry.* Unpublished data, Florida State University.

Tellegen, A. (1982). *Brief manual for the Multidimensional Personality Questionnaire.* Unpublished manuscript, University of Minnesota.

Teplin, L. A., Abram, K. M., & McClelland, G. M. (1996). Prevalence of psychiatric disorders among incarcerated women: I. Pretrial jail detainees. *Archives of General Psychiatry, 53,* 505–512.

Teplin, L. A., Abram, K. M., McClelland, G. M., Dulcan, M., & Mericle, A. (2002). Psychiatric disorders in youth in juvenile detention. *Archives of General Psychiatry, 59,* 1133–1143.

Tien, G., Lamb, D., Bond, L., Gillstrom, B., & Paris, F. (1993, May). *Report on the needs assessment of women at the Burnaby Correctional centre for women.* Burnaby, BC: BC Institute on Family Violence.

Tobin, R. M., Graziano, W. G., Vanman, E. J., & Tassinary, L. G. (2000). Personality, emotional experience, and efforts to control emotions. *Journal of Personality and Social Psychology, 79,* 656–669.

van Honk, J., Schutter, J. L. G., Hermans, E. J., Putman, P., Tuiten, A., & Koppeschaar, H., (2004). Testosterone shifts the balance between sensitivity for punishment and reward in healthy young women. *Psychoneuroendocrinology, 29,* 937–943.

van Honk, J., Tuiten, A., Verbaten, R., van den Hout, M., Koppeschaar, H., Thijssen, J., & de Haan, E. (1999). Correlations among salivary testosterone, mood, and selective attention to threat in humans. *Hormones and Behavior, 36,* 17–24.

Verona, E., & Carbonell, J. L. (2000). Female violence and personality: Evidence for a pattern of overcontrolled hostility among one-time violent female offenders. *Criminal Justice and Behavior, 27,* 176–195.

Verona, E., Hicks, B., & Patrick, C. J. (in press). Psychopathy and suicidal behaviors in female offenders: Mediating effects of temperament and abuse history. *Journal of Consulting and Clinical Psychology.*

Verona, E., Joiner, T. E., Johnson, F., & Bender, T. (in press). Gender specific gene-environment interactions on laboratory-assessed aggression. *Biological Psychology.*

Verona, E., Patrick, C. J., & Curtin, J. J., Lang, P. J., & Bradley, M. M. (2004). Psychopathy and physiological response to emotionally evocative sounds. *Journal of Abnormal Psychology, 113,* 99–108.

Verona, E., Patrick, C. J., & Joiner, T. T. (2001). Psychopathy, antisocial personality, and suicide attempt history risk. *Journal of Abnormal Psychology, 110,* 462–470.

Vitale, J. E., & Newman, J. P. (2001a). Response perseveration in psychopathic women. *Journal of Abnormal Psychology, 110,* 644–647.

Vitale, J. E., & Newman, J. P. (2001b). Using the Psychopathy Checklist—Revised with female samples: Reliability, validity, and implications for clinical utility. *Clinical Psychology: Science and Practice, 8,* 117–132.

Vitale, J. E., Newman, J. P. Bates, J. E., Goodnight, J., Dodge, K. A., & Pettit, G. S. (2004). *Deficient behavioral inhibition and anomalous selective attention in a community sample of adolescents with psychopathic and low-anxiety traits.* Manuscript under review.

Vitale, J. E., Smith, S. S., Brinkley, C. A., & Newman, J. P. (2002). The reliability and validity of the Psychopathy Checklist—Revised in a sample of female offenders. *Criminal Justice and Behavior, 29,* 202–231.

Walters, G. D. (2003). Predicting institutional adjustment and recidivism with the psychopathy checklist factor scores: A meta-analysis. *Law and Human Behavior, 27,* 541–558.

Warren, J. I., Burnette, M. L., South, S. C., Preeti, C., Bale, R., Friend, R., & Van Patten, I. (2003). Psychopathy in women: Structural modeling and comorbidity. *International Journal of Law and Psychiatry, 26,* 223–242.

Weiler, B. L., & Widom, C. S. (1996). Psychopathy and violent behavior in abused and neglected young adults. *Criminal Behavior and Mental Health, 6,* 253–271.

Werner, N. E., & Crick, N. R. (1999). Relational aggression and social–psychological adjustment in a college sample. *Journal of Abnormal Psychology, 108,* 615–623.

White, H. R., & Widom, C. S. (2003). Intimate partner violence among abused and neglected children in young adulthood: The mediating effects of early aggression, antisocial personality, hostility, and alcohol problems. *Aggressive Behavior, 29,* 332–345.

Widiger, T. A., Cadoret, R., Hare, R., Robins, L., Rutherford, M., Zanarini, M., et al. (1996). DSM-IV antisocial personality disorder field trial. *Journal of Abnormal Psychology, 105,* 3–16.

Widiger, T. A., & Spitzer, R. L. (1991). Sex bias in the diagnosis of personality disorders: Conceptual and methodological issues. *Clinical Psychology Review, 11,* 1–22.

Widom, C. S. (1978). An empirical classification of female offenders. *Criminal Justice and Behavior, 5,* 35–52.

Williamson, S., Harpur, T. J., & Hare, R. D. (1991). Abnormal processing of affective words by psychopaths. *Psychophysiology, 28,* 260–273.

Wilson, D. L., Frick, P. J., & Clements, C. B. (1999). Gender, somatization, and psychopathic traits in a college samples. *Journal of Psychopathology and Behavioral Assessment, 21,* 221–235.

Zagon, I. K., & Jackson, H. J. (1994). Construct validity of a psychopathy measure. *Journal of Personality and Individual Differences, 17,* 125–135.

22

Ethnic and Cultural Variations in Psychopathy

ELIZABETH A. SULLIVAN
DAVID S. KOSSON

Within psychopathology research, the term "psychopathy" is used to describe a constellation of affective, interpersonal, and behavioral symptoms that coalesce to form a stable, pervasive personality disorder. A great deal of empirical research supports the construct of psychopathy as a personality disorder with widespread psychological, social, and political implications within Western society. This cultural specificity, although frequently overlooked, cannot be treated lightly given that the majority of the research on psychopathy has been conducted in North America on European American prisoners. In fact, the leading tool for assessing psychopathy, the Psychopathy Checklist—Revised (PCL-R; Hare, 1991), was developed and normed almost exclusively on European Americans in prisons in Canada and the United States. Hare (1991) has acknowledged that there may be differences in the manifestations of psychopathy across ethnic and cultural groups. In the recent revision of the PCL-R manual, Hare advises that, although there is now more evidence for the reliability and validity of the PCL-R across ethnic and cultural groups, caution should be employed in interpreting scores in groups for which the PCL-R has not been validated (Hare, 2003).

Despite the potential ethnic and cultural limitations on the use and interpretation of the PCL-R, research on psychopathy using the PCL-R and its derivations has progressed rapidly. Several studies have examined how psychopathy manifests across different ethnicities, and the role it may play in serious criminal behavior in different cultures. These efforts should be encouraged as steps in the right direction that will aid in increasing our knowledge of the etiology of psychopathy and lead to a greater understanding of how cultural environments contribute to the manifestation and course of the psychopathic personality.

To understand how psychopathy may manifest differently across ethnic groups and cultures, we must first define culture and ethnicity. Anthony Marsella (1987), a cross-cultural psychologist, proposed that culture is represented in various artifacts, architectural and expressive forms, institutions, and role and behavior patterns. But culture is also represented internally, in the values, attitudes, beliefs, cognitive styles, and patterns of consciousness of an individual. As such, it is the primary mediator or filter for interacting with the world; it is the lens by which we experience and define our reality and orient ourselves to others, the unknown, and to our subjective experience. (p. 381)

Through his definition Marsella clearly demonstrates the importance of considering culture when attempting to assess and understand mental illness across cultural and ethnic groups.

The definition of ethnicity is based on the definition of culture in that ethnicity is typically distinguished on the basis of identifiable characteristics that imply a common cultural history. The term "ethnicity" is sometimes used interchangeably with "racial group." Although these are related terms, they are not identical. Racial group implies biologically based distinctions and is generally used to describe individuals with common physical characteristics. In contrast, members of an ethnic group *may* or may not share similar physical characteristics but *do* share the same cultural heritage. The frequency with which these terms are used interchangeably demonstrates how conceptual confusion can complicate examination of cultural and ethnic differences. Okazaki and Sue (1995) elegantly articulate this issue by asking: "Is the research concerned with race as a biological variable, ethnicity as a demographic variable, or some aspect of subjective cultural experience as a psychological variable?" (p. 368).

Current definitions of mental disorders recognize the importance of cultural and ethnic context. The fourth edition of *Diagnostic and Statistical Manual of Mental Disorders* (DSM-IV; American Psychiatric Association, 1994) specifies that mental disorders do not include "expectable or culturally sanctioned response[s] to an event," and "neither deviant behavior nor conflicts between the individual and society are mental disorders unless the deviance is a symptom of [behavioral, psychological, or biological] dysfunction in the individual" (p. xxi). Thus, understanding pathological behavior depends on an understanding of ethnic and cultural variety and norms. In this context, it is important to evaluate the construct of psychopathy in terms of ethnic and cultural variations, with the goal of expanding current conceptualizations of psychopathy beyond the bounds of Western society and taking a more critical and global perspective when applying the construct as it is currently measured.

CHAPTER GOALS

The primary goal of this chapter is to evaluate what has been learned about psychopathy in terms of cultural and ethnic differences by (1) examining the evidence for the universality of the construct; (2) reviewing current knowledge about the baserates and differential expression of psychopathic traits across cultures and ethnic groups; (3) addressing current methods that have impacted our understanding of ethnic and cultural variations in psychopathy; and (4) considering the controversies and debates that surround psychopathy and ethnicity.

ANECDOTAL EVIDENCE FOR PSYCHOPATHY ACROSS TIME AND CULTURES

A review of the historical and cultural literature suggests that the concept of psychopathy transcends both time and culture. For example, in his seminal book *The Mask of Sanity*, Cleckley described the behavior of the ancient Athenian general Alcibiades as that of a psychopath. Cleckley based his argument on many reported examples of Alcibiades's impulsive, irresponsible, and reckless behaviors. Driven primarily by self-interest and self-indulgence, these behaviors ultimately resulted in his failure as a leader (Cleckley, 1982).

Several other social scientists have provided additional evidence of psychopathy across cultures. Murphy (1976) examined abnormal behaviors across a variety of cultures in an attempt to evaluate the universality of various psychiatric diagnoses. Her research revealed syndromes similar to our conceptualization of psychopathy in two nonindustrialized indigenous cultures. Within the Yorubas, a rural tribe from Nigeria, she reported on a syndrome known as *aranakan*, which describes, "a person who always goes his own way regardless of others, who is uncooperative, full of malice, and bullheaded" (Murphy, 1976, p. 1026). Similarly, in the Alaskan Inuit Eskimos she described the concept of the *kunlangeta*, which refers to a person whose

mind knows what to do but he does not do it
. . . it might be applied to a man who, for example, repeatedly lies and cheats and steals

things and does not go hunting and, when the other men are out of the village, takes sexual advantage of many women- someone who does not pay attention to reprimands and who is always being brought to the elders for punishment. (Murphy, 1976, p. 1026)

Both of these syndromes appear to describe traits and behaviors consistent with our Western concept of psychopathy. Even further, Murphy reported that within these two ethnic groups, people who were seen as having these disorders were considered incapable of change and were often dealt with through extreme measures (e.g., a *kunlangeta* might be pushed off the ice by companions while hunting; Murphy, 1976). This belief in the intractable nature of such conditions is reminiscent of current views about the difficulty of treating psychopaths.

Additional evidence for the presence of psychopathy across cultures can be found in the religious and literary traditions of various cultural groups. For example, in both Southern African American literature and in many Native American religious myths a prominent theme is that of the trickster. The trickster is described as

at one and the same time creator and destroyer, giver and negator, he who dupes others and who is always duped himself. . . . He possesses no values, moral or social, is at the mercy of his passions and appetites. . . . He inflicts great damage on those around him and also suffers innumerable blows, defeats, indignities, and dangers resulting from his thoughtless, reckless forays. (Radin, 1972)

A similar archetype can be identified in ancient Greek myths about the messenger god Hermes, with whom "you'll get action, but it will be action with no moral strings attached, and no guarantees: Hermes goes in for one-night stands. He's also the patron of thieves, liars, crossroads, and footloose wandering" (Hyde, 1999). Carl Jung (1964) described the trickster as the first cycle in the hero myth, stating that the trickster is, "a figure whose physical appetites dominate his behavior; he has the mentality of an infant. Lacking any purpose beyond the gratification of his primary needs, he is cruel, cynical, and unfeeling" (Jung, 1964, p. 112).

The notion of the trickster as a character beyond law and morality, driven by impulses, is remarkably similar to modern concepts of the psychopath. Despite having evolved through myth and legend, the archetype of the trickster is present across many cultures. It may be argued that this shared concept of the trickster figure reflects a common understanding of a distinct syndrome that overlaps with what we currently know as psychopathy.

PSYCHOPATHY ACROSS CULTURES

Research examining the cross-cultural validity of psychopathy represents a relatively recent phenomenon within the field of psychopathy. This new emphasis appears to reflect the increasing acceptance of psychopathy within Western society as a syndrome with important implications for understanding criminality and violence and for predicting recidivism (Hare, 1999; Salekin, Rogers, & Sewell, 1996). As the North American legal and forensic communities have increasingly incorporated assessments of psychopathy into their evaluations for placement, treatment, and release, researchers and forensic professionals in other nations have begun to evaluate what role psychopathy may play in their criminal and forensic populations.

The leading instrument for assessing psychopathy is the PCL-R (Hare, 1991, 2003; Hare & Neumann, Chapter 4, this volume). Until recently, data addressing the cross-cultural reliability and validity of the PCL-R were unavailable. However, in the 2003 manual, data from British and Swedish samples are included in a separate appendix, which provides reliability data and discusses recent studies that have evaluated the cross-cultural applicability of the PCL-R (Hare, 2003). Despite these efforts, additional studies are needed to further explore how the construct of psychopathy as assessed by the PCL-R fits with different cultural conceptualizations of mental illness and criminality.

The majority of the research into cross-cultural applications of psychopathy, as measured by the PCL-R, has been conducted in European nations. In a recent review of findings on psychopathy across cultures, Cooke (1998) focused largely on research in European nations. In the sections that follow, we review research findings from European samples, as well as from other international research efforts to assess psychopathy and evaluate its utility of as a tool for understanding criminality. This review focuses on three broad areas relevant to the issue of psychopathy across cultures: (1) prevalence and baserates for comparing levels of psychopathy across cultures; (2) classical test theory, factor, and item response theory approaches to assessing reliability and generalizability of the PCL-R; and (3) construct validity.

The Prevalence of PCL-R Psychopathy across Cultures

An analysis of data from 19 samples of prisoners, psychiatric patients, and forensic offenders referred for evaluation in 10 countries outside North America, yielded a mean PCL-R total score of 18.7 (7.6) for 3,394 subjects (see Table 22.1). This average score is significantly lower than the overall mean 22.1 (7.9) reported in the 2003 PCL-R manual for both prisoners and psychiatric populations, $t(10,046) = 20.6$, $p < .001$, with a moderate effect size ($d = .43$). However, this average is significantly higher than the mean of 16.2 (8.4) reported by Cooke (1998) for a pooled European sample, which included 5 of the 19 samples listed in Table 22.1, $t(5,535) = 11.3$, $p < .001$. An important consideration in evaluating this difference is the heterogeneity of the samples and the loss of information arising from aggregating across potentially distinct populations. Indeed, Cooke acknowledged that sampling artifact may have affected the results of his comparisons, although he collapsed across samples of prisoners and "security patients."

The studies reviewed here used several terms to describe their samples. However, for the purposes of this review, the samples were classified into three categories: prisoners, psychiatric patients, and forensic participants. Prisoner samples were those for which participants were or had been incarcerated in a prison or correctional institution. Psychiatric samples were those describing participants as patients or inmates from a variety of psychiatric and secure hospitals. Forensic samples were those in which participants were court ordered for psychiatric evaluation but not yet convicted, and those including mixed samples of court evaluees, psychiatric patients, and prisoners. The 2003 PCL-R manual does not treat forensic samples separately but rather groups court-ordered

evaluation and mixed samples into the prisoner or psychiatric categories.

When the pooled international sample was divided into these more homogeneous samples and the means recalculated, the mean PCL-R score of 17.5 ($SD = 7.3$) for the combined international prisoner samples ($N = 2,046$) remained significantly lower than the mean for the normative North American prisoner sample listed in the manual, $t(7,452) = 23.2$, $p < .001$, with a moderate effect size ($d = .60$). This difference is similar to that reported by Cooke (1998), providing support for his assertion that representative international prison samples tend to have lower means when compared to North American samples.

However, as shown in Table 22.1, the mean PCL-R score for the international prisoner samples was in turn significantly lower than the mean of 22.5 (8.0) for the international psychiatric samples ($N = 440$), $t(2,484) = 13.1$, $p < .001$, and the mean of 19.5 (8.2) for the international forensic samples ($N = 908$), $t(2,952) = 6.9$, $p < .001$. In addition, a comparison of the North American and the international psychiatric samples revealed a significantly higher mean PCL-R score for the latter, $t(1,684) = 2.62$, $p < .025$, although the effect size for this difference was quite small ($d = .15$). The difference in mean scores for North American prisoners versus international psychiatric patients was not significant, $t(5,846) = 1.14$, $p > .1$ ($d = .06$). On the other hand, North American prisoners scored higher than international forensic offenders referred for evaluation, although the effect was relatively small, $t(6,314) = 9.0$, $p < .001$; $d = .32$. In summary, moderate differences were found between average PCL-R scores obtained in North American versus European prisons. However, such intercontinental differences appear to be larger for prisoner samples than for psychiatric or forensic samples.

Cooke (1998) argued that the differences in psychopathy scores between North American and international prison samples may reflect a lower prevalence of psychopathy in international samples due to cultural differences. However, an alternative possibility is that cultural differences exist in the way criminal justice systems identify and respond to mental illness across countries. For example, differences in national standards for in-

TABLE 22.1. PCL-R Psychopathy across Cultures

Research group	Population	Participants	PCL-R	Factor 1	Factor 2	Cutoff(s)	% psychopath
Cooke (1995)	Scottish	307 prisoners	13.8 (7.4)			≥ 30/ ≥ 25	3% / 8%
Hobson & Shine (1998)[a]	British	104 prisoners	24.2 (6.2)	8.1 (3.3)	12.4 (3.9)	≥ 30	26%
Hare et al. (2000)	British	728 prisoners	16.5 (7.8)	5.8 (3.7)	8.3 (4.5)	≥ 30/ ≥ 25	4.5% / 13%
Hare (2003)	British	448 prisoners	17.8 (7.1)	6.8 (3.1)	8.4 (4.3)	≥ 30	
Pham (1998)	Belgian	103 prisoners	18.8 (9.3)	7.4 (4.4)	9.5 (5.2)	≥ 30	5%
Rasmussen et al. (1999)	Norwegian	41 prisoners	22.6 (10.0)	9.3 (3.5)	11 (5.7)	≥ 26	49%
Molto et al. (2000)	Spanish	117 prisoners	22.4 (7.9)	9.5 (3.9)	10.4 (4.4)	≥ 30	18%
Pastor et al. (2003)	Spanish	48 prisoners	24.3 (1.6)	10.6 (1.6)	10.8 (1.7)	≥ 27.5	38%
Goncalves (1999)	Portuguese	150 prisoners	15.5 (1.8)			≥ 30	15%
Blackburn et al. (2003)	Scottish	60 psychiatric	16.6 (6.9)				
Blackburn & Coid (1998)[b]	British	167 psychiatric	26.1 (9.0)			≥ 30	47%
Blackburn et al. (2003)	British	115 psychiatric	21.6 (6.6)				
Hildebrand, de Ruiter, de Vogel, & van der Wolf (2002)	Dutch	98 psychiatric	21.3 (8.4)	9.4 (3.7)	9.1 (5.0)	≥ 30/ ≥ 26	20% / 33%
Nedopil et al. (1998)	German	131 forensic	18.1 (6.4)			≥ 25	23%
Stalenheim & van Knorring (1996)	Swedish	61 forensic	18.7 (11.9)			≥ 30	25%
Grann et al. (1999)	Swedish	352 forensic	20.7 (8.5)			≥ 26	32%
Tengstrom et al. (2000)[c]	Swedish	202 forensic	18.2 (7.5)			≥ 26	22%
Langstrom & Grann (2002)[d]	Swedish	97 forensic	19.8 (7.1)			≥ 26	24%
Folino, Marengo, Marchiano, & Ascazibar (2004)[e]	Argentinean	65 forensic	20.6 (9.1)				
International prisoners		2,046	17.5 (7.3)				
International psychiatric patients		440	22.5 (8.0)				
International forensic offenders		908	19.5 (8.2)				
All international samples		3,394	18.7 (7.6)				
Hare (2003)	North American	5,408 prisoners	22.1 (7.9)	8.5 (3.8)	10.5 (4.3)	≥ 30	20.5%
Hare (2003)	North American	1,246 psychiatric	21.5 (6.9)	8.0 (3.5)	10.9 (3.6)	≥ 30	13.4%
Hare (2003)	North American	6,654 all subjects	21.9 (7.2)				

Note. "Prisoners" refers to general prison population unless otherwise noted; "psychiatric" refers to forensic psychiatric patients in a mental hospital or similar facility; "forensic" refers to offenders court ordered for a forensic psychiatric evaluation.
[a] Prisoners at a therapeutic prison for a personality disorder or psychopathy.
[b] Combined sample of violent offenders from a maximum security hospital and special prison units for violent inmates.
[c] All in sample had a comorbid diagnosis of schizophrenia.
[d] Sample of young offenders, ages 15–20.
[e] Combined sample of prisoners and offenders court ordered for a forensic psychiatric evaluation.

sanity and placement practices have been discussed as a potential explanation for lower PCL-R total scores in Germany (Freese, Sommer, Muller-Isberner, & Ozokyay, 1999). Within the German courts a diagnosis of psychopathic disorder can result in a verdict of diminished responsibility and institutionalization in a forensic mental hospital instead of a standard correctional facility (Felthous & Sass, 2000). Similarly, "psychopathic disorder" and "dangerous as a result of severe personality disorder" (DSPD) are medicolegal designations in the United Kingdom that have implications for the placement of offenders (Blackburn, Logan, Donnelly, & Renwick, 2003). The United Kingdom has special placement facilities, such as Grendon therapeutic prison, that are designed to provide services for mentally disordered offenders detained under that nation's Mental Health Act (Doyle, Dolan, & McGovern, 2002). The Grendon facility requires a "personality disorder or psychopathy" as a prerequisite for admission (Hobson & Shine, 1998). In a study of prevalence rates, Hobson and Shine (1998) found higher base rates of psychopathy at Grendon (26%) than had been reported in traditional prisons in the United Kingdom—which they interpreted as reflecting these selection criteria (Hobson & Shine, 1998). Thus, differences in criminal classification policies may lead some psychopathic offenders who would be sentenced to prison in North America to instead be sent to forensic mental hospitals in other nations. This could be an important factor contributing to lower PCL-R scores in international versus North American prisons.

This explanation may also provide a framework for understanding the similarity of the North American prisoner and psychiatric samples with the international psychiatric and forensic samples. If a greater proportion of psychopathic offenders in other nations are being placed within psychiatric facilities, then the means for international psychiatric and forensic samples should be somewhat higher and more commensurate with those for North American prisons. As an example, the impact of differential classification practices is likely reflected in the high prevalence of psychopathy (47 %) in a sample of violent offenders described by Blackburn and Coid (1998). All participants in this sample had been sentenced to a spe-cial maximum security hospital after being detained under the nation's Mental Health Act and classified within the legal category of *psychopathic disorder* or special prison units for violent and disruptive inmates.

A third potential factor contributing to differences in mean PCL-R scores between international and North American samples is differences in incarceration rates across nations. In contrast to the policies in some nations of placing psychopaths (or DSPD) offenders in psychiatric facilities, the requirements for imprisonment in Norway are much higher regardless of diagnosis, especially when compared to the United States, where the rate of incarceration is 10 times that of Norway (Rasmussen, Storsaeter, & Levander, 1999). This difference may account for the extremely high base rates of psychopathy (49%, using a modified PCL-R cutoff score of ≥ 26) in a Norwegian prison sample, although a lower cutoff criterion would be expected to increase rates of psychopathy. Rasmussen and colleagues (1999) hypothesized that in a nation such as Norway, where imprisonment is less frequent, more severe offenders who would be incarcerated anywhere are likely to comprise a higher proportion of the inmate population. However, this explanation does not likely apply to Scotland: The incarceration rate for the United States is five to eight times that of Scotland, but the baserates of psychopathy in Scottish prisons are extremely low when compared to North American samples (i.e., 3% in Scotland vs. 28.4% in North America, applying the traditional PCL-R cutoff of ≥ 30; Cooke, 1995; Cooke & Michie, 1999; Hare, 1991).

This issue of baserates of psychopathy across international samples has received a great deal of attention in the literature. Based on a series of regression analyses addressing prevalence differences between North American and Scottish samples, Cooke and Michie (1999) suggested that the standard North American cutoff score for the PCL-R (≥ 30) was equivalent to a lower cutoff score in Scotland (≥ 25), although substantial differences in baserates between Scotland and North America still remained when the new cutoff was applied: 8% compared to 28.4% in North America (Cooke, 1998; Cooke & Michie, 1999). The results of this study paved the way for other European psychopathy researchers to use modified cutoff scores in their samples. Table 22.1 shows the range of baserates obtained at different cutoff scores across various international samples (see Table 22.1). The use of different cutoff scores makes it difficult to draw firm conclusions about the baserates of psychopathy across cultures. However, Table 22.1 illustrates that there is a great deal of variability in apparent baserates regardless of the cutoff scores used.

It remains unclear what accounts for apparent differences in baserates of psychopathy across settings and cultures; however, differences are not isolated to the international samples. There also appears to have been a change in psychopathy baserates within North America, from 28.4% in the 1991 PCL-R manual to 20.5% for North American prisoners in the 2003 manual— somewhat narrowing the gap between the North American sample and international samples. This apparent change in the North American baserates raises the possibility that the prevalence of psychopathy may be variable over time regardless of cultural context. Nevertheless, current evidence suggests that heterogeneity of samples, differences in legal classification and placement strategies across nations, and other as yet unaddressed cultural factors also contribute to observed differences in prevalence.

Classical Test Theory and Factor Analyses of PCL-R Psychopathy across Cultures

A more systematic approach to examining cross-cultural differences in psychopathy is to employ classical test theory techniques to examine reliability and the dimensions

underlying psychopathy ratings. The factor structure of the PCL-R has been extensively investigated in North American samples, revealing stable two-factor (Cooke & Michie, 1999; Hare et al., 1990; Harpur, Hakstian, & Hare, 1988; McDermott et al., 2000), three-factor (Cooke & Michie, 2001; Sullivan & Kosson, 2004), and, recently, four-factor (or facet) solutions (Hare, 2003). The differences between these models are less dramatic than may at first appear. As reviewed elsewhere in this volume (see Hare & Neumann, Chapter 4, and Cooke, Michie, & Hart, Chapter 5, this volume), across each of these solutions a similar constellation of symptoms has emerged, including affective expression, interpersonal style, impulsive/irresponsible behavior, and, in two of three models, antisocial behavior. Moreover, identical or nearly identical items load on each dimension across models.

Many attempts have been made by international investigators to validate the PCL-R as a tool for assessing psychopathy by examining the internal consistency and factor structure of the measure. An examination of Table 22.2 demonstrates the similarities in internal consistency across studies, with many of the samples showing similarly high alpha coefficients and item-to-total correlations. Factor analyses from these studies have also yielded generally similar findings for the two-factor solution across cultures, with a few exceptions, in both the proportion of variance explained and item loadings across factors (see Table 22.2). Whereas the similarities suggest that the PCL-R is internally consistent, with a largely replicable factor structure across international and North

TABLE 22.2. Classical Test Theory and Factor Analyses of PCL-R Psychopathy across Cultures

Research group	Cronbach's alpha	Item-to-total correlations	Factor 1 variance	Factor 2 variance	Differences in item loadings on factors
Cooke (1995)	.75	.30 to .71	16.15%	19.3%	No
Hobson & Shine (1998)	.82	.23 to .57	14.2%	24.4%	Item 11 on Factor 1 Item 20 on Factor 2
Molto et al. (2000)	.85	.18 to .62	12.6%	27%	Item 11 on Factor 1
Hildebrand et al. (2002)	.87	.26 to .64	14%	30%	Item 13 on Factor 1 Item 20 on Factor 2
Pham (1998)	.86	——	11%	35.7%	Item 15 both Factors Item 19 on Factor
Hare (1991)	.87	.30 to .61	17.15%	15%	

American samples, the minor differences suggest that in international samples, Factor 2 typically accounts for a greater proportion of the variance in total PCL-R scores than in North America. In addition, slight differences in factor loadings suggest the possibility of cultural variations in the most pertinent indicators of these dimensions of psychopathy.

Item Response Theory Analyses of PCL-R Psychopathy across Cultures

An alternative approach to evaluating the performance of the PCL-R is to employ item response theory (IRT) methods to examine relations between item scores and the underlying construct of psychopathy in international versus North American samples. Cooke and colleagues have argued that IRT methods have several advantages over classical test theory (CTT): (1) item response curves (IRC) are independent of the samples from which they are drawn; (2) representative samples are not required to gain unbiased estimates; (3) IRT methods can identify items that perform differently across samples; (4) IRT analyses can ensure measurement invariance; and (5) IRT analyses permit direct comparison of parallel items, both within the measure and across samples (Cooke, 1998; Cooke & Michie, 1999; Cooke et al., Chapter 5, this volume).

One of the major issues in comparing PCL-R scores across samples is whether the underlying construct of psychopathy is measured similarly in both samples. This issue is described in the IRT literature as the problem of measurement invariance. For performance of a measure to be considered comparable across distinct populations the measure must assess the trait on the same measurement scale (Reise, Widaman, & Pugh, 1993). IRT methods address this problem by examining whether there are items that perform similarly in both their ability to discriminate between individuals with differing levels of the underlying trait—as measured by slope—and difficulty or threshold (the level of the underlying trait at which the item is discriminating)—as measured by intercept. If such items can be used as anchors for estimating the latent trait in both samples on a common metric or scale, the remaining items may be compared across samples. Evidence of differ-

ential item functioning (DIF) for some items indicates that the measurement model is only partially invariant (Reise et al., 1993). However, a partially measurement invariant model is sufficient for comparing groups on a latent trait (Reise et al., 1993).

In one of the first cross-cultural IRT analyses, Cooke and Michie (1999) compared IRT results for the PCL-R across North American and Scottish samples. In basic terms, they found that the PCL-R items discriminated equally well (similar slopes) in both samples but that only three items were metrically equivalent (i.e., showed no DIF across the two samples). By using these items to develop a common metric for comparison, they found that the level of psychopathy, or threshold at which the items became discriminating, differed between the two samples, with a higher level of the trait being necessary in Scotland before 17 of the PCL-R items became maximally effective at discriminating among individuals (Cooke, 1998; Cooke & Michie, 1999). On the other hand, in a parallel series of analyses with an English prison sample, Hare (2003) reported that 10 of the PCL-R items performed in a similar manner in the English and North American samples, providing anchors for comparing the PCL-R items across these two samples. Results showed that of the 10 other items that exhibited DIF, 3 were from Factor 1 and 6 were from Factor 2. More important, aside from items that showed differences in the intercept parameter, five items appeared to exhibit differences in discriminating power: items 1 and 2 were less discriminating in the English sample; items 18–20 were more discriminating in the English sample (see Hare, 2003, Table B.6). Based on test characteristic curves, Hare concluded that moderate scores on the PCL-R may overestimate psychopathy in the English sample compared with the North American sample, but that higher scores appear to reflect the same latent trait of psychopathy across the two groups (Hare, 2003).

The findings from Hare's analysis are quite different from Cooke's findings in one important respect: Hare reported differences for both threshold and discrimination parameters, whereas Cooke reported differences only in threshold. As noted by Cooke and Michie (1999), a lack of differences in slope parameters suggests that psychopathy is defined by the same characteristics across North America and Scotland (Cooke & Michie, 1999). Conversely, the presence of differences in slope parameters across samples suggests that some items are "less relevant" to psychopathy in one group in comparison to another, suggesting that the functioning of those items is "culturally specific rather than culturally general" (Cooke & Michie, 1999, p. 65). Thus, Hare's recent analysis raises the possibility that some PCL-R items may in fact be less relevant to psychopathy outside North America. However, the conflicting evidence from these two IRT studies highlights the need for more studies using IRT methods to examine whether the differences across countries reflect the level of psychopathy at which the traits are relevant across cultures, the relevance of particular traits, or a combination of both.

Construct Validity of Psychopathy across International Samples

Another important consideration in assessing the cross-cultural validity of psychopathy is the construct validity of the syndrome across international samples. In North American samples, replicable patterns of associations between psychopathy and external variables have provided a framework for conceptualizing psychopathy. If psychopathy truly transcends cultural bounds, then similar patterns of relations should also be evident in international research.

Although international research on the construct validity of psychopathy is still in its early stages, the relations between psychopathy and comorbid psychiatric diagnoses, self-report personality traits, criminal behavior, prediction of violence and recidivism, and laboratory performance have received sufficient attention to warrant discussion here.

Relations between Psychopathy and Other Psychiatric Disorders

Studies examining the relationship between psychopathy and comorbid psychiatric diagnoses in international samples have demonstrated patterns very similar to those reported in North American samples. Some of the most commonly observed relationships between psychopathy and DSM disorders in the North American literature are for the

Axis II personality disorders, with antisocial personality disorder (APD) consistently revealing the greatest comorbidity, followed by other Cluster B disorders, and with some studies indicating small to moderate correlations with Cluster A diagnoses (Hart & Hare, 1989; Warren et al., 2003; Widiger, Chapter 8, this volume). Similarly, in a study of violent offenders in England, Blackburn and Coid (1998) found a high degree of comorbidity between Cluster B personality disorders of DSM-III and PCL-R psychopathy scores, along with moderate correlations for paranoid and passive–aggressive personality disorders (Blackburn & Coid, 1998). Stalenheim and von Knorring (1996), working in Sweden, reported that the greatest comorbidity for individuals high in psychopathy was APD, with strong correlations for other Cluster B personality disorders and smaller but significant correlations for Cluster A diagnoses. In a Spanish prison sample, Molto, Poy, and Torrubia (2000) replicated the relationship between APD and PCL-R psychopathy scores, which was largely attributable to Factor 2. Finally, in a study of German forensic patients, Nedopil, Hollweg, Hartmann, and Jaser (1998) found substantial comorbidity between psychopathy and other personality disorders.

Substance abuse/dependence disorders have also been extensively related to psychopathy in the North American literature (Hart & Hare, 1989; Hemphill, Hart, & Hare, 1994; Smith & Newman, 1990; Taylor & Lang, Chapter 25, this volume). In a Norwegian prison sample, Rasmussen and colleagues (1999) found that PCL-R-identified psychopaths demonstrated significantly more cannabis, inhalant, amphetamine and opiate abuse/dependency than did nonpsychopaths. High comorbidities between psychopathy and drug abuse/dependence have also been reported in samples of Swedish offenders (Stalenheim & von Knorring, 1996), U.K. special hospital patients (Blackburn et al., 2003), and a German forensic sample (Nedopil et al., 1998).

The relationship between psychopathy and other DSM Axis I diagnoses is less consistent. The North American literature contains conflicting reports, with some studies reporting negative associations between psychopathy and affective or anxiety disorders, and others reporting no relationship between psychopathy and these Axis I disorders (Hart & Hare, 1989; Rice & Harris, 1995). Studies outside North America appear similar, with one study reporting negative relationships between psychopathy and depression diagnoses but no relationship to anxiety disorder diagnoses (Stalenheim & von Knorring, 1996) and two studies reporting no relationships between psychopathy and Axis I disorders (other than substance use disorders: Nedopil et al., 1998; Rasmussen et al., 1999). More recently, Blackburn and colleagues (2003) found significant comorbidity between psychopathy in an offender sample (defined by overall scores ≥ 25 on the PCL-R) and the DSM-IV diagnosis of posttraumatic stress disorder (PTSD). Nevertheless, the overall pattern of findings is consistent with that reported in North American samples.

Relationships between Psychopathy and Self-Report Personality

Many international studies have also addressed the relationship between psychopathy and self-report measures of personality. In the North American literature, several studies corroborate positive relationships between psychopathy as indexed by overall scores on the PCL-R and impulsivity, aggression, sensation seeking (Hare, 2003; Verona, Patrick, & Joiner, 2001; Vitale, Smith, Brinkley, & Newman, 2002), and psychoticism (Hare, 2003; Kosson, Smith, & Newman, 1990; see Lilienfeld & Fowler, Chapter 6, and Lynam & Derefinko, Chapter 7, this volume). However, findings are mixed concerning extraversion, neuroticism, negative emotionality, and anxiety measures, with some studies suggesting that overall psychopathy is inversely or unrelated to these traits (Hare, 2003; Hart, Forth, & Hare, 1991; Schmitt & Newman, 1999) and others suggesting small to moderate positive relationships between total PCL-R scores and anxiety or negative affectivity (Hale, Goldstein, Abramowitz, Calamari, & Kosson, 2004; Hare, 2003; Verona et al., 2001; Vitale et al., 2002). In European samples, studies in both Denmark (Andersen, Sestoft, Lillebaek, Mortensen, & Kramp, 1999) and Sweden (af Klinteberg, Humble, & Schalling, 1992) have yielded positive correlations between overall psychopathy and

psychoticism. In the Swedish sample the high psychopathy group was also elevated on the Neuroticism scale of the Eysenck Personality Questionnaire (EPQ) and the Impulsiveness and Monotony Avoidance scales of the Karolinska Scales of Personality (KSP; af Klinteberg et al., 1992). Among Spanish prisoners, Molto and colleagues (2000) also reported significant correlations for PCL-R total (as well as Factor 2) scores with the Impulsiveness scale of the KSP as well as with the Hypomania scale of the Minnesota Multiphasic Personality Inventory (MMPI). In a U.K. sample of violent male offenders, Blackburn and Coid (1998) found that PCL-R Factor 1 was negatively related to anxiety and shyness but positively related to extraversion, whereas PCL-R total and Factor 2 scores were positively related to impulsivity. These results, similar to those in North American samples (Hare, 2003), provide further evidence of the cross-cultural construct validity of psychopathy.

Relationships between Psychopathy and Criminal Behavior

As reviewed elsewhere (see Douglas, Vincent, & Edens, Chapter 27, this volume), the majority of North American studies provide data corroborating the assumption that the psychopath's criminal career is typically longer, more severe, and more versatile than that of the nonpsychopath. In this section, we compare findings from studies in North America with those of other countries relating psychopathy to age of onset of criminal behavior, types of offenses, and institutional misconduct.

North American studies have commonly reported that psychopathy is inversely related to age of onset of criminal behavior—that is, higher PCL-R scores are associated with an earlier initiation of criminal behavior (Hemphill, Templeman, Wong, & Hare, 1998; Smith & Newman, 1990). Blackburn and Coid (1998) replicated this finding in their sample of British violent offenders. Similar findings for age of onset have been obtained in Danish (Andersen et al., 1999), Norwegian (Rasmussen et al., 1999), and Spanish samples (Molto et al., 2000).

Research in North American samples has suggested that psychopaths commit more violent and nonviolent crimes and have more versatile criminal careers than nonpsychopathic offenders (Hare & McPherson, 1984). In their Spanish prison sample, Molto and colleagues (2000) reported that PCL-R total scores were correlated with number of incarcerations, the number of violent and nonviolent crimes, and more types of crimes. Similar patterns were observed in samples of Norwegian prisoners (Rasmussen et al., 1999), British psychiatric patients (Blackburn & Coid, 1998), and Danish offenders (Andersen et al., 1999), with psychopaths consistently committing more violent and nonviolent crimes.

Finally, with respect to institutional misconduct, North American studies suggest that psychopaths commit both more frequent and more severe rule infractions while detained (Brandt, Kennedy, Patrick, & Curtin, 1997; Hare & McPherson, 1984; Heilbrun et al., 1998). This pattern was mirrored in a Dutch psychiatric sample, where psychopathy scores were significantly correlated with verbal abuse and threats, general violation of hospital rules, and the number of seclusions, although not with physical violence (Hildebrand, de Ruiter, & Nijman, 2004). In contrast, in a sample of Spanish prisoners, Molto and colleagues (2000) reported that psychopathy was correlated with both nonviolent and violent violations of prison rules. Similar findings were reported by Hare, Clark, Grann, and Thornton (2000) in a large sample of British prisoners, where PCL-R total scores were correlated with assaults on prison staff, assaults on inmates, and property damage (Hare et al., 2000). Thus, it appears that psychopathy is robustly related to multiple indices of criminal behavior, regardless of cultural differences. However, it should be noted that criterion contamination is often a problem when evaluating the relationship between psychopathy and criminal deviance, given that the extent and severity of criminal behavior are incorporated into the scoring of the PCL-R.

Psychopathy and Prediction of Violence and Recidivism

North American studies have consistently found that psychopathy scores are strongly predictive of both general and violent recidivism (Salekin et al., 1996; Serin, Peters, &

Barbaree, 1990). Among British prisoners, Hare and colleagues (2000) found that the PCL-R was a significant predictor of general reconviction and violent reconviction over a 2-year follow-up period. Several studies of violent recidivism in Sweden have reported that the PCL-R shows strong predictive utility in criminal offenders with personality disorders (Grann, Langstrom, Tengstrom, & Kullgren, 1999), in criminal offenders with schizophrenia (Tengstrom, Grann, Langstrom, & Kullgren, 2000), and in young offenders (Langstrom & Grann, 2002). Taken together, these studies suggest psychopathy is an excellent predictor of general and violent recidivism, both in North America and internationally.

Psychopathy and Psychophysiological and Behavioral Correlates

Experimental studies of the psychopath's ability to process cognitive and emotional material using North American samples have provided evidence suggesting that psychopathy is associated with deficits in emotional processing (e.g., Blair et al., 2002; Kosson, Suchy, Mayer, & Libby, 2002; Williamson, Harpur, & Hare, 1991) and with a specific deficit in defensive (fear) activation to emotional stimuli as evidenced by a lack of startle potentiation to negative affective pictures (Levenston, Patrick, Bradley, & Lang, 2000; Patrick, Bradley, & Lang, 1993; Patrick, Cuthbert, & Lang, 1994). Psychopathy has also been associated with deficits in response modulation (as assessed by behavior in reward–punishment tasks) and in performance on executive functioning tasks (LaPierre, Braun, & Hodgins, 1995; Newman, Patterson, & Kosson, 1987). If psychopathy is truly a syndrome that transcends cultural boundaries, then patterns of physiological and behavioral deficits should be replicable across international samples. Unfortunately, studies in other countries have only examined these issues to a limited degree. In a study of Spanish prisoners, Pastor, Moltó, Vila, and Lang (2003) reported that psychopaths displayed diminished startle response to negative affective pictures in comparison to nonpsychopaths. In contrast, a Belgian study failed to demonstrate significant differences between psychopaths and nonpsychopaths in physiological responses to emotional films, although it was found that psychopaths had significantly lower blood pressure throughout the study (Pham, Philippot, & Rime, 2000). In a separate study of Belgian prisoners, Pham, Vanderstukken, Philippot, and Vanderlinden (2003) found a pattern of performance consistent with impaired behavioral inhibition, similar to that reported in an earlier study by LaPierre and colleagues (1995). Thus, the few experimental studies conducted in international samples suggest that some cognitive and emotional processing deficits in psychopaths generalize across cultural differences. However, the small number of studies and inconsistencies emphasize the need for caution when drawing conclusions about the cross-cultural generality of mechanisms underlying psychopathy.

Is There Evidence for Psychopathy across Cultures?

A primary goal of this chapter has been to examine the evidence for the cross-cultural validity of psychopathy. Our systematic comparison of North American and international samples has yielded substantial evidence supporting the application and utility of the construct of psychopathy in international samples, with some provocative differences, and some notable gaps in the literature. One difference that has emerged across cultures is the replication of lower mean PCL-R scores in international prison populations and lower international baserates. We have discussed several potential explanations for this difference. Cultural differences also emerged in studies using IRT methods. Although the authors of these studies have suggested that the performance of the PCL-R is comparable across cultures, these investigations also provide preliminary evidence that there may be cultural variation in the relevance of some of the PCL-R indicators to the construct of psychopathy.

Despite these differences and a relative lack of research on mechanisms underlying psychopathy in international samples, the majority of findings provide compelling evidence that the construct of psychopathy as indexed by the PCL-R is valid across cultures. Studies employing CTT methods demonstrate that the leading measures of psychopathy can be reliably used to assess psychopathy in other cultures. Most important, international studies indicate similar patterns of relationships between psychopathy and comorbid psychiatric diagnoses, self-report personality traits, criminal behavior, prediction of violence and recidivism, and, to some extent, physiological and behavioral task performance, to those observed in North American samples. With so much evidence demonstrating parallels between North American and international samples, it is clear that psychopathy is similar in many respects across cultures. However, further research is needed to elucidate the basis of cross-cultural differences in mean scores and in the relevance of specific components of psychopathy.

PSYCHOPATHY ACROSS ETHNICITIES

The possibility of differences in the manifestation of psychopathy across ethnicities has been controversial for some time. The original PCL-R normative data (Hare, 1991) consisted largely of European Americans, despite the overrepresentation of African Americans in U.S. prisons. In the recent revision of the PCL-R manual, Hare (2003) reviewed findings regarding relationships between psychopathy and ethnicity and concluded that although there may be differences in the way individual items function across ethnicity, the PCL-R as a whole appears to provide a reliable and valid assessment of psychopathy in both African American and European American samples.

Several researchers have addressed this issue by including race or ethnicity as a variable in their analyses or by systematically analyzing their data with this question in mind. In this section we review empirical studies, address recent debates on this issue, and consider several potential mediating sociocultural factors. Throughout this section we use the terms "European American" and "African American" to refer to samples described elsewhere as "white" or "Caucasian," and "black." This difference in nomenclature reflects our emphasis on ethnic differences, not racial differences. Given our earlier discussion of the conceptual confusion in the use of these terms, and given that these studies were not designed to include representative sampling of individuals from distinct racial groups, it is more accurate to specify the cultural context from which the samples were derived.

In one of the first papers to examine this issue, Kosson and colleagues (1990) examined how the PCL functioned in samples of European American and African American prisoners. They demonstrated that psychopathy could be reliably assessed in African Americans but reported evidence of differences in the factor structure and patterns of construct validity across ethnicities. Moreover, this study demonstrated the importance of considering ethnicity in assessing psychopathy and served as a model for the systematic examination of this issue.

The Prevalence of PCL-R Psychopathy across Ethnicities

One important finding of Kosson and colleagues (1990) was that PCL total scores were found to be significantly higher in the African American than in the European American sample. Table 22.3 lists findings from seven additional studies that explicitly tested for differences in mean PCL scores between African American and European American samples, and in a few instances, samples with ethnicity classified as "Other." Five studies found no significant differences between African Americans and European Americans, and two studies reported higher PCL scores in African Americans than European Americans. Two studies also reported higher scores in African Americans than in the Other ethnic group. Taken together, these studies are inconclusive as to whether there are differences in mean level of PCL scores across ethnicity.

In an attempt to resolve this issue, Skeem, Edens, Camp, and Colwell (2004) used meta-analytic techniques to evaluate whether levels of psychopathy differ across ethnicity. These investigators compared mean PCL scores for African American and European American participants across 21 studies. They found a small but significant Cohen's *d* for PCL total scores and for scores on the Interpersonal and Affective Factors of the three-factor model but not for Factor 1 or Factor 2 of the two-factor model, for the Impulsive–Irresponsible Behavior factor of the three-factor model, or for Hare's Antisocial factor. They also assessed heterogeneity

of effect sizes and found evidence for variability in effect sizes across studies for the total score and for all the factors (from all models) except for Factor 1 of the two-factor model. Given the absence of ethnicity differences in effect sizes for Factor 1, and the homogeneity of Factor 1 scores across ethnicities, Skeem and colleagues (2004) concluded that there is no strong evidence that African Americans have higher levels of the core psychopathic traits than European Americans. However, because they obtained evidence for significant heterogeneity—and significant ethnicity differences—for both the Affective and Interpersonal factors that comprise Factor 1, it is difficult to accept this conclusion. More generally, Skeem and colleagues' review demonstrates substantial heterogeneity across samples for most components of psychopathy. Such heterogeneity and the variability in the range of differences in total PCL-R score across ethnic groups (from +3.3 to –4.7) indicate substantial ambiguity about the magnitude and direction of ethnicity differences in psychopathy.

Classical Test Theory and Factor Analyses of PCL-R Psychopathy across Ethnicities

As discussed earlier, Kosson and colleagues (1990) found adequate reliability for the PCL-R in their adult African American sample. Subsequent studies have also reported acceptable reliability figures for the PCL-R in adult African American samples (e.g., Abramowitz, Sullivan, Lopez, & Kosson, 2004; Toldson, 2002; Vitale et al., 2002). Likewise, the manual for the youth version of the PCL (PCL:YV; Forth, Kosson, & Hare, 2003) notes high internal consistency for adolescent samples of different ethnicities.

On the other hand, Kosson and colleagues (1990) found factor structure differences between European American and African American samples: Across the two samples, the congruence coefficient for Factor 1 failed to meet established criteria; moreover, a cross-comparison between Factor 2 for the African American sample and Factor 1 from the European American sample revealed a stronger relationship than expected, suggesting poorer differentiation between factors in the African American sample. Subsequent studies have corroborated this apparent dif-

TABLE 22.3. PCL Psychopathy across Ethnicities

Research group	Population	European American		African American		Other		Significance
		N	Mean (SD)	N	Mean (SD)	N	Mean (SD)	
Kosson et al. (1990)	Prisoners	232	25.74 (6.88)	124	28.04 (5.87)			AA > EA**
Thornquist & Zuckerman (1995)	Prisoners	26	15.96	32	23.5	21	15.43	AA > EA** AA > O**
Brandt et al. (1997)[a]	Prisoners	38	23.41 (5.0)	91	25.35 (5.29)			ns
Cooke & Michie (2001)	Federal prisoners	117	23.5	84	23.3			ns
Cooke & Michie (2001)	Jail inmates	247	24.1	267	25.7			AA > EA**
Toldson (2002)	Prisoners	130	22.65 (10.22)	121	24.52 (9.38)			ns
Vitale et al. (2002)[b]	Prisoners	248	18.44 (7.27)	280	19.13 (7.19)			ns
Abramowitz et al. (2004)	Prisoners	83	23.45 (7.18)	83	25.98 (7.16)	83	23.2 (7.57)	AA ns EA AA > O*
Hare (2003)	Prisoners	2119	23.2 (7.6)	932	22.8 (7.3)	114	24.5 (5.9)	
Hare (2003)	Psychiatric	765	21.1 (7.0)	329	22.9 (6.7)	148	20.8 (6.4)	

Note. "Prisoners" refers to general prison population unless otherwise noted; "psychiatric" refers to forensic psychiatric patients in a mental hospital or similar facility.
[a] Sample of adolescents at a residential training facility for severe juvenile delinquent boys.
[b] Sample of female prisoners.

ference in factor structure. Toldson (2002), using exploratory factor analysis (EFA), failed to find support for a two-factor model in a sample of African American federal prisoners. McDermott and colleagues (2000) also found, in a sample of African American substance abusers, that a cross-comparison between Factor 2 and Factor 1 of the PCL-R revealed a stronger relationship than was expected, suggesting poorer differentiation between factors. Thus, across studies, results from EFAs suggest that the commonly recognized dimensions of psychopathy may not manifest similarly in African American and European American samples.

In contrast, recent studies using confirmatory factor analysis (CFA) suggest comparable fit for the two-factor model of psychopathy across African American and European American adolescent prisoners (Brandt et al., 1997), and across African American, European American, and Puerto Rican alcoholic inpatients (Windle & Dumenci, 1999). Similarly, Cooke, Kosson, and Michie (2001) found that the three-factor model demonstrated a good fit in both African American and European American inmates. Finally, Sullivan and Kosson (2004) found that CFAs for both models provided adequate fit to the data in both African American and European American participants. Thus, in contrast to studies using EFA, results from CFA studies support the applicability of both the two- and three-factor models of psychopathy across ethnic groups.

Item Response Theory Analyses of PCL-R Psychopathy across Ethnicities

The advantages of IRT methods for examining latent constructs across groups were discussed earlier. Although there have been few applications of IRT to the question of ethnic differences in psychopathy, these studies are informative. Cooke and colleagues (2001) found that 8 of the 13 items of the three-factor model and 15 of the 20 items from the full PCL-R performed equivalently across the African American and European American samples. The five items that exhibited DIF were all associated with Factor 2 in the two-factor model and the Behavioral factor in the three-factor model. Moreover, in all five cases, the items differed only in threshold parameters, not in discrimination pa-

rameters. Two items were discriminating at lower levels of the underlying trait in African Americans than in European Americans; three, at higher levels of the underlying trait in African Americans (Cooke et al., 2001). Moreover, at the level of overall test functioning, Cooke and colleagues found no differences in the test characteristic curves across ethnicities. Consequently, they concluded that although there are minor differences in some of the behavioral item thresholds, these did not reduce the effectiveness of the PCL-R for assessing psychopathy in African American participants. The 2003 PCL-R manual also reported independent IRT analyses comparing African American and European American participants and reported a similar pattern, with DIF mainly for Factor 2 items (Bolt, Hare, & Newman, 2003, cited in Hare, 2003). Based on these two studies, it appears that the PCL-R measures psychopathy similarly across ethnicities, with equal discriminating power, although with differences in threshold for some behavioral items.

Nevertheless, two caveats should be kept in mind: First, differences in the behavioral items raise the possibility of ethnic differences in relationships between the behavioral or lifestyle dimension of psychopathy and various quasi-criteria. Second, as emphasized by Cooke and colleagues (2001), evidence that the PCL-R can be used in an unbiased way for assessing psychopathy does not imply that it is always used in an unbiased way. Researchers must remain alert to the possibility of biases in their use of the PCL-R with members of different ethnic groups. As a final comment, although IRT analyses can examine whether a measure is differentially assessing traits across groups, it is beyond the power of IRT to assess for global biases in the use of the PCL-R that may be contributing to ethnic differences in psychopathy.

Construct Validity of Psychopathy across Ethnicities

As noted previously, examining the relationship between psychopathy and its external correlates is central to understanding psychopathy. If there is a universal syndrome of psychopathy, its correlates should be similar across ethnic groups.

Unfortunately, much of the research on the construct validity of psychopathy has included ethnically diverse samples without explicitly examining ethnicity or race as a potential moderating variable. Among the few studies that have explicitly addressed this issue, analytic methods have varied substantially, from correlational and regression analyses to testing of main effects in analysis of variance models. In this section we review findings from studies addressing relationships between psychopathy and ethnicity for self-report measures of personality, criminal behavior indices, and experimental paradigms assessing cognitive and emotional processing.

As discussed earlier, relationships between self-report personality measures and psychopathy have been somewhat inconsistent, even in European Americans. To shed light on potential ethnic differences, Kosson and colleagues compared correlations between PCL-R psychopathy scores and various self-report criterion measures—the EPQ, the KSP, the Welsh Anxiety Scale (WAS), and the Socialization scale of the California Psychological Inventory—in African American versus European American male prisoners. Although most relationships were similar across ethnic groups, psychopathy was related to extraversion in African Americans but not in European Americans. Conversely, psychopathy was positively correlated with psychoticism, impulsiveness, and monotony avoidance in European Americans but not in African Americans—a finding that may imply differences in the relationship between impulsivity and psychopathy in African American prisoners. Thornquist and Zuckerman (1995) found a similar pattern, with a significant correlation between psychopathy and impulsiveness/sensation seeking in a European American sample that did not replicate in African American and Hispanic participants.

Vitale and colleagues (2002) also examined these relationships among female prisoners. Similar to Kosson and colleagues, they found a positive relationship between psychopathy and psychoticism in European Americans that did not replicate in African American participants. However, in contrast to Kosson et al., they found a similar negative correlation between PCL-R total scores and the Constraint factor of the Multidimensional Personality Questionnaire in both groups. For the remaining personality indices they also found similar patterns across African American and European American samples, including significant positive correlations between negative affectivity and Factor 2 psychopathy scores. Sullivan and Kosson (2004) also demonstrated similar relationships between negative affect and the behavioral aspects of psychopathy in African American and European American prisoners. Thus, current findings suggest that relationships between self-reported negative affect and psychopathy are similar across African American and European American participants, but inconsistent findings regarding impulsivity and psychoticism highlight the need for additional studies.

Another relationship that has been examined for ethnic differences is that between psychopathy and criminal behavior. Kosson and colleagues (1990) reported no psychopathy × ethnicity interactions for either number or versatility of criminal charges. In a study of groups of inmates matched on age, IQ, and years of education, Abramowitz and colleagues (2004) found parallel patterns of correlations between psychopathy and the number of violent and nonviolent charges across African American, European American, and Latino inmates. Vitale and colleagues (2002) also found similar patterns across African American and European American female prisoners for number and type of criminal charges. In contrast, Sullivan and Kosson (2004) found slightly different relationships between the PCL-R factors and the number of violent and nonviolent crimes. For African American participants, but not for European Americans, the number of nonviolent crimes was significantly related to the Behavioral factor in both the two- and three-factor models (Sullivan & Kosson, 2004). Number of violent crimes was also significantly related to the Interpersonal factor of the three-factor model in the European American sample, whereas for the African American participants it was significantly related to the Affective factor, a finding which tentatively suggests that different mechanisms may underlie violent crime in African American compared with European American inmates.

To date, only one study has addressed the role of psychopathy as a predictor of criminal behavior across ethnic groups. Walsh and Kosson (2004) demonstrated that PCL-R scores prospectively predicted both total and violent arrests over a 3-year follow-up period. However, when the effects of socio-economic status (SES) were considered, different patterns of association were found in African versus European American samples. Among African Americans, psychopathy remained a significant predictor of recidivism regardless of SES. However, among European Americans, the presence of a significant psychopathy × SES interaction indicated that psychopathy only predicted recidivism among low-SES European Americans. Because this appears to be the first study addressing interactive relationships between psychopathy and SES, caution is warranted. However, it is interesting that psychopathy was a more robust predictor of recidivism among African Americans than among European Americans. Clearly, additional investigations of interactions between psychopathy, SES, and ethnicity are needed. In summary, these studies provide important evidence for the construct validity of psychopathy in African American samples, although isolated findings suggest the possibility that the antisocial behavior of African American and European American psychopaths may reflect different aspects of psychopathy and be influenced by different moderating variables.

One of the few experimental domains in which the question of ethnic differences has been systematically examined is that of passive avoidance learning. Kosson and colleagues (1990) reported a similar pattern of passive avoidance learning deficits in African American and European American psychopaths, although the deficit was only a statistical trend in the former group. In contrast, two additional studies of passive avoidance learning in psychopaths reported weaker effects of psychopathy in African American samples than in European American samples (Newman & Schmitt, 1998), and in one case results for African American and Hispanic prisoners failed to even approach significance (Thornquist & Zuckerman, 1995). Nevertheless, it should be noted that Newman and Schmitt (1998), like Kosson and colleagues (1990), indicated no significant psychopathy × ethnicity interaction in passive avoidance errors. In addition to studies examining passive avoidance learning, different patterns of results have also emerged between African American and European American psychopaths in studies assessing response modulation (Newman, Schmitt, & Voss, 1997), responses to

distractors under divided visual attention (Kosson, 1998), Damasio's somatic marker hypothesis (Schmitt, Brinkley, & Newman, 1999), interpersonal and cognitive appraisals (Doninger & Kosson, 2001), and affective lexical decision (Lorenz & Newman, 2002). Although these studies have addressed different aspects of cognitive and emotional processing, the overall pattern of results suggests that there may be differences in the ways that African American and European American psychopaths process information. However, whether these differences reflect true neurocognitive differences as a function of ethnicity remains unclear.

At least one alternative possibility should be considered. Given the potential influence of antisocial behavior in rating several PCL-R items, a history of violent and criminal behavior can elevate scores on several PCL-R items. Thus, evidence that African Americans are arrested and convicted more often than European Americans, on average, and have more charges and convictions for violent offenses than European Americans (Abramowitz et al., 2004; Kosson et al., 1990) could contribute to African Americans earning higher PCL scores in some samples.[1] Even in the absence of evidence of DIF for PCL-R items related to antisocial behavior (Cooke et al., 2001; cf. Bolt et al., 2003, cited in Hare, 2003), ethnicity differences in criminal records may result in less effective differentiation between middle and high psychopathy groups in African American than in European American inmates. That is, among African American participants, there may be more "false positives" (i.e., individuals who are not truly psychopathic but receive PCL-R scores above 30). In this context, extreme group analyses may contribute to spurious differences between African American and European American psychopaths, and analysis of continuous data may be advantageous for investigating ethnicity effects.

The Controversy Surrounding the Question of Ethnic Differences in Psychopathy

Throughout this chapter we have attempted to provide a systematic review of the literature that has addressed the question of cultural and ethnic differences in psychopathy. Ours is not the first work that has attempted to review the issue of ethnic differences in a systematic way. Lynn (2002) recently addressed this issue and argued that there are higher levels of psychopathic personality among African Americans. In conducting his analysis, Lynn considered data using the MMPI Psychopathic-Deviate scale, disruptive behavior disorder diagnoses, and a variety of behavioral symptoms and statistics (school suspensions, credit ratings, crime rates, pregnancy rates, divorce rates, etc).

Lynn's approach to examining racial differences in psychopathic personality has drawn criticism from several researchers (Skeem, Edens, Sanford, & Colwell, 2003; Zuckerman, 2003). One of the strongest criticisms of Lynn's position stems from his failure to distinguish psychopathy from criminality and other behaviors merely associated with psychopathy. In a reply to Lynn, Skeem and colleagues (2003) emphasized Lynn's failure to review correlates of the interpersonal and affective dimensions sometimes considered to constitute the personality core of psychopathy. In addition, the failure to incorporate any of the research on PCL-based measures of psychopathy represents a serious limitation of Lynn's review.

Although there is substantial value in identifying links between behavioral anomalies and genetic and biological factors, it is also important to consider sociocultural mediating factors, such as poverty and SES, that may disproportionately contribute to ethnic differences in antisocial behaviors. Unfortunately, Lynn's discussion ignores the impact of racial biases and other sociocultural factors on the higher rates of arrest and conviction and the more severe sentences given to African Americans, factors which contribute to the overrepresentation of African Americans in jails and prisons (Skeem et al., 2003).

An additional concern is Lynn's generalization of statistics on ethnic differences to broad racial categories. Because the majority of the data Lynn reviewed was based on North American statistics, the samples are more appropriately distinguished in terms of ethnicity (i.e., as African Americans and European Americans) rather than being considered discrete racial groups. The thoughtful responses of both Skeem and colleagues (2003) and Zuckerman (2003) provide many additional points of criticism, which cannot be elaborated here due to space limitations.

However, these discussions provide a compelling refutation of the methods and claims of Lynn's paper and provide some constructive suggestions for the type of careful scientific exploration necessary to examine the question of ethnic differences in psychopathy.

Is There Evidence for Differences in Psychopathy across Ethnicities?

Although the majority of the North American psychopathy literature is based on samples that are ethnically diverse, very few studies have systematically examined the cross-ethnicity validity of psychopathy. Nevertheless, our review indicates substantial evidence for the application and utility of the construct of psychopathy across ethnicity. Psychopathy as assessed by the PCL-R appears to exhibit good internal consistency and a pattern of reliable relationships to several personality characteristics and to criminal behavior across ethnic groups. Thus it is clear that the psychopathy construct has utility among African Americans.

At the same time, our review has identified some important questions about potential differences in the nature of psychopathy across ethnicity. These questions fall into two major categories: (1) domains in which findings are inconsistent across studies and across methods, and (2) domains in which differences emerge consistently. The major areas of inconsistency are with respect to ethnic differences in mean PCL-R scores and the dimensions underlying psychopathy. Whether the differences in total scores sometimes reported reflect true differences in the level of psychopathy across ethnicity (in some settings), the influence of sociocultural factors on the scoring of specific items, or the impact of racial biases has yet to be disentangled. The other area of inconsistent findings is related to factor structure, where EFA findings suggest differences in factor structure, whereas CFA findings point to overall similarity of underlying structure. As a result, one of our chief conclusions is that more systematic studies of ethnicity and psychopathy in a variety of different settings are urgently needed.

Where differences across ethnicity have emerged more consistently, some of these appear relatively less serious than others. For example, IRT analyses suggest that the PCL-R as a whole is equally discriminating across ethnic groups. However, some behavioral items may discriminate at different levels of psychopathy in African Americans versus European Americans (see also Bolt et al., 2003). These differences suggest the possibility that sociocultural factors may contribute to behavioral differences in psychopathy across ethnicity. There also appear to be differences between African American and European Americans in relationships between psychopathy and self-reported impulsivity and psychoticism, and in laboratory paradigms assessing cognitive and emotional processing, raising the possibility of distinct mechanisms underlying psychopathy in European American and in African American prisoners. However, the small number of studies conducted in these areas precludes drawing firm conclusions about the stability or meaning of these differences. In summary, two conclusions appear warranted at this point: (1) there *is* evidence for the reliability and partial construct validity of psychopathy across ethnicities, and (2) there *may* be ethnic differences in the manifestations of psychopathy.

CONCLUDING REMARKS

Although not one of the stated goals of this chapter, questions regarding potential explanations for the observed differences across cultures and ethnicities have emerged through our review of the literature. At some points we have attempted to provide a framework for evaluating findings, without fully considering the wide array of possible mechanisms that may underlie these differences. More extensive discussions of factors contributing to differences in psychopathy across cultures are available in reviews by Cooke (1998) and Skeem and colleagues (2003). These discussions have focused on issues as diverse as sensation seeking and migration in Scottish psychopaths (Cooke, 1998), the impact of culture and ethnicity on early childhood environment and socialization in the etiology of psychopathy (Lykken, 1995; Mealey, 1995), and the role of differing cultural perspectives on the relationship of the individual to society (Cooke, 1998; Mealy, 1995; Reavis, 1998). The breadth of

explanations advanced to explain cultural and ethnic differences in psychopathy provides many avenues for future research into the complex factors that contribute to the development and maintenance of psychopathy.

In conclusion, our review has demonstrated the importance of considering ethnic and cultural factors when assessing and examining psychopathy. As the field of psychopathy research is rapidly expanding, we hope that the issues we have touched on will receive more systematic exploration. Considering ethnic and cultural variations in psychopathy is not merely a matter of practical significance. By exploring the ethnic and cultural similarities and differences that emerge we can gain greater insight into the etiology of the disorder and an improved understanding of the interplay of biological and social factors in psychopathy.

NOTE

1. The possibility that some behavioral PCL-R items are maximally discriminating at different levels of overall psychopathy in African Americans than in European Americans may also contribute to poorer discrimination between middle- and high-scoring African Americans. However, the one published study addressing this issue suggested that item differences cancel out at the level of the overall test (Cooke et al., 2001).

REFERENCES

Abramowitz, C. S., Sullivan, E. A., Lopez, M., & Kosson, D. S. (2004). *Reliability and validity of psychopathy in Latino, African-American, and Caucasian male inmates.* Manuscript in preparation.

af Klinteberg, B., Humble, K., & Schalling, D. (1992). Personality and psychopathy of males with a history of early criminal behaviour. *European Journal of Personality, 6,* 245–266.

American Psychiatric Association. (1994). *Diagnostic and statistical manual of mental disorders* (4th ed.). Washington, DC: Author.

Andersen, H. S., Sestoft, D., Lillebaek, T., Mortensen, E. L., & Kramp, P. (1999). Psychopathy and psychopathological profiles in prisoners on remand. *Acta Psychiatrica Scandinavica, 99,* 33–39.

Blackburn, R., & Coid, J. W. (1998). Psychopathy and the dimensions of personality disorder in violent offenders. *Personality and Individual Differences, 25,* 129–145.

Blackburn, R., Logan, C., Donnelly, J., & Renwick, S. (2003). Personality disorders, psychopathy and other mental disorders: Co-morbidity among prisoners at English and Scottish high-security hospitals. *Journal of Forensic Psychiatry and Psychology, 14*, 111–137.

Blair, R. J. R., Mitchell, D. G. V., Richell, R. A., Kelly, S., Leonard, A., Newman, C., & Scott, S. K. (2002). Turning a deaf ear to fear: Impaired recognition to vocal affect in psychopathic individuals. *Journal of Abnormal Psychology, 111*, 682–686.

Bolt, D., Hare, R. D., & Newman, J. P. (2003). *Multigroup IRT analyses of the Hare Psychopathy Checklist—Revised (PCL-R)*. Manuscript in preparation.

Brandt, J. R., Kennedy, W. A., Patrick, C. J., & Curtin, J. J. (1997). Assessment of psychopathy in a population of incarcerated adolescent offenders. *Psychological Assessment, 9*, 429–435.

Cleckley, H. (1982). *The mask of sanity.* St. Louis, MO: Mosby.

Cooke, D. J. (1995). Psychopathic disturbance in the Scottish prison population: Cross-cultural generalizability of the Hare Psychopathy Checklist. *Psychology, Crime and Law, 2*, 101–118.

Cooke, D. J. (1998). Psychopathy across cultures. In D. J. Cooke, A. E. Forth, & R. D. Hare (Eds.), *Psychopathy: Theory, research and implications for society* (pp. 13–45). Dordrecht, The Netherlands: Kluwer.

Cooke, D. J., Kosson, D. S., & Michie, C. (2001). Psychopathy and ethnicity: Structural, item and test generalizability of the Psychopathy Checklist—Revised (PCL-R) in Caucasian and African American participants. *Psychological Assessment, 13*, 531–542.

Cooke, D. J., & Michie, C. (1999). Psychopathy across cultures: North America and Scotland compared. *Journal of Abnormal Psychology, 108*, 58–68.

Cooke, D. J., & Michie, C. (2001). Refining the construct of psychopathy: Towards a hierarchical model. *Psychological Assessment, 13*, 171–188.

Doninger, N. A., & Kosson, D. S. (2001). Interpersonal construct systems among psychopaths. *Personality and Individual Differences, 30*, 1263–1281.

Doyle, M., Dolan, M., & McGovern, J. (2002). The validity of North American risk assessment tools in predicting in-patient violent behaviour in England. *Legal and Criminological Psychology, 7*, 141–154.

Felthous, A. R., & Sass, H. (2000). Introduction to this issue: International perspectives on psychopathic disorder. *Behavioral Sciences and the Law, 18*, 557–565.

Folino, J. O., Marengo, C. M., Marchiano, S. E., & Ascazibar, M. (2004). The risk assessment program and the court of penal execution in the province of Buenos Aires, Argentina. *International Journal of Offender Therapy and Comparative Criminology, 48*, 49–58.

Forth, A. E., Kosson, D. S., & Hare, R. D. (2003). *Hare Psychopathy Checklist: Youth Version (PCL:YV).* Toronto, ON, Canada: Multi-Health Systems.

Freese, R., Sommer, J., Muller-Isberner, R., & Ozokyay, K. (1999). *The PCL:SV as an instrument to predict violence in in-patients in a German hospital order institution.* Paper presented to the Conference on Risk Assessment and Risk Management: Implications for Prevention of Violence, Vancouver, BC.

Goncalves, R. A. (1999). Psychopathy and offender types: Results from a Portuguese prison sample. *International Journal of Law and Psychiatry, 22*, 337–346.

Grann, M., Langstrom, N., Tengstrom, A., & Kullgren, G. (1999). Psychopathy (PCL-R) predicts violent recidivism among criminal offenders with personality disorders in Sweden. *Law and Human Behavior, 23*, 205–217.

Hale, L. R., Goldstein, D. S., Abramowitz, C. S., Calamari, J. E., & Kosson, D. S. (2004). Psychopathy is related to negative affectivity but not to anxiety sensitivity. *Behaviour Research and Therapy, 42*, 697–710.

Hare, R. D. (1991). *Hare Psychopathy Checklist—Revised (PCL-R).* Toronto, ON, Canada: Multi-Health Systems.

Hare, R. D. (1999). Psychopathy as a risk factor for violence. *Psychiatric Quarterly, 70*, 181–197.

Hare, R. D. (2003). *Hare Psychopathy Checklist—Revised (PCL-R)* (2nd ed.). Toronto, ON, Canada: Multi-Health Systems.

Hare, R. D., Clark, D., Grann, M., & Thornton, D. (2000). Psychopathy and the predictive validity of the PCL-R: An international perspective. *Behavioral Sciences and the Law, 18*, 623–645.

Hare, R. D., Harpur, T. J., Hakstian, A. R., Forth, A. E., Hart, S. D., & Newman, J. P. (1990). The revised Psychopathy Checklist: Reliability and factor structure. *Psychological Assessment, 2*, 338–341.

Hare, R. D., & McPherson, L. E. (1984). Violent and aggressive behavior by criminal psychopaths. *International Journal of Law and Psychiatry, 7*, 35–50.

Harpur, T. J., Hakstian, A. R., & Hare, R. D. (1988). Factor structure of the Psychopathy Checklist. *Journal of Consulting and Clinical Psychology, 56*, 741–747.

Hart, S. D., Forth, A. E., & Hare, R. D. (1991). The MCMI-II as a measure of psychopathy. *Journal of Personality Disorders, 5*, 318–327.

Hart, S. D., & Hare, R. D. (1989). Discriminant validity of the Psychopathy Checklist in a forensic psychiatric population. *Psychological Assessment, 1*, 211–218.

Heilbrun, K., Hart, S. D., Hare, R. D., Gustafson, D., Nunez, C., & White, A. J. (1998). Inpatient and post-discharge aggression in mentally-disordered offenders: The role of psychopathy. *Journal of Interpersonal Violence, 13*, 514–527.

Hemphill, J. F., Hart, S. D., & Hare, R. D. (1994). Psychopathy and substance abuse. *Journal of Personality Disorders, 8*, 169–180.

Hemphill, J. F., Templeman, R., Wong, S., & Hare, R. D. (1998). Psychopathy and crime: Recidivism and criminal careers. In D. J. Cooke, A. E. Forth, & R. D.

Hare (Eds.), *Psychopathy: Theory, Research and Implications for Society* (pp. 375–399). Dordrecht, The Netherlands: Kluwer.

Hildebrand, M., de Ruiter, C., de Vogel, V., & van der Wolf, P. (2002). Reliability and factor structure of the Dutch language version Hare's Psychopathy Checklist—Revised. *International journal of Forensic Mental Health*, *1*, 139–154.

Hildebrand, M., de Ruiter, C., & Nijman, H. (2004). PCL-R psychopathy predicts disruptive behavior among male offenders in a Dutch forensic psychiatric hospital. *Journal of Interpersonal Violence*, *19*, 13–29.

Hobson, J., & Shine, J. (1998). Measurement of psychopathy in a UK prison population referred for long-term psychotherapy. *British Journal of Criminology*, *38*, 504–516.

Hyde, L. (1999). *Trickster makes this world: Mischief, myth, & art*. New York: North Point Press.

Jung, C. G. (1964). *Man and his Symbols*. Garden City, NY: Doubleday.

Kosson, D. S. (1998). Divided visual attention in psychopathic and nonpsychopathic offenders. *Personality and Individual Differences*, *24*, 373–391.

Kosson, D. S., Smith, S. S., & Newman, J. P. (1990). Evaluating the construct validity of psychopathy in African American and European American male inmates: Three preliminary studies. *Journal of Abnormal Psychology*, *99*, 250–259.

Kosson, D. S., Suchy, Y., Mayer, A. R., & Libby, J. (2002). Facial affect recognition in criminal psychopaths. *Emotion*, *2*, 398–411.

Langstrom, N., & Grann, M. (2002). Psychopathy and violent recidivism among young criminal offenders. *Acta Psychiatrica Scandinavica*, *106*, 86–92.

LaPierre, D., Braun, C. M. J., & Hodgins, S. (1995). Ventral frontal deficits in psychopathy: Neuropsychological test findings. *Neuropsychologia*, *33*, 139–151.

Levenston, G. K., Patrick, C. J., Bradley, M. M., & Lang, P. J. (2000). The psychopath as observer: Emotion and attention in picture processing. *Journal of Abnormal Psychology*, *109*, 373–385.

Lorenz, A. R., & Newman, J. P. (2002). Do emotion and information processing deficiencies found in Caucasian psychopaths generalize to African-American psychopaths? *Personality and Individual Differences*, *32*, 1077–1086.

Lykken, D. T. (1995). *The antisocial personalities*. Hillsdale, NJ: Erlbaum.

Lynn, R. (2002). Racial and ethnic differences in psychopathic personality. *Personality and Individual Differences*, *32*, 273–316.

Marsella, A. (1987). The measurement of depressive experience and disorder across cultures. In A. Marsella, R. M. Hirschfeld, & M. M. Katz (Eds.), *The measurement of depression* (pp. 376–397). New York: Guilford Press.

McDermott, P. A., Alterman, A. I., Cacciola, J. S., Rutherford, M. J., Newman, J. P., & Mulholland, E.

M. (2000). Generality of Psychopathy Checklist—Revised factors over prisoners and substance-dependent patients. *Journal of Consulting and Clinical Psychology*, *68*, 181–186.

Mealey, L. (1995). The sociobiology of sociopathy: An integrated evolutionary model. *Behavioral and Brain Sciences*, *18*, 523–599.

Molto, J., Poy, R., & Torrubia, R. (2000). Standardization of the Hare Psychopathy Checklist—Revised in a Spanish prison sample. *Journal of Personality Disorders*, *14*, 84–96.

Murphy, J. (1976). Psychiatric labeling in cross-cultural perspective. *Science*, *191*, 1019–1027.

Nedopil, N., Hollweg, M., Hartmann, J., & Jaser, R. (1998). Comorbidity of psychopathy with major mental disorders. In D. J. Cooke, A. E. Forth, & R. D. Hare (Eds.), *Psychopathy: Theory, research and implications for society* (pp. 257–268). Dordrecht, The Netherlands: Kluwer.

Newman, J. P., Patterson, C. M., & Kosson, D. S. (1987). Response perseveration in psychopaths. *Journal of Abnormal Psychology*, *96*, 145–148.

Newman, J. P., & Schmitt, W. A. (1998). Passive avoidance in psychopathic offenders: A replication and extension. *Journal of Abnormal Psychology*, *107*, 527–532.

Newman, J. P., Schmitt, W. A., & Voss, W. D. (1997). The impact of motivationally neutral cues on psychopathic individuals: Assessing the generality of the response modulation hypothesis. *Journal of Abnormal Psychology*, *106*, 563–575.

Okazaki, S., & Sue, S. (1995). Methodological issues in assessment research with ethnic minorities. *Psychological Assessment*, *7*, 367–375.

Pastor, M. C., Moltó, J., Vila, J., & Lang, P. J. (2003). Startle reflex modulation, affective ratings and autonomic reactivity in incarcerated Spanish psychopaths. *Psychophysiology*, *40*, 934–938.

Patrick, C. J., Bradley, M. M., & Lang, P. J. (1993). Emotion in the criminal psychopath: Startle reflex modulation. *Journal of Abnormal Psychology*, *102*, 82–92.

Patrick, C. J., Cuthbert, B. N., & Lang, P. J. (1994). Emotion in the criminal psychopath: Fear image processing. *Journal of Abnormal Psychology*, *103*, 523–534.

Pham, T. H. (1998). Evaluation psychométrique du questionnaire de la psychopathie de Hare auprès d'une population carcérale belge. *L'Encéphale*, *24*, 435–441.

Pham, T. H., Philippot, P., & Rime, B. (2000). Subjective and autonomic responses to emotion induction in psychopaths. *L'Encéphale*, *26*, 45–51.

Pham, T. H., Vanderstukken, O., Philippot, P., & Vanderlinden, M. (2003). Selective attention and executive functions deficits among criminal psychopaths. *Aggressive Behavior*, *29*, 393–405.

Radin, P. (1972). *The trickster, a study in American Indian mythology*. New York: Schocken Books.

Rasmussen, K., Storsaeter, O., & Levander, S. (1999).

Personality disorders, psychopathy, and crime in a Norwegian prison population. *International Journal of Law and Psychiatry, 22,* 91–97.

Reavis, J. A. (1998). *Individualist–collectivist cultures and psychopathy.* Unpublished doctoral dissertation, United States International University.

Reise, S. P., Widaman, K. F., & Pugh, R. H. (1993). Confirmatory factor analysis and item response theory: Two approaches for exploring measurement invariance. *Psychological Bulletin, 114,* 552–566.

Rice, M. E., & Harris, G. T. (1995). Psychopathy, schizophrenia, alcohol abuse, and violent recidivism. *International Journal of Law and Psychiatry, 18,* 333–342.

Salekin, R., Rogers, R., & Sewell, K. (1996). A review and meta-analysis of the Psychopathy Checklist and Psychopathy Checklist—Revised: Predictive validity of dangerousness. *Clinical Psychology: Science and Practice, 3,* 203–215.

Schmitt, W. A., Brinkley, C. A., & Newman, J. P. (1999). Testing Damasio's somatic marker hypothesis with psychopathic individuals: Risk takers or risk averse? *Journal of Abnormal Psychology, 108,* 538–543.

Schmitt, W. A., & Newman, J. P. (1999). Are all psychopathic individuals low-anxious? *Journal of Abnormal Psychology, 108,* 353–358.

Serin, R. C., Peters, R. D., & Barbaree, H. E. (1990). Predictors of psychopathy and release outcome in a criminal population. *Psychological Assessment, 2,* 419–422.

Skeem, J. L., Edens, J. F., Camp, J., & Colwell, L. H. (2004). Are there ethnic differences in levels of psychopathy? A meta-analysis. *Law and Human Behavior, 28,* 505–527.

Skeem, J. L., Edens, J. F., Sanford, G. M., & Colwell, L. H. (2003). Psychopathic personality and racial/ethnic differences reconsidered: A reply to Lynn (2002). *Personality and Individual Differences, 35,* 1439–1462.

Smith, S. S., & Newman, J. P. (1990). Alcohol and drug abuse/dependence disorders in psychopathic and nonpsychopathic criminal offenders. *Journal of Abnormal Psychology, 99,* 430–439.

Stalenheim, E. G., & von Knorring, L. (1996). Psychopathy and Axis I and Axis II psychiatric disorders in a forensic psychiatric population in Sweden. *Acta Psychiatrica Scandinavica, 94,* 217–223.

Sullivan, E. A., & Kosson, D. S. (2004). *A statistical comparison of the factor structure and construct validity of the two and three-factor models of PCL-R psychopathy.* Manuscript in preparation.

Tengstrom, A., Grann, M., Langstrom, N., & Kulgren, G. (2000). Psychopathy (PCL-R) as a predictor of violent recidivism among criminal offenders with schizophrenia. *Law and Human Behavior, 24,* 45–58.

Thornquist, M. H., & Zuckerman, M. (1995). Psychopathy, passive-avoidance learning and basic dimensions of personality. *Personality and Individual Differences, 19,* 525–534.

Toldson, I. A. (2002). *The relationship between race and psychopathy: An evaluation of selected psychometric properties of the Psychopathy Checklist—Revised (PCL-R) for incarcerated African American men.* Unpublished doctoral dissertation, Temple University, Philadelphia.

Verona, E., Patrick, C. J., & Joiner, T. E. (2001). Psychopathy, antisocial personality and suicide risk. *Journal of Abnormal Psychology, 110,* 462–470.

Vitale, J. E., Smith, S. S., Brinkley, C. A., & Newman, J. P. (2002). The reliability and validity of the Psychopathy Checklist—Revised in a sample of female offenders. *Criminal Justice and Behavior, 29,* 202–231.

Walsh, Z., Swogger, M. S., & Kosson, D. S. (2004). Psychopathy, IQ and violence in European American and African American county jail inmates. *Journal of Consulting and Clinical Psychology, 72*(6), 1165–1169.

Walsh, Z., & Kosson, D. S. (2004). *The impact of psychopathy, socioeconomic status, and ethnicity on recidivisim in a county jail population.* Manuscript in preparation.

Warren, J. L., Burnette, M., South, C. S., Chauhan, P., Bale, R., Friend, R., & Van Patten, I. (2003). Psychopathy in women: Structural modeling and co-morbidity. *International Journal of Law and Psychiatry, 26,* 223–242.

Webster, C. D., Douglas, K. S., Eaves, D., & Hart, S. D. (1997). *HCR-20: Assessing risk of violence* (version 2). Vancouver, BC: Mental Health, Law and Policy Institute, Simon Fraser University.

Williamson, S., Harpur, T. J., & Hare, R. D. (1991). Abnormal processing of affective words by psychopaths. *Psychophysiology, 28,* 260–273.

Windle, M., & Dumenci, L. (1999). The factorial structure and construct validity of the Psychopathy Checklist—Revised (PCL-R) among alcoholic inpatients. *Structural Equation Modeling, 6,* 372–393.

Zuckerman, M. (2003). Are there racial and ethnic differences in psychopathic personality? A critique of Lynn's (2002) racial and ethnic differences in psychopathic personality. *Personality and Individual Differences, 35,* 1463–1469.

23

The "Successful" Psychopath

Adaptive and Subclinical Manifestations of Psychopathy in the General Population

JASON R. HALL
STEPHEN D. BENNING

The "successful psychopath"—one who embodies the essential personality characteristics of psychopathy but who refrains from serious antisocial behavior—is a concept that has long held the interest of researchers and clinicians alike (Smith, 1978; Widom, 1977). The seemingly paradoxical designation of "successful" or noncriminal psychopathy has its modern roots in Cleckley's (1941/1988) landmark monograph, *The Mask of Sanity*. Cleckley documented several case studies of individuals who possessed the "core" personality features observed in criminal psychopaths (e.g., superficial charm, egocentricity, and guiltlessness) yet manifested those traits in ways that did not result in frequent arrests or convictions. Cleckley portrayed psychopathy as a personality disorder that did not necessarily entail severe criminal deviance, and he speculated that psychopaths could be found at nearly any occupation or level of society. Others have argued that certain psychopathic traits (e.g., glibness/charm and fearlessness) might in fact serve as valuable personal assets in some professions, such as law, politics, or business (Lykken, 1995).

The vast majority of research on psychopathy, however, has focused on samples of incarcerated male offenders. This tradition is problematic because the wealth of findings regarding incarcerated criminal psychopaths may not generalize to psychopaths (either criminal or noncriminal) residing in the community. Furthermore, as pointed out by Lilienfeld (1994), research on nonincarcerated psychopaths may contribute to the identification of protective factors that shield against chronic involvement in antisocial behavior. From a theoretical perspective, research on noncriminal psychopathy may help to address fundamental questions regarding the nature of psychopathy as a psychological disorder, such as the following: In the absence of criminal deviance, should the interpersonal–affective features of psychopathy be considered pathological? What is the true nature of the relationship between psychopathy and criminality? From a clinical standpoint, noncriminal psychopaths are of interest because they may engage in many behaviors that, although not formally illegal, represent significant breaches of social norms and the rights of others. For instance, they may achieve personal or professional successes at the expense of family, friends, and coworkers, leaving a swath of broken relationships in their wake. From this perspective, the "successful" psychopath may be well adapted in some spheres but less successful in other important domains. For this reason, the terms "noncriminal" or "nonincarcerated" psychopath will be used in lieu of "successful" in this chapter.

Despite longstanding interest in this topic, the noncriminal psychopath has proven to be an elusive target for research. Efforts to systematically study high-functioning psychopaths in the community have been greatly impeded by methodological obstacles. In particular, the identification and recruitment of psychopaths from the general population have presented an ongoing challenge, given the presumably low baserates of the disorder in noninstitutional settings. Another challenge has been the dearth of well-validated instruments for assessing psychopathy outside prisons. Furthermore, although recent years have seen notable advances in the assessment of psychopathy in community samples (for a review, see Lilienfeld, 1998), a number of questions remain concerning the basic conceptualization of noncriminal psychopaths. Specifically, are these individuals "subclinical" versions of incarcerated criminal psychopaths, representing less extreme examples of psychopathy? Or do they merely express their extreme personality tendencies in more adaptive ways, aided by compensatory mechanisms such as intelligence or socialization? To what extent does the etiology of noncriminal psychopathy overlap with its criminal expression?

The aim of this chapter is to review the existing literature concerning noncriminal psychopathy in an effort to clarify some of these issues. Specifically, we address three basic approaches to the conceptualization of the noncriminal psychopath and review both adaptive and maladaptive aspects of psychopathic personality. We then turn to a review of key methodological issues related to the study of psychopathy in noninstitutional settings. Special emphasis is placed on evaluating existing psychopathy assessment instruments with regard to their validity and appropriateness for use with nonincarcerated samples. This chapter also critically reviews the existing research literature on noncriminal psychopathy and concludes with recommendations for future research. First, however, we consider some key conceptual issues.

CONCEPTUALIZATION OF NONCRIMINAL PSYCHOPATHY

Case Studies, Fictional Illustrations, and Historical Examples

As a preface to our analysis of conceptual issues related to noncriminal psychopathy, we first highlight some illustrative examples of the phenotype. As alluded to previously, Cleckley (1988) presented several case histories exemplifying what he labeled "incomplete manifestations or suggestions of the disorder" (p. 188). Among these individuals were several prominent, high-functioning members of society, including physicians, businessmen, and aristocrats. Such cases were referred to as "psychopaths but in a milder degree" (p. 189) in that they were capable of functioning adaptively in society in spite of their underlying personality pathology. One such individual (the "Psychopath as Man of the World") was described as having connived, plagiarized, and cheated his way through several prestigious educational institutions. He was also regarded as a successful ladies' man, and was supported financially by the women he reportedly seduced. More recently, Babiak (1995) described the case of Dave, an individual who infiltrated a corporate organization and subsequently used flattery, manipulation, and backstabbing tactics to advance through the company ranks. Neither individual led a life marked by chronic antisocial behavior. Yet, both displayed many personality and behavioral features classically associated with psychopathy—superficial charm, egocentricity, parasitic lifestyle, manipulative nature, lack of remorse or empathy, irresponsibility, and so on.

Colorful examples of noncriminal psychopaths can also be found among the fictional villains (and heroes) of literature, film, and television. One vivid depiction of a successful psychopathic personality is Michael Douglas's portrayal of ruthless corporate raider Gordon Gekko in Oliver Stone's film *Wall Street*. Gekko is a cynical and callous, yet highly charismatic, leader of a Wall Street brokerage firm. His mantra, "Greed is good," underscores his ultimate devotion to personal profit at the expense of morality. The character J. R. Ewing from the television program *Dallas* (played by Larry Hagman) is another memorable example of an arrogant, remorseless, and cunning individual who casually exploits both family and business associates in order to advance his own interests. The character Alan Shore from the television legal drama *Boston Legal* (portrayed by James Spader) also presents as a charming, glib, yet quintessentially amoral individual who cons and manipulates his way into positions of power. Nevertheless, Shore, Ewing, and Gekko are all able to achieve great material and professional success while avoiding (for the most part) serious antisocial behavior.

History also provides us with numerous illustrative cases that embody the essence of the noncriminal psychopath. Lykken (1995) argued that many of history's leaders, heroes, and adventurers (such as Sir Richard Burton, Charles Yeager, and Lyndon Johnson) exhibited personality styles that, by virtue of their relatively fearless and daring natures, overlapped substantially with some of the most reviled psychopaths in recent memory (such as convicted murderers Ted Bundy and Gary Gilmore). Contemporary news headlines are also replete with accounts of brash corporate malfeasance on the part of high-functioning business leaders, such as former Enron executives Kenneth Lay and Andrew Fastow, both of whom were indicted as key figures in one of the largest bankruptcy scandals in history.

Two Sides of the Same Coin?: Adaptive and Maladaptive Manifestations of Psychopathic Traits

The aforementioned case examples illustrate the maladaptive aspects of psychopathic personality when it is found in the absence of severe criminality. Duplicitous (but not necessarily illegal) tactics such as deception, exploitation, and manipulation can have serious negative social consequences. Furthermore, as recent corporate scandals have demonstrated, these behaviors may sometimes cross over into the realm of formal criminal acts. Indeed, several studies have indicated that subclinical-range psychopathic traits are related to a range of maladaptive behaviors, including academic misconduct, major and minor legal infractions, and use of illicit substances (Benning, Patrick, Hicks, Blonigen, & Krueger, 2003; Forth, Brown, Hart, &

Hare, 1996; Gustafson & Ritzer, 1995; Levenson, Kiehl, & Fitzpatrick, 1995; Lynam, Whiteside, & Jones, 1999).

Some authors have suggested that subclinical psychopathy is one component of a "dark triad" of undesirable normal-range personality constructs that also includes subclinical narcissism and Machiavellianism (Paulhus & Williams, 2002). Narcissism in its subclinical form, as operationalized by the Narcissistic Personality Inventory (NPI; Raskin & Hall, 1979), involves a persistent pattern of self-aggrandizement and egocentricity, but at a severity that falls short of meeting formal criteria for narcissistic personality disorder (American Psychiatric Association, 1994). Machiavellianism (MACH), a construct derived from the writings of Niccolo Machiavelli (1513/1981), is intended to describe a propensity toward manipulation and instrumental use of others and is measured by the Mach-IV Inventory (Christie & Geis, 1970). The conceptual ties among these two constructs and psychopathy are nearly self-evident, lending face validity to the assertion that they share overlapping etiologies and may in fact be indicators of a common underlying construct. Indeed, empirical research has largely supported the proposed linkage of psychopathy to narcissism (Hart & Hare, 1998) and MACH (McHoskey, Worzel, & Szyarto, 1998), although the three may not represent isomorphic constructs (Paulhus & Williams, 2002).

Noncriminal psychopathy might also take the form of tactical impression management, a concept from social psychology that encompasses self-serving behaviors intended to curry favor with others and achieve social status; more devious forms of such tactics include ingratiation, intimidation, and self-promotion (Tedeschi & Melburg, 1984). Based on longitudinal–observational research in organizational settings, Babiak (1995, 2000) has described how psychopaths can function in business environments, coldly sizing up coworkers, then lying and manipulating their way into core power structures. Psychopaths may be particularly drawn to companies that are in a state of rapid or unstable transition, where they may take advantage of organizational chaos in order to profit at the expense of colleagues (Babiak, 2000).

Traits such as narcissism and MACH carry strong negative connotations that make them undesirable to possess. In contrast, Cleckley (1941/1988) described the typical psychopath as having a charming demeanor, above-average intelligence (or at least the appearance of such), an absence of delusions or neurotic behavior, and a reduced risk of (completed) suicide—all relatively desirable traits. In a similar vein, Lykken (1995) argued that the same fearless demeanor that makes the criminal psychopath so dangerous can also provide the raw psychological material for daring leadership or heroic behavior, assuming proper socialization. Others have contended that psychopathy is in fact a rational and adaptive survival strategy that is only defined as pathological when it occurs among the socially disadvantaged (Smith, 1999). Could it be that some aspects of psychopathy might imply or contribute to high levels of functioning and psychological health? Empirical evidence suggests that this may indeed be the case. For example, data from incarcerated samples indicate that the unique variance in Factor 1 of the Psychopathy Checklist—Revised (PCL-R; Hare, 1991, 2003) is negatively related to self-reported stress reactivity and positively associated with measures of trait positive emotionality, socioeconomic status, and verbal intelligence (Hall, Benning, & Patrick, 2004; Hare, 1991; Harpur, Hare, & Hakstian, 1989; Patrick, Zempolich, & Levenston, 1997; Verona, Patrick, & Joiner, 2001). In undergraduate samples, primary psychopathy as indexed by self-report is related to a highly competitive achievement orientation (Ross & Rausch, 2001), and subclinical narcissism is associated with heightened self-esteem (Raskin, Novacek, & Hogan, 1991; Watson, Little, Sawrie, & Biderman, 1992) and positive interpersonal evaluations based on first encounters (Paulhus, 1998). In addition, the fearless and socially dominant aspects of self-reported psychopathy are positively related to educational attainment and resilience against internalizing disorders such as depression and anxiety (Benning et al., 2003). Furthermore, recent data from an epidemiological twin sample indicate that self-reported psychopathic traits are negatively correlated with genetic risk for internalizing psychopathology (Blonigen, Hicks, Krueger, Patrick, & Iacono, 2005). Overall, these findings indicate that psychopathy, and in particular the fearless/interpersonally dominant features, may be related to a range of positive outcomes in the domains of cognitive and psychosocial functioning.

Synthesis: Three Conceptual Perspectives

The foregoing review of conceptual issues raises several questions that need to be addressed before a greater understanding of noncriminal psychopathy can be achieved. How can the adaptive and maladaptive aspects of psychopathy be reconciled? Do successful psychopaths share a common etiology with their criminal counterparts, distinguishable only in terms of severity? Or do they represent a separate breed? In what ways do noncriminal psychopaths resemble criminal psychopaths, and in what ways are they different? Without doubt, there is a pressing need for clarification in the conceptualization of noncriminal psychopathy. This state of affairs mirrors ongoing debate among psychopathy researchers regarding the structure and nature of the disorder in its criminal form. Nevertheless, the various conceptualizations of noncriminal psychopathy that have been proposed since the original publication of Cleckley's *Mask of Sanity* can be summarized in terms of three common themes:

1. Noncriminal psychopathy as a subclinical manifestation of the disorder.
2. Noncriminal psychopathy as a moderated expression of the full disorder.
3. Noncriminal psychopathy from a dual-process perspective.

In an effort to add clarity to the literature and to frame our subsequent discussion of empirical research on noncriminal psychopathy, we elaborate on these three conceptual motifs in turn. Examples of each perspective are provided, accompanied by a particular focus on assumptions regarding the etiology of psychopathy and its relationship to antisocial behavior and proposed differences between criminal and noncriminal psychopaths.

   1. *Noncriminal psychopathy as a subclinical manifestation of the disorder.* Central to the *subclinical process* perspective is the premise that noncriminal psychopaths

represent less extreme examples of psychopathy (i.e., "subclinical psychopaths"). From this perspective, these individuals evidence the same etiological process as incarcerated criminal psychopaths but at a reduced severity. The assumption inherent in this view is that the antisocial behaviors of incarcerated psychopaths stem directly from the core personality traits of psychopathy. Hence, the social transgressions of the less severely affected individual will be of a lesser magnitude and will occur at a lower frequency. This manner of conceptualizing noncriminal psychopathy descends directly from Cleckley's speculation that his noncriminal patients were "incomplete manifestations" of the disorder. In contemporary accounts, this perspective is perhaps best illustrated by the "aberrant self-promotion" theory of Gustafson and Ritzer (1995). Aberrant self-promoters (ASPs) are described as subclinical psychopaths who commit crimes only sporadically and possess narcissistic personality configurations. As Gustafson and Ritzer write, "the difference between the ASP and the psychopath is one of *degree*, not *kind*" (p. 148, original emphasis).

2. *Noncriminal psychopathy as a moderated expression of the disorder.* This approach proposes that criminal and noncriminal psychopaths share not only a common etiology but also equivalent severity of the basic underlying pathology. This *compensatory process* perspective also assumes that the antisocial behavior of incarcerated psychopaths is primarily a consequence of their psychopathic temperaments. However, this relationship is moderated by intervening variables. In this view, the critical difference between the two alternative manifestations (phenotypes) arises from moderating factors that shape the behavioral expression of the underlying trait disposition (genotype). For instance, the expression of psychopathy in its antisocial form might be attenuated or diverted by compensatory factors such as intelligence, exceptional talent, educational opportunity, socioeconomic status (SES), highly effective socialization, or independent aspects of temperament that constrain acting-out tendencies. Thus, bright or well-disciplined individuals may recognize and avoid the pitfalls of serious antisocial behavior and instead express their psychopathic tendencies via socially sanctioned outlets such as business, music, politics, athletics, and so on.

Such individuals may even excel in their licit pursuits, in which case they might be considered truly "successful" psychopaths.

This perspective is best exemplified by Lykken's (1957, 1995) fearlessness hypothesis of psychopathy, in which psychopaths are presumed to exhibit a specific deficit in fear reactivity. In the absence of exceptional parenting, the child with the relatively fearless temperament will be resistant to socialization and will likely evolve into an antisocial psychopath. However, Lykken (1982, 1995) argued that society's heroes, leaders, and adventurers are drawn from the same fearless stock as the psychopath, with the difference being adequate (vs. poor) socialization, and perhaps high intelligence, or the greater opportunities afforded by high SES.

3. *Noncriminal psychopathy from a dual-process perspective.* A third perspective stems from a *dual-process* model of psychopathy (cf. Patrick, 2001, in press). In this conceptualization, the interpersonal–affective features of psychopathy are considered to be etiologically distinct from the antisocial behavior component. Because these two trait dimensions are thought to reflect distinct etiologies, certain individuals could exhibit an elevation on one dimension but not the other. Thus, the noncriminal psychopath would present with elevated levels of interpersonal–affective traits but reduced or normal-range levels of traits related to antisocial deviance. This perspective draws from the tradition of research on the two-factor model of psychopathy (Hare et al., 1990; Harpur, Hakstian, & Hare, 1988; Harpur et al., 1989). Research in this area has demonstrated that the two facets of psychopathy indexed by the PCL-R (Hare, 1991) exhibit diverging (and often opposing) relations with a range of external criteria across domains of psychiatric symptoms, personality, antisocial behavior, substance use, psychophysiology, social functioning, and cognitive ability (Hall et al., 2004; Harpur et al., 1989; Patrick, 1994, 1995; Patrick, Bradley, & Lang, 1993; Patrick et al., 1997; Smith & Newman, 1990; Verona et al., 2001). Taken together, these findings have tended to indicate that an individual high in the interpersonal–affective facet of psychopathy but not the antisocial facet might have the potential to function adaptively in the community without experiencing significant legal problems.

It should be noted at this point that, while driven by differing assumptions, these three perspectives do not necessarily represent competing, mutually exclusive theories of nonincarcerated psychopathy. Rather, they can be viewed as research approaches that address different issues and potentially different target populations. For instance, the subclinical process perspective is primarily concerned with elucidating ways in which the etiologies of criminal and noncriminal psychopathy overlap and studying the characteristics and behavior of psychopaths outside of correctional settings. Research on such subclinical manifestations of psychopathy targets the population of nonincarcerated psychopaths who commit crimes sporadically or who commit crimes often but manage to escape legal detection and/or conviction. The compensatory process perspective, on the other hand, primarily seeks to detect characteristics that differentiate criminal from noncriminal psychopaths, in the interest of identifying possible protective factors. Thus, this approach involves the study of both noncriminal and nonincarcerated criminal psychopaths. Finally, the dual-process perspective is concerned with investigating potentially adaptive expressions of psychopathic traits and determining how differences in the constructs underlying psychopathy might give rise to a noncriminal subtype. Hence, this perspective is particularly focused on noncriminal manifestations of psychopathy, especially in high-functioning cases. Each of these perspectives entails different recruitment strategies, methods, and operational definitions of "successful" psychopathy. Thus, each of these conceptualizations is considered in turn in our review of empirical findings. However, before discussing this literature, we first turn to a review of methodological problems related to the study of psychopathy in community settings, with a particular focus on assessment.

ASSESSMENT OF THE NONINSTITUTIONALIZED PSYCHOPATH

A significant methodological problem in studying the noninstitutionalized psychopath involves the criteria for assessing psychopathy outside an institutional setting. At least two studies have used the PCL-R to examine psychopathy in a noninstitutional sample (Ishikawa, Raine, Lencz, Bihrle, & LaCasse, 2001; Vanman, Mejia, Dawson, Schell, & Raine, 2003). The PCL-R is widely regarded as the gold standard in psychopathy assessment; however, use of the PCL-R in nonforensic settings is problematic for several reasons. First, without the file information that is used in scoring the PCL-R in mental health and forensic settings, it is difficult or impossible to score certain items that rely on formal legal records (e.g., criminal versatility). Second, the PCL-R was intended for use with criminal populations, and consequently many (if not most) of the items are scored on the basis of information relating to antisocial deviance. Thus, the PCL-R may not be an appropriate instrument for measuring noncriminal manifestations of psychopathic traits. Third, scoring of the PCL-R requires a lengthy semistructured interview, making it a burdensome tool for studying psychopathy in community samples, where baserates of psychopathy are presumably low and large-scale screening would be needed to identify a sufficient number of psychopaths for study. Thus, alternative assessment strategies have been developed. Because the literature on self-report measures of psychopathy is reviewed elsewhere in this volume (see Lilienfeld & Fowler, Chapter 6, this volume), the major focus of this section is on observer-rating measures that may be useful in assessing noninstitutionalized individuals with psychopathy. However, recent self-report instruments that hold particular promise in assessing the two-factor conceptualization of psychopathy are also discussed briefly.

Observer Measures

Psychopathy Checklist: Screening Version

The screening version of the PCL-R (PCL:SV; Hart, Cox, & Hare, 1995) is a promising interview-based measure designed for assessing psychopathy in nonforensic samples. It consists of 12 items that are scored from 0 (not applicable) to 2 (definitely applicable) on the basis of a 30–60-minute interview (Forth et al., 1996). It has two factors that correspond to Factors 1 and 2 of the PCL-R. Forth and colleagues (1996) reported that total scores on this measure showed strong relations with child and adult symptoms of antisocial personality disorder (*r*'s ranged from .62 to .81), self-reported substance use problems (*r*'s = .47–.68), and antisocial behaviors (*r*'s = .22–.50). In this study, total scores on the PCL:SV were also positively related to scores on the arrogant-calculating octant of the interpersonal circumplex (*r*'s = .30–.50).

Interpersonal Measure of Psychopathy

The Interpersonal Measure of Psychopathy (IM-P; Kosson, Steuerwald, Forth, & Kirkhart, 1997) focuses on the interpersonal behaviors of psychopathic individuals. It comprises 18 items that are scored from 1 (not at all) to 4 (perfectly) on the basis of how descriptive each item is of a participant's behavior during a diagnostic interview. Kosson et al. (1997) noted that scores on this measure were correlated with age (*r*'s = .35–.37) and education (*r* = .34), and also preferentially with Factor 1 of the PCL-R (*r*'s = .33–.62 with Factor 1, vs. .15–.31 with Factor 2). After the influence of PCL-R Factors 1 and 2 were accounted for in regression analyses, IM-P scores uniquely predicted interviewer self-reports of trepidation and avoidance of conflict, observer ratings of interpersonal dominance, and history of adult fights (Kosson et al., 1997). These findings suggest that the IM-P captures variance in these interpersonal criterion measures that is distinct from that tapped by PCL-R Factors 1 and 2. Furthermore, after controlling for the influence of the PCL-R factors, IM-P scores were *negatively* associated with nonviolent disciplinary infractions, criminal and drug use versatility, and adult symptoms of antisocial personality disorder (Kosson et al., 1997). This finding is notable, as it implies that the interpersonal construct tapped by the IM-P is less rooted in antisocial deviance than the factors of the PCL-R, thereby suggesting that the IM-P may be a useful instrument for assessing noncriminal manifestations of psychopathy.

Psychopathy Q-Sort

The Psychopathy Q-Sort (PQS; Reise & Oliver, 1994) is an expert-generated prototype of psychopathy, derived from the 100 items of the California Q-Set (CAQ; Block, 1961). Each item is rated on a 9-point scale (1 = most uncharacteristic, 9 = most characteris-

tic), and item ratings are forced into a quasi-normal distribution. Items most characteristic of PQS psychopathy describe a charming, self-absorbed, deceitful, and hostile individual; those most uncharacteristic of PQS psychopathy reflect an anxious, reliable, submissive, and insightful person. Ratings on the PQS were found to correlate substantially (*r* = .51) with a CAQ narcissism prototype (Wink, 1992), but nonsignificantly (*r* = .16) with a CAQ hysteria prototype (Reise & Oliver, 1994). Furthermore, Reise and Wink (1995) reported that PQS profile scores were significantly and positively related to self-reported symptoms of most Cluster B personality disorders (*r*'s = .21–.33) and to scales loading on the "Externality, Social Poise, and Assurance" superfactor of Gough's (1987) California Psychological Inventory (CPI; *r*'s = .17–.33). In contrast, PQS scores correlated negatively with scales loading on the CPI "Normative Control of Impulse" superfactor (*r*'s = −.16– −.38).

Psychopathy-Scan

The Psychopathy-Scan (P-Scan; Hare & Herve, 1999) was designed to provide a rating scale for psychopathy that can be used by nonclinical raters. It comprises three factors (interpersonal, affective, and behavioral), with 30 items each, that mirror the three-factor structure of psychopathy proposed by Cooke and Michie (2001). Items are scored on a scale of 0 (item does not apply) to 2 (item definitely applies). Elwood, Poythress, and Douglas (2004) reported that total scores on this instrument significantly predicted self-reported antisocial behavior (*r*'s = .25–.28). However, when the influence of the other factors was controlled, none of the factors exhibited significant unique relations with antisocial behavior (Elwood et al., 2004), suggesting a lack of divergent validity among the three factors of the P-Scan—at least with respect to antisociality.

Business-Scan

The Business-Scan (B-Scan; Babiak & Hare, in press) is an instrument that permits supervisors and coworkers to assess psychopathic traits in business or occupational settings. It yields scores on four subscales (personal style, emotional style, organizational maturity, and antisocial tendencies) that parallel the factors of Hare's (2003) recent four-factor model of psychopathy. However, validity information has yet to be reported for this instrument.

Self-Report Measures

Self-Report Psychopathy–II

The Self-Report Psychopathy–II scale (SRP-II; Hare, 1991) is a 60-item measure that was designed to assess PCL-R psychopathy via self-report. It includes two correlated (r = .37; Zagon & Jackson, 1994), rationally derived factors designed to parallel Factors 1 and 2 of the PCL-R. Factor 1 of the SRP-II correlates negatively with measures of state and trait anxiety and personal distress, and positively with narcissism and positive self-presentation (Zagon & Jackson, 1994). SRP-II Factor 2 correlates positively with narcissism, as well as negative self-presentation (Zagon & Jackson, 1994) and MACH (Williams & Paulhus, 2004).

Levenson's Self-Report of Psychopathy

Similar in intent to the IM-P, Levenson's Self-Report of Psychopathy (LSRP; Levenson et al., 1995) was designed to assess a "protopsychopathic interpersonal philosophy." It comprises two correlated (r = .40; Levenson et al., 1995) factors, which putatively measure two distinct aspects of the interpersonal behavior of psychopathic individuals. The first factor, titled "primary psychopathy," consists of items describing a manipulative and exploitative interaction style; the second factor, titled "secondary psychopathy," consists of items describing an impulsive, alienated, and aggressive individual. Levenson and colleagues (1995) reported that primary psychopathy scores correlated preferentially with the boredom susceptibility and disinhibition facets of sensation seeking (Zuckerman, 1979) and were inversely related to scores on the Harm Avoidance subscale of Tellegen's (in press) Multidimensional Personality Questionnaire (MPQ). In contrast, secondary psychopathy scores correlated positively with scores on the Stress Reaction scale of the MPQ and inversely with academic grade point average, although both factors contributed independently to predicting self-reported antisocial behavior.

Five-Factor Model Psychopathy Prototype

Miller, Lynam, Widiger, and Leukefeld (2001) developed a prototypic psychopathic personality profile based on the personality dimensions of the five-factor model (FFM), as measured by the NEO Personality Inventory—Revised (NEO-PI-R; Costa & McCrae, 1992). This profile was marked by high overall scores on Extraversion and on the angry hostility and impulsivity facets of Neuroticism and by low scores on Agreeableness; the dutifulness and deliberation facets of Conscientiousness; and the anxiety, depression, and self-consciousness facets of Neuroticism. Scores on a prototypicality index of this profile correlated positively with antisocial behavior and substance misuse, and negatively with anxiety and depression.

Psychopathic Personality Inventory

The Psychopathic Personality Inventory (PPI; Lilienfeld & Andrews, 1996) is a 187-item measure that indexes the personality characteristics of psychopathy without explicit reference to antisocial/criminal behaviors. Its items are grouped into eight subscales: Machiavellian Egocentricity, Social Potency, Fearlessness, Coldheartedness, Impulsive Nonconformity, Blame Externalization, Carefree Nonplanfulness, and Stress Immunity. The PPI also includes validity scales designed to identify biased or inconsistent reporting. PPI total scores correlate positively with global observer ratings of Cleckley psychopathy as well as both self-report and interview measures of antisocial personality disorder and narcissism; total scores on the PPI correlate negatively with self-reported fears and anxiety (Lilienfeld & Andrews, 1996). Edens, Cruise, and Buffington-Vollum (2001) reported that PPI total scores also showed positive correlations with scores on the Antisocial Features scale of Morey's (1991) Personality Assessment Inventory. Lilienfeld and Andrews reported positive associations between PPI total scores and scores on the Psychopathic Deviate (Pd) scale of the Minnesota Multiphasic Personality Inventory (MMPI; Hathaway & McKinley, 1942), the Socialization (So) scale of the CPI, and total scores on both the SRP-II and the LSRP.

Recent work suggests that two broad, orthogonal (r = –.07) factors underlie the subscales of the PPI (Benning et al., 2003). One factor, termed "PPI-I" (Benning et al., 2003), or "fearless dominance" (Benning, Patrick, Blonigen, Hicks, & Iacono, 2005), comprises the Social Potency, Stress Immunity, and Fearlessness scales; the other, termed "PPI-II" (Benning et al., 2003), or "impulsive antisociality" (Benning et al., 2005), comprises the Impulsive Nonconformity, Machiavellian Egocentricity, Carefree Nonplanfulness, and Blame Externalization scales. Fearless dominance is associated positively with adult symptoms of antisocial personality disorder, educational attainment, and SES (Benning et al., 2003). In contrast, impulsive antisociality is associated positively with child and adult symptoms of antisocial personality disorder and alcohol/drug use, and negatively with IQ, educational attainment, and SES (Benning et al., 2003). In addition, Benning and colleagues (2003) found that the constructs associated with the two PPI factors were predicted well by the scales of an omnibus personality inventory, the MPQ. After disattenuating for loss of reliability associated with the lengthy interval (6 years) between administration of the MPQ and the PPI, multiple R's were .89 and .84 for fearless dominance and impulsive antisociality, respectively. Specifically, scores on the fearless dominance factor were significantly predicted by high Social Potency, low Stress Reaction, and low Harm Avoidance, whereas impulsive antisociality was significantly predicted by high Alienation, high Aggression, low planful Control, low Traditionalism, and low Social Closeness. As described later, this allows for investigation of the two PPI facets in existing datasets that include the MPQ (cf. Benning et al., in press).

LABORATORY STUDIES OF NONINCARCERATED PSYCHOPATHS

Early Research

In one of the first attempts to study psychopathy outside a prison setting, Widom (1977) recruited subjects from the community via newspaper advertisements requesting "adventurous" individuals leading "carefree" and "exciting, impulsive lives" who would "do almost anything on a dare" (p. 675). A later advertisement issued a call for "charming, aggressive, carefree people who are impulsively irresponsible but are good at handling people and looking out for number one" (p. 675). These advertisements were intended to attract individuals from the community who possessed psychopathic personality attributes but who were not extensively involved in criminal activity. Respondents were asked to submit brief autobiographical accounts, which were used to screen for the possible presence of psychopathic traits. Individuals who were invited to participate took part in an experiment consisting of a clinical interview and personality questionnaires, as well as two behavioral tasks. The first task was the Porteus Maze task (Porteus, 1965), a paper-and-pencil cognitive task that yields measures of accuracy as well as a Qualitative or Q-score, which is thought to index behavioral impulsivity or carelessness. The Q-score index has been associated with both delinquency and psychopathy in prior research (for a review, see Morgan & Lilienfeld, 2000). The second behavioral task was a test of delayed gratification, in which participants were given the option of receiving an extra $5 compensation if they elected to wait 2 weeks for payment rather than receiving it immediately.

Widom (1977) reported on the biographical, psychiatric, psychometric, and behavioral characteristics of the sample recruited via this novel method. Subjects ($N = 28$) were predominantly male (82%) and most were from lower SES backgrounds, although several reported holding jobs of considerable status and responsibility (business managers, investment bankers, etc.). Mean SES and level of education for this sample were higher than for comparison samples of incarcerated psychopaths. However, approximately one-fifth of the sample had received inpatient psychiatric care, and a similar proportion had official conviction records. Of note, nearly 65% of subjects in the Widom sample reported having an arrest record; almost half reported at least brief periods of incarceration. In addition, the majority of the sample (nearly four out of five) met or exceeded Robins's (1966) criteria for sociopathy, a diagnosis that relies heavily on the presence of chronic antisocial behavior (e.g., heavy alcohol/drug use, physical aggression, and repeated arrests). Taken together, these elevated indicators of criminality suggest that the sample was characterized more by evasion of conviction rather than avoidance of criminally deviant behavior.

As predicted, the mean MMPI profile for Widom's (1977) sample was marked by elevations on Scales 4 (*Psychopathic Deviate*) and 9 (*Hypomania*). Also consistent with prediction, this sample demonstrated elevated scores on the Extraversion scale of the Eysenck Personality Inventory (Eysenck & Eysenck, 1968), and low scores on the Hogan Empathy Scale (Hogan, 1969) and the *So* scale of the CPI. Thus, this community-recruited sample bore some psychometric similarity to incarcerated psychopaths. However, contrary to expectation, scores on the Machiavellianism Scale (Christie & Geis, 1970) and Porteus Maze Q-scores did not differ significantly from community norms. Furthermore, the majority of subjects chose to delay the delivery of their study compensation in order to obtain the additional $5 offered.

In a subsequent study, Widom and Newman (1985) collected personality, demographic, and behavioral data from a sample of 40 individuals recruited from the community using a similar strategy. Demographically and psychometrically, the sample for this study closely resembled the Widom (1977) group. On average, however, these participants were less antisocial than the Widom sample: Only one-third (N = 13) reported having an arrest record, and fewer than 10% had ever been incarcerated. Yet, nearly three-fourths of the sample (N = 29) met Robins's (1966) criteria for sociopathy. Widom and Newman (1985) found that the most severely antisocial participants who met the more stringent Research Diagnostic Criteria (RDC; Spitzer, Endicott, & Robins, 1975) for antisocial personality (N = 5) demonstrated the most interesting behavioral differences when compared with the rest of the sample. These subjects committed a greater number of passive avoidance errors during a successive go/no-go discrimination task, indicating that they were less able to inhibit responding when faced with cues indicating punishment. Newman and colleagues (Newman & Kosson, 1986; Newman, Patterson, Howland, & Nichols, 1990; Newman & Schmitt, 1998) have repeatedly demonstrated that incarcerated psychopaths show a deficit in the ability to withhold responses to stimuli that result in punishment,

especially when engaged in the active pursuit of reward. These findings thus extended prior work by demonstrating that in addition to their psychometric similarities, psychopaths recruited from the community also share some behavioral characteristics with incarcerated psychopaths in terms of performance on laboratory tasks.

Sutker and Allain (1983) attempted to avoid recruiting a highly antisocial sample by screening medical students (who were assumed to be high functioning) for psychopathic traits using the MMPI. A small sample of individuals (N = 8) with significant 4–9 elevations (labeled "adaptive sociopaths") and a matched sample of controls (N = 8) completed a brief interview along with personality questionnaires and the Porteus Maze task as part of the experiment. The adaptive sociopaths scored higher than controls on the Sensation Seeking Scale (SSS; Zuckerman, Kolin, Price, & Zoob, 1964) and lower on the CPI *So* scale. In contrast with Widom (1977), adaptive sociopaths produced higher Q-scores on the Porteus Maze task, suggesting greater behavioral impulsivity and carelessness than controls. However, they were not rated as lower in empathy by interviewers, and none were diagnosed with antisocial personality disorder (APD).

These three studies have been highly influential in that they represent the earliest attempts to systematically study psychopathy in community settings. Perhaps the most important finding to arise from these studies is that psychopathic individuals can indeed be recruited from the community, and that they resemble incarcerated psychopaths in some aspects of personality and behavior. However, these studies were limited in several notable ways.

First, well-validated and standardized assessments of psychopathy were not widely available at the time these studies were conducted. The interview assessments used to operationalize psychopathy in Widom's studies were heavily weighted toward the measurement of chronic antisocial behavior, with lesser emphasis on the core personality features of psychopathy. Sutker and Allain's (1983) use of MMPI profiles to identify psychopaths is also problematic, as the prototypically "psychopathic" 4–9 profile correlates robustly with the antisocial deviance component of psychopathy, but negligibly with the interpersonal–affective facet (Hare, 1991). Thus, the degree to which subjects in these two samples resemble psychopaths diagnosed using contemporary measures remains unclear.

Second, perhaps as a consequence of screening criteria, the prevalence of criminal behavior in the Widom (1977) study was significantly elevated above community base rates; furthermore, the majority of subjects in both the Widom and Widom and Newman (1985) samples met Robins's (1966) criteria for sociopathy, which, as noted earlier, rely heavily on the presence of chronic antisocial behavior. Thus, it is reasonable to question the extent to which these community psychopaths differed from their incarcerated counterparts. Widom speculated that the psychopaths recruited from the community differed from incarcerated psychopaths "not in terms of the frequency of arrests but in the *frequency of convictions*" (p. 681, original emphasis). From this standpoint, these two studies may be viewed as representations of the "subclinical" research strategy, in which individuals representing less severe manifestations of psychopathy are recruited for study. However, given the high rate of prior convictions for the nonincarcerated psychopaths in these two studies, an alternative possibility is that these individuals were quite similar to incarcerated psychopaths in terms of their antisocial deviance but were recruited and studied when they did not happen to be incarcerated.

Contemporary Research with the PCL-R in Community Samples

Since the publication of these landmark studies, several attempts have been made to extend initial findings on psychopathy to community samples using contemporary assessment techniques—namely, the PCL-R and its variants. Belmore and Quinsey (1994) recruited community subjects through the use of advertisements placed in newspapers and at a local unemployment office. Respondents were assessed using an abbreviated PCL-R measure supplemented by information regarding childhood behavior problems. Subjects also completed personality questionnaires and a card-playing task developed by Newman, Patterson, and

Kosson (1987), in which the odds of winning decreased incrementally over the course of the game. As predicted, subjects scoring high on the abridged PCL-R ($N = 15$) also scored high on the Kipnis (1971) Impulsiveness Scale, and low in CPI Socialization. In comparison with low scorers ($N = 15$), these high scorers also played more cards during the behavioral task, indicating a reduced ability to evaluate and incorporate loss feedback while engaged in approach behavior. These results are consistent with findings from the go/no-go task used by Widom and Newman (1985).

A sizable body of work exists concerning psychophysiological response characteristics of incarcerated psychopaths. Several studies have indicated that, compared to nonpsychopathic prisoners, psychopaths exhibit reduced physiological arousal during anticipatory anxiety (Hare, 1965; Hare, Frazelle, & Cox, 1978; Tharp, Maltzman, Syndulko, & Ziskind, 1980) and aberrant affective startle modulation (Levenston, Patrick, Bradley, & Lang, 2000; Patrick et al., 1993; Sutton, Vitale, & Newman, 2002). Researchers have recently begun to extend these findings to nonincarcerated psychopaths. Ishikawa and colleagues (2001) examined the psychophysiological correlates of psychopathy in a community sample recruited from temporary employment agencies and assessed using the PCL-R. Participants labeled "successful" psychopaths (those without a history of criminal conviction; $N = 13$) were compared with "unsuccessful" psychopaths (those with a conviction record; $N = 16$) and nonpsychopathic community controls (no criminal record; $N = 26$). Consistent with prior research, unsuccessful psychopaths demonstrated reduced cardiovascular reactivity during a social stressor task, relative to controls. The nonconvicted psychopaths, however, exhibited a pattern of *increased* cardiovascular response during the stressor, which consisted of giving a brief speech about one's faults. Relative to both comparison groups, these psychopaths also demonstrated a higher level of executive functioning, as measured by performance on the Wisconsin Card Sort Test (WCST; Heaton, Chelune, Talley, Kay, & Kurtis, 1993). Ishikawa and colleagues speculated that heightened autonomic reactivity to stress and relatively higher levels of executive functioning might act as protective factors for "successful" psychopaths, enabling them to avoid the riskiest of criminal activities that might result in arrest, conviction, and incarceration.

Vanman and colleagues (2003) examined patterns of affective startle modulation associated with psychopathy in the same community sample, although in this investigation, psychopaths were not divided into "successful" and "unsuccessful" groups. Startle blink responses, elicited by abrupt noise probes and measured via electromyographic recording from the *orbicularis occuli* muscle, were recorded while subjects viewed pleasant and unpleasant photographic stimuli. Whereas normal individuals show potentiated startle blinks while viewing negative emotional stimuli (Bradley, Cuthbert, & Lang, 1999), incarcerated psychopaths typically exhibit an abnormal pattern of *inhibited* startle amplitude while viewing negatively valenced stimuli (e.g., Patrick et al., 1993), implying a reduced reactivity to fearful or unpleasant emotional events. Vanman and colleagues replicated the findings of Patrick and colleagues (1993), demonstrating a similar pattern of reduced affective startle potentiation among psychopaths from the community. Furthermore, as in Patrick and colleagues this deficit in negative emotional reactivity was selectively associated with the interpersonal–affective facet of psychopathy; in contrast, the antisocial component of psychopathy was associated with significantly *greater* startle potentiation for negative stimuli. The Vanman and colleagues study thus successfully replicated prior findings from incarcerated samples and extended these findings to a community sample. However, unlike Ishikawa and colleagues (2001), this study did not separately examine psychopaths with and without criminal records, thus making the results difficult to interpret with regard to noncriminal manifestations of psychopathy.

Summary and Critique of Laboratory Research

To summarize, laboratory studies of psychopaths recruited from the community have demonstrated that these individuals tend to have higher arrest rates than the norm, but a slightly reduced rate of conviction relative to incarcerated psychopaths; they are psychometrically similar to incarcerated psychopaths in terms of self-reported personality (e.g., empathy, impulsivity, socialization, and MMPI profiles); and, like incarcerated psychopaths, they tend to demonstrate poor response modulation, careless motor behavior, and abnormal affective modulation of startle. Taken together, these findings point most notably to ways in which nonincarcerated psychopaths are phenotypically (and perhaps etiologically) similar to their incarcerated counterparts. Furthermore, these data suggest that at least a subset of nonincarcerated psychopaths manifest psychopathy at a reduced or subclinical level, insofar as their continued presence in the community is indicative of reduced severity of the process underlying their antisocial deviance. However, some nonincarcerated psychopaths (i.e., those without a history of conviction) may be differentiated on the basis of their increased autonomic responsiveness to stress and largely intact executive functioning, both of which could serve as protective factors against chronic antisocial behavior, as Ishikawa and colleagues (2001) speculate. Widom (1977) also noted that psychopaths from the community tend to come from higher socioeconomic backgrounds than incarcerated psychopaths. These findings have shed light on some compensatory processes that could potentially moderate the behavioral expression of psychopathic traits.

However, the issue of criminality among community samples remains a major interpretive challenge for researchers interested in the possibility of a noncriminal psychopathy subtype. Both Ishikawa and colleagues (2001) and Belmore and Quinsey (1994) reported high levels of antisocial behavior in their respective community samples, even among the "successful," never-convicted psychopaths. Samples such as these (in which both experimental and comparison groups exhibit histories of persistent antisocial behavior) do not permit inferences regarding noncriminal manifestations of psychopathy. These studies recruited subjects mainly from temporary employment agencies or unemployment offices, settings in which baserates of particular psychopathic traits (especially those traits linked to the antisocial–deviance component of psychopathy, e.g., irresponsibility, impulsivity, behavioral disinhibition, and parasitic lifestyle) are likely to be higher than in the general population. Consequently, recruitment of psychopathic subjects from such populations may be more tractable than in the larger community, where baserates of psychopathy are estimated to be low (approx. 1%; Hare, 2003).

The strategy of recruiting from high baserate settings has been viewed as a necessary measure due to the rigorous time demands of PCL-R assessment. However, while more efficient, pursuing a "high-risk" recruitment strategy also has the unfortunate effect of producing samples populated with both previously convicted and formally undetected criminals. This situation, although not an obstacle for those interested in studying subclinical manifestations of psychopathy, becomes problematic when the goal is to study psychopathy in the absence of chronic antisociality. To highlight the impact of this issue, it may be helpful to recall the noncriminal psychopaths described in the case studies cited previously: individuals who, although callous and manipulative, largely refrain from engaging in antisocial behavior, and may even achieve significant success in their legitimate pursuits (albeit via exploitative means). Clearly, the types of high-functioning individuals described by Cleckley and Lykken—slick but callous businessmen, smooth-talking and manipulative lawyers, arrogant and deceptive politicians—are likely to be missed by recruitment strategies that target high-risk populations. This is unfortunate, considering that these individuals could potentially yield the most information regarding protective factors and adaptive expressions of psychopathic traits. However, this methodological impediment can potentially be overcome through the use of self-report assessment of psychopathy, as described in the following section.

Laboratory Research Using Self-Report Assessments of Psychopathy

Recent years have seen a dramatic rise in the number of studies using self-report methods to study psychopathy among nonincarcerated samples. This assessment strategy offers a potential solution to the problem of criminality among community samples recruited from high-risk populations and assessed via the PCL-R. Self-report methods allow researchers to efficiently screen large numbers of potential research subjects from the general population and target high-scoring individuals for recruitment. In doing so, researchers may be more likely to encounter individuals with the core personality features associated with psychopathy but who have not engaged in repeated antisocial acts. Longstanding doubts regarding the effectiveness of self-report inventories for the assessment of psychopathy have begun to give way in the face of accumulating evidence supporting the validity of several self-report psychopathy measures (cf. Lilienfeld & Fowler, Chapter 6, this volume).

Two studies have investigated the hypothesis that noninstitutionalized psychopaths may have deficits in response modulation similar to those observed in incarcerated individuals with psychopathy. In a sample of 70 undergraduate males, Lynam and colleagues (1999) found that overall scores on the LSRP were related to commission errors in a go/no-go laboratory task, and to quickened reaction times to neutral cues previously associated with monetary punishment, implying impaired response modulation. Similarly, in a mixed sample of 211 undergraduates, participants whose personality profiles were most similar to the FFM psychopathy prototype identified by Miller and colleagues (2001) were found to be more impulsive, electing to receive smaller immediate rewards instead of greater delayed rewards (Miller & Lynam, 2003).

Self-report assessment methods have also been employed to test Blair's (2001) violence inhibition model of psychopathy in community samples. This theory posits that the destructive behaviors of psychopaths arise from a deficiency in evolutionary mechanisms responsible for cessation of aggression in the presence of distress signals from victims. Miller and Lynam (2003) reported that FFM psychopathy prototype scores were related to higher levels of aggression in a laboratory task. In addition, male undergraduate participants ($N = 100$) high on the primary psychopathy scale of the LSRP tended to perceive more positive consequences for aggression than those low in primary psychopathy, and they also tended to perceive fewer negative consequences for aggression after being primed by an aggressive film (Ferrigan, Valentiner, & Berman, 2000). However, participants high on the secondary psychopathy scale of the LSRP endorsed fewer positive consequences for aggression after being primed with an aggressive film (Ferrigan et al., 2000), suggesting that the two factors may give rise to separable types of aggressive behavior.

More recently, Benning, Patrick, and Iacono (in press) used the MPQ to estimate scores on the two factors of the PPI (fearless dominance and impulsive antisociality, cf. Benning et al., 2005) in order to investigate affective startle modulation among nonincarcerated individuals high in psychopathy. The sample consisted of a large number of young adult male twins (N = 353) recruited from the community. This study found that individuals demonstrating high trait levels of fearless dominance, relative to those who were low, exhibited attenuated startle potentiation and reduced skin conductance responses to aversive (vs. neutral) photographs. On the other hand, participant groups defined by high and low levels of impulsive antisociality showed equivalent physiological differentiation between aversive and neutral pictures. However, the high impulsive antisociality group showed reduced overall skin conductance response across all picture stimuli. The findings of this study replicate and extend the earlier findings of Patrick and colleagues (1993) and Vanman and colleagues (2003) by demonstrating that the two facets of psychopathy, as indexed by the PPI, exhibit distinct physiological correlates in a community sample. Specifically, the fearless dominance facet (akin to PCL-R Factor 1) is associated with attenuated physiological reactivity to aversive stimuli, whereas impulsive antisociality (akin to PCL-R Factor 2) may be associated with general sympathetic underarousal. These findings appear consistent with a dual-process model of psychopathy, which posits that separate underlying etiologies contribute to the psychopathy phenotype (Patrick, 2001, in press; see also Fowles & Dindo, Chapter 2, this volume). One facet—fearless dominance—appears to be manifested in terms of both adjustment (hardiness, resiliency) and maladjustment (narcissism, insensitivity), while the other—impulsive antisociality—is manifested more purely in terms of maladjustment (aggressive externalizing).

SUMMARY AND CONCLUSIONS

Noncriminal psychopathy is a conceptually complex phenomenon that has proven difficult to elucidate via empirical research. In this chapter we have endeavored to provide a cogent analysis of noncriminal psychopathy—a topic that has been marked by methodological challenges and differing conceptual definitions of the phenotype under consideration. In this final section we summarize the findings reviewed earlier, advance some conclusions regarding the nature of noncriminal psychopathy, and offer our recommendations for future research in this area.

Past research on noncriminal psychopathy has faced significant methodological challenges related to the recruitment and assessment of psychopaths in the community. Early recruitment strategies utilizing newspaper advertisements yielded promising results but have not been employed in more recent research. Broad screening efforts in the general population using interview assessments of psychopathy are relatively unfeasible, whereas targeted recruitment from "high-risk" populations may have the adverse effect of generating low-functioning samples characterized by high levels of antisocial deviance—an undesirable outcome when the goal is to study adaptive expressions of psychopathic traits or potential protective factors. An alternative strategy is to use self-report psychopathy inventories, which permit large-scale screening of participants from the general community. This approach may allow researchers to select a suitable number of psychopathic individuals from the community for study without resorting to high-risk recruitment strategies. However, the validation of these self-report psychopathy instruments remains an ongoing effort.

To date, research focusing on subclinical manifestations of psychopathy has revealed a number of similarities between incarcerated and nonincarcerated samples. Nonincarcerated antisocial psychopaths typically exhibit personality profiles similar to their incarcerated counterparts (i.e., high impulsivity, low empathy, low socialization, and similar MMPI profiles), implying that the same basic temperament disposition underlies manifestations of psychopathy in both populations. Nonincarcerated psychopaths in the community (particularly those possessing many of the interpersonal–affective features of the disorder) also consistently demonstrate abnormal patterns of affective startle modulation, implying a deficit in fearful or defensive reactivity paralleling that observed in psychopathic prisoners. Undergraduates with psychopathic personality profiles also tend to favor aggressive tactics in laboratory tasks and express positive attitudes toward aggressive behavior. In addition, mirroring results commonly obtained with incarcerated psychopaths, nonincarcerated psychopaths from undergraduate and community samples show deficits in response modulation, as indexed by tasks requiring inhibition of ongoing approach behavior in the face of cues signaling punishment. These similarities in personality, emotional responding, aggression, and response modulation all point to the conclusion that similar or overlapping etiological processes underlie psychopathy in both nonincarcerated and incarcerated populations.

On the other hand, research from a compensatory process perspective has identified a number of potentially meaningful distinctions between incarcerated and nonincarcerated psychopaths. For instance, while nonincarcerated psychopaths clearly show elevated arrest rates relative to the general population, they appear able to successfully avoid lengthy incarcerations for their criminal behavior. Psychopaths in the community also tend to hail from more advantaged socioeconomic backgrounds than psychopaths found in prison. Furthermore, when nonincarcerated psychopaths are separated into those with and without histories of criminal conviction, the nonconvicted group demonstrates higher levels of executive function and elevated physiological reactivity to social stress. The fact that nonconvicted psychopaths demonstrated elevated autonomic stress response seems to contradict the results of Benning and colleagues (in press), suggesting that the "successful" psychopaths in Ishikawa and colleagues (2001) may be distinguishable in terms of etiology from the high fearless–dominant group studied in Benning and colleagues. In fact, based on data suggesting greater parental absence among the families of nonconvicted psychopaths, Ishikawa and colleagues speculated

that the nonconvicted group may have been "pushed" toward psychopathic behavior by environmental circumstances rather than biological/temperament factors as specified by Benning and colleagues. Apparent conflicts such as these underscore the need for additional clarity in the conceptualization of psychopathy in noninstitutional settings.

Overall, however, these findings tend to bolster the notion that a subgroup of nonincarcerated psychopaths benefits from compensatory factors that mitigate the behavioral expression of the disorder. Nevertheless, given the high prevalence of self-reported criminal deviance among the "successful" psychopaths in the study by Ishikawa and colleagues (2001) and studies by Widom (1977) and Widom and Newman (1985), possible protective factors such as high SES, intact executive functioning, and autonomic hyperreactivity may serve to buffer against criminal conviction and incarceration but not necessarily antisocial behavior. Thus, without the inclusion of *noncriminal* psychopath groups, the findings of these studies are difficult to interpret with regard to protective or compensatory mechanisms that attenuate criminal manifestations of psychopathic attributes. Recently, the use of self-report assessments has allowed researchers to study psychopathy in community and undergraduate samples less characterized by prevalent antisocial behavior. Consistent with the dual-process perspective, there is some evidence to suggest that the two facets of self-reported psychopathy may reflect separate etiologies with distinct correlates in nonforensic samples (Benning et al., 2003, in press; Benning, Patrick, Salekin, & Leistico, in press; Blonigen et al., 2005; Levenson et al., 1995; Williams & Paulhus, 2004; Zagon & Jackson, 1994). Specifically, the two facets exhibit divergent correlations across domains of personality, psychiatric symptoms, psychosocial functioning, and physiological responding. Moreover, recent research using the PPI has indicated that the fearless dominance facet of self-reported psychopathy is uncorrelated with the impulsive antisociality facet and correlates only weakly with interviewer-rated adult antisocial behavior ($r = .15$), and negligibly with childhood behavior problems ($r = .02$; Benning et al., 2003).

These results suggest that the interpersonal–affective features of psychopathy, when measured via self-report and without specific reference to antisocial behavior, are essentially unrelated to most forms of criminal deviance. Furthermore, fearless dominance is positively associated with psychosocial resilience, SES, and academic achievement (Benning et al., 2003), suggesting some possible adaptive aspects of psychopathy. Those individuals who possess elevated trait levels of fearless dominance, but not impulsive antisociality, may be the quintessential high-functioning, noncriminal psychopaths of the type described by Lykken (1995). The dual-process perspective may thus be particularly well suited to the study of this type of individual. However, the strongest support for the dual-process perspective derives primarily from studies using a single instrument—the PPI—which appears to be unique among self-report psychopathy measures in that its two factors are uncorrelated, and only one of them relates to antisocial outcomes. Although there is some evidence pointing to the convergent validity of self-report psychopathy measures in community samples (Salekin, Trobst, & Krioukova, 2001), more work is needed to clarify the nature of the constructs measured by the different self-report instruments available at this time.

FUTURE DIRECTIONS

Despite significant advances in this area, a number of central questions remain regarding "successful" psychopathy. For instance, how is this phenomenon best defined? Three prominent conceptual definitions derived from previous work (subclinical, compensatory, and dual-process perspectives) have been reviewed here, but ultimately some synthesis of these perspectives may be achieved. Furthermore, although prior research has largely pointed to parallels or overlap in the etiologies of criminal and noncriminal/subclinical psychopathy, future research may reveal that there are in fact multiple etiological pathways to this phenotype—some involving genetic/temperamental factors (e.g., deficient fear response) and others involving environmental influences (e.g., parental absence and poor attachment).

Continuing research in this area will no doubt have implications for our conceptualizations of psychopathy generally, especially with regard to the diagnostic prominence of antisocial behavior within the syndrome. Traditional accounts of psychopathy have emphasized personality traits as central to the disorder, yet the most widely used instrument for assessing psychopathy, the PCL-R, virtually requires the presence of at least some antisocial features in order for a diagnosis of psychopathy to be made. The essential question, framed in the terminology of the PCL-R, is whether an individual who exhibits an elevation solely on Factor 1, and not Factor 2, can be considered a "true" psychopath or whether a separate clinical designation would be more useful. One possibility is to consider such cases to constitute a distinct subtype of psychopathy. Alternatively, it may be more appropriate to describe these individuals as merely having certain traits in common with criminal psychopaths. We strongly encourage ongoing debate and investigation to resolve this issue.

A separate, yet highly related question raised by research on noncriminal psychopathy is the issue of the relationship between Factor 1 traits and antisocial behavior. One prominent perspective is that the antisocial behavior observed in criminal psychopaths is in fact a consequence of "core" psychopathic personality traits (e.g., emotional detachment, arrogance, and manipulativeness), while others have suggested that both features arise from a single underlying construct. An alternative viewpoint holds that Factor 1 traits and antisocial behavior stem from separate etiological processes, and that these two processes may give rise to different types of behavioral deviance. Further research on nonincarcerated psychopathy can certainly contribute information relevant to this debate.

A final question concerns issues related to recruitment and assessment of psychopaths in community settings. As our review has illustrated, at the present time there is no single recruitment method or assessment instrument that has proven to be the most effective for studying nonincarcerated psychopathy. While self-report psychopathy inventories have made screening and recruitment efforts more feasible, we would note again that the construct validation of these instruments is an ongoing effort, and there appear to be notable differences among the constructs tapped by the various available measures. In conclusion, we offer the following four specific suggestions for future research on noncriminal psychopathy:

1. We suggest an enhanced focus on noncriminal, high-functioning manifestations of psychopathy to supplement existing work on nonincarcerated criminal psychopathy. Despite innovative efforts on the part of researchers, high-functioning psychopaths remain an understudied population. This is an unfortunate circumstance, as these individuals are likely to yield the most useful information regarding potential adaptive manifestations of psychopathic traits, as well as protective factors that shield against overt antisocial expressions. We therefore recommend the development and use of recruitment strategies that aim to minimize levels of antisocial behavior, and the use of analyses that control for the presence of criminal behavior whenever it is feasible to do so.

2. To help identify protective factors that might moderate the expression of psychopathic traits, we recommend a focus on those factors that differentiate incarcerated from nonincarcerated psychopaths. Such findings might ultimately inform treatment efforts intended to divert individuals with psychopathic personalities away from antisocial deviance and toward more prosocial outlets.

3. We strongly advocate the continuing validation of self-report instruments used to assess psychopathy. This assessment method offers a highly promising approach to studying noncriminal psychopathy, allowing for large-scale screening and epidemiological investigations of psychopathy and its correlates in the community. However, greater clarity is needed regarding the constructs measured by these various instruments and the relationships between them.

4. To gain greater insight regarding the processes underlying psychopathy in community samples, we suggest that researchers make greater use of laboratory tasks that measure the affective, behavioral, and physiological correlates of psychopathy. This recommendation is particularly relevant for research employing self-report assessments of psychopathy, as overreliance on self-report inventories as dependent variables may result in inflated correlations as a function of criterion contamination and method covariance.

Through continuing research efforts of this kind, we will ideally gain a greater understanding of psychopathy in both its criminal and noncriminal manifestations.

REFERENCES

American Psychiatric Association. (1994). *Diagnostic and statistical manual of mental disorders* (4th ed.). Washington, DC: Author.

Babiak, P. (1995). When psychopaths go to work: A case study of an industrial psychopath. *Applied Psychology: An International Review, 44*, 171–188.

Babiak, P. (2000). Psychopathic manipulation at work. In C. B. Gacono (Ed.), *The clinical and forensic assessment of psychopathy: A practitioner's guide* (pp. 287–311). Mahwah, NJ: Erlbaum.

Babiak, P., & Hare, R. D. (in press). *B-Scan: 360*. Toronto, ON, Canada: Multi-Health Systems.

Belmore, M. F., & Quinsey, V. L. (1994). Correlates of psychopathy in a noninstitutional sample. *Journal of Interpersonal Violence, 9*, 339–349.

Benning, S. D., Patrick, C. J., & Iacono, W. G. (in press). Fearlessness and underarousal in psychopathy: Startle blink modulation and electrodermal reactivity in a young adult male community sample. *Psychophysiology*.

Benning, S. D., Patrick, C. J., Blonigen, D. M., Hicks, B. M., & Iacono, W. G. (2005). Estimating facets of psychopathy from normal personality traits: A step toward community–epidemiological investigations. *Assessment, 12*, 3–18.

Benning, S. D., Patrick, C. J., Hicks, B. M., Blonigen, D. M., & Krueger, R. F. (2003). Factor structure of the Psychopathic Personality Inventory: Validity and implications for clinical assessment. *Psychological Assessment, 15*, 340–350.

Benning, S. D., Patrick, C. J., Salekin, R. T., & Leistico, A. R. (in press). Convergent and discriminant validity of psychopathy factors assessed via self-report: A comparison of three instruments. *Assessment*.

Blair, R. J. R. (2001). Neurocognitive models of aggression, the antisocial personality disorders, and psychopathy. *Journal of Neurology, Neurosurgery, and Psychiatry, 71*, 727–731.

Block, J. (1961). *The Q-sort method in personality research and psychiatric research*. Springfield, IL: Thomas.

Blonigen, D. M., Hicks, B. M., Krueger, R. F., Patrick, C. J., & Iacono, W. G. (2005). Psychopathic personality traits: Heritability and genetic overlap with internalizing and externalizing psychopathology. *Psychological Medicine, 35*, 637–648.

Bradley, M. M., Cuthbert, B. N., & Lang, P. J. (1999). Affect and the startle reflex. In M. E. Dawson, A. M. Schell, & A. H. Boemelt (Eds.), *Startle modification: Implications for neuroscience, cognitive science, and clinical science* (pp. 157–183). Cambridge, MA: Cambridge University Press.

Christie, R., & Geis, F. L. (1970). *Studies in Machiavellianism*. New York: Academic Press.

Cleckley, H. M. (1988). *The mask of sanity* (5th ed.). St. Louis, MO: Mosby. (Original work published 1941)

Cooke, D. J., & Michie, C. (2001). Refining the construct of psychopathy: Towards a hierarchical model. *Psychological Assessment, 13*, 171–188.

Costa, P. T., & McCrae, R. R. (1992). *NEO PI-R professional manual*. Lutz, FL: Psychological Assessment Resources.

Edens, J. F., Cruise, K. R., & Buffington-Vollum, J. K. (2001). Forensic and correctional applications of the Personality Assessment Inventory. *Behavioral Sciences and the Law, 19*, 519–543.

Elwood, C. E., Poythress, N. G., & Douglas, K. S. (2004). Evaluation of the Hare P-SCAN in a non-clinical population. *Personality and Individual Differences, 36*, 833–843.

Eysenck, H. J., & Eysenck, S. B. G. (1968). *Eysenck Personality Inventory (Form A)*. San Diego, CA: Educational and Industrial Testing Service.

Ferrigan, M. M., Valentiner, D. P., & Berman, M. E. (2000). Psychopathy dimensions and awareness of negative and positive consequences of aggressive behavior in a nonforensic sample. *Personality and Individual Differences, 28*, 527–538.

Forth, A. E., Brown, S. L., Hart, S. D., & Hare, R. D. (1996). The assessment of psychopathy in male and female noncriminals: Reliability and validity. *Personality and Individual Differences, 20*, 531–543.

Gough, H. G. (1987). *California Psychological Inventory: Administrator's guide*. Palo Alto, CA: Consulting Psychologists Press.

Gustafson, S. B., & Ritzer, D. R. (1995). The dark side of normal: A psychopathy-linked pattern called aberrant self-promotion. *European Journal of Personality, 9*, 147–183.

Hall, J. R., Benning, S. D., & Patrick, C. J. (2004). Criterion-related validity of the three-factor model of psychopathy: Personality, behavior, and adaptive functioning. *Assessment, 11*, 4–16.

Hare, R. D. (1965). Temporal gradient of fear arousal in psychopaths. *Journal of Abnormal Psychology, 70*, 442–445.

Hare, R. D. (1991). *The Hare Psychopathy Checklist—Revised*. Toronto, ON, Canada: Multi-Health Systems.

Hare, R. D. (2003). *The Hare Psychopathy Checklist—Revised* (2nd ed.). Toronto, ON, Canada: Multi-Health Systems.

Hare, R. D., Frazelle, J., & Cox, D. N. (1978). Psychopathy and physiological responses to threat of an aversive stimulus. *Psychophysiology, 15*, 165–172.

Hare, R. D., Harpur, T. J., Hakstian, A. R., Forth, A. E., Hart, S. D., & Newman, J. P. (1990). The revised psychopathy checklist: Reliability and factor structure. *Psychological Assessment, 2*, 338–341.

Hare, R. D., & Herve, H. F. (1999). *Hare P-SCAN*. Toronto, ON, Canada: Multi-Health Systems.

Harpur, T. J., Hakstian, A. R., & Hare, R. D. (1988). The factor structure of the Psychopathy Checklist. *Journal of Consulting and Clinical Psychology, 56*, 741–747.

Harpur, T. J., Hare, R. D., & Hakstian, A. R. (1989). Two-factor conceptualization of psychopathy: Construct validity and assessment implications. *Psychological Assessment, 1*, 6–17.

Hart, S. D., Cox, D. N., & Hare, R. D. (1995). *Hare Psychopathy Checklist: Screening Version (PCL:SV)*. Toronto, ON, Canada: Multi-Health Systems.

Hart, S., & Hare, R. D. (1998). Associations between psychopathy and narcissism: Theoretical views and empirical evidence. In E. F. Ronningstam (Ed.), *Disorders of narcissism: Diagnostic, clinical, and empirical implications* (pp. 415–436). Washington, DC: American Psychiatric Press.

Hathaway, S. R., & McKinley, J. C. (1942). *The Minnesota Multiphasic Personality Inventory*. St. Paul: University of Minnesota Press.

Heaton, R. K., Chelune, G. J., Talley, J. L., Kay, G. G., & Kurtis, G. (1993). *Wisconsin Card Sort Test manual—revised and expanded*. Odessa, FL: Psychological Assessment Resources.

Hogan, R. (1969). Development of an empathy scale. *Journal of Consulting and Clinical Psychology, 33*, 307–316.

Ishikawa, S. S., Raine, A., Lencz, T., Bihrle, S., & LaCasse, L. (2001). Autonomic stress reactivity and executive functions in successful and unsuccessful criminal psychopaths from the community. *Journal of Abnormal Psychology, 110*, 423–432.

Kipnis, D. (1971). *Character structure and impulsiveness*. New York: Academic Press.

Kosson, D. S., Steuerwald, B. L., Forth, A. E., & Kirkhart, K. J. (1997). A new method for assessing the interpersonal behavior of psychopathic individuals: Preliminary validation studies. *Psychological Assessment, 9*, 89–101.

Levenson, M. R., Kiehl, K. A., & Fitzpatrick, C. M. (1995). Assessing psychopathic attributes in a noninstitutional population. *Journal of Personality and Social Psychology, 68*, 151–158.

Levenston, G. K., Patrick, C. J., Bradley, M. M., & Lang, P. J. (2000). The psychopath as observer: Emotion and attention in picture processing. *Journal of Abnormal Psychology, 109*, 373–385.

Lilienfeld, S. O. (1994). Conceptual problems in the assessment of psychopathy. *Clinical Psychology Review, 14*, 17–38.

Lilienfeld, S. O. (1998). Methodological advancements and developments in the assessment of psychopathy. *Behaviour Research and Therapy, 36*, 99–125.

Lilienfeld, S. O., & Andrews, B. P. (1996). Development and preliminary validation of a self report measure of psychopathic personality traits in noncriminal populations. *Journal of Personality Assessment, 66*, 488–524.

Lykken, D. T. (1957). A study of anxiety in the sociopathic personality. *Journal of Abnormal and Social Psychology, 55*, 6–10.

Lykken, D. T. (1982). Fearlessness: Its carefree charm and deadly risks. *Psychology Today, 16,* 20–28.

Lykken, D. T. (1995). *The antisocial personalities.* Hillsdale, NJ: Erlbaum.

Lynam, D. R., Whiteside, S., & Jones, S. (1999). Self-reported psychopathy: A validation study. *Journal of Personality Assessment, 73,* 110–132.

Machiavelli, N. (1981). *The Prince (with selections from the Discourses)* (D. Donno, Trans.). New York: Bantam. (Original work published 1513)

McHoskey, J. W., Worzel, W., & Szyarto, C. (1998). Machiavellianism and psychopathy. *Journal of Personality and Social Psychology, 74,* 192–210.

Miller, J. D., & Lynam, D. R. (2003). Psychopathy and the Five-Factor Model of personality: A replication and extension. *Journal of Personality Assessment, 81,* 168–178.

Miller, J. D., Lynam, D. R., Widiger, T. A., & Leukefeld, C. (2001). Personality disorders as extreme variants of common personality dimensions: Can the five-factor model adequately represent psychopathy? *Journal of Personality, 69,* 253–276.

Morey, L. C. (1991). *Personality Assessment Inventory: A professional manual.* Odessa, FL: Psychological Assessment Resources.

Morgan, A. B., & Lilienfeld, S. O. (2000). A meta-analytic review of the relation between antisocial behavior and neuropsychological measures of executive function. *Clinical Psychology Review, 20,* 113–156.

Newman, J. P., & Kosson, D. S. (1986). Passive avoidance learning in psychopathic and non-psychopathic offenders. *Journal of Abnormal Psychology, 95,* 257–263.

Newman, J. P., Patterson, C. M., Howland, E. W., & Nichols, S. L. (1990). Passive avoidance in psychopaths: The effects of reward. *Personality and Individual Differences, 11,* 1101–1114.

Newman, J. P., Patterson, C. M., & Kosson, D. S. (1987). Response perseveration in psychopaths. *Journal of Abnormal Psychology, 96,* 145–148.

Newman, J. P., & Schmitt, W. A. (1998). Passive avoidance in psychopathic offenders: A replication and extension. *Journal of Abnormal Psychology, 107,* 527–532.

Patrick, C. J. (1994). Emotion and psychopathy: Startling new insights. *Psychophysiology, 31,* 319–330.

Patrick, C. J. (1995, Fall). Emotion and temperament in psychopathy. *Clinical Science,* pp. 5–8.

Patrick, C. J. (2001). Emotional processes in psychopathy. In A. Raine & J. Sanmartin (Eds.), *Violence and psychopathy* (pp. 57–77). New York: Kluwer.

Patrick, C. J. (in press). Getting to the heart of psychopathy. In H. Herve & J. C. Yuille (Eds.), *Psychopathy: Theory, research, and social implications.* Hillsdale, NJ: Erlbaum.

Patrick, C. J., Bradley, M. M., & Lang, P. J. (1993). Emotion in the criminal psychopath: Startle reflex modulation. *Journal of Abnormal Psychology, 102,* 82–92.

Patrick, C. J., Zempolich, K. A., & Levenston, G. K. (1997). Emotionality and violence in psychopaths: A biosocial analysis. In A. Raine, D. Farrington, P. Brennan, & S. A. Mednick (Eds.), *The biosocial bases of violence* (pp. 145–161). New York: Plenum Press.

Paulhus, D. L. (1998). Interpersonal and intrapsychic adaptiveness of trait self-enhancement: A mixed blessing? *Journal of Personality and Social Psychology, 74,* 1197–1208.

Paulhus, D. L., & Williams, K. M. (2002). The dark triad of personality: Narcissism, Machiavellianism, and psychopathy. *Journal of Research in Personality, 36,* 556–563.

Porteus, S. D. (1965). *Porteus Maze test: Fifty years' application.* Palo Alto, CA: Pacific Books.

Raskin, R., & Hall, C. S. (1979). A narcissistic personality inventory. *Psychological Reports, 45,* 590.

Raskin, R. N., Novacek, J., & Hogan, R. (1991). Narcissism, self-esteem, and defensive self-enhancement. *Journal of Personality, 59,* 19–38.

Reise, S. P., & Oliver, C. J. (1994). Development of a California Q-Sort indicator of primary psychopathy. *Journal of Personality Assessment, 62,* 130–144.

Reise, S. P., & Wink, P. (1995). Psychological implications of the Psychopathy Q-Sort. *Journal of Personality Assessment, 65,* 300–312.

Robins, L. N. (1966). *Deviant children grown up.* Baltimore: Williams & Wilkins.

Ross, S. R., & Rausch, M. K. (2001). Psychopathic attributes and achievement dispositions in a college sample. *Personality and Individual Differences, 30,* 471–480.

Salekin, R. T., Trobst, K. K., & Krioukova, M. (2001). Construct validity of psychopathy in a community sample: A nomological net approach. *Journal of Personality Disorders, 15,* 425–441.

Smith, R. J. (1978). *The psychopath in society.* New York: Academic Press.

Smith, R. J. (1999). Psychopathic behavior and issues of treatment. *New Ideas in Psychology, 17,* 165–176.

Smith, S. S., & Newman, J. P. (1990). Alcohol and drug abuse-dependence disorders in psychopathic and nonpsychopathic criminal offenders. *Journal of Abnormal Psychology, 99,* 430–439.

Spitzer, R. L., Endicott, J., & Robins, E. (1975). *Research diagnostic criteria.* New York: Biometrics Research, New York State Department of Mental Health.

Sutker, P. B., & Allain, A. N. (1983). Behavior and personality assessment in men labeled adaptive sociopaths. *Journal of Behavior Assessment, 5,* 65–79.

Sutton, S. K., Vitale, J. E., & Newman, J. P. (2002). Emotion among women with psychopathy during picture perception. *Journal of Abnormal Psychology, 111,* 610–619.

Tedeschi, J. T., & Melburg, V. (1984). Impression management and influence in the organization. *Research in the Sociology of Organizations, 3,* 31–58.

Tellegen, A. (in press). *Brief manual for the Multidimen-*

sional Personality Questionnaire. Minneapolis: University of Minnesota Press.

Tharp, V. K., Maltzman, I., Syndulko, K., & Ziskind, E. (1980). Autonomic activity during anticipation of an aversive tone in noninstitutionalized sociopaths. *Psychophysiology, 17,* 123–128.

Vanman, E. J., Mejia, V. Y., Dawson, M. E., Schell, A. M., & Raine, A. (2003). Modification of the startle reflex in a community sample: Do one or two dimensions of psychopathy underlie emotional processing? *Personality and Individual Differences, 35,* 2007–2021.

Verona, E., Patrick, C. J., & Joiner, T. E. (2001). Psychopathy, antisocial personality, and suicide risk. *Journal of Abnormal Psychology, 110,* 462–470.

Watson, P. J., Little, T., Sawrie, S. M., & Biderman, M. D. (1992). Measures of the narcissistic personality: Complexity of relationships with self-esteem and empathy. *Journal of Personality Disorders, 6,* 434–449.

Widom, C. S. (1977). A methodology for studying noninstitutionalized psychopaths. *Journal of Consulting and Clinical Psychology, 45,* 674–683.

Widom, C. S., & Newman, J. P. (1985). Characteristics of non-institutionalized psychopaths. In D. P. Farrington & J. Gunn (Eds.), *Aggression and dangerousness* (pp. 57–80). New York: Wiley.

Williams, K. M., & Paulhus, D. L. (2004). Factor structure of the Self-Report Psychopathy scale (SRP-II) in non-forensic samples. *Personality and Individual Differences, 37,* 765–778.

Wink, P. (1992). Three Narcissism scales for the California Q-Set. *Journal of Personality Assessment, 58,* 51–66.

Zagon, I. K., & Jackson, H. J. (1994). Construct validity of a psychopathy measure. *Personality and Individual Differences, 17,* 125–135.

Zuckerman, M. (1979). *Sensation seeking: Beyond the optimal level of arousal.* Hillsdale, NJ: Erlbaum.

Zuckerman, M., Kolin, E. A., Price, L., & Zoob, I. (1964). Development of a sensation-seeking scale. *Journal of Consulting Psychology, 28,* 477–482.

V

CLINICAL AND APPLIED ISSUES

24

Psychopathy and Aggression

STEPHEN PORTER
MICHAEL WOODWORTH

Psychopathy is a personality disorder characterized by a major affective deficit accompanied by a disregard for the rights of others and for societal rules in general (e.g., Hare, 1996). As defined by the well-validated Psychopathy Checklist—Revised (PCL-R; Hare, 1991), psychopaths are manipulative, callous, remorseless, impulsive, irresponsible individuals (e.g., Hare, 1996, 1998). In this chapter, we begin by outlining the contribution of psychopathy to the prediction of whether and the degree to which a person will engage in aggressive behavior. Our attention then turns to a much newer focus of research—the characteristics of violent actions by psychopaths. We review studies investigating the nature of their violence, examine the possible link between psychopathy and sadistic behavior, and consider how this work informs our understanding of their criminal motivations.

THE LINK BETWEEN PSYCHOPATHY AND AGGRESSION

Research has established a strong link between psychopathic traits and aggressive behavior in each of adult offenders, antisocial children and adolescents, and civil psychiatric patients.

Adult Offenders

A large number of studies have shown that the presence of psychopathic traits is associated with a propensity for violent behavior. In one of the earliest investigations of the relationship between psychopathy and violence, Hare and Jutai (1983) found that adult psychopathic offenders had been charged with violent crimes about twice as often as nonpsychopaths. Virtually all the psychopaths in their sample had perpetrated at least one violent crime compared to about half of the nonpsychopaths. Within a large sample of federal offenders (average age of 43.5 years), Porter, Birt, and Boer (2001) found that psychopaths had been convicted of an average of 7.32 violent crimes compared to 4.52 violent crimes by nonpsychopathic offenders. This pattern of a relatively high level of violence by psychopaths is witnessed throughout their criminal careers (e.g., Harpur & Hare, 1994; Porter, Birt, & Boer, 2001). Thus, it is clear that psychopaths are a highly aggressive group simply from examining the sheer number of violent crimes they have perpetrated.

Knowledge of the psychopathy/aggression link greatly aids in the prediction of future violent behavior in adult offenders (e.g., Harris, Rice, & Quinsey, 1993; Hemphill,

Hare, & Wong, 1998; Rice & Harris, 1997; Salekin, Rogers, & Sewell, 1996). For example, Serin and Amos (1995) found that psychopaths were about five times more likely than nonpsychopaths to engage in violent recidivism within 5 years of their release from prison. Recent meta-analyses indicate that psychopathy as measured by the PCL-R (Hare, 1991) shows an overall effect size of $r = .27–.37$ in predicting violence (e.g., Hemphill, Templeman, Wong, & Hare, 1998; Salekin et al., 1996).

Children and Adolescents with Conduct Problems

Although most research on psychopathy has focused on adults, growing evidence suggests that psychopathy is related to aggression much earlier in life. It appears that precursors to psychopathy emerge in early childhood in the form of "callous–unemotional" traits (e.g., Frick, Bodin, & Barry, 2000; Frick & Ellis, 1999; Lynam, 2002; Porter, 1996), which map closely onto adult psychopathic traits (especially Factor 1 features on the PCL-R). Such characteristics are associated with a pattern of serious aggressive behavior, and can signal a pattern of persistent antisocial and violent behavior (e.g., Dodge, 1991; Frick, 1998; Frick, O' Brien, Wooton, & McBurnett, 1994; Lynam, 2002; Waschbusch et al., 2004). During adolescence, psychopathic traits are associated with convictions for violent offenses (e.g., Campbell, Porter, & Santor, 2004; Forth, Hart, & Hare, 1990; Forth & Mailloux, 2000; Gretton, McBride, Hare, O'Shaughnessy, & Kumka, 2001), a high level of institutional aggression (Edens, Poythress, & Lilienfeld, 1999; Murdock, Hicks, Rogers, & Cashel, 2000; Rogers, Johansen, Chang, & Salekin, 1997), and increased violent recidivism (Brandt, Kennedy, Patrick, & Curtain, 1997; Gretton et al., 2001).

Psychiatric Patients

While the baserate of psychopathy in civil psychiatric patients is low relative to the rate in federal offenders (e.g., Douglas, Ogloff, Nicholls, & Grant, 1999), the association between psychopathy and aggression extends to this population. For example, in a study of 1,136 psychiatric patients from the MacArthur Violence Risk Assessment project, Skeem and Mulvey (2001) found that psychopathy scores predicted future serious violence, despite a psychopathy baserate of only 8%. During a 1-year follow-up period, 50% of psychopaths and 22% of nonpsychopaths committed violence. Furthermore, there was a 73% chance that a patient who became violent had scored higher on psychopathy than a patient who did not become violent (see also Douglas et al., 1999).

Overall, psychopathic features are associated with a high level of aggression in childhood, adolescence, and adulthood. Furthermore, psychopathy is a strong predictor of violent recidivism in both criminal offenders and civil psychiatric patients.

FLAWED PREDATORS: PSYCHOPATHIC AGGRESSION IN THE CLINICAL TRADITION

It has been long recognized that psychopaths expend much time and energy in exploiting others. With little empathy or remorse, they have few inhibitions against using other people for material gain, drugs, sex, or power. Accordingly, psychopaths are adept con artists, often with a long history of frauds and scams. Some may even become cult leaders, corrupt politicians, or successful corporate leaders. This proficiency as "intra-species predators" (Hare, 1993) is likely to derive from their superficially engaging personality and skilled use of deception through verbal and nonverbal communication. That is, their high level of psychological dangerousness to others is masked by well-planned, ill-intended social artistry. Thus, many nonviolent but pernicious actions of the psychopath involve forethought and are instrumental and skillfully orchestrated. In fact, most antisocial behavior by "white collar" psychopaths may be characterized in this way (e.g., Babiak, 2000).

Clinical and empirical observations suggest that some physically aggressive actions by psychopaths share these characteristics of premeditation and instrumentality. For example, psychopaths often perpetrate well-planned armed robberies or hostage takings (e.g., Hervé, Mitchell, Cooper, Spidel, & Hare, 2004). Even in adolescence, psychopathic individuals often plan aggressive acts from which they anticipate positive rewards (Pardini, Lochman, & Frick, 2003). However, most psychopaths have difficulty controlling themselves at times. Their actions may be highly spontaneous and foolhardy, facilitating their own arrest and incarceration. In other words, psychopaths sometimes show a violent temper that seems to be at odds with the obvious circumspection required for much of their crime. In this light, psychopaths are "flawed predators," frequently preying on others but unable to reliably control their behavior. One of us (first author) conducted a risk assessment on a psychopath named "Glen," who, according to his family members was a "likeable" child but had "lied to everyone" and was "like Jekyll and Hyde," quickly changing from being friendly to aggressive (see Porter & Porter, in press). Throughout adolescence and into adulthood, he had committed various types of violence, some highly premeditated and others unplanned and impulsive. In this respect, psychopaths might appear to others to have two "personalities." For example, Josef Stalin (who likely was a psychopath) was seen by many as having an engaging and charismatic personality. He maintained great power while continuing to dominate, intimidate, and deceive other people on a massive scale. Therefore, although psychopaths are dangerous individuals, their potential for uninhibited aggression and violence is disguised by charm (albeit, typically superficial), gregariousness, and an outward appearance of normalcy. Ishikawa, Raine, Lencz, Bihrle, and LaCasse (2001) have referred to those psychopathic individuals who manage to retain their veil of normalcy and function successfully (but unethically) in society, as "successful psychopaths" (see also Benning, Patrick, Hicks, Blonigen, & Krueger, 2003).

Research has begun to address more closely the consequences of these apparent paradoxical attributes of careful premeditation and poor behavioral controls for the violent conduct of psychopaths. Accumulating data are painting an interesting picture of how psychopaths perpetrate aggression and may provide a glimpse into the attitude of psychopaths themselves toward such behavior.

REACTIVE AND INSTRUMENTAL ASPECTS OF AGGRESSION BY PSYCHOPATHS

A key consideration in understanding violent behavior is whether the motivation of the perpetrator is "defensive" or "offensive." That is, was the perpetrator reacting aggressively to a desperate, emotional situation or, instead, was the aggressive action more volitional and instrumental? One longstanding view holds that aggression is founded in frustration and provocation. Berkowitz (1983) argued that aggression is best conceptualized as a hostile reaction to a perceived threat or dangerous situation. A second major view posits that aggression or violence involves goal-driven behavior with specific intended consequences (e.g., Bandura, 1983). As such, to understand the violent act, it is necessary to consider the external goals of the perpetrator. There appears to be merit in both of these perspectives (e.g., Stanford, Houston, Mathias, Villemarette-Pitman, & Greve, 2003). A consideration of both reactive and instrumental elements of aggression is essential toward understanding the motivations behind violent actions (e.g., Brown, Atkins, Osborne, & Milnamow, 1996; Dodge, 1991) and individual differences in the aggressors (e.g., Stanford, Houston, Villemarette-Pittman, & Greve, 2003). For example, instrumental aggression by children is associated with atypical affective functioning and foreshadows a pattern of long-term antisocial behavior (e.g., Pulkkinen, 1996; Vitaro, Gendreau, Tremblay, & Oligny, 1998). However, sometimes a violent act may contain elements of both reactivity and instrumentality (e.g., Bushman & Anderson, 2001). For example, Barratt, Stanford, Dowdy, Liebman, and Kent (1999) found that only 20–25% of the aggressive acts coded in their sample could be classified as either strictly premeditated or impulsive. Therefore, researchers of aggressive behavior must refine their operational definitions beyond simply "instrumental" or "reactive" in order to capture the complexities of motivations for violence.

Qualities of Psychopathic Violence in General

Given the concurrent attributes of callous premeditation and poor behavioral controls associated with the actions of psychopaths in general, predicting whether their violence will be primarily reactive or instrumental is not straightforward. However, according to Cleckley's (1976) anecdotal evidence, violence by psychopaths is more instrumental than violence by other offenders, who typically commit reactive violence because of rage or despair. In the first empirical test of this observation, Williamson, Hare, and Wong (1987) examined characteristics of violent offenses that had been committed by 101 Canadian offenders. They found that psychopaths were more likely (45.2% of the time) to have been motivated by an external goal such as material gain than were nonpsychopaths (14.6% of the time). In addition, psychopaths were less likely (2.4% of the time) to have experienced emotional arousal during their crimes than were nonpsychopaths (31.7% of the time). In the next study to examine the relationship between psychopathy and instrumental violence, Cornell and colleagues (1996) investigated the previous violent crimes of 106 male offenders incarcerated in a state prison. Adopting a different approach from Williamson and colleagues, they focused on whether offenders had committed one or more acts of instrumental violence during their criminal history. They found that psychopaths were more likely to have perpetrated an instrumental violent crime than were nonpsychopaths, who usually had committed reactive violence, as Cleckley had predicted. Furthermore, as with the finding by Williamson and colleagues, instrumental violence was associated with a self-reported lack of emotional arousal during the violent act. Chase, O'Leary, and Heyman (2001) found a relationship between psychopathy and the use of instrumental violence by male spousal assaulters. Within a sample of 60 abusive males, no men who were classified as being "reactively aggressive" were psychopathic, compared to 17% of those who were "instrumentally aggressive." Dempster and colleagues (1996) reviewed the files of 75 adult male violent offenders participating in an inpatient treatment program. Although psychopaths were found to have committed more instrumental violence, they also had displayed impulsive behavior in the context of their crimes. Hart and Dempster (1997) concluded that while psychopaths may be more likely to commit instrumental crimes, their behavior is best described as "impulsively instrumental."

From these studies, it became clear that violence by psychopaths was far more likely than violence by others to have an instrumental component. Nonetheless, for many of their documented acts of violence, there was no evidence of an external goal. For example, in the Williamson and colleagues (1987) study, the majority of violent acts by psychopaths in the sample were not instrumental. This supports the idea that poor behavioral controls or impulsivity in psychopaths contributes to their violence (also see Dempster et al., 1996). Overall, these data established that psychopaths engage in both major forms of aggression, whereas violent nonpsychopaths are unlikely to engage in instrumental violence.

Characteristics of Homicides by Psychopaths

Homicide is a heterogeneous crime, in terms of the characteristics of both the perpetrator and context. In particular, some homicides are highly planned, instrumental acts whereas others involve a lack of premeditation. The latter may occur in the context of an emotional dispute or in response to a situational provocation (a "crime of passion"). The most recent study to address the link between psychopathy and instrumental violence focused for the first time on the act of homicide. Woodworth and Porter (2002) reasoned that if the pattern for general violence held true, psychopathic murderers would perpetrate both types of homicides but would show a greater propensity toward reactive homicides. Nonpsychopaths, on the other hand, were expected to rarely perpetrate instrumental homicides. Porter, Birt, and Boer (2001) had previously reported that psychopaths who had killed showed higher scores on Factor 1 of the PCL-R than did other psychopathic offenders. This suggested that psychopathic murderers might be particularly ruthless individuals who would not be disinclined to commit instrumental violence. The opposite was true for nonpsychopaths; those who had committed murder showed higher Factor 2 scores than did their counterparts (Porter, Birt, & Boer, 2001), in line with individuals whose behavior could be more explosive or reactive.

The Woodworth and Porter (2002) study focused on 125 male homicide offenders incarcerated in one of two Canadian federal prisons. A "reactive" homicide was conceptualized as being unplanned and immediately preceded by a provocative situation. With this type of offense, the offender perceived that he was in a threatening , emotionally provoking, and perhaps inescapable situation before lashing out violently. On the other hand, it was possible for a homicide to be premeditated and not preceded by powerful affect. If the homicide had these characteristics and the perpetrator had an external incentive (such as material gain, drugs or sex) for committing the violent act, it was classified as "instrumental." To refine how the homicides were described, a Likert-type, 4-point scale (ranging from purely instrumental to purely reactive) was used. Offenses containing elements of both were classified as either instrumental with a reactive component or reactive with an instrumental component. The degree of instrumentality/reactivity of each homicide was rated by coders who were unaware of the offender's psychopathy rating. Results indicated that psychopaths were about twice as likely as nonpsychopathic offenders to have engaged in primarily instrumental homicides. In fact, nearly all (93.3%) of the homicides perpetrated by psychopaths were primarily instrumental, compared to 48.4% of the homicides by nonpsychopathic offenders.

Perhaps most surprising was the finding that psychopaths were unlikely to have perpetrated a reactive homicide, despite earlier findings that they often engage in reactive violence generally (Cornell et al., 1996; Williamson et al., 1987). These data called into question the assumption that the behavior of psychopaths is truly impulsive. Woodworth and Porter (2002) proposed a "selective impulsivity" explanation in which psychopaths' impulsive aggression in other contexts may not be as uncontrollable as it appears. Rather, it may reflect a choice not to inhibit such behavior when the perceived stakes are lower (see also Arnett, Smith, & Newman, 1997; Newman & Wallace, 1993). When they recognize that the consequences of such a response may be severe (e.g., life imprisonment), they are able to inhibit their behavior and/or delay their revenge (perhaps resulting in an instrumental homicide). Instead of using aggression impulsively, they are more likely to plan and execute an instrumental murder, perhaps with a belief that an arrest for this type of crime is less likely.

Another finding in the Woodworth and Porter (2002) study was that Factor 1 scores, but not Factor 2 scores, contributed to the instrumentality of the homicide. Therefore, it would appear that while Factor 2 behavioral features may have a more direct and obvious relationship with criminal offending and recidivism (e.g., Walters, 2003), the Factor 1 core emotional and interpersonal traits of psychopathy may help to better explain the specific types of violence in which psychopaths choose to engage (also see Skeem, Poythress, Edens, Lilienfeld, & Cale, 2003).

SELF-GRATIFYING ASPECTS OF AGGRESSION BY PSYCHOPATHS

The foregoing discussion establishes that psychopaths often use aggression for instrumental gain. Their violence can simply be a ruthless means to an end. However, there is recent evidence that psychopaths may derive gratification or enjoyment from their violent behavior. Analyses of their sexual violence, in particular, suggest that both thrill seeking and sadistic interests may play an important role in psychopathic crime.

Evidence for a Thrill-Seeking Motivation

It has been long recognized that psychopaths are thrill seekers and that this attribute may extend to crime (e.g., Hare, 1993), especially sexual violence. As with other forms of crime, psychopathy is associated with an increased risk for sexual aggression and recidivism (e.g., Kosson, Kelly, & White, 1997; Quinsey, Rice, & Harris, 1995). Recent work indicates that psychopathy is associated with particular types of sexual violence and particular types of target victims. This research suggests that psychopaths are both opportunists and thrill seekers in their sexual offending. For example, in a study of 456 sexual offenders, Forth and Kroner (1995) found that psychopathic rapists were more opportunistic in their offending than their nonpsychopathic counterparts. In both adolescent and adult offenders, psychopathy is associated with higher levels of violence in the commission of sexual offenses (e.g., Gretton, McBride, Lewis, O'Shaugnessy, & Hare, 1994), consistent with a thrill-seeking motivation (e.g., Porter, Campbell, Woodworth, & Birt, 2001; see also Hare, 1993).

If thrill seeking motivates psychopaths to commit sexual offenses, one might expect them to select a wider range of victims than other offenders who often "specialize" (especially paraphilic offenders). To examine this hypothesis, Porter and colleagues (2000) reviewed both the criminal records and PCL-R scores of a large sample of incarcerated Canadian offenders. They found a remarkably high baserate of psychopathy (64%) among those offenders who had targeted both child and adult victims. The baserate of psychopathy in the mixed group was higher than the prevalence in both rapists (35.9%) and child molesters (fewer than 10%). An unpublished analysis from that dataset indicated that the presence of psychopathy was associated with higher recidivism and poorer conditional release performance for all groups (mixed offenders, rapists, and molesters). Rice and Harris (1997) also found that offenders with multiple victim types showed the fastest rate of violent recidivism. It is likely that, in the absence of empathy or remorse, psychopathic offenders can move to a different victim type when the opportunity presents itself or when they become "bored," as one offender in the Porter and colleagues (2000) study reported (p. 229).

Additional research is needed to more fully examine the degree to which thrill seeking acts as a motivator for psychopathic violence. In particular, little work has addressed thrill seeking as a factor contributing to nonsexual violence or the possible interaction of thrill seeking and instrumental aggression.

Evidence for a Sadistic Motivation

The term "sadism" has been used to describe a range of cognitions and behaviors associated with the derivation of pleasure through inflicting physical or emotional pain on another person. Some authors have argued for a link between psychopathy and sadism (e.g., Hart & Hare, 1997). According to Krafft-Ebing's (1898/1965) classic study *Psychopathia Sexualis*, sadistic violence requires both sexual and personality pathology ("lust and cruelty") in the perpetrator. In his view, many individuals who experienced sadistic impulses did not act on them for "moral" reasons. Others who lacked morality acted on such impulses and derived enjoyment from perpetrating their violent acts. This consideration of both sexual and nonsexual elements in understanding sadism continued in the psychiatric literature. Sadism has referred to both a pathological personality structure (sadistic personality disorder in earlier editions of the *Diagnostic and Statistical Manual of Mental Disorders* (DSM; American Psychiatric Association, 1994) and pathological sexual functioning (sexual sadism).

Research has addressed the possible link between psychopathy and each of these conditions (Hare, Cooke, & Hart, 1999; Holt, Meloy, & Strack, 1999; Meloy, 2000). Using the Millon Clinical Multiaxial Inventory (MCMI-II; Millon, Davis, & Millon, 1997) and the Personality Disorder Examination items for sadistic personality traits, Holt and colleagues (1999) found that such traits were more common in violent psychopaths than violent nonpsychopaths in a maximum-security prison. Violent and sexually violent offenders did not differ in their level of sadistic personality traits, leading the authors to argue that the traits were not tied specifically to sexual pleasure. On the other hand, some studies have found that higher PCL-R scores are associated with sexual arousal to deviant visual and auditory stimuli. There is a significant but modest correlation (.21–.28) between PCL-R scores and deviant sexual arousal (Barbaree, Seto, Serin, Amos, & Preston, 1994; Quinsey et al., 1995; Serin, Malcolm, Khanna, & Barbaree, 1994).

As with instrumental aggression, an examination of the crime of homicide specifically may shed light on the nature of sadistic violence by psychopaths. A sexual homicide is one that includes sexual activity before, during, or after the commission of the crime. Unlike murderers in general (see, e.g., Porter, Birt, & Boer, 2001), sexual murderers are more likely than other violent offenders to be psychopathic. For example, Meloy (2000) found that about two-thirds of a sample of adult sexual homicide offenders scored in the moderate–high range on the PCL-R. A similar high baserate of psychopathic traits is seen in adolescent sexual homicide offenders (Myers & Blashfield, 1997).

Research examining offender behaviors exhibited in the context of sexual homicide would provide insight into this apparent link between psychopathy and sexual homicide. Porter, Woodworth, Earle, Drugge, and Boer (2003) examined the relationship between PCL-R scores and the types of aggression evidenced during the crime in a sample of 38 Canadian sexual murderers. The main source of information was the detailed file description of the crime known as the Criminal Profile Report, based on police, forensic/autopsy, and court information. Of major interest was the level of gratuitous and sadistic violence that had been perpetrated on the victim. Gratuitous violence was defined as excessive violence that went beyond the level that would be necessary to complete the homicide. Evidence for gratuitous violence included torture, beating, mutilation, and the use of multiple weapons from the crime scene. Evidence that the offender obtained enjoyment or pleasure from the violent acts was coded as sadistic violence (this was coded from self-report information or evidence from the crime scene). To avoid potential circularity in PCL-R scoring, a subsample of cases was coded by diagnosticians who had not read the descriptions of the violent crimes. Similarly, crime scene descriptions were coded by a coder who was unaware of the PCL-R score and other file information. One finding replicated the work mentioned previously: most offenders (84.7%) scored in the moderate to high range on the PCL-R (significantly higher than those of a group of nonsexual murderers). More important, homicides committed by psychopaths (n = 18) showed a significantly higher level of both gratuitous and sadistic violence than homicides by nonpsychopathic offenders (n = 20). Most psychopaths (82.4%) had committed sadistic acts on their victims, compared to 52.6% of the nonpsychopaths. In examining the offender files, it became clear that for many other offenders, the homicide was intended

to prevent the victim from reporting a sexual assault and did not serve the same "psychological" function that it seemed to for psychopaths.

Collectively, these findings suggest that psychopaths may be more likely than other offenders to derive pleasure from the suffering of others. The sadistic behavior perpetrated by psychopaths could relate to a thrill-seeking motive or sexual sadism, or both. However, we hypothesize that it reflects a generalized tendency toward callousness and thrill seeking (see Porter, Campbell, et al., 2001). Although there is a lack of research specifically in this area, the combination of these characteristics (and in particular, the thrill-seeking motivation) would suggest that there may be a link between psychopathy and serial homicide—particularly of the predatory sexual variety.

SELF-DIRECTED AGGRESSION

Does the propensity of psychopaths to perpetrate violence against others extend to self-directed aggression such as suicidal behaviors? Given the superficial affect, self-promoting tendencies, and grandiosity associated with psychopathy, such behavior may seem highly unlikely. As noted by Cleckley (1976), perhaps psychopaths never or rarely become sufficiently distressed to commit suicide. However, he observed that psychopaths frequently make empty threats of self-harm and engage in many bogus attempts characterized by "remarkable cleverness, premeditation, and histrionics" (p. 221). According to this view, self-directed aggression by psychopaths may occur but it is highly instrumental and rarely lethal, unlike the self-directed aggression by others which is associated with "internalizing" problems (e.g., depression). Verona, Patrick, and Joiner (2001) conducted one of the only studies to examine the relationship between psychopathy and self-harm in adult offenders. Using structured interviews and prison file records, they coded for a history of suicide attempts in a sample of 313 inmates. They found that there was a small but significant correlation (r = .11) between PCL-R scores and a history of suicidal behaviors. Suicidal behavior was mainly related to Factor 2 scores and to the presence of an antisocial personality disorder diagnosis but was unrelated to Factor 1 scores. Gretton (1998) found that within a group of male adolescent offenders, more psychopathic individuals (37%) had a history of self-injurious behavior than did nonpsychopaths (21%). Unfortunately, these studies relied heavily on self-report and did not examine the severity of the suicidal behavior. More research is needed to clarify the psychopathy/self-aggression relationship by coding self-harm incidents in terms of severity and motivation. Although the Verona and colleagues (2001) research indicated that suicide is related mainly to PCL-R Factor 2 scores, we think that psychopaths also engage in a substantial amount of insincere self-harm actions that are intended solely to manipulate others (which would be more consistent with higher scores on Factor 1).

Violence from the Psychopath's Perspective

Asking a psychopath to provide his or her view on violence is unlikely to elicit an honest response. Psychopaths long have been characterized as having a remarkable disregard for the truth (e.g., Cleckley, 1976; Hare, 1998; Meloy, 1988; Porter, Birt, Yuille, & Hervé, 2001), to the extent that deceit often is regarded as a defining characteristic of the disorder. A small number of empirical studies have also demonstrated a link between psychopathy and deceptive behavior (e.g., Lykken, 1957; Rogers et al., 2002; Seto, Khattar, Lalumiere, & Quinsey, 1997). Because psychopaths are known to lie frequently, recent studies have examined the psychopath's perspective on violence through less direct/more subtle means. One line of research has employed verbal stimuli to examine whether psychopaths view violence in a negative light. A second approach indicates that psychopaths use deception and minimize their role when they describe their violence, even in the context of a confidential research interview.

According to one view, psychopaths are more likely to engage in instrumental acts of aggression because they do not interpret their victims' emotional distress cues or violence as aversive (Blair, 2001; see also Nestor, Kimble, Berman, & Haycock, 2002). In line with this hypothesis, a recent British study suggests that psychopaths who have committed homicide do not view violence as unpleasant. Gray, Macculloch, Smith, Mossis, and Snowden (2003) measured implicit beliefs about murder in psychopathic and nonpsychopathic murderers, and psychopathic and nonpsychopathic offenders who had committed other offenses. Using a modified Implicit Association Test (IAT), the researchers presented participants with a word which they then had to associate with being either "unpleasant" or "pleasant" and either "peaceful" or "violent." In general, control participants take longer to respond to word stimuli with a right or left button press when words of contrasting valences require responses with the same button. For example, when the same response key is assigned for pleasant and violent words, participants usually find the task to be more difficult. Results indicated that psychopathic murderers did not display the same impairment in response time as nonpsychopaths when incongruent words (pleasant and violent words) called for equivalent responses. That is, they responded as if they did not associate violence and unpleasantness, and showed diminished negative reactions to violence compared with nonpsychopathic murderers.

A second line of work has recently examined the manner in which psychopaths describe their violent crimes. Porter and Woodworth (2005) interviewed 50 incarcerated offenders about their violent crimes. Naïve coders then rated either the offender's version or the official version of the crime in terms of the instrumentality or reactivity of the offense. When the self-reported and official descriptions of the violent offenses were compared, it was found that psychopaths were significantly more likely than nonpsychopaths to "reframe" the offenses in an exculpating way. That is, although nonpsychopaths also had a tendency to describe their offense as reactive (regardless of the actual nature of the violence), psychopaths were significantly more likely to downplay the level of instrumentality of their violence, describing it as more reactive than the official version of the offense. Furthermore, psychopaths were significantly more likely than nonpsychopaths to omit major details of the homicide offense. The results of this study further replicated Woodworth and Porter's

(2002) finding that instrumental violence was related to the Factor 1 interpersonal and affective features of psychopathy, and not to the Factor 2 social deviance/behavioral features (see also Patrick & Zempolich, 1998). In addition, results revealed that the tendency to exaggerate the reactivity of the homicides was strongly related to the Factor 1 scores but not the Factor 2 scores. Thus, it appears that the interpersonal and affective characteristics of psychopathy account for not only the type of violence used by offenders but also the manner in which they discuss it (for a further examination of how different the difference factors/facets of psychopathy may help to inform our understanding of the disorder, refer to Cooke, Michie, & Hart, Chapter 5, this volume).

Taken together, the evidence suggests that psychopaths may view aggression as a useful tool with which to satisfy a selfish need. They view violence "cognitively" as a means to an end, attach little emotion to such behavior, and see it as little different from other instrumental actions. With little remorse even years after the crime, psychopaths describe their violent actions as being more reactive and less planned than indicated by the official file.

Subtypes of Psychopathy

Clearly, there is much variation in the types and amount of aggression committed by different psychopaths. In observing the wide behavioral differences between individual psychopaths, some theorists have suggested the possibility of subtypes of the disorder. Cleckley (1976) himself questioned the validity of psychopathic subtypes, claiming that they potentially could serve to confuse the defining characteristics of psychopathy. However, more recently, some research may support the notion that there are separate subtypes that can be distinguished (and possibly lead to a more refined understanding of the disorder). For example, Millon and Davis (1998) concluded that there are 10 different subtypes of psychopathy. At the core of each of subtype was a marked self-centeredness and a disregard for the rights of others; however, Millon and Davis postulated that there were also unique characteristics that made each of these subtypes different and recognizable. Others have suggested that

psychopathy can be broken down into two main subtypes: primary and secondary psychopathy (e.g., Blackburn, 1998). Primary psychopathy is comprised of constitutional deficits that are not attributable to psychosocial learning; such individuals display the defining personality characteristics of psychopathy (such as grandiosity, lack of guilt or remorse, and callousness) from an early age. These individuals display low levels of anxiety and lack prosocial emotions (such as guilt and love) that would otherwise prevent them from engaging in extremely callous actions. On the other hand, secondary psychopaths do experience social emotions, and their hostile behavior is believed to be more a product of their negative life experiences and environment. Therefore, this behavior can be thought of as an adaptation to harsh environmental contingencies (such as bad parenting) and/or could be best explained in terms of some other pathology or syndrome (such as hysteria). Although research is needed, it is likely that that primary psychopathy would be more directly related to the type of instrumental violence observed in studies of homicidal aggression described previously.

Other researchers have also distinguished different subtypes of psychopathy based on separate etiological pathways. For example, Porter (1996) proposed that there were two main types of psychopathy with distinct causal factors. He suggested that primary psychopaths were born with a predisposition to the core interpersonal and affective features of psychopathy and that normal emotional development was not possible. However, Porter argued that secondary psychopaths acquired the affective deficits associated with psychopathy after experiencing long-term neglect or abuse (or other early traumatic experience) in early childhood. Furthermore, he suggested that this emotional detachment was spurred by dissociation and a more gradual blunting (or shutting down) of emotions. Although conducting the appropriate empirical test of this theory is difficult, recent innovative research has shown some support for this theory of secondary psychopathy (see Poythress & Skeem, Chapter 9, this volume).

In summary, any thorough consideration of the causes and types of psychopathic aggression should include a consideration of psychopathic subtypes as well as the etiological pathways. This is an area that will likely be the focus of much investigation in coming years.

Cognitive Ability as a Potential Moderator of the Psychopathy–Violence Association

Why is most of the ruthless conduct of some psychopaths nonviolent while others show a persistent pattern of violence? Perhaps some psychopaths view aggressive or violent behavior as being more necessary to achieve their goals than do other psychopaths. As noted earlier, some psychopaths, especially white-collar or corporate psychopaths, seem to rarely use physical aggression.

A potential moderator of the relationship between psychopathy and violence is intelligence. That is, more intelligent psychopaths may be less inclined to use aggression because they can they can use their cognitive resources to devise nonviolent means (such as conning and manipulation) to get what they want. Less intelligent psychopaths may resort to violence to compensate for their inferior abilities to manipulate others through language. Heilbrun (1982) found that past violent offending in a sample of 168 male inmates was influenced by the interaction of intellectual level and psychopathy. Less intelligent psychopaths were more likely to have a history of impulsive violence than more intelligent psychopaths (and than less intelligent nonpsychopaths). Heilbrun (1985) reported that the most dangerous offenders in a sample of 225 offenders were those with the following characteristics: psychopathic, low IQ, social withdrawal, and history of violence.

While these early studies offered some evidence for intelligence as a moderator of psychopathy and violence, little research has addressed the issue in recent years, largely due to methodological obstacles. Specifically, the most intelligent psychopaths in society may succeed in corporate or political circles and/or use violence less frequently and thus may be less likely to wind up in prison. As such, they would be less likely to be studied by psychological researchers, whereas less intelligent psychopaths are available in disproportionate numbers for research.

Another potential issue in this area is that psychopaths with higher cognitive functioning may be as likely to commit violence as other psychopaths but be much less likely to be apprehended for such acts. Ishikawa and colleagues (2001) tested a community sample of 16 "unsuccessful" and 13 "successful" psychopaths (classified based on their PCL-R scores and whether they had received criminal convictions) on measures of autonomic stress reactivity and executive functioning (referring to the capacity for initiation, planning, abstraction, decision making). The two groups had engaged in a substantial and similar amount of self-reported criminal behavior, including violence. The results indicated that the successful psychopaths exhibited greater autonomic reactivity to emotional stressors and stronger executive functioning than unsuccessful psychopaths. This suggested that psychopaths who are less likely to be caught and convicted for their violent acts have the capacity for better planning and decision making than their unsuccessful counterparts. While Ishikawa and colleagues did not address the type of violent acts perpetrated by successful and unsuccessful psychopaths, we hypothesize that successful psychopaths may have been more likely to use premeditated, instrumental violence than their counterparts.

CONCLUSION

There is a clear relation between psychopathy and aggressive behavior. In fact, psychopaths probably commit more nonsanctioned violence than any other members of society. Therefore, a critical agenda for researchers in forensic psychology should be to gain a better understanding of their violence. We have highlighted the need to examine more closely the quality (in addition to quantity) of their aggressive and violent behaviors. Our conclusion is that violence by psychopaths is multifaceted and very different from that of other offenders. For example, sexual violence by psychopaths in general seems to be motivated by sadistic interests and thrill seeking. Research has demonstrated that psychopaths are much more likely than other murderers to commit gratuitous and sadistic violence on their victims during a sexual homicide. Although some violence by psychopaths is reactive, this type of behavior is typically avoided when the stakes are the highest. Nearly all homicides by psychopaths tend to be highly premeditated and cold-blooded. We argued that impulsive behavior in psychopaths may have less to do with a lack of control than with a rapid, conscious consideration of the gravity of the consequences. Future research may also reveal that distinct manifestations of psychopathic violence are related to unique subtypes or facets of the disorder.

Perhaps the overriding problem is that psychopathic individuals have a wholly selfish orientation and a profound emotional deficit, as evidenced from studies of language, psychophysiology, neurology, and behavior. This translates into a pattern of ruthless aggressive and criminal actions. A major challenge for researchers in future work is to decipher the etiological factors contributing to the development of psychopathy and individual differences in psychopathic aggression.

REFERENCES

American Psychiatric Association. (1994). *Diagnostic and statistical manual of mental disorder* (4th ed.). Washington, DC: Author.

Arnett, P. A., Smith, S. S., & Newman, J. P. (1997). Approach and avoidance motivation in psychopathic criminal offenders during passive avoidance. *Journal of Personality and Social Psychology*, 72, 1413–1428.

Babiak, P. (2000). Psychopathic manipulation at work. In C. B. Gacono (Ed.), *The clinical and forensic as sessment of psychopathy: A practitioner's guide* (pp. 287–311). Mahwah, NJ: Erlbaum.

Bandura, A. (1983). Psychological mechanisms of aggression. In R. G. Green, & E. I. Donnerstein (Eds.), *Aggression: Theoretical and empirical views* (Vol. 1, pp. 1–40). New York: Academic Press.

Barbaree, H., Seto, M., Serin, R., Amos, N., & Preston, D. (1994). Comparisons between sexual and nonsexual rapist sub-types. *Criminal Justice and Behavior*, 21, 95–114.

Barratt, E. S., Stanford, M. S., Dowdy, L., Liebman, M. J., & Kent, T. A. (1999). Impulsive and premeditated aggression: A factor analysis of self-reported acts. *Psychiatry Research*, 86, 163–173.

Benning, S. D., Patrick, C. J., Hicks, B. M., Blonigen, D. M., & Krueger, R. F. (2003). Factor structure of the psychopathic personality inventory: Validity and implications for clinical assessment. *Psychological Assessment*, 15, 340–350.

Berkowitz, L. (1983). The experience of anger as a parallel process in the display of impulsive, "angry" aggression. In R. G. Green & E. I. Donnerstein (Eds.), *Aggression: Theoretical and empirical views* (pp. 103–134). New York: Academic Press.

Blackburn, R. (1998). Psychopathy and personality disorder: Implications of interpersonal theory. In D. J. Cooke, A. E. Forth, & R. D. Hare (Eds.) *Psychopathy: Theory, research, and implications for society* (pp. 269–301). Dordrecht, The Netherlands: Kluwer.

Blair, R. J. R. (2001). Neurocognitive models of aggression, the antisocial personality disorders, and psychopathy. *Journal of Neurology, Neurosurgery, and Psychiatry*, 71, 727–731.

Brandt, J. R., Kennedy, W. A., Patrick, C. J., & Curtain, J. J. (1997). Assessment of psychopathy in a population of incarcerated adolescent offenders. *Psychological Assessment*, 9, 429–435.

Brown, K., Atkins, M. S., Osborne, M. L., & Milnamow, M. (1996). A revised teacher rating scale for reactive and proactive aggression. *Journal of Abnormal Child Psychology*, 24, 473–480.

Bushman, B. J., & Anderson, C. A. (2001). Is it time to pull the plug on the hostile versus Instrumental aggression dichotomy? *Psychological Review*, 108, 273–279.

Campbell, M. A., Porter, S., & Santor, D. (2004). Psychopathic traits in adolescent offenders: An evaluation of criminal history, clinical, and psychosocial correlates. *Behavioral Sciences and the Law*, 22, 23–47.

Chase, K. A., O'Leary, K. D., & Heyman, R. E. (2001). Categorizing partner-violent men within the reactive–proactive typology model. *Journal of Consulting and Clinical Psychology*, 69, 567–572.

Cleckley, H. (1976). *The mask of sanity* (5th ed.). St. Louis, MO: Mosby.

Cornell, D. G., Warren, J., Hawk, G., Stafford, E., Oram, G., & Pine, D. (1996). Psychopathy in instrumental and reactive violent offenders. *Journal of Consulting and Clinical Psychology*, 64, 783–790.

Dempster, R. J., Lyon, D. R., Sullivan, L. E., Hart, S. D., Smiley, W. C., & Mulloy, R. (1996, August). *Psychopathy and instrumental aggression in violent offenders*. Paper presented at the annual meeting of the American Psychological Association, Toronto.

Dodge, K. A. (1991). The structure and function of reactive and proactive aggression. In D. J. Pepler & K. H. Rubin (Eds.), *The development and treatment of childhood aggression* (pp. 1–18). Hillsdale, NJ: Erlbaum.

Douglas, K., Ogloff, J., Nicholls, T., & Grant, I. (1999). Assessing risk for violence among psychiatric patients: The HCR-20, Violence Risk Assessment Scheme, and the Psychopathy Checklist: Screening Version. *Journal of Consulting and Clinical Psychology*, 67, 917–930.

Edens, J. F., Poythress, N. G., & Lilienfeld, S. O. (1999). Identifying inmates at risk for disciplinary infractions: A comparison of two measures of psychopathy. *Behavioral Sciences and the Law*, 17, 435–443.

Forth, A. E., Hart, S. D., & Hare, R. D. (1990). Assessment of psychopathy in male young offenders. *Psychological Assessment, 2,* 342–344.

Forth, A. E., & Kroner, D. (1995). *The factor structure of the Revised Psychopathy Checklist with incarcerated rapists and incest offenders.* Unpublished manuscript.

Forth, A. E., & Mailloux, D. L. (2000). Psychopathy in youth: What do we know? In C. B. Gacono (Ed.), *The clinical and forensic assessment of psychopathy: A practitioner's guide* (pp. 25–54). Mahwah, NJ: Erlbaum.

Frick, P. J. (1998). *Conduct disorders and severe antisocial behavior.* New York: Plenum Press.

Frick, P. J., Bodin, S. D., & Barry, C. T. (2000). Psychopathic traits and conduct problems in community and clinic-referred samples of children: Further development of the Psychopathy Screening Device. *Psychological Assessment, 12,* 382–393.

Frick, P. J., & Ellis, M. (1999). Callous-unemotional traits and subtypes of conduct disorder. *Clinical Child and Family Psychology Review, 2,* 149–168.

Frick, P. J., O'Brien, B. S., Wooton, J. M., & McBurnett, K. (1994). Psychopathy and conduct problems in children. *Journal of Abnormal Psychology, 103,* 700–707.

Gray, N., S., Macculloch, M. J., Smith, J., Mossis, M., & Snowden, R. J. (2003). Forensic psychology: Violence viewed by psychopathic murderers. *Nature, 423,* 497–98.

Gretton, H. M. (1998). *Psychopathy and recidivism in adolescence: A ten-year retrospective follow-up.* Unpublished doctoral dissertation. University of British Columbia, Vancouver.

Gretton, H. M., McBride, H. L., Hare, R. D., O'Shaughnessy, R., & Kumka, G. (2001). Psychopathy and recidivism in adolescent sex offenders. *Criminal Justice and Behavior, 28,* 427–449.

Gretton, H., McBride, M., Lewis, K., O'Shaugnessy, R., & Hare, R. D. (1994, March). *Patterns of violence and victimization in adolescent sexual psychopaths.* Paper presented at the biennial meeting of the American Psychology and Law Society, Santa Fe, NM.

Hare, R. D. (1991). *The Hare Psychopathy Checklist—Revised.* Toronto, ON, Canada: Multi-Health Systems.

Hare, R. D. (1993). *Without conscience: The disturbing world of the psychopaths among us.* New York: Simon & Schuster.

Hare, R. D. (1996). Psychopathy: A clinical construct whose time has come. *Criminal Justice and Behavior, 23,* 25–54.

Hare, R. D. (1998). Psychopathy and its nature: Implications for mental health and criminal justice systems. In T. Millon, E. Simonsen, M. Birkert-Smith, & R. D. Davis (Eds.), *Psychopathy: Antisocial criminal and violent behavior* (pp.188–212). New York: Guilford Press.

Hare, R. D., Cooke, D. J., & Hart, S. D. (1999). Psychopathy and sadistic personality disorder. In T. Millon, P. H. Blanney, & R. D. Davies (Eds.), *Oxford textbook of psychopathology* (pp. 555–584). New York: Oxford University Press.

Hare, R. D., & Jutai, J. (1983). Criminal history of the male psychopath: Some preliminary data. In K. T. Van Dusen & S. A. Mednick (Eds.), *Prospective studies of crime and delinquency* (pp. 225–236). Boston: Kluwer-Nijhoff.

Harpur, T. J., & Hare, R. D. (1994). Assessment of psychopathy as a function of age. *Journal of Abnormal Psychology, 103,* 604–609.

Harris, G., Rice, M., & Quinsey, V. (1993). Violent recidivism of mentally disordered offenders: The development of a statistical prediction instrument. *Criminal Justice and Behavior, 20,* 315–335.

Hart, S., & Dempster, R. (1997). Impulsivity and psychopathy. In C. Webster & M. Jackson (Eds.), *Impulsivity: Theory, assessment and treatment* (pp. 212–232). New York: Guilford Press.

Hart, S. D., & Hare, R. D. (1997). Psychopathy: Assessment and association with criminal behavior. In D. Stoff, J. Breiling, & J. D. Maser (Eds.), *Handbook of antisocial behavior* (pp. 22–35). New York: Wiley.

Heilbrun, K. (1982). Cognitive models of criminal violence based on intelligence and psychopathy levels. *Journal of Consulting and Clinical Psychology, 50,* 546–557.

Heilbrun, M. (1985). Psychopathy and dangerousness: Comparison, integration, and extension of two psychopathic typologies. *British Journal of Clinical Psychology, 24,* 181–195.

Hemphill, J. F., Hare, R. D., & Wong, S. (1998). Psychopathy and recidivism: A review. *Legal and Criminological Psychology, 3,* 139–170.

Hemphill, J., Templeman, R., Wong, S., & Hare, R. D. (1998). Psychopathy and crime: Recidivism and criminal careers. In D. Cooke, A. Forth, & R. D. Hare (Eds.), *Psychopathy: Theory, research, and implications for society* (pp. 374–399). Dordrecht, The Netherlands: Kluwer.

Hervé, H. M., Mitchell, D., Cooper, B. S., Spidel, A., & Hare, R. D. (2004). Psychopathy and unlawful confinement: An examination of perpetrator and event characteristics. *Canadian Journal of Behavioural Science, 36,* 137–145.

Holt, S. E., Meloy, J. R., & Strack, S. (1999). Sadism and psychopathy in violent and sexually violent offenders. *Journal of the American Academy of Psychiatry and Law, 27,* 23–32.

Ishikawa, S. S., Raine, A., Lencz, T., Bihrle, S., & LaCasse, L. (2001). Autonomic stress reactivity and executive functions in successful and unsuccessful criminal psychopaths from the community. *Journal of Abnormal Psychology, 110,* 423–432.

Kosson, D. S., Kelly, J. C., & White, J. W. (1997). Psychopathy-related traits predict self-reported sexual aggression among college men. *Journal of Interpersonal Violence, 12,* 241–254.

Krafft-Ebing, R. V. (1965). *Psychopathia sexualis* (H. Wedeck, Trans.). New York: Putnam. (Original work published 1898)

Lykken, D. T. (1957). A study of anxiety in the sociopathic personality. *Journal of Abnormal and Social Psychology, 55,* 6–10.

Lynam, D. R. (2002). Fledgling psychopathy: A view from personality theory. *Law and Human Behavior, 26,* 255–259.

Meloy, J. R. (1988). *The psychopathic mind: Origins, dynamics, and treatments.* Northvale, NJ: Jason Aronson.

Meloy, J. R. (2000). The nature and dynamics of sexual homicide: An integrative review. *Aggression and Violent Behavior, 5,* 1–22.

Millon, T., & Davis, R. D. (1998). Ten subtypes of psychopathy. In T. Millon, E. Simonson, M. Burket-Smith, & R. Davis (Eds.), *Psychopathy: Antisocial, criminal, and violent behavior* (pp. 161–170). New York: Guilford Press.

Millon, T., Davis, R. D., & Millon, C. (1997). *MCMI–III manual* (2nd ed.). Minneapolis, MN: National Computer Systems.

Murdock Hicks, M., Rogers, R., & Cashel, M. L. (2000). Predictions of violent and total infractions among institutionalized male juvenile offenders. *Journal of the American Academy of Psychiatry and the Law, 28,* 183–190.

Myers, W. C., & Blashfield, R. (1997). Psychopathology and personality in juvenile sexual homicide offenders. *Journal of the American Academy of Psychology and Law, 25,* 497–508.

Nestor, G., Kimble, M., Berman, I., & Haycock, J. (2002). Psychosis, psychopathy, and homicide: A preliminary neuropsychological inquiry. *American Journal of Psychiatry,1, 59,* 138–140.

Newman, J. P., & Wallace, J. F. (1993). Psychopathy. In P. C. Kendall & K. L. Ronnins (Eds.), *Psychopathology and cognition* (pp. 293–349). New York: Academic Press.

Pardini, D. A., Lochman, J. E., & Frick, P. J. (2003). Callous/unemotional traits and social–cognitive processes in adjudicated youths. *Journal of the American Academy of Child and Adolescent Psychiatry, 42,* 364–371.

Patrick, C. J., & Zempolich, K. A. (1998). Emotion and aggression in the psychopathic personality. *Aggression and Violent Behavior, 3,* 303–338.

Porter, S. (1996). Without conscience or without active conscience? The etiology of psychopathy revisited. *Aggression and Violent Behavior, 1,* 179–189.

Porter, S., Birt A. R., & Boer, D. P. (2001). Investigation of the criminal and conditional release histories of Canadian federal offenders as a function of psychopathy and age. *Law and Human Behavior, 25,* 647–661.

Porter, S., Birt, A. R., Yuille, J. C., & Hervé, H. (2001). Memory for murder: A psychological perspective on dissociative amnesia in forensic contexts. *International Journal of Law and Psychiatry, 24,* 23–42.

Porter, S., Campbell, M. A., Woodworth, M., & Birt, A. R. (2001). A new psychological conceptualization of the sexual psychopath. In F. Columbus (Ed.), *Advances in psychology research* (Vol. 7, pp. 21–36). New York: Nova Science.

Porter, S., Fairweather, D., Drugge, J., Herve, H., Birt, A. R., & Boer, D. P. (2000). Profiles of psychopathy in incarcerated sexual offenders. *Criminal Justice and Behavior, 27,* 216–233.

Porter, S., & Porter, S. (in press). Psychopathy and violent crime. In H. Hervé & J. C. Yuille (Eds.), *Psychopathy in the third millennium: Research and practice.* New York: Academic Press.

Porter, S., & Woodworth, M. (2005). *A comparison of self-reported and file descriptions of violent crimes as a function of psychopathy.* Manuscript under review.

Porter, S., Woodworth, M., Earle, J., Drugge, J., & Boer, D. P. (2003). Characteristics of violent behavior exhibited during sexual homicides by psychopathic and non-psychopathic murderers. *Law and Human Behavior, 27,* 459–470.

Pulkkinen, L. (1996). Proactive and reactive aggression in early adolescence as precursors to anti- and prosocial behaviors in young adults. *Aggressive Behavior, 22,* 241–257.

Quinsey, V. L., Rice, M. E., & Harris, G. T. (1995). Actuarial prediction of sexual recidivism. *Journal of Interpersonal Violence, 10,* 85–105.

Rice, M. E., & Harris, G. T. (1997). Cross-validation and extension of the Violence Risk Appraisal Guide for child molesters and rapists. *Law and Human Behavior, 21,* 231–241.

Rogers, R., Johansen, J., Chang, J. J., & Salekin, R. (1997). Predictors of adolescent psychopathy: Oppositional and conduct-disorders symptoms. *Journal of the American Academy of Psychiatry and Law, 25,* 261–270.

Rogers, R., Vitacco, M. J., Jackson, R. L., Martin, M., Collins, M., & Sewell, K. W. (2002). Faking psychopathy? An examination of response styles with antisocial youth. *Journal of Personality Assessment, 78,* 31–46.

Salekin, R. T., Rogers, R., & Sewell, K. W. (1996). A review and meta-analysis of the Psychopathy Checklist—Revised: Predictive validity of dangerousness. *Clinical Psychology Science and Practice, 3,* 203–215.

Serin, R. C., & Amos, N. L. (1995). The role of psychopathy in the assessment of dangerousness. *International Journal of Law and Psychiatry, 18,* 231–238.

Serin, R. C., Malcolm, P. B., Khanna, A., & Barbaree, H. E. (1994). Psychopathy and deviant sexual arousal in incarcerated sexual offenders. *Journal of Interpersonal Violence, 9,* 3–11.

Seto, M. C., Khattar, N. A., Lalumiere, M. L., & Quinsey, V. L. (1997). Deception and sexual strategy in psychopathy. *Personality and Individual Differences, 22,* 301–307.

Skeem, J. L., & Mulvey, E. P. (2001). Psychopathy and community violence among civil psychiatric patients: Results from the MacArthur violence risk assessment study. *Journal of Consulting and Clinical Psychology*, *69*, 358–374.

Skeem, J. L., Poythress, N., Edens, J. F., Lilienfeld, S. O., & Cale, E. M. (2003). Psychopathic personality or personalities? Exploring potential variants of psychopathy and their implications for risk assessment. *Aggression and Violent Behavior*, *8*, 513–546.

Stanford, M. S., Houston, R. J., Mathias, C. W., Villemarette-Pittman, N. R., Helfritz, L. E., & Conklin, S. M. (2003). Characterizing aggressive behavior. *Assessment*, *10*, 183–190.

Stanford, M. S., Houston, R. J., Villemarette-Pittman, N. R., & Greve, K. W. (2003). Premeditated aggression: clinical assessment and cognitive psychophysiology. *Personality and Individual Differences*, *34*, 773–781.

Verona E., Patrick C. J., & Joiner T. E. (2001). Psychopathy, antisocial personality, and suicide risk. *Journal of Abnormal Psychology*, *110*, 462–470.

Vitaro, F., Gendreau, P. L., Tremblay, R. E., & Oligny, P. (1998). Reactive and proactive aggression differentially predict later conduct problems. *Journal of Child Psychology and Psychiatry*, *39*, 377–385.

Walters, G. D. (2003). Predicting institutional adjustment and recidivism with the Psychopathy Checklist factor scores: A meta-analysis. *Law and Human Behavior*, *27*, 541–558.

Waschbusch, D., Porter, S., Carrey, N., Kazmi, O., Roach, K., & D'Amico, D. (2004). A comparison of conduct problems in elementary age children. *Canadian Journal of Behavioural Science*, *36*, 97–112.

Williamson, S. E., Hare, R. D., & Wong, S. (1987). Violence: Criminal psychopaths and their victims. *Canadian Journal of Behavioral Science*, *19*, 454–462.

Woodworth, M., & Porter, S. (2002). In cold blood: Characteristics of criminal homicides as a function of psychopathy. *Journal of Abnormal Psychology*, *111*, 436–445.

25

Psychopathy and Substance Use Disorders

JEANETTE TAYLOR
ALAN R. LANG

Substance use disorders (SUDs) such as abuse of, or dependence on, alcohol and/or illicit drugs affect 20–40% of the general population (e.g., Cottler et al., 1995; Grant, Harford, Dawson, & Chou, 1994), placing them among the most prevalent of mental disorders. Given such pervasiveness, it should not be surprising to find these problems occurring in the context of other diagnoses and, indeed, the comorbidity of SUDs and personality disorders has been reported at rates as high as 60% in outpatients (Skodol, Oldham, & Gallaher, 1999). More specifically, SUDs are often evident among individuals with externalizing disorders or behaviors of the sort marked by overt acting out and a general lack of behavioral control. Antisocial personality disorder (APD) and its precursor, conduct disorder (CD), are prototypical examples of externalizing disorders that are especially likely to be comorbid with SUDs (Strain, 1995). Similarly, delinquency and criminality frequently co-occur with substance use problems (Soderstrom, Sjodin, Carlstedt, & Forsman, 2004; Timmerman & Emmelkamp, 2001). Thus, the nature, implications, and management of the connection between various forms of antisocial behavior, including psychopathy, and SUDs appear to warrant further exploration.

The goal of this chapter is to enhance the understanding of psychopathy through an analysis of its relation to SUDs. One acknowledgement pertinent to this pursuit is the fact that considerably less is known about psychopathy—as compared to APD—as it relates to SUDs. Accordingly, we begin with a brief summary of the association between APD and SUDs and then touch on the distinctions between APD and psychopathy and the relevant assessment issues to set the stage for examination of psychopathy as a condition comorbid with SUDs. A description of the association between the key phenotypes of interest within various samples will then follow. The apparent close connections between antisocial behavior, psychopathy, and SUDs naturally set up the question of *why* these problems often manifest together. Consequently, an overview of prominent models purporting to explain this comorbidity is provided and one particularly promising model that ties various forms of externalizing behavior together is highlighted. Next, the clinical consequences of the comorbidity between SUDs and psychopathy is reviewed to elucidate and underscore the complications that can stem from the dual diagnosis. Finally, given these consequences, issues related to clinical management of individuals with both psychopathy and SUDs are discussed.

EPIDEMIOLOGY OF THE COMORBIDITY BETWEEN PSYCHOPATHY AND SUDs

Expectations of an association between psychopathy and substance (particularly alcohol) use problems emanate from Cleckley's (1976) comment that "although some psychopaths do not drink at all and others drink rarely, considerable overindulgence in alcohol is very often prominent in the life story" (p. 355). Furthermore, Cleckley listed "fantastic and uninviting behavior with drink" (p. 355) as a criterion for psychopathy indicating that psychopaths are not typical problem drinkers. They do not develop strong dependency and or experience much negative affect around their drinking. Rather, their problems with alcohol seem to arise from its ability to further dissolve the already weak restraints that characterize psychopaths. Research on the modern concept of psychopathy that has appeared since Cleckley described the syndrome tends to support his clinical observation regarding pathological alcohol involvement and extrapolates it to drug use disorders as well.

APD and SUDs

For nearly two decades, researchers have examined the issue of comorbidity between the diagnoses of APD and SUDs. Indeed, alcoholism researchers have consistently subscribed to a typology of alcohol use disorders in which the presence of APD is a major differentiating feature associated with characteristics such as higher heritability and childhood risk factors, earlier onset and greater alcohol-related symptom severity, more persistent and pervasive psychopathology and life stress, sensation seeking and impulsive drinking motives/styles, and poorer treatment outcome and general prognosis (e.g., Babor et al., 1992; Cloninger, 1987). In this connection, it is noteworthy that the APD diagnosis, introduced in the 1980 edition of the *Diagnostic and Statistical Manual of Mental Disorders* (DSM), borrowed heavily from Cleckley's notion of psychopathy. However, since then, the characterization of APD has been in terms of the criminal, externalizing aspects of psychopathy (lying, irritable aggression, etc.) with an attendant neglect of the emotional detachment element

of the syndrome (Moran, 1999). So defined, the prevalence of APD in the general population is about 2–3% (Moran, 1999). Controversy over the extent to which APD and psychopathy are the same, similar, or different constructs is addressed elsewhere in this volume and its discussion is beyond the scope of this chapter. However, we maintain that the APD diagnosis captures the part of the psychopathy construct that is most closely related to SUDs, and thus it is worthwhile to begin with a summary of evidence on the comorbidity of APD and SUDs.

The literature relevant to this comorbidity is sizable and has been reviewed several times over the past 20 years. In one of the first analyses, Grande, Wolf, Schubert, Patterson, and Brocco (1984) examined studies of APD, alcoholism, and drug abuse. They concluded that patients with drug use disorders (e.g., heroin addicts) consistently showed high rates of APD: from 16% to 55% (i.e., well above the 2–3% rate found in the general population). Similarly, studies of adult patients with alcohol use disorders indicated that 28% had APD as well and, in a juvenile delinquent sample, an astonishing 88% evidenced alcohol problems. In a subsequent reevaluation of the studies reviewed by Grande and colleagues that had reported statistical tests, Schubert, Wolf, Patterson, Grande, and Pendleton (1988) found that the association between APD and SUDs was significant enough that the presence of one diagnosis reliably predicted the presence of the other.

More recently, Moran (1999) examined the epidemiology of APD including an overview of its association with SUDs. As reported by Moran, data from community samples suggested that up to 80% of people with APD met lifetime criteria for at least one SUD. Similarly high rates of APD (as high as 70%) were found in substance-abusing populations—particularly illicit drug abusers. The consistency in the results reviewed by Moran and Grande and colleagues (1984) underscores the stability in the finding of high comorbidity of APD and SUDs. Furthermore, research on the association of APD and SUDs in women, though limited, indicates that the high rate of comorbidity of these diagnoses is apparent in both genders (e.g., Jordan, Schlenger, Fairbank, & Caddell, 1996; Mulder, Wells, Joyce, & Bushnell, 1994).

Assessment of Psychopathy in Individuals with SUDs

As detailed elsewhere, Cleckley's (1976) concept of the psychopath contained both overt antisocial behavior problems (reflected in the APD diagnostic criteria) and affective–interpersonal features such as emotional detachment, lack of empathy, and grandiosity (not reflected in the APD diagnostic criteria). The current standard for psychopathy assessment is Hare's Psychopathy Checklist (PCL; Harpur, Hakstian, & Hare, 1988) and its successor, the revised PCL (PCL-R; Hare, 1991, 2003). PCL-R scores, which are based on extensive interview data and a detailed review of criminal and social history records, can be understood in terms of two statistically derived factors: Factor 1, which taps the affective–interpersonal component of psychopathy, and Factor 2, which taps the antisocial behavior or social deviance component. Variants of this two-factor structure have been proposed recently by Cooke and Michie (2001) and Hare (2003). A total PCL score is also available to capture the broad construct of psychopathy.

Prior to the introduction of the PCL, researchers interested in psychopathy often relied on the Psychopathic Deviate (Pd) scale from the Minnesota Multiphasic Personality Inventory (MMPI) and the Socialization (So) scale from the California Psychological Inventory (CPI; Gough, 1986), both of which are still widely used as self-report measures of the psychopathy construct. In addition, DSM symptom scores for APD and some other self-report instruments have been used to index psychopathy-related traits such as detachment and socialization (e.g., the Karolinska Scales of Personality; KSP, Schalling & Edman, 1993). A limitation of these traditional self-report psychopathy measures is that they appear to index mainly the antisocial deviance facet of psychopathy (cf. Hare, 2003). A more recent alternative that appears to tap both the affective–interpersonal and antisocial behavior components is the Psychopathic Personality Inventory (PPI; Lilienfeld & Andrews, 1996; see also Benning, Patrick, Hicks, Blonigen, & Krueger, 2003).

These disparate approaches to assessment of psychopathy raise two related questions:

1. Does the PCL-R yield a comparable two-factor structure when applied to individuals with SUDs?
2. Are self-report instruments capable of detecting these same and/or additional factors worthy of consideration?

In one of the more sophisticated analyses of the factor structure of the PCL-R in SUD groups, Windle and Dumenci (1999) studied 740 inpatient alcoholics of both genders in three ethnic groups and found general support for the utility of the instrument in this population and showed that factors capturing the affective–interpersonal (Factor 1) and social deviance (Factor 2) aspects of psychopathy were robust, though intercorrelated. A study of APD and psychopathy in cocaine-dependent women (Rutherford, Cacciola, & Alterman, 1999) also yielded support for the notion that the two variants of antisociality should be considered separately and that the PCL-R can be useful in doing so.

Four of the half dozen PCL-R assessments of methadone patients done mainly by the same group (Alterman, Cacciola, & Rutherford, 1993; Rutherford, Alterman, Cacciola, & McKay, 1997; Rutherford, Cacciola, Alterman, & McKay, 1996; Rutherford, Cacciola, Alterman, McKay, & Cook, 1999) were likewise consistent in suggesting the applicability of the two standard PCL factors, which evidence reasonable psychometric properties in both institutionalized and community samples. For women, however, a dimensional approach sometimes seemed more appropriate than a categorical one for Factor 2, perhaps owing to the general lower levels of overt antisocial behavior in women. Results from another methadone maintenance sample (Darke, Kaye, Finlay-Jones, & Hall, 1998) were somewhat less consistent in that a five-factor solution fit the data on Australian men and women better than a two-factor approach, although the authors noted that three affective–interpersonal factors (glib/manipulative, callous, and irresponsible) and two social deviance factors (criminal behavior and promiscuous behavior) did emerge. A last study of methadone maintenance patients, using only men, incorporated DSM symptoms of APD and CD as well as the CPI So scale along with a PCL-R assessment and then compared clustered scores from these measures to external criterion variables tapping a variety of constructs (addiction severity, criminal history, DSM symptomatology, etc.). The results suggested that as many as six subtypes of addicts could be extracted from among the SUD sample. Even in this case, a psychopathy group that was relatively distinct from simple antisocials emerged among the subtypes.

Finally, McDermott and colleagues (2000) reported on the performance of the PCL-R in samples of male prisoners and substance-dependent patients of both sexes from three studies involving opioid, cocaine, and alcohol addicts. Their data were unusual in indicating that the usual two-factor solution evident in the prisoner group did not fit the data for SUD patients as well as a single factor. Taken together, the weight of evidence from these studies suggests that the PCL-R, with its distinct affective–interpersonal and social deviance factors, can make a useful contribution to assessment of psychopathy and APD in SUD populations. However, there are also indications that other assessment devices may have a place as well.

Cooney, Kadden, and Litt (1990) offered a comparison of PCL scores with DSM diagnoses and symptom counts for APD, the CPI *So* scale, and the MMPI Pd scale in an assessment of "sociopathy" in male and female alcoholics to evaluate the relative utility of these assessment approaches in a population with alcohol use disorders. They found that only the CPI *So* scale reliably distinguished between APD and non-APD diagnosed groups of alcoholics, suggesting that this self-report measure might continue to be a useful element of assessment in such samples. In another study designed to explore the psychometric properties of the CPI *So* in treatment-seeking alcoholics, Kadden, Litt, Donovan, and Cooney (1996) used a principal components analysis and found it yielded two dimensions of sociopathy that appeared to parallel the two standard factors derived from the PCL-R. Specifically, the negative affectivity subscale of the CPI *So* mapped onto the personality–affectivity factor of the PCL-R, whereas the childhood-socialization scale of the CPI *So* seemed to tap the PCL-R's antisocial behavior/social deviance factor. Such results lend support for concurrent analysis of these factors by the CPI *So* and

advocate for its use as both an adjunct and possible substitute for the PCL-R if the more elaborate protocol associated with the latter measure is impractical.

Psychopathy and SUDs

Although there are clearly indications of complexity in the assessment of externalizing features in SUD populations, consideration of the foregoing findings regarding methods for evaluation of psychopathy justifies focus of the present review primarily on studies that used the PCL or PCL-R. However, relevant studies applying other methods of psychopathy assessment are also included where useful in providing a more comprehensive overview of the literature on the comorbidity of psychopathy and SUDs. Whenever possible, results pertaining specifically to alcohol versus other drug use disorders are highlighted. Likewise, findings pertaining to possible gender differences are noted as appropriate to reveal any potentially important gender-based variations in the relationship between psychopathy and SUDs.

One important additional point needs to be made regarding terminology: In most of the studies reviewed, distinctions were not made between the technically different diagnoses of substance "abuse" and substance "dependence." Rather, it often appeared that the SUD variable under study either reflected both of these diagnoses (i.e., abuse and/or dependence) or perhaps just one of them. Hence, the term "SUD" as used in this review refers broadly to both substance abuse and/or dependence, without much distinction between them. However, this serves to underscore an important consideration for future study, as the current literature does not adequately address possible differences in the relationship of psychopathy to substance abuse versus substance dependence.

Criminal and Forensic Psychiatric Samples

Table 25.1 presents a summary of studies that provide evidence of the association between psychopathy as assessed by PCL methods and SUDs assessed by various means at a dimensional and/or categorical level. Three things are clear from these data. First, there is a moderate positive correlation between psychopathic traits and SUDs. Second, SUDs

TABLE 25.1. Correlations between SUDs and PCL-R Scores and Odds of Comorbidity between Psychopathy and SUDs in Criminal Samples

Study	Substance use disorder assessment	Alcohol use disorders				Drug use disorders			
		Total	Factor 1	Factor 2	Odds ratio	Total	Factor 1	Factor 2	Odds ratio
Hemphill, Hart, & Hare (1994)	PCL-R interview; collateral information	.13	.10	.03	0.97	.28**	.09	.35**	3.19
Hart, Forth, & Hare (1991)	MCMI-II	.17	−.04	.30**	—	.32**	.12	.41**	—
Hare & Hare (1989)[a]	Clinical rating from file	.24	.07	.26	2.33	.31**	.15	.40**	2.51
Smith & Newman (1990)	Semistructured interview	.34**	.14	.40**	5.09**	.33**	.13	.40**	2.74**
Blackburn & Coid (1998)	Structured interview	n.r.	n.r.	.22**	—	.30**	.22**	.32**	—
Reardon, Lang, & Patrick (2002)	SMAST	.07	−.04	.13*	—	—	—	—	—
Blackburn, Logan, Donnelly, & Renwick (2003)	Structured interview	—	—	—	1.29	—	—	—	2.16*

Note. MCMI-II, Millon Clinical Multiaxial Inventory–II; n.r., not reported; SMAST, Michigan Alcoholism Screening Test—Short; substance use disorder, abuse and/or dependence or, in the case of the MCMI-II and SMAST, substance use problems.

[a] Used PCL to assess psychopathy.

*$p < .05$; **$p < .01$.

are more strongly associated with the social deviance component of psychopathy (i.e., Factor 2) than with the affective–interpersonal component (i.e., Factor 1). It is this component of psychopathy (Factor 2) that accounts for the association between PCL-R scores and APD diagnoses, which as noted earlier are known to be highly comorbid with SUDs. Third, psychopathy is more strongly associated with illicit drug use problems than with alcohol use problems (although this may be confounded by the fact that illicit drug use is illegal and thus is, by definition, "antisocial"). Given the relative consistency of the findings across studies, which ranged from self-report to structured interview in their assessment of SUDs, the third conclusion does not appear to be attributable to methodological differences in the assessment of SUDs. However, it is noteworthy that all seven of the studies shown in Table 25.1 were conducted with male participants, leaving open the question of gender differences in the correlation between psychopathy traits and SUDs.

The odds ratios presented in Table 25.1 lend some support to the idea that psychopathy increases risk for SUDs—drug use disorders in particular—within criminal populations (where SUDs are already generally high). For example, Smith and Newman (1990) found a significant elevation in the rate of alcohol use disorders among male prisoners who were psychopathic (93%) versus those who were not psychopathic (65%). Similarly, their observed rate of drug use disorder was significantly higher among psychopaths (74%) than among nonpsychopaths (44%). However, another study found a significantly higher rate of drug abuse among psychopaths (31%) than among nonpsychopaths (13%) but no rate differences for alcohol use disorders (Blackburn & Coid, 1998). A similar pattern of findings was reported in a sample of 41 Swedish male prisoners (Rasmussen, Storsaeter, & Levander, 1999). In that study, psychopaths had significantly higher rates of cannabis, inhalant, amphetamine, and opiate use disorders than nonpsychopaths, but there was no difference between groups in rates of alcohol use disorders. In contrast, Hemphill, Hart, and Hare (1994) obtained a significant correlation between SUDs and continuous dimensions of psychopathic traits, but they

failed to find significant differences in rates of SUDs among psychopaths compared to nonpsychopaths in their prison sample. In both psychopathic and nonpsychopathic inmates, the rate of alcohol use disorders was high (around 57%) and the rate of drug use disorders was even higher (88–96%). Taken together, results from various studies seem to suggest that psychopathy increases the risk for drug use disorders and, to a lesser extent, alcohol use disorders in criminal populations.

The literature appears to support the idea that psychopathy predicts the presence of SUDs in criminal samples, but does the reverse hold true? Loza (1993) examined PCL-R scores in 163 Canadian male prisoners classified by interviews and file review as alcohol abusers, drug abusers, alcohol/drug abusers, and non-substance abusers. The mean total PCL-R score for the alcohol/drug abusers was 23.1 (a "middle" level of psychopathy according to the PCL-R), which was significantly higher than the mean for all other groups. With regard to Factor 1 scores, the alcohol/drug abusers had significantly higher scores than the non-substance abusers; there were no other group differences on Factor 1. For Factor 2, the alcohol/drug abusers had significantly higher scores than the alcohol abusers and the non-substance abusers (who were also significantly lower than the drug abusers). In another study, Neo, McCullagh, and Howard (2001) examined psychopathic male prisoners in Singapore who either did or did not have a history of alcohol dependence. The rate of psychopathy (assessed using the PCL screening version; Hart, Cox, & Hare, 1995) was significantly higher in the alcohol dependent group (83%) than in the group without an alcohol use disorder history (17%).

Among studies not using PCL methods, an evaluation of 58 male Swedish forensic psychiatric examinees by Stalenheim and von Knorring (1998) revealed significantly lower scores on the Socialization and Social desirability scales of the KSP among patients with an SUD than among those without an SUD (note that these KSP scales correlate significantly with PCL-R scores). In another study using the KSP, Finnish and Swedish men with criminal records that included two or more alcohol-related violations had significantly lower KSP Socialization scale scores than men without criminal histories but did not differ from criminal men without alcohol-related violations (Pulkkinen, Virtanen, Klinteberg, & Magnusson, 2000).

In sum, the literature suggests that criminals with SUDs—particularly drug use disorders—are more psychopathic than criminals without an SUD. Again, exclusive reliance on male samples leaves the literature uninformative about possible gender differences in the relationship between psychopathy and SUDs.

SUDs Samples

SUDs are found at high rates in criminal samples and psychopathy is, in turn, predictive of high rates of SUDs within these samples. Taking a different tack, Rutherford, Alterman, and Cacciola (2000) offer a summary, based largely in their own extensive work, of the rates of psychopathy found in SUD samples. In brief, they reported that psychopathy (defined by PCL-R scores of 30 or greater) is found in around 12% of SUD samples, which is near the low end of the range of base rates for psychopathy in prison samples (15–25%) but significantly higher than rates in the general population. Table 25.2 summarizes results from four additional relevant studies not covered in the summary reported by Rutherford and colleagues. The rate of psychopathy across the

different types of SUD samples varies widely and appears to be tied to the definition of psychopathy. Among studies that employed the traditional psychopathy definition (PCL-R score of 30 or greater), the highest rate was found among heroin-dependent criminals. When the definition of psychopathy was based on less extreme cutoffs (e.g., PCL-R score of 25 or greater), the rate climbed to as high as 37.5% among men and 23.3% in women with heroin dependence. The data in Table 25.2 suggest that up to one-quarter of drug- and alcohol-dependent populations show elevated levels of psychopathy, an effect that is of similar magnitude among both men and women with SUDs.

The idea that psychopathic traits appear at elevated levels among the SUD population is also supported by studies using another measure purported to capture psychopathy, the Pd scale from the MMPI, which is selectively associated with Factor 2 from the PCL-R (cf. Hare, 1991, 2003). For example, Hewett and Martin (1980) found that male alcoholics and narcotic addicts had clinically elevated Pd scale scores (mean T score of about 73) that were significantly higher than scores from men without a history of SUD treatment (mean T score of 58). In another study, men with alcohol dependence only evidenced significantly lower Pd scale scores (mean T score = 70) than men with drug dependence only (mean T score = 75) and men with both

TABLE 25.2. Rates of Psychopathy in SUD Treatment Samples

Study	Sample	% male	Psychopathy definition	Psychopathy rate (%)		
				All	Males	Females
Rutherford, Cacciola, & Alterman (1999)	Cocaine-dependent treatment seekers	0	PCL-R ≥ 30	1.5	—	1.5
			PCL-R ≥ 25	3.6	—	3.6
			PCL-R ≥ 20	19.1	—	19.1
Darke, Kaye, & Finlay-Jones (1998)	Methadone maintenance outpatients	55	PCL-R ≥ 30	4.0	7.0	0.0
	Methadone maintenance prisoners	81	As above	9.0	9.0	10.0
	Non-heroin-using prisoners	95	As above	4.0	4.0	0.0
Piotrowski, Tusel, Sees, Banys, & Hall (1996)	Methadone maintenance patients	70	PCL-R ≥ 25	26.5	37.5	23.3
Windle (1999)	Alcohol treatment inpatients	54	Score of 2 on 7+ PCL-R items	15.1	14.8	15.7

Note. PCL-R, Psychopathy Checklist—Revised.

alcohol and drug dependence (mean *T* score = 78) (Cannon, Bell, Fowler, Penk, & Finkelstein, 1990). More recently, Dush and Keen (1995) reported on a cluster analysis of 137 women and 388 men admitted to an inpatient alcohol treatment program. Prior to treatment, the sample was captured in five clusters, four of which were marked by an elevation on the Pd scale. This finding replicated an earlier study by Whitelock, Overall, and Patrick (1971) on 136 men admitted to a general psychiatric hospital. Interestingly, Dush and Keen also showed that the elevation on the Pd scale was the only elevation that remained posttreatment, indicating that antisocial personality features may be primary in the relationship between SUDs and antisocial behavior problems because Pd scores stayed high even after the alcohol dependence had remitted (at least temporarily). However, Whitelock and colleagues noted that alcohol use disorder in their general psychiatric sample was not related to Pd elevations but instead to elevations on scales tapping depression and anxiety, a fact that highlights the complexity of SUD populations and cautions against the assumption that antisociality underlies or is even present in all cases. Finally, Benning and colleagues (2003) recently reported on correlates of the two PPI factors in a sample of unselected adult males and found that the PPI-II (akin to the PCL-R Factor 2) correlated significantly with alcohol use problems but the PPI-I factor (akin to the PCL-R Factor 1) did not. Although not a report on a SUD sample, this recent study is notable in its consistency with findings from criminal and SUD samples.

Special Populations: Adolescents

A few studies have examined SUDs and psychopathy in adolescents, which may reveal something about the development of these problems. Results from investigations of adolescent samples are largely consistent with those from studies of adults in showing an association between psychopathy and SUDs. For example, Mailloux, Forth, and Kroner (1997) examined psychopathy (assessed using the youth version of the PCL) and self-reported substance use problems in adolescent male prisoners (mean age of 17). The

mean PCL total score was 25.9, quite close to that seen in adult prison samples. Significant correlations were found between PCL total score and self-reported alcohol ($r = .46$) and drug ($r = .42$) problems. This effect again appeared to be driven by Factor 2, which correlated significantly with both alcohol ($r = .41$) and drug ($r = .48$) problems, which, in turn, were not significantly associated with Factor 1. This pattern of results is strikingly similar—if not stronger in magnitude—to results observed in adult samples (see Table 25.1).

Also consistent with results found in adult samples, there appears to be a high rate of psychopathy in adolescents with SUDs. O'Neill, Lidz, and Heilbrun (2003b) examined psychopathy (assessed with the youth version of the PCL) in 64 males (mean age of 16) who had been court-ordered to SUD treatment (all met criteria for a SUD). The mean PCL total score for the sample was 25.5, quite close to that found in an adolescent prison sample (Mailloux et al., 1997). In a study of 52 adolescent males (mean age of 15.6) in a SUD treatment program, the rate of psychopathy (defined as a PCL-R score of 30 or more) was 9.6% (Toupin, Mercier, Dery, Cote, & Hodgins, 1996), a rate that is higher than that reported in adult samples using a similar definition of psychopathy (see Table 25.2).

Finally, Harvey, Stokes, Lord, and Pogge (1996) examined psychopathy in adolescent boys and girls (mean age of 15) in a treatment program for dual-diagnosed patients. Patients involved with alcohol plus at least one other drug had significantly higher PCL-R total scores than patients with only an alcohol use disorder. Furthermore, the PCL-R total score accounted for the most variance (36%) in predicting group membership. No information was provided on the performance of individual PCL factors, but the results for the total scores were nonetheless consistent with findings from adult samples showing a stronger association of psychopathy with drug use disorders alone or in combination with alcohol problems than with alcohol use disorders alone. Although Harvey et al. included girls in their sample, they did not report how gender affected their results. Thus, it may be that the association between psychopathy and SUDs was invariant across gender, but more information and more research are needed to have any confidence in such a conclusion.

The research on adolescent samples provides possible insights into the timing of the association between psychopathy and SUDs. Although the course and sequencing of each problem is not discernible from the extant literature, it does suggest that psychopathy and SUDs are comorbid prior to adulthood—at least by mid-adolescence. This could have important implications that call for further study using longitudinal designs that begin when participants are young children so that the developmental timing and conceptual connections of psychopathic traits and substance use problems can be accurately tracked and evaluated.

Conclusions

The empirical literature supports a moderate association between psychopathic personality traits and SUDs. Research on adult criminal/forensic clinical samples further suggests that psychopathy is associated more strongly with drug use disorders than with alcohol use disorders and that the association between SUDs and psychopathy is driven largely by the social deviance component dimension of psychopathy, not the affective–interpersonal dimension. The rate of SUDs is high in criminal samples in general and is particularly high in psychopathic criminals. The reverse (i.e., that psychopathy is predictable from SUD) is also true for such samples, but to a lesser degree. Adults in treatment for SUDs show a generally modest rate of psychopathy, indicating that antisocial behavior problems are probably not at the root of most SUDs. From a developmental perspective, there is evidence that the association between psychopathy and SUDs can manifest at least as early as adolescence, suggesting a fundamental and enduring connection. Finally, it is noteworthy that the vast majority of research examining psychopathy and SUDs has used exclusively male samples, but when girls and women were included, the relationship between psychopathy and SUDs appeared to be similar across gender. Similar trends were evident across racial/ethnic groups, but this conclusion also requires additional and elaborated replications.

UNDERSTANDING THE COMORBIDITY: ROLE OF A BROAD EXTERNALIZING VULNERABILITY FACTOR

The comorbidity between psychopathy and SUDs appears to rest heavily on the social deviance dimension of psychopathy, which overlaps to a large degree with the APD diagnosis. Accordingly, it is useful to consider the literature on APD and SUDs in an effort to understand the comorbidity of psychopathy and SUDs. Although there is still much to learn about why psychopathic traits are associated with SUDs, the available literature includes promising models that provide possible insights into the basis of this comorbidity and are generating the research necessary to gain a clearer understanding of the phenomena.

First, there is clearly an important role for biological factors in the apparent etiological underpinnings of the association between various features of antisociality, psychopathy, and SUDs. Indeed, a strong case can be made for the idea that a common genetic liability underlies them. In this connection, Waldman and Slutske (2000) and van den Bree, Svikis, and Pickens (1998) have provided comprehensive reviews of the behavioral genetic literature on antisocial behavior and SUDs. Although the adoption studies covered in their analyses suggest some specificity of transmission for APD and SUDs, twin studies clearly support a common genetic influence on these disorders. The pertinent evidence thus supports the notion that broad etiological factors are associated with both antisocial behavior and SUDs. However, the data do not suggest how genetic factors actually influence comorbidity. This vacuum has provided impetus for the development of models designed to address the link between SUDs and antisocial behavior in ways that are consistent with the idea that genetic factors make a contribution to the link.

For example, over two decades ago, Gorenstein and Newman (1980) proposed that psychopathy and alcoholism belong to a group of disorders now widely known as "disinhibitory psychopathology," which Gorenstein and Newman described as disorders marked by poor behavioral controls and hypothesized to emanate from a genetically mediated septal dysfunction in the brain. Later, Fowles (1988) outlined a motivational model of psychopathology based on the relative strengths of a behavioral inhibition system (BIS) and behavioral activation system (BAS) (cf. Gray, 1975). He proposed that psychopathy and SUDs stem, in part, from weak BIS (trouble inhibiting behavior in response to punishment or non-reward). In the last decade, Sher and Trull (1994) suggested that the link between alcohol use disorders and APD may stem from broad personality traits associated with those conditions (e.g., impulsivity). Patrick and Lang (1999) even drew parallels between psychopathic traits and intoxicated states, suggesting that disrupted cognitive/affective control associated with both phenomena may account for their attendant disinhibition of behavior and could act synergistically when psychopaths become intoxicated. Each of these models is compatible with the behavioral genetic data on SUDs and antisocial behavior in that the components (septal dysfunction, BIS strength, personality, affective/cognitive dysregulation, etc.) have been or could conceivably be associated with genetic factors. However, it is the recently introduced model of Krueger and colleagues (2002) that is perhaps the most promising account of the association between antisociality and SUDs because it attempts to account for the behavior genetic data in a more precise way.

Krueger and colleagues (2002) examined the etiological factors associated with the disorders of specific interest (viz., APD and alcohol and drug dependence) in the context of what is widely known as the "externalizing spectrum." Their access to twin data from a large epidemiological sample afforded the opportunity for a strong test of the fit of their proposed broad externalizing vulnerability factor. In this model, externalizing disorders such as APD and substance dependence are expected to covary because they are influenced by a latent vulnerability factor that is largely genetically mediated. This would be consistent with other twin data that have shown common genetic factors associated with APD and SUDs. Krueger and colleagues' model further allows for independent etiological factors to be associated with each disorder in the externalizing spectrum. This would be consis-

tent with adoption data that suggest independent etiologies for APD and SUDs. Finally, Krueger and colleagues included in the model a broad personality factor, Constraint, which reflects sensation seeking, behavioral control, and adherence to social norms. Pertinent analyses yielded support for a model in which APD, alcohol dependence, drug dependence, and Constraint were significantly associated with a latent externalizing vulnerability factor that was substantially influenced by genetic factors. Furthermore, analyses failed to find evidence of specific genetic influences on either APD or substance dependence but, instead, revealed specific environmental factors that were associated with each individual externalizing disorder. This is exciting in that it is indicative of how common genetic factors can influence the potential to exhibit APD and substance dependence and how environmental factors help shape the phenotypes that are actually expressed.

In sum, available models have generally agreed that antisocial behavior and substance use problems are etiologically linked and the behavioral genetic data largely support this proposition. Furthermore, pertinent analyses by Krueger and colleagues (2002) provided a convincing demonstration of a genetically mediated broad externalizing vulnerability factor that links various externalizing behaviors such as SUDs and APD. The comorbidity between psychopathy and SUDs thus appears to be driven by the social deviance dimension of psychopathy, which, in turn, suggests that the broad externalizing vulnerability factor model is potentially useful in understanding the comorbidity between psychopathy and SUDs. A recent analysis examining the association between the PCL-R factors and externalizing, defined as the common factor underlying conduct disorder/adult antisocial behavior, SUDs, and Constraint, demonstrated that PCL-R Factor 2 and externalizing tap essentially the same underlying construct, whereas the unique variance associated with PCL-R Factor 1 taps something entirely different (Patrick, Hicks, Krueger, & Lang, 2005). This suggests that one part of the psychopathy construct reflects a broad underlying constitutional vulnerability to externalizing disorders, including SUDs—and potentially other problems such as gambling, suicide, and other forms of disinhibited psychopathology.

CLINICAL CONSEQUENCES OF THE ASSOCIATION BETWEEN PSYCHOPATHY AND SUDs

The evidence for a meaningful relationship between psychopathy and SUDs highlights the importance of considering comorbidity in theory and research on these constructs. Nor should the clinical significance of this comorbidity be underestimated because it can have a profound impact on the course of both disorders and on treatment outcome, with SUD relapse and criminal recidivism as critical indices. In this connection, Gerstley, Alterman, McLellan, and Woody (1990) summarized the literature pertinent to various negative outcomes associated with ASPD in the treatment of SUDs and concluded that more attention should be paid to the construct of psychopathy and its components (personality vs. behavioral) in future efforts to understand the implications of antisocial behavior on SUD treatment outcomes. We strongly endorse this recommendation.

Table 25.3 summarizes the types of problems that the presence of psychopathic traits (as assessed by some version of the PCL) can pose for clinicians treating SUDs both in the prison system and in the community. In general, and not surprisingly, the presence of psychopathy or higher levels of psychopathic traits is often associated with poorer SUD treatment compliance and outcomes as well as a greater likelihood of criminal recidivism. Given the association of APD to SUDs, it is of particular interest to note that two studies examined the independent contributions of APD and psychopathy to outcomes. Tourian and colleagues (1997) found that HIV (human immunodeficiency virus) risk behaviors were more related to psychopathy scores (from the PCL-R) than to APD diagnosis in methadone maintenance patients. Similarly, PCL-R scores were also more predictive of positive drug urines and treatment noncompletion than APD features in methadone maintenance patients (Alterman, Rutherford, Cacciola, McKay, & Boardman, 1998).

The findings from Table 25.3 are supported by additional studies using other definitions of psychopathy or related constructs. For example, high Pd scores on the MMPI in men and women attending an alcohol treatment program was associated with more drinking relapse problems during the 4 years after treatment (Pettinati, Sugerman, & Maurer, 1982). Similarly, several reports have linked poorer alcohol and drug treatment outcomes (e.g., relapse) to the presence of APD symptoms (Cecero, Ball, Tennen,

TABLE 25.3. Clinical Impact of Psychopathy on SUD Treatment

Sample	Effects associated with psychopathy	Study
Methadone maintenance patients	Greater HIV risk behaviors (e.g., needle sharing)	Tourian et al. (1997)
	Poorer reality testing	Rutherford, Alterman, Cacciola, McKay, & Cook (1996)
	Positive cocaine and benzodiazapine urines during treatment	Alterman, Rutherford, Cacciola, McKay, & Boardman (1998)
	Lower likelihood of treatment completion	
Adolescents in treatment for substance use disorder	Higher arrest recidivism posttreatment	O'Neill, Lidz, & Heilbrun (2003a)
	Poorer treatment compliance and quality of participation	
	Positive drug urines during treatment	
	Less clinical improvement	
Prisoners in treatment for substance use disorder	Less change in response to treatment	Richards, Casey, & Lucente (2003)
	Longer time to treatment response	
	Recidivism after release	

Note. Psychopathy in each of the studies referenced was assessed with some version of the Psychopathy Checklist. Substance use disorder treatment refers to treatment for substance abuse and/or dependence.

Kranzler, & Rounsaville, 1999; Mather, 1987; Rounsaville, Dolinsky, Babor, & Meyer, 1987). Thus, clinicians who treat SUDs should be aware that the presence of psychopathy or persistent antisociality is likely to make attainment of successful treatment outcomes more challenging.

Effects of comorbid expression of psychopathy and SUD on antisocial behavior and criminal recidivism are also significant clinical concerns. Although relatively few studies have examined the impact of comorbid substance use problems and psychopathy on such outcomes, the small literature suggests that it is a difficult combination for clinicians. For instance, in a study of 55 male offenders in a state forensic hospital, high scores on the screening version of the PCL (Hart et al., 1995) and a SUD history combined to predict significant elevations in aggression during the hospitalization, and PCL score was a further predictor of treatment noncompliance (Hill, Rogers, & Bickford, 1996). Among a large group of male sex offenders, recidivism in problematic sexual behavior, recurrence of violence, and general criminal recidivism were all associated with a combination of alcohol use problems and high PCL-R score (Firestone et al., 1999). In another study, a higher proportion of violent criminal offenses was noted among psychopathic male alcoholic prisoners than in those without the psychopathy–alcohol combination (Walsh, 1999). However, Rice and Harris (1995) added a little equivocation to the prevailing trend when they observed that psychopathy was more related to violent recidivism than were alcohol use problems, which did not appear to add to risk for violent recidivism among psychopaths. In that study, however, alcohol use problem assessment depended solely on file information gathered at admission, an approach liable to yield less valid results than the more comprehensive SUD assessments used in the other studies, which typically included a self-report instrument and/or interview data in addition to case file information.

In summary, clinicians are liable to face substantial challenges when they treat patients or inmates with high levels of psychopathic traits coupled with SUDs. These will probably be most evident in lower treatment compliance, poorer treatment outcome, and reduced quality of overall treatment partici-pation, as well as a greater risk of violence. Further, the community at large may also pay a price for the comorbidity of psychopathy with SUDs, given the increased likelihood of criminal recidivism among people with this clinical combination.

PRACTICAL STRATEGIES FOR CLINICAL MANAGEMENT OF DUALLY DIAGNOSED PSYCHOPATHY AND SUDs

Detailed description of a program for the assessment and clinical management of individuals with comorbid psychopathy and SUD is far beyond the scope of this chapter, but interested readers are directed to relevant manuals by Wanberg and Milkman (1998) for excellent, comprehensive coverage of how one might effectively approach substance use problems in the context of criminal conduct. They lament the commonly compartmentalized treatment of the two oft-related classes of disorders and advocate for an integrated approach. Much of what we say in the brief coverage of general strategies offered here is consonant with their recommendations.

For any mental health intervention to succeed, clients first must be persuaded to answer two questions affirmatively: (1) "Will I be better off if I change?" and (2) "Can I change if I try?" In this connection, it should be noted that whereas many people with SUDs are, as the old adage goes, motivated to change by crises of "liver, lover, or livelihood" (i.e., health, relationship, or employment), the presence of psychopathic deviance in those with SUDs seems to dictate the need to develop other motives. This is because psychopaths tend to regard themselves as invincible and are relatively impervious to contrary evidence, by definition lack interest in and capacity for close relationships, and are not known for their commitment to employment. Indeed, the vast majority of persons meeting criteria for psychopathy or APD would probably never present themselves for mental health treatment of any kind unless coerced to do so. This is no less true of those with SUDs, who typically become involved in SUD treatment by way of the legal system, either as an alternative to jail time or in the context of criminal incarceration for substance-related offenses. Moreover, to the extent that the externalizing characteristics linking antisociality and SUD, as well as the very action of many psychoactive substances, represent disruption of brain systems involved in reliable regulation of affect, cognition, and behavior relevant to delay of gratification and to restraint (cf. Patrick & Lang, 1999), it is easy to see why individuals with such dispositions are not great candidates for sustained or total recovery. However, this need not lead to defeatism—only patience in the pursuit of realistic goals by the best available means.

The principal motivator at the disposal of those treating the typical client with comorbid psychopathy and SUD is most likely to be that individual's desire to escape and/or avoid further incarceration. With this in mind, the clinician conducting assessments of alcohol and other drug use (see Wanberg & Milkman, 1998, for suggested instruments) and evaluation of psychopathy and criminality via the PCL-R and perhaps the CPI *So* might be well advised to direct attention to the many obvious connections between substance use and crime. Interviews should be oriented toward developing a dispassionate summary of the evidence linking these two phenomena and showing how intoxication is often a catalyst for behavior that can lead to incarceration. The pertinent evaluation, discussed in a manner consistent with the motivational interviewing approach pioneered by Miller and his colleagues (Miller & Rollnick, 1991), may be the best bet to move antisocial SUD clients from the indifference of precontemplation or the ambivalence of contemplation into the action phase of change efforts (see DiClemente & Prochaska, 1998, for a discussion of the "stages of change" model as applied to addictive behaviors). Of course, more confrontational approaches such as those characteristic of 12-Step programs could also be tried, but psychopaths' dispositional lack of guilt or remorse and resistance to taking responsibility for their actions would seem to argue that such tactics are a poor fit for this population.

In connection with establishing motivation for change, selection of treatment goals and methods can be undertaken. The general observation that treatment success is more likely when clients participate in decision making on such matters should be applied here, especially given the self-centered nature of psychopathy, but with recognition that impulsivity and lack of realistic long-term planning are among the markers of APD and the social deviance factor in psychopathy. Accordingly, it might make most sense to focus on modest, short-term goals that are not overly restrictive or moralistic. This would be quite compatible with the notion of "harm reduction" (cf. Marlatt, 1998), wherein, given that at least some level of substance use is considered likely, one reasonable goal is to minimize its adverse consequences through educating people about and providing means for safer use practices (e.g., needle exchange and methadone maintenance for opiate addicts). This is not to say that abstinence is not still a highly desirable treatment target but, rather, that clients are best served when they are prepared for as many contingencies as possible. To accomplish this, more comprehensive and personally focused interventions have been developed using cognitive-behavioral methods (see Wanberg & Milkman, 1998, for a review). These are organized around cognitive restructuring of irrational ideas and behavioral coping skills training aimed at preventing and/or minimizing both relapses into problematic substance use patterns and recidivistic criminal behavior patterns. In the case of comorbid psychopathy and SUD, special attention may need to be directed at clear contingencies both within and outside treatment, given the relative dearth of functional, internally based restraints within such individuals. Obviously, incarceration and the conditions surrounding it will be a potentially powerful tool for change. In any case, the overarching principle in evaluating these endeavors is that treatment success is not an all-or-none enterprise but, rather, a continuum on which movement in a positive direction can be pursued and indexed.

CONCLUSIONS

Psychopathy has a moderate correlation with SUDs, particularly illicit drug use disorders. The association between SUDs and psychopathy appears to be driven largely by its social deviance component. A particularly promising model for explaining this association posits that antisocial behavior and SUDs arise from a broad, genetically mediated externalizing vulnerability factor. Evidence from twin data support this model, thus making it a compelling guide for future research into the etiology of the comorbidity between psychopathy and SUDs.

Research also suggests that the association of psychopathy and SUDs is evident at least as early as adolescence. Consequently, our understanding of this association should be further enlightened by developmental research examining the onset and course of each syndrome and of their sequencing and association. Pertinent evidence is scant but suggests—at least preliminarily—that the relationship between psychopathy and SUDs exists across gender and is not moderated by race or ethnicity. Future research should include large mixed-gender, mixed-race/ethnicity samples whenever feasible to allow for statistical evaluation of their potential effects. The negative consequences of psychopathy on SUD treatment are fairly well documented, and research also indicates that other outcomes (e.g., criminal recidivism) are negatively affected when psychopathy and one or more SUDs co-occur. These facts suggest the potential utility of adaptive clinical management strategies uniquely fitted to such dually diagnosed populations. An emphasis on the connection between the consequences of substance use in terms of risk for incarceration is one such strategy.

ACKNOWLEDGMENT

Preparation of this chapter was partially supported by Grant No. AA012164 from the National Institute on Alcohol Abuse and Alcoholism.

REFERENCES

Alterman, A. I., Cacciola, J. S., & Rutherford, M. J. (1993). Reliability of the Revised Psychopathy Checklist in substance abuse patients. *Psychological Assessment: A Journal of Consulting and Clinical Psychology, 5,* 442–448.

Alterman, A. I., Rutherford, M. J., Cacciola, J. S., McKay, J. R., & Boardman, C. R. (1998). Prediction of 7 months methadone maintenance treatment response by four measures of antisociality. *Drug and Alcohol Dependence, 49,* 217–223.

Babor, T. F., Hofmann, M., DelBoca, F. K., Hesselbrock, V., Meyer, R. E., Dolinsky, Z. S., & Rounsaville, B. (1992). Types of alcoholics: Evidence of an empirically derived typology based on indicators of vulnerability and severity. *Archives of General Psychiatry, 49,* 599–608.

Benning, S. D., Patrick, C. J., Hicks, B. M., Blonigen, D. M., & Krueger, R. F. (2003). Factor structure of the Psychopathic Personality Inventory: Validity and implications for clinical assessment. *Psychological Assessment, 15,* 340–350.

Blackburn, R., & Coid, J. W. (1998). Psychopathy and the dimensions of personality disorders in violent offenders. *Personality and Individual Differences, 25,* 129–145.

Blackburn, R., Logan, C., Donnelly, J., & Renwick, S. (2003). Personality disorders, psychopathy and other mental disorders: Co-morbidity among patients at English and Scottish high-security hospitals. *Journal of Forensic Psychiatry and Psychology, 14,* 111–137.

Cannon, D. S., Bell, W. E., Fowler, D. R., Penk, W. E., & Finkelstein, A. S. (1990). MMPI differences between alcoholics and drug abusers: Effect of age and race. *Psychological Assessment: A Journal of Consulting and Clinical Psychology, 2,* 51–55.

Cecero, J. J., Ball, S. A., Tennen, H., Kranzler, H. R., & Rounsaville, B. J. (1999). Concurrent and predictive validity of antisocial personality disorder subtyping among substance abusers. *Journal of Nervous and Mental Disease, 187,* 478–486.

Cleckley, H. (1976). *The mask of sanity* (5th ed.). St. Louis, MO: Mosby.

Cloninger, C. R. (1987). Neurogenetic adaptive mechanisms in alcoholism. *Science, 236,* 410–416.

Cooke, D. J., & Michie, C. (2001). Refining the construct of psychopathy: Toward a hierarchical model. *Psychological Assessment, 31,* 171–188.

Cooney, N. L., Kadden, R. M., & Litt, M. D. (1990). A comparison of methods for assessing sociopathy in male and female alcoholics. *Journal of Studies on Alcohol, 51,* 42–48.

Cottler, L. B., Schuckit, M. A., Helzer, J. E., Crowley, T., Woody, G., Nathan, P., & Hughes, J. (1995). The DSM-IV field trial for substance use disorders: Major results. *Drug and Alcohol Dependence, 38,* 59–69.

Darke, S., Kaye, S., & Finlay-Jones, R. (1998). Antisocial personality disorder, psychopathy and injecting heroin use. *Drug and Alcohol Dependence, 52,* 63–69.

Darke, S., Kaye, S., Finlay-Jones, R., & Hall, W. (1998). Factor structure of psychopathy among methadone maintenance patients. *Journal of Personality Disorders, 12,* 162–171.

DiClemente, C. C., & Prochaska, J. O. (1998). Toward a comprehensive, transtheoretical model of change: Stages of change and addictive behaviors. In W. Miller & N. Heather (Eds.), *Treating addictive behavior* (2nd ed., pp. 3–24). New York: Plenum Press.

Dush, D. M., & Keen, J. (1995). Changes in cluster analysis subtypes among alcoholic personalities after treatment. *Evaluation and the Health Professions, 18,* 152–165.

Firestone, P., Bradford, J. M., McCoy, M., Greenberg, D. M., LaRose, M. R., & Curry, S. (1999). Prediction of recidivism in incest offenders. *Journal of Interpersonal Violence, 14,* 511–531.

Fowles, D. C. (1988). Psychophysiology and psychopathology: A motivational approach. *Psychophysiology, 25,* 373–391.

Gerstley, L. J., Alterman, A. I., McLellan, A. T., & Woody, G. E. (1990). Antisocial personality disorder in substance abusers: A problematic diagnosis? *American Journal of Psychiatry, 147,* 173–178.

Gorenstein, E. E., & Newman, J. P. (1980). Disinhibitory psychopathology: A new perspective and a model for research. *Psychological Review, 87,* 301–315.

Gough, H. G. (1986). *California Psychological Inventory.* Palo Alto, CA: Consulting Psychologists Press.

Grande, T. P., Wolf, A. W., Schubert, D. S., Patterson, M. B., & Brocco, K. (1984). Associations among alcoholism, drug abuse, and antisocial personality: A review of the literature. *Psychological Reports, 55,* 455–474.

Grant, B. F., Harford, T. C., Dawson, D. A., & Chou, P. (1994). Epidemiologic Bulletin No. 35: Prevalence of DSM-IV alcohol abuse and dependence, United States 1992. *Alcohol Health and Research World, 18,* 243–248.

Gray, J. A. (1975). *Elements of a two-process theory of learning.* New York: Academic Press.

Hare, R. D. (1991). *Manual for the Hare Psychopathy Checklist—Revised.* Toronto, ON, Canada: Multi-Health Systems.

Hare, R. D. (2003). *The Hare Psychopathy Checklist* (2nd ed.). Toronto, ON, Canada: Multi-Health Systems.

Harpur, T. J., Hakstian, A. R., & Hare, R. D. (1988). Factor structure of the Psychopathy Checklist. *Journal of Consulting and Clinical Psychology, 56,* 741–747.

Hart, S. D., Cox, D. N., & Hare, R. D. (1995). *The Hare Psychopathy Checklist: Screening Version* (1st ed.). Toronto, ON, Canada: Multi-Health Systems.

Hart, S. D., Forth, A. E., & Hare, R. D. (1991). The MCMI-II as a measure of psychopathy. *Journal of Personality Disorders, 5,* 318–327.

Hart, S. D., & Hare, R. D. (1989). Discriminant validity of the Psychopathy Checklist in a forensic psychiatric population. *Psychological Assessment: A Journal of Consulting and Clinical Psychology, 1,* 211–218.

Harvey, P. D., Stokes, J. L., Lord, J., & Pogge, D. L. (1996). Neurocognitive and personality assessment of adolescent substance abusers: A multidimensional approach. *Assessment, 3,* 241–253.

Hemphill, J. F., Hart, S. D., & Hare, R. D. (1994). Psychopathy and substance use. *Journal of Personality Disorders, 8,* 169–180.

Hewett, B. B., & Martin, W. R. (1980). Psychometric comparisons of sociopathic and psychopathological behaviours of alcoholics and drug abusers versus a low drug use control population. *International Journal of the Addictions, 15,* 77–105.

Hill, C. D., Rogers, R., & Bickford, M. E. (1996). Predicting aggressive and socially disruptive behavior in a maximum security forensic psychiatric hospital. *Journal of Forensic Sciences, 41,* 56–59.

Jordan, B. K., Schlenger, W. E., Fairbank, J. A., & Caddell, J. M. (1996). Prevalence of psychiatric disorders among incarcerated women. *Archives of General Psychiatry, 53,* 513–519.

Kadden, R. M., Litt, M. D., Donovan, D., & Cooney, N. L. (1996). Psychometric properties of the California Psychological Inventory Socialization scale in treatment seeking alcoholics. *Psychology of Addictive Behaviors, 10,* 131–146.

Krueger, R. F., Hicks, B., Patrick, C. J., Carlson, S., Iacono, W. G., & McGue, M. (2002). Etiologic connections among substance dependence, antisocial behavior, and personality: Modeling the externalizing spectrum. *Journal of Abnormal Psychology, 111,* 411–424.

Lilienfeld, S. O., & Andrews, B. P. (1996). Development and preliminary validation of a self report measure of psychopathic personality traits in noncriminal populations. *Journal of Personality Assessment, 66,* 488–524.

Loza, W. (1993). Different substance abusing offenders require a unique program. *International Journal of Offender Therapy and Comparative Criminology, 37,* 351–358.

Mailloux, D. L., Forth, A. E., & Kroner, D. G. (1997). Psychopathy and substance use in adolescent male offenders. *Psychological Reports, 81,* 529–530.

Marlatt, G. A. (1998). *Harm reduction: Pragmatic strategies for managing high-risk behaviors.* New York: Guilford Press.

Mather, D. B. (1987). The role of antisocial personality in alcohol rehabilitation treatment effectiveness. *Military Medicine, 152,* 516–518.

McDermott, P. A., Alterman, A. I., Cacciola, J. S., Rutherford, M. J., Newman, J. P., & Mulholland, E. M. (2000). Generality of Psychopathy Checklist—Revised factors over prisoners and substance-dependent patients. *Journal of Consulting and Clinical Psychology, 68,* 181–186.

Miller, W. R., & Rollnick, S. (1991). *Motivational interviewing: Preparing people to change addictive behavior.* New York: Guilford Press.

Moran, P. (1999). The epidemiology of antisocial personality disorder. *Social Psychiatry and Psychiatric Epidemiology, 34,* 231–242.

Mulder, R. T., Wells, J. E., Joyce, P. R., & Bushnell, J. A. (1994). Antisocial women. *Journal of Personality Disorders, 8,* 279–287.

Neo, L. H., McCullagh, P., & Howard, R. (2001). An electrocortical correlate of a history of alcohol abuse in criminal offenders. *Psychology, Crime and Law, 7,* 105–117.

O'Neill, M. L., Lidz, V., & Heilbrun, K. (2003a). Adolescents with psychopathic characteristics in a substance abusing cohort: Treatment process and outcomes. *Law and Human Behavior, 27,* 299–313.

O'Neill, M. L., Lidz, V., & Heilbrun, K. (2003b). Predictors and correlates of psychopathic characteristics in substance abusing adolescents. *International Journal of Forensic Mental Health, 2,* 35–45.

Patrick, C. J., Hicks, B. M., Krueger, R. F., & Lang, A. R. (2005). Relations between psychopathy facets and externalizing in a criminal offender sample. *Journal of Personality Disorders, 19,* 339–356.

Patrick, C. J., & Lang, A. R. (1999). Psychopathic traits and intoxicated states: Affective concomitants and conceptual links. In M. Dawson, A. Schell, & A. Böhmelt (Eds.), *Startle modification: Implications for neuroscience, cognitive science, and clinical science* (pp. 209–230). Cambridge, UK: Cambridge University Press.

Pettinati, H. M., Sugerman, A. A., & Maurer, H. S. (1982). Four year MMPI changes in abstinent and drinking alcoholics. *Alcoholism: Clinical and Experimental Research, 6,* 487–494.

Piotrowski, N. A., Tusel, D. J., Sees, K. L., Banys, P., & Hall, S. M. (1996). Psychopathy and antisocial personality disorder in men and women with primary opioid dependence. In D. J. Cooke, A. E. Forth, J. P. Newman, & R. D. Hare (Eds.), *Issues in criminological and legal psychology: No. 24. International perspectives on psychopathy* (pp. 123–126). Leicester, UK: British Psychological Society.

Pulkkinen, L., Virtanen, T., Klinteberg, B. A., & Magnusson, D. (2000). Child behaviour and adult personality: Comparisons between criminality groups in Finland and Sweden. *Criminal Behaviour and Mental Health, 10,* 155–169.

Rasmussen, K., Storsaeter, O., & Levander, S. (1999). Personality disorders, psychopathy, and crime in a Norwegian prison population. *International Journal of Law and Psychiatry, 22,* 91–97.

Reardon, M. L., Lang, A. R., & Patrick, C. J. (2002). Antisociality and alcohol problems: An evaluation of subtypes, drinking motives, and family history in incarcerated men. *Alcoholism: Clinical and Experimental Research, 26,* 1188–1197.

Rice, M. E., & Harris, G. T. (1995). Psychopathy, schizophrenia, alcohol abuse, and violent recidivism. *International Journal of Law and Psychiatry, 18,* 333–342.

Richards, H. J., Casey, J. O., & Lucente, S. W. (2003). Psychopathy and treatment response in incarcerated female substance abusers. *Criminal Justice and Behavior, 30,* 251–276.

Rounsaville, B. J., Dolinsky, Z. S., Babor, T. F., & Meyer, R. E. (1987). Psychopathology as a predictor of treatment outcome in alcoholics. *Archives of General Psychiatry, 44,* 505–513.

Rutherford, M. J., Alterman, A. I., & Cacciola, J. S. (2000). Psychopathy and substance abuse: A bad mix. In C. B. Gacono (Ed.), *The clinical and forensic assessment of psychopathy: A practitioner's guide* (pp. 351–368). Mahwah, NJ: Erlbaum.

Rutherford, M. J., Alterman, A. I., Cacciola, J. S., & McKay, J. R. (1997). Validity of the Psychopathy Checklist—Revised in male methadone patients. *Drug and Alcohol Dependence, 44,* 143–149.

Rutherford, M. J., Alterman, A. I., Cacciola, J. S., McKay, J. R., & Cook, T. G. (1996). Object relations and reality testing in psychopathic and antisocial methadone patients. *Journal of Personality Disorders, 10,* 312–320.

Rutherford, M. J., Cacciola, J. S., & Alterman, A. I. (1999). Antisocial personality disorder and psychopathy in cocaine-dependent women. *American Journal of Psychiatry, 156,* 849–856.

Rutherford, M. J., Cacciola, J. S., Alterman, A. I., & McKay, J. R. (1996). Reliability and validity of the Revised Psychopathy Checklist in women methadone patients. *Assessment, 3,* 43–54.

Rutherford, M. J., Cacciola, J. S., Alterman, A. I., McKay, J. R., & Cook, T. G. (1999). Two-year test-retest reliability of the Psychopathy Checklist—Revised in methadone patients. *Assessment, 6,* 285–291.

Schalling, D., & Edman, G. (1993). *An inventory for assessing temperament dimensions associated with vulnerability for psychosocial deviance.* Stockholm, Sweden: Department of Psychiatry, The Karolinska Institute.

Schubert, D. S. P., Wolf, A. W., Patterson, M. B., Grande, T. P., & Pendleton, L. (1988). A statistical evaluation of the literature regarding the associations among alcoholism, drug abuse, and antisocial personality disorder. *International Journal of the Addictions, 23,* 797–808.

Sher, K. J., & Trull, T. J. (1994). Personality and disinhibitory psychopathology: Alcoholism and antisocial personality disorders. *Journal of Abnormal Psychology, 103,* 92–102.

Skodol, A. E., Oldham, J. M., & Gallaher, P. E. (1999). Axis II comorbidity of substance use disorders among patients referred for treatment of personality disorders. *American Journal of Psychiatry, 156,* 733–738.

Smith, S. S., & Newman, J. P. (1990). Alcohol and drug abuse/dependence disorders in psychopathic and nonpsychopathic criminal offenders. *Journal of Abnormal Psychology, 99,* 430–439.

Soderstrom, H., Sjodin, A., Carlstedt, A., & Forsman, A. (2004). Adult psychopathic personality with childhood-onset hyperactivity and conduct disorder: A central problem constellation in forensic psychiatry. *Psychiatry Research, 121,* 271–280.

Stalenheim, E. G., & von Knorring, L. (1998). Personality traits and psychopathy in a forensic psychiatric population. *European Journal of Psychiatry, 12,* 83–94.

Strain, E. C. (1995). Antisocial personality disorder, misbehavior, and drug abuse. *Journal of Nervous and Mental Disease, 183,* 162–165.

Timmerman, I. G. H., & Emmelkamp, P. M. G. (2001). The prevalence and comorbidity of Axis I and Axis II pathology in a group of forensic patients. *International Journal of Offender Therapy and Comparative Criminology, 45,* 198–213.

Toupin, J., Mercier, H., Déry, M., Côté, G., & Hodgins, S. (1996). Validity of the PCL-R for adolescents. In D. J. Cooke, A. E. Forth, J. P. Newman, & R. D. Hare (Eds.), *Issues in criminological and legal psychology: No. 24. International perspectives on psychopathy* (pp. 143–145). Leicester, UK: British Psychological Society.

Tourian, K., Alterman, A., Metzger, D., Rutherford, M., Cacciola, J. S., & McKay, J. R. (1997). Validity of three measures of antisociality in predicting HIV risk behaviors in methadone-maintenance patients. *Drug and Alcohol Dependence, 47,* 99–107.

van den Bree, M. B. M., Svikis, D. S., & Pickens, R. W. (1998). Genetic influences in antisocial personality and drug use disorders. *Drug and Alcohol Dependence, 49,* 177–187.

Waldman, I. D., & Slutske, W. S. (2000). Antisocial behavior and alcoholism: A behavioral genetic perspective on comorbidity. *Clinical Psychology Review, 20,* 255–287.

Walsh, T. C. (1999). Psychopathic and nonpsychopathic violence among alcoholic offenders. *International Journal of Offender Therapy and Comparative Criminology, 43,* 34–48.

Wanberg, K. W., & Milkman, H. B. (1998). *Criminal conduct and substance abuse treatment: Strategies for self-improvement and change.* Thousand Oaks, CA: Sage.

Whitelock, P. R., Overall, J. E., & Patrick, J. H. (1971). Personality patterns and alcohol abuse in a state hospital population. *Journal of Abnormal Psychology, 78,* 9–16.

Windle, M. (1999). Psychopathy and antisocial personality disorder among alcoholic inpatients. *Journal of Studies on Alcohol, 60,* 330–336.

Windle, M., & Dumenci, L. (1999). The factorial structure and construct validity of the Psychopathy Checklist—Revised (PCL-R) among alcoholic inpatients. *Structural Equation Modeling, 6,* 372–393.

26

The Role of Psychopathy in Sexual Coercion against Women

RAYMOND A. KNIGHT
JEAN-PIERRE GUAY

The hypothesis that there is a link between psychopathy and sexual aggression against women has a long and complex history. Early attempts to delineate the core characteristics of the psychopath (Cleckley, 1976) did not include the hypothesis that psychopaths would evidence a disproportionate proclivity to engage in sexually coercive behavior. Although Cleckley described the sexuality of psychopathic individuals as "abnormal," he characterized them as being disengaged from the emotional component of sexuality, not prone to sexual coercion. He noted that although the psychopath was disinhibited sexually and might seek sexual gratification with partners and in environments that would be avoided by others with greater discretion, he did not maintain that the psychopath was oversexualized. Although Cleckley believed that the psychopath was not disposed to consider the emotional state or level of engagement of his sexual partners—an attitude that might encourage seeking sexual gratification from someone who was distressed by sexual advances—he did not, however, hypothesize that this attitude increased the psychopath's proclivity to engage in sexually coercive behavior.

Despite Cleckley's speculations, evidence for a relation between the belief patterns and behaviors that characterize psychopaths and an increased risk for sexually coercive behavior has consistently emerged over the last half century in three somewhat independent research literatures. First, some indications of increased risk for sexual coercion among psychopathic criminals have been evident in the general criminal and clinical literatures, and recent research on the components of psychopathy has provided potential theoretical explanations for this increased risk. Second, in empirical studies of incarcerated rapists and in the clinical speculation about rapists, antisocial and psychopathic attitudes and behaviors have continually been identified as important constructs, at least for a significant subgroup of rapists. Moreover, in recent attempts to generate risk assessment instruments to predict recidivism among sexual offenders, psychopathy has emerged as a contributory construct. Third, from the beginning, research attempting to predict sexual coercion against women in noncriminal, community samples has found evidence that scales reflecting personal characteristics traditionally associated with delinquency, antisocial behavior, and psychopathy (e.g., lack of social conscience, irresponsibility, immaturity, poor internalization of prosocial attitudes) predicted self-reported sexually coercive behavior in community/college samples. Although early models based on research with community males moved away from the construct of psychopathy to focus on correlated but more proximal constructs that appeared to offer improved prediction (like negative masculinity and hostile attitudes toward women), more recent models have returned to incorporating the core aspects of psychopathy.

In this chapter we summarize the findings in each of these three literatures. The integration of components of psychopathy into a model for sexual coercion against women has recently yielded improved prediction of sexual coercion in both noncriminal and criminal samples and has led to a revision and restructuring of the only typology of rapists with demonstrated reliability and validity (Knight, 1999, 2002). We summarize both the etiological and typological models and the data supporting them, and we discuss their theoretical implications.

PREVALENCE OF SEXUAL COERCION IN PSYCHOPATHS

There are multiple definitions of psychopathy. Lilienfeld (1994) has characterized the two main conceptualizations. The first is the personality-based approach, inspired by Cleckley's work and operationalized in the Psychopathy Checklist—Revised (PCL-R; Hare, 1991, 2003). Here psychopathy is hypothesized to represent a constellation of personality traits. In contrast, the second conceptualization is a behavior-based approach that constitutes the core of the DSM-III and DSM-IV criteria for antisocial personality disorder (APD). This approach focuses predominantly on readily observable instances of antisocial behavior. The applications of these two conceptualizations do not identify coextensive groups (Hare, 1996, 1998). In our brief survey of the incidence of sexual coercion among psychopaths, we consider a broad range of definitions of psychopathy, with the hope that casting our diagnostic net widely will allow a more inclusive assessment of the level of sexually coercive behavior among psychopaths.

Presence of Sexual Coercion in Rating Scales and Diagnostic Criteria for Psychopathy

Psychopaths are noted for their criminal versatility (Hare, 1991, 2003), and sexual coercion has consistently been listed or implied among the variety of crimes they are hypothesized to commit. DSM-III (American Psychiatric Association, 1980) included in its diagnostic criteria for APD "repeated sexual intercourse in a casual relationship" before age 15. Both DSM-III-R (American Psychiatric Association, 1987) and DSM-IV-TR (American Psychiatric Association, 2000) criteria for APD do not specify in their diagnostic criteria the requisite antisocial behaviors before age 15. Rather they make the diagnosis of conduct disorder prior to age 15 a requirement for APD. In these versions of DSMs, the diagnosis of conduct disorder includes "forced someone into sexual activity" among the possible early violations of social norms. In the descriptive text accompanying the diagnostic criteria for APD in the DSM-IV, engaging in sexual behaviors with "a high risk for consequences" and "irresponsible and exploitative" sexual relationships are mentioned as associated features of the disorder along with having many sexual partners. Promiscuous sexual behavior is also one of the 20 items of the PCL-R. Notably, promiscuity, or the proclivity to engage in impersonal sexual behavior, is one of the characteristics associated with an increased probability of sexual coercion (Malamuth, 1998).

Empirical Correlates

Unfortunately, in studies examining the criminal correlates of psychopathy, rape is often grouped together with other violent crimes or crimes against persons (e.g., Heilbrun, 1979; Skeem & Mulvey, 2001), rather than being considered separately. Although psychopathy is associated with these violent- and person-crime composites in such studies (Hare, Clark, Grann, & Thornton, 2000), neither the comparative frequency of rape in psychopathic and nonpsychopathic criminals nor the strength of the specific association between psychopathy and sexually coercive behavior can be gleaned from such studies. One study directly compared the frequency of sexual assault convictions in male psychopaths and generic male prisoners (Coid, 1992). In the male psychopath category, 30% had an index offense of rape, buggery, or indecent assault, compared to 13% for the male prisoner subsample, supporting the hypothesis that psychopaths are at increased risk for sexual coercion.

Congruent Explanatory Constructs for Psychopathy and Rape

Recent research on psychopathy has identified potential explanatory links between psychopathy and sexually aggressive behavior. The two- (Harpur, Hakstian, & Hare, 1988; Harpur, Hare, & Hakstian, 1989), three- (Cooke & Michie, 2001), and four-factor (Hare, 2003) models of the PCL all identify two major components involving impulsivity–antisocial behavior and affective–interpersonal features. The disinhibitory tendencies associated with the impulsive–antisocial factor may contribute to maintaining appetitive drive and sexual behavior in circumstances in which victim noncompliance would normally act to inhibit such behavior (Knight & Sims-Knight, 2003, 2004).

Likewise, Blair's (Blair, 1995; James, Blair, Jones, Clark, & Smith, 1997) conceptualization of the affective–interpersonal factor of psychopathy also provides an alternative compelling hypothesis about how this component of psychopathy might function to increase the probability of sexually coercive behavior. He found data to support the hypothesis that a key component of the affective–interpersonal component (Factor 1) of the PCL-R is a hyporesponsivity to the distress of others (James et al., 1997). Blair hypothesized that the psychopath suffers from a lack of responsiveness to distress cues because of a deficit in the violence inhibition mechanism that humans and other animals have. This mechanism represents a narrower version of the general lack of defensive/fear reactivity posited by others (e.g., Lykken, 1995; Patrick, 1994). He argued further that it is the fostering of empathy (Blackburn, 1988; Blair & Morton, 1995; Hoffman, 1994; see also Miller & Eisenberg, 1988) rather than the development of conditioned emotional responses, as Eysenck (1964) and Patterson and Newman (1993) had main-

tained, that leads to such inhibition. He proposed that punishment leads to emotional detachment and deficient empathy (e.g., Brody & Shaffer, 1982).

Blair's notion about deficiencies in violence inhibition fits well with some earlier conceptual models of sexual aggression that emphasized deficiencies in such mechanisms (Marshall & Barbaree, 1990). Barbaree and Marshall (1991) proposed an inhibition model of sexual coercion to explain higher arousal to rape stimuli among sexually coercive males. This model provides a potential explanation of the role of affective–interpersonal features of psychopathy in sexual aggression. A consistent finding in phallometric studies of male sexual response has been that descriptions of foreplay and of the women's physical characteristics in consensual sex scripts increase sexual arousal of most men. The introduction of force and the consequent descriptions of pain, distress, and fear on the part of the woman in coercive scripts tend to inhibit sexual arousal for noncoercive males but not for coercive males (Bernat, Calhoun, & Adams, 1999; Lohr, Adams, & Davis, 1997). Males with more callous sexual beliefs also exhibit less inhibition to descriptions of force and distress (Bernat et al., 1999). In a subsequent section we present data from our structural equation modeling (SEM) studies supporting Blair's hypothesis that the affective–interpersonal component of psychopathy is associated with experiencing early physical abuse (Knight & Sims-Knight, 1999, 2003, 2004).

The hypothesis of a potential link between psychopathy and sexually coercive behavior has also been proposed in evolutionary models of psychopathy. For example, Mealey (1995) goes so far as to hypothesize that "it would be parsimonious to postulate that they [i.e., criminality/psychopathy and sexual coercion] might be expressions of a single sociopathy spectrum" (p. 527). Focusing on the primary psychopath's well-established "cheating strategies" aimed at short-term individual gains rather than long-term cooperative gains, evolutionary and game theoretic models have proposed that psychopathy may be an expression of a predatory and manipulative life strategy that is adaptive in particular environments and is thus naturally, but infrequently, selected (Mealey, 1995).

Evolutionary models of rape (e.g., Malamuth, 1998; Quinsey & Lalumière, 1995; Thornhill & Thornhill, 1992) have proposed that the proclivity for sexual coercion is related to particular divergent mating tactics, such as a preference for short-term relationships, a propensity for extra-pair romances, and a desire to engage in impersonal or uncommitted sexual behavior (i.e., sociosexuality). These mating strategies are hypothesized to provide a reproductive and therefore evolutionary benefit for males but not for females. Consequently, they are hypothesized to increase the potential for male sexual coercion. These theorists speculate that the proclivity for impersonal sex can be evolutionarily adaptive and therefore may be naturally selected for males. Alternative models are, of course, possible. For instance, Knight and Sims-Knight (2003) focus on sexual preoccupation, compulsivity, and drive rather than impersonal sex as the critical sexual behaviors in motivating coercion.

The congruence between the short-term, cheating strategies that have characterized the performance of psychopaths and the short-term relationship, high mating effort, low parental investment strategy proposed to explain rape provides a fecund source for evolutionary speculation (Lalumière & Quinsey, 1996). The link between these two domains could be explained by models involving a multitude of interpretive mechanisms—adaptation, which posits an effective trait that was naturally or sexually selected because of its evolutionary advantage; exaptation, which occurs when a trait that initially evolves as an adaptation for a one effect was subsequently exapted to another effect; and spandrel, which involves a trait selected not because of its particular adaptive advantage but because it was inextricably linked to another trait with reproductive advantages (Andrews, Gangestad, & Matthews, 2004). We do not have sufficient data to choose definitively among a variety of possible hypotheses, and it is not within the purview of the present chapter to delineate or discuss these various interpretations. It is sufficient for our purpose to note the important hypothesized evolutionary linkage between psychopathy and sexually coercive behavior as yet another indication of their covariation.

PERVASIVENESS, TAXONOMIC ROLE, AND PREDICTIVE VALIDITY OF PSYCHOPATHY AMONG RAPISTS

The Pervasiveness of Psychopathy and Antisocial Personality among Rapists

When clinicians and researchers first began assessing the characteristics of perpetrators of sexual aggression, the heterogeneity of these offenders was immediately recognized. Indeed, early research and theorizing about these offenders included a number of attempts to categorize the observed heterogeneity as a basis for deciding where such offenders should be placed within the judicial system and what types of interventions should be recommended. One attempt to parse this heterogeneity involved applying existing psychiatric diagnoses to these offenders (Knight, Rosenberg, & Schneider, 1985). Although differences in diagnostic criteria make cross-study comparisons difficult, the modal personality disorder reported for rapists has consistently been found to be some version of antisocial personality (e.g., Henn, Herjanic, & Vanderpearl, 1976; Prentky & Knight, 1991; Rada, 1978). Such diagnostic classifications were consistent with early Minnesota Multiphasic Personality Disorder (MMPI) studies that found that the modal MMPI profiles of rapists typically involved a high score on the Psychopathic Deviate (Pd) scale, with 4–3 (i.e., high Pd and Hysteria scale scores), 4–8 (high Pd–Schizophrenia), and 4–9 (high Pd–Mania) profiles most frequent (Armentrout & Hauer, 1978; Persons & Marks, 1971; Rader, 1977). Cluster-analytic studies (Anderson, Kunce, & Rich, 1979; Kalichman, Szymanowski, McKee, Taylor, & Craig, 1989) have also identified a substantial subgroup of sexual offenders with a prototypical MMPI 4–9 antisocial personality profile, often associated with individuals who show a marked disregard for social values and standards (Graham, 1990). More recent studies using the PCL-R (Hare, 1991) have found that between 12.1% and 40% of rapists (depending on the risk level of the sample) meet the criteria for a diagnosis of psychopathy (Brown & Forth, 1997; Prentky & Knight, 1991; Serin, Mailloux, & Malcolm, 2001). There is also evidence that mean PCL-R scores differ across sexual offender types. Higher PCL-R scores have been found among rapists than among child molesters, and still higher scores have been found among men who offend sexually against both adult and child victims (Porter, Campbell, Woodworth, & Birt, 2001; Porter et al., 2000; Quinsey, Rice, & Harris, 1995; Rice & Harris, 1997; Serin, Malcolm, Khanna, & Barbaree, 1994).

Role of Psychopathy in Rapist Typologies

An alternative approach to attempting to understand and describe the heterogeneity among rapists, which predominated in early clinical theorizing, was the generation of specific typologies for these offenders (cf. Knight et al., 1985). These early typological models were essentially global descriptions, representing clinicians' best guesses about the most important characteristics that discriminated among these offenders. These typologies also implicitly incorporated hypotheses about how these purportedly type-defining characteristics interrelated. Although each of the early classification schemes emphasized what was unique in its scheme for ordering sexual offenders, some clear consistencies emerged across these descriptive models (Knight et al., 1985). Consistent with the diagnostic and psychometric data just cited, many of the early rational typologies posited a rapist group for whom the defining characteristic was an antisocial lifestyle, with rape being only one of a large variety of antisocial behaviors (e.g., Amir, 1971; Cohen, Seghorn, & Calmus, 1969; Gebhard, Gagnon, Pomeroy, & Christenson, 1965; Guttmacher & Weihofen, 1952; Kopp, 1962; Seghorn & Cohen, 1980).

Investigations of typological issues among sexual offenders have remained disproportionately infrequent (Earls & Quinsey, 1985; Knight, 1999; Knight et al., 1985). This might be due in part to the "anticategory" bias that has dominated psychology, criminology, and sociology during the latter half of the last century (Meehl, 1999). Only two typological systems have received any empirical scrutiny—one is a variant of a system developed by Groth (Groth & Birnbaum, 1979; Groth, Burgess, & Holmstrom, 1977) and the other is a product of the Massachusetts Treatment Center (MTC) taxonomy program (Knight, 1999; Knight et al., 1985;

Knight & Prentky, 1990). For Groth's system, only global classification criteria that are inadequate for reliable classification have been provided, and no estimates of interrater reliability for type assignments have been generated. Moreover, this system has been subjected to minimal validity assessment (Hazelwood, 1987; Hazelwood & Burgess, 1987; Hazelwood, Reboussin, & Warren, 1989). Groth's system is almost identical to the adaptation of the four types described by Cohen et al. (1969) that was used as the original point of departure for the MTC taxonomy program (the Massachusetts Treatment Center Rapist typology, Version 1; MTC:R1), and there is reason to be skeptical of its potential utility. MTC:R1 was found to be riddled with reliability and validity problems to such a degree that it was deemed not to be a viable system, and thus in the course of the MTC taxonomy program it was displaced by subsequent typological revisions (cf. Knight & Prentky, 1990; Prentky, Knight, & Rosenberg, 1988).

The MTC typology has undergone two major data-driven overhauls. Both revisions involved changes that forced us to increase the role that the components of psychopathy play in identifying rapist types. The first revision (MTC:R2) attempted to address the reliability problems of MTC:R1 by explicitly introducing the construct of impulsivity as the third decision level in a three-tier hierarchical decision tree (Knight et al., 1985). Subsequent research indicated that this third level, which correlated highly with juvenile and adult antisocial behavior and criminality (Prentky et al., 1988), increased classification reliability in MTC:R2 and showed retrospective (Rosenberg, Knight, Prentky, & Lee, 1988), concurrent (Prentky & Knight, 1986), and predictive validity (Prentky & Knight, 1986). Unfortunately, significant validity problems still plagued MTC:R2 and another revision was necessary (Knight & Prentky, 1990).

The second revision was more extensive than the first. It relied on an inductive, bottom-up strategy involving multiple cluster and multivariate profile analyses of an extensive sexual offender database (for details, see Knight & Prentky, 1990). The resultant structure of MTC:R3 is presented in Figure 26.1. It is noteworthy that our empirically driven strategy increased the role of psy-

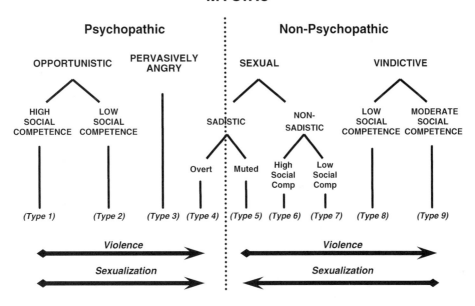

FIGURE 26.1. A depiction of the structure of the MTC:R3 typology with indicators of the embedded distinctions among psychopathy, violence, and sexualization. Comp, competence.

chopathy in the typology. It isolated and grouped four types (the two Opportunistic, the Pervasively Angry, and the Overt Sadistic on the left side of Figure 26.1) that comprise individuals who are more psychopathic than the remaining groups (Brown & Forth, 1997; Prentky & Knight, 2000). At the bottom of Figure 26.1, two sets of arrows illustrate how types similar in "sexualization" and violence were also juxtaposed in this typology.

MTC:R3 remains the best available published typological model for discriminating among rapists. It solved significant problems of the prior systems (Knight & Prentky, 1990) and subsequent studies by our research group have supported the validity of many of its components (Knight, 1999; Knight, Warren, Reboussin, & Soley, 1998; Prentky & Knight, 2000). Independent researchers have also investigated the model, and these studies have provided partial support for its categorization of rapists (Barbaree, Seto, Serin, Amos, & Preston, 1994; Brown & Forth, 1997; Guay, 2001; Polascheck, 1997; Preston, 1996; Proulx, 2001; Smith, 2000).

Although MTC:R3 represented a marked improvement over it predecessors, validity

analyses revealed two major flaws in its structure (Knight, 1999). Moreover, SEM studies of the developmental antecedents of sexual coercion against women (Knight, 1998; Knight & Sims-Knight, 2003, 2004) have yielded a promising three-path causal model involving sexual drive/preoccupation and the two aforementioned facets of psychopathy (impulsivity–antisocial behavior and affective–interpersonal features). Clearly, it would be ideal if dimensional and taxonomic models could be integrated and the similarities of the role of psychopathy in both elucidated. A recent restructuring of MTC:R3 (Knight, 2002), which attempted to solve the two major identified validity problems, also provides a theoretical integration of the typological and dimensional models. We describe this restructuring effort after we present the SEM dimensional model.

Psychopathy and Risk Assessment for Sexual Coercion

The role of PCL-R psychopathy in predicting recidivism among generic, nonsexual criminals has been well established (Hemphill, Hare, & Wong, 1998), with a large and growing body of empirical research supporting its validity in predicting both general (Hart, Kropp, & Hare, 1988) and violent recidivism (Hare, 2001; Rice, Harris, & Quinsey, 1990). More recently, the predictive validity of psychopathy and its components have been explored among sexual offenders. Although the PCL-R's prediction of general and violent recidivism among sexual offenders would simply be consistent with its demonstrated predictive validity among generic criminals, the specific prediction of sexual reoffending would suggest a more distinct role of psychopathy in sexually coercive behavior. In a meta-analysis of 61 longitudinal follow-up studies of sexual offenders, Hanson and Bussière (1998) found that measures related to antisocial personality (i.e., criminal history, diagnosis of antisocial personality disorder, elevated scores on the MMPI Psychopathic–Deviate subscale, and scores on psychopathy rating scales) were consistently related to general, violent, *and* sexual recidivism. In a 25-year follow-up of sexual offenders committed as sexually dangerous, Prentky, Knight, Lee, and Cerce (1995) found that measures of impulsivity predicted both general and sexual recidivism.

Although PCL-R scores have repeatedly been found to predict both general (Harris, Rice, & Cormier, 1991; Harris, Rice, & Quinsey, 1993; Hart et al., 1988; Serin, 1996; Serin & Amos, 1995; Serin et al., 2001) and violent (including sexual) recidivism (Quinsey et al., 1995; Rice et al., 1990; Seto & Barbaree, 1999) among sexual offenders, the results of specifically predicting sexual recidivism among these offenders have not always been consistent. Rice and colleagues (1990) found that PCL-R scores predicted both sexual and nonsexual recidivism among adjudicated rapists, over and above variables such as age, offense history, and psychiatric history. Quinsey and colleagues (1995) also found that scores on the PCL-R predicted sexual recidivism in a sample of 178 rapists and child molesters. Rice and Harris (1997) reported that the interaction of high PCL-R scores and indices of penile tumescence to sexual deviance was particularly predictive of sexually aggression recidivism. Consequently, Quinsey, Harris, Rice, and Cormier (1998) hypothesized that the addition of a tumescence index to the Violence Risk Appraisal Guide (VRAG), which

already included the PCL-R total score as a heavily weighted item, would improve predictive validity for sexual recidivism. This revised assessment instrument was named the Sex Offender Risk Appraisal Guide (SORAG).

In their study of six risk assessment instruments for predicting general, violent, and sexual recidivism in sex offenders, Barbaree, Seto, Langton, and Peacock (2001) found that although the PCL-R total score significantly predicted both general and serious recidivism, neither the PCL-R itself nor the VRAG, which includes the PCL-R, contributed significantly to prediction of sexual recidivism. In contrast, the SORAG predicted sexual recidivism in addition to general and violent recidivism. Langton (2003) found comparable results with a larger sample ($n = 468$). Specifically, he found that whereas both PCL-R total and Factor 2 scores predicted general recidivism, only Factor 2 scores predicted sexual recidivism for the entire sample. The predictive validity of Factor 2 for sexual recidivism was consistent with Serin and colleagues' (2001) finding of significantly higher Factor 2 scores for sexual recidivists than for nonrecidivists and with Prentky and colleagues' (1995) results on the predictive validity of impulsivity cited earlier. In an analysis, however, of a subset of sexual offenders for whom predictive accuracy could be considered optimized (i.e., all participants both had ratings for all items on all assessment instruments and had been available for the full follow-up period), Langton found that the validity of Factor 2 for predicting sexual recidivism fell slightly below the acceptable level of significance. Within this optimized sample, the SORAG predicted sexual recidivism but the VRAG did not. Taken as a whole, these results suggest that aspects generally associated with Factor 2 (difficulties modulating inappropriate behavior and loss of behavioral control and chronically unstable and antisocial lifestyle) may make a moderate contribution to disinhibiting sexually coercive behavior and may predict the proclivity of subsequent sexual aggression better than the total PCL-R. Although SORAG was superior to VRAG in predicting sexual recidivism in these studies, this superiority has not always been found (Harris et al., 2003; Hanson & Morton-Bourgon, 2004), even though survival analyses have demonstrated that offenders who are high in both psychopathy and sexual deviance constitute an especially high-risk group (Harris et al., 2003).

Consistent with the results using adult sex offenders, the association between PCL-R scores and general and violent recidivism has also emerged in studies of juvenile sex offenders. In a follow-up study of juvenile sex offenders, Auslander (1998) found that whereas total PCL-R scores predicted violent nonsexual recidivism, the affective–interpersonal factor of the PCL-R was related to *lower* sexual recidivism. In a study of young sex offenders ages 15–20 years old, PCL-R scores predicted general but not sexual recidivism (Långström & Grann, 2000). Similarly, using file information to score the Youth Version of the PCL (PCL:YV), Gretton, McBride, Hare, Shaughnessy, and Kumka (2001) found an association between psychopathy scores and general and violent reoffending but not between psychopathy and sexual reoffending. In a 4½-year follow-up study (range = 1–134 months) of 156 adolescent sexual offenders, Parks (2004) found that whereas the Interpersonal factor of the PCL:YV predicted sexual recidivism, the Affective and Antisocial factors predicted nonsexual recidivism.

Studies comparing juvenile sexual offenders to nonsexual offenders have also found differences in psychopathy-related scales. Caputo, Frick, and Brodsky (1999) compared a group of juvenile sex offenders to a group of violent juvenile nonsexual offenders and a group of juvenile offenders with only "noncontact" property and drug offenses on the Psychopathy Screening Device (PSD), a youth version of the PCL-R (cf. Salekin, Chapter 20, this volume). Compared to the nonsexual offenders, the juvenile sexual offenders had higher scores on the "callous–unemotional" factor (the counterpart to the affective–interpersonal factor of the PCL-R), reflecting less guilt and empathy and greater emotional restriction. Knight and Zakireh (2005) obtained contrasting results in a study that compared subgroups of residential and outpatient juvenile offenders with and without a history of sexual offending on the Multidimensional Assessment of Sex and Aggression (MASA; Knight, Prentky, & Cerce, 1994), a computerized inventory. Substantial differences were found between the sexual offender groups (especially residential sexual offenders) and the nonsexual delinquents in sexual behavior, fighting, and aggressive fantasies, but no differences were found on scales that assessed the two PCL-R factors.

In sum, measures of psychopathy have consistently been found to predict subsequent general and violent behavior in both adult and juvenile sexual offender samples. Although there are exceptions (e.g., Parks, 2004), when components of psychopathy do predict sexual recidivism, it is the impulsive–antisocial component that has most often been found predictive. Moreover, in some (but not all) studies, the inclusion of assessments of deviant sexual arousal along with psychopathy measures increased the ability to predict sexual recidivism. Most of these studies must be interpreted cautiously, however, because they analyze generic sexual offenders, and they do not differentiate rapists from child molesters. They might be underestimating the specific relevance of psychopathy to rapists.

PSYCHOMETRIC CORRELATES OF RAPE IN NONCRIMINAL SAMPLES

Early studies attempting to identify the correlates of sexually coercive behavior against women among college students took some guidance from the criminological literature and examined the contributions of various components of psychopathy and antisocial behavior. Rappaport and Burkhart (1984) found a significant correlation between Gough's (1956) Socialization (*So*) Scale and sexually coercive behavior. This scale, which assesses asocial tendencies (with lower scores indicative of greater deviance), has been found to correlate with substance abuse and criminal behavior in college students (Kosson, Steuerwald, Newman, & Widom, 1994), and to covary with the impulsive–antisocial behavior factor of the PCL-R (Factor 2; Harpur et al., 1989). Using discriminant function analysis to predict college male's self-reported sexually coercive behavior (five groups ranging from nonaggressive through sexual coercion by verbal pressure and authority to rape), Koss and Dinero (1988) found that although Scale 4 of the MMPI (Pd) was related to sexually coercive behavior in the zero-order correlations, it did not contribute independently to discrimination beyond the contribution of higher correlating scales (e.g., Sexual Conservatism and Rape Myths). The slightly higher predictive validity and apparently greater explanatory potential of these alternative scales led subsequent researchers studying noncriminal samples to focus their predictive models on these more sexual-aggression-congruent attitudes and behaviors (Malamuth, 1986, 2003) and to speculate that different models might be appropriate for criminal and noncriminal populations.

Using SEM, Malamuth, Sockloskie, Koss, and Tanaka (1991) developed and tested a two-factor confluence model of sexually coercive behavior in a large sample of college men. They predicted that hostile childhood experiences would affect involvement in delinquency and lead to sexual aggression through the confluence of two paths: negative or hostile masculinity, in which individuals espouse "macho" attitudes (e.g., risk taking, power seeking, overly competitive behavior, callous attitudes toward women, and grandiosity); and sexual promiscuity, supported by attitudes emphasizing sexuality and sexual conquest. Malamuth's model exhibited an excellent fit to the data within this college student sample, and confirmation of the model was replicated within a sample of men followed longitudinally for 10 years (Malamuth, Linz, Heavey, Barnes, & Acker, 1995).

Knight (1993) replicated Malamuth's two-factor confluence model in a sample of college males. He used data gathered using Version 2 of the MASA, an inventory developed in the late 1980s (cf. Knight et al., 1994; Knight & Cerce, 1999) to assess all the dimensions necessary for classifying rapists in the MTC:R3 typology, described earlier. In the MASA-2, scales assessing analogues of Malamuth's negative masculinity were introduced as well as items intended to measure aspects of the affective–interpersonal factor of the PCL-R (cf. Knight & Cerce, 1999). Knight used parallel constructs of sexual drive/sexual fantasy and negative masculinity as the two intervening variables that defined Malamuth's two paths. In place of Malamuth's cursory measures of early developmental antecedents, Knight introduced more detailed assessments of childhood physical and verbal abuse, corresponding to Malamuth's parental violence and generic child abuse antecedents. He also added a measure of sexual abuse as a potential early antecedent of sexual drive. In Malamuth's model he measured "delinquency" by two items—having "friends who are delinquent" and "running away." Knight substituted more detailed retrospective self-reports of juvenile antisocial behavior and aggression. Although significant correlations in the expected directions were found in this replication, Knight noted that the model accounted for only a relatively small percent of the sexually coercive behavior variance (16%).

Holmes and Knight (1994) subsequently examined the role of alcohol use and abuse in sexual aggression. They found that when scales assessing childhood and adolescent alcohol abuse were added to the model examined by Knight (1993), the percent of variance accounted for in predicting sexual coercion increased substantially. Because it was known that alcohol and drug use were correlated with the Factor 2 of the PCL-R (e.g., Hart & Hare, 1989; Smith & Newman, 1990), Knight (1995) substituted this more generic index of impulsivity–antisocial behavior for the alcoholism measure included in the Holmes–Knight model. In addition, because the scales measuring negative masculinity correlated substantially with MASA-2 scales developed to index Factor 1 of the PCL, Knight incorporated negative masculinity into the broader construct of the affective–interpersonal features of psychopathy. The resulting model, which yielded improved predictive validity and superior indices of SEM fit, constituted the basis for the three-factor model presented in Figure 26.2.

The model in Figure 26.2 depicts the first application of this three-path model, tested on 275 sexually aggressive offenders (Johnson & Knight, 1998). In addition to replications of this model in a second sample of sexual offenders, in college students, and in generic non-sex offending criminals (Knight & Sims-Knight, 1999), the model was recently replicated in juvenile sexual offenders (Knight & Sims-Knight, 2004) and blue-collar community controls (Knight & Sims-Knight, 2003). In these last two studies, the three-path model was found to yield better fit indices than those for Malamuth's two-path confluence model.

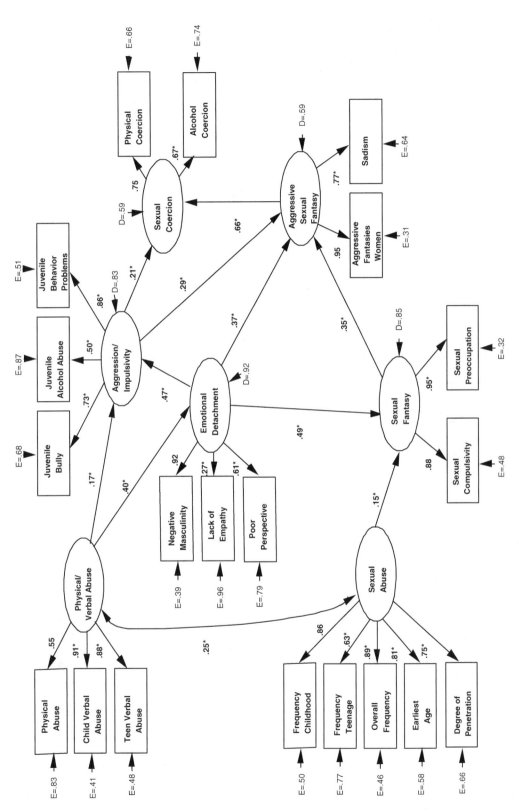

FIGURE 26.2. Adjusted three-path structural model predicting sexual coercion against women, tested in a sample of 275 adult male sexual offenders.

The three-path model modified Malamuth's model in two important ways. First, it expanded the number of the intervening paths leading to sexually coercive behavior against women by adding an impulsivity–antisocial behavior path. Malamuth did not include impulsivity–antisocial behavior as a prominent causal path. Its role was only implied in "delinquency," which was hypothesized to be an antecedent of sexual promiscuity. Second, we reconceptualized negative masculinity as an element of the affective–interpersonal factor of psychopathy. These modifications yielded a more powerful model with intriguing theoretical links to the personality and psychopathy literature. The three-path model suggests an important role for the two broad components of psychopathy in predicting rape across multiple populations. The importance of psychopathy in predicting sexual aggression in noncriminal samples has been supported in a number of other studies (Calhoun, Bernat, Clum, & Frame, 1997; Kosson, Kelly, & White, 1997; Lalumière & Quinsey, 1996). There are multiple advantages to the model. We briefly discuss these advantages in the following section.

Advantages of the Three-Path Model of Sexual Coercion

When we restructured the path model to include the domain of impulsive–antisocial deviance as a third path, the R^2 for predicting sexually coercive behavior and the fit indices for the entire model increased substantially over those parameters for the two-path model (Knight & Sims-Knight, 2003, 2004). Recent data suggest that impulsive–antisocial deviance is a phenomenon with a strong underlying genetic basis (Krueger et al., 2002; Mason & Frick, 1994), with correlated cognitive deficits (Iacono, Malone, & McGue, 2003; Morgan & Lilienfeld, 2000), neuroanatomical underpinnings (Blair, 2004), and neurochemical correlates (Coscina, 1997). Our strategy of creating and assessing models using the variance accounted for in dependent measures and improved fit indices has been criticized (Rice & Harris, 2003). The data we have reviewed indicate, however, that not only has the addition of this neurodevelopmental path improved predictive potency and model fit, but also there is

strong empirical and theoretical support for its inclusion in a model of sexually coercive behavior.

Another benefit of the proposed three-path model is that it permits integration of findings about sexual coercion with psychometric research on psychopathy, and with the experimental literatures on basic processes underlying personality traits. Ultimately, the determination of the number of "paths" that are necessary and sufficient to explain and predict sexual coercion will not depend on the covariation between traits and the identification of independent paths in SEM, as Malamuth (2003) proposes, but on the isolation of the basic processes involved (Depue & Lenzenweger, 2001; Tellegen & Waller, in press). Specific etiologies, including particular genetic origins; prenatal, perinatal, and postnatal biological determinants; and specific life experiences impacting on causal neurobiological influences within personality structure will determine the relevant processes contributing to sexual aggression. As Malamuth suggests, it is also important to link such "broad-band" process components to more "narrow-band" characteristics with the demonstrated potential to specify rape as opposed to other forms of aggression. Because of its link to extant, well-developed experimental literatures, the proposed three-path model provides not only an avenue to advance the search for a universal theory of sexual coercion and a potential road map with well-validated measures to explore more differentiated and specific alternative formulations of the proposed constructs but also a speculative template for integrating basic broad-band processes with more proximal narrow-band predictors.

Finally, the introduction of impulsive–antisociality provides a factor that differentiates criminal rapists from noncriminal rapists. Knight (1997) compared noncriminal, self-admitted rapists (college students and community controls) to convicted rapists and to criminal and noncriminal nonrapists on MASA measures of impulsivity–antisocial and affective–interpersonal characteristics of psychopathy. He found that noncriminal, self-admitted rapists were significantly lower than criminals in their reported antisocial deviance, but they did not differ from criminal rapists in the affective–interpersonal features of psychopathy, and indeed they were significantly higher in these features than all nonrapists. Self-admitted, noncriminal rapists were still significantly higher than noncriminal, nonrapists in their antisocial behavior, but their impulsivity had not been sufficiently high to result in involvement with the criminal justice system. Therefore, the impulsivity–antisocial path not only appears to be important in sexually coercive behavior but also differentiates criminal from noncriminal rapists.

INTEGRATING TYPOLOGICAL AND DIMENSIONAL MODELS OF RAPE

We have demonstrated the importance of the components of psychopathy both in our classification of rapist types and in the proposed three-path dimensional model predicting sexual coercion against women in multiple criminal and noncriminal samples. Ideally, if both the taxonomic and dimensional models are reflections of the same core underlying processes, they should coalesce. Fortunately, a recent attempt to solve the two major structural problems identified in the research on MTC:R3 has led to a reconfiguration of MTC:R3 that is amenable to such an integration (Knight, 2002). In this section we briefly present the new structure of the rapist typology, illustrate its potential consistency with the three-path model, and highlight the prominence of the components of psychopathy in both. A more detailed description and justification of the integration of the two models is forthcoming (Knight, 2005).

Structural Problems of MTC:R3

Although MTC:R3 was a vast improvement over its predecessors, and several aspects of the model showed substantial concurrent and predictive validity (Knight, 1999), nonetheless two serious, nagging problems were evident in the empirical research on the typology—the "sexualization" and the "Vindictive types" problems.

Sexualization had been operationalized in MTC:R3 as a combination of sexual preoccupation, a frequent need for sexual activity (i.e., a high total sexual outlet), extensive use of pornography, and the presence of paraphilic fantasies and behavior. In both

MTC:R2 and MTC:R3, sexualization and expressive aggression (i.e., violence in sexually coercive acts) were hypothesized to be independent constructs (Knight, 1999). The arrows in the bottom of Figure 26.1 illustrate this hypothesis. Note that in this model low sexualization was hypothesized to co-occur with both low (Opportunistic Types 1 & 2) and high (Vindictive Types 8 and 9) sexual violence. Likewise, high sexualization was typologically linked to both low (Muted and Non-Sadistic Types 5, 6, and 7) and high (Sadist Type 4) sexual violence, indicating that sexualization and sexual violence yielded independent types in the model and consequently their criteria should not be correlated. In our validation studies, however, sexualization was not found to distribute across types as predicted (Knight, 1999, 2002); indeed, evidence from studies using the scales of the MASA indicated that within adult and juvenile samples, both criminal and noncriminal, sexualization consistently and substantially correlated with aggressive sexual fantasies and expressively aggressive behavior in sexual crimes (Knight, 1999; Knight & Cerce, 1999). This covariation is also reflected in the relation between Sexual Fantasies and Aggressive Sexual Fantasies in our SEM models (e.g., see Figure 26.2). The covariation of sexualization and affective–interpersonal features (labeled Emotional Detachment in the figure) was also not expected but has been apparent in every SEM model we have tested (e.g., Knight & Sims-Knight, 2003, 2004).

The second structural problem involved the relative position of the Vindictive types in the MTC:R3 rapist typology. As can be seen by their typological location in Figure 26.1, Sexualized types (Types 6 and 7) were hypothesized to be more like the Sadistic types (Types 4 and 5) than were the Vindictive types (Types 8 and 9). The results of several studies indicated that this was not the case. Compared to the Non-Sadistic Sexual types, Vindictive offenders showed (1) greater similarity to the Sadists on the sadistic and expressive aggression scales of the MASA (Knight, 1999); (2) a closer similarity to the Sadists in their phallometric responsivity, when more violent audio stimuli (Quinsey, Chaplin, & Upfold, 1984) were used as stimuli (Preston, 1996; Proulx, 2001); and (3) a closer similarity to the Sadists than the Non-

Sadistic Sexual types on the PCL:SV ratings of the affective–interpersonal features factor (Prentky & Knight, 2000). Thus, it is not surprising that MTC:R3 classification disagreements were more common between the Vindictive types and the Sadist types than between the Sadist and the Non-Sadistic Sexual types. The high correlations we found across samples between sexualization and expressive aggression were also consistent with the higher than anticipated sexualization levels we found among Vindictive types (Knight, 1999).

Solving the Structural Problems of MTC:R3

All these data suggested that the structure of MTC:R3 would improve if the relative positions of the Vindictive and Sexual types were switched and the Vindictive types were juxtaposed to the Overt Sadistic type. Because our studies had not supported the existence of the Muted Sadistic type, this type was dropped, and the remaining four nonpsychopathic types were flipped and rearranged, so that the Vindictive types were positioned closer to the Overt Sadists (see Figure 26.3).

This new structure revealed an interesting phenomenon. Although the Non-Sadistic Sexual types were never confused with the Sadistic types in the classification process, they had been at times confused with the Opportunistic types. Both constitute low violence types. Their similarity suggested that the goal of the juxtaposition of similar types could be more accurately achieved if we moved from a linear to a circular configuration. The arrows at the bottom of Figure 26.3 indicate the direction of the linear to circular modification. The proposed new circumplex configuration is presented in Figure 26.4. Here, types that are adjacent to each other in the circle are hypothesized to be more similar than types that are separated from each other.

Relating the New Circumplex Model to the SEM Model

The restructuring of MTC:R3 provides a framework to reconcile the typological model with our SEM three-path model. Figure 26.5 graphically illustrates how the constructs defining the three paths in the SEM model can now be superimposed on the new circumplex structure as major characteristics for discriminating among rapist types. The three lines indicate the cutoffs that differentiate types high and low on the three major etiological components—sexualization,

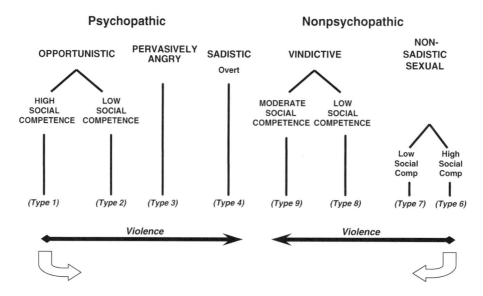

FIGURE 26.3. A depiction of the structure of the rapist typology after the nonpsychopathic side of MTC:R3 was flipped so that the Vindictive types (Types 9 and 8) juxtaposed the Overt Sadists (Type 4). Comp, competence.

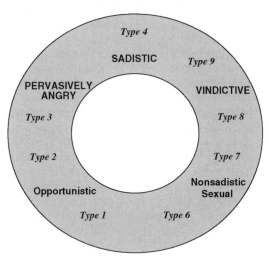

FIGURE 26.4. A depiction of the revised structure of the rapist typology after the linear structure of types in Figure 26.3 had been transformed into a circular structure.

impulsivity–antisocial behavior, and affective–interpersonal features. Most of the defining characteristics for the individual types remain quite similar to those in MTC:R3 and preserve the aspects of that typology that were validated. The major changes involve the addition of the affective–interpersonal characteristics as more explicit type discriminators, the incorporation of the higher correlation of sexualization with violence, and the reconceptualization of the Vindictive types as more sexualized.

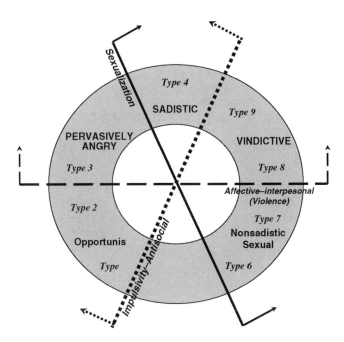

FIGURE 26.5. A depiction of the revised structure of the rapist typology indicating speculative cutoffs for the three major components of the typology (impulsivity–antisocial, sexualization, and affective–interpersonal [violence]).

The speculative integration of the restructured MTC:R3 typology with the SEM model requires three core assumptions. First, the Non-sadistic Sexual types in the lower right quadrant of the circumplex are conceptualized as the purest manifestation in the typology of hypersexual motivation with the lowest complication of the other contributing factors. Although hypersexuality does not appear to be sufficient by itself to produce sexual coercion (Malamuth, 1998; Malamuth, Heavey, & Linz, 1993) and can lead to other forms of sexual pathology (Kafka, 1997, 2000), offenders of this type apparently have the minimal amounts of poor impulse control and affective–interpersonal features conducive to sexual coercion. Second, the Opportunistic types in the lower left quadrant are conceptualized as the purest manifestations of the impulsivity–antisocial factor in the typology. Third, to these two predispositions we add the affective–interpersonal features, which in all our SEM models has been found to be predicted by physically abusive histories. In the revised model these features are hypothesized to correlate with a proclivity to increased violence.

These three components, which are equivalent to the three paths in the SEM model, are hypothesized to combine to yield the more aggressive rapist types. The combination of hypersexuality and affective–interpersonal features yields the Vindictive type, whom our MASA data have revealed is high on both of these factors. The combination of the impulsivity–antisocial factor and affective–interpersonal features increases general violence and leads to the Pervasively Angry type. This is consistent with research that has found that whereas high scores on PCL-R Factor 2 (Impulsivity–Antisocial Behavior) predict general recidivism more strongly than high scores on Factor 1 (Affective–Interpersonal Features), the combination of high scores on both PCL-R factors predicts violence (Harpur & Hare, 1991; Hemphill & Hare, 1995; Hemphill et al., 1998). Pervasively Angry offenders are among the most violent individuals in the rapist typology in both sexual and nonsexual behavior. Finally, the combination of all three components increases the probability of the Sadistic type, here defined as the high-violence, psychopathic offender, as it had been in MTC:R3.

The placement of the dividing lines among the three components in Figure 26.5 (both their relative angle to each other and the portion of the circle designated as high for each component) is clearly not final, and substantial research will be required to establish empirically based classification criteria for the proposed types. In an attempt to facilitate and inform this process, we have been applying taxometrics (Meehl, 1995; Ruscio, Ruscio, & Keane, 2004) to the three components of the typology to determine whether identification of latent taxons for each of the three components would facilitate the establishment of maximal categorical cutoffs (Guay & Knight, 2003; Guay, Ruscio, Knight, & Hare, 2004; Knight & Guay, 2003). The consistent and clear result of these analyses has been that each of the components appears to be distributed as a dimension, suggesting that the circumplex model might ultimately best be conceived as a dimensional model with "types" representing extreme manifestations of the confluence of components. The dimensionality of these components is also consistent with their predictive potency across such a wide range of samples, from college students to committed, sexually dangerous criminals.

CONCLUSIONS

In each of the three research areas we examined—the prevalence of sexual coercion among psychopaths, the presence of psychopathy among rapists and the role of its components in differentiating among rapists, and the role of the components of psychopathy in predicting rape in noncriminal samples—evidence of a relation between psychopathy and sexual coercion against women was found. Psychopaths appear to be more likely than nonpsychopathic criminals to rape. Psychopaths are overrepresented in samples of sexual offenders and appear to constitute a coherent subgroup of rapists, and the components of psychopathy—especially the impulsive–antisocial deviance component—have been found to predict subsequent sexually aggressive behavior in convicted offenders. Moreover, the proposed underlying processes that contribute to psychopathy also have some theoretical congruence with and explanatory potential for the phenomenon of sexually coercive behavior. Finally, the components of psychopathy predict sexually coercive behavior against women in noncriminal samples.

The proposed integration of explanatory constructs across typological and dimensional models, as well as across criminal and noncriminal samples, suggests the potential universality of the identified components in accounting for sexual coercion against women. These converging lines of evidence provide convincing support for the proposed typological and SEM models, encourage the creation of a unified theory of sexual coercion, and hold promise for generating and testing strong, precise, falsifiable theoretical predictions across diverse samples (Meehl, 1978, 1990). As we have described in this review, the links between sexual coercion and components of the psychopathy construct also point to promising avenues for exploring the core processes underlying the proclivity to aggress sexually. The empirical evidence for the covariation between psychopathy and sexually aggressive behavior also affords a solid basis for theorizing about the reasons for this linkage (e.g., Wiebe, 2004).

ACKNOWLEDGMENTS

The recent SEM and taxometric research from our lab, reported in this chapter, was supported by research Grant Nos. MH54263-01 from the National Institute of Mental Health and 94-IJ-CX-0049 from the National Institute of Justice.

REFERENCES

American Psychiatric Association. (1980). *Diagnostic and statistical manual of mental disorders* (3rd ed.). Washington, DC: Author.

American Psychiatric Association. (1987). *Diagnostic and statistical manual of mental disorders* (3rd ed., rev.). Washington, DC: Author.

American Psychiatric Association. (2000). *Diagnostic and statistical manual of mental disorders* (4th ed., text rev.). Washington, DC: Author.

Amir, M. (1971). *Patterns in forcible rape*. Chicago: University of Chicago Press.

Anderson, W. P., Kunce, J. T., & Rich, B. (1979). Sex offenders: Three personality types. *Journal of Clinical Psychology, 35*, 671–676.

Andrews, P. W., Gangestad, S. W., & Matthews, D. (2002). Adaptationism—How to carry out an exaptationist program. *Behavioral and Brain Sciences, 25*, 489–553.

Armentrout, J. A., & Hauer, A. L. (1978). MMPI's of rapists of children, and non-rapist sex offenders. *Journal of Clinical Psychology, 34*, 330–332.

Auslander, B. A. (1998). *An exploratory study investigating variables in relation to juvenile sexual reoffending*. Unpublished doctoral dissertation, Florida State University, Tallahassee.

Barbaree, H. E., & Marshall, W. L. (1991). The role of male sexual arousal in rape: Six models. *Journal of Consulting and Clinical Psychology, 59*, 621–630.

Barbaree, H. E., Seto, M., Langton, C. M., & Peacock, E. J. (2001). Evaluating the predictive accuracy of six risk assessment instruments for adult sex offenders. *Criminal Justice and Behavior, 28*, 490–521.

Barbaree, H., Seto, M. C., Serin, R. C., Amos, N. L., & Preston, D. L. (1994). Comparisons between sexual and nonsexual rapist subtypes: Sexual arousal to rape, offence precursors, and offense characteristics. *Criminal Justice and Behavior, 21*, 95–114.

Bernat, J. A., Calhoun, K. S., & Adams, H. E. (1999). Sexually aggressive and nonaggressive men: Sexual arousal and judgments in response to acquaintance rape and consensual analogues. *Journal of Abnormal Psychology, 108*, 662–673.

Blackburn, R. (1988). Psychopathy and personality disorder. In E. Miller & P. J. Cooper (Eds.), *Adult abnormal psychology* (pp. 218–244). Edinburgh, Scotland: Churchill Livingstone.

Blair, R. J. R. (1995). A cognitive developmental approach to morality: investigating the psychopath. *Cognition, 57*, 1–29.

Blair, R. J. R. (2004). The roles of orbital frontal cortex in the modulation of antisocial behavior. *Brain and Cognition, 55*, 198–208.

Blair, R. J. R., & Morton, J. (1995). Putting cognition in sociopathy. *Behavioral and Brain Sciences, 18*, 548.

Brody, G. H., & Shaffer, D. R. (1982). Contributions of parents and peers to children's moral socialization. *Developmental Review, 2*, 31–75.

Brown, S. L., & Forth, A. E. (1997). Psychopathy & sexual assault: Static risk factors, emotional precursors, and rapist subtypes. *Journal of Consulting and Clinical Psychology, 65*, 848–857.

Calhoun, K. S., Bernat, J. A., Clum, G. A., & Frame, C. L. (1997). Sexual coercion and attraction to sexual aggression in a community sample of young men. *Journal of Interpersonal Violence, 12*, 392–406.

Caputo, A. A., Frick, P. J., & Brodsky, S. L. (1999). Family violence and juvenile sex offending: The potential mediating role of psychopathic traits and negative attitudes toward women. *Criminal Justice and Behavior, 26*, 338–356.

Cleckley, H. (1976). *The mask of sanity* (5th ed.). St. Louis, MO: Mosby.

Cohen, M. L., Seghorn, T., & Calmas, W. (1969).

Sociometric study of sex offenders. *Journal of Abnormal Psychology, 74,* 249–255.

Coid, J. W. (1992). DSM-III diagnosis in criminal psychopaths: A way forward. *Criminal Behaviour and Mental Health, 2,* 78–94.

Cooke, D. J., & Michie, C. (2001). Refining the construct of psychopathy: Towards a hierarchical model. *Psychological Assessment, 13,* 171–188.

Coscina, D. V. (1997). The biopsychology of impulsivity: Focus on brain serotonin. In C. D. Webster & M. A. Jackson (Eds.), *Impulsivity: Theory, assessment, and treatment* (pp. 95–115). New York: Guilford Press.

Depue, R. A., & Lenzenweger, M. F. (2001). A neurobehavioral dimensional model. In W. John Livesley (Ed.), *Handbook of personality disorders: Theory, research, and treatment* (pp. 136–176). New York: Guilford Press.

Earls, C. M., & Quinsey, V. L. (1985). What is to be done? Future research on the assessment and behavioral treatment of sex offenders. *Behavioral Sciences and the Law, 3,* 377–390.

Eysenck, H. J. (1964). *Crime and personality.* London: Routledge & Kegan Paul.

Gebhard, P. H., Gagnon, J. H., Pomeroy, W. B., & Christenson, C. V. (1965). *Sex offenders: An analysis of types.* New York: Harper and Row.

Gough, H. G. (1956). *California Psychological Inventory.* Palo Alto, CA: Consulting Psychologists Press.

Graham, J. R. (1990). *MMPI-2: Assessing personality and psychopathology.* New York: Oxford University Press.

Gretton, H. M., McBride, M., Hare, R. D., O'Shaughnessy, R., & Kumka, G. (2001). Psychopathy and recidivism in adolescent sex offenders. *Criminal Justice and Behavior, 28*(4), 427–449.

Groth, A. N., & Birnbaum, H. J. (1979). *Men who rape.* New York: Plenum Press.

Groth, A. N., Burgess, A. W., & Holmstrom, L. L. (1977). Rape: Power, anger, and sexuality. *American Journal of Psychiatry, 134,* 1239–1243.

Guay, J. P. (2001, November). *Intelligence scores of MTC:R3 rapist subtypes.* Symposium presented at the 20th annual meeting of the Association for the Treatment of Sexual Abusers, San Antonio, TX.

Guay, J. P., & Knight, R. A. (2003, July). *Taxometric analyses of psychopathy.* Poster presented at the conference on Developmental and Neuroscience Perspectives on Psychopathy, Madison, WI.

Guay, J. P., Ruscio, J. P., Knight, R. A., & Hare, R. D. (2004, October). *The latent structure of psychopathy: When more is simply more.* Poster presented at the 19th annual meeting of the Society for Research in Psychopathology, St. Louis, MO.

Guttmacher, M. S., & Weihofen, H. (1952). *Psychiatry and the law.* New York: Norton.

Hanson, R. K., & Bussière, M. T. (1998). Predicting relapse: A meta-analysis of sexual offender recidivism studies. *Journal of Consulting and Clinical Psychology, 66,* 348–362.

Hanson, R. K., & Morton-Bourgon, K. (2004). *Predictors of sexual recidivism: An updated meta-analysis 2004-02.* Ottawa: Public Works and Government Services Canada. (Cat. No. PS3-1/2004-2E-PDF)

Hare, R. D. (1991). *Manual for the Revised Psychopathy Checklist.* Toronto, ON, Canada: Multi-Health Systems.

Hare, R. D. (1996). Psychopathy: A clinical construct whose time has come. *Criminal Justice and Behavior, 23,* 25–54.

Hare, R. D. (1998). Psychopaths and their nature: Implications for mental health and criminal justice systems. In T. Millon, E. Simonsen, M. Birket-Smith, & R. D. Davis (Eds.), *Psychopathy: Antisocial, criminal, and violent behavior* (pp. 188–212). New York: Guilford Press.

Hare, R. D. (2001). Psychopaths and their nature: Some implications for understanding human predatory violence. In A. Raine & J. Sanmartin (Eds.), *Violence and psychopathy* (pp. 5–34). New York: Kluwer/Plenum Press.

Hare, R. D. (2003). *Hare Psychopathy Checklist—Revised (PCL-R): 2nd Edition, Technical Manual.* Toronto, ON, Canada: Multi-Health Systems.

Hare, R. D., Clarke, D., Grann, M., & Thornton, D. (2000). Psychopathy and the predictive validity of the PCL-R: An international perspective. *Behavioral Sciences and the Law, 18,* 623–645.

Harpur, T. J., Hakstian, A., & Hare, R. D. (1988). Factor structure of the Psychopathy Checklist. *Journal of Consulting and Clinical Psychology, 56,* 741–747.

Harpur, T. J., & Hare, R. D. (1991, August). *Psychopathy and violent behavior: Two factors are better than one.* Paper presented at the 9th annual meeting of the American Psychological Association, San Francisco.

Harpur, T. J., Hare, R. D., & Hakstian, A. (1989). Two-factor conceptualization of psychopathy: Construct validity and assessment implications. *Psychological Assessment: A Journal of Consulting and Clinical Psychology, 1,* 6–17.

Harris, G. T., Rice, M. E., & Cormier, C. A. (1991). Psychopathy and violent recidivism. *Law and Human Behavior, 15,* 625–637.

Harris, G. T., Rice, M. E., & Quinsey, V. L. (1993). Violent recidivism of mentally disordered offenders: The development of a statistical prediction instrument. *Criminal Justice and Behavior, 20,* 315–335.

Harris, G. T., Rice, M. E., Quinsey, V. L., Lalumière, M. L., Boer, D., & Lang, C. (2003). A multisite comparison of actuarial risk instruments for sex offenders. *Psychological Assessment, 15,* 413–425.

Hart, S. D., & Hare, R. D. (1989). Discriminant validity of the Psychopathy Checklist in a forensic psychiatric population. *Psychological Assessment: A Journal of Consulting and Clinical Psychology, 1,* 211–218.

Hart, S. D., Kropp, P. R., & Hare, R. D. (1988). Performance of male psychopaths following conditional release from prison. *Journal of Consulting and Clinical Psychology, 56,* 227–232.

Hazelwood, R. R. (1987). Analyzing the rape and profiling the offender. In R. R. Hazelwood & A. W. Burgess (Eds.), *Practical aspects of rape investigation: A multidisciplinary approach* (pp. 169–199). New York: Elsevier.

Hazelwood, R. R., & Burgess, A. W. (1987). The behavioral-oriented interview of rape-victims: The key to profiling. In R. R. Hazelwood & A. W. Burgess (Eds.), *Practical aspects of rape investigation: A multidisciplinary approach* (pp. 151–168). New York: Elsevier.

Hazelwood, R. R., Reboussin, R., & Warren, J. I. (1989). Serial rape: Correlates of increased aggression and the relationship of offender pleasure to victim resistance. *Journal of Interpersonal Violence, 4*, 65–78.

Heilbrun, A. B. (1979). Psychopathy and violent crime. *Journal of Consulting and Clinical Psychology, 47*, 509–516.

Hemphill, J. F., & Hare, R. D. (1995). Psychopathy checklist factor scores and recidivism. *Issues in Criminological and Legal Psychology, 24*, 68–73.

Hemphill, J. F., Hare, R. D., & Wong, S. (1998). Psychopathy and recidivism: A review. *Legal and Criminological Psychology, 3*, 139–170.

Henn, R. A., Herjanic, M., & Vanderpearl, R. H. (1976). Forensic psychiatry: Profiles of two types of sex offenders. *American Journal of Psychiatry, 133*, 694–696.

Hoffman, M. L. (1994). Discipline and internalization. *Developmental Psychology, 30*, 26–28.

Holmes, K. N., & Knight, R. A. (1994, April). *Exploring an interaction model of the etiology of sexual coercion.* Paper presented at the 65th annual meeting of the Eastern Psychological Association, Providence, RI.

Iacono, W. G., Malone, S. M., & McGue, M. (2003). Substance use disorders, externalizing psychopathology, and P300 event-related potential amplitude. *International Journal of Psychophysiology, 48*, 147–178.

James, R., Blair, R., Jones, L., Clark, F., & Smith, M. (1997). The psychopathic individual: A lack of responsiveness to distress cues? *Psychophysiology, 34*, 192–198.

Johnson, G. M., & Knight, R. A. (1998). *Developmental antecedents of sexual coercion in adult sex offenders.* Unpublished manuscript.

Kafka, M. P. (1997). Hypersexual desire in males: An operational definition and clinical implications for males with paraphilias and paraphilia-related disorders. *Archives of Sexual Behavior, 26*, 505–526.

Kafka, M. P. (2000). The paraphilia-related disorders: Nonparaphilic hypersexuality and sexual compulsivity/addiction. In S. R. Lieblum & R. C. Rosen (Eds.), *Principles and practice of sex therapy* (pp. 471–503). New York: Guilford Press.

Kalichman, S. C., Szymanowski, D., McKee, G., Taylor, J., & Craig, M. (1989). Cluster analytically derived MMPI profile subgroups of incarcerated adult sex offenders. *Journal of Clinical Psychology, 45*, 149–155.

Knight, R. A. (1993, November). *The developmental and social antecedents of sexual aggression.* Invited presentation to the 12th annual conference of the Association for the Treatment of Sexual Abusers, Boston.

Knight, R. A. (1995, October). *A unified developmental theory of sexual aggression: Models in the making.* Paper presented at the 14th annual meeting of the Association for the Treatment of Sexual Abusers, New Orleans, LA.

Knight, R. A. (1997, October). *A unified model of sexual aggression: Consistencies and differences across noncriminal and criminal samples.* Paper presented at the 16th annual meeting of the Association for the Treatment of Sexual Abusers, Arlington, VA.

Knight, R. A. (1998, October). *Using a new computerized developmental inventory to examine the family and early behavioral antecedents of sexual coercion.* Paper presented at the 17th annual meeting of the Association for the Treatment of Sexual Abusers, Vancouver.

Knight, R. A. (1999). Validation of a typology for rapists. *Journal of Interpersonal Violence, 14*, 297–323.

Knight, R. A. (2002, September). *Hunting snarks and battling jabberwocks: A Knight's quest for etiology and typology in sexual aggression against women.* Presidential address at the 17th annual meeting of the Society for Research in Psychopathology, San Francisco.

Knight, R. A. (2005). *Integrating dimensional and taxonomic models of rape: A circumplex proposal.* Manuscript in preparation.

Knight, R. A., & Cerce, D. D. (1999). Validation and revision of the Multidimensional Assessment of Sex and Aggression. *Psychologica Belgica, 39–2/3*, 187–213.

Knight, R. A. & Guay, J. P. (2003, October). *Assessing the underlying constructs of a rapist typology using the MASA.* Paper presented at the 22nd annual meeting of the Association for the Treatment of Sexual Abusers, St. Louis, MO.

Knight, R. A., & Prentky, R. A. (1990). Classifying sexual offenders: The development and corroboration of taxonomic models. In W. L. Marshall, D. R. Laws, & H. E. Barbaree (Eds.), *The handbook of sexual assault: Issues, theories, and treatment of the offender* (pp. 27–52). New York: Plenum Press.

Knight, R. A., Prentky, R. A., & Cerce, D. (1994). The development, reliability, and validity of an inventory for the multidimensional assessment of sex and aggression. *Criminal Justice and Behavior, 21*, 72–94.

Knight, R. A., Rosenberg, R., & Schneider, B. (1985). Classification of sexual offenders: Perspectives, methods and validation. In A. Burgess (Ed.), *Rape and sexual assault: A research handbook* (pp. 222–293). New York: Garland.

Knight, R. A., & Sims-Knight, J. E. (1999, November). *Family and early behavioral antecedents of sexual coercion.* Paper presented at the 14th annual meeting of the Society for Research in Psychopathology, Montreal.

Knight, R. A., & Sims-Knight, J. E. (2003). Developmental antecedents of sexual coercion against women: Testing of alternative hypotheses with structural equation modeling In R. A. Prentky, E. S. Janus, & M. C. Seto (Eds.), *Sexually coercive behavior: Understanding and management* (Vol. 989, pp. 72–85). New York: Annals of the New York Academy of Sciences.

Knight, R. A., & Sims-Knight, J. E. (2004). Testing an etiological model for male juvenile sexual offending against females. *Journal of Child Sexual Abuse, 13,* 33–55.

Knight, R. A., Warren, J. I., Reboussin, R., & Soley, B. J. (1998). Predicting rapist type from crime-scene variables. *Criminal Justice and Behavior, 25,* 46–80.

Knight, R. A., & Zakireh, B. (2005). *Bootstrapping recidivism risk indicators for juvenile sexual offenders: The convergence of dual strategies.* Manuscript submitted for publication.

Kopp, S. B. (1962). The character structure of sex offenders. *American Journal of Psychotherapy, 16,* 64–70.

Koss, M. P., & Dinero, T. E. (1988). Predictors of sexual aggression among a national sample of male college students. In R. A. Prentky & V. L. Quinsey (Eds.), *Human sexual aggression: Current perspectives* (pp. 133–147). New York: New York Academy of Sciences.

Kosson, D. S., Kelly, J. C., & White, J. W. (1997). Psychopathy-related traits predict self-reported sexual aggression among college men. *Journal of Interpersonal Violence, 12,* 241–254.

Kosson, D. S., Steuerwald, B. L., Newman, J. P., & Widom, C. S. (1994). The relation between socialization and antisocial behavior, substance use, and family conflict in college students. *Journal of Personality Assessment, 63,* 473–488.

Krueger, R. F., Hicks, B. M., Patrick, C. J., Carlson, S. R., Iacono, W. G., & McGue, M. (2002). Etiologic connections among substance dependence, antisocial behavior, and personality: Modeling the externalizing spectrum. *Journal of Abnormal Psychology, 111,* 411–424.

Lalumière, M. L., & Quinsey, V. L. (1996). Sexual deviance, antisociality, mating effort, and the use of sexually coercive behaviors. *Personality and Individual Differences, 21,* 33–48.

Långström, N., & Grann, M. (2000). Risk of recidivism among young sex offenders. *Journal of Interpersonal Violence, 15*(8), 855–871.

Langton, C. M. (2003). *Contrasting approaches to risk assessment with adult male sexual offenders: An evaluation of recidivism prediction schemes and the utility of supplementary clinical information for enhancing predictive accuracy.* Unpublished doctoral dissertation, University of Toronto.

Lilienfeld, S. O. (1994). Conceptual problems in the assessment of psychopathy. *Clinical Psychology Review, 14,* 17–38.

Lohr, B. A., Adams, H. E., & Davis, J. M. (1997). Sexual arousal to erotic and aggressive stimuli in sexually coercive and noncoercive men. *Journal of Abnormal Psychology, 106,* 230–242.

Lykken, D. T. (1995). *The antisocial personalities.* Hillsdale, NJ: Erlbaum.

Malamuth, N. M. (1986). Predictors of naturalistic sexual aggression. *Journal of Personality and Social Psychology, 5,* 953–962.

Malamuth, N. M. (1998). An evolutionary-based model integrating research on the characteristics of sexually coercive men. In J. Adair, K. Deon, & D. Belanger (Eds.), *Advances in psychological science. Vol. 1: Social, personal, and developmental aspects* (pp. 151–184). Hove, UK: Psychology Press/Erlbaum.

Malamuth, N. M. (2003). Criminal and noncriminal sexual aggressors: Integrating psychopathy in a hierarchical-mediational confluence model. In R. A. Prentky, E. S. Janus, & M. C. Seto (Eds.), *Sexually coercive behavior: Understanding and management* (Vol. 989, pp. 33–58). New York: Annals of the New York Academy of Sciences.

Malamuth, N. M., Heavey, C. L., & Linz, D. (1993). Predicting men's antisocial behavior against women: The interaction model of sexual aggression. In G. C. Nagayama Hall, R. Hirschman, J. R. Graham, & M. S. Zaragoza (Eds.), *Sexual aggression: Issues in etiology and assessment, treatment and policy* (pp. 63–97). Washington, DC: Hemisphere.

Malamuth, N. M., Linz, D., Heavey, C. L., Barnes, G., & Acker, M. (1995). Using the confluence model of sexual aggression to predict men's conflict with women: A 10-year follow-up study. *Journal of Personality and Social Psychology, 69,* 353–369.

Malamuth, N. M., Sockloskie, R. J., Koss, M. P., & Tanaka, J. S. (1991). Characteristics of aggressors against women: Testing a model using a national sample of college students. *Journal of Consulting and Clinical Psychology, 59,* 670–681.

Marshall, W. L., & Barbaree, H. E. (1990). An integrated theory of the etiology of sexual offending. In W. L. Marshall, D. R. Laws, & H. E. Barbaree (Eds.), *The handbook of sexual assault: Issues, theories, and treatment of the offender* (pp. 257–275). New York: Plenum Press.

Mason, D. A., & Frick, P. J. (1994). The heritability of antisocial behavior: A meta-analysis of twin and adoption studies. *Journal of Psychopathology and Behavioral Assessment, 16,* 301–323.

Mealey, L. (1995). The sociobiology of sociopathy: An integrated evolutionary model. *Behavioral and Brain Sciences, 18,* 523–599.

Meehl, P. E. (1978). Theoretical risks and tabular asterisks: Sir Karl, Sir Ronald, and the slow progress of soft psychology. *Journal of Consulting and Clinical Psychology, 46,* 806–834.

Meehl, P. E. (1990). Appraising and amending theories:

The strategy of Lakatosian defense and two principles that warrant it. *Psychological Inquiry, 1,* 108–141.

Meehl, P. E. (1995). Bootstraps taxometrics: Solving the classification problem in psychopathology. *American Psychologist, 50,* 266–275.

Meehl, P. E. (1999). Clarifications about taxometric method. *Applied and Preventive Psychology, 8,* 165–174.

Miller, P. A., & Eisenberg, N. (1988). The relation of empathy to aggressive and externalizing/antisocial behavior. *Psychological Bulletin, 103,* 324–344.

Morgan A. B., & Lilienfeld, S. O. (2000). A meta-analytic review of the relation between antisocial behavior and neuropsychological measures of executive function. *Clinical Psychology Review, 20,* 113–136.

Parks, G. A. (2004). *Juvenile sex offender recidivism: An examination of typological differences in risk assessment.* Unpublished doctoral dissertation, Walden University.

Patrick, C. J. (1994). Emotion and psychopathy: Startling new insights. *Psychophysiology, 31,* 319–330.

Patterson, C. M., & Newman, J. P. (1993). Reflectivity and learning from aversive events: Toward a psychological mechanism for the syndromes of disinhibition. *Psychological Review, 100,* 716–736.

Persons, R. W., & Marks, P. A. (1971). The violent 4–3 M.M.P.I. personality type. *Journal of Consulting and Clinical Psychology, 36,* 189–196.

Polascheck, D. L. L. (1997). New Zealand rapists: An examination of subtypes. In G. M. Habermann (Ed.), *Looking back and moving forward: Fifty years of New Zealand Psychology* (pp. 224–231). Wellington: New Zealand Psychological Society.

Porter, S., Campbell, M. A., Woodworth, M., & Birt, A. R. (2001). A new psychological conceptualization of the sexual psychopath. In F. Columbus (Ed.), *Advances in psychology research* (Vol. VII, pp. 21–36). New York: Nova Science.

Porter, S., Fairweather, D., Drugge, J., Hervé, H., Birt, A., & Boer, D. P. (2000). Profiles of psychopathy in incarcerated sexual offenders. *Criminal Justice and Behavior, 27,* 216–233.

Prentky, R. A., & Knight, R. A. (1986). Impulsivity in the lifestyle and criminal behavior of sexual offenders. *Criminal Justice and Behavior, 13,* 141–164.

Prentky, R. A., & Knight, & R. A. (1991). Identifying critical dimensions for discriminating among rapists. *Journal of Consulting and Clinical Psychology, 59,* 643–661.

Prentky, R. A., & Knight, R. A. (2000, November). *Psychopathy baserates among subtypes of sex offenders.* Paper presented at the 19th annual meeting of the Association for the Treatment of Sexual Abusers, San Diego, CA.

Prentky, R. A., Knight, R. A., Lee, A. F. S., & Cerce, D. D. (1995). Predictive validity of lifestyle impulsivity for rapists. *Criminal Justice and Behavior, 22,* 106–128.

Prentky, R. A., Knight, R. A., & Rosenberg, R. (1988). Validation analyses on a taxonomic system for rapists: Disconfirmation and reconceptualization. In R. A. Prentky & V. E. Quinsey (Eds.), *Human sexual aggression: Current perspectives* (pp. 21–40). New York: New York Academy of Sciences.

Preston, D. L. (1996). Patterns of sexual arousal among rapist subtypes. *Dissertation Abstracts International: Section B: The Sciences and Engineering, 56*(11-B), 6445.

Proulx, J. (2001, November). *Sexual preferences and personality disorders of MTC:R3 rapist subtypes.* Symposium presented at the 20th annual meeting of the Association for the Treatment of Sexual Abusers, San Antonio, TX.

Quinsey, V. L., Chaplin, T. C., & Upfold, D. (1984). Sexual arousal to nonsexual violence and sadomasochistic themes among rapists and non-sex-offenders. *Journal of Consulting and Clinical Psychology, 52,* 651–657.

Quinsey, V. L., Harris, G. T., Rice, M. E., & Cormier, C. A. (1998). *Violent offenders: Appraising and managing risk.* Washington, DC: American Psychological Association.

Quinsey, V. L., & Lalumière, M. L. (1995). Psychopathy is a non-arbitrary class. *Behavioral and Brain Sciences, 18,* 571.

Quinsey, V. L., Rice, M. E., & Harris, G. T. (1995). Actuarial prediction of sexual recidivism. *Journal of Interpersonal Violence, 10,* 85–105.

Rada, R. T. (1978). Psychological factors in rapist behavior. In R. T. Rada (Ed.), *Clinical aspects of the rapist* (pp. 21–58). New York: Grune & Stratton.

Rader, C. M. (1977). MMPI profile types of exposers, rapists, and assaulters in a court service population. *Journal of Consulting and Clinical Psychology, 45,* 61–69.

Rappaport, K., & Burkhart, B. R. (1984). Personality and attitudinal characteristics of sexually coercive college males. *Journal of Abnormal Psychology, 93,* 216–221.

Rice, M. E., & Harris, G. T. (1997). Cross-validation and extension of the Violence Risk Appraisal Guide for child molesters and rapists. *Law and Human Behavior, 21,* 231–241.

Rice, M. E., & Harris, G. T. (2003). Overview of the session. In R. A. Prentky, E. S. Janus, & M. C. Seto (Eds.), *Sexually coercive behavior: Understanding and management* (Vol. 989, pp. 144–146). New York: Annals of the New York Academy of Sciences.

Rice, M. E., Harris, G. T., & Quinsey, V. L. (1990). A follow-up of rapists assessed in a maximum-security psychiatric facility. *Journal of Interpersonal Violence, 5,* 435–448.

Rosenberg, R., Knight, R. A., Prentky, R. A., & Lee, A. (1988). Validating the components of a taxonomic system for rapists: A path analytic approach. *Bulletin of the American Academy of Psychiatry and the Law, 16,* 169–185.

Ruscio, J., Ruscio, A. M., & Keane, T. M. (2004). Using taxometric analysis to distinguish a small latent taxon from a latent dimension with positively skewed indicators: The case of involuntary defeat syndrome. *Journal of Abnormal Psychology, 113,* 145–154.

Seghorn, T. K., & Cohen, M. (1980). The psychology of the rape assailant. In W. Cerran, A. L. McGarry, & C. Perry (Eds.), *Modern legal medicine, psychiatry, and forensic science.* Philadelphia: F. A. Davis.

Serin, R. C. (1996). Violent recidivism in criminal psychopaths. *Law and Human Behavior, 20,* 207–217.

Serin, R. C., & Amos, N. L. (1995). The role of psychopathy in the assessment of dangerousness. *International Journal of Law and Psychiatry, 18,* 231–238.

Serin, R. C., Malcolm, P. B., Khanna, A., & Barbaree, H. E. (1994). Psychopathy and deviant sexual arousal in incarcerated sex offenders. *Journal of Interpersonal Violence, 9,* 3–11.

Serin, R. C., Mailloux, D. L., & Malcolm, P. B. (2001). Psychopathy, deviant sexual arousal, and recidivism among sexual offenders. *Journal of Interpersonal Violence, 16,* 234–246.

Seto, M. C., & Barbaree, H. E. (1999). Psychopathy, treatment behavior, and sex offender recidivism. *Journal of Interpersonal Violence, 14,* 1235–1248.

Skeem, J. L., & Mulvey, E. P. (2001). Psychopathy and community violence among civil psychiatric patients: Results from the MacArthur violence risk assessment study. *Journal of Consulting and Clinical Psychology, 69,* 358–374.

Smith, A. D. (2000). Motivation and psychosis in schizophrenic men who sexually assault women. *Journal of Forensic Psychiatry, 11,* 62–73.

Smith, S. S., & Newman, J. P. (1990). Alcohol and drug abuse/dependence in psychopathic and nonpsychopathic criminal offenders. *Journal of Abnormal Psychology, 99,* 430–439.

Tellegen, A., & Waller, N. G. (in press). *Exploring personality through test construction: Development of the multidimensional personality questionnaire.* Minneapolis: University of Minnesota Press.

Thornhill, R., & Thornhill, N. W. (1992). The evolutionary psychology of men's coercive sexuality. *Behavioral and Brain Sciences, 15,* 363–421.

Wiebe, R. P. (2004). Psychopathy and rape: A Darwinian analysis. *Counseling and Clinical Psychology Journal, 1,* 23–41.

27

Risk for Criminal Recidivism

The Role of Psychopathy

KEVIN S. DOUGLAS
GINA M. VINCENT
JOHN F. EDENS

There is a spirited debate over the usefulness and appropriate role of psychopathy—and its primary measurement tools such as the Hare Psychopathy Checklist—Revised (PCL-R; Hare, 1991, 2003)—in decision making regarding people's liberty on the basis of their likelihood of future criminal behavior and violence (Gendreau, Goggin, & Smith, 2002; Hemphill & Hare, 2004). There is immense pressure within criminal justice, forensic, and psychiatric settings to "make the right decision" about which persons are safe to release into the community or require extra management within an institution. There are at least 15 points within the mental health, criminal justice, and family law realms that require decisions about risk for crime and violence to be made (Lyon, Hart, & Webster, 2001; Shah, 1978). Decision makers, policymakers, clinicians, and researchers alike have been searching—more fervently within the past two decades or so, since a series of studies concluded that mental health professionals were unable to predict violence (see Monahan, 1981)—for something to help raise predictions of violence and crime to "respectable" levels of accuracy. Early research showing that diagnoses of psychopathy might help achieve this

goal (Hart, Kropp, & Hare, 1988) served as an impetus for research on psychopathy and violence and strengthened the consumer demand for predictions of violence and crime (by parole boards, courts, clinicians responsible for releasing patients, etc.).

In addition to numerous studies that have investigated the predictive utility of psychopathy vis-à-vis violence and crime, there have been many past reviews of this issue (Hart, 1998; Hart & Hare, 1997; Hemphill, Hare, & Wong, 1998; Hemphill & Hart, 2003). We do not intend to catalogue every study on psychopathy and criminal recidivism; rather, we hope to draw out important overarching issues in this area of investigation. Specifically, we (1) provide a synthesis and interpretation of criminal recidivism prediction studies, focusing on recent meta-analytic studies and the impact of methodological and measurement factors; (2) evaluate the generalizability of the predictive utility of psychopathy across medicolegal contexts, settings, and important demographics (country, gender, ethnicity, and age); (3) compare the predictive utility of psychopathy to that of other risk factors; (4) explore the relevance of theories and models of psychopathy to the connection between psychopathy and violence; and (5) discuss the role of psychop-athy within, and its comparison to, contem-porary risk assessment instruments.

CRIMINAL RECIDIVISM PREDICTION STUDIES

Evidence from Meta-Analyses

Salekin, Rogers, and Sewell (1996) con-ducted the first meta-analysis of 18 psychop-athy–crime studies, and reported mean effect sizes (Cohen's d) of .79 for violent institu-tional and community behavior (based on 13 of 18 studies) and .55 for general (violent or nonviolent) criminal recidivism (10 of 18 studies). Although widely cited, concerns have been expressed about the Salekin and colleagues meta-analysis, particularly in rela-tion to the combination of both prospective and retrospective data, from both institu-tional and community studies (Gendreau et al., 2002; Hemphill, Hare, & Wong, 1998).[1] More recent meta-analyses of this literature have focused on studies that appear free of the specter of criterion contamination, and of the potential "apples and oranges" prob-lem (Lipsey & Wilson, 2001) associated with combining effects across disparate contexts (e.g., institutional and community settings). Using a somewhat larger sample of prospec-tive studies than Salekin and colleagues, Hemphill, Hare, and Wong (1998) examined the recidivism rates of offenders released into the community, and obtained weighted cor-relations of .27 for general recidivism (total $N = 1,275$), .27 for violent recidivism (total $N = 1,374$), and .23 for sexual recidivism (total $N = 178$). PCL-R Factor 2 (antisocial deviance features) was more predictive of general recidivism than was Factor 1 (affec-tive–interpersonal features), although nei-ther factor was more strongly correlated than the other with violent recidivism. (For a discussion of the PCL-R factors, see Hare & Neumann, Chapter 4, and Cooke, Michie, & Hart, Chapter 5, this volume.)

Following the review by Hemphill, Hare, and Wong (1998), two other published meta-analyses (Gendreau et al., 2002; Walters, 2003a; see also Walters, 2003b) provided coverage of an even larger number of studies examining the relationship between psy-chopathy and criminal behavior. In a com-parison of the PCL-R total score and the Level of Service Inventory—Revised (LSI-R; Andrews & Bonta, 1995), the latter an index of risk for recidivism within correctional samples, Gendreau et al. reported a weighted effect size for the PCL-R of $\Phi = .23$ (95% confidence interval [CI] = .17–.28) for gen-eral recidivism ($k = 33$ studies) and .21 (95% CI = .17–.25) for violent recidivism ($k = 26$ studies). It should be noted that considerable heterogeneity was observed among these ef-fects (Gendreau, Goggin, & Smith, 2003), and several relevant studies of the PCL were apparently not included in this review (see Hemphill & Hare, 2004). Using somewhat different measures of effect size, Walters re-ported a weighted point biserial correlation of .26 (95% CI = .24–.29) for prediction of general recidivism by the PCL-R across 33 studies. Subsequently, Walters (2003b) re-ported that Factor 1 showed lower predictive relations with general ($r = .15$) and violent ($r = .18$) recidivism than Factor 2 ($r = .32$ and .26, respectively, for these same outcome variables). However, considerable heteroge-neity in coefficients across studies was noted here as well.

The magnitude of the mean effects re-ported in these meta-analyses clearly sup-ports the presence of a general relationship between psychopathy and future criminal conduct, particularly when contrasted with the lower relative magnitude of association reported for most risk factors in other meta-analyses of the recidivism literature (Bonta, Law, & Hanson, 1998; Gendreau, Little, & Goggin, 1996). Despite this general conclu-sion, the heterogeneity evident in these meta-analyses raises some concerns about the ag-gregation of very diverse effect sizes across available studies and suggests that there may be factors that significantly moderate the as-sociation between psychopathy and recidi-vism. We address this issue in detail in the sections that follow.

Impact of Methodological Factors

Basic research methods can vary substan-tially across recidivism studies, and we be-lieve that some of the heterogeneity across studies in the meta-analyses discussed earlier is attributable to this. Thus, it is important to be aware of the limitations of alternative methodological approaches when evaluating and interpreting the results of different studies. We categorize these methodological factors into (1) design variation, (2) variation in measurement of psychopathy, and (3) variation in measurement of recidivism and testing of outcomes.

Design Variation

The most important point to make with respect to design variation is that postdictive studies of the psychopathy–crime relationship (correlating psychopathy with previous crime) are inherently limited because most measures of psychopathy contain items relating to criminal behavior. As such, the risk of criterion contamination (i.e., correlating something with itself) and spurious inflation of effect sizes is great. More informative are prospective studies in which the scoring of the psychopathy measure precedes the outcome of interest, hence eliminating the probability that the same episode of criminal behavior is used to score both the predictor and the predictand. In postdictive analyses, it is very important to remove items from the psychopathy measure that focus squarely on criminal behavior in order to avoid criterion contamination. This can also be important in prospective designs if the researcher wishes to test whether the aspects of psychopathy that are not dependent on criminal behavior predict recidivism.

Variation in Measurement of Psychopathy

It is quite interesting to note that self-report measures historically have shown only modest correlations with the PCL measures, particularly their affective and interpersonal features (for an overview, see Hare, 2003). There are multiple reasons why this may be the case, ranging from a "method–mode mismatch" to outright deceptiveness among psychopathic offenders (see Edens, Hart, Johnson, Johnson, & Olver, 2000, for a review; see also Lilienfeld & Fowler, Chapter 6, this volume). However, these relatively modest correlations do not preclude the possibility that such measures might provide useful information in the prediction of future behavior, as there is considerable unexplained variance when using PCL-defined

psychopathy to forecast such outcomes. Walters (in press) recently has examined the utility of "content relevant" self-report measures in relation to more widely accepted measures of risk that minimize or exclude self-report information, such as the PCL-R or the Violence Risk Appraisal Guide (VRAG; Quinsey, Harris, Rice, & Cormier, 1998), a 12-item actuarial violence prediction instrument that relies primarily on static risk factors that can be scored from file information. Perhaps somewhat surprisingly, there was no appreciable difference in the magnitude of the effects reported across these types of assessment procedures (weighted r of .28 for self-report vs. .31 for risk measures), although the total number of direct comparisons was relatively small ($k = 12$).

Although meta-analyses can be informative in terms of the absolute magnitude of associations between predictor and criterion variables, it does not inform our understanding of the incremental validity (Sechrest, 1963) of one predictor versus another—unless those predictors have been directly compared in a sufficient number of studies to warrant aggregation of effect sizes that represent the unique variance attributable to each measure (e.g., a meta-analysis of partial correlations). Direct comparisons of self-report measures to the PCL family of measures have generally suggested that both may account for unique variance in predicting recidivism beyond the other. The aforementioned study by Walters (in press) provided the most extensive examination of this issue to date by comparing the incremental validity of various self-report scales to the PCL family of measures in relation to various outcome criteria, such as criminal recidivism and institutional misconduct (see Walters, in press, Table 6). In 10 of the 19 comparisons, self-report measures accounted for additional variance beyond the PCL measures, whereas in 8 of the 19 comparisons PCL-defined psychopathy explained variance beyond the self-report scales. In two comparisons, both explained unique variance. Moreover, several of the nonsignificant comparisons were based on relatively small samples, which obviously constrains the likelihood of obtaining statistically significant effects unless the amount of unique variance explained is rather large.

Variation in Measurement of Outcomes

Recidivism studies vary widely in how they operationalize outcomes (i.e., reoffense behavior). Some make a distinction between *general* and *violent* recidivism, while others consider only "any recidivism." Some define violence broadly to include verbal aggression, threats, and arson, whereas others define violence narrowly (i.e., only as physical harm to a person). Some researchers define recidivism narrowly, according to postrelease community incidents only, whereas others include institutional misconduct and conditional release violations as well. Most studies employ a single method for measuring recidivism—most typically, official criminal records (although even here studies differ in terms of their use of arrests vs. convictions as outcomes). However, some studies use multimethod measures in which official records are supplemented with self-reports and collateral informants. In general, *broader definitions of violence* and *longer follow-up periods* will lead to higher base rates of recidivism and more powerful statistical predictions (Hemphill, Hare, & Wong, 1998). Furthermore, *self-report measures* of violence will generate significantly greater and ostensibly more accurate reports of violent incidents (e.g., Lahey et al., 1998; Monahan et al., 2001; Silverthorn, Frick, & Reynolds, 2001). For example, in their community follow-up of civil psychiatric patients, Monahan et al. found that the baserate for violent incidents identified via self-reports significantly exceeded the baserate for violent incidents identified via official records. Applying a principle of forensic assessment, it is reasonable to assume that self-reports of negative behaviors, being statements against self-interest, are accurate unless there are external reasons to portray oneself in a negative light.

Additional variability is associated with the metric used to quantify recidivism (Hart, 1998), which is dependent on the outcome of interest. Generally, statistics that use dichotomous outcomes (e.g., χ^2, Φ) will underestimate predictive accuracy because these do not reflect the full complexity of the data (Hart, 1998). On the other hand, statistical techniques that *incorporate time at risk* prior to reoffending, such as survival or Cox regression analysis, can improve the sensitivity of outcome measures and thereby enhance predictive accuracy. As an illustration of this, Richards, Casey, and Lucente (2003) reported that although the PCL-R was not related to the simple dichotomous occurrence of postrelease recidivism among a sample of female offenders, it was strongly related to the time to ("hazard for") recidivism in survival analyses (e.g., each 1-point increase on Factor 1 was associated with an 11% increase in the hazard for recidivism).

GENERALIZABILITY

In the previous section, we reviewed meta-analytic evidence for the ability of psychopathy to predict criminal recidivism and discussed methodological factors that might influence the association. Given the heterogeneity observed in meta-analyses, we evaluate the extent to which the predictive utility of psychopathy does or does not generalize across the many important contexts in which it has been studied, including medicolegal settings, institutional settings, and the gender, country, race, age, and of origin of the participants.

Medicolegal Settings

Prison and Correctional Settings

Most early research evaluated psychopathy in prison samples. Hence, we might consider prison research findings a benchmark against which generalizability to other settings can be evaluated. Most of the early foundational studies on the validity of the PCL and PCL-R in predicting criminal recidivism were conducted on male offenders released from prisons and yielded quite favorable results. For instance, Hart and colleagues (1988) conducted a prospective study of 231 offenders, and reported that persons scoring high on the PCL were four times more likely to recidivate violently. Overall, 65% of high scorers violated release terms, compared to 24% of the low scorers. The PCL was predictive beyond a variety of other potential risk factors. In this study, PCL Factor 2 ($r = .38$) was more strongly related to overall failure than was Factor 1 ($r = .18$).

This study, along with a number of other early studies (Serin, 1991; Serin, Peters, &

Barbaree, 1990; Wong, 1984), established the PCL as an important predictor of a variety of criminal recidivism indices, typically with moderate to large effect sizes. This finding has not been seriously challenged by subsequent research with prison samples, at least when community recidivism comprises the outcome variable. More recent research has confirmed that psychopathy tends to predict general and violent recidivism of criminal offenders with at least moderate strength (Douglas, Yeomans, & Boer, in press; Hare, Clark, Grann, & Thornton, 2000; Porter, Birt, & Boer, 2001; Serin, 1996; Serin & Amos, 1995). Later work has sought to determine whether the predictive accuracy of the PCL and PCL-R would generalize to other samples. In particular, researchers turned their attention to forensic psychiatric samples, owing to the fact that risk for violence is a determining factor in decisions about which insanity acquittees can be discharged into the community.

Forensic Psychiatric Settings (Insanity Acquittees)

The presence of major mental disorder as a possible competing risk factor introduces the interesting possibility that psychopathy might be less relevant in terms of understanding and predicting criminal behavior in forensic samples. In forensic settings, risk assessment is relevant to decisions within the institution for determining appropriate security levels, and to decisions (defined by statute) about whether a patient is safe to release into the community, either with or without conditions. A series of studies emanating from Penetanguishene Mental Health Centre in Ontario, Canada, confirmed the findings of prior prison studies using samples of insanity acquittees and offenders with mental disorders receiving treatment. In a representative retrospective follow-up study, Harris, Rice, and Cormier (1991) reported that among a group of 169 forensic patients, 77% of those who scored 25 and above on the PCL (coded from file records only) recidivated violently, compared to 21% of those scoring below 25. The correlation between the PCL and violent recidivism was .42. In later work involving 800-plus patients and offenders in a forensic setting, the PCL-R remained the strongest predictor of

violence among more than 50 risk factors, with a standardized beta of .34 (Quinsey et al., 1998). Several studies conducted within Swedish forensic samples have reported that the PCL-R or PCL:Screening Version (PCL:SV; Hart, Cox, & Hare, 1995) is associated with future recidivism, with moderate to large effects (AUCs [area under the curve] = .64 to .75; Dernevik, Grann, & Johansson, 2002; Strand, Belfrage, Fransson, & Levander, 1999), even after controlling for numerous other predictors such as substance abuse, prior violence, and age (Tengström, Hodgins, Grann, Långström, & Kullgren, 2004).

Some studies have focused on offenders with mental disorders, many of whom differ from forensic patients only as a function of a legal decision about criminal responsibility. In a British sample, for example, Doyle, Dolan, and McGovern (2002) reported that the PCL:SV was more strongly related (AUC = .76) to institutional physical violence over 12 weeks than were the VRAG or the Historical/Clinical/Risk Management–20 (HCR-20; Webster, Douglas, Eaves, & Hart, 1997), a 20-item violence risk assessment measure. In a small prospective study in the United Kingdom, Gray and colleagues (2003) reported that the PCL-R was strongly predictive of inpatient physical violence and destruction of property (AUCs = .70–.76), with PCL-R Factor 2 being more strongly predictive than Factor 1 of property damage (AUCs = .87 and .60, respectively), and to a lesser degree physical violence (AUCs = .69 and .63). Although some studies have reported smaller predictive effects for the PCL-R or PCL:SV (Douglas, Strand, Belfrage, Fransson, & Levander, 2005; Heilbrun et al., 1998) or no significant association with violence (Dernevik et al., 2002, for inpatient violence; Douglas, Ogloff, & Hart, 2003, for community violence), it is fair to conclude that most published investigations have supported the PCL-R as a meaningful predictor of criminal recidivism among forensic patients.

Civil Psychiatric Settings

Compared with research on prisoners and forensic samples, there is substantially less research on the predictive validity of psychopathy among civil or general psychiatric patients. Typically, a person must be seriously mentally ill, be in need of treatment, and pose a risk of serious harm to self or others in order to be committed involuntarily to a psychiatric facility. In a retrospective follow-up study of 193 patients, Douglas, Ogloff, Nicholls, and Grant (1999) reported that PCL:SV scores were strongly related to violent criminal behavior (odds ratio [OR] = 13.6; AUC = .79) over 2 years in the community, with Part 2 of the PCL:SV (analogous to PCL-R Factor 2) being slightly more predictive than Part 1 (analogous to PCL-R Factor 1): AUCs = .76 versus .72, respectively, for violent crime, and .68 versus .62 for any violence. In a later expansion of this sample (N = 268), Nicholls, Ogloff, and Douglas (2004) reported that the PCL:SV also predicted general criminal offending (AUCs = .70 for males and .92 for females). In an unpublished study, Ross, Hart, and Webster (1998) reported AUC values of .65 and .70 for the PCL:SV's relationship to community physical violence and violence leading to criminal arrest or charge, respectively. Using data from the MacArthur risk assessment study of 1,136 civil psychiatric patients (Monahan et al., 2001), Skeem and Mulvey (2001) reported a significant OR of 3.6 (AUC = .73) for the association between the PCL:SV and violent behavior in the community. Unlike Douglas and colleagues, however, the PCL:SV was not predictive of less serious forms of aggression (AUC = .50). Nevertheless, Steadman and colleagues (2000) reported that the PCL:SV was the strongest predictor—of 134 in all—of serious violence in the MacArthur study.

Findings are somewhat inconsistent for inpatient violence. Among 100 inpatients, PCL:SV scores were related to physical aggression (median follow-up = 9.5 days) in bivariate analyses (r's = .16–.27), although associations became nonsignificant after two other risk measures were entered into multivariate analyses (McNiel, Gregory, Lam, Binder, & Sullivan, 2003). Nicholls and colleagues (2004) reported that the PCL:SV predicted inpatient violence for female patients only, with small effects for physical aggression. In Ross and colleagues' (1998) unpublished report, the AUC between PCL:SV total score and inpatient violence (.61) was smaller than values reported for community violence in the above-mentioned studies.

In summary, the PCL:SV predicts community crime and violence among civil psychiatric patients with, on average, moderate effect sizes (ranging from small to large across study samples) that are diminished—sometimes to the point of nonsignificance—in multivariate analyses that incorporate other predictor variables (Douglas et al., 1999). The implication is that psychopathy may not serve as a unique predictor of violent behavior among such patients. Effects for institutional aggression are variable (AUCs range from .58 to .72) and also may vary by gender (Nicholls et al., 2004). The vast minority of persons with mental illness display marked levels of psychopathic personality, and therefore small effects could be attributable to restricted range. For instance, Skeem and Mulvey (2001) reported that 8% (72/871) of civil psychiatric patients met criteria for psychopathy on the PCL:SV, and Douglas and colleagues (1999) reported an even lower percentage (2%). Furthermore, there likely are a number of mental illness-specific pathways to violence among civil psychiatric samples, such as acute, positive psychotic symptoms (Douglas & Webster, 1999), which may reduce the salience of psychopathy as a predictor of violent behavior.

Institutional Settings

Because of the importance of context (Edens, Buffington-Vollum, Keilen, Roskamp, & Anthony, 2005; Edens, Petrila, & Buffington-Vollum, 2001), examination of the utility of psychopathy in institutional settings is critical in order to gauge the absolute and relative utility of the PCL measures in environments where there may be fewer opportunities to act out, such as controlled institutional settings. In a narrative review focused on the application of the PCL-R to death penalty litigation, Edens, Petrila, and Buffington-Vollum (2001) concluded that the PCL generally was associated with various forms of institutional misconduct but asserted that its relationship with violent acts appeared to be much more modest, particularly among U.S. samples, and hence its application to death penalty litigation (about whether a person would commit future criminal violent acts) was questionable (also see Edens et al., 2005, for a similar conclusion incorporating a much larger number of relevant U.S. prison studies).

More recently, Walters (2003a) published two meta-analyses bearing on these issues. Across 14 studies, he reported a moderate association (r = .27) between PCL-R total scores and a broad "institutional adjustment" criterion measure; however, analyses specific to violent misconduct were not reported. In subsequent analyses aggregating effects from seven analyses of the PCL-R, Walters (2003b) reported that PCL-R Factor 1 correlated only modestly with nonviolent misconduct (r = .14), whereas Factor 2 correlated more strongly (r = .21). Aggregating across 14 effects related to "violent" infractions (e.g., verbal aggression, hostility, destruction of property, fighting, and assault), Walters reported mean correlations of .12 and .22 for Factors 1 and 2, respectively. It is worth mentioning that Walters identified significant heterogeneity in the magnitude of these effects and examined several moderators in an attempt to explain this variability but was unable to identify any variables that accounted for the diversity of the effects. In sum, the predictive utility of psychopathy within institutions appears comparable to community studies, especially for broad categories such as "institutional infractions." However, its relationship to violent infractions might be weaker, especially within U.S. institutions (see also Guy, Edens, Anthony, & Douglas, in press).

Gender

Commentators have queried whether the disorder might manifest itself differently across genders as a function of socialization (see Cale & Lilienfeld, 2002, and Verona & Vitale, Chapter 21, this volume, for summaries). If this were true, contemporary measurement procedures might not optimally capture the essence of the construct in women. However, in general, construct validity studies suggest that psychopathy measures capture an underlying disorder in women similar to that in men (Cale & Lilienfeld, 2002; Jackson, Rogers, Neumann, & Lambert, 2002; Skeem, Mulvey, & Grisso, 2003), although some unexpected divergences have been noted (Vitale, Smith, Brinkley, & Newman, 2002). With respect to risk, there are gender differences in the development and phenomenology of violence that may interfere with the usefulness of psychop-

athy measures. Women tend to engage more in "relational aggression," defined as indirect forms of subterfuge within the context of interpersonal relationships, whereas men tend to act in a more physically aggressive manner (Crick & Grotpeter, 1995).

Few prediction studies have taken gender differences into account, and hence the base of research from which to generalize is small. In two prospective studies, Salekin and colleagues (1996; Salekin, Rogers, Ustad, & Sewell, 1998) found that the accuracy of the PCL-R for classifying women as recidivists versus nonrecidivists was "moderate to poor." Alternatively, Loucks and Zamble (2000) found a strong relationship (r = .45; d = .82) between PCL-R scores and general recidivism among 81 female offenders. Nicholls and colleagues (2004) found that the PCL:SV was *more* predictive of inpatient aggression and community violent criminal recidivism for female than male psychiatric patients. Douglas and colleagues (2005) reported similar findings for forensic inpatient violence. Richards and colleagues (2003) reported that Factor 1 was more predictive of inpatient violence among female offenders during a pretreatment phase, but Factor 2 was more predictive during an "in-program" phase. Two recent meta-analyses reported that, on average, Factor 2 is more predictive than Factor 1 for both sexes, with no mean gender differences in terms of predictive utility emerging across studies (Guy et al., in press; Walters, 2003a). In summary, there are differential findings across studies, and this leaves the status of psychopathy and its factors as predictors of recidivism in women unclear. Although there are a handful of studies that support the predictive utility of risk assessment instruments in adult women (e.g., Nicholls et al., 2004; Strand & Belfrage, 2001), the availability of research on violence prediction in women is extremely limited and the findings are unclear at best. We agree with Vitale and Newman (2001) that the PCL-R is in need of much further predictive research with women.

Race and Country of Study

Cross-cultural research and theory hold that societal and contextual forces can shape the manifestation of symptoms of mental or personality disorder across cultures or ethnicities (Berry, Poortinga, Segall, & Dasen, 1992; Robins, Tipp, & Przybeck, 1991). There is reasonable evidence from item response theory (IRT) analyses that the PCL-R total score shows metric equivalence (i.e., the items are equally responsive to the underlying trait of psychopathy across race) between African American and white samples, despite some differential item functioning among several Factor 2 items with respect to the level of the underlying trait at which items are most discriminating (Cooke, Kosson, & Michie, 2001; Sullivan & Kosson, Chapter 22, this volume). However, IRT analyses have revealed metric nonequivalence between North American and Scottish offenders, prompting a recommendation that cut scores be reduced by approximately 5 points for Scottish examinees (Cooke & Michie, 1999).

With respect to predictive validity, it appears that for some forms of institutional misconduct, U.S. samples produce substantially lower validity coefficients than non-U.S. samples. In Guy and colleagues (in press), the mean weighted r for the "general infraction" category was .13 for U.S. studies ($k = 6$) versus .35 for non-U.S. samples ($k = 11$). Reasons for this are not clear, but the disparity could stem from tighter security or greater ethnic/racial heterogeneity in U.S. institutions (e.g., Hicks, Rogers, & Cashel, 2000). Hare and colleagues (2000) concluded that the PCL-R has "considerable cross-cultural generalizability" (p. 623), although the data in this paper were reviewed in a narrative fashion only. Although available information attests to the predictive utility of psychopathy outside North America (Hare, 2003; Hare et al., 2000), most U.S. predictive studies with both African American and white participants unfortunately tend not to report predictive statistics separately by race, nor do they use race as a moderating factor or covariate. Several studies have investigated potential ethnicity differences as a function of *past* indices of criminal behavior, with most reporting minimal or no differences (Cornell et al., 1996; Kosson, Cyterski, Steuerwald, Neumann, & Walker-Matthews, 2002; Kosson, Smith, & Newman, 1990; but see Brinkley, Schmitt, Smith, & Newman, 2001), although *prospective* studies are rare.

Richards and colleagues (2003) reported that the PCL-R was strongly associated with the time to first general reoffense among a sample of 239 female offenders, 65% of whom were African American. However, the role of ethnicity was not directly examined. Heilbrun and colleagues (1998), although generally finding only small predictive effects, reported that the PCL was predictive of institutional and community violence among forensic patients, and race was neither a significant predictor of violence nor a moderator of the relationship between psychopathy and violence. Vitacco, Neumann, and Jackson (in press) reported that minority race (primarily African American) was correlated (r's = .15–.20) with the PCL:SV in the MacArthur dataset. Minority race was inconsistently and weakly associated with violence in this study; it bore no relationship to violence when the four-factor model was used but was significantly though weakly (.04) related to community violence when Cooke and Michie's (2001) three-factor model was used. By contrast, Hicks and colleagues (2000) reported that the PCL:SV was substantially more accurate in predicting institutional violent and nonviolent infractions among adolescent African Americans compared to whites or Hispanics, although the sample sizes of these racial/ethnic groups were relatively small.

Most studies that have investigated ethnicity/race as a moderator of the association between psychopathy and recidivism have reported weak or negligible effects. However, such studies are admittedly few, and in particular, there is a scarcity of data from large-scale prospective studies that would be needed to draw firm conclusions. The existing evidence seems to favor the utility of psychopathy measures across at least African Americans and whites within the United States and within Western Europe. Nevertheless, data showing that the disorder may manifest itself at different levels of the underlying trait across groups (Cooke et al., 2001; Cooke & Michie, 1999) and that some etiological-relevant findings (i.e., passive avoidance errors) might not generalize across groups (Newman & Schmitt, 1998) suggest the possibility that race might moderate the psychopathy–violence association in some as yet undetermined way. Research with Asian, Hispanic, Pacific Islander, Middle Eastern and other groups is essentially lacking, and hence generalizability should not be assumed.

Age

The absence of long-term longitudinal studies does not allow us to draw strong conclusions about changes in the PCL-R scores of individuals across the lifespan. However, cross-sectional data for adults suggest that there is an age-related reduction ("burnout") in PCL-R Factor 2 scores between the ages of 35 and 40, which is not evident for Factor 1 scores (Harpur & Hare, 1994). Some studies using mixed retrospective and prospective designs report that when mapping trends of recidivism, the rate of nonviolent crime appears to plummet *among psychopaths* between ages 41 and 50, during which time the rate of violent crime remains fairly constant (Hare, Forth, & Strachan, 1992). However, this result should be interpreted with caution because existing studies have employed very small samples of older adult psychopaths, of whom only a small proportion actually had the opportunity for reconviction in the community. Furthermore, rates of nonviolent recidivism for older psychopaths in these studies did not significantly differ from those of nonpsychopathic offenders. Rates of violent recidivism did not differ significantly either, but this null result was likely a product of very low baserates for this outcome measure (i.e., only 4 [13.3%] psychopaths and 2 [4.5%] nonpsychopaths were reconvicted for violent acts). As such, use of the PCL-R as a risk assessment tool with older inmates is questionable given that only 11.6% of older (i.e., 41 to 50 years old) psychopaths in the Hare and colleagues sample were reconvicted for violent crime, versus 7.4% of nonpsychopaths (see Edens, Petrila, & Buffington-Vollum, 2001). In general, any conclusions about "burnout" among psychopaths are extremely tentative given the absence of prospective studies with sufficient sample sizes and analyses weighting differential times at risk.

With respect to preadult years,[2] a number of studies show that adults and youth high on psychopathy measures have more serious and persistent criminal histories (Blackburn & Coid, 1998; Brandt, Wallace, Patrick, & Curtin, 1997; Hemphill, Templeman, Wong, & Hare, 1998; Toupin, Mercier, Déry, Côté, & Hodgins, 1996; see Forth, Kosson, & Hare, 2003, for a review), even after removing the criminal behavior items from the

PCL-R or the Hare Psychopathy Checklist: Youth Version (PCL:YV; Forth et al., 2003) (Vincent, Vitacco, Grisso, & Corrado, 2003). Similar results have been reported for children ages 6–13, with those exhibiting more callous–unemotional traits showing stronger histories of police contacts and conduct problems (Christian, Frick, Hill, Tyler, & Frazer, 1997). Longitudinally, retrospective studies of adolescents spanning periods of 5–10 years generally have reported strong associations between PCL:YV scores and general and violent recidivism (for reviews, see Edens, Skeem, Cruise, & Cauffman, 2001; Forth et al., 2003). For example, in a "retrospective follow-up" study (i.e., the PCL:YV was coded retrospectively from files as of a certain date, and violence was measured after this date) spanning an average of 4.6 years, Gretton, McBride, Hare, O'Shaughnessy, and Kumka (2001) found that the upper third of PCL:YV scorers were four times more likely to recidivate and three times more likely to violently recidivate than the lower third of PCL:YV scorers, and they did so sooner after release. Prospective studies have found that scores on the PCL:YV strongly predict violent recidivism in most cases (e.g., Catchpole & Gretton, 2003 [AUC = .73]; Vincent et al., 2003), and general recidivism in some cases (Corrado, Vincent, Hart, & Cohen, 2004; Ridenour, Marchant, & Dean, 2001; Toupin et al., 1996).

Although the association between psychopathy and recidivism appears to generalize to youth, published prospective studies with adolescents have been rare, have used short follow-up periods averaging only 12–27 months, and have yet to systematically track recidivism into adulthood—although several retrospective and prospective studies would have included early adult offenses for older members of the baseline sample (e.g., Gretton et al., 2001). Furthermore, aside from the Brandt and colleagues (1997) study, there has been minimal evaluation of youth psychopathy measures with respect to their incremental validity over other risk factors. Distinct factors of psychopathy (e.g., affective–interpersonal vs. antisocial deviance) have also been considered only rarely (Brandt et al., 1997; Corrado et al., 2004). In one study that did examine psychopathy factors, Corrado and colleagues (2004) found that prediction of general recidivism was attributable exclusively to the antisocial deviance features of the PCL:YV, whereas violent recidivism was predicted by both the affective–interpersonal features and the antisocial deviance features. Finally, there have been no true prospective studies to date examining the prediction of socially deviant outcomes in children (< 12) on the basis of psychopathic traits.

COMPARISON OF PSYCHOPATHY TO OTHER RISK FACTORS

Incremental Validity

There can be little argument that psychopathy predicts both violent and general recidivism, broadly speaking. Less clear is whether there is anything unique about the predictive utility of psychopathy once other risk factors are taken into account. Hemphill and colleagues (1998) reviewed a number of studies that investigated the predictive utility of the PCL-R relative to other predictors such as demographics, criminal history variables, and personality disorder. Based on studies reporting comparative univariate statistics and the few studies reporting actual tests of incremental validity, the PCL-R was more strongly predictive or added incrementally to these other factors. More recently, others have similarly reported that the PCL-R retains its predictive validity even after variables such as substance abuse, criminal history, and demographics are controlled (Tengström et al., 2004).

In perhaps the most thorough investigation to date of the incremental validity of psychopathy in predicting violent behavior, Skeem and Mulvey (2001) conducted both traditional incremental predictive analyses (i.e., comparing the PCL:SV to various criminal history, personality, substance misuse, mental health, and psychosocial variables) and propensity score analyses, in which nonspecific antisocial behavior was removed from the estimate of the relationship between psychopathy and violence. On the basis of hierarchical logistic regression analyses, the PCL:SV (Part 2 in particular) added to the model fit produced by 15 covariates alone. On the basis of propensity score analyses holding nonspecific psychopathy-related variance constant, the correlation between the PCL:SV and violence was reduced from .26 to .12. The authors considered this to represent the "unique" predictive effect of psychopathy for violence.

What these studies suggest is that the predictive contribution of psychopathy remains quite robust in the face of competing factors. Although its association with violence was reduced to .12 in Skeem and Mulvey's (2001) analyses, this was after controlling for 15 other variables that were theoretically and empirically related to psychopathy and violence. Hence, it was a highly conservative test of the incremental validity of the PCL:SV. Other studies that have focused on single or smaller sets of competing predictors have also tended to support the incremental utility of the PCL measures. However, as we report later, this apparent unique predictive contribution of the PCL-R may not hold in relation to contemporary risk assessment measures.

Interaction Effects

The interaction between psychopathy and other risk factors has not been an area of extensive research, although one particular topic has received a good deal of attention. There is some evidence that high psychopathy scores combined with deviant sexual arousal may portend a significantly elevated risk for sexual reoffending among convicted rapists. Rice and Harris (1997) reported that phallometric measures of sexual deviance and psychopathy were both modestly correlated with sexual recidivism in a sample of 288 Canadian sex offenders followed for an average of 10 years, but the interaction of these two variables was much more informative regarding increased violence risk: Approximately 70% of sex offenders who exhibited both elevated PCL scores and deviant sexual arousal were convicted of a new sexual offense after release, compared to only 40% of offenders in the other groups (also see Hildebrand, de Ruiter, & de Vogel, 2004). In contrast, Gretton and colleagues (2001) reported that the interaction between deviant sexual arousal and psychopathy scores was predictive of general and violent recidivism but *not* sexual recidivism per se. However, participants in the Gretton and colleagues study were adolescents with prior sex offenses, a group that is thought to differ dramatically from adults in their motivations for sex crimes (e.g., Hunter, Figueredo, Malamuth, & Becker, 2003; Pithers, Gray, Busconi, & Houchens, 1998).

RELEVANCE OF THEORIES AND MODELS TO THE PSYCHOPATHY–VIOLENCE RELATIONSHIP

The vast majority of research on psychopathy's prediction of recidivism is atheoretical—unless one considers psychopathy itself a "mini-theory" of violence, as some have (Steadman et al., 1994). More specifically, until recently, most studies have not been situated within a larger theoretical framework *either* of psychopathy *or* of crime and violence. Recent conceptual work, based on seminal theories of psychopathy, has explored the possibility that different variants of psychopathic personality may exist (Poythress & Skeem, Chapter 9, this volume; Skeem, Poythress, Edens, Lilienfeld, & Cale, 2003). Skeem et al. reviewed several theories of psychopathy (e.g., Cleckley, 1941/1976; Fowles, 1980; Gray, 1987; Karpman, 1941; Mealey, 1995; Porter, 1996) along with recent cluster-analytic research in an attempt to discern trait dimensions along which so-called primary and secondary psychopaths might vary. Primary psychopaths, for example, are more likely to show true affective deficits (i.e., lack of conscience and lack of guilt), a lack of trait anxiety, and overt narcissism. Secondary psychopaths, though appearing at times not to show these features, do in fact have the capacity for social emotions. They are also more likely to be characterized by anxiety and perhaps negative emotionality, as well as traits consistent with borderline personality disorder (e.g., anger, impulsivity, and primitive defense mechanisms such as splitting).

The notion of different phenotypical variants of psychopathy gives rise to hypotheses about different types of criminal and violent behavior that might be associated with each. We may see more elements of instrumentality among primary psychopaths and less reactive, angry violence, or violence in response to provocation or insult (Patrick & Zempolich, 1998; Skeem et al., 2003). Indeed, there is some evidence to support this

hypothesis, insofar as the Factor 1/Part 1 component of the PCL measures tends to correlate more strongly with indices such as planning and material gain than Factor 2 and less strongly with emotional arousal (Cornell et al., 1996; Porter & Woodworth, Chapter 24, this volume; Williamson, Hare, & Wong, 1987). We also may see some persons with high levels of "primary symptoms" who are not physically violent because they are able to meet their needs through manipulation rather than through force. Consistent with the idea that the primary (affective–interpersonal) features of psychopathy are more associated with the use of guile and manipulation, Moltó, Poy, and Tourrubia (2000) reported that Factor 1 of the PCL-R was more strongly associated with fraud-related offenses than Factor 2.

Closely related to this theoretical discussion is ongoing debate about the most appropriate conceptualization of psychopathy as measured by the Hare family of measures. Two alternative structural models of PCL-R psychopathy have been proposed: (1) the traditional two-factor model (Harpur, Hare, & Hakstian, 1989) and its recent four-facet extension (which parses each of the original factors into two nested facets; Hare, 2003), and (2) an alternative three-factor model advanced by Cooke and Michie (2001). These models are described in detail elsewhere in this volume (see Hare & Neumann, Chapter 4, and Cooke et al., Chapter 5). For present purposes, it is sufficient to note that the main difference between these models centers on how they deal with antisocial, criminal behavior in relation to psychopathy. Hare's (2003) position is that antisocial behavior defines part of the construct of psychopathy, and items relating to overt behavioral deviance are explicitly represented in his fourth (Antisocial) facet. On the other hand, Cooke and Michie (2001) excluded these items from their three-factor model on the grounds that they did not provide unique information about the underlying trait of psychopathy according to item response theory and confirmatory factor analyses, and subsequently, Cooke, Michie, Hart, and Clark (2004) conceptualized antisocial behaviors as *consequences* of psychopathy rather than as part of the constellation of personality traits that combine to define the disorder.

Regardless of how this conceptual debate

is ultimately resolved, there is an obvious tautology inherent in using a personality measure that contains items dealing with past socially deviant acts to predict future social deviance (see Cooke et al., 2004, for a review). Because of this, the traditional approach to PCL-R recidivism research cannot answer the question whether psychopathy is a causal risk factor or whether its connection to future antisocial acts simply reflects the inclusion of items relating to past criminal behavior. Psychopathic personality may be one causal contributor to violence, but some psychopaths will not be violent or criminal, possibly due to an increased capacity for inhibiting such responses or the presence of internal motivations that compete with criminal activity (cf. Hall & Benning, Chapter 23, this volume). In this regard, Cooke and colleagues (2004) argued compellingly that use of a more "pure" measure of psychopathy (i.e., one that excludes indicators of overt antisocial deviance) could increase the specificity of risk assessments and advance understanding of pathways to various forms of social deviance, such as sexual violence, spousal violence, and parasitic but nonaggressive white-collar crimes.

With respect to sex offenders, the balance of research suggests that (1) psychopathy predicts the *nonsexual violence* and general criminality of sex offenders (Gretton et al., 2001; Hildebrand et al., 2004; Quinsey, Rice & Harris, 1995), and (2) some types of sex offenses are less strongly related to psychopathy than others. Studies are divided in terms of whether psychopathy predicts sexual recidivism, with several finding a significant predictive effect (Firestone, Bradford, Greenberg, & Serran, 2000; Hanson & Harris, 2000; Quinsey et al., 1995) and others not, despite finding predictive effects for violent or general recidivism (Barbaree, Seto, Langton, & Peacock, 2001; Hildebrand et al., 2004; Långström & Grann, 2000). Sex offenses involving physical force and violence—such as rape—are more strongly related to psychopathy than offenses such as incest, and perpetrators of more than one type of sexual crime are more likely to be psychopathic (Porter et al., 2000). Research reviewed earlier suggests that the combination of psychopathy and deviant sexual arousal markedly enhances risk for sexual recidivism.

The role of psychopathy in partner violence is not well researched. One study found that it predicted spousal violence (Grann & Wedin, 2001); another found that it predicted the *general violence* of spousal assaulters, although the authors had no data specifically on reoffenses involving spousal violence (Hilton, Harris, & Rice, 2001). In a retrospective study, Hervé, Vincent, Kropp, and Hare (2001) reported that high PCL-R scoring inmates were more likely than other inmates to have at least one documented incident of spousal violence; however, most psychopaths did not have histories of spousal violence. Conceptually, the two factors of psychopathy might be expected to show opposing relations with some types of partner violence, such as stalking and violence against ex-intimate partners. Primary (affective–interpersonal) deficits might ironically protect against this type of aggression because of an absence of normal affectional ties, whereas the antisocial deviance component, which includes items reflecting impulsiveness, reactive aggression, and delinquency (and which is selectively associated with borderline personality traits; cf. Poythress & Skeem, Chapter 9, this volume) would likely be positively predictive of stalking and related violence. The only direct evidence on this issue is an unpublished study by Dempster, Hart, and Boer (1997) that reported a substantially lower overall mean PCL-R score among stalkers (15) than among sexual, violent, and general offenders (21–23). Indirectly, there is meta-analytic evidence that personality disorder is predictive of stalking-related violence (Rosenfeld, 2004), and that it is most likely to be of the borderline variety (Douglas & Dutton, 2001; Meloy & Gothard, 1995).

PSYCHOPATHY AND RISK ASSESSMENT

General Considerations Regarding Psychopathy and Risk Assessment

First, neither the PCL-R nor any other measure of psychopathy can be considered a risk assessment instrument. They are instruments used to measure a personality construct and, as such, were not designed specifically to predict crime or violence. In the risk assessment context, they index a single risk factor. Second, it follows that psychopathy instruments should never be used in isolation without consideration of other risk factors, and, where available and appropriate, comprehensive evidence-based risk assessment instruments. There are multiple pathways to violence—psychopathy is but one. As some commentators have noted (Hart, 1998), an extreme score on the PCL-R may be sufficient for a decision of high risk (although perhaps not in some contexts, such as estimating risk of institutional violence among life-sentenced offenders; Edens, Petrila, & Buffington-Vollum, 2001), but it is not necessary. Third, although there is general support for the predictive utility of psychopathy, it remains important to garner empirical support for its utility within the specific setting in which it is to be used, particularly in view of the heterogeneity of findings reported in the meta-analyses reviewed earlier.

Inherent Difficulties in Prediction

We wish to draw attention to several points, highlighted by limitations inherent in many existing recidivism studies, that should be considered in attempting to interpret findings emerging from predictive studies of psychopathy. First, readers should bear in mind that if there is a low baserate of either psychopathy or crime in a sample, then effect sizes will be attenuated. This has led to the use of ROC (Receiver Operator Characteristics) analysis, which is less sensitive to low baserates than other statistics. However, from a practical perspective, even if low correlations appear attributable in part to low baserates, it would be a mistake to assert that these baserates should be ignored. When it comes to making predictions about individual offenders, low positive predictive power is low positive predictive power, regardless of its cause, and this greatly constrains what legitimately can be claimed about risk for acting out in such circumstances.

An associated problem with outcome variables pertains to the procedure used to measure recidivism. Sole reliance on official criminal records will invariably underestimate actual criminal behavior. In addition to reducing accuracy through artificially inflating the false-positive rate, this also can reduce accuracy by lowering baserates. Supplementing criminal records with archival data from other sources (e.g., psychiatric hospital records, and forensic psychiatric hospital records) and with self- and collateral reports

will increase the baserate and permit a truer estimate of predictive utility. A prospective study of 629 psychiatric patients by Mulvey, Shaw, and Lidz (1994) provides an illustration of the impact on baserates of using archival records alone versus supplementing records with self- and collateral reports. These investigators reported a 12% baserate of violence by using official records only, compared to 47% when self- and collateral reports were included. Similarly, in a sample of 193 psychiatric patients, Douglas and Ogloff (2003) reported that when criminal records alone were used to measure recidivism, the baserate was 10%. Just by supplementing these records with data from two other *archival* sources (i.e., general and psychiatric hospital records), the baserate rose to 38%. Furthermore, the accuracy of the PCL:SV varied tremendously across the three sources of outcome data (AUCs = .55 to .83)—such that if only one of these sources were used, conclusions could range from psychopathy being a *noncorrelate* to a *very strong correlate* of violence among psychiatric patients. By using multiple sources of outcome data, the AUCs (.67 to .73) were predictably more stable across different types of violence and, arguably, more representative of the "true" effect size than the estimates from any one source alone.

Further, statistical procedures that optimize predictive strategies (e.g., cutoff scores on the PCL-R) within single samples may face generalizability problems when applied to new contexts. For instance, a decision rule derived from a sample of offenders specifying that scores of 18 and above on the PCL:SV (a diagnosis of psychopathy) indicate high risk would simply not be useful in a setting with a 2% baserate of psychopathy (i.e., Douglas et al., 1999). With these issues as background, we next discuss the role of psychopathy in contemporary risk assessment.

The Empirical Relationship between Psychopathy and Formal Risk Assessment Instruments

Given its reputation as a robust predictor of recidivism, it is not surprising that psychopathy—usually as measured by the Hare family of measures—plays a prominent role in contemporary (post-1990) risk assessment instruments. This is true of measures from the "structured professional judgment" model of risk assessment (e.g., the HCR-20 [Webster et al., 1997], Sexual Violence Risk-20 [SVR-20; Boer, Hart, Kropp & Webster, 1998], and Risk for Sexual Violence Protocol [RSVP; Hart et al., 2003]), in which psychopathy was chosen by their authors because of its importance across multiple studies, as well as actuarial instruments in which psychopathy was chosen because it entered a statistical predictive model within a given sample (i.e., the VRAG; Harris, Rice, & Quinsey, 1993; Quinsey et al., 1998). In fact, in the VRAG, the inclusion of 11 risk factors in addition to the PCL-R only raised its predictive validity from .34 to .44. An early version of the Iterative Classification Tree, a risk assessment instrument developed as part of the MacArthur project on mental disorder and violence, included the PCL:SV because it proved to be the strongest ($r = .26$) risk factor (of 134 candidate indicators) in a sample of close to 1,000 civil psychiatric patients (Steadman et al., 2000).

Psychopathy—typically as measured by the PCL-R—correlates moderately to highly with various risk assessment instruments, demonstrating that it is related to indices designed to predict general or violent criminal recidivism. For instance, Hemphill and colleagues (1998) reviewed the relationship between the PCL measures and several correctional prediction instruments, and reported absolute correlations ranging from .41 to .70. The PCL measures also correlate with more contemporary risk assessment instruments such as the HCR-20 and VRAG. For instance, the PCL-R correlated .85 with the HCR-20 total score and .65 with the VRAG in a sample of 188 criminal offenders (Douglas, Yeomans, & Boer, in press). The PCL-R also correlated highly with the VRAG (.70) and with Quinsey and colleagues' (1998) Sex Offender Risk Appraisal Guide (SORAG; $r = .72$) in a sample of sexual offenders (Barbaree et al., 2001). The PCL:SV's correlation with the HCR-20 was smaller though still substantial ($r = .68$) in a sample of 560 offenders and forensic patients (Douglas, Strand, et al., 2005), and also in a sample of 100 civil psychiatric patients ($r = .61$; McNiel et al., 2003). Often, correlations are smaller (typically .30–.50) between Factor/Part 1 of psychopathy and HCR-20 indices, and for the Clinical and

Risk Management scales of the HCR-20 (Douglas, Strand, et al., 2005; Douglas, Yeomans, & Boer, in press; Gray et al., 2004; McNiel et al., 2003)—understandably so, given the relatively less similar item content of these various scales to one another. Similarly, the PCL-R does not correlate as strongly with actuarial sexual recidivism instruments (range of .13–.45) (Barbaree et al., 2001).

Comparison of Psychopathy Measures to Risk Assessment Instruments in the Prediction of Criminal Behavior

How have psychopathy measures compared to measures designed specifically to assess risk? Until fairly recently, the evidence on the prediction of general and violent recidivism seemed to indicate a draw, or perhaps a slight advantage, for the PCL measures (for a review, see Hemphill et al., 1998). However, more recent meta-analytic studies comparing the PCL-R to contemporary risk assessment instruments have yielded somewhat different conclusions. Before reviewing these findings, it should be noted that questions have been raised about the meaningfulness of such comparative validity studies. For example, Hemphill and Hare (2004) asserted that PCL-R should not be evaluated against risk assessment measures because it provides "unique information" regarding an offender. However, if the question at hand is purely risk prediction (Heilbrun, 1997), then the issue of incremental validity is of practical importance (Sechrest, 1963). Put simply, if two measures correlate significantly with a criterion of interest, the question becomes whether they provide unique or simply redundant information.

Walters (2003a) recently asserted that the PCL-R had no greater validity for predicting general recidivism than the Lifestyle Criminality Screening Form (LCSF; Walters, White, & Denney, 1991), based on a meta-analysis of seven studies with a mean weighted effect size of .31 (95% CI = .23–.39) for the LCSF compared to a mean effect size of .26 (95% CI = .24–.29) for the PCL-R. However, there was a trend for the PCL-R to correlate more highly with "minor" institutional misconduct ($r = .39$, vs. .21 for the LCSF) and release revocations ($r = .37$ vs. .28), although formal statistical tests of the difference in correlations for the two measures were not reported. The relative absence of studies examining the predictive validity of the LCSF in relation to violent recidivism specifically also raises serious cautions with regard to interpreting these findings.

In another meta-analytic study mentioned earlier, Gendreau and colleagues (2002; see also Gendreau et al., 2003) found that the LSI-R outperformed the PCL substantially in relation to general recidivism and modestly in the prediction of violent recidivism, thus challenging Salekin and colleagues' (1996) assertion that psychopathy is "unparalleled" as a measure of risk. Hemphill and Hare (2004; see also Hare, 2003) responded by noting various concerns about the Gendreau and colleagues meta-analysis, such as heavy reliance on unpublished LSI papers of unknown methodological rigor, failure to include relevant articles examining other Hare instruments, questionable selection of appropriate effect sizes from studies with multiple outcomes of interest, and reliance on phi coefficients that may underestimate the magnitude of effects that would be obtained with noncategorical predictor and criterion measures. Of particular interest is Hemphill and Hare's reanalysis of most of the studies directly comparing the LSI and the PCL, which yielded markedly different results regarding the relative superiority of the LSI. Unfortunately, neither meta-analysis reported tests of incremental validity for the two measures.

Some research *has* tested the incremental validity of the PCL-R against other risk assessment instruments. The evidence from this research tends to indicate that the risk assessment instruments predict violence more accurately, even though the difference between the PCL-R and its competitors often appears small when compared in terms of simple univariate effect sizes. For example, Douglas, Yeomans, and Boer (in press) reported a correlation of .42 between the PCL-R and subsequent violent recidivism in a sample of 188 offenders. The correlation between Factor 2 of the PCL-R and later violence was larger (.50). In comparison, the HCR-20 correlated .51 with violence, and the VRAG correlated .47. Presented in this format, Factor 2 of the PCL-R predicts just as strongly as the HCR-20 or VRAG. However, in multivariate analyses that included all three measures (with the psychopathy

items removed from the HCR-20 and VRAG), the PCL-R total or factor scores failed to enter the regression models (see Douglas et al., 1999, for a similar finding among civil psychiatric patients, and Douglas, Ogloff, & Hart, 2003, for a similar finding among forensic psychiatric patients). In our view, such a multivariate, incremental analysis is necessary to reach conclusions about how well the PCL-R predicts criminal behavior in relation to formal risk assessment instruments. To be fair, this pattern of results is not always obtained; sometimes the PCL-R predicts as well as the risk assessment instruments (see Hare, 2003, for a review). However, in general, an edge can be given to contemporary risk assessment instruments whose design purpose was predictive accuracy.

Psychopathy and Violence Risk Management

There has been a decided conceptual movement in the risk assessment field toward increased focus on the reduction and management of future violence as the primary goal of risk assessment, rather than mere prediction per se (Hart, 1998; Heilbrun, 1997). Many commentators have called for the inclusion of so-called dynamic or changeable risk factors within risk assessment procedures (Douglas & Skeem, in press). Although we are in general agreement with this position, we believe that jettisoning "static" or (relatively) unchanging risk factors (which arguably includes psychopathy) from risk assessment would be a mistake, given the extent of research in support of their predictive validity (for reviews, see Douglas & Webster, 1999; Monahan & Steadman, 1994), and their importance for establishing the appropriate level or intensity of intervention and informing the selection of appropriate treatment and risk management strategies. Effective treatment strategies for psychopaths will require significant departures from traditional approaches with violent offenders (Hemphill & Hart, 2003). For example, as pointed out by Hare (1998b; see also Harris & Rice, Chapter 28, this volume), empathy training is not highly recommended for psychopathic individuals, whereas it may be effective with other high-risk offenders.

There are special circumstances that arise

in relation to psychopathy/risk management when the population of interest is youthful offenders. Forth (2005) has described the role of the PCL:YV in risk management as follows: "This information may be useful in identifying youth who represent a more serious management problem within institutions, who need intensive intervention, and who require more resources for risk management in the community. . . . " However, Forth cautioned that the PCL:YV is *not* appropriate as a basis for decisions regarding transfer to adult court or restricting treatment access. Furthermore, the manual for the PCL:YV explicitly states that "it is inappropriate for clinicians or other professionals to label a youth as a psychopath" (Forth et al., 2003, p. 17). However, a problem in deciding what interventions are appropriate for youthful offenders with psychopathic features is that there are no long-term longitudinal data tracking the course and stability of psychopathic traits. Hence, we are unable to distinguish between "phenotypically" psychopathic youth who actually have or do not have psychopathy (Hart, Watt, & Vincent, 2002; Salekin, Chapter 20, this volume). Although retrospective studies provide evidence that most psychopathic adults exhibit affiliated traits by ages 6–10 (Widiger et al., 1996), prospective data suggest that at least 50% of children with serious, pervasive antisocial traits do not develop into antisocial adolescents or adults (Moffitt & Caspi, 2001), much less PCL-defined "psychopaths."

We noted earlier in regard to adult populations that psychopathy as indexed by the PCL-R represents only one risk factor, not a comprehensive assessment of risk. This point is perhaps even more important with respect to youth. In predicting violent behavior in younger samples, it is important for measures of psychopathy to be used in conjunction with other environmental, individual, and familial risk indicators as well as established protective factors (Herrenkohl, Hawkins, Chung, Hill, & Battin-Pearson, 2001; Reppucci, Fried, & Schmidt, 2002; U.S. Department of Health and Human Services, 2001). Given that adolescence is a time of extreme developmental change, clinicians should routinely reassess psychopathic characteristics and affiliated risk in samples of problem youth to determine if maturation attenuates risk. Furthermore, there is some evidence that individuals exhibiting only behavioral (Factor 2) features of psychopathy are more likely to desist than youth with high overall scores on the PCL:YV (Vincent et al., 2003), implying they may be more amenable to treatment.

SUGGESTIONS FOR FURTHER INVESTIGATION

There has been a plethora of research on the relationship of psychopathy measures—particularly from the PCL family of instruments—to future criminal recidivism (and institutional misconduct). With some disclaimers, it is fair to state that psychopathy is an important and meaningful risk factor for subsequent antisocial behavior of many types, across many contexts, by many different types of people. In fact, the field may have reached asymptote in terms of novel information to be gleaned from studies that simply address the question whether an association exists between psychopathy and recidivism. For this reason, we advocate a shift of emphasis toward other research questions in order to move the psychopathy–recidivism research literature forward.

First, there remain certain settings and samples in which the predictive validity of psychopathy remains understudied. These include civil psychiatric settings, nonoffender and nonpatient community samples, offenders sentenced to life in prison rather than death, female and youthful offender samples, and ethnic and racial minority groups. With regard to population subgroups, studies that cross demographic factors such as ethnicity/race and gender (and even age) are particularly needed. More pragmatically, we advocate a continuation of research on the predictive utility of self-report psychopathy inventories. Irrespective of debates regarding what such inventories actually measure and whether self-reports could conceivably be valid for the assessment of psychopathy (Hart & Hare, 1997; Lilienfeld, 1994), the question whether self-report psychopathy inventories can be of practical utility for making decisions about future crime and violence remains an empirical one.

In addition, we advocate further exploration of the relevance of contemporary theories and models of psychopathy, described elsewhere in this volume, to the nature and prediction of criminal and violent behavior. In our view, conceptually informed studies are more likely than atheoretical endeavors to lead to better prediction of specific categories of crime and violence. In this regard, further exploration of sexual crimes and crimes against former intimate partners within the context of a theoretical framework that emphasizes the affective and interpersonal deficits of psychopathy would be fruitful. Similarly, further investigation of the potentially (and ironically) protective nature of Factor 1 items in relation to crimes against current or former intimate partners is recommended. Aside from improving the prediction of outcomes, theory-based risk assessments would likely contribute to risk management and treatment efforts aimed at violence reduction by better aligning appropriate interventions with particular variants of psychopathy. In a reciprocal fashion, the development of effective treatment for even one variant of psychopathy could influence predictions of criminal behavior. That is, risk levels would be estimated to be lower among those who completed the treatment and higher among those who did not.

CONCLUSION

Psychopathy has been described as a "socially devastating disorder" (Hare, 1998b, p. 188). A large part of its devastating impact stems from the increased likelihood that psychopathic individuals will harm others and generally violate others' rights. For this reason, psychopathy has played a prominent role in the literature on criminal and violent recidivism. Although we advocate continued investigation of the psychopathy–recidivism association along the lines described in the preceding section, we caution against considering psychopathy a harbinger of ineluctable danger—automatically elevating risk for all types of criminal and violent behavior—or its absence an indication of the absence of risk. We believe it is equally misguided to adopt an attitude of resignation toward the treatment of psychopathy, for ultimately our job when making a prediction of high likelihood of criminal recidivism is to prove ourselves wrong and prevent what we have predicted (Hart, 1998).

NOTES

1. Although Salekin et al. (1996) reported that their test of the heterogeneity of the obtained effects was not significant, a small k can oftentimes obscure meaningful differences (Lipsey & Wilson, 2001).
2. We are aware of the controversy surrounding the "youth psychopathy" issue (well discussed in other chapters in this volume—see Frick & Marsee, Chapter 18; Salekin, Chapter 20; and Edens & Petrila, Chapter 29), and we do not assume here that psychopathy exists as a stable personality trait in preadult years. We are referring merely to scores on measures of psychopathic features in younger participant samples.

REFERENCES

Andrews, D. A., & Bonta, J. (1995). *The Level of Service Inventory—Revised* (LSI-R). Toronto, ON, Canada: Multi-Health Systems.

Barbaree, H. E., Seto, M. C., Langton, C. M., & Peacock, E. J. (2001). Evaluating the predictive accuracy of six risk assessment instruments for adult sex offenders. *Criminal Justice and Behavior, 28,* 490–521.

Berry, J. W., Poortinga, Y. H., Segall, M. H., & Dasen, P. R. (1992). *Cross-cultural psychology: Research and applications.* Cambridge, UK: Cambridge University Press.

Blackburn, R., & Coid, J. W. (1998). Psychopathy and the dimensions of personality disorders in violent offenders. *Personality and Individual Differences, 25,* 129–145.

Boer, D. P., Hart, S. D., Kropp, P. R., & Webster, C. D. (1998). *Manual for the Sexual Violence Risk—20.* Vancouver, BC, Canada: British Columbia Institute against Family Violence.

Bonta J., Law, M., & Hanson K. (1998). The prediction of criminal and violent recidivism among mentally disordered offenders: A meta-analysis. *Psychological Bulletin, 123,* 123–142.

Brandt, J. R., Wallace, A. K., Patrick, C. J., & Curtin, J. J. (1997). Assessment of psychopathy in a population of incarcerated adolescent offenders. *Psychological Assessment, 9,* 429–435.

Brinkley, C. A., Schmitt, W. A., Smith, S. S., & Newman, J. P. (2001). Construct validation of a self-report psychopathy scale: Does Levenson's self-report psychopathy scale measure the same constructs as Hare's psychopathy checklist-revised? *Personality and Individual Differences, 31,* 1021–1038.

Cale, E. M., & Lilienfeld, S. O. (2002). Sex differences in psychopathy and antisocial personality disorder: A review and integration. *Clinical Psychology Review, 22,* 1179–1207.

Catchpole, R. E. H., & Gretton, H. M. (2003). The predictive validity of risk assessment with violent young offenders. *Criminal Justice and Behavior, 30,* 688–708.

Christian, R. E., Frick, P. J., Hill, N. L., Tyler, L., & Frazer, D. R. (1997). Psychopathy and conduct problems in children: II. Implications for subtyping children with conduct problems. *Journal of the American Academy of Child and Adolescent Psychiatry, 36,* 233–241.

Cleckley, H. (1976). *The mask of sanity* (5th ed.). St. Louis, MO: Mosby. (Original work published 1941)

Cooke, D. J., Kosson, D. S., & Michie, C. (2001). Psychopathy and ethnicity: Structural, item, and test generalizability of the Psychopathy Checklist—Revised (PCL-R) in Caucasian and African American participants. *Psychological Assessment, 13,* 531–542.

Cooke, D. J., & Michie, C. (1999). Psychopathy across cultures: Scotland and North America compared. *Journal of Abnormal Psychology, 108,* 58–68.

Cooke, D. J., & Michie, C. (2001). Refining the construct of psychopathy: Towards a hierarchical model. *Psychological Assessment, 13,* 171–188.

Cooke, D. J., Michie, C., Hart, S. D., & Clark, D. A. (2004). Reconstructing psychopathy: Clarifying the significance of antisocial and socially deviant behavior in the diagnosis of psychopathic personality disorder. *Journal of Personality Disorders, 18,* 337–357.

Cornell, D. G., Warren, J., Hawk, G., Stafford, E., Oram, G., & Pine, D. (1996). Psychopathy in instrumental and reactive violent offenders. *Journal of Consulting and Clinical Psychology, 64,* 783–790.

Corrado, R. R., Vincent, G. M., Hart, S. D., & Cohen, I. M. (2004). Predictive validity of the Psychopathy Checklist: Youth Version for general and violent recidivism. *Behavioral Sciences and the Law, 22,* 5–22.

Crick, N. R., & Grotpeter, J. K. (1995). Relational aggression, gender, and social–psychological adjustment. *Child Development, 66,* 710–722.

Dempster, R. J., Hart, S. D., & Boer, D. P. (1997, August). *Psychopathy and violent criminal histories in male inmates.* Paper presented at the annual meeting of the American Psychological Association, Chicago.

Dernevik, M., Grann, M., & Johansson, S. (2002). Violent behaviour in forensic psychiatric patients: Risk assessment and different risk management levels using the HCR-20. *Psychology, Crime, and Law, 8,* 83–111.

Douglas, K. S., & Dutton, D. G. (2001). Assessing the link between stalking and domestic violence. *Aggression and Violent Behavior, 6,* 519–546.

Douglas, K. S., & Ogloff, J. R. P. (2003). Violence by psychiatric patients: The impact of archival measurement source on violence prevalence and risk assessment accuracy. *Canadian Journal of Psychiatry, 48,* 734–740.

Douglas, K. S., Ogloff, J. R. P., & Hart, S. D. (2003). Evaluation of a model of violence risk assessment among forensic psychiatric patients. *Psychiatric Services, 54,* 1372–1379.

Douglas, K. S., Ogloff, J. R. P., Nicholls, T. L., & Grant, I. (1999). Assessing risk for violence among psychiatric patients: The HCR-20 violence risk assessment scheme and the Psychopathy Checklist: Screening Version. *Journal of Consulting and Clinical Psychology, 67,* 917–930.

Douglas, K. S., Strand, S., Belfrage, H., Fransson, G., & Levander, S. (2005). Reliability and validity evaluation of the Psychopathy Checklist: Screening Version (PCL:SV) in Swedish correctional and forensic psychiatric samples. *Assessment, 12,* 145–161.

Douglas, K. S., & Skeem, J. L. (in press). Violence risk assessment: Getting specific about being dynamic. *Psychology, Public Policy, and Law.*

Douglas, K. S., & Webster, C. D. (1999). Predicting violence in mentally and personality disordered individuals. In R. Roesch, S. D. Hart, & J. R. P. Ogloff (Eds.), *Psychology and law: The state of the discipline* (pp. 175–239). New York: Plenum Press.

Douglas, K. S., Yeomans, M., & Boer, D. P. (in press). Comparative validity analysis of multiple measures of violence risk in a general population sample of criminal offenders. *Criminal Justice and Behavior.*

Doyle, M., Dolan, M., & McGovern, J. (2002). The validity of North American risk assessment tools in predicting in-patient violent behaviour in England. *Legal and Criminological Psychology, 7,* 141–154.

Edens, J. F., Buffington-Vollum, J. K., Keilen, A., Roskamp, P., & Anthony, C. (2005). Predictions of future dangerousness in capital murder trials: Is it time to "disinvent the wheel"? *Law and Human Behavior, 29,* 55–86.

Edens, J. F., Hart, S. D., Johnson, D. W., Johnson, J., & Olver, M. E. (2000). Use of the Personality Assessment Inventory to assess psychopathy in offender populations. *Psychological Assessment, 12,* 132–139.

Edens, J. F., Petrila, J., & Buffington-Vollum, J. K. (2001). Psychopathy and the death penalty: Can the Psychopathy Checklist—Revised identify offenders who represent "an ongoing threat to society"? *Journal of Psychiatry and the Law, 29,* 433–481.

Edens, J. F., Skeem, J. L., Cruise, K. R., & Cauffman, E. (2001). Assessment of "juvenile psychopathy" and its association with violence: A critical review. *Behavioral Sciences and the Law, 19,* 53–80.

Firestone, P., Bradford, J. M., Greenberg, D. M., & Serran, G. A. (2000). The relationship of deviant sexual arousal and psychopathy in incest offenders, extrafamilial child molesters, and rapists. *Journal of the American Academy of Psychiatry and the Law, 28,* 303–308.

Forth, A. E. (2005). Hare Psychopathy Checklist: Youth Version. In T. Grisso, G. Vincent, & D. Seagrave (Eds.), *Mental health screening and assessment in juvenile justice* (pp. 324–338). New York: Guilford Press.

Forth, A. E., Kosson, D. S., & Hare, R. D. (2003). *Hare Psychopathy Checklist: Youth Version.* Toronto, ON, Canada: Multi-Health Systems.

Fowles, D. (1980). The three arousal model: Implications for Gray's two-factor learning theory for heart rate, electrodermal activity, and psychopathy. *Psychophysiology, 17,* 87–104.

Gendreau, P., Goggin, C., & Smith, P. (2002). Is the PCL-R really the "unparalleled" measure of offender risk? A lesson in knowledge cumulation. *Criminal Justice and Behavior, 29,* 397–426.

Gendreau, P., Goggin, C., & Smith, P. (2003). Erratum. *Criminal Justice and Behavior, 30,* 722–724.

Gendreau, P., Little, T., & Goggin, C. (1996). A meta-analysis of the predictors of adult offender recidivism: What works! *Criminology, 34,* 575–607.

Grann, M., & Wedin, I. (2001). Risk factors for recidivism among spousal assault and spousal homicide offenders. *Psychology, Crime, and Law, 8,* 1–19.

Gray, J. (1987). *The psychology and fear and stress* (2nd ed.). Cambridge, UK: Cambridge University Press.

Gray, N. S., Snowden, R. J., MacCulloch, S., Phillips, H., Taylor, J., & MacCulloch, M. J. (2004). Relative efficacy of criminological, clinical, and personality measures of future risk of offending in mentally disordered offenders: A comparative study of HCR-20, PCL:SV, and OGRS. *Journal of Consulting and Clinical Psychology, 72,* 523–530.

Gretton, H. M., McBride, M., Hare, R. D., O'Shaughnessy, R., & Kumka, G. (2001). Psychopathy and recidivism in adolescent sex offenders. *Criminal Justice and Behavior, 28,* 427–449.

Guy, L. S., Edens, J. F., Anthony, C., & Douglas, K. S. (in press). Does psychopathy predict institutional misconduct among adults? A meta-analytic investigation. *Journal of Consulting and Clinical Psychology.*

Hanson, R. K., & Harris, A. J. R. (2000). Where should we intervene? Dynamic predictors of sexual offense recidivism. *Criminal Justice and Behavior, 27,* 6–35.

Hare, R. D. (1991). *The Hare Psychopathy Checklist—Revised.* Toronto, ON, Canada: Multi-Health Systems.

Hare, R. D. (1998a). The Hare PCL-R: Some issues concerning its use and misuse. *Legal and Criminological Psychology, 3,* 101–122.

Hare, R. D. (1998b). Psychopaths and their nature: Implications for the mental health and criminal justice systems. In T. Millon, E. Simonson, M. Burket-Smith, & R. Davis (Eds.), *Psychopathy: Antisocial, criminal, and violent behavior* (pp.188–212). New York: Guilford Press.

Hare, R. D. (2003). *The Hare PCL-R* (2nd ed.). Toronto, ON, Canada: Multi-Health Systems.

Hare, R. D., Clark, D., Grann, M., & Thornton, D. (2000). Psychopathy and the predictive validity of the PCL-R: An international perspective. *Behavioral Sciences and the Law, 18,* 623–645.

Hare, R. D., Forth, A. E., & Strachan, K. E. (1992). Psychopathy and crime across the life span. In R. D. Peters & R. J. McMahan (Eds.), *Aggression and violence throughout the life span* (pp. 285–300). Thousand Oaks, CA: Sage.

Harpur, T. J., & Hare, R. D. (1994). The assessment of psychopathy as a function of age. *Journal of Abnormal Psychology, 103,* 604–609.

Harpur, T. J., Hare, R. D., & Hakstian, A. R. (1989). Two-factor conceptualization of psychopathy: Construct validity and assessment implications. *Psychological Assessment: A Journal of Consulting and Clinical Psychology, 1,* 6–17.

Harris, G. T., Rice, M. E., & Cormier, C. A. (1991). Psychopathy and violent recidivism. *Law and Human Behavior, 15,* 625–637.

Harris, G. T., Rice, M. E., & Quinsey, V. L. (1993). Violent recidivism of mentally disordered offenders: The development of a statistical prediction instrument. *Criminal Justice and Behavior, 20,* 315–335.

Hart, S. D. (1998). The role of psychopathy in assessing risk for violence: Conceptual and methodological issues. *Legal and Criminological Psychology, 3,* 121–137.

Hart, S. D., Cox, D. N., & Hare, R. D. (1995). *Manual for the Psychopathy Checklist: Screening Version (PCL:SV).* Toronto, ON, Canada: Multi-Health Systems.

Hart, S. D., & Hare, R. D. (1997). Psychopathy: Assessment and association with criminal conduct. In D. M. Stoff, J. Brieling, & J. Maser (Eds.), *Handbook of antisocial behavior* (pp. 22–35). New York: Wiley.

Hart, S. D., Kropp, P. R., & Hare, R. D. (1988). Performance of psychopaths following conditional release from prison. *Journal of Consulting and Clinical Psychology, 56,* 227–232.

Hart, S. D., Kropp, P. R., Laws, D. R., Klaver, J., Logan, C., & Watt, K. A. (2003). *The risk for sexual violence protocol.* Burnaby, BC, Canada: Simon Fraser University.

Hart, S. D., Watt, K. A., & Vincent, G. M. (2002). Commentary on Seagrave and Grisso: Impressions of the state of the art. *Law and Human Behavior, 26*(2), 241–245.

Heilbrun, K. (1997). Prediction versus management models relevant to risk assessment: The importance of legal decision-making context. *Law and Human Behavior, 21,* 347–359.

Heilbrun, K., Hart, S. D., Hare, R. D., Gustafson, D., Nunez, C., & White, A. (1998). Inpatient and post-discharge aggression in mentally disordered offenders: The role of psychopathy. *Journal of Interpersonal Violence, 13,* 514–527.

Hemphill, J. F., & Hare, R. D. (2004). Some misconceptions about the Hare PCL-R and risk assessment: A reply to Gendreau, Goggin, and Smith. *Criminal Justice and Behavior, 31,* 203–243.

Hemphill, J. F., Hare, R. D., & Wong, S. (1998). Psychopathy and recidivism: A review. *Legal and Criminological Psychology, 3,* 141–172.

Hemphill, J. F., & Hart, S. D. (2003). Forensic and clinical issues in the assessment of psychopathy. In I. B. Weiner (Series Ed.) & A. M. Goldstein (Vol. Ed.), *Comprehensive handbook of psychology: Vol. 11. Forensic psychology.* New York: Wiley.

Hemphill, J. F., Templeman, R., Wong, S., & Hare, R. D. (1998). Psychopathy and crime: Recidivism and behavior. In D. J. Cooke, A. E. Forth, & R. D. Hare (Eds.), *Psychopathy: Theory, research, and implications for society* (pp. 375–399). Dordrecht, The Netherlands: Kluwer.

Herrenkohl, T. I., Hawkins, J. D., Chung, I. J., Hill, K. G., & Battin-Pearson, S. (2001). School and community risk factors and interventions. In R. Loeber & D. P. Farringon (Eds.), *Child delinquents: Development, intervention, and service needs* (pp. 211–246). Thousand Oaks, CA: Sage.

Hervé, H., Vincent, G. M., Kropp, P. R., & Hare, R. D. (2001, April). *Psychopathy and spousal assault.* Paper presented at the 2001 founding conference of the International Association of Mental Health Services, Vancouver, BC.

Hicks, M. M., Rogers, R., & Cashel, M. (2000). Predictions of violent and total infractions among institutionalized male juvenile offenders. *Journal of the American Academy of Psychiatry and the Law, 28,* 183–190.

Hildebrand, M., de Ruiter, C., & de Vogel, V. (2004). Psychopathy and sexual deviance in treated rapists: Association with sexual and non-sexual recidivism. *Sexual Abuse: A Journal of Research and Treatment, 16,* 1–24.

Hilton, N. Z., Harris, G. T., & Rice, M. E. (2001). Predicting violence by serious wife assaulters. *Journal of Interpersonal Violence, 16,* 408–423.

Hunter, J. A., Figueredo, A. J., Malamuth, N. M., & Becker, J. V. (2003). Juvenile sex offenders: Toward the development of a typology. *Sex Abuse: Journal of Research and Treatment, 15,* 27–47.

Jackson, R. L., Rogers, R., Neumann, C. S., & Lambert, P. L. (2002). Psychopathy in female offenders: An investigation of its underlying dimensions. *Criminal Justice and Behavior, 29,* 692–704.

Karpman, B. (1941). On the need of separating psychopathy into two distinct clinical types: The symptomatic and the idiopathic. *Journal of Criminal Psychopathology, 3,* 112–137.

Kosson, D. S., Cyterski, T. D., Steuerwald, B. L., Neumann, C. S., & Walker-Matthews, S. (2002). The reliability and validity of the Psychopathy Checklist: Youth Version (PCL:YV) in nonincarcerated adolescent males. *Psychological Assessment, 14,* 97–109.

Kosson, D. S., Smith, S. S., & Newman, J. P. (1990). Evaluating the construct validity of psychopathy in black and white male inmates: Three preliminary studies. *Journal of Abnormal Psychology, 99,* 250–259.

Lahey, B .B., Loeber, R., Quay, H., Applegate, B., Shaffer, D., Waldman, I., et al. (1998). Validity of DSM-IV subtypes of conduct disorder based on age of onset. *Journal of the American Academy of Child and Adolescent Psychiatry, 37,* 435–442.

Långström, N., & Grann, M. (2000). Risk for criminal recidivism among young sex offenders. *Journal of Interpersonal Violence, 15,* 856–872.

Lilienfeld, S. O. (1994). Conceptual problems in the assessment of psychopathy. *Clinical Psychology Review, 14,* 17–38.

Lipsey, M. W., & Wilson, D. B. (2001). *Practical meta-analysis.* (Applied Social Research Methods Series, Vol. 49). Thousand Oaks, CA: Sage.

Loucks, A. D., & Zamble, E. (2000). Predictors of criminal behavior and prison misconduct in serious female offenders. *Empirical and Applied Criminal Justice Review* [Online], *1*(1), 1–47.

Lyon, D. R., Hart, S. D., & Webster, C. D. (2001). Violence risk assessment. In R. Schuller & J. R. P. Ogloff (Eds.), *Law and psychology: Canadian perspectives* (pp. 314–350). Toronto, ON, Canada: University of Toronto Press.

McNiel, D. E., Gregory, A. L., Lam, J. N., Binder, R. L., & Sullivan, G. R. (2003). Utility of decision support tools for assessing acute risk of violence. *Journal of Consulting and Clinical Psychology, 71,* 945–953.

Mealey, L. (1995). The sociobiology of sociopathy: An integrated evolutionary model. *Behavioral and Brain Sciences, 18,* 523–599. Reprinted in S. Baron-Cohen (Ed.). (1997). *The maladapted mind.* Hillsdale, NJ: Erlbaum/Taylor & Francis.

Meloy, J. R., & Gothard, S. (1995). Demographic and clinical comparison of obsessional followers and offenders with mental disorders. *American Journal of Psychiatry, 152,* 258–263.

Moffitt, T. E., & Caspi, A. (2001). Childhood predictors differentiate life-course persistent and adolescence-limited antisocial pathways among males and females. *Development and Psychopathology, 13,* 355–375.

Moltó, J., Poy, R., & Tourrubia, R. (2000). Standardization of the Hare Psychopathy Checklist—Revised in a Spanish prison sample. *Journal of Personality Disorder, 14,* 84–96.

Monahan, J. (1981). *Predicting violent behavior: An assessment of clinical techniques.* Beverly Hills, CA: Sage.

Monahan, J., & Steadman, H. J. (Eds.). (1994). *Violence and mental disorder: Developments in risk assessment.* Chicago: University of Chicago Press.

Monahan, J., Steadman, H. J., Silver, E., Appelbaum, P. S., Robbins, P. C., Mulvey, E. P., et al. (2001). *Rethinking risk assessment: The MacArthur study of mental disorder and violence.* New York: Oxford University Press.

Mulvey, E. P., Shaw, E., & Lidz, C. W. (1994). Why use multiple sources in research on patient violence in the community? *Criminal Behaviour and Mental Health, 4,* 253–258.

Newman, J. P., & Schmitt, W. (1998). Passive avoidance in psychopathic offenders: A replication and extension. *Journal of Abnormal Psychology, 107,* 527–532.

Nicholls, T. L., Ogloff, J. R. P., & Douglas, K. S. (2004). Assessing risk for violence among male and female civil psychiatric patients: The HCR-20, PCL:SV, and VSC. *Behavioral Sciences and the Law, 22*, 127–158.

Patrick, C. J., & Zempolich, K. A. (1998). Emotion and aggression in the psychopathic personality. *Aggression and Violent Behavior, 3*, 303–338.

Pithers, W. D., Gray, A., Busconi, A., & Houchens, P. (1998). Five empirically-derived subtypes of children with sexual behaviour problems: Characteristics potentially related to juvenile delinquency and adult criminality. *Irish Journal of Psychology, 19*, 49–67.

Porter, S. (1996). Without conscience or without active conscience? The etiology of psychopathy revisited. *Aggression and Violent Behavior, 1*, 179–189.

Porter, S., Birt A. R., & Boer, D. P. (2001). Investigation of the criminal and conditional release profiles of Canadian federal offenders as a function of psychopathy and age. *Law and Human Behavior, 25*, 647–661.

Porter, S., Fairweather, D., Drugge, J., Hervé, H., Birt, A., & Boer, D. P. (2000). Profiles of psychopathy in incarcerated sexual offenders. *Criminal Justice and Behavior, 27*, 216–233.

Quinsey, V. L., Harris, G. T., Rice, M. E., & Cormier, C. (1998). *Violent offenders: Appraising and managing risk*. Washington, DC: American Psychological Association.

Quinsey, V. L., Rice, M. E., & Harris, G. T. (1995). Actuarial prediction of sexual recidivism. *Journal of Interpersonal Violence, 10*, 85–105.

Reppucci, N. D., Fried, C. S., & Schmidt, M. G. (2002). Youth violence: Risk and protective factors. In R. R. Corrado, R. Roesch, S. D. Hart, & J. Gierowski (Eds.), *Multi-problem violent youth: A foundation for comparative research on needs, interventions, and outcomes* (pp. 3–22). Amsterdam: IOS Press.

Rice, M. E., & Harris, G. T. (1997). Cross-validation and extension of the Violence Risk Appraisal Guide for child molesters and rapists. *Law and Human Behavior, 21*, 231–241.

Richards, H. J., Casey, J. O., & Lucente, S. W. (2003). Psychopathy and treatment response in incarcerated female substance abusers. *Criminal Justice and Behavior, 30*, 251–276.

Ridenour, T. A., Marchant, G. J., & Dean, R. S. (2001). Is the revised psychopathy checklist clinically useful for adolescents? *Journal of Psychoeducational Assessment, 19*, 227–238.

Robins, L. N. (1978). Etiological implications in studies of childhood histories relating to antisocial personality. In R. D. Hare & D. Schalling (Eds.), *Psychopathic behavior: Approaches to research* (pp. 255–271). Chichester, UK: Wiley.

Robins, L. N., Tipp, J., & Przybeck, T. (1991). Psychiatric disorders in America. In L. N. Robins & D. A. Reiger (Eds.), *Antisocial personality disorder* (pp. 258–290). New York: Free Press.

Rosenfeld, B. (2004). Violence risk factors in stalking and obsessional harassment: A review and preliminary meta-analysis. *Criminal Justice and Behavior, 31*, 9–36.

Ross, D. J., Hart, S. D., & Webster, C. D. (1998). *Aggression in psychiatric patients: Using the HCR-20 to assess risk for violence in hospital and in the community*. Unpublished manuscript.

Salekin, R. T., Rogers, R., & Sewell, K. W. (1996). A review and meta-analysis of the Psychopathy Checklist and Psychopathy Checklist—Revised: Predictive validity of dangerousness. *Clinical Psychology: Science and Practice, 3*, 203–215.

Salekin, R., Rogers, R., Ustad, K. L., & Sewell, K. (1998). Psychopathy and recidivism among female inmates. *Law and Human Behavior, 22*, 109–128.

Sechrest, L. (1963). Incremental validity: A recommendation. *Educational and Psychological Measurement, 23*, 153–158.

Serin, R. C. (1991). Psychopathy and violence in criminals. *Journal of Interpersonal Violence, 6*, 423–431.

Serin, R. C. (1996). Violent recidivism in criminal psychopaths. *Law and Human Behavior, 20*, 207–217.

Serin, R. C., & Amos, N. L. (1995). The role of psychopathy in the assessment of dangerousness. *International Journal of Law and Psychiatry, 18*, 231–238.

Serin, R. C., Peters, R. D., & Barbaree, H. E. (1990). Predictors of psychopathy and release outcome in a criminal population. *Psychological Assessment: A Journal of Consulting and Clinical Psychology, 2*, 419–422.

Shah, S. A. (1978). Dangerousness and mental illness: Some conceptual, prediction, and policy dilemmas. In C. Frederick (Ed.), *Dangerous behavior: A problem in law and mental health* (pp. 153–191). Washington, DC: U.S. Government Printing Office.

Silverthorn, P., Frick, P. J., & Reynolds, R. (2001). Timing of onset and correlates of severe conduct problems in adjudicated girls and boys. *Journal of Psychopathology and Behavioral Assessment, 23*, 171–181.

Skeem, J. L., & Mulvey, E. P. (2001). Psychopathy and community violence among civil psychiatric patients: Results from the MacArthur Violence Risk Assessment study. *Journal of Consulting and Clinical Psychology, 69*, 358–374.

Skeem, J. L., Mulvey, E. P., & Grisso, T. (2003). Applicability of the traditional and revised models of psychopathy to the Psychopathy Checklist: Screening Version (PCL:SV). *Psychological Assessment, 15*, 41–55.

Skeem, J. L., Poythress, N., Edens, J. F., Lilienfeld, S. O., & Cale, E. M. (2003). Psychopathic personality or personalities? Exploring potential variants of psychopathy and their implications for risk assessment. *Aggression and Violent Behavior, 8*, 513–546.

Steadman, H. J., Monahan, J., Appelbaum, P. S., Grisso, T., Mulvey, E. P., Roth, L. H., et al. (1994). Designing a new generation of risk assessment research. In J. Monahan & H. J. Steadman (Eds.), *Violence and mental disorder: Developments in risk assessment* (pp. 297–318). Chicago: University of Chicago Press

Steadman, H. J., Silver, E., Monahan, J., Appelbaum, P. S., Clark Robbins, P., Mulvey, E. P., Grisso, T., et al. (2000). A classification tree approach to the development of actuarial violence risk assessment tools. *Law and Human Behavior, 24,* 83–100.

Strand, S., & Belfrage, H. (2001). Comparison of HCR-20 scores in violent mentally disordered men and women: Gender differences and similarities. *Psychology, Crime and Law, 7,* 71–79.

Strand, S., Belfrage, H., Fransson, G., & Levander, S. (1999). Clinical and risk management factors in risk prediction of mentally disordered offenders—more important than historical data? *Legal and Criminological Psychology, 4,* 67–76.

Tengström, A., Hodgins, S., Grann, M., Långström, N., & Kullgren, G. (2004). Schizophrenia and criminal offending: The role of psychopathy and substance use disorders. *Criminal Justice and Behavior, 31,* 367–391.

Toupin, J., Mercier, H., Déry, M., Côté, G., & Hodgins, S. (1996). Validity of the PCL-R for adolescents. In D. J. Cooke, A. E. Forth, J. P. Newman, & R. D. Hare (Eds.), *Issues in criminological and legal psychology: No. 24, International perspectives on psychopathy* (pp. 143–145). Leicester, UK: British Psychological Society.

U.S. Department of Health and Human Services. (2001). *Mental health: A report of the Surgeon General.* Rockville, MD: U.S. Department of Health and Human Services, Substance Abuse and Mental Health Services Administration, Center for Mental Health Services, National Institutes of Health, National Institute of Mental Health.

Vincent, G. M., Vitacco, M. J., Grisso, T., & Corrado, R. R. (2003). Subtypes of adolescent offenders: Affective traits and antisocial behavior patterns. *Behavioral Sciences and the Law, 21,* 695–712.

Vitacco, M. J., Neumann, C. S., & Jackson, R. L. (in press). Testing a four-factor model of psychopathy and its association with ethnicity, gender, intelligence, and violence. *Journal of Consulting and Clinical Psychology.*

Vitale, J. E., & Newman, J. P. (2001). Response perseveration in psychopathic women. *Journal of Abnormal Psychology, 110,* 644–647.

Vitale, J. E., Smith, S. S., Brinkley, C. A., & Newman, J. P. (2002). The reliability and validity of the Psychopathy Checklist—Revised in a sample of female offenders. *Criminal Justice and Behavior, 29,* 202–231.

Walters, G. D. (2003a). Predicting criminal justice outcomes with the Psychopathy Checklist and Lifestyle Criminality Screening Form: A meta-analytic comparison. *Behavioral Sciences and the Law, 21,* 89–102.

Walters, G. D. (2003b). Predicting institutional adjustment and recidivism with the Psychopathy Checklist factor scores: A meta-analysis. *Law and Human Behavior, 27,* 541–558.

Walters, G. D. (in press). Risk-appraisal versus self-report in the prediction of criminal justice outcomes: A meta-analysis. *Criminal Justice and Behavior.*

Walters, G. D., White, T. W., & Denney, D. (1991). The Lifestyle Criminality Screening Form: Preliminary data. *Criminal Justice and Behavior, 18,* 406–418.

Webster, C. D., Douglas, K. S., Eaves, D., & Hart, S. D. (1997). *HCR-20: Assessing Risk for Violence* (Version 2). Burnaby, BC, Canada: Mental Health, Law, and Policy Institute, Simon Fraser University.

Widiger, T. A., Cadoret, R., Hare, R. D., Robins, L., Rutherford, M., Zanarini, M., et al. (1996). DSM-IV antisocial personality disorder field trial. *Journal of Abnormal Psychology, 105,* 3–16.

Williamson, S. E., Hare, R. D., & Wong, S. (1987). Violence: Criminal psychopaths and their victims. *Canadian Journal of Behavioural Science, 19,* 454–462.

Wong, S. (1984). *Criminal and institutional behaviors of psychopaths.* Ottawa, ON, Canada: Programs Branch Users Report, Ministry of the Solicitor General of Canada.

28

Treatment of Psychopathy

A Review of Empirical Findings

GRANT T. HARRIS
MARNIE E. RICE

Can psychopaths be treated? In this chapter, we evaluate the empirical evidence on the treatment of psychopaths. We concentrate on treatment for criminal psychopaths and intervention strategies in which efforts to reduce criminal and violent behavior are at least part of the protocol. Without denying the importance of other psychopathic characteristics, criminal and violent behaviors are clearly the most important outcomes from a social policy perspective.

We do not discuss treatment for various types of psychopaths, although there has been considerable discussion about the clinical and theoretical significance of psychopathy subtypes. Prototypical (sometimes called primary) psychopaths present as callous and unemotional, whereas secondary psychopaths seem more emotionally labile, angry, or anxious (Poythress & Skeem, Chapter 9, this volume; Skeem, Poythress, Edens, Lilienfield, & Cale, 2002). It has been hypothesized that one form of psychopathy is primarily a heritable condition while another is due mainly to environmental influences, particularly abuse during childhood (Mealey, 1995). Whether the primary–secondary distinction maps onto the genetic–environmental distinction is unclear. Nevertheless, subtypes of psychopathy might require different therapies (Skeem, Poythress, et al., 2002). However, until there is more evidence that it matters to prognosis (criminal outcome, response to treatment), the existence of subtypes cannot have much relevance to treatment.

TREATMENT OF PSYCHOPATHIC OFFENDERS AND PSYCHOPATHIC FORENSIC PSYCHIATRIC PATIENTS

The clinical literature has been quite pessimistic about the outcome of therapy for psychopaths. Hervey Cleckley, in his several editions of *The Mask of Sanity* (1941, 1982), described psychopaths as neither benefiting from treatment nor capable of forming the emotional bonds required for effective therapy. In contrast, some early studies claimed positive effects of psychotherapy (Beacher, 1962; Corsini, 1958; Rodgers, 1947; Rosow, 1955; Schmideberg, 1949; Showstack, 1956; Szurek, 1942; Thorne, 1959). However, all these were uncontrolled case reports. Reviewers before 1990 concluded, as had Cleckley, that there was no evidence for the efficacy of treatment with adult psychopaths (Hare, 1970; McCord, 1982).

Therapeutic Communities

One of the most popular treatments for psychopathy has been the therapeutic community. Hare (1970) suggested that the reshaped social milieu of a therapeutic community might alter the basic personality characteristics and social behavior of psychopaths. Although lacking comparative data for untreated psychopaths, there were several early positive reports (Barker & Mason, 1968; Copas, O'Brien, Roberts, & Whiteley, 1984; Copas & Whiteley, 1976; Kiger, 1967). Based on these, Rice, Harris, and Cormier (1992) evaluated an intensive therapeutic community for mentally disordered offenders thought to be especially suitable for psychopaths. It operated for over a decade in a maximum security psychiatric hospital and drew worldwide attention for its novelty. The program was described at length by Barker and colleagues (e.g., Barker, 1980; Barker & Mason, 1968; Barker, Mason, & Wilson, 1969; Barker & McLaughlin, 1977) and elsewhere (Harris, Rice, & Cormier, 1994; Maier, 1976; Nielson, 2000; Weisman, 1995). Briefly, the program was based on one developed by Maxwell Jones (1956, 1968). It was largely peer operated and involved intensive group therapy for up to 80 hours per week. The goal was an environment that fostered empathy and responsibility for peers.

The evaluation (Rice et al., 1992) was quasi-experimental in which 146 treated offenders were matched with 146 untreated offenders on variables related to recidivism (age, criminal history, and index offense). Almost all offenders had a history of violent crime and were scored on the Psychopathy Checklist—Revised (PCL-R; Hare, 1991, 2003). Although the two groups were not explicitly matched on the PCL-R, the average score in each was 19. Because the PCL-R was scored using file information only, the cutoff score for classifying offenders as psychopaths was set at 25 rather than the customary 30. The results of a follow-up conducted an average of 10.5 years after completion of treatment showed that, compared to no program (in most cases, untreated offenders went to prison), treatment was associated with lower violent recidivism for nonpsychopaths but *higher* violent recidivism for psychopaths. Psychopaths showed poorer adjustment in terms of problem behaviors while in the program, even though they were just as likely as nonpsychopaths to achieve positions of trust and early recommendations for release.

Why did the therapeutic community program have such different effects on the two offender groups? We speculated that both the psychopaths and nonpsychopaths who participated in the program learned more about the feelings of others, taking others' perspective, using emotional language, behaving in socially skilled ways, and delaying gratification. For the nonpsychopaths, these new skills helped them behave in prosocial and noncriminal ways. For the psychopaths, however, the new skills emboldened them to manipulate and exploit others.

In another therapeutic community, Ogloff, Wong, and Greenwood (1990) reported on the behavior of psychopaths and nonpsychopaths defined by criteria outlined in an early version of the Psychopathy Checklist (Hare & Frazelle, 1985). Compared to nonpsychopaths, psychopaths showed less motivation, were discharged earlier (usually because of lack of motivation or security concerns), and showed less improvement. Similar results were reported for a therapeutic community in England's Grendon prison in (Hobson, Shine, & Roberts, 2000), where poor adjustment to the program was likewise associated with higher PCL-R scores. A recent study of a therapeutic community for female substance abusers (Richards, Casey, & Lucente, 2003) reported that, although none of the offenders scored over 30 on the PCL-R, higher psychopathy scores were nevertheless associated with poorer treatment response indicated by failing to remain in the program, rule violations, avoiding urine tests, and sporadic attendance.

Despite evidence that therapeutic communities are ineffective with psychopaths, they remain popular in prisons, secure hospitals, and other institutions in Europe in which some participants are likely to be psychopaths (Dolan, 1998; McMurran, Egan, & Ahmadi, 1998; Reiss, Meux, & Grubin, 2000). Even in North America, therapeutic communities are advocated for people with substance abuse problems (e.g., Knight, Simpson, & Miller, 1999; Wexler, Melnick, Lowe, & Peters, 1999), some of whom are likely to be psychopaths. Few studies of therapeutic communities outside North America, and only one for substance abusers (Richards et al., 2003), have used PCL measures that would allow estimating the prevalence of psychopathy.

Other Treatment Approaches

Besides therapeutic communities, cognitive-behavioral therapy is often recommended for psychopathic offenders. Andrews and Bonta (1994), Brown and Gutsch (1985), Serin and Kurychik (1994), and Wong and Hare (2005) all suggested that intensive cognitive-behavioral programs targeting "criminogenic needs" (i.e., personal characteristics correlated with recidivism) might be effective. For example, Wong and Hare recommended relapse prevention in combination with cognitive-behavioral programs. However, doubts as to the efficacy of this treatment with psychopaths arose from an evaluation of a cognitive-behavioral and relapse prevention program for sex offenders conducted by Seto and Barbaree (1999). High psychopathy offenders who were rated as having shown the most improvement (as measured by conduct during the treatment sessions, quality of homework, and therapists' ratings of motivation and change) were more likely to reoffend than other participants, particularly in violent ways. The treatment followed the principles of good correctional treatment (Andrews & Bonta, 1994; Andrews et al., 1990): It was highly structured and cognitive-behavioral, best matching the learning style of most offenders, including psychopaths. Moreover, psychopaths are high-risk offenders with many criminogenic needs (Zinger & Forth, 1998), and thus the program targeted deviant sexual preferences and antisocial attitudes (Barbaree, Peacock, Cortini, Marshall, & Seto, 1998). In view of these features, the results pertaining to psychopaths are especially notable.

Further doubts regarding the efficacy of cognitive-behavioral treatment for psychopaths emerge from other outcome studies. Among participants in a program for mentally disordered offenders in a secure psychiatric hospital, Hughes, Hogue, Hollin, and Champion (1997) found that PCL-R score was inversely correlated with therapeutic gain, even though patients with PCL-R

scores over 30 were excluded. In another study, Hare, Clark, Grann, and Thornton (2000) evaluated cognitive-behavioral prison programs for psychopathic and nonpsychopathic offenders. After short-term anger management and social skills training, 24-month reconviction rates for 278 treated and untreated offenders yielded an interaction between psychopathy and treatment outcome similar to that reported by Rice and colleagues (1992). Whereas the program had no demonstrable effect on nonpsychopaths, treated offenders who scored high on Factor 1 of the PCL-R had significantly higher rates of recidivism than high-scoring but untreated offenders.

In short, the few available empirical results regarding the effectiveness of treatment with psychopathic offenders are dismal, leading some to suggest that one should discuss management rather than treatment for psychopathic offenders (see Lösel, 1998). It may be that the very highest-risk offenders (i.e., psychopaths) might not be treatable even with very intensive and carefully designed and implemented programs. Of even more concern, perhaps, is the possibility that programs that might be beneficial for other offenders actually increase the risk represented by psychopaths.

Meta-Analysis of Research on the Treatment of Psychopathy

Traditionally, in a review of the evidence pertaining to a particular question, commentators summarize studies and derive an informal summary of the state of knowledge. This summary is usually accompanied by speculation about possible sources of apparent conflict in findings across studies. However, a more systematic way to resolve apparent inconsistencies in research findings is to use meta-analysis. This statistical approach allows the combination of research results from many studies, permitting conclusions about the likelihood that a group difference or relationship exists, how large it is, and why some studies find it and others do not. Research on the treatment of psychopathic offenders might seem particularly fruitful for meta-analysis because studies in this area often use small samples, such that effects might go undetected due to low statistical power. Studies also differ in the measures of psychopathy, kinds of treatment provided, criteria by which candidates are assigned to treatments, and procedures used to evaluate outcomes. Meta-analysis offers a solution to the problem of small sample sizes in individual studies, as well as a methodology for testing hypotheses about the sources of differences in findings across studies.

Of course, meta-analysis cannot overcome general deficits. For example, if very few studies of psychopathy treatment used the PCL-R, meta-analysis could not examine it in moderating treatment effects. A meta-analysis also cannot make up for methodological inadequacies in the literature as a whole. For example, one of the most serious problems in this literature is the scarcity of well-controlled studies, especially those using random assignment. By contrast, there is an increasing trend toward evidence-based medicine in the treatment of physical and mental health problems in general, which has resulted in the Cochrane Database of systematic reviews—a collection of methodologically adequate studies on various diseases and conditions (www.update-software.con/cochrane/). Studies using random assignment are heavily weighted in this database and few other designs are considered strong enough to be informative.

A good illustration of the limitations of meta-analysis was afforded by a recent meta-analysis of research findings on the treatment of psychopathy (Salekin, 2002).[1] Salekin provided a quantitative review of 42 studies he identified as having evaluated the effectiveness of some form of therapy for psychopaths. Salekin reported that the mean rate of successful intervention across all treatment studies was .62, $p < .01$. This was the proportion of treatment candidates judged to have "improved"[2] minus the proportion expected to have improved without treatment (the latter proportion was calculated, according to the author, by averaging the improvement of untreated subjects in eight studies identified as including comparison or control groups). Salekin concluded that the prevailing pessimism about the treatment of psychopaths was unfounded.

Several aspects of this meta-analysis are noteworthy: The mean intensity of treatment was approximately four sessions per week over a year; only four studies employed the Hare PCL-R; only eight studies included comparison subjects[3]; few studies (< 20%) assessed outcome in terms of criminal behavior, and even fewer (< 10%) mentioned violence or aggression; the most effective treatment was found to be psychodrama; and the evaluation of effectiveness was most often (> 70%) based on therapists' impressions. In an effort to improve the rigor of studies without control groups, Salekin stated that he used averaged data from the "controlled" studies to estimate an effect of nontreatment for all studies. However, for reasons articulated later, we consider this method of calculating the improvement of control subjects to be problematic.

Our opinion, based on a variety of considerations, is that no firm conclusions can be drawn from this meta-analysis. In particular, we maintain that only controlled studies can be informative regarding treatment efficacy, and no conclusions can be drawn from uncontrolled studies. Because we consider control groups to be essential, we turn our attention first to the eight studies Salekin identified as controlled. We begin with Rice and colleagues (1992), which was discussed at some length earlier in this chapter, and then consider each of the other seven studies in turn. Rice and colleagues reported that 78% of the treated psychopaths committed a new violent offense during the follow-up compared to 55% of untreated psychopaths. Salekin's summary of Rice and colleagues stated that 22% of the psychopaths "benefited" from treatment compared to 20% who would have "benefited" without the program, for a net benefit of 2%. Salekin considered that psychopaths who did not violently reoffend during the follow-up "benefited" from treatment even though untreated psychopaths exhibited less violent recidivism. The 20% figure was the weighted average proportion of psychopaths he calculated as having improved without treatment from the eight studies considered to be controlled. For each study in the meta-analysis, he subtracted this 20% figure from the percentage he considered to have benefited from treatment to compute net benefit. We believe the Rice and colleagues study shows why this method is problematic.

Craft, Stephenson, and Granger (1964) compared 50 severely delinquent boys alternately assigned to either a group psychotherapy unit or an "authoritarian" unit. No accepted measure of psychopathy was used.

The former program was new and incorporated many components of Jones's therapeutic community. In the latter, "authoritarian" program, patients were told on admission that "noise and disarray would not be tolerated and peace and quiet would be enforced by putting offenders to bed, fines, [and] deprivation of privileges . . . [combined with] "superficial psychotherapy" (p. 546). It was described as "standard" treatment at the time (1958). The authors had clearly expected that group psychotherapy would emerge as the superior program, but the results favored the authoritarian program. Significantly fewer offenses were committed by boys from that program in the follow-up period than by boys from the group psychotherapy program. Psychological test results also clearly favored the authoritarian program. The authors concluded that no conclusions could be drawn about the effectiveness of either treatment, as there was no untreated control group. They stressed that their study yielded no evidence to support the prevalent view among therapists that psychotherapy was more effective than standard treatment.

Salekin categorized this study as containing two treated groups—"therapeutic community" (the group psychotherapy program) and "cognitive-behavioral" (the authoritarian regime). The term "cognitive-behavioral" did not appear in the original study and cognitive-behavioral therapy was not developed until approximately a decade after this study was completed (Friedman, 1970). Salekin reported that this study showed positive results for both programs because 63% benefited (i.e., had no convictions in the follow-up) from the cognitive-behavioral program, and 43% benefited from the therapeutic community program. However, a different interpretation was given by the study's original authors: "Both treatments may have been better than nothing; both . . . may have worsened the boys—we do not know" (Craft et al., 1964, p. 553). We think a fairer interpretation is that this study yielded results similar to those of Rice and colleagues (1992), inasmuch as the therapeutic community increased recidivism relative to a standard, more custodial, approach.

Ingram, Gerard, Quay, and Levinson (1970) compared 20 juvenile delinquents treated in an "action-oriented" program

with 41 youths admitted either before the program began or after it ended. All were categorized as psychopathic according to an instrument developed by one of the authors. Treated youths had fewer assaultive offenses during the program (.25 per youth) compared to controls (.50 per youth), although the difference was nonsignificant. None of the treated youths were reported to have made a negative institutional adjustment after transfer to another institution, compared to 21% of controls. Salekin reported this study as demonstrating that 75% of treatment participants had benefited in terms of reduction of institutional aggression, and 100% had benefited in terms of improvement in community adjustment.

Korey (1944) studied delinquent boys in a training school. No objective measure of psychopathy was used, although all participants were diagnosed as "constitutional psychopathic inferiors" with "severe delinquent and behavior problems" (p. 127). Seven boys (the experimental group) received benzedine sulfate, and five boys (the controls) received a placebo. Outcome was measured by therapist opinion regarding improvement in various aspects of institutional adjustment. Significantly more ($N = 4$) boys given the drug were judged to have improved than boys given placebo (none of whom were judged to have improved). Korey cautioned that benzedine left the boys' underlying personalities untouched and that it should be part of a more comprehensive treatment. Salekin reported that 57% of the treated boys in this study benefited.

Maas (1966) studied 46 adult female offenders classified as unsocialized on Gough's socialization continuum. Half were assigned to group therapy emphasizing psychodrama, and the others were assigned to an untreated control group. The outcome measure was self-reported ego identity. No actual data were presented indicating how many offenders improved, but the authors stated that there was a significant difference in favor of the psychodrama group. Salekin summarized this study, stating that 63% of the treated subjects improved.

Persons (1965) compared 12 inmates randomly assigned to treatment with 40 inmates randomly assigned to no treatment. Treatment was eclectic counseling twice a week for 10 weeks. All 52 inmates were psychopaths according to a self-report questionnaire. Self-report and therapist ratings showed significantly more improvement for treated offenders. Treated offenders also had significantly fewer disciplinary reports over the 10 program weeks. Salekin reported that 92% of the treated inmates benefited, although (as is the case with the Maas study described previously) it is unclear how this figure was obtained, as no such data were in the original article.

Skolnick and Zuckerman (1979) compared 59 male drug abusers treated in a therapeutic community with 37 untreated male drug abusers of similar IQ who spent an equivalent period in prison. The article neither mentions psychopathy nor how many subjects were classified as psychopaths. The main outcome variables were changes on Minnesota Multiphasic Personality Inventory (MMPI) scales and three other self-report personality measures administered upon admission and again 6 to 8 months later. Although treated subjects decreased significantly more than controls on several measures of psychopathology, Salekin reported a negative effect of treatment in this study, presumably because the number of treated subjects who had 49 or 94 high peak codes on the MMPI increased significantly, whereas there was no increase in the comparison group. The authors pointed out that the increase in treatment participants with 49 or 94 high peak codes was due to decreases in the other scales rather than the result of an absolute increase in four and nine scale scores.

Finally, Woody, McLellan, Luborsky, and O'Brien (1985) studied 30 opium-dependent men diagnosed with personality disorder. Some (N = 17) had an additional diagnosis of depression. Some received drug counseling alone while others received counseling plus professional psychotherapy. The outcome variable was change in problem severity measured before and after treatment via structured clinical interviews. Some positive changes were reported for the depressed men, but the other men "showed little evidence of improvement" (Woody et al., 1985, p. 1064). No comparison of the two treatments was reported, and it is unclear how Salekin could have considered this a controlled study. Nevertheless, he reported that

80% of the treated men benefited from treatment.

One study in Salekin's meta-analysis was not classified as controlled, but we believe it should have been. Miles (1969) compared 40 male adolescents admitted to a therapeutic community with 20 control patients in the same hospital (described as a "psychiatric hospital for the subnormal," p. 23) who were not offered the therapeutic community. The two patient groups were similar on age, IQ, and social class. Although Cleckley's work is cited, no mention is made of how many patients were psychopaths. Sociometry was used to measure outcome, and there was a net improvement in acceptance in 70% of the therapeutic community subjects compared to 10% of the comparison subjects. The authors concluded that the therapeutic community "increased the ability of the patients to accept their fellows more than did the traditional treatment" (p. 35). Salekin reported that the therapeutic community benefited 65% of the patients on measures that included "improved empathy," although the authors stressed that they used no measure of empathy.

How can we summarize these "controlled" studies of treatment outcome? We note that only one study (Rice et al., 1992) used the PCL-R, which is the contemporary standard (and most empirically valid) measure of psychopathy. Only two employed objective measures of criminal recidivism (Craft et al., 1964; Rice et al., 1992). Interestingly, our interpretation of both of these is that the treated group exhibited higher rates of recidivism than the control group. Our reading of the "controlled" studies in the Salekin meta-analysis is that there is absolutely no basis for optimism regarding treatment to reduce the risk of criminal or violent recidivism.

Other problematic aspects of the meta-analysis cast further doubt on the author's optimistic conclusion. As mentioned earlier, most studies in the meta-analysis relied on therapists' ratings to measure outcome. We consider this inadequate, especially for psychopaths. Note that Seto and Barbaree (1999) examined the recidivism of sex offenders as a function of psychopathy and progress in treatment, with progress assessed via eight structured therapist ratings. Based on these ratings, which showed good interrater agreement and were undoubtedly more reliable than unstructured impressions of therapeutic progress, those offenders with better than average progress were more likely to recidivate violently, and this was especially true for psychopaths. In our opinion, therapists' impressions of clinical progress cannot be defended as an index of treatment effectiveness for offenders, especially psychopaths. Independently measured criminal conduct must be at least part of the outcome for an evaluation of treatment for psychopaths. This requirement eliminates all but a handful of the studies in the Salekin meta-analysis.

Several other categorizations in the Salekin meta-analysis were problematic. For example, Salekin categorized a study by Glaus (1968) as involving cognitive-behavioral therapy, with three psychopaths (defined by Cleckley's criteria) all reported to have improved as a function of the therapy. Compared to the 20% Salekin estimated would have improved without treatment, this was reported as a net treatment benefit of 80%. However, a careful reading of Glaus reveals that the author reported on the history and follow-up of 1,000 criminal psychopaths, of which 31 were "fully recovered and socialized" (p. 30). Glaus reported that many more might have improved, but he was unable to find more information (presumably despite follow-up efforts). Glaus described the three aforementioned positive-outcome cases in detail but made no claim that these were representative. Cleckley's criteria were never mentioned, nor was cognitive-behavioral therapy (which was only in its infancy in 1968; see Friedman, 1970); the therapy provided was so briefly described that it is impossible to categorize it. The journal editor noted that "the percentage of favorable results observed is low (over 3 percent), but the author's standards of follow-up and cure are unusually high" (p. 35). There is a huge discrepancy between the original author's report of just above 3% benefit and Salekin's report of 100%. In sum, close scrutiny of the studies in the Salekin (2002) meta-analysis reveals a variety of methodological weaknesses that cast serious doubt on its salutary conclusions. Most important, we think more random as-

signment treatment studies are required before meta-analysis can be informative.

Treatment for Nonforensic Psychopaths

Few studies reviewed by Salekin (2002) included offenders or forensic patients. Even if one could overlook the methodological weaknesses of the meta-analysis and studies included therein and accept its conclusions, it cannot tell us much about the population of primary interest—psychopathic offenders. Nonetheless, to be complete, we describe here findings from a recent evaluation of treatment for nonforensic "potentially psychopathic" patients (Skeem, Monahan, & Mulvey, 2002) not available at the time of the Salekin meta-analysis. Data from the MacArthur Risk Assessment Study were used to examine the interrelationships among psychopathy (assessed by the PCL-SV), self-reported involvement in treatment (mostly unspecified verbal therapy with or without drugs), and serious subsequent violence (almost all of which was undetected by the criminal justice system). The MacArthur methodology entailed interviews conducted every 10 weeks over a period of 1 year during which released civil psychiatric patients were asked about their involvement with treatment and violent behavior in the preceding period. Skeem and colleagues examined the relationship between violence in each target period and self-reported treatment in the previous period. They concluded that, in the first 10 postdischarge weeks, potentially psychopathic patients (> 12 on the PCL: Screening Version [PCL:SV]) who participated in more than 6 sessions of therapy (with an average of 11) exhibited less subsequent violence than those who participated in fewer sessions (the average was 3).

Recognizing that treatment was not assigned at random, the authors attempted to compensate by deriving a multivariate "propensity for treatment score" based on nine variables associated with the likelihood that subjects would report they had attended more treatment. This score was used as covariate in the aforementioned analysis. The inclusion of the "propensity score" attenuated the apparent treatment effect, but it remained statistically significant. While acknowledging several limitations of this study,

Skeem and colleagues (2002) inferred that the results provided evidence of an effect of mental health treatment as usual on reducing the violence associated with psychopathy, thus supporting the conclusions of Salekin's (2002) meta-analysis.

In our view, several methodological problems compromise the conclusions of this study regarding the effectiveness of treatment for psychopaths, despite efforts to correct for nonrandom assignment. First, psychopathy, treatment involvement, and violence were all assessed in the same interviews, leaving open the possibility of unintended measurement bias in all three constructs. A second issue concerns the number of bivariate comparisons performed in seeking evidence of a treatment effect. Skeem and colleagues reported 10 bivariate comparisons (two cutoff scores for psychopathy by four time periods, plus the entire follow-up period, presumably), only one of which yielded a statistically significant ($p < .10$) result[4] after the incorporation of the "propensity" covariate. One significant result in 10 is exactly as anticipated by chance alone.

Moreover, Skeem and colleagues' (2002) use of a "treatment propensity" covariate is questionable in its own right. Miller and Chapman (2001) critiqued the use of covariance analysis on the grounds that it capitalizes on regression to the mean, and they asserted that its use as a method to equate nonrandomly assigned groups was inappropriate. They did acknowledge that a *propensity score* approach (Rosenbaum & Rubin, 1984) might be of assistance but noted that it could not address unobserved differences between groups. Skeem and colleagues cited Rubin (1997) as a source for "propensity" analysis, but did not employ a key aspect of the method, which involves disaggregating the subjects into subgroups defined by the propensity variable or function.

In our view, the Skeem and colleagues (2002) study probably exhibits "creaming intervention selection bias" (Larzelere, Kuhn, & Johnson, 2004), whereby patients of lower risk are more likely to receive treatment. Moreover, even if one accepts its findings, there are other concerns. Skeem and colleagues acknowledged that the civil patients scoring over 12 on the PCL:SV were only "potentially" psychopathic. The study provided no information about effective components of treatment, and the conclusion that a dozen hours of unspecified therapy reduced serious violence by psychopaths seems highly questionable. We conclude that this study offers little guidance to those wondering about the efficacy of treatment for psychopathy or what therapy is indicated.

ALTERNATIVE CONCLUSIONS REGARDING THE EFFECTS OF TREATMENT

Given that it is such a serious and long-recognized problem, it is surprising that there has been so little good evaluation research on the treatment of psychopathy. Considering the available treatment literature, several alternative conclusions might be entertained:

- *Alternative Conclusion 1.* There have already been satisfactory demonstrations of effective treatment(s) for psychopaths (i.e., therapy that causes decreases in criminal and violent behavior), and the appropriate course is to provide such treatment(s) with intensity and integrity to as many psychopaths as possible. From this perspective, pressing research questions would pertain to the investigation of the conditions that ensure the successful export and adoption of such treatment(s) throughout the world's criminal justice systems, and modifications required to apply such treatment to noncriminal and youthful psychopaths.
- *Alternative Conclusion 2.* There have not been any satisfactory demonstrations, but only because adequate and persuasive evaluation work has yet to be done. Effective interventions for psychopaths have already been discovered and applied; it is the persuasive demonstrations that are lacking. For example, psychopathic offenders benefit from treatments already shown to be effective for offenders in general, but they require unusually high doses and intensities of such treatments in order for them to be effective. From this perspective, the obvious research priority is for rigorous and persuasive empirical demonstrations of the effectiveness of available treatments with psychopaths (with the next step being broader dissemination; viz. Alternative Conclusion 1).
- *Alternative Conclusion 3.* There have

been no satisfactory demonstrations because an effective clinical intervention is lacking. Psychopaths are fundamentally different even from other serious offenders, so that—despite available knowledge of what methods are effective for getting nonpsychopathic offenders to desist—no effective interventions yet exist for psychopaths. Indeed, some treatments that are effective for nonpsychopaths actually increase the risk of represented by psychopaths. Furthermore, the fact that psychopaths and nonpsychopaths are mixed together in most studies is the main reason why it has been so difficult to demonstrate effective treatment for adult offenders overall (i.e., positive treatment effects for nonpsychopaths are diluted or even negated by null or negative effects for the psychopaths). From this perspective, detailed analysis of the characteristics of psychopaths (inside and outside the laboratory) is needed to inform the design of new and effective interventions tailored to this unique population.

• *Alternative Conclusion 4.* No clinical intervention will ever be effective. Psychopaths are qualitatively different from other offenders but do not have deficits or impairment in any standard clinical sense. From this standpoint, the entire clinical enterprise is fundamentally unsuited to interventions to reduce the harm perpetrated by psychopaths. All that can be hoped for is a set of strategies to limit the harm by psychopaths by constraining their activities and opportunities.

It should be noted that these alternatives are not entirely mutually exclusive. For example, even if one concluded that a dozen sessions of mental health service as usual (Skeem et al., 2002) had actually reduced psychopathic violence (Alternative Conclusion 1), one would be unable specify the operative elements of that treatment, which would necessitate following the implications of Alternative Conclusion 2. Similarly, the enterprise that follows from Alternative Conclusion 3 of finding new therapies founded on an examination of the fundamental features of psychopathy could still be worthwhile even if some effective treatments had already been discovered. However, to the extent that one accepts Alternative Conclusions 1 or 2, one would probably assign lower priority to this task of developing new therapies.

In the final analysis, we adopt a blend of Alternative Conclusions 3 and 4. We believe, as outlined in Alternative Conclusion 4 (and explained further later), that the available evidence implies that psychopaths do not have deficits in the biological or medical sense. We propose that findings from outside the literature on treating psychopathy warrant serious consideration in designing interventions for psychopaths. We believe the evidence favors applying behavioral principles to reducing the harm occasioned by psychopathy. Our belief is based partly on empirical evidence that this approach has worked with some offender and violent populations (although effectiveness with psychopaths remains to be demonstrated). Our belief in the value of behavioral strategies for treating psychopaths also reflects a theoretical perspective that views psychopathy as a nonpathological condition, a reproductively viable life strategy. Next, we outline our evolutionary perspective on psychopathy to highlight implications for interventions.

A NONPATHOLOGICAL, SELECTIONIST ACCOUNT OF PSYCHOPATHY

There is evidence that psychopathy, unlike many psychological constructs, is underlain by a natural discontinuity or taxon (Ayers, 2000; Harris, Rice, & Quinsey, 1994, Haslam, 2003; Skilling, Harris, Rice, & Quinsey, 2002; Skilling, Quinsey, & Craig, 2001). By this view, scores on the best measure of psychopathy, the PCL-R, appear continuous because the identification of indicators and scoring are imperfect. Perfect measurement would, in theory, reveal just two possibilities—an individual either is or is not a true psychopath. Although not unanimous (Marcus, John, & Edens, 2004), the evidence supports the idea that psychopathy is a taxon.

The evidence on taxonicity, our research on treatment and the prediction of recidivism (Harris & Rice, in press; Harris, Rice, & Cormier, 1991; Rice & Harris, 1995) all suggest to us that psychopathy exists because it was a reproductively viable life strategy during human evolution. Adaptations (including those with psychological effects) were selected because they increased inclusive fitness in ancestral environments. For example, being in a cohesive, mutually supportive ("reciprocally altruistic") group was adaptive and heritable inclinations favoring group solidarity and adherence to rules have been associated with human reproductive success (Dawkins, 1978; Ridley, 1997). However, we (Harris, Skilling, & Rice, 2001; see also Mealey, 1995; Seto & Quinsey, Chapter 30, this volume) hypothesize that such a general strategy created a niche for an alternative cheating (i.e., psychopathic) strategy. When effective, this strategy is especially selfish, callous, manipulative, and lacking in empathy. If many people were cheaters, however, the strategy would lose its effectiveness due to the difficulty finding cooperators to exploit and the increased vigilance of remaining cooperators. Thus, the two strategies are expected to be frequency dependent, with cheating/psychopathy at low prevalence.

We hypothesize that high mating effort (i.e., promiscuous sexual behavior and many short-term marital relationships), and especially the willingness to employ deception and coercion, glibness, and charm, were (and are) also part of the psychopathic life strategy. Belsky, Steinberg, and Draper (1991) argued that a high mating effort life strategy is characterized by insecure attachment to parents and childhood behavior problems, followed by early puberty and precocious sexual behavior, and then unstable adult pair bonding and low parental investment. Psychopathy, we suggest, represents a genetically determined life strategy that has been maintained in the population through its relationship with reproductive success (Barr & Quinsey, 2004; Harris, Skilling, & Rice, 2001; Lalumière, Harris, Quinsey, & Rice, 2005; Rice, 1997).

The evidence on the neurocognitive characteristics of psychopaths (reviewed in this volume) reveals the condition to be an enduring set of traits that can be conceived of as aspects of personality or as differences in the form, manner, and relative speed of processing information. Key for this selectionist account is that these traits endure from situation to situation across the lifespan. Situations vary in the degree to which they differentiate between psychopaths and nonpsychopaths, but, by this account, reinforcement and punishment operate for psycho-paths as they do for everyone else, although what constitute reinforcers and punishers might differ.

Because psychopathy exhibits substantial heritability (reviewed in Waldman & Rhee, Chapter 11, this volume), the most straightforward and parsimonious version of the evolutionary account is that psychopaths have executed a "healthy" (in the biomedical[5] but not moral sense) obligate strategy. Subtle neuroanatomical and neurochemical differences (without gross lesions) are consistent with this hypothesis. As well, it is expected that special tests would reveal that psychopaths act relatively impulsively, fearlessly, and unempathically and are resistant to punishment under some laboratory conditions but are not grossly disadvantaged. Psychopathy should also be associated with enhanced performance on some tasks. This account of psychopathy is consistent with the observation that it is peculiar for disorders to enhance any ability (such as conning and manipulation, Blair, personal communication, May 2000).

We have tested this account by examining several indicators of neurodevelopmental problems associated with psychiatric disorders (obstetrical and perinatal problems, medical problems in infancy, learning disability, etc.) and found them to be related to violent crime but unrelated or inversely related to violent offenders' PCL-R scores (Harris, Rice, & Lalumière, 2001; Lalumière, Harris, & Rice, 2001). Although each of neurodevelopmental problems and psychopathy were associated with having had antisocial, negligent, and abusive parents, each appeared to be an independent cause of violent crime. Nonpsychopathic offenders exhibited more fluctuating asymmetry (an index of biomedical health) than psychopaths who themselves were not different from healthy volunteers (Lalumière et al., 2001). Finally, among sex offenders, those who preferentially target "reproductively viable" victims (i.e., postpubertal females) have significantly higher PCL-R scores than those who target all other classes of people (Harris, Hilton, Lalumière, Quinsey, & Rice, 2004). We are unaware of another hypothesis about sex offenders or psychopathy that accounts for this widely known difference.

Thus, there might be two distinct paths to serious, chronic criminality—one associated with psychopathy and one (associated with less extensive crime and for which some treatments are effective) caused by developmental neuropathology and low embodied capital. If this nonpathological interpretation of psychopathy is correct, there are implications for intervention.

INTERVENTIONS FOR PSYCHOPATHS?

Is psychopathy likely to respond to very intense forms of the treatment that works with nonpsychopaths? The most straightforward implication of a dimensional view of psychopathy is that a high-intensity version of what has been shown to be effective with offenders in general would be effective for psychopaths. This would amount to a cognitive-behavioral program incorporating relapse prevention to combat substance abuse, anger management to control expressive aggression, prosocial modeling to break down antisocial thinking and values, and motivational interviewing to enhance commitment to treatment (Wong & Hare, 2005). The empirical literature supporting this approach for seriously violent adult offenders (Rice & Harris 1997) is as yet quite limited (and nonexistent for psychopaths). Thus, this approach needs to be further implemented and evaluated, specifically with psychopathic offenders. However, by our taxonic, nonpathological account of psychopathy, we believe more success might come from identifying different approaches. These are described in the remaining subsections in this chapter.

Behavior Modification

Meta-analyses of intervention studies have been informative with regard to the treatment of offenders. Lipsey (1992; see also Lipsey & Wilson, 1998) examined almost 400 evaluations of interventions for juvenile delinquency and reported a small statistically significant effect. Effects were larger to the extent that interventions were behavioral and oriented toward building skills. Even more broadly, Lipsey and Wilson (1993) conducted a meta-analysis of over 300 meta-analytic evaluations of human service interventions. Again, there was a moderate significant overall effect size, and, as far as can be

determined, behavioral interventions yielded effects larger than average and larger than the average for medical interventions. That properly implemented behavioral contingencies cause parallel changes in behavior is incontrovertible.[6] There are debates concerning the mechanisms underlying punishment, the best ways to promote generalization, the effect of reinforcement on intrinsically rewarding behavior, and so on, but there is no doubt that behavior (whether pathological or not) responds predictably to its consequation (e.g., Corrigan & Muesser, 2000; Foxx, 2003; LePage et al., 2003; Lovaas, 1987; Paul & Lentz, 1977; Stein, 1999; Wong, Woolsey, Innocent, & Liberman, 1988; a longer list is available from the authors) while contingencies are in effect.

In no sense are we arguing that any of the foregoing provides evidence for a treatment effect among psychopaths. However, in general, behavioral treatments have the virtue of being explicitly designed for use under conditions in which the cause of the distressing behavior is unknown or cannot be specified (or is known, but cannot be altered). Furthermore, there is a technology that facilitates the implementation of behavioral treatment across an entire facility or agency—namely, the token economy system (Morris & Braukmann, 1987). Unlike other therapeutic approaches, psychopathy does not appear to present special problems for the effectiveness of a token economy (Pickens, Erickson, Thompson, Heston, & Eckert, 1979).

Multisystemic Therapy

The second impressive and persuasive literature on interventions for offenders concerns multisystemic therapy (MST) for juvenile delinquents (Brown, Borduin, & Henggeler, 2001; Brown et al., 1997; Randall & Cunningham, 2003). Theoretically, adolescent criminality is a systems problem: Adolescents engage in crime when responding naturally to the systems in which they operate. Dysfunctional families, ineffective schools, and antisocial peers combine to produce the obvious result—delinquency. MST seeks to alter each system to build functional school and family systems. In practice, MST is very individual and flexible with several general features: building skills, especially for parents; emphasis on monitoring and consequation both for adolescents and parents; behavioral principles (positive reinforcement; promoting behaviors incompatible with antisociality; emphasizing specific, observable, active behaviors; concern with generalization); and ensuring therapeutic integrity and adherence (Henggeler, Cunningham, Pickrel, Schoenwald, & Brondino, 1996; Henggeler, Melton, Brondino, Scherer, & Hanley, 1997; Henggeler, Schoenwald, & Pickrel, 1995). Most important, MST has yielded large treatment effects in randomized controlled trials (Borduin et al., 1995; Borduin, Schaeffer, Ronis, & Scott, 2003).

For our present purposes, we recognize that the work on MST provides no evidence of a treatment effect for psychopaths or for adult offenders. In fact, its developers acknowledge that it cannot easily be applied to adults (Borduin, personal communication, August 2003). Moreover, our selectionist hypothesis about psychopathy (Harris, Skilling, & Rice, 2001) assigns little direct causal influence to antisocial peers: Psychopaths have more antisocial friends, but as a result of psychopathy, not as a cause. However, our hypothesis does maintain that psychopathic behavior is occasioned by opportunities favorable for its occurrence and that behavioral monitoring and consequation could reduce antisocial conduct by psychopaths by reducing its payoff. Our point here is that the evidence supporting MST as a treatment for delinquency is so promising that we can look past its theoretical underpinnings (Burns, Schoenwald, Burchard, Faw, & Santos, 2000; Huey, Henggeler, Brondino, & Pickrel, 2000) and move on to evaluate its efficacy when applied to offender groups for which it was not specifically designed.

Institutional and Community Programs

Where psychopaths have already committed serious offenses and exhibit evidence of high risk for future violence, we favor the use of selective incapacitation in the form of long-term institutionalization. Regardless of the duration of incapacitation, some organizational system must be in place within the institution. To this end, we favor the application of a sophisticated token economy incorporating four main features. First, the program is completely explicit and concentrates on reinforcement of behaviors incompatible with psychopathic conduct (i.e., delaying gratification, telling the truth, being responsible, being helpful and cooperative—each tied to an appropriate operational definition) and penalties for impulsive, dishonest, aggressive, irresponsible, and, of course, criminal actions. Second, there is no expectation that the program will be completed or withdrawn; the program is only expected to be efficacious under conditions of continuous administration. Third, contingencies are tightly monitored by institutional staff, based only on observed, overt behavior, and never based on what inmates report about thoughts, feelings, or conduct. Fourth, systems are in place to monitor and consequate performance by front-line and supervisory program staff.

It must be recognized that societal and economic conditions would permit use of this incapacitation strategy with a minority of psychopaths (and a small minority of offenders). For most psychopathic offenders, release to the community in the form of parole or probation is inevitable. In our opinion, greater prospects for effective intervention lie in applying continuing behavioral principles to psychopaths under conditional release. Quite clearly, it will not be easy to design and implement a behavioral program for the institutional management of psychopathic offenders. It is to be expected that psychopathic offenders would resist such a program, break the rules in unexpected ways, seek to undermine institutional security, and engage in attempts to deceive and manipulate staff, supervisors, volunteers, the media, and members of the public.

The challenges associated with operating a program for psychopathic offenders should not be underestimated, but implementing an institutional program will be straightforward compared to delivering a similar behavioral intervention for psychopathic offenders under community supervision. We suggest, however, that the same principles should apply to community-release programs—behavioral monitoring, positive consequation, ensuring program integrity, and an emphasis on observable behavior. Participation in such programs would need to be a condition for release; otherwise, few psychopaths would volunteer for and persist in such a program. We anticipate that programs of this sort will require more resources than customary parole or probation services, especially because the program is expected to be efficacious only as long as it continues to be administered. Nevertheless, given the broad societal harm caused by psychopaths, we believe an evaluation of such a program could show it to be cost-effective.

Protecting Potential Victims

The aforementioned suggested interventions are expected to reduce the violent and criminal behavior of psychopaths by shrinking the behavioral niche. By our selectionist account, psychopaths (like everyone) are sensitive to the features of the interpersonal environment favoring one behavior over another. To the extent that a particular behavior does not (or appears unlikely to) pay off, we expect its frequency to decline. Because humans exhibit excellent discrimination, we do not expect such behavioral changes to generalize to a postprogram environment because it would be obvious that the niche had changed. However, one might also ask: Rather than simply addressing the behavior of psychopaths, why not change the social environment itself? Some approaches of this kind have been tried with other populations.

Wassermann and Miller (1998; see also Catalano, Arthur, Hawkins, Berglund, & Olson, 1998) evaluated outcome data for several universal programs for preschool and school-age children and concluded that such programs can positively affect outcomes plausibly or empirically related to later antisociality. Programs targeting at-risk adolescents appear to reduce delinquent conduct (e.g., Tolan & Guerra, 1994). Similarly, increasing school supervision, boosting police patrols, installing surveillance cameras, using metal detectors, promoting neighborhood watch and citizen patrols, restricting access to firearms, increasing access to abortion, restricting citizens' freedom to move to relocate, and so on (cf. Catalano et al., 1998) can all be expected to shrink the opportunity for harm due to psychopathy. Of course, no one can say whether the reductions in antisocial conduct achieved by such broad-based

interventions reflect differences in the small minority of youth who become psychopaths. Nevertheless, on theoretical grounds, population-based interventions that (whatever else they do) decrease the opportunity for psychopathic aggression and exploitation can be expected to be worthwhile.

Finally, one might advocate explicit teaching about psychopathy in school and in public education campaigns. Such campaigns do appear to have had salutary effects in improving safety-related behaviors (safe sex, seatbelt use, decreasing smoking, increasing cancer screening, etc.). What is somewhat less obvious, however, is the specific content of training aimed at reducing the harm caused by psychopaths. For example, effectively instructing people to distrust strangers, telling young women that young men only want one thing, and advising everyone that leopards never change their spots are all approaches that might decrease the niche for psychopathy, but at such large social costs that benefits would be outweighed. More focused instructional approaches are probably desirable. Of course, similar concerns apply to tactics described in the previous paragraph. For example, how much police surveillance should law-abiding citizens tolerate in order to diminish the harm caused by psychopaths and other offenders? In our view, there is probably a trade-off in that restrictions on law enforcement agencies' security precautions necessarily increase the niche favorable to psychopathy.

Perhaps the following words of guidance, which we would give to novice forensic clinicians, could be a starting point for all safe relationships:

1. Read Hare (1998).
2. Reputation matters; leopards seldom change their spots.
3. Never take an offender's word at face value; always check his assertions against the record and with other informants.
4. Don't just attend to how he behaves toward you; carefully observe how he treats everyone—peers and other staff.
5. Beware of flattery.
6. Be very suspicious if an offender asks you to break a rule, no matter how minor, or to keep an illicit confidence.
7. Talk to a colleague about your rela-

tionship with him; if your trusted colleague says things don't sound right, beware.

CONCLUSIONS

We believe there is no evidence that any treatments yet applied to psychopaths have been shown to be effective in reducing violence or crime. In fact, some treatments that are effective for other offenders are actually harmful for psychopaths in that they appear to promote recidivism. We believe that the reason for these findings is that psychopaths are fundamentally different from other offenders and that there is nothing "wrong" with them in the manner of a deficit or impairment that therapy can "fix." Instead, they exhibit an evolutionarily viable life strategy that involves lying, cheating, and manipulating others.

Although no therapy has yet been shown to reduce the likelihood of future violence or crime among psychopaths, this does not mean that nothing can help. The best available evidence for effective intervention comes from the application of social learning principles in the form of behavioral programs and from MST. We believe that the strongest evidentiary support exists for institutional incapacitation where practical, and in tightly controlled behavioral programs with contingencies that remain in effect both inside and outside the institution. We can also conceive of societal changes that might reduce the behavioral niche for psychopathy, but such changes inevitably carry some negative impact with respect to the personal liberty of all citizens. Finally, none of these ideas comes close to a solution or cure for the societal harm caused by psychopathy. It is to be expected from our nonpathological, selectionist perspective that psychopaths will attempt to subvert harm reduction strategies employed by nonpsychopaths. In the ongoing arms race, the existing literature only suggests ways to limit psychopaths' advantages. More complete solutions lie in interventions based on future advances in basic neuroscience and molecular genetics (see MacDonald & Iacono, Chapter 19, and Seto & Quinsey, Chapter 30, this volume).

NOTES

1. One other study reported a meta-analysis of treatment for psychopaths (Garrido, Esteban, & Molero, 1995). The authors said there were two separate meta-analyses. The first included 34 studies that examined treatment outcomes for psychopaths compared to nonpsychopaths and purportedly showed that outcomes for psychopaths were worse than those for nonpsychopaths. The second included 19 studies that examined pre- and posttreatment studies of psychopaths and purportedly showed that psychopaths "are able to improve in behavioral and psychological functioning" (p. 59). Because no references were included in the article, there is no way to critically examine the methodology.

2. Salekin's definition of "improved" was somewhat unusual. For example, in the case of criminal behavior, he counted those who did not recidivate in the follow-up period as having "improved" regardless of how long the follow-up period was.

3. Salekin does not name the eight studies he counted as "controlled" in the meta-analysis. In a personal communication (May 2004), he advised that the eight were Craft, Stephenson, and Granger (1964); Ingram, Gerard, Quay, and Levinson (1970); Korey (1944); Maas, (1966); Persons (1965); Rice et al. (1992); Skolnick and Zuckerman (1979); and Woody, McLellan, Luborsky, and O'Brien (1985).

4. Skeem et al. reported a chi-square value of 3.31 as significant, $p < .05$. However, the use of a one-tailed procedure is clearly unwarranted in examining therapy that according to the authors themselves is of doubtful effectiveness, and might even in some instances be harmful.

5. This argument relies on a particular definition of pathology or "disorder" (Wakefield, 1992) which says disorders involve the failure of a mechanism to perform as designed by natural selection. Because this account asserts that it exists because it has been reproductively successful (i.e., it was designed by natural selection) psychopathy is, by definition, not a disorder.

6. Readers might wonder why we consider single case studies persuasive regarding the effects of behavior modification but not with respect to the benefits of psychodrama. The reason is that single-case designs typical of the evaluation of behavioral treatment incorporate considerable methodological control (e.g., objective measurement, multiple baselines, and reversal designs) rarely seen in the informal, impressionistic evaluation of nonbehavioral therapies.

REFERENCES

Andrews, D. A., & Bonta, J. (1994). *The psychology of criminal conduct.* Cincinnati, OH: Anderson.

Andrews, D. A., Zinger, I., Hoge, R. D., Bonta, J., Gendreau, P., & Cullen, F. T. (1990). Does correctional treatment work? A clinically relevant and psychologically informed meta-analysis. *Criminology, 28,* 369–404.

Ayers, W. A. (2000). Taxometric analysis of borderline and antisocial personality disorders in a drug and alcohol dependent population. *Dissertation Abstracts International: Section B: The Sciences and Engineering, 61,* 1684.

Barbaree, H. E., Peacock, E. J., Cortini, F., Marshall, W. L., & Seto, M. (1998). Ontario penitentiaries' program. In W. L. Marshall, Y. M. Fernandez, S. M. Hudson, & T. Ward (Eds.), *Sourcebook of treatment programs for sexual offenders.* New York: Plenum Press.

Barker, E. (1980). The Penetanguishene Program: A personal review. In H. Toch (Ed.), *Therapeutic communities in corrections* (pp. 73–81). New York: Praeger.

Barker, E. T., & Mason, M. H. (1968). Buber behind bars. *Canadian Psychiatric Association Journal, 13,* 61–72.

Barker, E. T., Mason, M. H., & Wilson, J. (1969). Defence-disrupting therapy. *Canadian Psychiatric Association Journal, 14,* 355–359.

Barker, E. T., & McLaughlin, A. J. (1977). The total encounter capsule. *Canadian Psychiatric Association Journal, 22,* 355–360.

Barr, K. N., & Quinsey, V. L. (2004). Is psychopathy a pathology or a life strategy? Implications for social policy. In C. Crawford & C. Salmon (Eds.), *Evolutionary psychology, public policy, and personal decisions* (pp. 293–317). Hillsdale, NJ: Erlbaum.

Beacher, A. I. (1962). Psychoanalytic treatment of a sociopathy in a group situation. *American Journal of Psychotherapy, 16,* 278–288.

Belsky, J., Steinberg, L., & Draper, P. (1991). Childhood experience, interpersonal development, and reproductive strategy: An evolutionary theory of socialization. *Child Development, 62,* 647–670.

Borduin, C. M., Mann, B. J., Cone, L. T., Henggeler, S. W., Fucci, B. R., Blaske, D. M., et al. (1995). Multisystemic treatment of serious juvenile offenders: Long-term prevention of criminality and violence. *Journal of Consulting and Clinical Psychology, 63,* 569–578.

Borduin, C. M., Schaeffer, C. M., Ronis, M., & Scott, T. (2003). Multisystemic treatment of serious behavior in adolescents. In C. A. Essau (Ed.), *Conduct and oppositional defiant disorders: Epidemiology, risk factors, and treatment* (pp. 299–318). Mahwah, NJ: Erlbaum.

Brown, H. J., & Gutsch, K. U. (1985). Cognitions associated with a delay of gratification task: A study with psychopaths and normal prisoners. *Criminal Justice and Behavior, 12,* 453–462.

Brown, T. L., Borduin, C. M., & Henggeler, S. W. (2001). Treating juvenile offenders in community settings. In J. B. Ashford, B. D. Sales, & W. H. Reid, *Treating adult and juvenile offenders with special needs* (pp. 445–464). Washington, DC: American Psychological Association.

Brown, T. L., Swenson, C. C., Cunningham, P. B., Henggeler, S. W., Schoenwald, S. K., & Rowland, M. D. (1997). Multisystemic treatment of violent and chronic juvenile offenders: Bridging the gap between research and practice. *Administration and Policy in Mental Health, 25,* 221–238.

Burns, B. J., Schoenwald, S. K., Burchard, J. D., Faw, L., & Santos, A. B. (2000). Comprehensive community-based interventions for youth with severe emotional disorders: Multisystemic therapy and the wraparound process. *Journal of Child and Family Studies, 9,* 283–314.

Catalano, R. F., Arthur, M. W., Hawkins, D. J., Berglund, L., & Olson, J. J. (1998). Comprehensive community-and school-based interventions to prevent antisocial behavior. In R. Loeber & D. P. Farrington (Eds.), *Serious and violent juvenile offenders: Risk factors and successful interventions* (pp. 248–283). Thousand Oaks, CA: Sage.

Cleckley, H. (1941). *The mask of sanity.* St. Louis, MO: Mosby.

Cleckley, H. (1982). *The mask of sanity* (6th ed., rev.). St. Louis, MO: Mosby.

Copas, J. B., O'Brien, M., Roberts, J., & Whiteley, J. S. (1984). Treatment outcome in personality disorder: The effect of social psychological and behavioural variables. *Personality and Individual Differences, 5,* 565–573.

Copas, J. B., & Whiteley, J. S. (1976). Predicting success in the treatment of psychopaths. *British Journal of Psychiatry, 129,* 388–392.

Corrigan, P. W., & Mueser, K. T. (2000). Behavior therapy for aggressive psychiatric patients. In M. L. Crowner (Ed.), *Understanding and treating violent psychiatric patients* (pp. 69–85). Washington, DC: American Psychiatric Association.

Corsini, R. J. (1958). Psychodrama with a psychopath. *Group Psychotherapy, 11,* 33–39.

Craft, M., Stephenson, G., & Granger, C. (1964). A controlled trial of authoritarian and self- governing regimes with adolescent psychopaths. *American Journal of Orthopsychiatry,* 543–554.

Dawkins, R. (1978). *The selfish gene.* London: Paladin Books.

Dolan, D. (1998). Therapeutic community treatment for severe personality disorders. In T. Millon, E. Simonsen, M. Birket-Smith, & R. D. Davis (Eds.), *Psychopathy: Antisocial, criminal and violent behavior.* New York: Guilford Press.

Foxx, R. M. (2003). The treatment of dangerous behavior. *Behavioral Interventions, 18,* 1–21.

Friedman, P. H. (1970). Limitations in the conceptualization of behavior therapists: Toward a cognitive-behavioral model of behavior therapy. *Psychological Reports, 27,* 175–178.

Garrido, V., Esteban, C., & Molero, C. (1995). The effectiveness in the treatment of psychopathy: A meta-analysis. *Issues in Criminological and Legal Psychology, 24,* 57–59.

Glaus, A. (1968). The handling of criminal psychopaths in Switzerland. *International Journal of Offender Therapy, 12,* 29–36.

Hare, R. D. (1970). *Psychopathy: Theory and research.* New York: Wiley.

Hare, R. D. (1991). *The Psychopathy Checklist—Revised.* Toronto, ON, Canada: Multi-Health Systems.

Hare, R. D. (1998). *Without conscience: The disturbing world of the psychopaths among us.* New York: Guilford Press.

Hare, R. D. (2003). *The Psychopathy Checklist—Revised* (2nd ed.). Toronto, ON, Canada: Multi-Health Systems.

Hare, R. D., Clark, D., Grann, M., & Thornton, D. (2000). Psychopathy and the predictive validity of the PCL-R: An international perspective. *Behavioral Sciences and the Law, 18,* 623–645.

Hare, R. D., & Frazelle, J. (1985). *Some preliminary notes on a research scale for the assessment of psychopathy in criminal populations.* Unpublished manuscript, University of British Columbia, Vancouver.

Harris, G. T., Hilton, N. Z., Lalumière, M. L., Quinsey, V. L., & Rice, M. E. (2004). *Precocious coercive sexuality in life course persistent antisociality.* Manuscript in preparation.

Harris, G. T., & Rice, M. E. (in press). Psychopathy research at Oak Ridge: Skepticism overcome. In H. Herve & J. C. Yuille (Eds.), *Psychopathy: Theory, research, and implications for society.* Mahwah, NJ: Erlbaum.

Harris, G. T., Rice, M. E., & Cormier, C. A. (1991). Psychopathy and violent recidivism. *Law and Human Behavior, 15,* 625–637.

Harris, G. T., Rice, M. E., & Cormier, C. A. (1994). Psychopaths: Is a therapeutic community therapeutic? *Therapeutic Communities, 15,* 283–300.

Harris, G. T., Rice, M. E., & Lalumière, M. (2001). Criminal violence: The roles of psychopathy, neurodevelopmental insults and antisocial parenting. *Criminal Justice and Behavior, 28,* 402–426.

Harris, G. T., Rice, M. E., & Quinsey, V. L. (1994). Psychopathy as a taxon: Evidence that psychopaths are a discrete class. *Journal of Consulting and Clinical Psychology, 62,* 387–397.

Harris, G. T., Skilling, T. A., & Rice, M. E. (2001). The construct of psychopathy. In M. Tonry (Ed.), *Crime and justice: An annual review of research* (pp. 197–264). Chicago: University of Chicago Press.

Haslam, N. (2003) The dimensional view of personality disorders: A review of the taxometric evidence. *Clinical Psychology Review, 23,* 75–93.

Henggeler, S. W., Cunningham, P. B., Pickrel, S. G., Schoenwald, S. K., & Brondino, M. J. (1996). Multisystemic therapy: An effective violence prevention approach for serious juvenile offenders. *Journal of Adolescence, 19,* 47–61.

Henggeler, S. W., Melton, G. B., Brondino, M. J., Scherer, D. G., & Hanley, J. H. (1997). Multisystemic therapy with violent and chronic juvenile offenders and their families: The role of treatment fidelity in successful dissemination. *Journal of Consulting and Clinical Psychology, 65,* 821–833.

Henggeler, S. W., Schoenwald, S. K., & Pickrel, S. G. (1995). Multisystemic therapy: Bridging the gap between university- and community-based treatment. *Journal of Consulting and Clinical Psychology, 63,* 709–717.

Hobson, J., Shine, J., & Roberts, R. (2000). How do psychopaths behave in a prison therapeutic community? *Psychology, Crime and Law, 6,* 139–154

Huey, S. J., Henggeler, S. W., Brondino, M. J., & Pickrel, S. G. (2000). Mechanisms of change in multisystemic therapy: Reducing delinquent behavior through therapist adherence and improved family and peer functioning. *Journal of Consulting and Clinical Psychology, 68,* 451–467.

Hughes, G., Hogue, T., Hollin, C., & Champion, H. (1997). First-stage evaluation of a treatment programme for personality disordered offenders. *Journal of Forensic Psychiatry, 8,* 515–527.

Ingram, G. L., Gerard, R. E., Quay, H. C., & Levinson, R. B. (1970). An experimental program for the psychopathic delinquent: Looking in the "correctional wastebasket." *Journal of Research in Crime and Delinquency, 7,* 24–30.

Jones, M. (1956). The concept of the therapeutic community. *American Journal of Psychiatry, 112,* 647–650.

Jones, M. (1968). *Social psychiatric in practice,* Harmondsworth, UK: Penguin Books.

Kiger, R. S. (1967). Treating the psychopathic patient in a therapeutic community. *Hospital and Community Psychiatry, 18,* 191–196.

Knight, K., Simpson, D. D., & Miller, M. L. (1999). Three-year incarceration outcomes for in-prison therapeutic community treatment in Texas. *The Prison Journal, 79,* 337–351.

Korey, S. R. (1944). The effects of Benzedine sulfate on the behavior of psychopathic and neurotic juvenile delinquents. *Psychiatric Quarterly, 18,* 127–137.

Lalumière, M. L., Harris, G. T., Quinsey, V. L., & Rice, M. E. (2005). *The causes of rape: Understanding individual differences in the male propensity for sexual aggression.* Washington, DC: American Psychological Association.

Lalumière, M. L., Harris, G. T., & Rice, M. E. (2001). Psychopathy and developmental instability. *Evolution and Human Behavior, 22,* 75–92.

Larzelere, R. E., Kuhn, B. R., & Johnson, B. (2004). The intervention selection bias: An underrecognized confound in intervention research. *Psychological Bulletin, 130,* 289–303.

LePage, J. P., DelBen, K., Pollard, S., McGhee, M., VanHorn, L., Murphy, J., et al. (2003). Reducing assaults on an acute psychiatric unit using a token economy: A 2-year followup. *Behavioral Interventions, 18,* 179–190.

Lipsey, M. W. (1992). The effect of treatment on juvenile delinquents: Results from meta-analysis. In F. Loesel & D. Bender (Eds.), *Psychology and law: International perspectives* (pp. 131–143). Oxford, UK: Walter De Gruyter.

Lipsey, M. W., & Wilson, D. B. (1993). The efficacy of psychological, educational, and behavioral treatment: Confirmation from meta-analysis. *American Psychologist, 48,* 1181–1209.

Lipsey, M. W., & Wilson, B. D. (1998). Effective intervention for serious juvenile offenders: A synthesis of research. In R. Loeber & D. P. Farrington (Eds.), *Serious and violent juvenile offenders: Risk factors and successful interventions* (pp. 313–345). Thousand Oaks, CA: Sage.

Lösel, F. (1998). Treatment and management of psychopaths. In D. J. Cooke, R. D. Hare, & A. E. Forth (Eds.), *Psychopathy: Theory, research, and implications for society.* Dordrecht, The Netherlands: Kluwer.

Lovaas, O. I. (1987). Behavioral treatment and normal educational and intellectual functioning in young autistic children. *Journal of Consulting and Clinical Psychology, 55,* 3–9.

Maas, J. (1966). The use of actional procedures in group psychotherapy with sociopathic women. *International Journal of Group Psychotherapy, 16,* 190–197.

Maier, G. J. (1976). Therapy in prisons. In J. R. Lion & D. J. Madden (Eds.), *Rage, hate, assault and other forms of violence* (pp. 113–133). New York: Spectrum.

Marcus, D. K., John, S. L., & Edens, J. F. (2004). A taxometric analysis of psychopathic personality. *Journal of Abnormal Psychology, 113,* 626–635.

McCord, J. (1982). Parental behavior in the cycle of aggression. *Psychiatry, 51,* 14–23.

McMurran, M., Egan, V., & Ahmadi, S. (1998). A retrospective evaluation of a therapeutic community for mentally disordered offenders. *Journal of Forensic Psychiatry, 9,* 103–113.

Mealey, L. (1995). The sociobiology of sociopathy: An integrated evolutionary model. *Behavioral and Brain Sciences, 18,* 523–599.

Miles, A. E. (1969). The effects of therapeutic community on the interpersonal relationships of a group of psychopaths. *British Journal of Criminology, 9,* 22–38.

Miller, G. A., & Chapman, J. P. (2001). Misunderstanding analysis of covariance. *Journal of Abnormal Psychology, 110,* 40–48.

Morris, E. K., & Braukmann, C. J. (Eds.). (1987). *Behavioral approaches to crime and delinquency: A handbook of application, research, and concepts.* New York: Plenum Press.

Nielsen, R. F. (2000). *Total encounters: The life and times of the Mental Health Centre Penetanguishene.* Hamilton, ON, Canada: McMaster University Press.

Ogloff, J., Wong, S., & Greenwood, A. (1990). Treating criminal psychopaths in a therapeutic community program. *Behavioral Sciences and the Law, 8,* 81–90.

Paul, G. L., & Lentz, R. J. (1977). *Psychosocial treatment of chronic mental patients: Milieu versus social learning programs.* Cambridge, MA: Harvard University Press.

Persons, R. W. (1965). Psychotherapy with sociopathic offenders: An empirical evaluation. *Journal of Clinical Psychology, 21,* 205–207.

Pickens, R., Errickson, E., Thompson, T., Heston, L., & Eckert, E. D. (1979). MMPI correlates of performance on a behavior therapy ward. *Behavior Research and Therapy, 17,* 17–24.

Randall, J., & Cunningham, P. B. (2003). Multisystemic therapy: A treatment for violent substance-abusing and substance-dependent juvenile offenders. *Addictive Behaviors, 28,* 1731–1739.

Reiss, D., Meux, C., & Grubin, D. (2000). The effect of psychopathy on outcome in high security patients. *Journal of the American Academy of Psychiatry and Law, 28,* 309–314.

Rice, M. E. (1997). Violent offender research and implications for the criminal justice system. *American Psychologist, 52,* 414–423.

Rice, M. E., & Harris, G. T. (1995). Psychopathy, schizophrenia, alcohol abuse and violent recidivism. *International Journal of Law and Psychiatry, 18,* 333–342.

Rice, M. E., & Harris, G. T. (1997). Treatment of adult offenders. In D. Stoff, J. Breiling, & J. D. Maser (Eds.), *Handbook of antisocial behavior* (pp. 425–435). New York: Wiley.

Rice, M. E., Harris, G. T., & Cormier, C. (1992). A follow-up of rapists assessed in a maximum security psychiatric facility. *Journal of Interpersonal Violence, 5,* 435–448.

Richards, H. J., Casey, J. O., & Lucente, S. W. (2003). Psychopathy and treatment response in incarcerated female substance abusers. *Criminal Justice and Behavior, 30,* 251–276.

Ridley, M. (1997). *The origins of virtue.* New York: Viking Press.

Rodgers, T. C. (1947). Hypnotherapy in character neuroses. *Journal of Clinical Psychopathology, 8,* 519–524.

Rosenbaum, P. R., & Rubin, D. B. (1984). Reducing bias in observational studies using subclassification on the propensity score. *Journal of the American Statistical Association, 79,* 516–524.

Rosow, H. M. (1955). Some observations on group

therapy with prison inmates. *Archives of Criminal Psychodynamics, 1,* 866–897.

Rubin, D. B. (1997). Estimating causal effects from large data sets using propensity scores. *Annals of Internal Medicine, 127,* 757–763.

Salekin, R. T. (2002). Psychopathy and therapeutic pessimism clinical lore or clinical reality? *Clinical Psychology Review, 22,* 79–112.

Schmideberg, M. (1949). Psychology and treatment of the criminal psychopath. *International Journal of Psychoanalysis, 20,* 197.

Serin, R. C., & Kuriychuk, M. (1994). Social and cognitive processing deficits in violent offenders: Implications for treatment. *International Journal of Law and Psychiatry, 17,* 431–441.

Seto, M. C., & Barbaree, H. (1999). Psychopathy, treatment behavior, and sex offender recidivism. *Journal of Interpersonal Violence, 14,* 1235–1248.

Showstack, N. (1956). Treatment of prisoners at the California medical facility. *American Journal of Psychiatry, 112,* 821–824.

Skeem, J. L., Monahan, J., & Mulvey, E. P. (2002). Psychopathy, treatment involvement, and subsequent violence among civil psychiatric patients. *Law and Human Behavior, 26,* 577–603.

Skeem, J. L., Poythress, N., Edens, J. F., Lilienfeld, S. O., & Cale, E. M. (2002). Psychopathic personality or personalities? Exploring potential variants of psychopathy and their implications for risk assessment. *Aggression and Violent Behavior, 8,* 513–546.

Skilling, T. A., Harris, G. T., Rice, M. E., & Quinsey, V. L. (2002). Identifying persistently antisocial offenders using the Hare Psychopathy Checklist and DSM antisocial personality disorder criteria. *Psychological Assessment, 14,* 27–38.

Skilling, T. A., Quinsey, V. L., & Craig, W. A. (2001). Evidence of a taxon underlying serious antisocial behavior in boys. *Criminal Justice and Behavior, 28,* 450–470.

Skolnick, N. J., & Zuckerman, M. (1979). Personality change in drug abusers: A comparison of therapeutic community and prison groups. *Journal of Consulting and Clinical Psychology, 47,* 768–770.

Stein, D. B. (1999). Outpatient behavioral management of aggressiveness in adolescents: A response cost paradigm. *Aggressive Behavior, 25,* 321–330.

Szurek, S. A. (1942). Notes on the genesis of psychopathic personality trends. *Psychiatry, 5,* 1–6.

Thorne, F. C. (1959). The etiology of sociopathic reactions. *American Journal of Psychotherapy, 13,* 319–330.

Tolan, P. H., & Guerra, N. G. (1994). Prevention of delinquency: Current status and issues. *Applied and Preventive Psychology, 3,* 251–273.

Wakefield, J. C. (1992). The concept of mental disorder: On the boundary between biological facts and social values. *American Psychologist, 47,* 373–388.

Wasserman, G. A., & Miller, L. S. (1998). The prevention of serious and violent juvenile offending. In R. Loeber & D. P. Farrington (Eds.), *Serious and violent juvenile offenders: Risk factors and successful interventions* (pp. 197–247). Thousand Oaks, CA: Sage.

Weisman, R. (1995). Reflections on the Oak Ridge experiment with mentally disordered offenders, 1965–1968. *International Journal of Law and Psychiatry, 18,* 265–290.

Wexler, H. K., Melnick, G., Lowe, L., & Peters, J. (1999). Three-year reincarceration outcomes for amity in-prison therapeutic community and aftercare in California. *The Prison Journal, 79,* 321–336.

Wong, S., & Hare, R. D. (2005). *Guidelines for a psychopathy treatment program.* Toronto, ON, Canada: Multi-Health Systems.

Wong, S. E., Woolsey, J. E., Innocent, A. J., & Liberman, R. P. (1988). Behavioral treatment of violent psychiatric patients. *Psychiatric Clinics of North America, 11,* 569–581.

Woody, G. E., McLellan, T. A., Luborsky, L., & O'Brien, C. P. (1985). Sociopathy and psychotherapy outcome. *Archives of General Psychiatry, 42,* 1081–1086.

Zinger, I., & Forth, A. E. (1998). Psychopathy and Canadian criminal proceedings: The potential for human rights abuses. *Canadian Journal of Criminology, 40,* 237–276.

29

Legal and Ethical Issues in the Assessment and Treatment of Psychopathy

JOHN F. EDENS
JOHN PETRILA

"Psychopathy" is a term that is becoming pervasive in law. It is increasingly found in both judicial opinions and legislation, and it also has been the focus of expert testimony in numerous types of criminal and civil cases (Hare, 1998; Lyon & Ogloff, 2000; Ogloff & Lyon, 1998). Although the legal system often appears to use the term uncritically, "psychopathy" lies at the heart of some of the most contentious debates in criminal and mental health law. Those debates embrace fundamental legal questions such as the restraint of liberty and imposition of the death penalty, as well as professional issues such as the proper role of mental health expertise, diagnoses, and labels in legal proceedings. This chapter discusses core issues in assessing and treating individuals labeled "psychopaths," focusing both on the legal contexts in which this construct may be introduced and on the ethical issues that arise when mental health examiners choose (or are obligated by statute) to assess psychopathy for purposes of addressing legal questions (e.g., treatment amenability, violence risk).

In the first part of this chapter ("The Role of Psychopathy in the Legal System"), we provide a brief overview of the legal contexts in which the term "psychopath" has been used. We also note a number of threshold issues, including questions of language, proba-bilistic versus individual decision making in legal settings, and general questions of admissibility. The second part of the chapter ("Assessing Psychopathy: Ethical Standards and Guidelines") discusses the specific role of the mental health examiner in assessing psychopathy, focusing on ethical issues related to the assessment itself, controversies regarding what types of conclusions and inferences should be made regarding the results of these assessments, and how to best communicate these conclusions and inferences to nonclinicians in the legal system who may be unfamiliar with this construct and its implications. In particular, we review contexts in which we believe the relevance of psychopathy data has been or can be overstated, such as in relation to violence risk issues and perceived lack of treatment amenability.

THE ROLE OF PSYCHOPATHY IN THE LEGAL SYSTEM

The Legal Contexts in Which "Psychopathy" Is Used

The use of the term "psychopath" in legal settings has a long history. Civil commitment and mental health statutes used the word liberally in the past. For example, in England, the Mental Deficiency Act (1913) used the term "moral imbecile," which eventually began to be equated by psychiatrists with "psychopathic personality" (cited in Reed, 1996). The Mental Health Act (1959) adopted the label "psychopathic disorder," defining it as "a persistent disorder or disability of mind (whether or not including subnormality of intelligence) which results in abnormally aggressive or seriously irresponsible conduct on the part of the patient, and requires or is susceptible to medical treatment" (cited in Reed, 1996, p. 4). In the United States, the term could also be found in civil commitment statutes, though it was most frequently used in "first-generation" sexual psychopath statutes that were rehabilitative in nature and assumed that treatment could reduce recidivism among sexual offenders (Fitch & Ortega, 2000).

Today the term, or something that effectively becomes an analogue, is much more likely to be used in statutes that are designed to further the long-term confinement of certain classes of individuals. These uses include preventive detention, sex offender civil commitment hearings, and waiver hearings to determine whether a juvenile should be tried in adult court. For example, the sexual offender statutes found today in the United States permit the indefinite confinement of individuals, often at the end of a prison sentence; the individual cannot be released absent a showing that he or she will not be dangerous in the future. Such legislation assumes a *lack* of treatability. For example, the Washington statute asserts that "in contrast to persons appropriate for civil commitment . . . sexually violent predators generally have antisocial personality features which are unamenable to existing mental illness treatment modalities . . . the prognosis for curing sexually violent predators is poor . . ." (Wash Laws Sec 71-09-010 [2000]). In Texas, an assessment to determine whether an individual suffers from a "behavioral abnormality" that makes the person more likely to engage in predatory sexual violence must include "testing for psychopathy, a clinical interview, and other appropriate assessments and techniques" (Tex. Health & Safety Code Sec. 841.023 [2004]). In the United Kingdom, legislation is being considered that would permit the preventive detention of persons with "dangerous severe personality disor-

ders" (Parliamentary Office of Science and Technology, 2004); in Scotland, proposed legislation would permit indeterminate imprisonment or detention for individuals meeting certain criteria under risk assessment procedures that would be codified (Scottish Executive, 2000). In Canada, a finding of psychopathy is considered an aggravating factor in sentencing, permitting imposition of a longer sentence than otherwise would be available (Zinger & Forth, 1998), and in the United States, prosecutors have used "psychopathy" to support a finding that a defendant will be dangerous in the future, a necessary element to impose capital punishment in some jurisdictions (Cunningham & Reidy, 2002; Edens, Petrila, & Buffington-Vollum, 2001).

Some statutory provisions explicitly use the term "psychopathy," whereas others invite application of the construct in determining which individuals qualify for long-term confinement, including preventive detention in the case of the U.K. proposal. Although the term is becoming pervasive, there are still differences in how it is used in particular settings, an issue with ramifications for clinicians, policymakers, and legal decision makers.

Issues of Language and "Fit"

The term "psychopath" when used in a statute typically does not mean the same thing as the term "psychopath" as used throughout this volume. For example, "sexual psychopath" statutes in the United States tend to emphasize a requirement that an individual lack control over his or her behavior; this is because of concerns that failing to emphasize volition would invite the courts to rule that such statutes were unconstitutional (Janus, 1998; see also *Kansas v. Crane*, 2002). A lack of control—at least in regard to how the legal concept of *volitional impairment* typically is construed in relation to criminal cases—arguably is not a defining characteristic of psychopathy as it is commonly conceptualized by clinicians, although research in this area ultimately may provide more support for the idea that a diagnosis of psychopathy does reflect a disturbance in behavioral control that is relevant to legal definitions of volitional impairment. At present, however, it seems that the same term is used to describe quite different individuals and groups with quite diverse characteristics.

There is also a larger debate regarding whether terms such as psychopathy and personality disorder are primarily legal or diagnostic categories, or neither (Ogloff & Lyon, 1998; Reed, 1996). John Gunn, for example, in commenting on the term "dangerous severe personality disorders" in the proposed aforementioned U.K. legislation, observed, "The English have invented a new disease" and that "another unusual feature is that this disease was invented by politicians"(Gunn, 2000, p. 73). There is also general debate regarding whether personality disorders should be regarded as mental illnesses, with one commentator noting that the development of effective treatments for personality disorders would influence psychiatrists to conclude that such disorders were illnesses (Kendell, 2002; see also Krober & Lau, 2000, for a discussion of the use of personality disorders in German criminal law). In addition, terms such as antisocial personality disorder, psychopathy, sociopathy, and dissocial personality disorder are often used interchangeably, despite the different criteria for each label (Ogloff & Lyon, 1998).

This difference in nomenclature has important ramifications for mental health professionals performing assessments in legal settings. The same term may carry different meanings for mental health professionals, attorneys, judges, and legislators, and examiners should be careful not to present data regarding their psychological measures as dispositive of the legal definition of what constitutes "a psychopath." In relation to legal decision making, it has been argued (Otto & Heilbrun, 2002) that the Psychopathy Checklist—Revised (PCL-R; Hare, 1991, 2003) is best construed as a "forensically relevant instrument" (FRI), in the sense that it measures a construct that, although not specifically psycholegal in nature, may be pertinent to consider in relation to various legal questions, such as whether a sex offender is at increased risk to engage in predatory sexual crimes in the future if released back into the community.

On a related note, mental health professionals may also use terms interchangeably that do not have the same meaning. Zinger and Forth (1998) in a review of Canadian cases observed, much like Ogloff and Lyon

(1998), that "antisocial personality disorder (APD)" and "sociopath" were often used by mental health professionals in testimony as if they were identical to "psychopathy." This practice was particularly troubling because of the much higher rates of APD among offender populations (Zinger & Forth, 1998). It is axiomatic that mental health professionals should be precise in their testimony. With stakes as high as indefinite confinement or the death penalty, precision in the use of language is both a legal and ethical imperative. We return to these issues in greater detail in subsequent sections.

Probabilistic versus Individualized Decision Making

The law traditionally addresses individual cases and relies on evidence regarding the individual. However, statutes such as those discussed previously invite evidence (e.g., that a person is likely to be a danger because of a particular score on the PCL-R) that is essentially probabilistic in nature. This has been a source of significant debate among legal decision makers, as illustrated by the majority and dissenting opinions in the decision by the Minnesota Supreme Court in the case *In re Linehan* (1994). This was one of a series of cases in which the court considered the constitutionality of the Minnesota sexual psychopathic personality statute as well as whether sufficient evidence had been produced to label Linehan a sexual psychopath. The majority opinion, in upholding the statute, indicated that trial courts were to consider the following factors in determining whether an individual had an "uncontrollable" impulse and therefore could be properly adjudicated a "sexual psychopath": (1) the person's relevant demographic characteristics (e.g., age, education); (2) the person's history of violent behavior (paying particular attention to recency, severity, and frequency of violent acts); (3) the baserate statistics for violent behavior among individuals of this person's background (e.g., data showing the rate at which rapists recidivate, the correlation between age and criminal sexual activity); (4) the sources of stress in the environment (cognitive and affective factors indicating that the person may be predisposed to cope with stress in a violent or nonviolent manner); (5) the similarity of the present or future context to those contexts in which the person has used violence in the past; and (6) the person's record with respect to sex therapy programs (*In re Linehan*, 1994, at 614).

A dissenting judge quarreled with the majority's insistence on the use of baserate statistics, writing:

> I am at a loss to understand what "the base rate statistics for violent behavior among individuals of this person's background (e.g., data showing the rate at which rapists recidivate, the correlation between age and criminal sexual activity, etc.)" . . . can possibly contribute with respect to predicting the seriousness of the danger to the public posed by the release of a certain person. It is the habitual course of criminal sexual conduct revealed by the record of the person in question which provides a basis for predicting serious danger to the public, not the course of misconduct committed by other persons. Not only are the statistics concerning the violent behavior of others irrelevant, but it seems to me wrong to confine any person on the basis not of that person's own prior conduct but on the basis of statistical evidence regarding the behavior of other people. (*In re Linehan* [1994], dissenting opinion, at 616)

Although the dissenting opinion seems to reflect a fundamental misconception about the most accurate predictors of future behavior, it is in fact truer to the traditional stance of the law, which is idiographic and prescriptive in nature rather than nomothetic and probabilistic (see Brigham, 1999; Melton, Petrila, Poythress, & Slobogin, 1997). Although the courts struggle to incorporate probabilistic testimony into a conceptual framework that focuses on the individual, it seems clear that there is an increasing focus on the empirical foundation on which mental health professionals base their opinions and testimony.

General Questions of Legal Admissibility

In the United States, questions regarding the admissibility of expert testimony historically were governed by the *Frye* rule (*Frye v. United States*, 1923). Scientific evidence would be admitted if it had gained "general acceptance" in the scientific community of interest. In the federal courts, this test was superseded by the decision of the U.S. Supreme Court in *Daubert v. Merrell-Dow*

Pharmaceuticals (1993). The Court ruled that the Federal Rules of Evidence, particularly Rule 702, governed the decision of a trial court regarding the acceptance of scientific evidence. The trial court was to consider a variety of factors in its decision, including whether the testimony's underlying reasoning or methodology is scientifically valid and properly can be applied to the facts at issue in the case. The Court suggested that the trial judge should consider a number of factors in making this decision, including the testability of the theory or technique in question, whether peer review has been applied, the known or potential error rate, presence and use of standards controlling its operation, and whether the theory or technique had attracted widespread acceptance within a relevant scientific community. In Canada, the courts examine four factors in determining whether to admit expert evidence, including relevance, whether the evidence is necessary to assist the trier of fact, the presence or absence of an exclusionary rule, and an expert who is qualified (Ogloff & Lyon, 1998).

In general, courts have accepted the use of actuarial risk assessment instruments, as well as the PCL-R, under any of these tests. Most of the cases in the United States have involved hearings under sexual offender statutes, with one court commenting that "our research has revealed no state appellate court decision which has found actuarial instruments inadmissible at SVP (sexual violent predator) proceedings" (*In re Commitment of R.S.*, 2001, at 96; *In re Detention of Holtz*, 2002; *Garcetti v. Superior Court*, 2000, upholding the admissibility of the PCL-R among other instruments). There have occasionally been rulings to the contrary (*In re Valdez*, 2000). However, admissibility appears not to be a significant question in most courts at this time, at least when the issue relates to violence risk assessment.

We believe that questions of admissibility, particularly on the ground of relevance, should be examined more closely (see, e.g., the discussion of capital cases later). It may be that the PCL-R, as an example, is germane to many contexts in which violence risk is at issue and has achieved general acceptance within a comparatively broad scientific community. However, the fact that the instrument is generally relevant to issues of violence risk does *not* mean that it is relevant to *all* legal proceedings in which future dangerousness may be at issue (Hare, 1998; cf. Hart, 1998). Given this, more analytic precision by the courts in assessing the question of admissibility would be welcome and would sharpen the inquiry into not only the strengths but the limitations of the assessment of psychopathy.

Absent greater scrutiny by the courts, however, it may fall primarily to the forensic examiner to make informed decisions regarding the proper uses of the PCL-R in legal settings and to then draw defensible inferences regarding exactly what these scores mean in relation to a given examinee. Noted previously, we believe psychopathy has an important role to play in many contexts, but the nature of the construct also raises several concerns about the potential for "overreaching" and/or misapplication in various circumstances. We summarize several of these concerns in the following sections.

ASSESSING PSYCHOPATHY: ETHICAL STANDARDS AND GUIDELINES

The recent publication of the American Psychological Association's (2002) revised ethical guidelines and code of conduct provides an occasion to review the standards to which examiners should adhere when conducting any type of psychological evaluation (e.g., Ethical Standards 9.1–9.11), as well as the general guidelines to which examiners should aspire when engaged in such work (e.g., Justice, Nonmaleficence). In addition, the Specialty Guidelines for Forensic Psychologists (Committee on Ethical Guidelines for Forensic Psychologists, 1991), which are currently being revised (Otto, 2004), also should be given careful consideration when engaged in forensic work. As a general comment, although one might assume that many of the issues addressed below are not particularly likely to be "troublespots" for most examiners, it is surprising to see how often they become a point of contention in legal cases. Moreover, there is ample anecdotal evidence (e.g., Edens, in press; Hare, 1998; Ogloff & Lyon, 1998; Zinger & Forth, 1998) to suggest that these issues are not given sufficient attention by at least some examiners working in the legal system.

In this section, we specifically consider ethical issues related to (1) when assessments of psychopathy may and may not be justifiable to conduct; (2) what measures should be used to operationalize psychopathy when the construct is considered appropriate to assess; (3) qualifications to use the PCL-R and its derivatives; and (4) information and data sources needed to score these measures adequately. We conclude with a discussion of specific concerns we have about how this information is used in various settings and presented by examiners to nonclinicians who may know little or nothing about this complex construct.

In What Contexts Are Assessments of Psychopathy Justifiable?

Given the influential and potentially prejudicial nature of the term "psychopath" (see below) and the items comprising the PCL-R (e.g., Lack of Remorse, Superficial Charm), it is incumbent upon the examiner to consider closely what types of contexts do and do not warrant the potential introduction of such terms (see American Psychological Association, 2002, Standard 1.01: Misuse of Psychologists' Work; Standard 3.04: Avoiding Harm). Although space constraints preclude an exhaustive review of this subject, we believe that examiners should consider as a primary issue whether there is empirical support to justify the introduction of the construct to address whatever the particular question is to be answered. In more legalistic terminology, does psychopathy have any demonstrated "probative" value in relation to the issue(s) to be addressed by the evaluation? As the American Psychological Association ethics code clearly dictates, "Psychologists administer, adapt, score, interpret, or use assessment techniques, interviews, tests, or instruments in a manner and for purposes that are appropriate *in light of the research on or evidence of the usefulness and proper application of the techniques*" (Standard 9.02(a), p. 1071; emphasis added).

To the extent that examiners are willing to make inferential leaps regarding the application of psychopathy and related diagnoses to a particular question where its relevance is questionable, then they are treading into much more ethically questionable generalizations from their assessment data. For example, on more than one occasion the *absence* of psychopathic traits has been used to justify expert testimony that a criminal defendant was unlikely to have committed a particular offense (Edens, 2001; Hare, 1998). This is a conclusion that most psychology–law scholars would consider problematic on both legal and empirical grounds. Although it is beyond the scope of this chapter to review all the types of cases in which attempts have been made to introduce psychopathy or APD testimony where it would seem to be tangential at best (see Lyon & Ogloff, 2000, for several examples), suffice it to say that both prosecutors and defense attorneys have attempted to bolster their legal arguments by using experts who are willing to interpret the relevance of psychopathy in "novel" or creative ways.

As a general guideline we would offer that there are three broad domains in which psychopathy *may be* relevant to consider in legal settings: (1) risk assessment, (2) mental or behavioral "abnormality" issues, and (3) treatment amenability. Despite our identification of these broad areas of relevance, however, we do not mean to imply that psychopathy will be germane in all (or even most) specific contexts within these broader domains. For example, we have written extensively (Edens, 2001; Edens, Buffington-Vollum, Keilen, Roskamp, & Anthony, 2005; Edens, Colwell, Fernandez, & Desforges, in press; Edens, Desforges, Fernandez, & Palac, 2004; Edens, Guy, & Fernandez, 2003; Edens, Petrila, & Buffington-Vollum, 2001; Guy, Edens, Anthony, & Douglas, in press) about the limited probative value of psychopathy to inform questions of "future dangerousness" in death penalty cases in the United States. Despite the general association between psychopathy and aggression, the specific (and relatively rare) types of violence at issue in capital cases (i.e., violent recidivism following at least 30 years of incarceration, violence committed while incarcerated in a U.S. prison) are not meaningfully informed by knowledge of whether a capital defendant is a PCL-R-defined psychopath (for a more detailed review, see Edens et al., 2001, 2005; for a slightly different perspective, see Hare, 2003, p. 15).

As another example, although using psychopathy to inform issues of "mental disease or defect" or "behavioral abnormality" may

be considered justifiable in relation to the civil commitment of sexual predators, courts historically have taken a rather dim view of the applicability of this construct to adjudicative competence and insanity issues. This is quite curious, as the concept of "volitional control" over one's behavior has lost favor in relation to insanity standards over the years (see Melton et al., 1997, for a more detailed review) but is quite prominent in the adjudication of recent sexual predator cases (e.g., *Kansas v. Crane*, 2002; *Kansas v. Hendricks*, 1997). Nevertheless, if examiners attempt to introduce psychopathy or APD evidence in criminal cases to support arguments that defendants are less capable of exercising volitional control over their actions or are less likely to appreciate the wrongfulness of their behavior, then they are likely to be met with legal definitions that preclude such evidence and/or a judiciary that is generally unreceptive to such information (Lyon & Ogloff, 2000).

As another caveat, simply because psychopathy has an empirically demonstrated association with a particular outcome of interest (e.g., community violence committed by released psychiatric patients [Skeem & Mulvey, 2001]), one should also consider whether there may be equally (or more) empirically defensible assessment methods that are also less likely to be as stigmatizing to the examinee in question. For example, it has been argued (Gendreau, Goggin, & Smith, 2002) that the Level of Service Inventory—Revised (LSI-R; Andrews & Bonta, 1995) is a better predictor of criminal recidivism than is the PCL-R. If this were in fact the case (see Hemphill & Hare, 2004, for a highly critical review of the conclusions drawn by Gendreau et al., 2002), it raises the question whether it is justifiable to label someone "a psychopath" if another assessment methodology works better for the same purpose. Of course, it may be that unique variance in recidivism outcomes is explained by each measure, which actually argues for the use of both to maximize predictive accuracy. If, however, the PCL-R demonstrates no incremental validity over the LSI-R (or other risk measures), then it becomes exceedingly difficult to justify its inclusion in a risk assessment if a less stigmatizing instrument can be administered. Although it has previously been asserted that it may be unethical to conduct a risk assessment *without* assessing for psychopathy (Hart, 1998), this position appears to be driven by the presumption that psychopathy will *always* improve the validity of extant violence risk assessment methods. If in fact this were not the case, then this argument would seem to be untenable.

Finally, in relation to determinations of when or if psychopathy should be assessed, it is important to address the burgeoning research base on "juvenile" psychopathy (see, e.g., two recent special issues of *Behavioral Sciences and the Law* on this topic) and the plethora of instruments ostensibly measuring these traits in children and adolescents (cf. Salekin, Chapter 20, this volume). Their widespread applied use in legal contexts is likely to be forthcoming in the near future, at least for the now commercially available Psychopathy Checklist: Youth Version (PCL:YV; Forth, Kosson, & Hare, 2003). Legal and ethical issues related to assessments of psychopathy in young people could fill an entire chapter itself, but we restrict our comments here to a few key issues that we believe are central to determining whether to use any of these measures in a given case (see also Frick & Marsee, Chapter 18, this volume). First, although it is frequently argued that psychopathic traits can be identified in childhood and that these traits are highly stable over the lifespan (e.g., Harris, Skilling, & Rice, 2001), relatively little is known about the long-term stability of measures used to assess these traits and whether youths who appear relatively psychopathic at one point will continue to do so even a few years later. Preliminary evidence (Cauffman & Skeem, 2004) suggests that more extreme scores will decrease significantly over time, which has obvious implications for any conclusions (e.g., in juvenile waiver evaluations) regarding the likelihood that a child or adolescent is amenable to rehabilitation or is too dangerous for the juvenile justice system.

A second and related point is that research on the predictive validity of the youth psychopathy construct is in a nascent state, particularly in relation to U.S. samples. Although much of the extant research is encouraging regarding modest to moderate associations with short-term juvenile or criminal justice outcomes (e.g., recidivism and institutional conduct), it is by no means uniformly positive (Campbell, Porter, & Santo,

2004; Edens, Skeem, Cruise, & Cauffman, 2001; Forth et al., 2003; Marcyzk, Heilbrun, Lander, & DeMatteo, 2003; Ponder, 1998). Moreover, it is unclear to what extent the psychopathy construct evinces incremental validity beyond conduct disorder diagnoses or other measures of externalizing psychopathology when predicting these outcomes (Brandt, Kennedy, Patrick, & Curtin, 1997; Hicks, Rogers, & Cashel, 2000). It is also unknown to what extent the prediction of criminal justice outcomes is improved by the inclusion of affective–interpersonal items (e.g., Pathological Lying and Lack of Remorse) in the PCL:YV (see Corrado, Vincent, Hart, & Cohen, 2004), which arguably have a greater likelihood of biasing decision makers than do factors that might seem more consistent with a "typical" adolescent offender (e.g., impulsivity, irresponsibility). Our concerns about the likely prejudicial impact of identifying adults as evincing psychopathic traits (described in greater detail later) extend even more so to children and adolescents, where such traits are likely to promote more punitive responses (Edens, Guy, & Fernandez, 2003). In summary, given this brief review of concerns surrounding the construct of "youth psychopathy," we believe examiners should be exceedingly cautious regarding what circumstances warrant the introduction of these instruments and labels.

How Should Psychopathy Be Operationalized?

When the examiner has determined that it is justifiable to use psychopathy to inform an assessment question (or it is required to be assessed by statute), the question then becomes one of how exactly to measure it. The long history of difficulty in assessing psychopathic traits reliably is well documented (see Part II, "Issues in Conceptualization and Assessment," this volume). Although rather critical reviews of the PCL-R have appeared in the literature recently (Edens, Petrila, & Buffington-Vollum, 2001; Gendreau et al., 2002; Walters, 2003), at the current state of knowledge it would seem difficult to justify use of something *other* than the PCL-R once it has been determined that the construct of psychopathy per se is relevant (e.g., in Texas sexual predator evaluations where "psychopathy" assessments are mandated by statute). Arguably one of the greatest contributions of the PCL-R is the wealth of reliability data suggesting that it can serve as a reasonably stable estimate of psychopathic traits, at least in offender populations where there is adequate file data to supplement information obtained by interview (see below). Although several promising alternative assessment procedures are in various stages of development (Kosson, Steuerwald, Forth, & Kirkhart, 1997; Lilienfeld & Andrews, 1996), none seems sufficiently well validated at this point to warrant inclusion in forensic evaluations where the assessment of psychopathy is meant to inform legal questions such as violence risk or treatment amenability. Their use in applied settings at this time would appear to be ethically questionable at best, given the current dearth of information needed to evaluate their utility in forensic contexts (e.g., normative data, professional manuals; see Heilbrun, 1992).

That is not to imply, however, that some alternative scales may not be relevant to address particular issues where there is sufficient empirical justification for their inclusion. For example, although the Antisocial Features (ANT) scale of the Personality Assessment Inventory (PAI; Morey, 1991) does not correlate exceedingly highly with the PCL-R (Edens, Hart, Johnson, Johnson, & Olver, 2001; Walters, Duncan, & Geyer, 2003), it does seem to correlate at least as well as the PCL-R with indicators of institutional misconduct, at least in U.S. samples of offenders in which the two measures have been compared directly (Buffington-Vollum, Edens, Johnson, & Johnson, 2002; Salekin, Rogers, & Sewell, 1997; Walters et al., 2003). As such, if examiners are expected to comment on the likelihood of misconduct while an offender is institutionalized, then the ANT scale may in fact provide relevant information.

However, our general support for the utility of the PCL-R at present should not be taken as a blanket endorsement of all assessment procedures in the "Hare family," some of which have limited or inconsistent empirical support at this time. For example, the Hare P-Scan (Hare & Hervé, 1999) is a commercially available scale that ostensibly allows mental health and criminal justice personnel "to make reasonably informed evaluations and judgments" (Hare, 2003, p. 13) regarding the presence of psychopathic traits among offenders, patients, suspects, and other individuals of interest. The items comprising the P-Scan are scored on the familiar 0–2 PCL-R scale and are classified into interpersonal, affective, and lifestyle facets (30 items each). A total score can be derived as well, based on the average of the three facet scores. Total scores range from 0 to 60 and fall into one of three general levels: high, moderate, and low. Scores greater than 30 are noted as a "cause for serious concern" (Hare & Hervé, 1999, p. 11) and those who obtain such scores "should be referred for a professional evaluation and opinion by a psychologist or psychiatrist" (p. 7). There is a dearth of published research in peer-reviewed journals on the P-Scan at present (Elwood, Poythress, & Douglas, 2004), however, and there is little evidence to suggest that when completed by nonclinicians, this instrument assesses a construct at all similar to that indexed by the PCL-R when used by a trained diagnostician (Warren, Chauhan, & Murrie, 2004). In addition, although the P-Scan has been described as appropriate for use with adolescents (Hare & Hervé, 1999), there are several reasons to question its applicability to this age group (Edens, Skeem, et al., 2001).

Aside from the P-Scan, there are two other PCL-R related measures that are designed for use with children or adolescents. The Antisocial Process Screening Device (APSD; Frick & Hare, 2001) is another relatively new assessment procedure that, similar to the P-Scan, deviates from the typical interview and file review format of the PCL measures. The item content of this measure is similar to that of the PCL-R, but the items are rated by parents and teachers rather than by a trained examiner; a self-report version of this instrument also exists. Although considerable data have accumulated on the *concurrent* validity of the APSD, one of the more curious findings to emerge thus far (Lee, Vincent, Hart, & Corrado, 2003; Murrie & Cornell, 2002) is that it does not correlate very highly with the PCL:YV (Forth et al., 2003). As such, it is hard to argue that the two instruments are measuring the same construct. More important, recent evidence suggests that extreme scores on the APSD may not be particularly stable over time (Frick, Kimonis, Dandreaux, & Farell, 2003). Aside from having important theoretical and psychometric implications (see Johnstone & Cooke, 2004), this finding calls into question the extent to which scores on this instrument should be considered when making choices that affect the long-term placement and treatment of youths.

Who Is Qualified to Assess Psychopathy via PCL Measures?

The question of what constitutes "adequate" training to administer, score, and interpret (as well as potentially testify about) the PCL-R is a complicated topic that goes beyond the issue of psychopathy itself and raises more general ethical issues related to forensic examiner competence and certification, as well as legal questions regarding credentialing as an expert witness (Melton et al., 1997). The ethics code of the American Psychological Association (2002) notes that competence is based on relevant "education, training, supervised experience, consultation, study, or professional experience" (p. 1063) but offers little in the way of specific recommendations as to what thresholds need to be achieved in these diverse areas.

The PCL-R manual (Hare, 2003) provides recommendations regarding qualifications for clinical use (e.g., possession of an advanced degree in the social, medical, or behavioral sciences and completion of graduate coursework in psychometrics and psychopathology; see pp. 16–17), although the author also notes that he has "no professional or legal authority to determine who can and cannot use the PCL-R, or to provide judgments about the adequacy of specific clinicians and their assessments" (p. 16). Despite this assertion, a review of Canadian cases suggests that the recommended qualifications listed in the PCL-R manual are given substantial weight when considering examiner competence. Similar to the recommendations in the PCL manuals, our position is that before assessing psychopathy in "real-world" contexts, an examiner should have knowledge of psychopathology and psychometric theory, possess some type of advanced degree in the social/medical/behavioral sciences, have familiarity with both the relevant empirical literature and the population being assessed (e.g., sexual offenders, female offenders), and have training and experience in administering and scoring the PCL specifically (Forth et al., 2003; Hare, 2003). Although it may seem obvious that examiners should be competent to administer and score the PCL-R and *interpret* (see below) the results, there are ample anecdotal examples of use of the PCL measures by individuals who appear to be lacking in these basic qualifications (Edens, 2001; Hare, 1998).

Regarding the extensiveness of training itself, the PCL-R (Hare, 2003) and PCL:YV (Forth et al., 2003) manuals note that a formal series of basic and advanced workshops (with optional post-workshop evaluations of scoring accuracy) is provided by Darkstone Research Group. It is also noted, however, that these workshops are *not* the exclusive means by which examiners can become competent to administer and score the PCL-R and that some institutions have established their own in-house programs for training staff. It is also asserted that "most clinicians who participate in this [in-house] training should have little difficulty in conducting reliable PCL-R assessments" (Hare, 2003, p. 18), although we are aware of no published research specifically examining the efficacy of any particular training program.

What Type and How Much Information Is Needed to Score PCL Measures?

The newly revised manual (Hare, 2003) describes in detail the assessment procedures required to score the PCL-R (pp. 18–22), with considerable attention given to item-level ratings (see chap. 3). Ideally, scoring is based on information gleaned from semistructured interviews together with reviews of collateral data from institutional files and other sources. The manual specifies that PCL-R ratings should never be based on interview data alone, although scoring on the basis of collateral information alone is permitted. There is ample evidence that PCL-R scores based on collateral information alone are systematically lower than those based on interview plus collateral data (see, e.g., Hare, 2003, Table 4.7), perhaps due to the greater difficulty in gleaning information regarding affective and interpersonal features without conducting an interview.

One rather large area of ambiguity related to PCL assessments is exactly *how much* file and collateral data are needed when attempting to rate the individual items. Here again American Psychological Association (2002) guidelines offer little in the way of specific instruction other than that psychologists should base their opinions on information and techniques sufficient to substantiate their findings (p. 1071). The PCL-R manual (Hare, 2003) notes (in boldface) that ratings "should not be made in the absence of adequate collateral information" (p. 19), but exactly what constitutes "adequate" information is left undefined. Although the manual describes several types of collateral information that would be useful to complete the PCL-R (e.g., arrest reports, institutional adjustment data, prior psychological evaluations, interviews with family members and friends), there is no "minimal threshold" that one can readily point to as a benchmark for declining to complete the PCL-R. It is certainly possible to omit specific items that lack adequate information to score, with the manual recommending that as many as five can be deleted—with scores subsequently being prorated to account for this modification. Although helpful in dealing with specific items, this recommendation does not really address the broader question, "How much is enough?" This would seem to be an even greater concern in relation to the PCL:YV, in that less collateral information is likely to be available for making informed decisions regarding the scoring of items with adolescents. An important and (as best we can discern) unexamined area of research is the extent to which examiners agree or differ in terms of exactly how much information they believe is needed to rate these measures reliably and validly.

Communicating about Psychopathy: Caveats and Qualifiers

At various points in this chapter we have stressed the potentially "prejudicial" nature of psychopathy, with no real evidence reviewed to bolster such claims. As a background for considering some of our concerns about the introduction of PCL scores or other psychopathy-related diagnostic information into legal proceedings, we next review data consistent with our concerns that

psychopathy has the potential to "trump" other sources of information and unduly bias nonclinicians (e.g., judges, jurors) who are the "consumers" of these evaluations.

Among laypersons, the term "psychopath" brings to mind images of serial killers and mass murderers, and the traits associated with psychopathy can have a pronounced impact on attitudes regarding criminal offenders. For example, in a telephone survey of community residents, Helfgott (1997) reported that more than 60% of respondents identified Ted Bundy, Jeffery Dahmer, or Charles Manson when asked to name someone whom they believed to be a psychopath. More recently, in a series of studies manipulating the presence/absence of testimony related to psychopathy in death penalty and sexual predator cases (Edens, Desforges, Fernandez, & Palac, 2004; Edens et al., 2003, in press; Guy & Edens, 2003), it has been demonstrated that psychopathic offenders generally are viewed more negatively and treated more severely by mock jurors than offenders identified as not mentally ill or identified as having a different type of disorder (e.g., schizophrenia). Perhaps even more interesting, support for the death penalty in these studies has been relatively strongly associated with perceptions of the defendant as exhibiting psychopathic traits. That is, the greater the extent to which mock jurors construe the defendant as being a "prototypical psychopath," the higher is the likelihood they will support a death verdict—regardless of whatever testimony or case information they review (see also Guy & Edens, in press). Real-world evidence also supports a similar conclusion, in that surveys of actual jurors in capital murder cases have identified perceived defendant traits such as remorselessness and egocentricity as being influential in jurors' decisions to support a death verdict (Sundby, 1998). As such, unlike many psychological labels that may invoke sympathy (e.g., posttraumatic stress disorder, mental retardation) or at least indifference (e.g., generalized anxiety disorder, schizoid personality disorder), labeling someone a "psychopath" or as possessing psychopathic traits carries a negative connotation that may fundamentally alter how others view and respond to him or her.

Given this brief overview of the potential stigma associated with a diagnosis of psychopathy, we now turn to a discussion of some of the ethical challenges associated with attempting to convey the results of a psychopathy assessment in a manner that comports with professional standards and ethical guidelines. We should note that other commentators might strongly disagree with some of our conclusions and suggestions. We hope, however, that some of our points will at least stimulate further discussion of what we believe to be very important issues.

How "Valid" Is Psychopathy?

It is common in legal case summaries to see assessment measures globally described as "reliable and valid." Although somewhat understandable, we believe such encompassing assertions typically are off point because they ignore what is usually a context-specific question about the utility of a measure as it relates to a particular legal question. For example, when psychopathy is used in relation to violence risk assessments, we would argue that the question of its validity primarily revolves around its predictive utility in relation to the criterion of interest. As such, discussions of the validity of the PCL should be framed in terms of the particular question(s) it is intended to inform (e.g., violence risk of a released sex offender). In authoritative and adversarial legal settings, it is widely known that decision makers often dislike and devalue *"It depends"* answers that reflect probabilistic reasoning and equivocation (Brigham, 1999). However, blanket statements that overgeneralize about complex concepts such as validity for the sake of simplicity (e.g., *"the PCL-R is valid"*) seem less defensible than more exacting and appropriately constrained assertions about the meaning of psychopathy scores in relation to particular legal questions (e.g., *"PCL-R scores can reliably differentiate between those released offenders who are at higher versus lower risk for community violence"*). Moreover, admissibility standards such as the Daubert criteria would seem to compel a careful examination of the validity of any assessment technique in relation to the case at hand.

Two areas in which the issue of validity comes clearly to the fore are violence risk and treatment amenability. Particularly in these areas, we believe the construct of psychopa-

thy lends itself to considerable overreaching by the courts, perhaps with the implicit or explicit support of forensic examiners. In relation to risk assessment issues, a few key areas are worth highlighting beyond those already noted earlier. First, although the use of standardized inventories represents an improvement over unaided clinical judgment, a diagnosis of psychopathy should not be equated with a designation of "dangerousness," nor should it foster any particular level of confidence regarding dichotomous predictions of violence for a specific offender. Although in many contexts a high score on the PCL-R identifies someone who is *probabilistically more likely* to engage in violence than someone with a lower score, this is not the functional equivalent of a "dangerous offender" or "sexual psychopath" classification. These are legal categories that may be informed by expert mental health testimony but are ultimately decided by the trier-of-fact. Moreover, separate from the legal issue is the empirical fact that the baserates of criminal recidivism for psychopathic offenders over relatively long followup periods are quite variable and sometimes relatively low (Freedman, 2001). Although this does not preclude the use of the PCL-R to inform risk assessments, it does raise complicated questions regarding the merits of categorical claims regarding an offender's degree of risk (e.g., *"offender X is at 'high risk' to reoffend"*) (for a more detailed review, see Heilbrun, Dvoskin, Hart, & McNiel, 1999).

More generally, one might question whether it is defensible to use the categorical label "psychopath" at all, particularly in adversarial legal settings. Zinger and Forth (1998), for example, support the use of dimensional measures rather than categorical terminology because it provides more precision in testimony and lessens the chance for judicial misunderstanding. A similar position has been advanced by the American Psychological Association (2001, pp. 63–65), which advises against the labeling of individuals by their disorder or disability (e.g., "schizophrenics," "paraplegics," and "psychopaths"). Conversely, one argument in favor of such a dichotomization would be that there is evidence that a latent taxon may underlie psychopathy (Harris, Rice, & Quinsey, 1994) and that "psychopaths comprise a *dis-*

crete natural class" (Harris et al., 2001, p. 197, emphasis added). Despite this assertion, more recent evidence using more advanced taxometric procedures has suggested that psychopathy is dimensional in nature (Edens, Marcus, Lilienfeld, & Poythress, 2005; Guay, Ruscio, Hare, & Knight, 2004; Marcus, John, & Edens, 2004; see also Bucholz, Hesselbrock, Heath, Kramer, & Schuckit, 2000; Osgood, McMorris, & Potenza, 2002). The implication is that any categorization of "psychopath" versus "nonpsychopath" is an arbitrary cut point on a scale that reflects differences in *degree* rather than in *kind*. As such, qualitative references to whether an individual is "a psychopath," which appear frequently in Canadian cases, would seem to characterize needlessly PCL-R "high scorers" as a unique subgroup of individuals. Although it is conceivable that research will ultimately provide support for etiological theories that might warrant classifying them as fundamentally distinct from the rest of society (e.g., Mealey, 1995), the current state of evidence does not justify such claims in legal settings.

This same concern arises in relation to the relevance of psychopathy to the question of treatment amenability, in that "psychopaths" are often viewed as a class of individuals who are "untreatable." Despite such assertions, the degree to which psychopathy is in fact amenable to intervention remains an area of open inquiry. The available research does clearly suggest that individuals high in psychopathic traits have been *less likely* to benefit from the types of interventions that have been investigated. In our view, however, these findings do *not* support a conclusion that psychopathy is "untreatable." Similar to the findings of recidivism studies, such results indicate a *probabilistic difference* in treatment outcome rather than a categorical distinction between high and low PCL scorers in terms of treatability (Edens, Petrila, & Buffington-Vollum, 2001; Edens, Skeem, et al., 2001). As such, we believe that examiners should scrupulously avoid misinterpreting the results of extant studies to conclude that psychopathy is immutable.

Moreover, based on such nomothetic findings, examiners frequently are asked to draw idiographic conclusions about particular individuals. Again, there is the legal determination that a fact-finder must address that may

be informed by mental health evidence or testimony. Such testimony in turn should be informed by a critical understanding of the strengths and limitations of the extant treatment literature. The relative absence of controlled studies examining treatment approaches that are known to decrease recidivism among offender populations would seem to militate against drawing categorical conclusions that a particular psychopathic offender would not respond to correctional interventions that work with other offenders. Perhaps even more important is to be aware of the limitations of earlier treatment research, which in some instances involved interventions that were ethically questionable and unlikely to result in improvement (e.g., Harris, Rice, & Cormier, 1994). In addition, it is noteworthy that the pessimistic outlook of some commentators (e.g., Kernberg, 1998) is being challenged by recent reviews and newer data that provide some evidence of treatment effects (Salekin, 2002; Skeem, Monahan, & Mulvey, 2002).

How "Reliable" Is a Diagnosis of Psychopathy?

Although much of this chapter has dealt with issues of predictive validity, and a corresponding appeal to examiners to base their conclusions and interpretations on relevant empirical data, a few caveats related to the reliability of psychopathy assessments are in order as well. It is quite interesting to review court cases in which PCL-R ratings become a point of contention. In some instances it seems that there is a strong focus on a specific score (or the concomitant percentile rank at which this score falls), with almost no consideration given to the reliability estimates of the instrument and its standard error of measurement. Although on one level it is heartening to see a critical analysis of the scores, in some instances this seems driven mostly by a desire to support categorical placements (e.g., a 29 is a "nonpsychopath" and a 31 is a "psychopath"). One wonders if such debates would occur if examiners were more prone to report 95% confidence intervals for PCL-R scores rather than (or at least in addition to) the scores themselves. One could easily argue that confidence intervals are a more defensible method of reporting results than discrete scores, as they represent the likely range in which an individual offender's "true" score actually falls and also make clearer some of the intrinsic limitations of psychological assessment data.

As a final issue related to reliability, it is also worth noting that the standard errors of measurement reported in the PCL manuals almost certainly should be considered a "best case" scenario, in that they typically have been derived from controlled studies in nonadversarial circumstances using examiners with extensive training. This may be a far cry from some "real-world" contexts involving less optimal data or less well-trained examiners, such as one recent case in which examiners hired separately by the defense and by the prosecution (both of whom were credentialed as "experts" by the court) differed by 11 points on their PCL-R ratings of the defendant (*R. v LaRue*, 2003; for a more extreme example, see *R. v K.S.*, 2004, where one examiner suggested the offender's score fell at the 32nd percentile, whereas the other examiner scored him at the 91st percentile). We are unaware of any studies examining the reliability of psychopathy scores by prosecution versus defense experts, but anecdotal evidence from several Canadian and U.S. cases suggests that discrepancies often exceed the standard error of difference that would be expected on the basis of data reported in the PCL-R manual.

SUMMARY

In this chapter, we have reviewed several areas in which various legal systems may (and may not) consider psychopathy to be important in terms of addressing issues such as violence risk potential and treatment amenability. We also have noted that it is clear the term "psychopath" in legal contexts often is not synonymous with current clinical definitions. Mental health professionals have contributed to this confusion by using various terms and labels to describe constructs that may be only loosely related, such as sociopathy and APD (Ogloff & Lyon, 1998; see section "Issues of Language and 'Fit,'" earlier in this chapter). Despite these nosological inconsistencies, however, a review of admissibility standards and cases suggests that assessments of psychopathy

tend to survive legal challenges to their introduction and use. As such, examiners are likely to have considerable latitude in terms of the opinions and conclusions they offer regarding the relevance of psychopathy assessments.

As noted earlier, the term "psychopath" is a powerful label that can have a profound impact on how individuals are perceived and treated within the legal system. In this chapter, we have identified several ethical issues that may arise when mental health examiners bring this complex psychological construct "out of the lab" and into the real world, and we have discussed the legal climate related to psychopathy as it is construed by the criminal justice system. There are clearly instances in which the PCL-R and its derivatives have "probative" value, in that scores from these instruments are meaningfully associated with important outcomes (e.g., violent recidivism), and their appropriate use may lead to socially desirable outcomes (e.g., reduced victimization). However, there is also growing anecdotal evidence regarding misuses of these instruments, some of which may be attempts to capitalize on its face validity as a label typically associated with "bad" or "evil" individuals such as Charles Manson or Ted Bundy (Helfgott, 1997) for purposes of stigmatizing criminal defendants (Edens, Petrila, & Buffington-Vollum, 2001). Finally, there remain areas in which we simply do not know what the ultimate implications of psychopathy will be for the legal system. It is conceivable, for example, that advances in our understanding of the etiology and biological bases of psychopathy may some day legitimize it as an exculpatory factor in criminal proceedings, or at least justify its relevance in relation to diminished capacity issues. The current legal climate, however, offers little to suggest that such evidence would be well received in the post-Hinckley era, in which sanity statutes and the courts typically have shunned volitional impairment as a legal defense. In fact, such evidence probably would be more likely to be used to support further deprivations of liberty (e.g., civil commitment) because it would bolster legal claims that such persons are suffering from a "behavioral abnormality" characterized by volitional impairment (e.g., *Kansas v. Crane*, 2002).

We have offered some general suggestions and comments regarding what we believe to be ethically defensible uses of the psychopathy construct in legal settings. Some of these are relatively banal (e.g., know the data supporting its relevance to the case at hand), whereas others are likely to be more controversial (e.g., abandon the use of the diagnostic label "psychopath"). We hope that, regardless of the ultimate merits of some of our suggestions, they will at least spark further discussion of how best to use psychopathy measures in settings in which they can have life-altering (or perhaps even life-ending) consequences.

REFERENCES

American Psychological Association. (2001). *Publication manual of the American Psychological Association* (5th ed.). Washington, DC: Author.

American Psychological Association. (2002). Ethical principles of psychologists and code of conduct. *American Psychologist, 57,* 1060–1073.

Andrews, D. A., & Bonta, J. L. (1995). *The Level of Service Inventory—Revised (LSI-R): User's manual.* Toronto, ON, Canada: Multi-Health Systems.

Brandt, J. R., Kennedy, W. A., Patrick, C. J., & Curtin, J. J. (1997). Assessment of psychopathy in a population of incarcerated adolescent offenders. *Psychological Assessment, 9,* 429–435.

Brigham, J. (1999). What is forensic psychology anyway? *Law and Human Behavior, 23,* 273–298.

Bucholz, K. K., Hesselbrock, V. M., Heath, A. C., Kramer, J., & Schuckit, M. (2000). A latent class analysis of antisocial personality disorder symptom data from a multi-centre family study of alcoholism. *Addiction, 95,* 553–567.

Buffington-Vollum, J. K., Edens, J. F., Johnson, D. W., & Johnson, J. (2002). Psychopathy as a predictor of institutional misbehavior among sex offenders: A prospective replication. *Criminal Justice and Behavior, 29,* 497–511.

Campbell, M. A., Porter, S., & Santor, D. (2004). Psychopathic traits in adolescent offenders: An evaluation of criminal history, clinical, and psychosocial correlates. *Behavioral Sciences and the Law, 22,* 23–48.

Cauffman, E., & Skeem, J. L. (2004, March). The developmental (in)appropriateness of assessing juvenile psychopathy. In J. Skeem (Chair), *Contemporary issues in juvenile psychopathy.* Symposium conducted at the biennial meeting of the American Psychology–Law Society, Scottsdale, AZ.

Committee on Ethical Guidelines for Forensic Psychologists. (1991). Specialty guidelines for forensic psychologists. *Law and Human Behavior, 15,* 655–665.

Corrado, R. R., Vincent, G. M., Hart, S. D., & Cohen, I. M. (2004). Predictive validity of the Psychopathy Checklist: Youth Version for general and violent recidivism. *Behavioral Sciences and the Law, 22,* 5–22.

Cunningham, M. D., & Reidy, T. J. (2002). Violence risk assessment at federal capital sentencing: Individualization, generalization, relevance, and scientific standards. *Criminal Justice and Behavior, 29,* 512–537.

Daubert v. Merrell-Dow Pharmaceuticals, Inc. 113 S.Ct. 2786 (1993).

Edens, J. F. (2001). Misuses of the Hare Psychopathy Checklist—Revised in court: Two case examples. *Journal of Interpersonal Violence, 16,* 1082–1093.

Edens, J. F. (in press). Unresolved controversies concerning psychopathy: Implications for clinical and forensic decision-making. *Professional Psychology: Research and Practice.*

Edens, J. F., Buffington-Vollum, J. K., Keilen, A., Roskamp, P., & Anthony, C. (2005). Predictions of future dangerousness in capital murder trials: Is it time to "disinvent the wheel"? *Law and Human Behavior, 29,* 55–86.

Edens, J. F., Colwell, L. H., Desforges, D. M., & Fernandez, K. (in press). The impact of mental health evidence on support for capital punishment: Are defendants labeled psychopathic considered more deserving of death? *Behavioral Sciences and the Law.*

Edens, J. F., Desforges, D. M., Fernandez, K., & Palac, C. A. (2004). Effects of psychopathy and violence risk testimony on mock juror perceptions of dangerousness in a capital murder trial. *Psychology, Crime, and Law, 10,* 393–412.

Edens, J. F., Guy, L. S., & Fernandez, K. (2003). Psychopathic traits predict attitudes toward a juvenile capital murderer. *Behavioral Sciences and the Law, 21,* 807–828.

Edens, J. F., Hart, S. D., Johnson, D. W., Johnson, J., & Olver, M. E. (2000). Use of the Personality Assessment Inventory to assess psychopathy in offender populations. *Psychological Assessment, 12,* 132–139.

Edens, J. F., Marcus, D. K., Lilienfeld, S. O., & Poythress, N. G. (2005). *Psychopathic, not psychopath: Taxometric evidence for the dimensional structure of psychopathy.* Manuscript submitted for publication.

Edens, J. F., Petrila, J., & Buffington-Vollum, J. K. (2001). Psychopathy and the death penalty: Can the Psychopathy Checklist—Revised identify offenders who represent "a continuing threat to society"? *Journal of Psychiatry and Law, 29,* 433–481.

Edens, J. F., Skeem, J. L., Cruise, K. R., & Cauffman, E. (2001). Assessment of "juvenile psychopathy" and its association with violence: A critical review. *Behavioral Sciences and the Law, 19,* 53–80.

Elwood, C. E., Poythress, N. G., & Douglas, K. S. (2004). Evaluation of the Hare P-SCAN in a non-clinical population. *Personality and Individual Differences, 36,* 833–843.

Fitch, W. L., & Ortega, R. J. (2000). Law and the confinement of psychopaths. *Behavioral Sciences and the Law, 18*, 663–678.

Forth, A. E., Kosson, D., & Hare, R. D. (2003). *Psychopathy Checklist: Youth Version technical manual.* Toronto, ON, Canada: Multi-Health Systems.

Freedman, D. (2001). False prediction of future dangerousness: Error rates and Psychopathy Checklist—Revised. *Journal of the American Academy of Psychiatry and Law, 29*, 89–95.

Frick, P. J., & Hare, R. D. (2001). *Antisocial Process Screening Device.* Toronto, ON, Canada: Multi-Health Systems.

Frick, P. J., Kimonis, E. R., Dandreaux, D. M., & Farell, J. M. (2003). The 4 year stability of psychopathic traits in non-referred youth. *Behavioral Sciences and the Law, 21*, 713–736.

Frye v. United States 293 F. 1013 (D.C. Cir. 1923).

Garcetti v. Superior Court, 85 Cal. App. 4th 508 (2000).

Gendreau, P., Goggin, C., & Smith, P. (2002). Is the PCL-R really the "unparalleled" measure of risk? A lesson in knowledge cumulation. *Criminal Justice and Behavior, 29*, 397–426.

Guay, J., Ruscio, J., Hare, R., & Knight, R. A. (2004, October). *The latent structure of psychopathy: When more is simply more.* Paper presented at the annual meeting of the Society for Research in Psychopathology, St. Louis, MO.

Gunn, J. (2000). A millennium monster is born. *Criminal Behaviour and Mental Health, 10*, 73–76.

Guy, L. S., & Edens, J. F. (2003). Juror decision-making in a mock sexually violent predator trial: Gender differences in the impact of divergent types of expert testimony. *Behavioral Sciences and the Law, 21*, 215–237.

Guy, L. S., & Edens, J. F. (in press). Gender differences in attitudes toward psychopathic sexual offenders. *Behavioral Sciences and the Law.*

Guy, L. S., Edens, J. F., Anthony, C., & Douglas, K. S. (in press). Does psychopathy predict institutional misconduct among adults? A meta-analytic investigation. *Journal of Consulting and Clinical Psychology.*

Hare, R. D. (1991). *Hare Psychopathy Checklist—Revised manual.* Toronto, ON, Canada: Multi-Health Systems.

Hare, R. D. (1998). The Hare PCL-R: Some issues concerning its use and misuse. *Legal and Criminological Psychology, 3*, 99–119.

Hare, R. D. (2003). *Hare Psychopathy Checklist—Revised manual* (2nd ed.). Toronto, ON, Canada: Multi-Health Systems.

Hare, R. D., & Hervé, H. F. (1999). *Hare P-Scan: Research Version manual.* Toronto, ON, Canada: Multi-Health Systems.

Harris, G. T., Rice, M. E., & Cormier, C. A. (1994). Psychopaths: Is a therapeutic community therapeutic? *Therapeutic Communities, 15*, 283–299.

Harris, G., Rice, M., & Quinsey, V. (1994). Psychopathy as a taxon: Evidence that psychopaths are a discrete class. *Journal of Consulting and Clinical Psychology, 62*, 387–397.

Harris, G., Skilling, T., & Rice, M. (2001). The construct of psychopathy. *Crime and Justice, 28*, 197–264.

Hart, S. D. (1998). Psychopathy and risk for violence. In D. J. Cooke, A. E. Forth, & R. D. Hare (Eds.), *Psychopathy: Theory, research, and implications for society* (pp. 355–373). Dordrecht, The Netherlands: Kluwer.

Heilbrun, K. (1992). The role of psychological testing in forensic assessment. *Law and Human Behavior, 16*, 257–272.

Heilbrun, K., Dvoskin, J., Hart, S., & McNeil, D. (1999). Violence risk communication: Implications for research, policy, and practice. *Health, Risk, and Society, 1*, 91–106.

Helfgott, J. B. (1997, March). *The popular conception of the psychopath: Implications for criminal justice policy and practice.* Paper presented at the annual convention of the Academy of Criminal Justice Sciences, Louisville, KY.

Hemphill, J. F., & Hare, R. D. (2004). Some misconceptions about the Hare PCL-R and risk assessment. *Criminal Justice and Behavior, 31*, 203–243.

Hicks, M., Rogers, R., & Cashel, M. (2000). Predictions of violent and total infractions among institutionalized male juvenile offenders. *Journal of the American Academy of Psychiatry and the Law, 28*, 183–190.

In re Commitment of R.S., 773 A.2d 72 (N.J. Super. 2001).

In re Detention of Holtz, 653 N.W.2d 613 (Iowa App. 2002).

In re Linehan, 518 N.W.2d 609; 1994 Minn. LEXIS 501.

In re Valdez, No. 99-000045C1 (unpub. op., Pinellas County, 6th Cir., Aug. 21, 2000).

Janus, S. (1998). Hendricks and the moral terrain of police power civil commitment. *Psychology, Public Policy, and Law, 4*, 297–322.

Johnstone, L., & Cooke, D. J. (2004). Psychopathic-like traits in childhood: Conceptual and measurement concerns. *Behavioral Sciences and the Law, 22*, 103–126.

Kansas v. Crane, 122 S. Ct. 867 (2002).

Kansas v. Hendricks, 117 S. Ct. 2072 (1997).

Kendell, R.E. (2002). The distinction between personality disorder and mental illness. *British Journal of Psychiatry, 180*, 110–115.

Kernberg, O. (1998). The psychotherapeutic management of psychopathic, narcissistic, and paranoid transferences. In T. Millon, E. Simonsen, M. Birket-Smith, & R. D. Davis (Eds.), *Psychopathy: Antisocial, criminal, and violent behavior* (pp. 372–382). New York: Guilford Press.

Kosson, D. S., Steuerwald, B. L., Forth, A. E., & Kirkhart, K. J. (1997). A new method for assessing the interpersonal behavior of psychopathic individuals: Preliminary validation studies. *Psychological Assessment, 9*, 89–101.

Krober, H. L., & Lau, S. (2000). Bad or mad? Personality disorders and legal responsibility—The German situation. *Behavioral Sciences and the Law, 18*, 679–690.

Lee, Z., Vincent, G. M., Hart, S. D., & Corrado, R. R. (2003). The validity of the Antisocial Process Screening Device as a self-report measure of psychopathy in adolescent offenders. *Behavioral Sciences and the Law, 21*, 771–786.

Lilienfeld, S. O., & Andrews, B. P. (1996). Development and preliminary validation of a self-report measure of psychopathic personality traits in noncriminal populations. *Journal of Personality Assessment, 66*, 488–524.

Lyon, D. R., & Ogloff, J. R. P. (2000). Legal and ethical issues in psychopathy assessment. In C. Gacono (Ed.), *The clinical and forensic assessment of psychopathy* (pp. 139–173). Mahwah, NJ: Erlbaum.

Marcus, D. K., John, S., & Edens, J. F. (2004). A taxometric analysis of psychopathic personality. *Journal of Abnormal Psychology, 113*, 626–635.

Marcyzk, G. R., Heilbrun, K., Lander, T., & DeMatteo, D. (2003). Predicting juvenile recidivism with the PCL:YV, MAYSI, and YLS/CMI. *Journal of Forensic Mental Health, 2*, 7–18.

Mealey, L. (1995). The sociobiology of sociopathy: An integrated evolutionary model. *Behavioral and Brain Sciences, 19*, 523–540.

Melton, G. B., Petrila, J., Poythress, N. G., & Slobogin, C. (1997). *Psychological evaluations for the courts* (2nd ed.). New York: Guilford Press.

Morey, L.C. (1991). *Personality Assessment Inventory manual.* Odessa, FL: PAR.

Murrie, D. C., & Cornell, D. G. (2002). Psychopathy screening of incarcerated juveniles: A comparison of measures. *Psychological Assessment, 14*, 390–396.

Ogloff, J. R. P., & Lyon, D. R. (1998). Legal issues associated with the concept of psychopathy. In D. J. Cooke, A. E. Forth, & R. D. Hare (Eds.) *Psychopathy: Theory, research, and implications for society* (pp. 401–422). Dordrecht, The Netherlands: Kluwer.

Osgood, D. W., McMorris, B. J., & Potenza, M. T. (2002). Analyzing multiple-item measures of crime and deviance I: Item response theory scaling. *Journal of Quantitative Criminology, 18*, 267–296.

Otto, R. K. (2004, March). *Committee to revise Div. 41/ ABFP specialty guidelines.* Presentation at the biennial meeting of the American Psychology–Law Society, Scottsdale, AZ.

Otto, R. K., & Heilbrun, K. (2002). The practice of forensic psychology: A look toward the future in light of the past. *American Psychologist, 57*, 5–18.

Parliamentary Office of Science and Technology. (2003). *Reform of mental health legislation.* Postnote: October 2003, Number 04. Retrieved from www.parliament.uk/post.

Ponder, J. I. (1998). *An investigation of psychopathy in a sample of violent juvenile offenders.* Unpublished doctoral dissertation, University of Texas at Austin.

R. v. K.S., O.J. No. 3826; ON.C. LEXIS 4498 (2004).

R. v. LaRue, B.C.D. Crim.J. 14785 (2003).

Reed, J. (1996). Editorial: Psychopathy—A clinical and legal dilemma. *British Journal of Psychiatry, 168*, 4–9.

Salekin, R. T. (2002). Psychopathy and therapeutic pessimism: Clinical lore or clinical reality? *Clinical Psychology Review, 22*, 79–112,

Salekin, R. T., Rogers, R., & Sewell, K. W. (1997). Construct validity of psychopathy in a female offender sample: A multitrait–multimethod evaluation. *Journal of Abnormal Psychology, 106*, 576–585.

Scottish Executive. (2000). *Report of the Committee on Serious Violent and Sexual Offenders.* Edinburgh: Author.

Skeem, J. L., Monahan, J., & Mulvey, E. P. (2002). Psychopathy, treatment involvement, and subsequent violence among psychiatric patients. *Law and Human Behavior, 26*, 577–603.

Skeem, J. L., & Mulvey, E. P. (2001). Psychopathy and community violence among civil psychiatric patients: Results from the MacArthur Violence Risk Assessment Study. *Journal of Consulting and Clinical Psychology, 69*, 358–374.

Sundby, S. E. (1998). The capital jury and absolution: The intersection of trial strategy, remorse, and the death penalty. *Cornell Law Review, 83*, 1557–1598.

Tex. Health & Safety Code, § 841.023 (Vernon 2004).

Walters, G. D. (2003). Predicting criminal justice outcomes with the Psychopathy Checklist and Lifestyle Criminality Screening Form: A meta-analytic comparison. *Behavioral Sciences and the Law, 21*, 89–102.

Walters, G. D., Duncan, S., & Geyer, M. (2003). Predicting disciplinary adjustment in inmates undergoing forensic evaluation: A direct comparison of the PCL-R and PAI. *Journal of Forensic Psychiatry and Psychology, 14*, 382–292.

Warren, J. I., Chauhan, P., & Murrie, D. (2004). *Screening for psychopathy among incarcerated women: Psychometric properties and construct validity of the Hare P-SCAN.* Manuscript submitted for publication.

Wash. Laws SECTION SIGN 71-09-010 (2000).

Zinger, I., & Forth, A. E. (1998). Psychopathy and Canadian criminal proceedings: The potential for human rights abuses. *Canadian Journal of Criminology, 40*, 237–277.

30

Toward the Future

Translating Basic Research into Prevention and Treatment Strategies

MICHAEL C. SETO
VERNON L. QUINSEY

Such men are *born criminals by nature*, and are only distinguished from ordinary criminals by the great extent of their moral incapacity, by their having wills completely unaffected by the restraining experiences of life, and by their being *fundamentally incorrigible*. . . . There is, therefore, as a rule, no other course to be taken, for their own sake, and for the sake of those around them, than to isolate them as being unfit for society, and as far as possible to find them occupation.
—KRAEPELIN (1904/1968, p. 289; original emphasis)

Harris and Rice (Chapter 28, this volume) review the treatment outcome research on psychopathic offenders. As those authors point out, this research has been hampered by methodological limitations, including different operationalizations of psychopathy, the absence of objective outcome measures, and the absence of randomized clinical trials. Only a few evaluation studies are informative about treatment outcomes for psychopathic offenders. One matched-comparison study found that psychopathic offenders were more likely to reoffend after participating in a therapeutic community program, whereas nonpsychopathic offenders were less likely to reoffend (Rice, Harris, & Cormier, 1992). A more recent matched-comparison study found that participation in education or vocational training programs reduced recidivism in nonpsychopathic offenders but had no effect on psychopathic offenders (Hare, Clark, Grann, & Thornton, 2000). The same investigators also found that among offenders who scored high on Factor 1 (interpersonal and affective features) of the Psychopathy Checklist—Revised (PCL-R), those who participated in short-term psychotherapy were more likely to reoffend than those who did not participate, while there was no difference between treated and untreated groups among those who were low on Factor 1.

Because the principal problem in interpreting the efficacy of interventions for psychopathic offenders is the absence of randomized clinical trials, we examined the outcomes of randomized clinical trials involving offenders diagnosed with antisocial personality disorder (APD; American Psychiatric Association, 2000). These outcome studies are germane because there is a strong correlation ($r \approx .85$) between the number of diagnostic features of APD that a person exhibits and his or her PCL-R score, and both APD features and PCL-R items are good indicators of an antisocial taxon (Skilling, Harris, Rice, & Quinsey, 2002).

Two randomized clinical trials investigating the effect of substance abuse treatment found no difference between the treatment and comparison groups for those diagnosed with APD, while those who did not have the diagnosis and were assigned to treatment were less likely to relapse than those assigned to the comparison group (Leal, Ziedonis, & Kosten, 1994; Messina, Wish, & Nemes, 1999). Again, this suggests that individuals who are likely to be psychopaths (by virtue of having many features of APD) do not appear to benefit from treatment that is effective for nonpsychopaths.

There is also indirect evidence for the lack of positive treatment effects on psychopathic offenders from work done on offender risk assessment. Offenders in many follow-up studies have received treatment of some sort prior to their release from custody. Thus, risk appraisal scales designed on the basis of these follow-up studies are crude measures of treatment efficacy. These scales often include measures of psychopathy or proxies of psychopathic traits such as early behavior problems, substance abuse, and criminal history; very few valid risk appraisal scales contain treatment-related items, and these items are generally less predictive than items reflecting psychopathic traits. Moreover, as the accuracy of predictors pertaining to psychopathy and its proxies increases, the variance that could be potentially accounted for by existing interventions necessarily decreases.

In the following sections, we consider the potential problems for current interventions, the relevance of basic research for prevention and intervention efforts, and the relevance of a developmental understanding of psychopathy in thinking about how to intervene. We conclude with a summary of research that can inform the design of future interventions and describe features of treatment that may increase their effectiveness.

DESIGNING FUTURE INTERVENTIONS

Clinicians who have worked with psychopaths commonly believe that they are untreatable. One reason for this pessimism—which is based on only a few empirical evaluations of interventions for psychopathic offenders—is the observation that the personal characteristics associated with recidivism in follow-up studies are also related to poor treatment response. We discuss this notion in greater detail in the next section. Nonetheless, this clinical pessimism raises several important questions: How broadly can our inductive net from previous treatment trials be cast? Can we generalize previous failures only to particular treatments delivered in particular venues or can we write off entire classes of interventions, such as any psychotherapeutic program that requires interpersonal influence? If we accept the proposition that psychopaths are not going to benefit from current interventions, does this apply only to adults? Are "fledgling psychopaths" (at-risk children and youths; Lynam, 1996) unlikely to be affected by intervention? The treatment outcome literature suggests that programs to reduce crime are more successful with children than with adults (Aos, Phipps, Barnoski, & Lieb, 2001), so it is not unreasonable to expect the same to be true among psychopaths.

Another fundamental question is how to judge the impact of an intervention; in other words, what represents a successful outcome? For professionals working in the criminal justice system and for many people in the public, an intervention must lead to a reduction in criminal recidivism in order to be successful. However, success is a relative term and depends on how we measure the reduction in recidivism. For example, in a comparison between treated and nontreated psychopaths, we might find a substantial and statistically significant difference in favor of the treated group even when the majority of both groups recidivated. The goal of a relative reduction in recidivism is much less ambitious and more realistic than requiring an intervention to reduce the recidivism rate of psychopaths to that of all offenders (much less to the offending rate of the general population).

There are different ways in which a hypothetical intervention for psychopaths could reduce criminal recidivism. One way in which an intervention could work is by preventing psychopathic offenders from reoffending by altering the environment in substantial and ongoing ways (e.g., 24-hour monitoring by supervisory staff, restricted mobility, and teaching the public to protect itself better from psychopaths they encounter). Such an intervention could reduce recidivism but would not alter psychopathic traits, at least directly. One could consider this a form of harm reduction, but one that focuses on harm resulting from criminal behavior and not harm resulting from noncriminal exploitation in interpersonal relationships. An alternative possibility is that a treatment would achieve a reduction in recidivism by altering one or more psychopathic traits. Such a treatment would reduce both the harm associated with crime as well as the personal and social harm caused by psychopaths' tendencies to engage in selfish, short-sighted noncriminal behaviors.

Treatments that target psychopathic characteristics not only permit the social harm associated with psychopathy to be reduced but also broaden the population of individuals to which the treatment could be applied to include noncriminal psychopaths. However, it is worthwhile to contemplate the outcome literature on the treatment of attention-deficit/hyperactivity disorder (ADHD) when thinking about the potential efficacy of prevention efforts for psychopathy. Children with ADHD are at greater risk than children without ADHD for antisocial outcomes as adults, including psychopathy (Frick & Marsee, Chapter 18, this volume). One might think that interventions might be more profitably directed toward at-risk children. The most effective interventions for ADHD are known to involve psychostimulants, behavior modification, or their combination. Unfortunately, these treatments, while efficacious during the time they are administered, appear to have little or no long-term effect (Waschbusch & Hill, 2003). One could imagine that prevention efforts directed at psychopathy might have short-term effects on relevant behaviors (e.g., aggression, noncompliance, and lying), but that such effects would dissipate over time so that adolescent and adult psychopaths would continue to cause harm in both criminal and noncriminal ways.

Psychopathic Features That Might Interfere with Treatment

Given the lack of empirical support for current treatment approaches, how do we proceed from what we know after several decades of basic research on psychopathy? We use a simple model of therapeutic relationships to organize some of the relevant research (see Figure 30.1). This model of treatment effects recognizes that client characteristics, therapist characteristics, therapeutic alliance, and the specific mechanisms of a particular psychotherapy approach can all contribute to outcome.

Client Characteristics

Many psychopathic characteristics are likely to limit the potential for interventions to reduce recidivism. For example, most psychotherapeutic approaches are predicated on the individual's motivation to change, because effort is required to participate in individual or group therapy sessions, complete in-session and homework assignments, and comply with any program requirements. Psychopathic offenders are more likely to be disruptive and noncompliant during therapy sessions than nonpsychopathic offenders

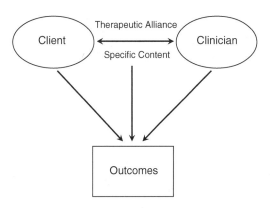

FIGURE 30.1. Simple model of factors associated with outcome for one-on-one treatment relationship.

(e.g., Hobson, Shine, & Roberts, 2000; Ogloff, Wong, & Greenwood, 1990; Seto & Barbaree, 1999) and thus are less likely to be able to benefit fully from their participation in these sessions.

Cleckley (1976) and Hare (1991, 2003) have commented at length on the core interpersonal and affective features of psychopathy, including lack of remorse, guilt, callousness, and shallow affect (loading onto Factor 1). Can these aspects of psychopathy be altered? If psychopaths are callous in the sense that they truly do not care about the well-being of other people, and are not motivated to change their interpersonal styles, how would a psychotherapy technique increase empathy? Research on the differences in psychopaths' processing of verbal and emotional information suggests that any psychotherapies that focus on inducing remorse or guilt, increasing empathy, and accepting personal responsibility for offenses and other antisocial behavior are very unlikely to be successful. For example, the emotional valence of target words in lexical tasks appears to have a smaller effect on psychopaths, such that strong emotional words enhance task performance among nonpsychopaths but do not do so among psychopaths (Williamson, Harpur, & Hare, 1991; Newman, Lorenz, & Schmitt, 1998, cited in Steuerwald & Kosson, 2000). However, psychopaths do show affective facilitation in lexical tasks if provoked by a confederate prior to the task, suggesting that psychopaths have a higher threshold rather than a lack of this capacity in processing emotional information (Steuerwald, 1996). There is also some evidence that psychopaths do not differ from nonpsychopaths in their ability to correctly label affective words (Forth, 1992; Patterson, 1991). Based on these findings, Steuerwald and Kosson (2000) have suggested that, "psychopaths may be characterized by a lack of insight into their affective state and may have difficulty accessing affective material when in nonaffective states" (p. 129).

Psychopaths also appear to be less affected by emotionally neutral distractions (Newman, Schmitt, & Voss, 1997), and individuals with psychopathic traits are less sensitive to nondominant cues when engaged in goal-directed behavior (Newman, Patterson, & Kosson, 1987; O'Brien & Frick, 1996). In other words, psychopaths pay less attention to peripheral cues once their attention is focused on the reward associated with task success (e.g., winning money for being correct on a computer game trial). This tendency toward a dominant response style among psychopaths could interfere with psychotherapies that focus on problem-solving or relapse prevention skills, because the use of these skills requires an awareness of the costs as well as the benefits of a particular course of action.

Although psychopathic offenders make more errors than nonpsychopathic offenders in tasks in which correct responses are rewarded, they do not differ in conditions when errors are concomitantly punished (Newman & Kosson, 1986). Moreover, psychopathic offenders do not differ in their performance when both reward and punishment contingencies are manipulated so that they are obvious, or when there is a long enough interval between trials to allow the participants to consider their options (Newman, Patterson, Howland, & Nichols, 1990). These studies suggest that, as in the laboratory research on emotional information processing, psychopaths differ from nonpsychopaths in their threshold for response modulation but do not lack this ability.

Although psychopaths do respond to punishments, they appear to be less reactive than nonpsychopathic offenders to aversive stimuli; for example, they do not show the same startle potentiation during exposure to aversive stimuli as nonpsychopathic offenders or control volunteers show in the laboratory (Levenston, Patrick, Bradley, & Lang, 2000; Patrick, Bradley, & Lang, 1993). Again, this suggests that the threshold of psychopaths for shifting their attention from goal seeking is higher. There is also some evidence that noncriminal psychopaths do not show conditioned aversive responding (Flor, Birbaumer, Hermann, Ziegler, & Patrick, 2002), a finding that could not be explained by psychopaths having a lower sensitivity to aversive or noxious stimuli because there was no group difference in responses to the unconditioned stimuli.

Another obstacle to therapies that focus on developing relapse prevention strategies and other cognitive skills is the tendency of psychopathic offenders to be more impulsive, unrealistic in their long-term planning, and disorganized in their lifestyles. Thus, it may not be surprising that more positive ratings of offenders' understanding of the antecedents of their offenses and ability to describe relapse prevention strategies do not appear to be related to a reduction in recidivism, at least among sex offenders scoring higher in psychopathy (Looman, Abracen, Serin, & Marquis, 2005; Seto, 2003; Seto & Barbaree, 1999). In fact, there appears to be a critical conceptual problem with relapse prevention models, because these models are predicated on the assumption that the person undergoing therapy is motivated to avoid offending. What about offenders (psychopaths or otherwise) who seek opportunities to offend and are primarily motivated by a desire to engage in criminal behaviors without getting caught? We would argue that interventions that rely on psychopathic offenders' motivation to change are less likely to be successful than those interventions, such as behavior modification regimens, that do not.

Finally, many proximal treatment outcome measures are based on offender self-report (e.g., acceptance of responsibility, expressions of remorse or guilt, and awareness of offense antecedents or relapse prevention strategies). Psychopathic offenders engage in much more deception than nonpsychopathic offenders, although (fortunately, for treatment providers and supervisory staff) much of this deception is in implausible forms (Rogers & Cruise, 2000). Psychopathic offenders may be more likely to attempt to deceive treatment providers than nonpsychopathic offenders, creating a demand for proximal treatment outcome measures that are not based on self-report. Importantly, ultimate treatment outcome measures such as recidivism and other antisocial behavior are not based on self-report.

To summarize, many defining characteristics of psychopaths may impede the ability of interventions to reduce recidivism or other harm. These characteristics include psychopaths' lack of remorse or guilt, callousness, irresponsibility, impulsivity, unrealistic long-term planning, unstable lifestyles, and dominant response styles. Other obstacles to many contemporary psychotherapy approaches are the therapeutic alliance (or lack thereof) and the identification of suitable treatments.

Therapist Characteristics and Alliance

Meta-analytic studies demonstrating relatively few or no differences in the success of various psychotherapeutic approaches have stimulated research on the nonspecific factors that affect treatment outcome. There is good evidence that aspects of the therapeutic alliance are particularly important, with a recent meta-analysis of 79 studies finding a reliable, moderate relationship between measures of therapeutic alliance and outcome (Martin, Garske, & Davis, 2000). According to Martin and colleagues, the common elements across different definitions of therapeutic alliance are the collaborative nature of the therapeutic relationship, the affective bond between therapist and client, and the therapist's and client's agreement on treatment goals and tasks.

Developing a therapeutic alliance with psychopathic clients could be quite challenging because of their defining characteristics and because of therapists' reaction to noncompliance; disruptive behavior; the nature of psychopaths' offenses; and concerns about possible exploitation, manipulation, and deception. One could imagine that there is a great deal of potential for therapist mistrust, suspicion, and more confrontational or hostile interactions with psychopathic clients (these therapist behaviors are sometimes referred to as countertransference in the clinical literature). Consistent with this hypothesis, Taft, Murphy, Musser, and Remington (2004) found that self-reported psychopathic characteristics were significantly and negatively associated with therapeutic alliance in a sample of men in treatment for partner abuse. Psychopathic characteristics were also negatively associated with motivation for change, and motivation for change mediated the relationship between psychopathic characteristics and therapeutic alliance.

Treatment Content

Research on criminogenic needs (changeable factors associated with a greater likelihood of reoffending; see Andrews & Bonta, 1998) has lagged behind the research advancing actuarial assessment methods for predicting recidivism. The most important issue here is that psychopathy may be a moderator of treatment effects: What works for nonpsychopathic offenders might not work for psychopathic offenders. For example, substance abuse predicts recidivism among nonpsychopathic offenders but not among psychopathic offenders, even though psychopathic offenders often abuse substances. This suggests that reducing substance abuse would not concomitantly reduce recidivism among psychopaths. This is an empirical question, of course, but studies examining the impact of substance abuse interventions on individuals diagnosed with antisocial personality disorder do not suggest a positive outcome. Our brief review of research on information processing among psychopaths suggests that they differ in terms of their *thresholds* for affective facilitation, fearfulness, response modulation, and startle reflex potentiation, rather than in their absolute capacity to engage in the cognitive and affective processes that underlie these phenomena. The major applied question arising from this basic research concerns how treatment might be designed to lower or normalize these thresholds, and how changing these thresholds might affect recidivism and other behaviors of interest.

The Relevance of Basic Research for Designing Interventions

Little is known about the proximate causes of psychopathy. Although treatments can be effective without addressing causes (e.g., the impact of behavior modification on symptoms displayed by institutionalized schizophrenic patients; Paul & Lentz, 1977), understanding the proximal causes of psychopathy may help us identify the most promising avenues to pursue in intervention. Of particular interest to us is the literature on neuroscientific findings comparing psychopathic and nonpsychopatic offenders.

Raine and Yang (Chapter 14, this volume) provide an extensive review of the neuroscientific literature on psychopathy. There have been very few such investigations of psychopathic offenders per se; most of the extant studies have examined violent or persistent offenders. These studies have consistently identified the prefrontal and temporal lobes as key areas in understanding violent offending and persistent criminality. Raine and Yang note that identifying areas that differ between psychopaths and controls may

eventually lead to stem cell therapies that would target the neuropsychological substrate of psychopathy. Although this represents an exciting possibility, we expect that such endeavours will need to distinguish between primary and secondary psychopathy (see Poythress & Skeem, Chapter 9, this volume) in order to achieve success. Much of the research reviewed by Raine and Yang may apply only to secondary psychopaths (i.e., those who display psychopathic traits and behavior as a result of neurodevelopmental problems). From the developmental account described later, we would predict that primary psychopaths do not show evidence of neuropsychological deficits when compared to normal volunteers (although there might be *differences* in both brain structure and function), whereas secondary psychopaths would show evidence of neuropsychological deficits.

A rodent model is germane in thinking about how neuroscientific research on psychopaths can help advance clinical practice. The hormone vasopressin facilitates pair bonding and paternal care in the monogamous prairie vole (*Microtus ochrogaster*) but has no such effect on the closely related polygamous montane vole (*Microtus montanus*). The different effects of vasopressin in these two species are associated with different patterns of vasopressin receptors in the brain, and these receptor patterns are in turn related to differences in the DNA sequence of vasopressin receptor genes (Young, Wang, & Insel, 1998). Specifically, there is a long DNA sequence in the promoter region of the vasopressin receptor gene of the gregarious but monogamous prairie voles that is absent in the promiscuous montane voles.

Young, Nilsen, Waymire, MacGregor, and Insel (1999) inserted the long promoter sequence into the genome of mice. The vasopressin receptor gene was expressed in the brains of these transgenic mice in a pattern like that naturally found in the prairie vole brain. Although mice are normally much less social than prairie voles, the transgenic mice responded to vasopressin injections with increased social behavior. The transgenic mice were not monogamous but engaged in more social contact with females than either normal mice or montane voles.

The importance of these experiments on rodents is not that vasopressin receptor genes are necessarily involved in psychopathy, although it is possible that they are, but rather that a change in the promoter region of a single gene can lead to a change in complex social behavior. Advances in neuroscience, together with the results of the Human Genome Project and transgenic research on nonhuman species, may very well lead to the development of genetic and neurohormonal interventions for psychopathy. Further elucidation of the phenotypical characteristics of psychopathy (including the issue of psychopathy subtypes; Poythress & Skeem, Chapter 9, this volume) can be expected both to facilitate and be facilitated by advances in neuroscientific and genetic investigations of antisocial behavior.

The Relevance of a Developmental Understanding of Psychopathy

We have elsewhere described a taxonomy of delinquents comprised of Moffitt's (1993) adolescence-limited offenders and two types of life-course-persistent offenders: a neurodevelopmentally impaired type and a primary psychopathic type (Quinsey, Skilling, Lalumière, & Craig, 2004; see also Harris & Rice, Chapter 28, this volume). Evidence reviewed in this volume (Waldman & Rhee, Chapter 11) and elsewhere (Quinsey et al., 2004) suggests that there are substantial genetic influences on the etiology of psychopathy. This fact has the same implications regardless of whether genes directly cause the condition (so that psychopathy is relatively unaffected by environmental influence, or obligate) or act only under certain environmental conditions (so that psychopathy is facultative), and regardless of whether psychopathy is conceptualized as pathological or not. Because it is certain that some genes contribute to the development of psychopathy, we may speculate about what characteristics these genes might produce. The close association of antisocial conduct with early high mating effort (allocating energy toward short-term, uncommitted relationships with multiple sexual partners) and lack of parental investment (allocating energy toward taking care of one's mate and one's offspring) suggest that genes connected with these characteristics are of particular interest (see below).

Barr and Quinsey (2004) have compared

the implications of the view that psychopathy represents a life history strategy and the view that psychopathy represents a pathology (see also Harris & Rice, Chapter 28, this volume). A life history strategy, from a Darwinian or selectionist perspective (for a brief introduction, see Quinsey, 2002), is a particular pattern of energy and resource allocation to species-typical problems of survival and reproduction. From this life history perspective, psychopathic traits such as risk taking, aggressiveness, early reproduction, and social manipulativeness were selected for in ancestral environments because of their positive effects on fitness (relative reproductive success in terms of number and quality of offspring, or their modern proxy in terms of access to potentially fertile sexual partners). Thus, the life history view requires that psychopathy is at least partly heritable and that it did not incur fitness costs in the environment in which the psychopathic traits were selected. According to this view, psychopathic traits were selected because they were designed to solve problems of survival or reproduction in ancestral environments. Like the pathology view, the life history view requires that the brains of psychopaths be different in some way from those of nonpsychopaths, but it is silent about the nature of the differences and does not specify a proximal causal mechanism.

The life history view is also silent about whether particular environmental events are causally related to the development of psychopathic traits. With respect to genotype–environment interactions, it could be argued that psychopathic traits are species-typical characteristics that develop in any person exposed to particular environmental events. In this case, psychopathy would be inherited but its coefficient of heritability would be zero, there being no genetically caused variation among individuals (heritability is the proportion of phenotypical variance attributable to genetic influence). Because we know that psychopathy does not show zero heritability, this view is certainly false. The life history view, therefore, asserts that the alleles responsible for psychopathic characteristics have been maintained in the population through frequency-dependent selection. In this form of selection, the traits confer a fitness advantage if they are uncommon in the population—for example, a small group of cheaters prospering in a large crowd of co-operators (see Frank, 1988).

The pathology view—which appears to be more commonly held than the life history view—asserts that the differences observed between psychopaths and nonpsychopaths reflect abnormalities in psychopaths' emotional information processing, impulse control, and so forth. These deficits are presumably the result of disturbances in development; candidate causes include prenatal insults, adverse early environments, childhood infections, and head injuries. The deficits result in serious disturbances in the individual's functioning, which in turn lead to the commission of crimes (e.g., callousness and poor impulse control impair interpersonal relationships, and this increases the likelihood of violent behavior). Thus, the pathology view suggests that interventions should redress the deficits of psychopaths in order to improve their functioning and thereby reduce recidivism.

Because the conceptualization of psychopathy as a pathology deals entirely with proximal causes (the mechanisms by which psychopathic traits are caused in current environments) and a life history view is concerned with ultimate causes (the selection pressures that caused the traits to develop in ancestral environments), strong inference tests of the relative merits of these two views are not straightforward. Nevertheless, the two views do lead to some different empirical predictions. The life history view would be falsified if it were to be shown that psychopathy was not inherited, that the constellation of psychopathic traits inevitably led to fitness losses (e.g., death before reaching sexual maturity or decreased reproductive success), that psychopathic traits were not present across cultures and historical time, that psychopathy was an extremely rare condition, or that psychopathic traits only occurred as a result of pathological agents (illness or injury). In contrast, the view that psychopathy is a pathology requires that the traits arise from injury or disease, have neutral or negative fitness consequences, and—if psychopathy is inherited—that it be a very rare condition. From a Darwinian viewpoint, a pathological condition that led to increased reproductive success would raise questions about the meaningfulness of the definition of pathology being employed (see Wakefield, 1992).

What few data are available support a life history view of psychopathy. Highly antisocial males exhibit a unique constellation of traits marking them as a discrete natural class (taxon) both as adults (Harris, Rice, & Quinsey, 1994; Skilling et al., 2002) and as children (Skilling, Quinsey, & Craig, 2001). (For an alternative perspective, see Krueger, Markon, Patrick, & Iacono, in press.) A substantial literature demonstrates that antisocial traits show a strong genetic influence by themselves (e.g., Slutske et al., 1997; Waldman & Rhee, Chapter 11, this volume) and in combination with early environmental influences (Cadoret, Yates, Troughton, Woodworth, & Stewart, 1995; Caspi et al., 2002). High levels of antisocial traits are associated with high mating effort in men (Rowe, Vazsonyi, & Figueredo, 1997) and early reproductive activity in samples of men (Capaldi, Crosby, & Stoolmiller, 1996; Fagot, Pears, Capaldi, Crosby, & Leve, 1998; Stouthamer-Loeber & Wei, 1998), women (Lanctôt & Smith, 2001; Quinsey, Book, & Lalumière, 2001; Serbin et al., 1998) and both sexes (Bingham & Crockett, 1996; Jessor, Costa, Jessor, & Donovan, 1983; Rowe, Rodgers, Meseck-Bushey, & St. John, 1989). High mating effort and age at first intercourse also show strong genetic influences (Bailey, Kirk, Zhu, Dunne, & Martin, 2000; Dunne et al., 1997). Of particular importance, psychopathy does not appear to be associated with pathological agents or neurodevelopmental anomalies (Harris, Rice, & Lalumière, 2001; Lalumière, Harris, & Rice, 2001). In fact, in a study by Hare (1984), individuals scoring very high on the PCL-R were found to have fewer neuropsychological deficits than those scoring in the midrange.

Furthermore, although psychopaths have been described as affectively impoverished—for example, being less responsive to distress cues than nonpsychopaths (Blair, Jones, Clark, & Smith, 1997)—they do not appear to have deficits in the recognition of emotional states in others. Book, Quinsey, Cooper, and Langford (2004) studied the relationship between psychopathy and accuracy in perceiving the emotional meaning of facial expressions and body language in a sample of 59 male prison inmates and 60 men recruited from the community. Psychopathy was measured by the Self-Report Psychopathy Scale (Levenson, Kiehl, & Fitzpatrick, 1995) for all participants, and by the PCL-R for the inmates. The inmates' PCL-R scores were not correlated with the number of errors in categorizing posed facial expressions and were positively but not significantly correlated with the inmates' accuracy in rating emotional intensity of posed facial photographs. All participants rated the assertiveness of confederates from a brief, spontaneous videotaped social interaction between the confederate and one of the confederate's friends. The Self-Report Psychopathy Scale was positively correlated with the accuracy of participants' ratings of the friend's level of assertiveness, as measured by both the confederate's rating and the friend's self-rating.

In a companion study involving a subset of the same sample, Book, Quinsey, and Langford (2004) examined the relationship between psychopathy and the accuracy of posed facial expressions of emotion. Thirty-one inmates and 50 community volunteers agreed to be videotaped while attempting to mimic prototypical facial expressions (happy, sad, fearful, disgusted, and angry). PCL-R scores were positively associated with increased intensity of fear in the posed fearful faces, as measured by Ekman and Friesen's (1978) Facial Action Coding System. Undergraduate students gave higher believability and intensity ratings to fearful faces posed by participants who had higher scores on the Primary Psychopathy subscale of the Self-Report Psychopathy Scale. A similar trend was observed for Factor 1 of the PCL-R. Taken together with other research showing that psychopathy is associated with deceptiveness (Seto, Khattar, Lalumière, & Quinsey, 1997), lack of response to distress cues (Blair et al., 1997), and an adequate theory of mind (Richell et al., 2003), these results indicate that psychopaths lack feelings for others but do understand their mental states; in other words, they know but they do not care. This does not seem to be much of a deficit if part of a socially manipulative and exploitative life history strategy.

As we noted earlier, the life history conceptualization of psychopathy has implications for psychotherapies that aim to address "deficits" in psychopathic offenders. These deficits might in fact be differences (and the differences might be in kind rather than degree; Harris et al., 1994; Skilling et al.,

2001). For example, the absence of startle potentiation to the presence of aversive stimuli could be seen as a deficit in fearfulness or defensive reactivity, but it could also be viewed as an adaptation for an antisocial lifestyle in which the individual needs to be relatively fearless in order to pursue his goals in a chaotic and difficult environment. Other authors have recognized this alternative interpretation as well: "From this viewpoint, psychopaths are predatory individuals . . . who are uniquely adapted to survive in settings in which resources are scarce and goal-seeking behavior must persist in the face of all but imminent danger" (Levenston et al., 2000, p. 382).

CONCLUSIONS AND RECOMMENDATIONS

There have been few studies of the impact of currently available interventions on psychopathy, and none of the adequately controlled studies are encouraging. In this chapter, we reviewed the reasons why current psychotherapies can probably be ruled out as a class of interventions that are likely to reduce recidivism among psychopathic offenders. These reasons include the obstacles posed by psychopaths' characteristics, the interaction of psychopaths' characteristics with therapist factors, the collaborative nature of typical psychotherapeutic processes, and the content of treatment. Based on our analysis, we do not have much confidence in psychotherapies that emphasize motivation to change, long-term thinking, and rational analyses of costs and benefits, given psychopaths' known difficulties with motivation to change, response modulation, and noncompliance. Beyond the obvious call for more evaluation research to guide our thinking about interventions for psychopathic offenders, we have suggested that several areas of basic research might shed light on how to proceed with future intervention and prevention efforts. These include laboratory studies of psychopaths' emotional information processing, neuroscientific and genetic research, and studies of developmental trajectories in antisocial and criminal behaviors.

Future interventions can be broadly divided into those that try to target (putative) proximal causes and those that focus on psychopathic traits or behavior without specifically targeting proximal causes. Examples of the former are stem cell graft or gene therapies to address brain differences in structure or function (Raine & Yang, Chapter 14, this volume), if indeed these brain differences cause the psychopathic phenotype; examples of the latter are behavior modification regimens that should be able to have an effect regardless of the individual's level of psychopathy.

What is to be done while we await explication of the causal mechanisms of psychopathy? Long-term incapacitation may be required for some offenders, but it is not an option for many psychopathic offenders for a variety of legal, moral, social, and practical reasons. Prevention efforts may be part of the solution, even if current prevention methods are associated with only modest effect sizes in reducing crime (e.g., Aos et al., 2001). Most of these efforts target high-risk youth, many of whom would not turn out to be psychopathic adults even in the absence of an intervention. Nevertheless, a reduction of crime among disadvantaged groups is a worthy goal. Moreover, many prevention efforts promote social justice and thus are laudable in and of themselves, even if unaccompanied by a reduction in crime. Many of the correlates of antisocial behaviors are familial, including single parenthood, teenage parenthood, poverty, parental antisocial characteristics, parental alcoholism and drug abuse, and so forth. Policies regarding family planning, delayed parenthood, access to abortion, and improved health and education of mothers are therefore likely to produce benefits in the form of reduced crime and fewer psychopaths. Donohue and Levitt (2001), for example, have documented a reduction in American crime rates associated with improved access to abortion resulting from the 1973 *Roe v. Wade* decision. They argue that the reduction in crime rate occurred because the liberalization of U.S. abortion laws was associated with a differentially increased abortion rate among high-risk mothers.

Even with the best prevention efforts, adult psychopaths are not about to stop engaging in crime soon. What might future interventions look like? We can get some ideas from research in support of behavioral modification of symptoms exhibited by individuals with severe chronic schizophrenia. Although schizophrenia is a genetically caused brain disease, the most effective treatment discovered to date for its most severe manifestations is a rigorously implemented and very carefully planned behavioral program (Paul & Lentz, 1977). The thoroughness and integrity of implementation of this program seem to be the keys to its success.

The implications for treatments of psychopathic offenders are clear (see also Harris & Rice, Chapter 28, this volume). Interventions to reduce recidivism among psychopathic offenders will need to be provided on an ongoing basis, although the intensity of service may vary over time with changing circumstances. These interventions will likely involve high staff-to-client ratios in order to provide sufficient supervision, to protect therapists from being deceived or manipulated, and to help them refrain from negative reactions to psychopaths that might interfere with intervention efficacy. Moreover, the interventions will focus on shaping behavior in desired directions, rather than more abstract concepts such as responsibility, empathy, and relapse prevention, with substantial attention devoted to program fidelity and a reliance on measures other than self-report. Given the evidence for psychopaths' dominant response styles and differing response thresholds, increasing the salience and consistency of punishments would be important elements in these interventions. Other important intervention targets would include increasing delay of gratification and compliance with program rules and reducing aggression and associations with antisocial peers.

To summarize, major progress in the near future is likely to be dominated by advances in neuroscience associated with better neuroimaging technologies, a better understanding of how and where neurotransmitters work, and the knowledge produced by the Human Genome Project. The prospects for progress in the treatment of psychopathy are likely similar to those for other major conditions, such as schizophrenia, that are known to be at least partly heritable, to arise during development, and to have neurological correlates. Only basic research can provide insight into the etiology of psychopathy, but such investigations, even when successful, require applied and evaluative research to transform the resulting etiological insights into practical interventions. The interplay between basic and applied investigations is likely to be a major theme in fostering productive future research on psychopathy.

ACKNOWLEDGMENTS

We would like to thank Meredith Chivers, Grant Harris, Martin Lalumière, Marnie Rice, and Tracey Skilling for their helpful comments on an earlier version of this chapter.

REFERENCES

American Psychiatric Association. (2000). *Diagnostic and statistical manual of mental disorders* (4th ed., text rev.). Washington, DC: Author.

Andrews, D. A., & Bonta, J. (1998). *The psychology of criminal conduct* (2nd ed.). Cincinnati, OH: Anderson.

Aos, S., Phipps, P., Barnoski, R., & Lieb, R. (2001, May). *The comparative costs and benefits of programs to reduce crime* (Version 4, Research Report #01-05-1201). Olympia: Washington State Institute for Public Policy.

Bailey, J. M., Kirk, K. M., Zhu, G., Dunne, M. P., & Martin, N. G. (2000). Do individual differences in sociosexuality represent genetic or environmentally contingent strategies? Evidence from the Australian twin registry. *Journal of Personality and Social Psychology, 78,* 537–545.

Barr, K. N., & Quinsey, V. L. (2004). Is psychopathy a pathology or a life strategy? Implications for social policy. In C. Crawford & C. Salmon (Eds.), *Evolutionary psychology, public policy, and personal decisions* (pp. 293–317). Hillsdale, NJ: Erlbaum.

Bingham, C. R., & Crockett, L. J. (1996). Longitudinal adjustment patterns of boys and girls experiencing early, middle, and late sexual intercourse. *Developmental Psychology, 32,* 647–658.

Blair, R., Jones, L., Clark, F., & Smith, M. (1997). The psychopathic individual: A lack of responsiveness to distress cues? *Psychophysiology, 34,* 192–198.

Book, A. S., Quinsey, V. L., Cooper, A. K., & Langford, D. (2004). *The mask of sanity revisited: Psychopathy and feigned fear.* Manuscript submitted for publication.

Book, A. S., Quinsey, V. L., & Langford, D. (2004). *Psychopathy and perception of affect and vulnerability.* Manuscript submitted for publication.

Cadoret, R. J., Yates, W. R., Troughton, E., Woodworth, G., & Steward, M. A. (1995). Genetic–environmental interaction in the genesis of aggressivity and conduct disorders. *Archives of General Psychiatry, 52,* 916–924.

Capaldi, D. M., Crosby, L., & Stoolmiller, M. (1996). Predicting the timing of first sexual intercourse for adolescent males. *Child Development, 64,* 344–359.

Caspi, A., McClay, J., Moffitt, T. E., Mill, J., Martin, J., Craig, I. W., et al. (2002). Role of genotype in the cycles of violence in maltreated children. *Science, 297,* 851–854.

Cleckley, H. (1976). *The mask of sanity* (5th ed.). St. Louis, MO: Mosby.

Donohue, J. J., III, & Levitt, S. D. (2001). The impact of legalized abortion on crime. *Quarterly Journal of Economics, 116,* 379–420.

Dunne, M. P., Martin, N. G., Statham, D. J., Slutske, W. S., Dinwiddie, S. H., Bucholz, K. K., et al. (1997). Genetic and environmental contributions to variance in age at first sexual intercourse. *Psychological Science, 8,* 211–216.

Ekman, P., & Friesen, W. V. (1978). *Facial action coding system: A technique for the measurement of facial movement.* Palo Alto, CA: Consulting Psychologists Press.

Fagot, B. I., Pears, K. C., Capaldi, D. M., Crosby, L., & Leve, C. S. (1998). Becoming an adolescent father: Precursors and parenting. *Developmental Psychology, 34,* 1209–1219.

Flor, H., Birbaumer, N., Hermann, C., Ziegler, S., & Patrick, C. J. (2002). Aversive Pavlovian conditioning in psychopaths: Peripheral and central correlates. *Psychophysiology, 39,* 505–518.

Forth, A. (1992). *Emotion and psychopathy: A three-component analysis.* Unpublished doctoral dissertation, University of British Columbia, Vancouver.

Frank, R. H. (1988). *Passions within reason: The strategic role of the emotions.* New York: Norton.

Hare, R. D. (1984). Performance of psychopaths on cognitive tasks related to frontal lobe function. *Journal of Abnormal Psychology, 93,* 133–140.

Hare, R. D. (1991). *Manual for the Hare Psychopathy Checklist—Revised.* Toronto, ON, Canada: Multi-Health Systems.

Hare, R. D. (2003). *The Hare Psychopathy Checklist—Revised* (2nd ed.). Toronto, ON, Canada: Multi-Health Systems.

Hare, R. D., Clark, D., Grann, M., & Thornton, D. (2000). Psychopathy and the predictive validity of the PCL-R: An international perspective. *Behavioral Sciences and the Law, 18,* 623–645.

Harris, G. T., Rice, M. E., & Lalumière, M. L. (2001). The roles of psychopathy, neurodevelopmental insults and antisocial parenting. *Criminal Justice and Behavior, 28,* 402–406.

Harris, G. T., Rice, M. E., & Quinsey, V. L. (1994). Psychopathy as a taxon: Evidence that psychopaths are a discrete class. *Journal of Consulting and Clinical Psychology, 62,* 387–397.

Hobson, J., Shine, J., & Roberts, R. (2000). How do psychopaths behave in a prison therapeutic community? *Psychology, Crime and Law, 6,* 139–154.

Jessor, R., Costa, F., Jessor, L., & Donovan, J. E. (1983). Time of first intercourse: A prospective study. *Journal of Personality and Social Psychology, 44, 608–626.

Kraepelin, E. (1968). Lectures on Clinical Psychiatry (T. Johnstone, Trans. & Ed.). London: Baillière. (Original work published 1904)

Krueger, R. F., Markon, K. E., Patrick, C. J., & Iacono, W. G. (in press). Externalizing psychopathology in adulthood: A dimensional-spectrum conceptualization and its implications for DSM-V. Journal of Abnormal Psychology.

Lalumière, M. L., Harris, G. T., & Rice, M. E. (2001). Psychopathy and developmental instability. Evolution and Human Behavior, 22, 75–92.

Lanctôt, N., & Smith, C. A. (2001). Sexual activity, pregnancy, and deviance in a representative urban sample of African American girls. Journal of Youth and Adolescence, 30, 349–372.

Leal, J., Ziedonis, D., & Kosten, T. (1994). Antisocial personality disorder as a prognostic factor for pharmacotherapy of cocaine dependence. Drug and Alcohol Dependence, 35, 31–35.

Levenson, M. R., Kiehl, K. A., & Fitzpatrick, C. M. (1995). Assessing psychopathic attributes in a non-institutionalized population. Journal of Personality and Social Psychology, 68, 151–158.

Levenston, G. K., Patrick, C. J., Bradley, M. M., & Lang, P. J. (2000). The psychopath as observer: Emotion and attention in picture processing. Journal of Abnormal Psychology, 109, 373–385.

Looman, J., Abracen, J., Serin, R., & Marquis, P. (2005). Psychopathy, treatment change and recidivism in high-risk high-need sexual offenders. Journal of Interpersonal Violence, 20, 549–568.

Lynam, D. R. (1996). Early identification of chronic offenders: Who is the fledgling psychopath? Psychological Bulletin, 120, 209–234.

Martin, D. J., Garske, J. P., & Davis, M. K. (2000). Relation of the therapeutic alliance with outcome and other variables: A meta-analytic review. Journal of Consulting and Clinical Psychology, 68, 438–450.

Messina, N. P., Wish, E. D., & Nemes, S. (1999). Therapeutic community treatment for substance abusers with antisocial personality disorder. Journal of Substance Abuse Treatment, 17, 121–128.

Moffitt, T. E. (1993). Adolescence-limited and life-course-persistent antisocial behavior: A developmental taxonomy. Psychological Bulletin, 100, 674–701.

Newman, J. P., & Kosson, D. S. (1986). Passive avoidance learning in psychopathic and nonpsychopathic offenders. Journal of Abnormal Psychology, 95, 257–263.

Newman, J. P., Patterson, C. M., Howland, E. W., & Nichols, S. L. (1990). Passive avoidance in psychopaths: The effects of reward. Personality and Individual Differences, 11, 1101–1114.

Newman, J. P., Patterson, C. M., & Kosson, D. S. (1987). Response perseveration in psychopaths. Journal of Abnormal Psychology, 96, 145–148.

Newman, J. P., Schmitt, W. A., & Voss, W. (1997). The impact of motivationally neutral cues on psychopathic individuals: Assessing the generality of the response modulation hypothesis. Journal of Abnormal Psychology, 106, 563–575.

O'Brien, B. S., & Frick, P. J. (1996). Reward dominance: Associations with anxiety, conduct problems, and psychopathy in children. Journal of Abnormal Child Psychology, 24, 223–240.

Ogloff, J. R., Wong, S., & Greenwood, A. (1990). Treating criminal psychopaths in a therapeutic community program. Behavioral Sciences and the Law, 8, 81–90.

Patrick, C. J., Bradley, M. M., & Lang, P. J. (1993). Emotion in the psychopath: Startle reflex modulation. Journal of Abnormal Psychology, 102, 82–92.

Patterson, C. M. (1991). Emotion and interpersonal sensitivity in psychopaths. Unpublished doctoral dissertation, University of Wisconsin–Madison.

Paul, G. L., & Lentz, R. J. (1977). Psychosocial treatment of chronic mental patients: Milieu versus social learning programs. Cambridge, MA: Harvard University Press.

Quinsey, V. L. (2002). Evolutionary theory and criminal behavior. Legal and Criminological Psychology, 7, 1–13.

Quinsey, V. L., Book, A. S., & Lalumière, M. L. (2001). A factor analysis of traits related to individual differences in antisocial behavior. Criminal Justice and Behavior, 28, 522–536.

Quinsey, V. L., Skilling, T. A., Lalumière, M. L., & Craig, W. M. (2004). Juvenile delinquency: Understanding the origins of individual differences. Washington, DC: American Psychological Association.

Rice, M. E., Harris, G. T., & Cormier, C. (1992). Evaluation of a maximum security therapeutic community for psychopaths and other mentally disordered offenders. Law and Human Behavior, 16, 399–412.

Richell, R., Mitchell, D., Newman, C., Leonard, A., Baron-Cohen, S., & Blair, R. (2003). Theory of Mind and psychopathy: Can psychopathic individuals read the "language of the eyes"? Neuropsychologia, 41, 523–526.

Rogers, R., & Cruise, K. R. (2000). Malingering and deception among psychopaths. In C. B. Gacano (Ed.), The clinical and forensic assessment of psychopathy: A practitioner's guide (pp. 269–284). Mahwah, NJ: Erlbaum.

Rowe, D. C., Rodgers, J. L., Meseck-Bushey, S., & St. John, C. (1989). Sexual behavior and nonsexual deviance: A sibling study of their relationship. Developmental Psychology, 25, 61–69.

Rowe, D. C., Vazsonyi, A. T., & Figueredo, A. J. (1997). Mating-effort in adolescence: A conditional or alternative strategy. Personality and Individual Differences, 23, 105–115.

Serbin, L. A., Cooperman, J. M., Peters, P. L., Lehoux, P. M., Stack, D. M., & Schwartzman, A. E. (1998). Intergenerational transfer of psychosocial risk in women with childhood histories of aggression, withdrawal, or aggression and withdrawal. *Developmental Psychology, 34*, 1246–1262.

Seto, M. C. (2003). Interpreting the treatment performance of sex offenders. In A. Matravers & R. Lieb (Eds.), *Managing sex offenders in the community: Contexts, challenges, and responses* (Cambridge Criminal Justice Series, pp. 125–143). London: Willan.

Seto, M. C., & Barbaree, H. E. (1999). Psychopathy, treatment behavior, and sex offender recidivism. *Journal of Interpersonal Violence, 14*, 1235–1248.

Seto, M. C., Khattar, N. A., Lalumière, M. L., & Quinsey, V. L. (1997). Deception and sexual strategy in psychopathy. *Personality and Individual Differences, 22*, 301–307.

Skilling, T. A., Harris, G. T., Rice, M. E., & Quinsey, V. L. (2002). Identifying persistently antisocial offenders using the Hare Psychopathy Checklist and DSM antisocial personality disorder criteria. *Psychological Assessment, 14*, 27–38.

Skilling, T. A., Quinsey, V. L., & Craig, W. M. (2001). Evidence of a taxon underlying serious antisocial behavior in boys. *Criminal Justice and Behavior, 28*, 450–470.

Slutske, W. S., Heath, A. C., Dinwiddie, S. H., Madden, P. A. F., Bucholz, K. K., Dunne, M. P., et al. (1997). Modeling genetic and environmental influences in the etiology of conduct disorder: A study of 2,682 adult twin pairs. *Journal of Abnormal Psychology, 106*, 266–279.

Steuerwald, B. L. (1996). *Anger following provocation in individuals with psychopathic characteristics*. Unpublished doctoral dissertation, University of North Carolina at Greensboro.

Steuerwald, B. L., & Kosson, D. S. (2000). Emotional experiences of the psychopath. In C. B. Gacano (Ed.), *The clinical and forensic assessment of psychopathy: A practitioner's guide* (pp. 111–135). Mahwah, NJ: Erlbaum.

Stouthamer-Loeber, M., & Wei, E. H. (1998). The precursors of young fatherhood and its effect on delinquency of teenage males. *Journal of Adolescent Health, 22*, 56–65.

Taft, C. T., Murphy, C. M., Musser, P. H., & Remington, N. A. (2004). Personal, interpersonal, and motivational predictors of the working alliance in group cognitive-behavioral therapy for partner violent men. *Journal of Consulting and Clinical Psychology, 72*, 349–354.

Wakefield, J. C. (1992). The concept of mental disorder: On the boundary between biological facts and social values. *American Psychologist, 47*, 373–388.

Waschbusch, D. A., & Hill, G. P. (2003). Empirically supported, promising, and unsupported treatments for children with attention-deficit/hyperactivity disorder. In S. O. Lilienfeld, S. J. Lynn, & J. M. Lohr (Eds.), *Science and pseudoscience in clinical psychology* (pp. 333–362). New York: Guilford Press.

Williamson, S., Harpur, T. J., & Hare, R. D. (1991). Abnormal processing of affective words by psychopaths. *Psychophysiology, 28*, 260–273.

Young, L. J., Nilsen, R., Waymire, K. G., MacGregor, G. R., & Insel, T. R. (1999). Increased affiliative response to vasopressin in mice expressing the V-1a receptor from a monogamous vole. *Nature, 400*, 766–768.

Young, L. J., Wang, Z., & Insel, T. R. (1998). Neuroendocrine bases of monogamy. *Trends in Neurosciences, 21*, 71–75.

VI

CONCLUSIONS AND FUTURE DIRECTIONS

31

Back to the Future

Cleckley as a Guide to the Next Generation of Psychopathy Research

CHRISTOPHER J. PATRICK

As the many outstanding contributions to this volume clearly illustrate, the study of psychopathy is alive and well and numerous significant advances have been made in the field in recent years. A good deal of the continuing interest and progress in this area owes to the availability of a well-established system for the clinical diagnosis of psychopathy in offender samples—namely, Hare's (1991, 2003) Psychopathy Checklist—Revised (PCL-R), and its variants. Vigorous research continues to be done on the content and structure of the PCL-R (cf. Hare & Neumann, Chapter 4; and Cooke, Michie, & Hart, Chapter 5), and on the applicability of the PCL-R conceptualization of psychopathy to populations including women, children, and various ethnic and cultural groups (Verona & Vitale, Chapter 21; Salekin, Chapter 20; and Sullivan & Kosson, Chapter 22, respectively). Much has been learned about the personality correlates of PCL-R psychopathy and its relations with other forms of psychopathology (Lynam & Derefinko, Chapter 7; and Widiger, Chapter 8), and there is a growing literature on the linkages between psychopathy and specific problem behaviors including aggression, substance abuse, sexual offending, and recidivism (Porter & Wood-worth, Chapter 24; Taylor & Lang, Chapter 25; Knight & Guay, Chapter 26; and Douglas, Vincent, & Edens, Chapter 27). Moreover, important advances have been made toward an understanding of the roots and developmental course of psychopathy (cf. chapters in Part III)—with recent studies beginning to address the role of genetic and familial–environmental influences (Waldman & Rhee, Chapter 11; Farrington, Chapter 12) and specific brain neurotransmitters and systems (Minzenberg & Siever, Chapter 13; Raine & Yang, Chapter 14; Blair, Chapter 15; Rogers, Chapter 16) in the disorder.

Nevertheless, as highlighted within several of the chapters in this volume, there are a number of important and basic questions that have yet to be resolved—some of which are crucial to continuing progress in the area. These include questions about the scope of the psychopathy construct—in particular, how central aggression and anxiety are to the disorder; whether antisocial behavior is a defining feature of psychopathy; whether the construct should be viewed as unitary or configural; what mechanism or mechanisms underlie the disorder; whether distinct subgroups of psychopathic individuals exist; what procedures should be used to assess psychopathy in nonoffender (community) samples; and how "successful" psychopathy (if it exists) should be defined. Several of these key issues have been addressed in the integrative summary chapters that close each major section of the current volume. The valuable points expressed in these excellent commentaries will not be reiterated here. Instead, the goal of the present chapter is to look to Cleckley's (1941/1976) classic monograph *The Mask of Sanity* for insights into these vexing questions.

Published in its initial edition in 1941, Cleckley's book continues to provide a vital point of reference for contemporary researchers in the field of psychopathy as well as clinicians in a range of settings. Its enduring impact is traceable to a number of factors. The volume as a whole is rich in detail and written in a sophisticated and engaging style. Its vivid case illustrations remain the definitive clinical portrayals of the psychopath. In addition, based on the details of these case studies, Cleckley formulated a set of diagnostic criteria that served as the foundation for Hare's (1980, 1991) development of the Psychopathy Checklist. He also proposed an etiological model of the disorder that inspired Lykken's (1957) seminal study of "anxiety in the sociopathic personality." In the sections that follow, I summarize perspectives on key issues in contemporary psychopathy research that can be gleaned from Cleckley's work and identify important directions for future research that can be derived from these perspectives.

ARE PSYCHOPATHS HOSTILE AND AGGRESSIVE?

Cleckley's (1976) 15 case descriptions of psychopaths certainly include examples of individuals who exhibited tendencies toward aggression and interpersonal antagonism. Three of these individuals ("Frank," "Walter," and "Gregory") are described as generally belligerent and aggressive. For example, Cleckley says of Frank: "He has been consistently arrogant and aggressive toward his neighbors and acquaintances, usually over trifling matters. After taking a few drinks, he has often threatened others, claimed things that were not his own, and made such a nuisance of himself that local police would be

called to deal with him. . . . He is boastful and histrionic, more eloquently and aggressively so with a few highballs, and much given to temper tantrums" (p. 96).

Four other case descriptions ("Max," "George," "Chester," and "Stanley") include notable evidence of verbal or physical aggression, but contrary indications of affability and cooperativeness are also strongly evident in these cases. For example, on one hand, Max is described as: making "dramatically aggressive gestures" toward police at the time of an arrest (p. 29); engaging in street brawls (p. 30); insulting staff members and encouraging other patients to fight with one another and to disobey hospital personnel (p. 30); being restless in hospital settings and demanding of staff (p. 32); and fighting with hospital attendants and with other patients (p. 32). However, at other times, Max is described as: "friendly and even flattering" toward hospital personnel (p. 29); "cooperative and agreeable" (p. 30); "happily adjusted on the admission ward, busy doing small favors for the physician, congenial with all the personnel, and helpful and kindly toward psychotic patients" (p. 32); and "friendly, cooperative, and apparently content" (p. 37). Furthermore, according to Cleckley, Max's periodic aggressive displays seemed to stem from a desire to show off rather than from cruelty or vindictiveness: "[His] fights always started over trifles. . . . He never attacked others suddenly or incomprehensibly. . . . The causes of his quarrels were readily understandable and were usually found to be similar to those which move such types as the familiar schoolboy bully. . . . No signs of towering rage appeared or even of impulses too strong to be controlled by a very meager desire to refrain. . . . The desire to show off appeared to be a strong motive behind many of his fights" (pp. 32–33). Cleckley was also careful to note that Max had never, to his knowledge, deliberately injured anyone.

Three other cases ("Tom," "Joe," and "Anna") include limited mention of aggressive acts—but Cleckley makes it clear that interpersonal antagonism is not characteristic of these individuals. Of Tom, Cleckley writes: "He did not every day or every week bring attention to himself by major acts of mischief or destructiveness. He was usually polite, often considerate in small, appealing ways" (pp. 65–66); "He gave the impression of a young man fresh and unhardened, in no respect brutalized or worn by his past experiences. He also seemed a poised fellow, one who would make his decisions not in hot-headed haste but calmly" (p. 70). Of Joe, Cleckley states: "He was cheerful, convivial, alert, and energetic. He asked for work and at once made himself useful, checking laundry, typing various lists, helping psychotic patients, and performing many other duties. ... He was at all times in perfect contact, reasonable, optimistic, and plainly intelligent" (p. 147). Anna is described as: "urbane and gracious" (p. 102), "poised, polite, and a paragon of happy behavior" (p. 119), and "courteous, composed, undemanding, and cheerful" (p. 119).

Five of Cleckley's case examples ("Roberta," "Arnold," "Pierre," "Jack," and "Milt") include no mention of verbal or physical aggressiveness. These individuals— while impulsive, deceitful, and emotionally shallow—are portrayed as generally personable and agreeable (and even kind!) in their direct interactions with others. For example, Cleckley says of Roberta: "One of this girl's most appealing qualities is, perhaps, her friendly impulse to help others. In the hospital she showed tact and kindness in doing small favors for seriously troubled patients. This did not seem pretentious or in any way staged. At home she had for years shown similar traits. She often went to sit with an ill neighbor, watched the baby of her mother's friend, and rather patiently helped her younger sister with her studies. An easy kindness seemed also to mark her attitude toward small animals" (p. 49). Her parents describe her as naively oblivious to personal obligations and to the feelings of others, rather than callous or mean-spirited: " 'I can't understand the girl, no matter how hard I try,' said the father, shaking his head in genuine perplexity. 'It's not that she seems bad or exactly that she means to do wrong.' " (p. 47) " 'She has such sweet feelings,' Roberta's mother said, 'but they don't amount to much. She's not hard or heartless, but she's all on the surface. I really believe she means to stop doing all these terrible things, but she doesn't mean it enough to matter' " (p. 49).

In summary, a careful review of Cleckley's 15 prototypical cases yields consistent evidence of petulance and aggression in only 3

cases, mixed evidence of aggressiveness in 4 cases, minor evidence of aggression in 3 cases, and no evidence of aggressive behavior in 5 cases. From this, one is led to conclude that aggressive behavior is not central to Cleckley's conception of psychopathy—and indeed, Cleckley's criteria for the disorder do not include specific indicators of hostility or aggression. Only three of his criteria ("unreliability," "general poverty in major affective reactions," and "fantastic and uninviting behavior under the influence of alcohol") include reference to aggressive behavior as a potential manifestation. In contrast with this, the first of Cleckley's criteria ("superficial charm and good 'intelligence' ") includes some distinctly nonaggressive content: "More often than not, the typical psychopath will seem particularly agreeable and make a distinctly positive impression when he is first encountered. Alert and friendly in his attitude, he is easy to talk with and seems to have a good many genuine interests" (p. 338).

Moreover, Cleckley explicitly notes that serious violent behavior is not a characteristic feature of psychopathy: "Of course I am aware of the fact that many persons showing the characteristics of those here described do commit major crimes and sometimes crimes of maximal violence. There are so many, however, who do not, that such tendencies should be regarded as the exception rather than as the rule, perhaps, as a pathologic trait independent, to a considerable degree, of the other manifestations which we regard as fundamental" (p. 262). Instead, Cleckley maintained that the psychopath's underlying affective disposition mitigated against angry, vengeful displays: "It is my opinion that when the typical psychopath ... occasionally commits a major deed of violence, it is usually a casual act done not from tremendous passion or as a result of plans persistently followed with earnest compelling fervor. ... The psychopath is not volcanically explosive, at the mercy of irresistible drives and overwhelming rages of temper. Often he seems scarcely wholehearted, even in wrath or wickedness" (p. 263). Further relevant to this, Cleckley noted: "Many people, perhaps most, who commit violent and serious crimes fail to show the chief characteristics which so consistently appear in the cases we have considered. Many, in fact, show features that make it very difficult to identify them with this group" (pp. 262–263).

It is notable that Cleckley's perspective on psychopathy and aggression is at odds with empirical data indicating that PCL-R psychopathy shows its strongest associations with personality traits of aggression and antagonism (Lynam & Derefinko, Chapter 7), and that PCL-R scores are reliably predictive of aggressive behavior and violent recidivism in criminal offenders (Douglas et al., Chapter 27). The implication that overall scores on the PCL-R, which was developed to identify psychopathic individuals within prison settings, index a somewhat different construct than that portrayed by Cleckley—one in which aggression and cold-heartedness occupy a more central role.

ARE PSYCHOPATHS NONANXIOUS?

There is little doubt that Cleckley considered a lack of anxiety to be central to the syndrome of psychopathy. Twelve of his 15 illustrative cases are described as characteristically calm, poised, or lacking in nervousness, concern, tension, anxiety, stress, or "psychoneurosis." In another case, low anxiety is not specifically mentioned, but the individual in question (Joe) is described as having "complete confidence in himself" (p. 157). There are only two cases among the 15 (Frank and Gregory) in which calmness or marked self-assurance is not cited as a distinguishing feature; interestingly, these represent two of the three cases in which consistent tendencies toward aggressiveness and interpersonal antagonism are also evident.

Consistent with this analysis, Cleckley explicitly included "absence of 'nervousness' or psychoneurotic manifestations" (p. 339) as one of his 16 criteria for the disorder: "There are usually no symptoms to suggest a psychoneurosis in the clinical sense. . . . It is highly typical for him not only to escape the abnormal anxiety and tension fundamentally characteristic of this whole diagnostic group but also to show a relative immunity from such anxiety and worry as might be judged normal or appropriate in disturbing situations. . . . Within himself he appears almost as incapable of anxiety as of profound remorse" (p. 340). Elsewhere in his book, dis-

tinguishing between the psychopathic and the psychoneurotic patient, Cleckley states: "Those called psychopaths *are very sharply characterized by the lack of anxiety* (remorse, easy anticipation, apprehensive scrupulousness, the sense of being under stress or strain) and, *less than the average person*, show what is widely regarded as basic in the neurotic" (p. 257; emphasis added).

As with aggressiveness, it is notable that Cleckley's position that low anxiousness is central to psychopathy runs contrary to empirical findings for the PCL-R. Existing data indicate that overall PCL-R scores are negligibly related to indices of trait anxiety (Hare, 1991, 2003) and, if anything, somewhat positively (albeit weakly) to the construct of Neuroticism (Lynam & Derefinko, Chapter 7). Again, the implication is that overall scores on the PCL-R index a construct somewhat different from that of Cleckley—one in which deficient anxiety is not a core element.

IS ANTISOCIAL BEHAVIOR A DEFINING FEATURE OF PSYCHOPATHY?

There is no question that Cleckley considered persistent antisocial deviance to be characteristic of psychopaths. Without exception, all the individuals represented in his case histories engage in repeated violations of the law—including truancy, vandalism, theft, fraud, forgery, fire setting, drunkenness and disorderly conduct, assault, reckless driving, drug offenses, prostitution, and escape. (Notably, the only major crimes not featured in Cleckley's prototype case examples are robbery, rape, and murder.) Furthermore, Cleckley listed antisocial behavior as one of his 16 diagnostic criteria for psychopathy. However, he described this behavior as being of a distinctive sort, that is, as being "inadequately motivated": "He will commit theft, forgery, adultery, fraud, and other deeds for astonishingly small stakes and under much greater risks of being discovered than will the ordinary scoundrel. He will, in fact, commit such deeds in the absence of any apparent goal at all" (p. 343).

That is, Cleckley viewed the antisocial behavior of psychopaths as symptomatic of a pervasive whimsicality that he saw as fundamental to the disorder: "Objective stimuli (value of the object, specific conscious need) are, as in compulsive (or impulsive) stealing, inadequate to account for the psychopath's acts. Evidence of any vividly felt urge symbolizing a disguised but specifically channelized, instinctive drive is not readily available in the psychopath's wide range of inappropriate and self-defeating behavior" (p. 344). This quality of capriciousness is also a salient theme in the descriptions of several other of Cleckley's diagnostic criteria (i.e., "unreliability," "untruthfulness and insincerity," "poor judgment and failure to learn by experience," "general poverty in major affective reactions," "unresponsiveness in general interpersonal relations," "fantastic and uninviting behavior with drink and sometimes without," and "sex life impersonal, trivial, and poorly integrated").

Cleckley further clarifies his position with regard to antisocial behavior among psychopaths in a section in which he distinguishes the psychopathic individual from the "ordinary" (i.e., career) criminal. Specifically, he identifies four key differences between the two groups:

1. The antisocial behavior of ordinary criminals, in contrast with the psychopath, is generally goal oriented: "The criminal usually works consistently and with what abilities are at his command toward obtaining his own ends. . . . The psychopath very seldom takes much advantage of what he gains and almost never works consistently in crime or in anything else to achieve a permanent position of power or wealth or security" (p. 261).
2. The motives of the ordinary criminal are discernible to the average observer.
3. "The criminal usually spares himself as much as possible and harms others. The psychopath, though he heedlessly causes sorrow and trouble for others, usually puts himself also in a position that would be shameful and most uncomfortable for the ordinary man. . . . In fact, his most serious damage to others is often largely through their concern for him and their efforts to help him" (p. 262).
4. In contrast with ordinary criminals, psychopaths rarely commit major crimes such as murder that result in major prison

sentences. Instead: "A large part of his antisocial activity might be interpreted as purposively designed to harm himself if one notices the painful results that so quickly overtake him" (p. 262).

The upshot of these distinctions is that antisocial deviance in psychopaths, according to Cleckley, has a peculiarly aimless quality—symptomatic, in his view, of a fundamental underlying defect (discussed further below): "If there is no positive motivation toward major goals, no adequate inhibition by revulsion from what is horrible or sordid, it is perhaps more understandable that the rudderless and chartless facsimile of a full human being may flounder about in trivialities or in tragic blunders and see little distinction between them" (p. 267). According to Cleckley, it is the presence of this core inner defect that also distinguishes the psychopath from the persistent delinquent: "In repetitive delinquent behavior the subject often seems to be going a certain distance along the course that a full psychopath follows to the end. . . . Although anxiety, remorse, shame, and other consciously painful subjective responses to undesirable consequences are deficient in both as compared to normal, this callousness or apathy is far deeper in the psychopath. The deficiency is also far more successfully masked" (p. 268).

ARE THERE DIFFERENT SUBTYPES OF PSYCHOPATHS?

Cleckley's *Mask of Sanity* was intended as an effort to refine and narrow the concept of psychopathy—to reverse historic trends that had broadened the term to encompass a wide range of disparate conditions. In a section of his book titled "Conceptual Confusions Which Cloud the Subject," Cleckley highlighted two trends in particular that had promoted confusion: "One of these tendencies arose from efforts to group these patients with many other types by no means similar. The other seems to have proceeded from ambitious attempts to break down the psychopath's disorder by fine and largely imaginary distinctions, by all sorts of descriptive nuances and diagnostic legerdemain, into theoretical entities to be differentiated and classified under many subheadings" (p. 229). For Cleckley, the main order of business was to reorient professionals toward a more precise meaning of the term—one revealed through the rich details of his clinical case studies, his formulation of specific diagnostic indicators, and the distinctions he drew between psychopathy and other conditions previously classed with it. Consequently, limited attention is devoted in his book to the possibility of distinctive subtypes among individuals he regarded as truly psychopathic. Nevertheless, Cleckley did allude to the possibility that subtypes might be detected once the basic boundaries of the syndrome had been clarified: "Before these fine distinctions can be made to any good purpose, there must first appear some recognition of the basic group that is to be further differentiated" (p. 229).

Some distinctions among psychopathic individuals can indeed be found in the biographical material included in Cleckley's case histories. One distinction relates to the degree of aggressiveness shown by these individuals. As noted earlier, a small number of the individuals Cleckley described as prototypical psychopaths appear highly aggressive and antagonistic. The clearest examples of this sort are Frank, Walter, and Gregory. These individuals appear routinely brash, arrogant, and domineering in their interactions with others, and they engage repeatedly in fights, threats against others, and physical assaults. Two of these three cases (Frank and Gregory) do not include specific reference to the "absence of nervousness" highlighted in other case descriptions. A history of suicidal threats or gestures is evident in these same two cases; although Cleckley characterizes the episodes in question as primarily manipulative, they are nonetheless salient given their rarity in the sample as a whole and the fact that Cleckley listed "suicide rarely carried out" as one of his diagnostic criteria for psychopathy. Moreover, a history of alcohol abuse is reported in all three of these cases, with drug addiction also noted in one (Frank). The picture that emerges from these cases is one of an antagonistic, belligerent, and reckless individual prone to abuse of substances. Notably, overall scores on the PCL-R, besides exhibiting marked associations with traits of aggression and antagonism, show a robust association with alcohol

and drug problems (cf. Hare, 2003) and a positive (albeit weak) association with suicidal behavior (Verona, Hicks, & Patrick, in press; Verona, Patrick, & Joiner, 2001). The implication is that higher PCL-R scorers identified within prison settings are more predominantly of this type.

In contrast, a larger subgroup of individuals among Cleckley's prototype cases (8 of the 15) are described as cheerful, affable, and agreeable in interactions with others and generally nonaggressive. Extreme confidence or an absence of neurosis, anxiety, or worry is noted in all these cases. Evidence of suicidal behavior (again characterized as manipulative) is noted in only one of these cases (Joe). Four cases include no mention of heavy drinking or drunkenness, and a fifth (Tom) is described as "not a very regular drinker or one who characteristically drank to sodden confusion or stupefaction" (p. 68). No history of drug abuse is evident in any of these cases. The picture that emerges here is one of a personable and psychologically well adjusted but untrustworthy and behaviorally unpredictable individual. The behavioral profile of these individuals seems less compatible with the correlates of the PCL-R taken as a whole.

Cleckley's remaining four cases do not fall clearly into either of the aforementioned subgroups. In these individuals, episodes of petulance and aggression are intermingled with periods of geniality and cooperativeness. Heavy drinking is evident in three of these cases (Max, George, and Chester), accompanied by drug abuse in one case. A history of suicidal behavior is also present in one of these cases (Chester). The behavioral profile of these four cases seems at least somewhat compatible with the empirical correlates of the PCL-R taken as a whole—although less so than the first group of prototype cases ($n = 3$).

DO "SUCCESSFUL" PSYCHOPATHS EXIST?

Cleckley characterized psychopathy in its full form as a severely debilitating condition: "The persons already described are regarded as typical examples showing the disorder in its distinct clinical manifestations of disability. Many of them are plainly unsuited for life in any community; some are as thoroughly incapacitated, in my opinion, as most patients with unmistakable schizophrenic psychosis" (p. 188). Nevertheless, he also presented case examples of psychopathic individuals who managed to achieve and maintain successful functioning in the community (e.g., "The psychopath as businessman"; "The psychopath as scientist"; "The psychopath as physician"; and "The psychopath as psychiatrist"). However, he referred to such cases as "incomplete manifestations or suggestions of the disorder" (p. 188). By this, did he mean to imply that these individuals do not qualify as psychopaths? Almost certainly not—as indicated in the preceding quotation, he simply meant that (in line with the current DSM perspective) the concept of "disorder" entails significant disability, so that the presence of successful functioning denotes a subclinical condition: "In the reports that follow, an effort has been made to present persons who are able to make some sort of adjustment in life and who may perhaps be regarded as less severely incapacitated, and in varying degrees. . . . The psychopathologic process, the deviation (or the arrest), is, as with the others, a process affecting basic personal reactions; but here it has not altogether dominated the scene. It has not crowded ordinary successful functioning in the outer aspects of work and social relations entirely out of the picture" (p. 189).

In subsequent passages, Cleckley makes it clear that he views these "successful" cases as alternative manifestations of the same underlying pathology evident in his 15 prototypical clinical cases: "There are many patients who show relatively circumscribed antisocial behavior or temporary episodes of gross, general delinquency, who have, I feel, much less in common with the obvious psychopath than those who make a better outward impression but who consistently show signs of inner subjective reactions typical of the clinically disabled patient. . . . I believe that in these personalities designated as partially or inwardly affected, a deepseated disorder often exists. The true difference between them and the psychopaths who continually go to jails or to psychiatric hospitals is that they keep up a far better and more consistent outward appearance of being normal" (pp. 190–191).

IS PSYCHOPATHY A UNITARY CONSTRUCT?

Differing structural models of the PCL-R have recently been proposed. Initial research on the structure of the PCL/PCL-R (Hare et al., 1990; Harpur, Hakstian, & Hare, 1988) emphasized a two-factor model. More recently, four-factor (Hare & Neumann, Chapter 4) and three-factor models (Cooke et al., Chapter 5) have been proposed. However, in all these models the distinctive factors of the PCL-R are viewed as elements of a broader underlying entity presumed to reflect psychopathy: The two factors reported initially by Harpur et al. were oblique factors. The four factors in the Hare–Neumann model are depicted as intercorrelated with one another, and in the model of Cooke and colleagues, the three factors are represented as loading on a common, superordinate factor. The implication is that psychopathy as indexed by the PCL-R is a unitary but multifaceted construct (cf. Lilienfeld & Fowler, Chapter 6), analogous to general intelligence with its verbal and performance facets.

In contrast with this, Cleckley characterized psychopathy as an inherently paradoxical syndrome—one in which severe behavioral maladjustment and positive psychological adjustment go hand in hand: "I find it necessary . . . to postulate that the psychopath has a genuine and very serious disability, disorder, defect, or deviation . . . [but] a different kind of abnormality from all those now recognized as seriously impairing competency. . . . The first and most striking difference is this: In all the orthodox psychoses . . . , there is a more or less obvious alteration of reasoning processes or of some other demonstrable personality feature. In the psychopath, this is not seen. The observer is confronted with a convincing mask of sanity" (p. 368).

In considering what Cleckley meant by this, it is useful to group his 16 diagnostic criteria for psychopathy into three distinctive categories (see Table 31.1). One category comprises explicit indicators of positive psychological adjustment—including good intelligence and social charm, absence of delusions/irrationality, absence of nervousness, and suicide rarely carried out. With regard to these indicators, it is important to note that Cleckley was not referring merely to the ab-

TABLE 31.1. Categorization of Cleckley's (1976) 16 Diagnostic Criteria for Psychopathy

Item category	Item Number and Descriptive Label
Positive adjustment	1. Superficial charm and good "intelligence" 2. Absence of delusions and other signs of irrational thinking 3. Absence of "nervousness" or psychoneurotic manifestations 14. Suicide rarely carried out
Chronic behavioral deviance	7. Inadequately motivated antisocial behavior 8. Poor judgment and failure to learn by experience 4. Unreliability 13. Fantastic and uninviting behavior with drink and sometimes without 15. Sex life impersonal, trivial, and poorly integrated 16. Failure to follow any life plan
Emotional–interpersonal deficits	5. Untruthfulness and insincerity 6. Lack of remorse or shame 10. General poverty in major affective reactions 9. Pathologic egocentricity and incapacity for love 11. Specific loss of insight 12. Unresponsiveness in general interpersonal relations

sence of other significant mental illness but the presence of resiliency and good adjustment: "The surface of the psychopath . . . shows up as equal to or better than normal and gives no hint at all of a disorder within. Nothing about him suggests oddness, inadequacy, or moral frailty. His mask is that of robust mental health" (p. 383). The paradoxical aspect of the disorder lies in the fact that this overt appearance of robust mental health is accompanied by severe behavioral maladjustment: "Yet he has a disorder that often manifests itself in conduct far more seriously abnormal than that of the schizophrenic" (p. 383). "The psychopath, however perfectly he mimics man theoretically, that is to say, when he speaks for himself in words, fails altogether when he is put into the practice of actual living. His failure is so complete and so dramatic that it is difficult to see how such a failure could be achieved by anyone less defective than a downright madman" (p. 370). This aspect of the disorder is captured by indicators of overt behavioral deviance, including impulsive antisocial acts, irresponsibility (unreliability), promiscuity, and an absence of any clear life plan. A third category includes items reflecting the emotional impoverishment and lack of

genuine interpersonal relations that Cleckley viewed as the core of the syndrome (see next section below).

It is notable that the emotional–interpersonal and behavioral deviance features described by Cleckley are well represented in the PCL-R. On the other hand, the positive adjustment features are not. Although it could be argued that the first part of Cleckley's "superficial charm and 'good intelligence' " criterion is captured by item 1 of the PCL-R ("glibness and superficial charm"), a comparison of the wording of Cleckley's criterion with that of PCL-R item 1 reveals a key difference. PCL-R item 1 includes reference to excessive talkativeness, insincerity, slickness, and a lack of believability in the target individual's social presentation. Related to this, the instructions for scoring call for an intermediate rating of "1" in cases in which the individual presents with a "macho" or "tough guy" image, whereas a rating of "0" is called for if the individual presents as sincere and straightforward. Thus, the emphasis is on a somewhat deviant ("too good to be true") or hypermasculine self-presentation. The wording of Cleckley's criterion has a notably different flavor: "There is nothing at all odd or queer about him, and in every respect he tends to embody the concept of a well-adjusted, happy person. Nor does he, on the other hand, seem to be artificially exerting himself like one who is covering up or who wants to sell you a bill of goods. ... Signs of affectation or excessive affability are not characteristic. He looks like the real thing" (p. 338). The inclusion of "good intelligence" (reflecting good sense, intact reasoning, and above-average or superior intellect) as part of this diagnostic criterion reinforces the impression that Cleckley intended this to be an indicator of positive psychological adjustment.

What might account for the absence of pure indicators of adjustment among the items of the PCL-R? Although information in the PCL-R manual (Hare, 1991, 2003) and in the initial report on the development of the PCL (e.g., Hare, 1980) is somewhat unclear as to what precise criteria were used to select items, these sources do indicate that indicators were retained if they discriminated low- versus high-psychopathy groups defined on the basis of "global ratings" (i.e., reflecting degree of match with Cleckley's case examples) and if they showed "good psychometric properties." The latter implies that indicators were chosen that contributed to the reliability (internal consistency) of the overall scale, as well as helping to discriminate extreme groups. This item selection strategy, which fits with the aim of indexing a unitary construct, would operate to homogenize the item set: indicators similar to most other indicators in the candidate pool would be retained while those differing most from the others would be dropped. Because the greater majority of Cleckley's diagnostic criteria (12 of 16) reflect tendencies toward deviance as opposed to adjustment, the initial candidate pool would almost certainly have included more indicators of deviance. Indicators of positive adjustment presumably dropped out because they failed to coalesce with the larger proportion of (pathological) indicators. This would yield a final item set more uniformly indicative of deviance and maladjustment than Cleckley's original criterion set.

Some of the data contained in the initial report on the development of the PCL (Hare, 1980) appear consistent with this account. Of particular interest are data for a sample of 143 prison inmates who were rated on

Cleckley's 16 criteria for psychopathy as well on the 22 items of the original PCL. A principal components analysis of the Cleckley items in this sample yielded five components, accounting for 64% of the total variance. The largest of these was an emotional–interpersonal component (marked by pathological egocentricity, poverty of affect, unresponsiveness in interpersonal relations, untruthfulness, and lack of remorse), accounting for 29.3% of the variance, and a behavioral deviance component (marked by absence of life plans, unreliability, and failure to learn by experience) that accounted for 12% of the variance. In addition, a psychological adjustment component clearly emerged (marked by charm and good intelligence, absence of delusions/irrationality, and absence of nervousness), but this accounted for a smaller proportion of the variance (7.1%). A principal components analysis of the PCL items also yielded five components, accounting for approximately 61% of the overall variance. However, in this case the dominant component, accounting for 27.3% of the total variance, was one reflecting behavioral deviance (proneness to boredom, lack of realistic plans, parasitic lifestyle, and impulsivity). The second component, reflecting the emotional–interpersonal features of psychopathy (lack of remorse, failure to accept responsibility, conning, grandiosity, glibness, and callousness), accounted for only 13% of the variance. These findings are consistent with the idea that the effort to operationalize Cleckley's criteria as a unitary construct in the PCL resulted in an item set that was generally more reflective of deviance and maladjustment.

Nevertheless, it is important to note that the PCL/PCL-R, while developed to assess a putatively unitary construct, does include distinctive factors that exhibit discriminant validity in their relations with external criterion variables. A substantial body of evidence, most of it conducted from the standpoint of the two-factor model, indicates that the emotional–interpersonal and behavioral deviance components of the PCL-R show differential associations with a wide range of variables including aggression, social dominance, trait anxiety, alcohol and drug abuse, and suicidal behavior (Hare, 2003; Patrick, in press). These differential associations tend to be accentuated when the unique variance in each factor is examined (i.e., after removing overlap between the factors using partial correlation or hierarchical regression techniques). For example, some work has shown that the unique variance in the emotional–interpersonal component of the PCL-R (Factor 1) is negatively associated with trait anxiety, whereas the behavioral deviance component (Factor 2) is positively associated with trait anxiety (Patrick, 1994; Verona et al., 2001). This suggests that the positive adjustment component of psychopathy might be tapped to some extent by the unique variance in Factor 1 (i.e., that that part which is unrelated to behavioral deviance).

As noted previously, the empirical correlates of overall scores on the PCL-R are somewhat at odds with Cleckley's portrayal of the prototypical psychopath. In particular, overall scores on the PCL-R show marked positive associations with measures of aggression, interpersonal antagonism, and alcohol and drug problems and weak positive associations with anxiety/neuroticism and suicidal behavior. Thus, the focus on psychopathy as a unitary construct leads to a picture of the psychopath as more aggressive and psychologically maladjusted than the majority of Cleckley's case examples. If, as Cleckley implied, the syndrome of psychopathy represents a unique blend (or configuration; Lilienfeld & Fowler, Chapter 6) of distinctive trait dispositions—reflecting positive adaptation on one hand, and maladjustment on the other—it may be important to isolate these distinctive components in order to better understand the overall syndrome and its variants, and to elucidate the etiological mechanisms that underlie it (cf. Fowles & Dindo, Chapter 2).

WHAT CAUSES PSYCHOPATHY?

Cleckley hypothesized that the symptoms of psychopathy arise from a core underlying "defect or deviation," and one of the later sections of his book is devoted to clarifying the nature of this underlying deviation. However, some confusion exists as to the nature of the underlying mechanism postulated by Cleckley. This confusion exists because of an analogy that Cleckley drew between the underlying deviation in psychopathy and that associated with a brain disorder termed "semantic aphasia" (or "semantic dementia" in the initial, 1941 edition of his book). This disorder, documented by neurologist Henry Head, entailed a selective impairment in language production—one in which the logical meaningfulness of speech is absent or defective. Cleckley made it clear that he regarded the language impairment associated with semantic dementia as merely an analogy for the deficit he theorized to underlie psychopathy: "We need not assume Head's interpretation of the aphasias to be entirely and finally correct if it will by analogy help us formulate and clarify a concept of personality disorder, a concept in which the deeper and less obvious levels of function can be compared and contrasted with more superficial aspects of behavior. Let us use the analogy not as evidence for the concept but only as a means of stating it." (p. 379) Nevertheless, some investigators have erroneously interpreted Cleckley as suggesting that psychopathy reflects an underlying impairment in language processing.

Instead, what Cleckley proposed was that psychopaths are fundamentally deficient in the capacity for emotional experience: "Behind the exquisitely deceptive mask of the psychopath the emotional alteration we feel appears to be primarily one of degree, a consistent leveling of response to petty ranges and an incapacity to react with sufficient seriousness to achieve much more than pseudoexperience or quasi-experience. ... Just as meaning and the adequate sense of things as a whole are lost with semantic aphasia in the circumscribed field of speech although the technical mimicry of language remains intact, so in most psychopaths the purposiveness and the significance of all life-striving and of all subjective experience are affected without obvious damage to the outer appearance or superficial reactions of the personality" (p. 383).

According to Cleckley, this underlying weakness in the capacity for emotional response, referenced directly in his "poverty in major affective reactions" criterion, accounts for the superficiality and manipulativeness of the psychopath's relations with other people as well as the feckless nature of his behavior in other spheres. The psychopath's characteristic "mask of sanity," in Cleckley's view, arises from a natural tendency to simulate the emotional reactions of others in order to "fit in" and to attain everyday goals, without any true awareness of the simulated quality of these reactions: "Let us assume, as a hypothesis, that the psychopath's disorder, or defect, . . . consists of an unawareness and a persistent lack of ability to become aware of what the most important experiences of life mean to others. By this is not meant an acceptance of the arbitrarily postulated values of any particular theology, ethics, esthetics, or philosophic system . . . but rather the common substance of emotion or purpose . . . from which the various loyalties, goals, fidelities, commitments, and concepts of honor and responsibility of various groups and various people are formed. . . . Let us say that, despite his otherwise perfect functioning, the major emotional accompaniments are absent or so attenuated as to count for little. Of course, he is unaware of this, just as everyone is bound, except theoretically, to be unaware of that which is out of his scale or order or mode of experience" (p. 371).

It is important to note that although Cleckley viewed this underlying deficiency in emotional response as disposing the individual toward impulsive antisocial deviance, he also acknowledged that this deviation could exist in the absence of marked or disabling levels of behavioral maladjustment. For example, in discussing examples of "successful psychopaths" (i.e., businessman, scientist, and physician), Cleckley notes: "The chief difference between the patients already discussed and some of those to be mentioned lies perhaps in whether the mask or façade of psychobiologic health is extended into superficial material success. I believe that the relative state of this outward appearance is not necessarily consistent with the degree to which the person is really affected by the essential disorder" (pp. 191–192). Cleckley also identifies characters from history (e.g., the Greek military leader and statesman, Alcibiades; pp. 327–336) and fiction (e.g., the character Scarlett O'Hara in the novel Gone with the Wind; p. 321) as other examples of this type. The implication is that other etiological factors interact with this underlying emotional deviation to determine the manner of its overt phenotypic expression. An obvious, key objective in the scientific study of psychopathy is to elucidate the nature and origins of these intersecting etiological mechanisms. In this regard, individuals who exhibit the core affective features of psychopathy in the absence of severe behavioral maladjustment are likely to provide a unique source of information.

THE ROAD AHEAD

Over six decades have now passed since the first edition of the Mask of Sanity was published, but Cleckley's classic volume remains a rich source of information about the characteristics of psychopathic individuals, as well as a valuable reference point for theorizing about the nature and mechanisms of this disorder. The foregoing analysis of Cleckley's historic work suggests a number of important, interrelated directions for future research.

First, systematic efforts are needed to investigate distinctive components of the psychopathy construct. One strategy for doing this will be to further explore the differential correlates of the various facets of psychopathy embodied in the PCL-R, particularly the unique (nonoverlapping) variance associated with each, and to study subgroups of high PCL-R scorers who differ in terms of their behavioral or personality profiles. For example, recent research by our laboratory (Patrick, Hicks, Krueger, & Lang, 2005) has shown that the PCL-R as a whole, and in particular the antisocial deviance component (Factor 2 in the two-factor model), is substantially related to the externalizing factor of psychopathology—a latent variable that accounts for the systematic comorbidity among syndromes of disinhibition (conduct disorder, adult antisocial behavior, alcohol dependence, and drug dependence) within DSM (Krueger, 1999; Krueger, Caspi, Moffitt, & Silva, 1998). On the other hand, the unique variance associated with the emotional–interpersonal component of the PCL-R is essentially unrelated to this externalizing factor. Together with other research demonstrating that this broad factor represents a common, highly heritable vulnerability to disorders within the externalizing spectrum (Krueger et al., 2002), the implication is that the behavioral deviance component of the PCL-R (Factor 2) taps this same underlying vulnerability. On the other hand, the variance in the emotional–interpersonal (Factor

1) component that is separate from Factor 2 taps something completely different, perhaps something more related to the adjustment component of psychopathy (absence of nervousness, social poise, etc.) emphasized by Cleckley.

With regard to subgroups of high PCL-R scorers, another recent study by our laboratory (Hicks, Markon, Patrick, Krueger, & Newman, 2004) used model-based cluster analysis to classify the personality profiles of 96 male prison participants who achieved scores of 30 or higher on the PCL-R (i.e., the standard cutoff for a research diagnosis of psychopathy). Two subgroups were identified with markedly different personality profiles. One was characterized by extremely high aggression and alienation and very low constraint (i.e., impulsiveness, rebelliousness, and risk taking). The other group showed a markedly normal personality profile, distinguished primarily by low anxiousness and high agency (i.e., dominance and well-being). Notably, the proportion of individuals in the first group ($N = 66$, or 68.8%) exceeded that in the second ($N = 30$, or 31.2%). This finding coincides with the suggestion that the PCL-R as a whole tends to identify more aggressive, behaviorally maladjusted individuals as psychopaths—but at the same time, it suggests that individuals resembling Cleckley's psychologically well-adjusted prototype are also represented among high PCL-R scorers. Further research is needed to confirm the existence of distinctive subgroups among individuals with very high PCL-R scores, and to examine how these subgroups differ on other measures aside from personality variables (e.g., physiological and behavioral measures). Also valuable will be studies that examine differences between subgroups of individuals scoring very high on one factor of the PCL-R but comparatively low on the other (cf. Patrick, 1994). Studies of this kind would help to elucidate causal factors underlying different phenotypic variants of psychopathy, as well as contributing to an understanding of etiological mechanisms associated with the two distinctive components of the PCL-R (cf. Fowles & Dindo, Chapter 2).

Another strategy for studying distinctive components of psychopathy will be to employ alternative assessment instruments that tap these components as separate constructs rather than as facets of a single higher-order construct. One example of such an instrument in the domain of self-report is Lilienfeld's Psychopathic Personality Inventory (PPI; cf. Lilienfeld & Fowler, Chapter 6), which was developed to comprehensively assess traits of psychopathy in nonoffender samples. Recent factor-analytic research (Benning, Patrick, Hicks, Blonigen, & Krueger, 2003) indicates that seven of the eight subscales of the PPI map onto two broad factors, one (PPI-I) reflecting tendencies toward social dominance, low stress reactivity, and fearlessness, and the other (PPI-II) reflecting impulsivity, rebelliousness, alienation, and aggressiveness (the eighth subscale of the PPI, "coldheartedness," did not load appreciably on either factor). In contrast with the factors of the PCL-R, the two broad factors of the PPI are uncorrelated with one another. Nevertheless, both show relations with indices of psychopathy: PPI-I shows strong positive associations with measures of narcissism and thrill seeking and negative associations with indices of anxiousness and empathy; PPI-II shows robust positive associations with measures of child and adult antisocial behavior, alcohol and drug abuse, and boredom susceptibility, as well as being negatively related to empathy (Benning, Patrick, Blonigen, Hicks, & Iacono, 2005). Interestingly, the first of these factors is also associated *positively* with measures of adjustment such as educational attainment, sociability, and executive functioning, whereas the second factor is associated *negatively* with such criterion measures (Benning et al., 2003; Benning, Patrick, Blonigen, Hicks, & Iacono, 2005; Ross, Benning, Patrick, Thompson, & Thurston, 2005).

Besides contributing to an understanding of distinctive elements of psychopathy as conceptualized by Cleckley, personality-based instruments such as the PPI will also facilitate the study of psychopathy in community samples because they are not specifically tailored to offenders and because they can be administered efficiently to very large samples of participants. For example, recent studies of monozygotic and dizygotic twins recruited from the community have begun to elucidate genetic and environmental contributions to these PPI factor constructs, as well as examining their etiological associations with other forms of psychopathology (e.g., Blonigen et al., 2005). Other recent research has begun to examine differences in affective physiological response associated with these factor constructs in community samples (Benning, Patrick, & Iacono, in press). Such research should contribute to an understanding of manifestations of psychopathy in non-criminal samples (including the phenomenon of the "successful psychopath") as well as advancing our knowledge of etiological mechanisms associated with different components of the psychopathy construct. As a function of increased knowledge in these areas, it should be possible to devise improved methods of intervention that directly target the essential processing impairments underlying this important and intriguing disorder (cf. Seto & Quinsey, Chapter 30).

ACKNOWLEDGMENTS

Preparation of this chapter was supported by Grant Nos. MH52384 and MH65137 from the National Institute of Mental Health, Grant No. R01 AA12164 from the National Institute on Alcohol Abuse and Alcoholism, and funds from the Hathaway endowment at the University of Minnesota.

REFERENCES

Benning, S. D., Patrick, C. J., Blonigen, D. M., Hicks, B. M., & Iacono, W. G. (2005). Estimating facets of psychopathy from normal personality traits: A step toward community-epidemiological investigations. *Assessment, 12,* 3–18.

Benning, S. D., Patrick, C. J., Hicks, B. M., Blonigen, D. M., & Krueger, R. F. (2003). Factor structure of the Psychopathic Personality Inventory: Validity and implications for clinical assessment. *Psychological Assessment, 15,* 340–350.

Benning, S. D., Patrick, C. J., & Iacono, W. G. (in press). Fearlessness and underarousal in psychopathy: Startle blink modulation and electrodermal reactivity in a young adult male community sample. *Psychophysiology.*

Blonigen, D. M., Hicks, B. M., Patrick, C. J., Krueger, R. F., Iacono, W. G., & McGue, M. K. (2005). Psychopathic personality traits: Heritability and genetic overlap with internalizing and externalizing psychopathology. *Psychological Medicine, 35,* 1–12.

Cleckley, H. (1976). *The mask of sanity* (5th ed.). St. Louis, MO: Mosby. (Original work published 1941)

Hare, R. D. (1980). A research scale for the assessment of psychopathy in criminal populations. *Personality and Individual Differences, 1,* 111–119.

Hare, R. D. (1991). *The Hare Psychopathy Checklist—Revised.* Toronto, ON, Canada: Multi-Health Systems.

Hare, R. D. (2003). *The Hare Psychopathy Checklist—Revised* (2nd ed.). Toronto, ON, Canada: Multi-Health Systems.

Hare, R. D., Harpur, T. J., Hakstian, A. R., Forth, A. E., Hart, S. D., & Newman, J. P. (1990). The Revised Psychopathy Checklist: Reliability and factor structure. *Psychological Assessment, 2,* 338–341.

Harpur, T. J., Hakstian, A. R., & Hare, R. D. (1988). Factor structure of the Psychopathy Checklist. *Journal of Consulting and Clinical Psychology, 56,* 741–747.

Hicks, B. M., Markon, K. E., Patrick, C. J., Krueger, R. F., & Newman, J. P. (2004). Identifying psychopathy subtypes based on personality structure. *Psychological Assessment, 16,* 276–288.

Krueger, R. F. (1999). The structure of common mental disorders. *Archives of General Psychiatry, 56,* 921–926.

Krueger, R. F., Caspi, A., Moffitt, T. E., & Silva, P. A. (1998). The structure and stability of common mental disorders (DSM-III-R): A longitudinal–epidemiological study. *Journal of Abnormal Psychology, 107,* 216–227.

Krueger, R. F., Hicks, B., Patrick, C. J., Carlson, S., Iacono, W. G., & McGue, M. (2002). Etiologic connections among substance dependence, antisocial behavior, and personality: Modeling the externalizing spectrum. *Journal of Abnormal Psychology, 111,* 411–424.

Lykken, D. T. (1957). A study of anxiety in the sociopathic personality. *Journal of Abnormal and Clinical Psychology, 55,* 6–10.

Patrick, C. J. (1994). Emotion and psychopathy: Startling new insights. *Psychophysiology, 31,* 319–330.

Patrick, C. J. (in press). Getting to the heart of psychopathy. In H. Herve & J. C. Yuille (Eds.), *Psychopathy: Theory, research, and social implications.* Hillsdale, NJ: Erlbaum.

Patrick, C. J., Hicks, B. M., Krueger, R. F., & Lang, A. R. (2005). Relations between psychopathy facets and externalizing in a criminal offender sample. *Journal of Personality Disorders, 19,* 339–356.

Ross, S. R., Benning, S. D., Patrick, C. J., Thompson, A., & Thurston, A. (2005). *Factors of the Psychopathic Personality Inventory: Criterion-related validity and relationships with the Five-Factor Model of personality.* Manuscript submitted for publication.

Verona, E., Patrick, C. J., & Joiner, T. T. (2001). Psychopathy, antisocial personality, and suicide risk. *Journal of Abnormal Psychology, 110,* 462–470.

Verona, E., Hicks, B. M., & Patrick, C. J. (in press). Psychopathy and suicidal behavior in female offenders: Mediating influences of temperament and abuse history. *Journal of Consulting and Clinical Psychology.*

Author Index

Damasio, A. R., 279, 284, 286, 287, 296, 299, 300, 319, 325
Damasio, H., 286, 287, 299, 300, 319, 325
Dandreaux, D. M., 74, 354, 362, 397, 405, 581
Dane, H. A., 355, 405
Dann, M., 323
Darby, A., 286
Darke, S., 497, 501
Dasen, P. R., 540
Dash, L., 11
Daugherty, T. K., 16
Davidson, R. J., 279, 282, 287, 344, 348
Davis, C. G., 377
Davis, J. M., 514
Davis, M., 18, 20, 21, 297, 299, 349
Davis, M. H., 119
Davis, M. K., 593
Davis, P., 319
Davis, R., 51
Davis, R. D., 177, 178, 186, 188, 486, 489
Dawkins, R., 564
Dawson, D. A., 495
Dawson, M. E., 22, 464
Dax, E., 263
Day, D. M., 356
Day, R., 39, 303, 348
Deakin, F. W., 253
Deakin, J. F. W., 280
Deakin, W. J., 253
Dean, R. S., 405, 541
Dearing, M. F., 298
Deater-Deckard, K., 242
Dedrick, R. F., 81
DeGarmo, D. S., 27
Dehaene, S., 326
De Jong, J., 253
DeJonge, S., 257
Deka, R., 258
Delaney, M. A., 266
DeLion, S., 265
Delizonna, L., 299
Delong, M. R., 315
DeLuca, D., 220
DelVecchio, W. F., 353, 367
DeMatteo, D., 579
Dempster, R. J., 177, 252, 484, 544
Denenberg, V. H., 287
Denney, D., 546
Depue, R. A., 22, 30, 44, 45, 122, 136, 522
De Raad, B., 136
Dernevik, M., 537
de Ruiter, C., 441, 447, 542

Déry, M., 363, 405, 502
Derzon, J. H., 232, 239
Desforges, D. M., 578, 582
Desimone, R., 302
De Vet, K., 306
de Vogel, V., 441, 542
Devonshire, P. A., 322
Devor, E. J., 254
de Vries, H., 16
Diamond, R., 318
Dias, R., 317, 324, 325
Diaz, A., 44
DiCicco, T. M., 76, 389
Dick, D. M., 196
Dickinson, A., 298
Dickson, N., 357
DiClemente, C. C., 507
Diener, E., 220
Digman, J. M., 135, 197
Dikman, Z. V., 327
DiLalla, L. F., 209, 215, 216, 220, 376
Dimitrov, M., 285
Dimond, S. J., 287
Dindo, L., 24
Dinero, T. E., 519
Dinitz, S., 176
Dinn, W. M., 320
Dinov, I. D., 281
Dion, K. L., 61, 97
Dishion, T. J., 27, 239, 243, 357, 391
Dmitrieva, T. N., 263, 264
Dodge, K. A., 184, 239, 242, 354, 355, 356, 403, 482, 483
Dolan, D., 556
Dolan, M. C., 73, 95, 159, 251, 253, 254, 280, 281, 291, 320, 421, 442, 537
Dolan, R. J., 296, 302, 318
Dolinsky, Z. S., 506
Doninger, N. A., 453
Donnelly, J. P., 184
Donnelly, J., 161, 442, 499
D'Onofrio, B. M., 222
Donohue, J. J., III, 598
Donovan, D., 498
Donovan, J. E., 596
Donovan, S. J., 266
Doolan, M., 243
Doren, D. M., 38, 59
Dorr, D., 160
Doty, R. L., 323
Dougherty, D. M., 254, 430
Douglas, D., 400
Douglas, K. S., 114, 115, 124, 398, 446, 465, 537, 538, 539, 544, 545, 546, 547, 578, 580

Douglas, K., 101, 177, 482
Douglas, V., 26
Dowdy, L., 483
Doyle, A. E., 223, 376
Doyle, M., 421, 442, 537
Draguns, J. G., 93
Draper, P., 564
Drevets, W. C., 317, 318
Drewe, E. A., 323
Driver, J., 302
Dror, S., 265
Drugge, J., 487
Du, L., 427
Dulawa, S. C., 222, 259
Dulcan, M., 422
Dumenci, L., 451, 497
Dunbar, S. B., 72
Duncan, J., 302, 317
Duncan, S., 580
Dunn, G., 75, 77
Dunn, J., 175, 393
Dunne, M. P., 422, 596
Durant, S. L., 405
Durbin, C. E., 19
Duros, R. L., 76, 389
Durrett, C. A., 74
Dush, D. M., 502
Dutton, D. G., 544
Dvoskin, J., 583
Dyce, J. A., 164

E

Earle, J., 487
Earls, C. M., 516
Earls, F., 240
Eaves, D., 537
Eaves, L. J., 19, 136, 208
Ebmeier, K. P., 382
Ebstein, R. P., 257, 259
Eckert, E. D., 565
Edelbrock, C. S., 206
Edelmann, R. J., 116
Edens, J. F., 24, 59, 65, 83, 94, 111, 112, 115, 116, 122, 123, 125, 126, 157, 173, 176, 186, 363, 366, 367, 396, 403, 405, 446, 449, 454, 466, 482, 485, 535, 538, 539, 541, 543, 545, 549, 555, 563, 574, 577, 578, 579, 580, 581, 582, 584, 585
Edman, G., 254, 497
Edvardsen, J., 212
Edwards, D. W., 300
Edwards, J., 424
Egan, V., 556

Subject Index